COMPANION ENCYCLOPEDIA
OF THE
HISTORY OF MEDICINE

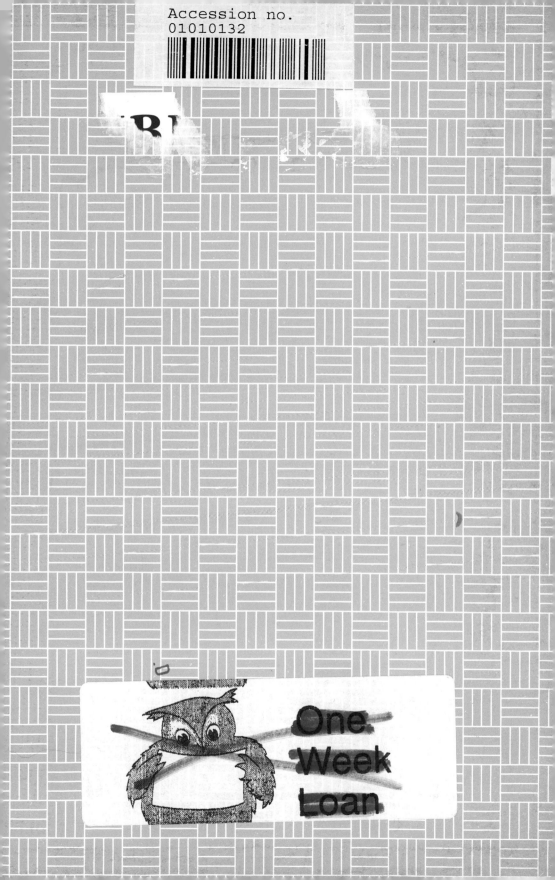

COMPANION ENCYCLOPEDIA
OF THE
HISTORY OF MEDICINE

Volume 2

Edited by

W. F. BYNUM AND ROY PORTER

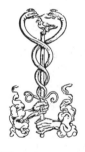

London and New York

First published in 1993
Reprinted in 1994
by Routledge
11 New Fetter Lane, London EC4P 4EE

Simultaneously published in the USA and Canada
by Routledge
a division of Routledge, Chapman and Hall, Inc.
29 West 35th Street, New York, NY 10001

Phototypeset in 10/12½ Ehrhardt Linotronic 300 by Intype, London
Printed in Great Britain by T.J. Press (Padstow) Ltd, Cornwall
Printed on acid-free paper

British Library Cataloguing in Publication Data

A catalogue record for this book is available from the British Library

Library of Congress Cataloging-in-Publication Data

A catalog record for this book is available on request.
ISBN 0-415-04771-4 (set)
ISBN 0-415-09242-6 (Volume 1)
ISBN 0-415-09243-4 (Volume 2)

CONTENTS

VOLUME 1

Notes on contributors	xi
Note to the reader	xxv
Acknowledgements	xxvi

Introduction

1 The art and science of medicine 3
  Roy Porter and W. F. Bynum

Part I   The place of medicine

2 What is specific to Western medicine? 15
  Arthur Kleinman

3 The historiography of medicine 24
  Gert Brieger

4 Medical care 45
  Guenter B. Risse

Part II   Body systems

5 The anatomical tradition 81
  Roger French

6 The microscopical tradition 102
  Brian Bracegirdle

7   The physiological tradition   120
    E. M. Tansey

8   The biochemical tradition   153
    W. H. Brock

9   The pathological tradition   169
    Russell C. Maulitz

10 The immunological tradition   192
    Paul Weindling

11 Clinical research   205
    Christopher C. Booth

Part III   Theories of life, health, and disease

12 The concepts of health, illness, and disease   233
    Arthur L. Caplan

13 Ideas of life and death   249
    W. R. Albury

14 Humoralism   281
    Vivian Nutton

15 Environment and miasmata   292
    Caroline Hannaway

16 Contagion/germ theory/specificity   309
    Margaret Pelling

17 Nosology   335
    W. F. Bynum

18 The ecology of disease   357
    Kenneth F. Kiple

19 Fevers   382
    Leonard G. Wilson

20 Constitutional and hereditary disorders   412
    Robert C. Olby

21 Mental diseases   438
    Theodore M. Brown

22 Nutritional diseases   463
    Kenneth J. Carpenter

23 Endocrine diseases   483
    R. B. Welbourn

24 Tropical diseases   511
    Michael Worboys

25 Cancer   536
    David Cantor

26 Sexually transmitted diseases   561
    Allan M. Brandt

27 Diseases of civilization   584
    Roy Porter

Part IV Understanding disease

28 Unorthodox medical theories   603
    Norman Gevitz

29 Non-Western concepts of disease   634
    Murray Last

30 Folk medicine   661
    Françoise Loux

31 Arab-Islamic medicine   676
    Lawrence I. Conrad

32 Chinese medicine   728
    Francesca Bray

33 Indian medicine   755
    Dominik Wujastyk

VOLUME 2

Part V Clinical medicine

34 The history of the doctor–patient relationship   783
    Edward Shorter

35 The art of diagnosis: medicine and the five senses   801
    Malcolm Nicolson

36 The science of diagnosis: diagnostic technology   824
    Stanley Joel Reiser

37 The history of medical ethics   852
    Robert Baker

38 Women and medicine   888
    Johanna Geyer-Kordesch

39 Drug therapies   915
    Miles Weatherall

40 Physical methods   939
    Harold J. Cook

41 Surgery (traditional)   961
    Ghislaine Lawrence

42 Surgery (modern)   984
    Ulrich Tröhler

43 Psychotherapy   1029
    Sander Gilman

44 Childbirth   1050
    Irvine S. L. Loudon

45 Childhood   1072
    Debórah Dwork

46 Geriatrics   1092
    Pat Thane

Part VI Medicine in society

47 The history of the medical profession   1119
    Toby Gelfand

48 Medical education   1151
    Susan Lawrence

49 The hospital   1180
    Lindsay Granshaw

50 The medical institutions and the state   1204
    Daniel M. Fox

51 Public health   1231
    Dorothy Porter

52 Epidemiology   1262
    Lise Wilkinson

53 The history of personal hygiene   1283
    Andrew Wear

54 A general history of nursing: 1800–1900   1309
    Christopher Maggs

55 The emergence of para-medical professions   1329
    Gerald Larkin

56 Psychiatry   1350
    Jan Goldstein

57 Health economics: finance, budgeting, and insurance   1373
    Nick Bosanquet

Part VII Medicine, ideas, and culture

58 Medicine and colonialism   1393
    David Arnold

59 Internationalism in medicine and public health   1417
    Milton I. Roemer

60 Medicine and anthropology   1436
    Carol MacCormack

61 Religion and medicine   1449
    Roy Porter

62 Charity before *c.*1850   1469
    Colin Jones

63 Medical philanthropy after 1850   1480
    W. F. Bynum

64 Medicine and architecture   1495
    Christine Stevenson

65 Medicine and literature   1520
    Michael Neve

66 War and modern medicine   1536
    Roger Cooter

67 Pain and suffering   1574
    Roy Porter

68 Medical technologies: social contexts and consequences   1592
    Harry M. Marks

69 Medicine and the law   1619
    Catherine Crawford

70 Medical sociology   1641
    David Armstrong

71 Demography and medicine   1663
    Richard M. Smith

72 Medicine, mortality, and morbidity   1693
    Stephen J. Kunitz

Index   1713

PART V

CLINICAL MEDICINE

34

THE HISTORY OF THE DOCTOR–PATIENT RELATIONSHIP

Edward Shorter

The history of the doctor–patient relationship since the eighteenth century may be divided into three phases: traditional, modern, and post-modern. Each is characterized by a distinctive level of scientific accomplishment on the doctor's part, and a distinctive psychological attitude toward the doctor on the patient's part. Much of the modern social history of medicine may be understood as what happens to these two actors in the psychodrama, doctor and patient, as these three phases unfold.

THE TRADITIONAL PERIOD

From the viewpoint of the history of medical theories, it would be incorrect to talk about a single 'traditional' period, for over the centuries many modifications had been carved into the basic trunk of Galenic humoralism. (➤ Ch. 14 Humoralism) Indeed in the eighteenth century, several rival 'schools' threw humoralism overboard. Yet over this long haul the structure of the consultation itself remained relatively unchanged. Thus, while we would not be entitled to talk about 'traditional' theories of patho-physiology, we take only a few liberties in speaking of the constant nature of the doctor–patient relationship before the nineteenth century: hence the term 'traditional', or that which existed before the infusion of science into medical practice.

These 'traditional' physicians may in most countries be divided into two groups: the élite consultant physicians of the cities, and the great mass of starveling practitioners elsewhere. This distinction cleaved traditional physicians into those of high or low social standing, the bearers of the 'gold-headed canes' and the country apothecaries. In England, the fellows of the

Royal College of Physicians stood out clearly against the surgeon-apothecaries who were the forebears of the nineteenth-century 'general practitioner'. On the continent of Europe, the professors of medicine in the university towns contrasted starkly with the second- and third-class barber-surgeons and *Wundärzte* of the countryside, though there were gradations in between. In the United States, the majority of health-care providers to the people were 'frontier doctors' whose formal medical training might have been limited to a brief apprenticeship. While all of these second-class medical attendants dispensed 'physic', so did a variety of other paramedical practitioners, such as midwives, apothecaries, corn-removers, and the like. What we therefore understand by 'doctor' before the early nineteenth century had little to do with university-trained physicians, implicating instead a wide variety of professions whose essential preparation had been the apprenticeship. (➤ Ch. 47 History of the medical profession; Ch. 55 The emergence of para-medical professions)

What characterized the structure of the traditional consultation? If we break a consultation into its component parts – history-taking, observation and examination, drawing up a differential diagnosis with accompanying prognosis, and treatment – we may claim that traditional physicians:

1   did fairly well in history-taking;
2   virtually omitted any kind of clinical investigation, in the sense of observing and examining the patient;
3   had almost no sense of differential diagnosis; and
4   did – by their own lights – spectacularly at treatment. (➤ Ch. 4 Medical care)

It is clear from eighteenth- and early nineteenth-century case histories that these doctors spent considerable time upon the past medical history of the patient and the history of the present illness; they hoped thereby to cast some light upon the patient's 'constitution'. As for the perfunctoriness of the clinical investigation, a still quite traditional physician, Bernhard Liehrsch of Dresden, advised colleagues in 1842 on the physical examination: 'You should never omit feeling the pulse, and looking at the urine and the tongue. These are the three matters to which every patient attaches value.' Do it even if unnecessary, he urged, so that you will not be accused of forgetting anything.[1] (➤ Ch. 35 The art of diagnosis: medicine and the five senses) The very nature of traditional medical nosology, which offered diagnoses in the form of descriptions of symptoms ('putrid malignant fever' and the like) meant that little differential diagnosis was occurring. (➤ Ch. 17 Nosology) There was no 'differential' list of competing diagnoses to be got through. Finally, the overwhelming therapeutic confidence of the traditional doctor rested upon endless lists of syrups, spirits, infusions, and extracts in a traditional pharmacopoeia, each with its own indications. The *Pharmacopoeia* of the Royal College of Physicians of London of 1824, for example, mentions forty different tinctures, twenty-three spirits, and fourteen syrups, all based upon different plants.[2] These physicians believed they had tremendous therapeutic power at their disposal.

Familiar with plant parts though they may have been, traditional doctors enjoyed little social status in the eyes of their patients. An English surgeon-apothecary named Popjay had this sign in front of his house, 'I Popjay, Surgeon Apotecary [sic] and Midwife etc; draws teeth and bleeds on lowest terms. Confectionary Tobacco Snuff Tea Coffee Sugar and all sorts of perfumery sold here. NB New laid eggs every morning by Mrs. Popjay.'[3] These surgeon-apothecaries in Britain and their equivalents on the European continent were not seen as 'gentlemen', that is to say, they did not have Latin, the mark of the qualified physician. Looking back over a lifetime of medical practice, the German surgeon Georg Stromeyer (1804–76) wrote in 1875:

> The rights and privileges of a Doctor of Medicine were more fancy than fact in those days. It was hard to succeed even to the pretension of being considered as a man of good breeding, although Latin did help out some. My colleague [Adolph] Henke in Erlangen used to say, Latin was the only means of telling us apart from the barbers.[4] (➤ Ch. 48 Medical education)

As for aspiring to go to medical school, commerce was often seen as a preferable career choice. Elias Canetti (b. 1905), who grew up in a quite traditional Jewish community in Bulgaria, rememberd the opinions of his Uncle Solomon, whose own world-views had been forged many decades earlier, about the undesirability of medicine as a career. 'What are you going to do?' he asked young Canetti. Canetti's aunt volunteered, 'He wants to go to university.' 'Oh no way,' said Uncle Solomon, 'He's going to be a business-man.' The only member of the family who had gone into medicine, a cousin, had soon regretted it. 'A doctor doesn't earn anything,' said Uncle Solomon. 'He's the errand boy of the rich and has to come for every little thing, and then it turns out there's nothing wrong with the people at all.'[5] The Uncle Solomons of this world reflected the low opinion in which the doctor was traditionally held.

These traditional doctors often lived in a poverty as dire as that of the patients themselves. What were the prospects of becoming rich from medical practice in Germany? In 1804, Johann Rademacher (1772–1850) advised his fellow physicians that any doctors who looked prosperous had probably inherited money:

> But around here, even if you made so much that you could live from it, you still wouldn't be able to save anything. And then what will you live from when you get weak from age, or you get an ulcer on your foot or a hernia, or some

other condition which would keep you from horseback, or from travelling about, or from the privilege of immersing yourself in storm and tempest.

If you ask me how an impoverished physician is supposed to get on in this land and prepare himself for the future, I say, if you don't have any money marry a rich girl. If you're an ugly devil whom no one will have, maybe you can win the lottery a couple of times.

And if that failed, Dr Rademacher advised emigrating to America.[6] Unless one was a member of the medical élite, such as the Royal College of Physicians, and could profit from the consulting fees of the wealthy, the lowly income of the traditional physician corresponded roughly to his reduced status.

Lay people mixed into medical matters with a blithe disregard of 'medical authority'. Medical learning counted for little; for example, at the Julius Hospital in Würzburg early in the nineteenth century, lay administrators summoned the doctors to stand at attention alongside the servants. Anton Müller (1755–1827), the psychiatrist, recalled the obstetrician Professor Elias von Siebold (1775–1826) in full uniform and ceremonial dagger, lined up beside the chambermaids for inspection.

> A certain clerical member of the hospital would come into the pharmacy, ask for the prescription books and page through them, indicating approval with a nod of his head or disapproval with a headshake. This individual even dared, after reading [Philippe] Pinel's work on the treatment of the insane, to draft a long set of guidelines about how the insane in our ward were to be treated.[7]

For their modest social standing these doctors paid the therapeutic price of patients' non-compliance. It was, perhaps, just as well anyway that patients often refused the courses of bleeding, vomiting, and purgation that represented the therapeutic armamentarium of traditional medicine. Yet frequent refusal to follow the doctor's orders indicates how little those orders meant in lay eyes. For example, physicians obliged to control the spread of epidemic disease late in the eighteenth century in Brittany deplored the reluctance of peasants to accept medical authority. In 1786, one rural physician, attempting to cope with malarial fevers in some provincial nest said, 'It happened often that patients omitted to use the prescribed medications nor did they want to use the emetics. Usually a stubborn constipation would ensue, followed by dropsy.'[8] Henry Sutler, who lived towards the middle of the nineteenth century in Pittsfield, Illinois, was one such disobedient patient, in the days when small-town frontier physicians such as Thomas Shastid (1866–1947) had improved but little in status. Shastid's son, a boy at the time accompanying his father on house calls, tells the story. Although Henry Sutler was a kind man and successful in business, his weak point was that 'he never liked anybody to tell him what to do'. But when he came down with typhoid fever he had to obey his wife and his doctor, up to a certain point:

> Then Henry Sutler's condition began to improve. Henry did not understand typhoid fever, but he thought that he did. After the fourth week, when he had no more fever and scarcely any pain, *he* informed *my father* that he was all right now, that he was going to get up shortly, dress himself and set about his work. [Shastid demurred and said Henry risked the danger of haemorrhaging from the bowels if he were to get up.]
>
> Henry persisted. My father resisted. Henry begged his wife to bring him his shoes, his shirt, his trousers. Father told her not to bring them. [Unless Henry promised not to get up, Dr Shastid threatened to] gather up every particle of clothing that you have in the house, take it away home with me and burn it. [Henry promised.]
>
> Father and I then went away happy. Scarcely, however, had we driven half a quarter when we heard behind us a woman's shrill screaming. Turning, we saw Mrs. Sutler standing on her front porch, crying and frantically gesturing to us to come back.
>
> At the house again we arrived just in time to see Henry Sutler faint and fall to the floor. Yes, he was dead, and his trousers were full of blood.[9]

Beneath this non-compliance lay patients' fundamental disbelief in the doctor as a professional who understood the secrets of Nature. Two thousand years of traditional humoral diagnosis and therapeutics, with their consistently poor, counter-therapeutic results, had sapped the willingness of the population to believe implicitly in the enterprise of medicine itself. For the traditional patient, therefore, access to medicine meant really procuring a prescription for some complex purgative the patient could not compound or as a last desperate resort in terminal illness.

THE MODERN PERIOD

What distinguishes the modern from the traditional period is the establishment of patho-physiology in the nineteenth century as a *method* of investigation – in contrast to being yet another doctrine, or 'school'. In the nineteenth century, three crucial events infused the scientific method into the practice of medicine.

First, the clinical investigation started to become both art and science, in the form of percussion, palpation, and auscultation, permitting the physical examination of the patient to go beyond merely looking at the tongue and urine, and feeling the radial pulse. Although the description of percussion technically belongs to the Viennese physician Leopold Auenbrugger (1722–1809) in 1761, the components of the physical examination were really only put into practice early in the nineteenth century by the Parisian clinical school, of which René Laënnec (1781–1826) was the most notable member.

It is interesting to contrast the traditional dismissal of the physical examination with the method of Professor Franz Volhard (1872–1950) of teaching medical students to examine patients in the Frankfurt university clinic in the early 1930s. One young staff-member later recalled that at first in the session students were not permitted to touch the patients at all, merely to say what they observed by looking at them:

> After the students had observed the most minute details, including the pulse of the carotid and the appearance of the nail-bed, and duly described what they had seen, they were allowed to feel the radial pulse. After they had seen asymmetries in the expansion of the chest, they were permitted to feel the circumference of the ribs. . . . It was quite extraordinary to experience the varieties of tactile sensation. There was, quite aside from the world of sight, an entire world of touch which we had never perceived before. In feeling differences of radial pulse you could train yourself to feel dozens of different waves with their characteristic peaks, blunt and sharp, steep and slanting, and the corresponding valleys. There were so many ways in which the margin of the liver came up towards your palpating finger. There were extraordinary varieties of smell. There was not just pallor but there seemed to be hundreds of hues of yellow and gray.[10]

It was an added benefit that the modern physician, in this kind of observing and examining, also established a close physical rapport with the patient.

A second contribution was the development of the science of pathological anatomy which, in combination with the close clinical observation of patients ante-mortem, would make possible the accurate diagnosis of disease, replacing traditional symptomatic diagnoses. Notable milestones in the unfolding of the science of pathology were the refinement of the microscope in the 1820s, the introduction of the microtome by C. M. Topping in the 1840s, and the discovery of various histological stains, notably haematoxylin from the heartwood of the American *Haematoxylon* tree in 1865 and eosin from aniline dye in 1876.[11] (➤ Ch. 6 The microscopical tradition) Accurate clinical data, together with microscopic pathological findings, resulted in the 'anatomical-clinical method', which was the great motor of progress in clinical medicine during the nineteenth century. Although this great accumulation in knowledge of pathological anatomy caused little improvement in therapy, it did establish the image of the physician as a scientist, able to give patients a reliable diagnosis and prognosis. (➤ Ch. 9 The pathological tradition)

Finally came the germ theory of disease late in the century, putting an end to centuries-old notions about 'miasmas' and 'evil west winds'. (➤ Ch. 15 Environment and miasmata) The diagnostic capabilities of medicine advanced enormously with the science of microbiology. Establishing that symptoms resulted from infection, and then being able to differentiate microscopically and with serum cultures among the varieties of infective organisms, repre-

sented a leap towards science comparable to the introduction of the anatomical-clinical method early in the century. (➤ Ch. 11 Clinical research) The discovery by Robert Koch (1843–1910) in 1882 of the bacillus that caused
tuberculosis was the main scientific landmark in establishing microbiology.
But the demonstration by Louis Pasteur (1822–95) of the therapeutic effectiveness of the rabies vaccine in 1885 and the preparation by Emil von
Behring (1854–1917) of the diphtheria antitoxin in 1890 confirmed in the
public mind the status of the doctor as a scientist who could actually cure
disease. (➤ Ch. 16 Contagion/germ theory/specificity)

The result of these three advances – the clinical examination, pathological
anatomy, and microbiology – was to place medical diagnosis upon a scientific
footing. By the end of the nineteenth century, the doctor could, for the first
time in history, diagnose successfully the most important disease conditions
of humankind. Similarly, the doctor was in a position to make reasonably
confident prognoses of the disease course, now that tuberculosis had been
differentiated from pneumonia, typhus from typhoid fever, and so forth.
(➤ Ch. 19 Fevers; Ch. 36 The science of diagnosis: diagnostic technology)

In therapeutics, the gains from infusing science into medicine were modest:
a handful of new vaccines; salvarsan for syphilis patented in 1909 by Paul
Ehrlich (1854–1915); and a scattering of sedatives and analgesics. Quinine
for malaria and digitalis for congestive heart failure were already present in
the pre-1850 pharmacopoeia (or rather, the plants from which they were
extracted were present). The gains which these few new drugs represented
did greatly impress the public, but their limited nature must be emphasized.
In view of the vast gamut of bacterial and viral infections that remained
untreatable, in view of the array of degenerative diseases such as arthritis,
coronary artery disease, and cancer whose palliation was scarcely possible,
the 'therapeutic nihilism' of the late nineteenth century was not unjustified.
(➤ Ch. 20 Constitutional and hereditary disorders; Ch. 25 Cancer)

How did the structure of the modern medical consultation differ from the
traditional? The modern consultation may be characterized as:

1 excellent in history-taking, for the anatomical-clinical method attached
   great importance to the chart, the course of the illness;
2 excellent in clinical investigation, especially in the physical examination
   of the patient;
3 excellent in diagnosis, genuine differential diagnoses organized about
   elucidating a 'chief complaint' appearing now for the first time;
4 terrible in therapeutics, there being few effective medications. (➤ Ch. 67
   Pain and suffering)

The new scientific basis of medicine lent enormous prestige to the physician
in the eyes of the patient. First, the physical examination encouraged a laying-

on of hands, a gesture with ritual as well as practical import, suggesting to the patient that he or she was being cared for. Establishing this kind of physical rapport became almost a code of honour with the physicians of a certain generation. Michael Lepore (b. 1910), a New York internist, looked back at this clinical style as taught before the Second World War at the College of Physicians and Surgeons at Columbia University: 'Who will ever forget having witnessed the aristocratic and fastidious Hugh Auchincloss Sr (1878–1947), Professor of Surgery at Columbia Presbyterian, clearing a patient's "intestinal obstruction" on rounds by rolling up his gold cuff-linked shirtsleeves and digging out by hand, a large fecal impaction!'[12] The men of his generation – there were as yet few women – attached great importance to communicating to the patient a physical sense of care.

Second, pathological anatomy, whose source of knowledge is the laboratory and the autopsy suite, may not greatly have affected the psychodrama of the doctor–patient relationship. But it did generate a public image of the doctor as a scientist poring at all hours over his heavy tomes. This image was used to great effect by the drug companies in the 1920s and 1930s in advertisements featuring, not various prescription drugs ('ethical specialties'), but clean-shaven, lantern-jawed physicians reading the latest pathology journals at a time of night when the rest of the population was at play.[13]

Third, the science of microbiology had a great effect upon opinion. After the drama of the rabies vaccine in 1885, Louis Pasteur (1822–95) started to become a household name. The work of Paul de Kruif (1890–1971) published in 1926, *Microbe Hunters*, inspired a whole generation with the nobility of microbiology as a calling. On its title-page stood the quotation, 'The gods are frankly human, sharing in the weaknesses of mankind, yet not untouched with a halo of divine Romance.' The 'gods' were the physicians![14] As for 'germs' themselves, their impact upon public consciousness is evident in the neurotic vogue of the 1920s for opening door-handles with pieces of tissue and indulging in compulsive hand-washing. Without the prestige of 'medical science' in the background, the neuroses driving these deformed precautions would have taken other forms.

The image of the physician as a demi-god possessed of boundless authority over patients dates from the late nineteenth century. Female patients, for example, became willing to submit to pelvic examinations and to give birth in the lithotomy position mainly because they had acquired an implicit belief in the doctor as a scientist. (➤ Ch. 38 Women and medicine) As Worthington Hooker (1806–67), a physician in Norwich, Connecticut, and later a professor at Yale, said in 1849, the doctor acted not merely as clinician but as a 'confidential friend'.

If he has been the physician of the family for any length of time . . . this feeling of affectionate reliance is deep and ardent; so much so that it is a severe trial to the sensitive mind to be obliged to consult a stranger. . . . Especially this is so when the patient is a female.[15]

Similarly, doctors in the modern period often involved themselves in counselling patients in intimate problems, indeed presuming to advise society as a whole in a wholly unfamiliar extension of this new medical authority.

The great irony of the modern phase of the doctor–patient relationship is that the prestige of the doctor rested not upon his improved ability to cure, but rather to understand disease and to establish an accurate prognosis. Nineteenth-century physicians cast their therapeutic helplessness in the Viennese doctrine of 'therapeutic nihilism', the view of both Joseph Skoda (1805–81) and Carl Rokitansky (1804–78) that doctors did far better in investigating basic disease mechanisms than in curing. Psychoanalyst Fritz Wittels (1880–1950), reflecting about his medical training in late nineteenth-century Vienna, wrote:

> In contradistinction to the naive faith of the romantic epoch, the medical school in Vienna fostered a notorious nihilism in therapeutics. . . . The order of the day was to cleanse the temple of science of superstitions, some of them thousands of years old. Such a cleansing had to precede any scientific therapy of the future.[16]

But the lecturers did ignore therapeutics. 'They frequently seemed to forget that sick people want to regain their health.[17]

Because therapeutic horizons were so limited, these modern physicians needed everything they had going for them, and that meant relying therapeutically upon the psychological dimension of the doctor–patient relationship, trying with the force of the doctor's personality, and the quality and closeness of concern, to 'suggest' the patient into a cure. This is why modern doctors were so mindful of the notion of the 'great physician', the commanding personality whose bedside manner worked in and of itself, in the words of Michael Balint, 'as a pill'.[18] One thinks of such well-known internists and neurologists as Hermann Nothnagel (1841–1905) and Carl von Noorden (1858–1944) in Vienna, Jean-Martin Charcot (1825–93) in Paris, Hermann Weber (1823–1918) and his son Frederick Parkes Weber (1863–1962) in London, and Silas Weir Mitchell (1829–1914) the inventor of the 'rest cure', in Philadelphia. None of these physicians could do much for patients but prescribe placebos and send them off to spas, yet all possessed powerful personalities and were acknowledged in their day to be great healers.

From these turn-of-the century internists and neurologists we first encounter admonitions to 'treat the patient as a person', meaning to consider the patient's personal history and social situation in diagnosing and treating organic disease. Valentin Holst (1839–1904), a neurologist with forty years of experience, said in 1897, that one had to treat the whole person:

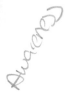

> And the patient must be able to feel this. He should approach the physician with a feeling of trust, he should have the confident feeling of being entirely understood by his doctor. It is precisely these patients who suffer most from the feeling that [no one understands them].[19] (➤ Ch. 43 Psychotherapy)

What gave doctors of this modern period their distinctive therapeutic skill was the ability, based on the patients' implicit confidence in 'science', to inspire them into a cure. Although increasing the patient's morale plays a role in treating all disease conditions, the inspirational aspects of the doctor–patient relationship were especially important in the treatment of the psychogenic physical symptoms associated with 'hysteria' and 'neurasthenia'. Somatizing patients often benefited from the opportunity to experience a 'catharsis' in the presence of a respected figure. And the modern doctor's newly acquired social status had resulted in such respect.

There is much evidence that somatizing patients obtained relief from the sheer opportunity to tell the doctor their stories at their own pace (rather than responding to a series of 'yes–no'-style questions). Already at the end of the eighteenth century, this was clear to forward-looking physicians such as Jacob Isenflamm (1726–93), Professor of Medicine at Erlangen:

> Not without reason does one give patients full reign to tell their stories. It is the more important for patients [with psychological problems] that precisely this manner of letting them ramble on about their histories and leaving nothing out – sometimes even putting the whole affair down on paper then reading it aloud to the doctor – be allowed, for in doing so they believe they receive marked relief.[20]

Although not unknown in traditional medicine, this cathartic benefit of the consultation was more commonly obtained in the modern style of medical practice. John Horder (b. 1919) recalled in 1967, 'My partner, Dr M. Modell, had a classic example of a quick consultation: a woman came for the first time, sat down, began to cry, did so for four minutes, said "Thank you, doctor, you have helped me a lot" – and left.'[21] This kind of confidence is conferred only upon physicians whom patients regard as healers.

THE POST-MODERN PERIOD

The post-modern period is characterized by an overweening confidence on the physician's part in medications which, for the first time in history, really do heal or ameliorate a vast range of disease conditions. It is this confidence that makes the psychological benefits that flow from the consultation seem secondary. But post-modern patients respond to what they perceive as the physician's lack of interest with anger and withdrawal, ultimately with malpractice suits and recourse to alternative healers.

The advent of drugs that could cure a wide range of disorders began in 1935 with Prontosil, or benzenesulphonamide. The first of the sulpha drugs, it gave way to a cascade of medications for bacterial infections. Penicillin, for example, became available to the civilian population in 1945. These new drugs enabled physicians to treat successfully such nightmares of previous medical practice as post-partum sepsis, and vastly reduced the mortality from bacterial disease. (➤ Ch. 39 Drug therapies)

The success of these 'wonder drugs' prompted research into biochemical and pharmacological mechanisms, as opposed to pathological anatomy, which had dominated the previous period. A whole new line of scientific investigation, beginning with biochemistry and terminating in clinical applications in the field of internal medicine, thus opened up. (➤ Ch. 8 The biochemical tradition) The post-modern period therefore may be said to have begun as this new line of biochemistry/internal medicine started to be taught in medical schools in the years after the Second World War. For only via the medical schools would it truly be introduced into medical practice. The dominant approach to medical education in the 1950s was to treat medical students as mini-scientists rather than as physicians-to-be. This tilt towards science in the curriculum was rationalized on the grounds that the physician must understand the scientific mechanisms underlying the drugs prescribed. (This apparently sensible rationale ignored the realities that, first, it is not at all necessary to understand basic metabolic pathways in order to prescribe successfully; and second, most doctors forget this information anyway after they leave medical school.) The impression thus arose in medical education that 'legitimate' symptoms stemmed only from organic diseases, the mechanisms of whose biochemistry and whose pharmacological treatment may be understood and memorized. Other kinds of symptoms were deemed to come mainly from 'crocks', and were really most suitable for the psychiatrist to treat. (➤ Ch. 56 Psychiatry)

Thus, in the 1950s, a new generation of ultra-scientifically trained physicians, truly prepared to take on the classic killers of humankind, burst into the doctor–patient relationship. For this generation, most of that 'psychological stuff' had been dismissed. The great internist of Columbia University, Robert Loeb (1895–1973), coolly pronounced its last rites in 1953, when he complained to the administration that he had heard enough about training pre-meds in 'social sciences' and experimental 'home care programs in which medical students would participate even during their first year'. From now on at Columbia, only standards of 'the highest possible scientific level' would prevail.[22]

How did this new emphasis upon disease mechanisms affect the consultation? For one thing, it precipitated a loss of interest in the whole 'patient-as-a-person' approach, which had hallmarked much of medicine before the

Second World War. The doctor did not now have to exhibit interest in the patient's overall life, given drugs that really cured disease. It must be emphasized that it was the *appearance* of caring that tended to be withdrawn. It would be ridiculous to argue that doctors actually became somehow less caring or less humane, since the character attributes of physicians have probably not changed over thousands of years. Merely the show of concern, the stage presence of a trained physician, came to seem less therapeutically important, simply because the doctor now handed out effective medications.

For another thing, advances in clinical investigation since the Second World War entailed the downgrading of careful history-taking and physical examination. Patients once experienced a catharsis in being able to tell their stories at their own pace, and felt a thorough physical examination to be an expression of the doctor's concern for them. With the advent of such post-modern techniques of investigation as computerized blood tests, computerized tomography scans, magnetic resonance imaging, and ultrasonography, old-fashioned percussing, palpating, and auscultating seemed increasingly irrelevant, for the new techniques yielded far more information. The 'history' too became downplayed, and letting the patient talk was perceived as a waste of the busy physician's time. (➤ Ch. 68 Medical technologies: social contexts and consequences)

The structure of the post-modern consultation may accordingly be classed as:

1 limited to an impatient and abbreviated style of history-taking;
2 cursory attention to physical examination while giving painstaking attention to laboratory data and diagnostic imaging;
3 concern with differential diagnosis unchanged;
4 enormous therapeutic power by the standards of double-blind controlled studies.

One of the great ironies of the social history of medicine is that, at the supreme moment of achieving this therapeutic power, the crown of glory was snatched from the doctor's head. In the last quarter of the twentieth century, as an ever-broader stream of antibacterial, anti-inflammatory and antineoplastic medications became available, patients became increasingly alienated from the former 'demigods in white'. Recent statistics illustrate these changes. For example, rising numbers of malpractice suits point to growing alienation: one half of all surgeons in Florida had been sued for malpractice within the period 1975–80, and the better trained the surgeons were, the greater the number of suits.[23] Between 1975 and 1985, claims per 100 physicians in the United States as a whole more than doubled. Some specialities were exceedingly vulnerable: over the five-year period 1976–81, claims against obstetricians tripled. The average claim itself climbed from $18,000 in 1975 to almost $100,000 in 1988.[24] (➤ Ch. 69 Medicine and the law; Ch. 37 History of medical ethics)

Second, patients responded to their perception of physicians' coolness and lack of interest with a lack of loyalty. Several different American polls commissioned in the mid-1980s found that two-thirds of all patients would be willing to 'change their provider in an attempt to find more satisfactory medical care'.[25] One contrasts this high volatility with patients in the days before the Second World War who, with their families, would often develop lifelong attachments to the same family doctor.

The whole persona of the 'family doctor', the elderly pipe-puffing figure present both at birth and death, is now disappearing, both in fact and in the minds of patients. In the United States in 1988, only slightly more than one doctor in ten was in 'general family practice'.[26] Nor were American patients particularly interested in the advice of their physicians: the percentage of patients willing to use the family doctor as a source of 'local health care information' declined from 46 per cent in 1984 to 21 per cent in 1989.[27] How did families select which hospital to attend? More than 50 per cent of patients polled in 1989 said that 'they or their family have the most influence in selection of a hospital' – as opposed to listening to the doctor – up from 40 per cent in previous years.[28] (Non-American readers will recall that private American hospitals compete for patients.)

This alienation from the doctor–patient relationship has diminished the public's former hero-worship of the doctor. According to a Gallup poll in 1989, 26 per cent of patients said they respected doctors less now than ten years ago (14 per cent said more). And of those who respected doctors less, 26 per cent said, 'they [the doctors] are in it for the money'. Seventeen per cent claimed that doctors 'lack rapport and concern'.[29]

Alienation is also apparent in a flight to alternative therapies such as naturopathy, iridology, reflexology, and the like. Lacking any scientific basis, these represent a return to the eighteenth century, when all therapies, medical and non-medical alike, were based upon anecdotal results rather than quantitative demonstrations of efficacy. For example, in the United Kingdom: in 1981, alternative practitioners were 27 per cent as numerous as the total number of general practitioners; the number of acupuncturists doubled between 1978 and 1981; and the consultation of such non-orthodox practitioners increased by 42 per cent from 1981 to 1985.[30] (➤ Ch. 28 Unorthodox medical theories)

Post-modern physicians, wounded and estranged by this lack of patient trust, often respond with a similar emotional withdrawal from the doctor–patient relationship. In a nationwide American survey in 1989, 63 per cent of the physicians polled said they felt their control over patient treatment decisions had decreased (up from 54 per cent in 1987). In the same poll, four doctors in ten said they would be unlikely to go to medical school if they had their lives over again, and only one in four said that he or she would definitely go.[31] A decline of 23 per cent in the number of applicants to American medical schools between 1978 and 1987 suggests that fewer young people look forward to being doctors.[32]

Thus, at the very moment of triumph, the post-modern doctor is rewarded with snarls of rage rather than praise from the patient. What lies behind this paradoxical reaction? Most important, in my opinion, has been the effect of the media on patients' knowledge of medicine and medical practice. In former times, patients acquired their medical knowledge from the experience of their families and communities. Within this rather folkloric knowledge base, the image of the doctor as kindly general practitioner, with an office piled high with books of learning, loomed prominently. The knowledge base of the post-modern patient, by contrast, is heavily informed by the media. Family and community sources of information recede. The world-view of medicine that patients receive from the media is a highly Manichean one, in which the miracle of virtually eternal life through Medical progress is extended on the one hand, horror stories of malpractice brandished on the other. Unlike family or village knowledge, medical knowledge disseminated in the post-modern world is assessed by editors primarily by its sensational value. It is this sensationalizing of all medical stories that creates a climate in which any unfavourable outcome is seen as the incompetent denial of the hope proffered in the press. Thus a flood of malpractice suits, eroding the goodwill between doctor and patient, is the result.

One may read this larger chronicle of changes in the relationship between doctor and patient in two ways. One group of scholars has been inclined to see these changes as evidence of 'medicalization', arguing that the autonomous attitude of traditional patients towards their bodies and their healthy collaboration with non-professional healers became replaced by a toxic kind of hero-worship in which patients sacrificed their own judgement to place themselves in the thrall of the experts. This disdainful assessment of the physician's increasing role in patients' lives thus sees them as ever more passive objects of professionalization. The account offered in this chapter is flavoured, of course, by quite different value judgements, interpreting the doctors' growing influence upon the patients as positive, and celebrating the scientific basis of modern medicine. I would modify the received wisdom on medicalization in two ways.

First, one forgets how much power the patient has in the doctor–patient relationship when choice among physicians prevails. Rather than being a passive recipient of authoritarian medical commands, the patient has beliefs that set limits on the range of procedures and medications available to the doctor. The post-modern triumph of the consumers' movement in obstetrics

offers an example, forcing doctors to admit husbands to the delivery suite
and to desist from automatically administering analgesia and anaesthesia.[33] A
historic example was the shift in psychiatric terminology from 'mental disease'
to 'nervous disease' at the end of the nineteenth century, as wealthy patients,
dreading the familial stigma of insanity, insisted on their symptoms being
seen as an organic affection of the nevous system.[34] (➤ Ch. 21 Mental diseases)

The rapport of forces in the doctor–patient relationship is the result, in
other words, of the play between medical supply and patient demand.
Science-driven changes in technology, pharmacology, and concepts of patho-
physiology affect the supply, or what doctors wish to offer. Larger cultural
and social trends affect the demand, or what patients are willing to accept.
As George Bernard Shaw said in his preface to *The Doctor's Dilemma* in
1911:

> [Doctors] must believe, on the whole, what their patients believe, just as they
> must wear the sort of hat their patients wear. The doctor may lay down the
> law despotically enough to the patient at points where the patient's mind is
> simply blank; but when the patient has a prejudice the doctor must either keep
> it in countenance or lose his patient. If people are persuaded that night air is
> dangerous to health and that fresh air makes them catch cold, it will not be
> possible for a doctor to make his living in private practice if he prescribes
> ventilation.[35] (➤ Ch. 65 Medicine and literature):

Second, the modern style of medical practice may be said to have offered
some therapeutic benefits for the patient. The distinctive accomplishment of
the modern doctor was the ability to relieve psychogenic conditions, or
somatization. Lacking an organic basis, such complaints responded to the
informal kind of psychotherapy conferred by the doctor–patient relationship
itself. Such somatoform problems represent at least 30 per cent of all complaints seen in primary care today.[36] Only one person in ten in the general
population does not experience symptoms in a given two-week period, and
the average adult has fully four symptoms of illness on one out of every four
days.[37] Stripping the doctor–patient relationship of its intrinsic healing qualities in the post-modern period cannot be said to represent a therapeutic
advance in the management of such complaints.

NOTES

1 Bernard Liehrsch, *Bilder des ärztlichen Lebens, oder: die wahre Lebenspolitik des
   Arztes für alle Verhältnisse*, Berlin, 1842, p. 148.

2 Richard Phillips, *A Translation of the Pharmacopoeia of the Royal College of Physicians
   of London*, 1824; 2nd edn, London, 1831.

3 Quoted in Irvine Loudon, 'Two thousand medical men in 1847', *Society for the
   Social History of Medicine Bulletin*, 1983, 33: 8.

4   Georg Friedrich Louis Stromeyer, *Erinnerungen eines deutschen Arztes*, 2 vols, 2nd edn, Hanover, n.d [1873], Vol. I, p. 206.

5   Elias Canetti, *Die gerettete Zunge: Geschichte einer Jugend*, Frankfurt, Fischer, 1977, pp. 234–5.

6   Johann Gottfried Rademacher, *Briefe für Ärzte und Nichtärzte über die Aftermedizin und deren Nothwendigkeit im Staate*, Cologne, [1804], pp. 89–90.

7   Anton Müller, *Die Irren-Anstalt in dem königlichen Julius-Hospitale zu Würzburg*, Würzburg, 1824, p. 61.

8   Quoted in Jean-Pierre Goubert, *Malades et Médecins en Bretagne, 1770–90*, Rennes, Université de Haute-Bretagne, 1974, p. 232.

9   Thomas H. Shastid, *My Second Life*, Ann Arbor, MI, G. Wahr, 1944, pp. 226–7.

10   Karl Stern, *The Pillar of Fire*, New York, Harcourt, Brace, 1951, pp. 102–3.

11   W. D. Foster, *A Short History of Clinical Pathology*, Edinburgh, Livingstone, 1961, p. 20, *passim*.

12   Michael J. Lepore, *Death of the Clinician: Requiem or Reveille?* Springfield, IL, C. C. Thomas, 1982, p. 272.

13   Such drug companies as Merck and Parke-Davis ran numerous such advertisements in the American Medical Association's popular magazine *Hygeia* in the 1920s and 1930s.

14   Paul de Kruif, *Microbe Hunters*, New York, 1926. The chapter on Walter Reed was subtitled, 'In the interest of science – and for humanity!' (p. 311).

15   Worthington Hooker, *Physician and Patient*, New York, 1849, p. 384.

16   Fritz Wittels, 'Freud's scientific cradle', *American Journal of Psychiatry*, 1943–4, 100: 521–8, quote on p. 522.

17   Ibid.

18   Michael Balint, *The Doctor, his Patient and the Illness*, rev. edn, New York, International Universities Press, 1972; orig. pub. 1957.

19   Valentin Holst, *Erfahrungen aus einer vierzigjährigen neurologischen Praxis*, Stuttgart, 1903, p. 24; reprint of a lecture given in 1897. See also George Canby Robinson, *The Patient as a Person: a Study of the Social Aspects of Illness*, New York, 1939; Francis Weld Peabody, *The Care of the Patient*, Cambridge, MA, 1927.

20   Jacob Friedrich Isenflamm, *Versuch einiger praktischen Anmerkungen über die Nerven zur Erläuterung . . . hypochondrisch- und hysterischer Zufälle*, Erlangen, 1774, p. 182.

21   John Horder, 'The role of the general practitioner in psychological medicine', *Royal Society of Medicine, London, Proceedings*, 1967, 60: 261–70, quote on pp. 267–8.

22   Robert Loeb and Dana W. Atchley, letter, *Journal of Medical Education*, 1953, 28: 87–8.

23   Frank A. Sloan *et al.*, 'Medical malpractice experience of physicians: predictable or haphazard?', *Journal of the American Medical Association*, 1989, 262: 3291–7, quote on p. 3291. Some of these statistics are also cited in the new preface of Edward Shorter, *Doctors and Patients in Historical Perspective*, New Brunswick, NJ, Transaction Books, 1991.

24   Peter Jacobson, 'Medical malpractice and the tort system', *Journal of the American Medical Association*, 1989, 262:, 3320–7.

25   Cited in Alan H. Rosenstein, 'Consumerism and health care: will the traditional

patient–physician relationship survive?, *Postgraduate Medicine*, 1986, 79: 13–18, quote on p. 16.

26 *New York Times*, 18 February 1990, p. 20.

27 Maggie Christensen, 'Smart consumers present a marketing challenge', *Hospitals*, 1989, 63: 42–47, quote on p. 44.

28 Ibid., p. 42.

29 American Medical Association, *Surveys of Physicians and Public Opinion*, Chicago, IL, American Medical Association, 1989; Commissioned Gallup pol. These data represent a continuation of trends that had begun at least as soon as the early 1980s. See George D. Lundberg, 'Medicine – a profession in trouble?', *Journal of the American Medical Association*, 1985, 253: 2879–80; on survey data for the years 1982–5 showing declines in the percentage of the public who believe that 'physicians explain things well', and that 'physicians' fees are reasonable'.

30 Joanna Murray and Simon Shepherd, 'Alternative or additional medicine? A new dilemma for the doctor', *Journal of the Royal College of General Practitioners*, 1988, 38: 511–14.

31 op. cit. (n. 29). American Medical Association, Doctors were asked 'whether they would go to medical school if they were in college now, knowing what they now know about medicine'. Fourteen per cent said they would definitely not go, and 25 per cent said they would probably not go.

32 Victor R. Neufeld *et al.*, 'Optimal outcomes of clinical education', in Barbara Gastel *et al.*, (eds), *Clinical Education and the Doctor of Tomorrow*, New York, New York Academy of Medicine, 1989, p. 13.

33 As evidence of this change see Iain Chalmers, Murray Enkin and Marc J. N. C. Keirse (eds), *Effective Care in Pregnancy and Childbirth*, 2 vols, Oxford, Oxford University Press, 1989.

34 See Edward Shorter, 'Private clinics in central Europe, 1870–1933', *Social History of Medicine*, 1990, 3, no. 2: 159–95.

35 Bernard Shaw, *The Doctor's Dilemma: a Tragedy*, Harmondsworth, Penguin, 1957, p. 67; orig. pub. 1911.

36 Z. J. Lipowski, 'Somatization: medicine's unsolved problem', *Psychosomatics*, 1987, 28: 294–7; Lipowski, 'Somatization: the concept and its clinical application', *American Journal of Psychiatry*, 1988, 145: 1358–68.

37 Donna E. Stewart, 'The changing faces of somatization', *Psychosomatics*, 1990, 31: 153–8.

FURTHER READING

Goubert, Jean-Pierre, *Malades et médecins en Bretagne, 1770–90*, Rennes, Université de Haute-Bretagne, 1974.

Huerkamp, Claudia, *Der Aufstieg der Ärzte im 19. Jahrhundert*, Göttingen, Vandenhoeck & Ruprecht, 1985.

Lesky, Erna, *Die Wiener medizinische Schule im 19. Jahrhundert*, Graz, Hermann Böhlaus, 1978.

Loudon, Irvine, *Medical Care and the General Practitioner, 1750–1850*, Oxford, Clarendon Press, 1986.

Pendleton, David and Hasler, John (eds), *Doctor–Patient Communication*, London, Academic Press, 1983.

Porter, Dorothy and Porter, Roy, *Patient's Progress: Doctors and Doctoring in Eighteenth-Century England*, Cambridge, Polity Press, 1989.

Porter, Roy (ed.), *Patients and Practitioners: Lay Perceptions of Medicine in Pre-industrial Society*, Cambridge, Cambridge University Press, 1985.

Ramsey, Matthew, *Professional and Popular Medicine in France, 1770–1830: the Social World of Medical Practice*, Cambridge, Cambridge University Press, 1988.

Shorter, Edward, *Bedside Manners: the Troubled History of Doctors and Patients*, New York, Simon & Schuster, 1985; repub. with a new preface as *Doctors and Patients in Historical Perspective*, New Brunswick, NJ, Transaction Books, 1991.

Spree, Reinhard, *Health and Social Class in Imperial Germany*, New York, Berg, 1988; Eng. trans. of 1981 German edn. New York, Berg, 1988.

Warner, John Harley, *The Therapeutic Perspective: Medical Practice, Knowledge, and Identity in America, 1820–85*, Cambridge, MA, Harvard University Press, 1986.

THE ART OF DIAGNOSIS: MEDICINE AND THE FIVE SENSES

Malcolm Nicolson

... having entered the sick room the physician should view the body of the patient, palpate it with his hands, and enquire about his complaint ... the five sense organs of hearing, touch, sight, smell and taste, as well as oral inquiry, materially contribute to a better diagnosis.

(*Súsruta Saṃhitā*)

The term 'diagnosis' may refer to the identification of the specific disease from which an individual is suffering. Or it may have a more general meaning, as in the above quotation, referring to the overall process of consultation and inquiry whereby the problems which the patient presents to his or her medical attendant are elucidated.[1] It is a truism to say that, in the latter sense, diagnosis has always been a central element of the practice of medicine. However, the particular means by which medical attendants address the problems of their patients have varied from culture to culture and from one historical era to another. In one society, the identification of disease may be accomplished by a formal interrogation of the spirit world;[2] (➤ Ch. 60 Medicine and anthropology) in another, by the sending of samples of tissue to a diagnostic laboratory. Even within the mainstream of Western medicine there has been much temporal and geographical variation in how the challenge posed by the need to diagnose has been addressed. Moreover, what the doctor does at the bedside of the patient tells us a great deal about the status and power of the practitioner and about the social context within which medical knowledge is produced.[3] The history of diagnosis is thus an important aspect of the wider history of patient–practitioner relationships. The purpose of this essay is to provide a broad overview of the changing character of diagnostic practice, mainly within the context of the development of Western medicine, up until the end of the eighteenth century. (➤ Ch. 34 History of the doctor–patient relationship)

EARLY HISTORY

Within the Western tradition, the historical antecedents of a naturalistic attitude to disease and its diagnosis are usually traced back to the authors of the Hippocratic Corpus (fifth to third centuries BC). The Hippocratic approach to disease was characterized by a lack of emphasis upon supernatural causation and by a matter-of-fact empiricism within the consultative encounter. 'It is the business of the physician to know in the first place, things . . . which are to be perceived by the sight, touch, hearing, the nose, and the tongue, and the understanding.'[4] The Hippocratic physician was particularly concerned to ascertain the patient's way of life, habitation, work, diet, and so on. Verbal inquiry was combined with careful and systematic examination:

> When you examine the patient, inquire into all particulars; first how the head is . . . then examine if the hypochondrium and sides be free of pain, for . . . if there be pain in the side, and along with the pain either cough, tormina or bellyache, the bowels should be opened with clysters. . . . The physician should ascertain whether the patient be apt to faint when he is raised up, and whether his breathing is free; and examine the discharges from the bowels. . . . Attention should also be paid to the hands . . . and observe the nostrils . . . if the tongue be rough, and if there be swoonings, it is likely to be a remission of fever.[5]

As well as palpating the abdomen, the Hippocratic physician listened carefully to any sounds emanating from within the thorax. Sometimes, the patient might be shaken in order to ascertain whether splashing noises could be elicited within the chest. He or she might be set exercises to do, such as climbing or running, and their effect observed. In a practice similar in principle to the modern concept of diagnostic therapeutics, the patient might be fed certain foods to see how he or she reacted to them. This process of observation often continued over a period of days.[6]

It is important to emphasize that the Hippocratic physician set out principally to investigate and comprehend the individuality of the patient rather than to identify a specific disease entity with which he or she might be affected. In other words, the Hippocratic consultation was a patient-oriented, rather than a nosography-oriented, form of diagnostic inquiry. This was because Hippocratic medicine, although recognizing the existence of a number of definite diseases, conceived of disease in terms of its expression within suffering individuals. There were, in effect, as many diseases as there were patients. And therapy had to be tailored precisely to the individual circumstances of the patient, if it were to be effective. The aim of diagnosis was accurately to know the person with whom the physician was presented.

It has sometimes been argued that the sophistication of Hippocratic consultative inquiry was causally related to their rejection of supernatural aetiology.[7] It was their commitment to a naturalistic cosmology that allowed them to depend upon the evidence of their senses. It should, however, be noted that, remarkable as the diagnostic acumen of the Hippocratic physician undoubtedly was, Greek medicine was not the only system in the ancient world in which considerable importance was accorded to the patient's physical appearance in disease. The ancient Hindu physicians, for instance, took astrological and supernatural influence very seriously. Yet they also placed great stress upon the evidence available to the physician from the direct examination of the patient. The passage quoted at the beginning of this essay is from the *Suśruta Saṃhitā*. (➤ Ch. 33 Indian medicine) It continues:

> By the sense of hearing we can ... determine whether the contents of an abscess are frothy and gaseous, for the emptying of such is attended with noise. By the sense of touch we may know whether the skin is hot or cold, rough or smooth. ... By the sense of sight we can determine corpulence or emaciation, vital power ... and change of colour. By the sense of taste we can assure ourselves concerning the state of the urine in diabetes. ... And by the sense of smell we can recognise the peculiar perspiration of many diseases.[8]

The real reason why Hipocratic physicians developed such acute procedures of diagnostic observation would seem to lie in the uncertain nature of their employment. It should be remembered that the Hellenic physician had only the social status of a craftsperson.[9] No formal qualification or professional accreditation was possessed, and the physician was very often itinerant. Therefore, it was necessary to be resourceful in devising means of quickly making a favourable impression upon potential clients.[10] One way of displaying skill and knowledge was accurately to foretell the development of patient's complaints. Acuity in prognosis also enabled the physician to distinguish between those patients who would recover and those who would not, so that the latter could be avoided in order to preserve reputation.

The Hindu physician's well-developed interest in diagnostic observation would seem to have sprung from very similar considerations. The physician's social position was also insecure, and there was great concern to distinguish between patients who would or would not recover. As a result, the Hindu diagnostic process began, in effect, with a scrutiny of the sick person's messenger. Undue agitation in the messenger could indicate that a terminal crisis was imminent.[11] There might therefore be little to gain for the physician in getting involved with the case.

With their stress upon careful observation, the diagnostic practices of both the Hippocratic and the Hindu physicians may seem to resemble, in some respects, a modern consultation. That similarity should not, however, be attributed to any anticipation of the Western clinical perspective, far less to a timeless scientific impulse. As we have seen, Hippocratic diagnostics served purposes specific to the social role and status of the Hellenic physician. It is in this light that the character of diagnostics should always be interpreted. Diagnostic practices are a product both of the cultural context of medicine in any period and of the specific interests of particular groups of medical practitioners. In many respects, Hippocratic diagnosis was very different from modern modes of clinical thinking, notably in its lack of distinction between diagnosis and prognosis and the absence of a concept of 'differential diagnosis'.

The Hippocratic texts do not mention the taking of the peripheral pulse in diagnosis. However, observations upon the quality of the pulse as an aid to understanding the patient's condition had entered Greek medical texts by about 300 BC.[12] The study of the pulse was accorded great importance during the later evolution of Greek medicine, as exemplified by the writings of Galen (AD c.129–200/210). Galen's diagnostic practice represents a development of the Hippocratic doctrines, reflecting the greater knowledge of anatomy, physiology, and logic in the Hellenistic period.

Like the Hippocratics, Galen was concerned to ascertain the patient's milieu, age, way of life, and so on.[13] On occasion, he seems to have spent many hours in conversation with his patients. Sometimes, he felt able to diagnose the illness purely by this means. But generally, he used his senses to complement the information gained from the patient. During direct examination of his patients, Galen gave pride of semiological place to the pulse. He also studied the urine, as an indication of the inner state of the humours, (➤ Ch. 14 Humoralism) noting variations of colour, density, and composition through the course of the disease:

> One generally obtains the major indications in fevers from the pulse and the urine. It is essential to add to these the other signs, as Hippocratics taught, such as those that appear in the face, the posture the patient adopts in bed, the breathing, the nature of the upper and lower excretions ... presence or absence of headache ... prostration or good spirits in the patient ... the appearfance of the body.[14]

Galen knew, for instance, the value of Hippocratic observations such as the characteristic colouring of the cheeks in cases of inflammation of the lungs, and the curvature of the nails in consumption. He also followed the progress of fever by noting changes in the intensity of shivering, sweating and heat, and paid particular attention to the presence or absence of vomiting, as an expression of disturbance of the humours. (➤ Ch. 19 Fevers) He inspected the faeces, their colouring, consistency, and composition. He noted the appearance of the blood, if bleeding had taken place. He inspected the nasal passages and the fauces, as far back as the tonsils, positioning the patient so as to get maximum illumination from sunlight. He palpated the abdomen over the liver, spleen, and bladder and was able, in thin persons, to take the pulse from the abdominal artery in the epigastrium.

Galen's knowledge of anatomy aided his diagnostic acumen, enabling him, for example, to trace the cause of numbness in the extremities to localized damage to the spinal column. To Galen, the best diagnoses were those that united the experience of the senses with functional anatomical knowledge and the exercise of inductive reasoning. His methods were more formalized than the Hippocratics', expressing the influence of philosophy, especially that of Aristotle, upon medicine. (➤ Ch. 5 The anatomical tradition)

Many other Greek authors compiled descriptions of clinical syndromes from which it is clear that they employed inspection, palpation, abdominal percussion, and auscultation. Here, for instance, a contemporary of Galen, Aretaeus the Cappadocian (*fl.* second century AD), describes the recognition of ascites and tympanites:

> Ascites is easy to see by the tumidity of the abdomen . . . the face . . . and other parts are slender, but the scrotum and prepuce swell. . . . Ascites is easy to . . . palpate by strongly applying the hand and compressing the lower belly, for the fluid will pass to other parts. But when the patient turns to this side or that, the fluid . . . occasions swelling and fluctuation, the sound of which may be heard. . . . Tympanites may be recognized not only from the sight of the swelling, but also by the sound which is heard on percussion . . . if you tap with the hand the abdomen resounds.[15]

THE MIDDLE AGES AND RENAISSANCE

The diagnostic practices of the medieval physician have received relatively little attention from historians. However, as in other fields of medicine, diagnosis in the Middle Ages was probably dominated by the classical legacy, somewhat attenuated and with Islamic additions and influences. (➤ Ch. 31 Arab-Islamic medicine) Urinoscopy and pulse-lore, based upon Galenic precepts, seem to have been very important, and an elaborate practice of astrological diagnosis was developed.[16] On the other hand, medieval and Renaissance physicians do not seem to have adopted many of the Greek techniques of physical examination. Abdominal palpation was undoubtedly practised, but how frequently remains unclear.[17]

As medicine became dominated, at least in its higher echelons, by university-educated physicians, so it took upon itself the general characteristics of medieval scholarship, including a disdain for manual work and a deference to textual authority. For the medieval and Renaissance physician, authority lay with the works attributed to Galen.[18] (➤ Ch. 48 Medical education) But this exemplar was developed selectively, so as to endorse reason over observation, book learning over sensory experience. This association of medicine with prevailing notions of the dignity of mental, as against physical, activity was to cast a long shadow. Although there were doubtless many exceptions, the physicians of the sixteenth, seventeenth, and even eighteenth centuries seem to have been more interested in what their patients said about their diseases than they were in investigating the physical signs and symptoms associated with the various conditions.

THE EIGHTEENTH CENTURY

In the wake of the Scientific Revolution, new elements were introduced into the diagnostic repertoire, such as the counting of the pulse and the measurement of body temperature.[19] But neither the pulse-watch nor the thermometer came into general use. One reason for the neglect of the latter was that no consistent association could be found between measured body temperature and the patients' subjective accounts of warmth or cold.[20] In fever, for example, a patient might shiver and complain of feeling cold, although the thermometer recorded an elevated temperature. However, there was, at least in the hospital setting, a definite trend toward a more quantitative form of diagnostics as the eighteenth century progressed, as evidenced by James Gregory (1753–1821) in his careful measurements of ingesta and urine of diabetic patients in the Edinburgh Royal Infirmary.[21]

Pre-modern diagnostic practice reached its fullest expression in the eighteenth century, and it is with this period that the remainder of this essay is concerned. The eighteenth-century physician seems to have relied upon four basic diagnostic techniques.[22] First and foremost, the patient's own descriptions of his or her complaint were listened to. Second, the patient's general appearance was noted, especially around the face, and behaviour – whether the patient tended to favour one side or the other when lying in bed, whether he or she was calm or confused, and so on. Third, the pulse was taken. Fourth, a visual inspection of the patient's urine, faeces, sputum, and pus was performed. Only relatively rarely would the physician examine the patient's body manually or even visually inspect those parts of the body normally covered by clothes or bedclothes.

Touching the patient's wrist to take the pulse might allow the physician to gain other information. The patient's bodily heat might thereby be ascertained. To the pre-modern physician, body temperature did not lie along a simple linear scale. Rather, there were different qualities or types of heat. For example in the putrid fevers:

the heat is . . . sharp, so as to . . . seem uneasy to the touch. . . . In other fevers, though there is an intense heat perceived immediately . . . yet it is soon overcome by the heat of the finger touching . . . but in these continual putrid fevers, the heat often seems mild in the beginning when the patient's hand is felt; yet the heat is increasing . . . every minute, so that it pricks or excites an uneasiness to the touch of the physician, as if the heat came from a deep part of the body.[23]

Observation of facial appearance required considerable care – as the Dutch physician Gerhard van Swieten (1700–72) acknowledged when advising how to position oneself at the bedside:

the physician should sit neither in darkness nor far from the patient's head; but opposite to him, in a light place, that he may perceive all the signs that can be taken from the countenance of the patient. But the eyes usually afford . . . many of the most certain signs in diseases; and no wonder since even in healthy people they point out the various affections of the mind, and often the first attack of diseases appear earliest in the eyes. When the fit or a quatrain first invades, there is a paleness of the eyes; when a person suddenly faints away, the usual brightness of the eyes is first diminished.[24]

Van Swieten also recommended that: 'A prudent physician never leaves a patient till he has inspected his tongue and the inside of his mouth, which so fairly shows the state of the viscera . . . as also of the lungs.'[25]

The Edinburgh sources tell a similar story. For example, John Rutherford (1695–1779), Professor of the Practice of Medicine, frequently impressed upon his students the value of closely inspecting the patient's facial appearance. The following quotation is from a lecture upon the case of a young woman newly admitted to his clinical ward:

If it had been daylight, I would have examined her gums and the internal canthus of her eyes for without bloodletting, which is not proper in her case, one may give a tolerable guess by inspecting these for by looking into the internal canthus and the gums and finding them in a florid state then the blood is in a good state but if they are pale or livid it is a sign that blood is dissolved and watery, if they have a yellowish cast it is frequently attended with a degree of acrimony, but when the cast is of a greenish colour, the acrimony is much greater as we see in scorbutick people.[26]

Rutherford's careful visual examination did not, however, extend to other parts of the patient's body. His conclusion was that, 'The disease seems to be owing to the mismanagement she underwent in childbed. She says she was lacerated and probably it was her vagina.'[27] But he made no attempt to check this supposition of physical damage for himself, nor, it seems, did any other of the hospital's staff. This case vividly exemplifies the generally circumscribed extent of eighteenth-century physical examination.

The clinical lectures of William Cullen (1710–90) likewise provide no direct evidence that he ever touched the bodies of his hospital patients.[28] The clinical procedure in the Infirmary in Cullen's time seems to have been that the clinical clerk took down a written account of the patient's complaint, elicited verbally through systematic and standardized questioning. The clerk's account was read to the physician as he came to each patient on his rounds. He observed the patient's general appearance and asked him or her if the clerk's account was an accurate one. The only occasion on which the patient's body was routinely handled by the physician or the clinical clerk seems to have been at the taking of the pulse.[29]

Cullen's important text *First Lines of the Practice of Physic* provides further insight into his clinical procedures. In it, he described how to identify and treat a wide variety of diseases, virtually all being characterized in terms of symptoms observable either to the patient him- or herself or to a physician standing near the bed. The following account of how to assess the seriousness of chronic menorrhagia is very typical:

> When in consequence of the circumstances ... the face becomes pale; the pulse grows weak; ... the breathing is hurried by moderate exercise; when also the back becomes pained from any continuance in an erect posture; when the extremities become frequently cold; and when in the evening the feet appear affected with oedematous swelling; we may ... conclude, that the flow of menses has been immoderate, and has induced a dangerous state of debility.[30]

Cullen's interest in nosology caused him to attend very carefully to the distinctions to be made between diseases. (➤ Ch. 17 Nosology) Yet he seems to have employed physical signs very rarely indeed in differential diagnosis. There are only two examples of physical examination in the whole of the lengthy *First Lines*. Cullen wrote that tympanites was distinguishable from anasarca partly by the fact that in the former 'the swelling does not readily yield to any pressure' and 'being struck, it gives a sound like a drum';[31] whereas, in the latter, the swelling, when pressed with the finger, 'forms a hollow that remains for some little time after the pressure is removed'.[32] In ascites, 'the fluctuation of the water ... may be perceived by the practitioner's feeling, and sometimes by his hearing'.[33] Similarly, Cullen held the 'most decisive' symptom in the recognition of hydrothorax to be fluctuation of water, 'perceived by the patient himself, or by the physician, upon certain movements of the body'.[34]

Cullen denied, however, that fluctuation noises in the chest could allow the physician to distinguish exactly where the fluid was situated.[35] This view was widely shared. When Greatzius (*fl.* 1740), a student of Friedrich Hoffmann (1660–1742) in Halle, considered the problem of distinguishing between 'dropsy of the pericardium' and 'dropsy of the thorax', he decided that the best distinguishing criteria were those revealed by the patient's general behaviour or by listening to his experiential testimony:

> the faintings were more frequent in the dropsy of the pericardium, than that of the thorax, and the difficulty of breathing more mild; and besides, that the patient affected with a dropsy of the pericardium, does not feel the fluctuation of the water so distinctly, in turning himself from side to side, as ... they are accustom'd to do, who labour under a dropsy of the thorax.[36]

It would seem likely that Edinburgh diagnostic practice was more or less typical of Britain as a whole. We have recently been provided with a fascinating account of the consultations between the philosopher David Hume (1711–76), and his doctors during his terminal illness in 1776.[37] Hume was seen by a number of leading physicians, including Sir John Pringle (1707–82). They were unable to agree upon the nature of his complaint. The issue was not resolved until Hume was physically examined. This, however, was eventually undertaken not by a physician, but by a surgeon: 'John Hunter ... coming accidentally to Town ... Dr Gusthart proposed that I should be inspected by him: He felt very sensibly [that is, palpably] as he said, a Tumor or swelling in my Liver'.[38]

A similar attitude to physical diagnosis seems also to have been prevalent in late eighteenth-century France and Italy. The Parisian physician Antoine Portal (1742–1832) was, by his own account, accomplished in the diagnostic use of palpation. However, he lamented that only four other physicians in the whole of Paris could apply the technique.[39] He had, therefore, actively to proselytize for it. Likewise, Loris Premuda has documented the absence of physical examination in Padua from 1770 until 1830.[40]

Reiser has argued, moreover, that, even if the eighteenth-century physician did occasionally palpate, he would attach far less weight to the information obtained by his sense of touch than to the patient's narrative.[41] The frequency with which many eighteenth-century practitioners gave advice by letter is also good evidence that actual examination of the patient's body was not considered essential in forming a clinical opinion. As Bynum has put it, 'the patient's own description of his illness was the pivotal point in the diagnostic process'.[42]

The patient would tell the doctor how and when the complaint had started, how it progressed, what its peculiar discomforts were. He or she would also describe his or her way of life and constitution, diet, sleeping habits, bowel movements, and so on. Some physicians became famous for their special skill in 'history-taking'. Roy Porter has noted how Erasmus Darwin (1731–1802) was renowned for his acumen in cross-examining the patient until a satisfactory clinical judgement was arrived at.[43] Equal verbal skill might be required to persuade the patient to accept the diagnosis, once the doctor had decided upon one.[44]

However, widespread as the antipathy to physical examination undoubtedly was, it should not be assumed that there was complete uniformity of diagnostic practice throughout Western Europe during the entire eighteenth century. If we look at the great Dutch physician Hermann Boerhaave (1668–1738), we find that his practice broadly conforms to the above description of typical diagnostic behaviour. When advising how to distinguish ascites from tympanites, Boerhaave suggested neither palpation nor percussion, but the taking of the patient's weight. If he or she were abnormally heavy, that would indicate the presence of water rather than gas in the abdomen.[45] However, it seems that on occasion, in especially interesting or unusual cases, Boerhaave was prepared to examine the patient directly with his hands.[46] Furthermore, he refined the normal procedure of visually inspecting the fauces by employing a technological aid:

> To examine the eyes, tongue and lips of the patients I use a microscope made from a lens. . . . You know how the naked vessels in these parts – in the eye and eyelids in particular – reveal the humours which are visible and not covered by a skin. These lenses are best enclosed in a tube so that it is not necessary to bring ones face too close to these parts of the patient.[47]

Boerhaave also used this 'new instrument' to examine wounds and ulcers. (➤ Ch. 6 The microsopical tradition)

PHYSICAL EXAMINATION IN THE PRACTICE OF VAN SWIETEN AND MORGAGNI

Boerhaave's compatriot, Gerhard van Swieten, provides us with rather more striking exceptions to the accepted picture of eighteenth-century diagnostic procedures. His great book, *Commentaria in Hermanni Boerhaave Aphorismes de Cognoscendis et Curandis Morbis*, was published between 1742 and 1772. One of its most remarkable passages contains a description of the swelling of the lymphatic glands in the groin shortly after infection with venereal disease:

> I have often and carefully observed buboes at their rise. The patients begin to complain of a certain tension in the groin; sometimes of a dull obtuse pain; then I could feel the glands deep down, as yet but a little increased, distinct, and ranged lengthwise along the groin; they are soon increased in bulk, and unite almost into one mass; which afterwards rises into a tumour, often very great.[48]

This passage is ample evidence that van Swieten did not entirely rely upon the verbal testimony and general appearance of his patients. Here, we have a physician not merely examining the body of his patient directly with his hands, but palpating firmly and determinedly in that part of the body which might be imagined to be the most strictly guarded by a taboo against physical contact between physician and patient. It is noteworthy that van Swieten claimed to have undertaken this procedure with many patients, and several times with each.

Most of van Swieten's venereal patients appear to have been male. But not all of them. He made it very clear that his experience had not been confined to a single sex: 'I have often been an eye-witness of the external skin of the penis, and the exterior parts of the pudenda in women, having been attacked by venereal shankers'.[49] (➤ Ch. 26 Sexually transmitted diseases) His examination of the pelvic region of the female body was not confined to venereal cases, nor was it exclusively visual:

> I myself saw an inflammatory tumour . . . mistaken for a luxation of the femur; when at the same time, the girl being of lean habit, one might easily perceive by the touch that the articulation was right, and that there was no preternatural cavity.[50]

I give especial prominence to the above passages because they provide the most dramatic evidence that van Swieten, unlike many of the other eighteenth-century physicians named thus far, examined the bodies of his patients directly, on occasion at least. It was not, however, only in the genital area that van Swieten inspected and palpated:

> [I]t is . . . very difficult to distinguish disorders of the pancreas, since it is not so easily rendered the object of our touch as the spleen, and whenever it is swelled must of necessity compress the stomach and the duodenum. Therefore an inflammation of the pancreas may sometimes be confounded with a malady of the stomach or duodenum.[51]

As this passage indicates, the information gained from physical examination aided van Swieten in making crucial diagnostic discriminations.[52]

Van Swieten is not the only prominent exception to the general rule that eighteenth-century diagnostic practice was a hands-off activity. Giovanni Battista Morgagni (1682–1771) was Primary Professor of Anatomy at the University of Padua from 1715 until the year of his death. His major text, *De Sedibus et Causis Morborum per Anatomen Indagatis* (*The Seats and Causes of Diseases as Investigated by Anatomy*), was published in 1761.[53] It contains many passages in which Morgagni clearly and explicitly described his diagnostic procedures. Moreover, he frequently recorded laying his hands upon the living bodies of his patients. The following passage is worth quoting at length because of the vivid picture it provides of Morgagni in action at the bedside:

> I happen'd . . . to go up to the hospital . . . and being asked to feel the man's

belly, I scarcely perceiv'd any particular tumour elsewhere than in the scrobiculus cordis, the abdominal cavity being so greatly distended with water. The tumour was very hard ... but free from pain, even when you press'd upon it. I inquir'd whether it was troublesome by its weight? whether there was any pain which was produc'd quite to the throat? and whether he was ever troubled with a cough? To all which queries the patient answer'd in the negative. But when I asked him whether the tumour increas'd at that time? he not only answer'd negatively, but even asserted that it had subsided ... I suppose because it was in great measure obscur'd by the increasing water.... The face of the man was somewhat pale but not yellow, nor of a cineritous colour; and even the white parts of the eyes, though I examin'd them very attentively, did not appear to me to have the least yellowness.[54]

By his own account, Morgagni was regarded by his colleagues as having particular acumen in the practice of palpation. However, palpation in early eighteenth-century Padua should not be thought of as something peculiar to Morgagni. There are many references in De Sedibus to the technique being used by his contemporaries. Morgagni mentions being taught particular aspects of palpation by one of his professors in Bologna, Ippolito Francesco Albertini (1662–1738).[55] It seems likely that palpation was an unremarkable element of the clinical procedures employed by élite physicians in Padua and Bologna at this time. Furthermore, Morgagni appears to have robustly palpated in what might be thought of as a delicate area, given accepted standards of behaviour between non-intimates: 'And although it is very difficult in very fat and full-breasted women ... to distinguish this disorder; unless ... by pressing your fingers very strongly against the chest, at the sides of the breasts'.[56] Morgagni and his colleagues also palpated in the groins of both male and female patients. A woman with a tumour in the groin seems to have been examined by several physicians: 'All signs of a hernia were absent; except that immediately upon applying their hands to that part, the woman discharged wind'.[57]

Morgagni also valued auscultation, pointing out that attending to the noises made by fluid fluctuating in the abdomen or thorax was useful in the identification of dropsy. The precise location and character of the noises sometimes enabled differentiation between the various forms of dropsy. For instance, the difficult diagnosis of 'dropsy of the pericardium' was made confidently in a case where the physician 'could very distinctly hear the agitation of the water itself in the pericardium, when the heart was pulsating'.[58] This may be contrasted with the criteria employed by Greatzius, as quoted on p. 809, to make the same diagnosis. Morgagni also employed percussion to distinguish whether a swollen abdomen contained water or gas.

Morgagni's palpation and percussion were accompanied by a visual scrutiny of the whole surface of the body, extending into the body orifices. As we have seen, eighteenth-century physicians routinely examined their patients' eyes and mouth. But Morgagni also inspected the auditory meatus, using an apparatus of lenses and candles, to determine the position of foreign bodies. *De Sedibus*, moreover, contains detailed accounts, observed in life, of pathological and congenital abnormalities of both male and female genitalia. He also undertook, on occasion, internal vaginal examinations, diagnosing pregnancy by digital examination of the os uteri. There is, on the other hand, no unequivocal evidence that Morgagni did internal rectal examinations, although his mentor, Antonio Maria Valsalva (1666–1723), did undertake such examinations of both men and women. On one occasion, for example, Valsalva demonstrated how to differentiate between piles and a rectal ulcer:

> For ... having introduc'd his finger, pretty high up in the rectum, he point'd out to the others, the certain situation of the ulcer as the apex of his finger being receiv'd into the orifice of it, seem'd to be embrac'd around, with a kind of ring as it were; for in this manner he assur'd them, that the ulcers of the rectum, or vagina, were frequently found, so that a narrow mouth is dilated into a more capacious sinus.[59]

Physical examination offered Morgagni and his colleagues a means of making informed decisions as to what the precise prognostic significance of abnormal structure might be. (➤ Ch. 9 The pathological tradition) Whether or not a tumour adhered to underlying tissue could be of crucial importance:

> When we had withdrawn from the patient, one of the physicians, under whose care he had been, gave us a long dissertation upon the nature and seat of the tumour ... he believed the tumour to be scirrhous; but a spurious one, because it was painful when compress'd: and that it had its seat in the omentum, because it was movable and external.[60]

It is noteworthy that, for Morgagni, the patient's testimony, or a written account derived from it, was not always an adequate basis on which to form a clinical opinion. Like most eighteenth-century physicians, he conducted a considerable consultation correspondence. In the majority of cases, he felt able to rely on the information provided by the patient or the attending physician. Sometimes, however, he wrote back that he was unable to form a full opinion without having examined the patient: 'I would not dare to assert that such was the case ... without having first made an exact inspection of the injured place, in order to ascertain whether the sign mentioned by Bassio was encountered.'[61] On occasion it was necessary for the physician to see for himself.

The above description of eighteenth-century diagnostic practice begs two questions. First, why did so many physicians neglect the Greek legacy of techniques of physical examination, or palpation, succussion, auscultation, and abdominal percussion? Second, why were Morgagni and van Swieten different, apparently out of step with the majority of their counterparts in Scotland, England, France, and even Italy, later in the century?

Taking the more general question first – as we have already noted, diagnostic techniques are component parts of the totality of medical discourse in any historical period. Jewson has argued that the most important feature of the eighteenth-century physician's social context was the power of the individual patient.[62] The dominant mode of eighteenth-century medicine was private practice for a negotiated fee. Under such circumstances, the patient was autonomous and authoritative. The reliance of diagnosis on the patient's verbal account of his or her disease reflected this autonomy. The patient's own experience of his or her illness constituted the primary reality of the medical encounter, the essential phenomena with which the physician had to deal.

A conceptualization of disease in terms of unique qualitative differences between individuals accorded only limited meaning to physical signs. In Charles Newman's more down-to-earth vocabulary, 'the doctors in those days lived in a different world'[63] – a world in which disease did not have to follow the localized laws of organs and tissues as it did in the nineteenth century. In the eighteenth century, the seat of a disease need not be an essential part of its nature. Diseases could move from site to site, according to their own natural history, the individual characteristics of the patient, or the effects of medical management.[64]

As we have seen, the lack of epistemological significance granted to physical examination neatly harmonized with the widely prevalent prejudice against manual work. The eighteenth-century élite physician was keenly concerned with questions of professional dignity and status. Preferred clientele were from the upper strata of society, and the physician aspired to be accepted as a gentleman. Part of the rationale behind this claim to exalted status was scholarship. A scholar worked with the mind, not with the hands; the important skills were verbal and rational. As Porter points out, the Hume episode indicates that evidence provided by the sense of touch was not necessarily dismissed. Dr Gusthart did not oppose physical examination nor did he dispute the validity of Hunter's findings. Palpation was not, however, a procedure that he was himself prepared to undertake. Manual procedures were the business of surgeons, not of eminent physicians.[65] (➤ Ch. 47 History of the medical profession)

These conventions whereby physicians did not routinely handle or examine too closely the bodies of their patients appear to have been an important aspect of their professional mores. We can see this from the reception given to Leopold Auenbrugger's (1722–1809) diagnostic innovation, thoracic percussion. His colleagues in Vienna responded with indifference to this novel technique.[66] At least part of the explanation for this attitude seems to lie in an antipathy toward handling the bodies of their patients directly. Indeed, such a reluctance seems to characterize certain features of Auenbrugger's own work. He recommended that the percussing physician should don a glove of fine leather or that the patient should wear a thin shirt.[67] We have already seen how Boerhaave preferred to remain a little distance away from his patients while examining their mouths. Similarly, many older practitioners in England, in the first decades of the nineteenth century, vigorously opposed the introduction of physical methods of diagnosis such as stethoscopy, apparently because they were unwilling to compromise their professional dignity by employing a manual procedure.[68]

Furthermore, as noted on p. 814, the behaviour of the eighteenth-century physician was constrained by the authority of the patient within the consultative encounter. The patient could insist that, unless he or she specifically decreed otherwise, the physician should abide by the normal social conventions governing physical intimacy. Even surgeons might have their professional activities constrained by a patient's unwillingness to submit to direct visual or manual examination of the affected parts, and might have to rely on the patient's own testimony. The Portsmouth surgeon James Douglas (1675–1742) had been treating a woman for eight days when she: 'now informed me of a tumor she had . . . in the right groin; she would not allow me to see it, but told me it was as big as a small hen's egg, and by gentle pressure of the hand receded, and never gave her any pain.'[69] Douglas diagnosed a hernia and prescribed appropriate remedies. It was not until four days later, with the pain much worse, that Douglas 'prevailed upon her to let me see it'.

However, real as the effect of the patients' authority undoubtedly was in modulating the behaviour of the eighteenth-century practitioner, the importance of the social conventions governing physical contact can be exaggerated. Patients did frequently consent to being examined very intimately indeed by surgeons, if not by physicians. Otherwise, no operations for hernia, bladder-stone or anal fistula would ever have been done. Yet these operations were quite common, as was bladder catheterization.[70] (➤ Ch. 41 Surgery (traditional)) Thus, if social constraints did limit physicians' diagnostic behaviour, the explanation must lie, to some extent, in physicians and patients choosing to be bound by social conventions. In other words, the physicians' utilization of physical examination was circumscribed by their cultivation of a social role distinct from that of other medical practitioners.

If physicians' use of physical examination was indeed hindered by the cultivation of a distinctive social role, then we might expect the exact configuration of the physicians' choices and the patients' expectations to be a cultural variable. The fact that, in the eighteenth century, the professional boundaries between physician and surgeon were often not clear-cut reinforces this expectation. We ought therefore to be alert to the possibility of a finely textured pattern of variation in diagnostic practice, corresponding to the wide range of different cultural and professional contexts within which the physician worked.

Along these lines, I shall pursue an answer to the more specific of the two questions posed on p. 814 of why Morgagni and van Swieten cultivated procedures and skills that most of their contemporaries neglected. Temkin has argued that much of the novel character of nineteenth-century medicine arose as the result of a process of cross-fertilization between surgery and internal physic.[71] This process started in the latter half of the eighteenth century and was intensified with the work of the Paris School. In France, reforms consequent upon the Revolution abolished the professional and educational distinctions between surgery and physic and created a unified medical profession. The cognitive consequence of this union was a body of medical knowledge in which internal disease was newly conceived of from a surgical prespective. That is to say, internal disease was reconceptualized in localized, structural terms, as opposed to the whole-body humoral pathology of eighteenth-century physic. This new outlook found expression in an upsurge of interest in both pathological anatomy, which could reveal the structural expressions of disease in the corpse, and physical examination, which could reveal them at the bedside.[72] Percussion and auscultation were revived. The stethoscope was invented. The foundations of the modern pattern of clinical diagnosis were established.

It might be conjectured that where physic and surgery were close together, socially, educationally, and institutionally, one might expect to find, in the eighteenth century, forms of practice more like those that were to become dominant in the nineteenth.[73] It is interesting, therefore, to note that, in Padua and indeed in Italy generally, throughout the first half of the eighteenth century, physicians and surgeons were not so rigidly separated from one another as they were elsewhere. Trainee surgeons attended classes at the medical schools; surgery was taught by professors who were also professional surgeons; and people who had the right to call themselves physicians and who actively practised physic also practised surgery. One could find no such distinguished coterie of dual practitioners in contemporary Edinburgh, Paris, or London.[74]

Although he did not undertake operative surgery, Morgagni performed many other procedures which would have been regarded as falling within the normal repertoire of the eighteenth-century surgeon. Moreover, physicians in Bologna and Padua often undertook the overall supervision of surgical cases, even though the cutting and mending were done by specialist operators. Morgagni did not confine himself to advising whether or not an operation was required. Using his great knowledge of human anatomy, he made detailed suggestions as to what especial precautions the operator should take, and so on. Thus, Morgagni's professional situation allowed and required him to be capable of surgical modes of thought.

Morgagni, moreover, undertook a great deal of post-mortem dissection and championed a view of pathology that entailed considerable structural localization.[75] In other words, in Morgagni's case, as in the case of the Parisian physicians of the early nineteenth century, pathological anatomy and physical examination may be seen as the joint expressions of a single tenet of pathology – that the internal disease process is somehow associated with perceivable structural changes, the sort of pathology with which surgeons are familiar. The abscesses, tumours, and gangrenes that Morgagni found on the internal surfaces of the body were precisely the same phenomena as surgeons were accustomed to seeing on the external surface of the body.

Van Swieten also worked in a professional context in which physic and surgery were closely associated. There had long been, in the Netherlands, a superior class of surgeon and, as in northern Italy, many graduated doctors of medicine cultivated and practised surgery. The example of 'Dr Paul de Wind, who practised physic with great applause ... and who is no less eminent for his dexterity in the most important operations of surgery' is, as Daniel de Moulin has recently shown, a very typical one.[76] Boerhaave generally confined himself merely to supervising surgical operations, but even he, on at least one occasion, apparently picked up the knife himself.[77] Van Swieten was regarded by his contemporaries as having taken an especially active interest in surgery.[78] He certainly performed many procedures which would ordinarily have been regarded as lying within the province of the surgeon:

A youth ... came to me ... shewing me a little fungous lump of grown flesh, about the distance of one twelfth of an inch from the orifice of the urethra; and which, upon gently dilating the urethral orifice, I saw to adhere to the internal membrane. . . . I touched the caruncle with some lapis infernalis; and it quickly subsided. . . . But lest the caruncle, thus seared by the caustic, should immediately touch the opposite side of his urethra, I held the orifice of the urethra for some minutes dilated, and fomented the cauterised part with a little sponge.[79]

It is difficult to imagine John Rutherford or Sir John Pringle undertaking such a procedure.[80] But one should remember that the Netherlands was, compared with Britain or France, a society with a high degree of social mobility and a narrow range of disparity between the social strata.[81] Artisans shared in the general prosperity of the country, and there was less stigma associated with skilled manual labour. Temkin has correlated the Dutch physician's close involvement in surgery with the great achievements in anatomy, both normal and pathological, which were a feature of academic medicine in the Low Countries in the seventeenth and eighteenth centuries.[82]

Thus it was the existence of a close social and professional association between physic and surgery in the Netherlands and in northern Italy that stimulated the interest shown by van Swieten and Giovanni Morgagni in physical examination. However, in arguing that Morgagni and van Swieten represent an eighteenth-century corollary of the Temkin thesis, I am not suggesting that their diagnostic practice was identical with that which was to become standard in the nineteenth century. In many other respects, their consultative behaviour is perfectly typical of the pre-modern physician. For example, before inspection or palpation of the body could take place, the physician had first to gain the permission of the patient. Morgagni recommended the following procedure, if a pulse could not be felt at the wrists: 'other arteries are to be examined ... the temporal arteries and the carotids; and finally also, *when it is permitted*, the crural arteries, which have a pulsation in the groins.'[83] Morgagni did not have absolute licence to conduct physical examinations: his diagnostic practice was finely modulated and controlled by social convention and by the authority of the patient. Certain parts of the patients' bodies were more easily touchable than others; the patient might allow certain procedures and not others. Vaginal examination was often problematic. Morgagni recalled that he made use of this procedure 'when it was in my power; but I have it in my power very seldom; the women of our country being for the most part repugnant to an examination of that kind'.[84] (➤ Ch. 38 Women and medicine)

Van Swieten's freedom to employ physical examination was circumscribed in exactly the same way. He too was always dependent upon his patients' forbearance. Some co-operated eagerly: 'A man ... flew to me from a neighbouring village, to show me a swelling ... in his right testicle.'[85] But others did not. Like Morgagni, van Swieten found that gaining permission for vaginal examination was particularly difficult.[86]

NINETEENTH-CENTURY COMPARISONS

In the nineteenth century, by contrast, the intensity of physical examination which was routinely accepted by patients greatly increased. Being examined by the doctor became identified as a special form of interpersonal interaction – no longer constrained by normal social conventions, but controlled by ethical standards and modes of conduct established and maintained by the medical profession itself.[87] (➤ Ch. 37 History of medical ethics) Physical examination still required the patient's consent, but effective departure from the normal procedure depended not upon the patient granting additional consent, but upon the patient withdrawing consent. Morgagni or van Swieten would have expanded the extent of their physical examination when additional permission was forthcoming; a modern hospital doctor would contract his normal diagnostic procedure when permission for certain forms of examination was withdrawn.

Another systematic difference between Morgagni's approach to physical examination and that of his nineteenth-century counterpart may be found in the fact that Morgagni only very occasionally used the evidence gained by examination to contradict the patient's account. In general, the two sources of information complemented each other. In the nineteenth and twentieth centuries, by contrast, the information that the doctor gathered in the process of direct physical examination was given epistemological priority and could make the patient's testimony redundant. Complaints by the patient not supported by clinical signs might be dismissed as merely 'functional'. The doctor's expertise might routinely negate the patient's understanding of his or her own disease.[88]

Morgagni and van Swieten should thus be seen both as pioneers of physical examination and as typical eighteenth-century physicians. The same might be said of other innovators in the field of physical diagnosis. Auenbrugger, the pioneer of thoracic percussion, for example, was as concerned as any of his contemporaries with the general behaviour of his patients and the appearance of their waste products:

> The urine rarely presents any deviation from the natural state; sometimes, however, it is red and with a sediment . . . of a cinnabar colour. The stools are of natural character, except under the influence of medicine. The extremities, even when of a livid colour, are never hotter than natural, until a few days before death; the affected side is, moreover, observed to swell, and the hand and foot in the first place. The patient now suffers from frequent sinkings and faintings; and from having hitherto been able to lie easily on either side, he is able to remain on the affected side only.[89]

As a case description, this would not have been wholly out of place in the Hippocratic Corpus.

Likewise, when thoracic percussion was taken up by British physicians in the early nineteenth century, its initial function was to complement, not to displace, older diagnostic procedures. One of the first occasions on which thoracic percussion was employed in Britain was by Andrew Duncan Jr (1773–1832), in the Edinburgh Royal Infirmary. The patient, Mary Rickman, entered the Infirmary on 11 March 1815, complaining of 'pain in the thorax, more particularly referred to the sternum'.[90] Duncan diagnosed pleuritis. The patient continued to complain of severe pain in the centre of the chest. On 5 April, Duncan decided to try the experiment of percussing the thorax. He noted that the 'sternum, when struck, does not emit a hollow sound and the pulsation of the heart is very distinctly felt lower than the ensiform cartilage'.

However, he continued to treat her for pleuritis. Rickman died on 13 April. Autopsy revealed enlargement of the heart and inflammation of the pericardium. Duncan explained his failure to apprehend the true nature of the case in terms of its not exhibiting the recognized signs and symptoms of carditis: 'Rickman had not the *pulsus inequalis, palpitatio et syncope* of Cullen; nor the constant vomiting of Darwin; nor the palpitation, faintings, quick and unequal pulse of Sauvages; nor the very intense thirst of Burserius . . . nor the delirium of Davis'.[91] In other words, even as he began to experiment with percussion, Duncan still sought to base diagnosis principally upon gross observation of the patient's behaviour. It would be many years before the new physical techniques were granted full epistemological and practical priority over more-traditional clinical methods.

CONCLUSION

This essay should be regarded as a preliminary sketch. Medical historians are still some distance from being able to provide a fully satisfactory description of the pre-modern consultative encounter. In the seventeenth- and eighteenth-century literature, precise descriptions of clinical procedures tend to occur, if at all, only incidentally to accounts of other matters. Perhaps simply because of their routine everyday nature, diagnostic procedures seem not to have been readily incorporated into the written record. It must also be admitted that our ignorance is not wholly due to any inadequacy in the sources but to the fact that historians have tended to ignore, at least until quite recently, the practical aspects of medicine. Medical historians have concerned themselves excessively with the theoretical writings of a tiny literary élite.[92] Thus comparatively little attention has been paid to how medicine was actually practised at the bedside of the patient.

This sin of omission cannot be complacently excused as merely involving the neglect of one part of medicine (practice) at the expense of another (theory). An overweening preoccupation with theory must necessarily distort our image of the medical enterprise as a whole. Medicine is a practical goal-oriented activity – or it is not medicine. As Canguilhem reminds us, it is the responsive attempt to help the sufferer that is the defining characteristic of medicine, both as an art and a science.[93] Moreover, what the doctor does at the bedside is the aspect of medicine that most immediately and importantly impinges upon the patient. Fortunately, there have recently been many encouraging signs that scholars are finally rising to the challenge posed by the elucidation of the pre-modern consultative encounter. (➤ Ch. 36 The science of diagnosis: diagnostic technology; Ch. 68 Medical technologies; social contexts and consequences)

NOTES

1 For a modern discussion of the meaning of diagnosis, see R. L. Engle and B. J. Davis, 'Medical diagnosis, present, past and future', *Archives of Internal Medicine*, 1963, 102: 512–43.

2 E. Evans-Pritchard, *Witchcraft, Oracles and Magic among the Azande*, Oxford, Clarendon Press, 1937, p. 91.

3 See, for example, Dorothy Porter and Roy Porter, *Patient's Progress: Doctors and Doctoring in Eighteenth-Century England*, Cambridge, Polity Press, 1989.

4 F. Adams, 'The surgery', *The Genuine Works of Hippocrates*, 2 vols, London, Sydenham Society, 1849, Vol. II, p. 474.

5 Ibid., 'Appendix to the regimen in acute diseases', Vol. I, pp. 321–2.

6 L. G. Ballester, 'Galen as a medical practitioner: problems in diagnosis', in V. Nutton (ed.), *Galen: Problems and Prospects*, London, Wellcome Institute for the History of Medicine, 1981, pp. 13–46.

7 See L. Edelstein, 'Greek medicine in its relation to religion and magic', in O. Temkin and C. L. Temkin (eds), *Ancient Medicine: Selected Papers of Ludwig Edelstein*, Baltimore, MD, Johns Hopkins University Press, 1967, pp. 205–46.

8 K. K. L. Bhishagratna, *An English Translation of the Sushruta Samhita Based on an Original Sanskrit Text*, 3 vols, Calcutta, Bhaduri, 1907–16, Vol. I, p. 74.

9 L. Edelstein, 'The Hippocratic physician', in Temkin and Temkin, op. cit. (n. 7), pp. 87–110.

10 G. E. R. Lloyd (ed.), *Hippocratic Writings*, London, Penguin, 1973, p. 16.

11 Bhishagratna, op. cit. (n. 8), p. 74.

12 Lloyd, op. cit. (n. 10), p. 31.

13 My account of Galen's diagnostics is largely based on Ballester, op. cit. (n. 6).

14 Quoted in Ballester, op. cit. n. 6), p. 26.

15 F. Adams, *The Extant Works of Aretaeus the Cappadocian*, London, Sydenham Society, 1856, p. 334.

16 K. D. Keele, *The Evolution of Clinical Methods in Medicine*, pp. 22–9.

17 See E. Wickersheimer (ed.), *Anatomies de Mondino dei Luzzi et de Guido de Vigevano*, Paris, Droz, 1926.

18 O. Temkin, *Galenism: the Rise and Decline of a Medical Philosophy*, Ithaca, NY, Cornell University Press, 1973.

19 Keele, op. cit. (n. 16), pp. 31–41.

20 J. Worth Estes, 'Quantitative observations of fever and its treatment before the advent of short clinical thermometers', *Medical History*, 1991, 35: 189–216.

21 J. Worth Estes, 'Drug usage at the Infirmary: the example of Dr. Andrew Duncan, Sr.', appendix D in G. B. Risse, *Hospital Life in Enlightenment Scotland: Care and Teaching at the Royal Infirmary of Edinburgh*, Cambridge, Cambridge University Press, 1986, pp. 361–4.

22 C. Newman, 'Physical signs in the London hospitals', *Medical History*, 1958, 2: 195–201.

23 G. van Swieten, *Commentaria in Hermanni Boerhaave Aphorismes de Cognoscendis et Curandis Morbis*, 5 vols, Leyden, 1742–72; trans. as *Commentaries on Boerhaave's Aphorisms Concerning the Knowledge and Cure of Diseases*, 17 vols, Edinburgh, Elliot, 1776, Vol. VII, p. 20.

24 Ibid., p. 45.

25 Van Swieten, op. cit. (n. 23) Vol. I, p. 225.

26 J. Rutherford, 'Clinical lectures', student's MS notes, Edinburgh University Library, Dc.10.28, p. 20.

27 Ibid.

28 For example, W. Cullen, 'Clinical lectures', notes taken by Sir Charles Blagden, Wellcome Institute Library, MS 1948.

29 My picture of the clinical practice at the Edinburgh Royal Infirmary is a composite one, drawn from Risse, op. cit. (n. 21); G. Stewart, 'Sketch of the history of the Royal Infirmary and the development of clinical teaching', *Edinburgh Hospital Records*, Edinburgh, Pentland, 1893, pp. 1–17; J. Struthers, *Historical Sketch of the Edinburgh Anatomical School*, Edinburgh, MacLachlan & Stewart, 1867 and M. Barfoot, personal communication.

30 W. Cullen, *First Lines on the Practice of Physic*, 4th edn, 4 vols, Edinburgh, Elliot, 1784, Vol. III, pp. 13–14.

31 Ibid., Vol. IV, p. 228.

32 Cullen, op. cit. (n. 30), Vol. IV, p. 277.

33 Cullen, op. cit. (n. 30), Vol. IV, p. 323.

34 Cullen, op. cit. (n. 30), Vol. IV, p. 314.

35 Cullen, op. cit. (n. 28), p. 40.

36 Quoted in G. B. Morgagni, *De Sedibus et Causis Morborum per Anatomen Indagatis*, Venice, Remondini, 1761; pub. as *The Seats and Causes of Diseases Investigated by Anatomy*, by B. Alexander 3 vols, London, Millar & Cadell, 1769, Vol. I, p. 391.

37 Porter and Porter, op. cit. (n. 3), pp. 59–60.

38 Quoted in Porter and Porter, op. cit. (n. 3), p. 60.

39 E. Ackerknecht, *Medicine at the Paris Hospital, 1794–1848*, Baltimore, MD, Johns Hopkins University Press, 1967, p. 26.

40 L. Premuda. 'Die anatomisch-klinische Methode: Padua-Paris-Wien-Padua', *Gesnerus*, 1987, 44: 15–32.

41 S. J. Reiser, *Medicine and the Reign of Technology*, Cambridge, Cambridge University Press, 1978, pp. 5–6.

42 W. F. Bynum, 'Health, disease and medical care', in G. Rousseau and R. Porter (eds), *The Ferment of Knowledge: Studies in the Historiography of Eighteenth-Century Science*, Cambridge, Cambridge University Press, 1980, pp. 211–54.

43 Roy Porter, 'The rise of physical examination', in W. F. Bynum and R. Porter (eds), *Medicine and the Five Senses*, Cambridge, Cambridge Univeristy Press, 1978.

44 Porter and Porter, op. cit. (n. 3), pp. 78–9.

45 G. A. Lindeboom, *Boerhaave's Correspondence*, Leiden, Brill, 1962–79, Vol. II, p. 79; Vol. III, p. 195.

46 L. S. King, 'Description of another dreadful and unusual disease drawn up by Hermann Boerhaave', *Journal of the History of Medicine*, 1968, 23: 331–48; W. J. Derbes and R. E. Mitchell, 'Hermann Boerhaave's *Atroci, nec Descripti Morbi Historia*, the first translation of the classic case report of rupture of the esophagus, with annotations', *Bulletin of the Medical Libraries Association*, 1955, 43: 217–40.

47 Lindeboom, op. cit. (n. 45), Vol. III, p. 257.

48 Van Swieten, op. cit. (n. 23), Vol. XVII, p. 113.

49 Van Swieten, op. cit. (n. 23), Vol. XVII p. 65.

50 Van Swieten, op. cit. (n. 23), Vol. III, p. 219.

51 Van Swieten, op. cit. (n. 23), Vol. IX, p. 287.

52 See also Van Swieten, op. cit. (n. 23), Vol. XV p. 116.

53 Morgagni, op. cit. (n. 36).

54 Alexander (trans.), op. cit. (n. 36), Vol. II, p. 206.

55 Morgagni, op. cit. (n. 36) 1769, Vol. II, pp. 178–9.

56 Morgagni, op. cit. (n. 36) 1769, Vol. II, pp. 638–9.

57 Morgagni, op. cit. (n. 36) 1769, Vol. II, p. 556.

58 Morgagni, op. cit. (n. 36) 1769, Vol. I, pp. 394–7.

59 Morgagni, op. cit. (n. 36) 1769, Vol. II, p. 109.

60 Morgagni, op. cit. (n. 36) 1769, Vol. II, p. 382.

61 S. Jarcho, *The Clinical Consultations of Giambattista Morgagni*, Charlottesville, University Press of Virginia, 1984, p. 4.

62 N. D. Jewson, 'Medical knowledge and the patronage system in eighteenth-century England', *Sociology*, 1974, 8: 369–85.

63 C. Newman, 'Diagnostic investigation before Laennec', *Medical History*, 1960, 4: 322–9.

64 M. Nicolson, 'The metastatic theory of pathogenesis and the professional interests of the eighteenth-century physician', *Medical History*, 1988, 32: 277–300.

65 Porter, op. cit. (n. 43).

66 J. B. Herrick. 'A note concerning the long neglect of Aucnbrugger's *Inventum Novum*', *Archives of Internal Medicine*, 1943, 71: 741–8.

67 L. Auenbrugger, '*On Percussion of the Chest*, translated by John Forbes', *Bulletin of the Institute of the History of Medicine*, 1936, 4: 373–403, see p. 382.

68 M. Nicolson, 'The introduction of percussion and stethoscopy to early nineteenth-century Edingburgh', in Bynum and Porter, op. cit. (n. 43).

69 J. Douglas, 'Worms evacuated at an ulcer of the groin', *Medical Essays and Observations*, 1733, 1: 222–6.

70 O. H. Wangensteen and S. D. Wangensteen, *The Rise of Surgery: from Empiric Craft to Scientific Discipline*, Folkestone, Dawson, 1978.

71 O. Temkin, 'The role of surgery in the rise of modern medical thought', *Bulletin of the History of Medicine*, 1951, 25: 248–59.

72 Ackerknecht, op. cit. (n. 39); M. Foucault, *The Birth of the Clinic*, London, Tavistock, 1973.

73 See T. Gelfand, *Professionalizing Modern Medicine: Paris Surgeons and Medical Science and Institutions in the Eighteenth Century*, Westport, CT, Greenwood Press, 1980; and O. Keel, 'Les rapports entre médecine et chirurgie dans la grande école anglaise de William et John Hunter', *Gesnerus*, 1988, 45: 323–41.

74 M. Nicolson, 'Giovanni Battista Morgagni and eighteenth-century physical examination', in C. Lawrence (ed.), *Surgical Practice; Medical Theory*, London, Routledge, 1992.

75 S. Jarcho, 'Giovanni Battista Morgagni; his interests, ideas and achievement', *Bulletin of the History of Medicine*, 1948, 22: 503–24.

76 Van Swieten, op. cit. (n. 23), Vol. X, p. 15; D. de Moulin, *A History of Surgery with Emphasis on the Netherlands*, Dordrecht, Martinus-Nijhoff, 1988.

77   G. A. Lindeboom, *Hermann Boerhaave: the Man and his Work*, London, Methuen, 1968, p. 302.

78   Erna Lesky, 'Van Swieten und die Chirurgie', in G. A. Lindeboom (ed.), *Circa Tiliam, Studia Historiae Medicinae*, Leiden, Brill, 1974, pp. 140–9.

79   Van Sweiten, op. cit. (n. 23), Vol. XVII, p. 137.

80   W. F. Bynum, 'Treating the wages of sin: venereal disease and specialism in eighteenth-century Britain', in W. F. Bynum and R. Porter (eds), *Medical Fringe and Medical Orthodoxy, 1750–1850*, London, Croom Helm, 1987, p. 12.

81   The best starting-point for the Dutch background is S. Schama, *The Embarrassment of Riches: an Interpretation of Dutch Culture in the Golden Age*, London, Collins, 1987.

82   Temkin, op. cit. (n. 71), p. 488.

83   Morgagni, op. cit. (n. 36), Vol. I, p. 718; emphasis added.

84   Morgagni, Vol. II, p. 696.

85   Van Swieten, op. cit. (n. 23), Vol. XVII, p. 127.

86   Van Swieten, Vol. XIII, p. 301.

87   P. Strong, *The Ceremonial Order of the Clinic*, London, Routledge & Kegan Paul, 1979.

88   Newman, op. cit. (n. 63), p. 323.

89   Auenbrugger, op. cit. (n. 67), p. 397.

90   A. Duncan, 'Three cases of inflammation of the heart, with appearances on dissection', *Edinburgh Medical and Surgical Journal*, 1816, 16: 43–71, see p. 59.

91   Ibid., p. 66.

92   E. H. Ackerknecht, 'A plea for a "behaviorist" approach in writing the history of medicine', *Journal of the History of Medicine*, 1967, 22: 211–4.

93   G. Canguilhem, *The Normal and the Pathological*, New York, Zone Books, 1989.

FURTHER READING

Galdston, I., 'Diagnosis in historical perspective', *Bulletin of the History of Medicine*, 1941, 9: 367–84.

Keele, K. D., *The Evolution of Clinical Methods in Medicine*, London, Pitman, 1963.

King, L. S., 'What is a diagnosis?', *Journal of the American Medical Association*, 1967, 202: 714–17.

——, 'Signs and symptoms', *Journal of the American Medical Association*, 1968, 206: 1063–5.

Newman, C., 'Physical signs in the London hospitals', *Medical History*, 1958, 2: 195–201.

——, 'Diagnostic investigation before Laennec', *Medical History*, 1960, 4: 322–9.

Nicolson, M., 'Giovanni Battista Morgagni and eighteenth-century physical examination', in C. Lawrence (ed.), *Surgical Practice; Medical Theory*, London, Routledge, 1992.

Porter, Dorothy and Porter, Roy, *Patient's Progress: Doctors and Doctoring in Eighteenth-Century England*, Cambridge, Polity Press, 1989.

Porter, Roy, 'The rise of physical examination', in W. F. Bynum and Roy Porter (eds), *Medicine and the Five Senses*, Cambridge, Cambridge University Press, 1993.

Reiser, S. J., *Medicine and the Reign of Technology*, Cambridge, Cambridge University Press, 1978.

——, 'The decline of the clinical dialogue', *Journal of Medicine and Philosophy*, 1978, 3: 305–13.

Ryle, J. A. *The Natural History of Disease*, 2nd edn, London, Keynes Press, 1988.

Shorter, E., *Bedside Manners: the Troubled History of Doctors and Patients*, New York, Simon & Schuster, 1986.

36

THE SCIENCE OF DIAGNOSIS: DIAGNOSTIC TECHNOLOGY

Stanley Joel Reiser

The introduction of instrumental technology as a basic, common, and significant feature of the diagnosis of disease began in 1816 with the invention of the stethoscope. Before this time, instruments to extend the senses were not a feature of diagnostic investigations. The key antecedent circumstances that produced this innovation were the rise of anatomical perspective on illnesses, and flaws in the techniques commonly used to make diagnostic evaluations. Comments on each are necessary to understand not only the innovative act of creating the stethoscope, but also the subsequent development and use of diagnostic technologies generally.

DIAGNOSTIC TECHNOLOGY AND ANATOMICAL THINKING

In 1761, the Italian anatomist G. B. Morgagni (1682–1771) published his treatise, *The Seats and Causes of Diseases Investigated by Anatomy*.[1] It was the culmination of several centuries of work exploring the structural changes in the fabric of the body produced by diseases. The work draws physicians into considering the links between symptoms found in the living patient and lesions discovered by an autopsy. Morgagni demonstrated that only by understanding the nature and site of these lesions could a clear and accurate picture emerge of the nature of the illnesses and the symptoms that accompanied them. This proof was developed by studying bedside cases, reporting their autopsy findings, and then comparing the two for interconnections. This tripartite scheme of analysis dominates Morgagni's book. (➤ Ch. 9 The pathological tradition)

By invoking the image of site-specific lesions as the hallmark of pathology, Morgagni helped radically to transform conceptual thinking about illness from that previously dominant. The common medical view about what illness was had been shaped by the humoral concept of physiological function, which had dominated medicine for several millennia. (➤ Ch. 14 Humoralism) It postulated the existence of four fluid-like humours as the basic substances of the body, which in health existed in a stable equilibrium. Change in the proportion of any one of them caused the balance to break down and illness to ensue. Restoring health required re-establishing the equilibrium. Thus the focus of this theory of health and illness was the whole person. The physiological system of a person, and the exquisite interlinking of its humoral parts was kept at the centre of medical analysis. (➤ Ch. 7 The physiological tradition)

The anatomical viewpoint on illness caused directly opposite thinking. It drew medical observers into a focus on parts, not wholes; on the site of the illness, not the system it affected. (➤ Ch. 5 The anatomical tradition) Morgagni epitomized his message in the second word of his book's title, where he used the term 'seats'. He was concerned with showing the locus of illness: he was a guide leading with his scalpel to the place where illness resided – the pathological lesion. In the half-century between the publication of Morgagni's work and the invention of the stethoscope, anatomical thinking was adopted by a widening medical audience.

Among them was the French clinician Nicholas Corvisart (1755–1821), who in 1806 published *An Essay on the Organic Diseases and Lesions of the Heart and Great Vessels*. At its beginning, he asked why physicians had been so inattentive to learning of and properly treating these diseases. He located the problem in the doctors' still inadequate knowledge of anatomy: 'By abstaining carefully from finding in the dead body, the mistakes which their ignorance of anatomy caused them to commit',[2] physicians misdiagnosed patients, treated alike those that had different ailments, and prescribed therapies either useless or harmful. Corvisart, physician to Napoleon, was among the growing number of medical leaders who now urged colleagues to integrate anatomical thought into their practice. However, he recognized that even a precise anatomical knowledge could not prevent grievous errors of treatment. The doctor was still faced with the problem of understanding the symptoms displayed at the bedside by the patient. These must be compared with their expression as lesions in the body after death to comprehend disease fully. Here a major problem existed: 'the motions which are produced in the inside of the viscera, and which are consequently out of the reach of our senses' concealed from doctors knowledge essential to uncovering 'the secret foundation of organic diseases'.[3] Thus, completing the revolution promised by anatomical exploration required a complementary revolution in learning how the tissues and organs functioned during life. It would be one of Corvisart's pupils, just ten years after his essay on organic diseases appeared, who would provide a crucial answer.

THE SCIENCE OF DIAGNOSIS: THE SOUND

René Laënnec (1781–1826), a physician at the Necker Hospital in Paris, was consulted in 1816 by a young female patient with the symptoms of heart disease. Laënnec and his contemporaries learned of symptoms and evaluated disease, chiefly through the medium of the patients' subjective accounts of the events and experiences connected with their illnesses. Neither physical examination of the patient nor the use of technology to diagnose disease were common to practice. Soon after the establishment of universities in Europe in the thirteenth century, medical training began to move from apprenticeship to an academic curriculum. A set of mores then developed that viewed manual examination and the use of tools as antithetical to the dignity of a learned doctor. This led to the expulsion of surgery from the medical curricula of universities, and to a discouraging of physicians from applying hands and tools at the bedside. (➤ Ch. 35 The art of diagnosis: medicine and the five senses; Ch. 48 Medical education)

However, by the nineteenth century, doctors were being encouraged by forceful advocates such as Corvisart to go to the autopsy room to examine and dissect dead patients as an extension of clinical learning. Such an exercise directly challenged the saliency of the constraint on physicians toward the use of hands or tools because, as the view of Corvisart shows, encouraging physicians to evaluate lesions in the dead as a crucial feature of understanding illness inevitably led them to seek ways to discern lesions in the living patient.

With this as a backdrop, we return to Laënnec's diagnostic puzzle, the illness of his young female patient. Laënnec attempted to apply the technique of percussion to her. It involved rapping the chest with the fingers of one hand to attempt to get it to produce sounds that indicated the state of the organs within. The inhibitions of doctors against physical examintion had limited the diffusion of this technique, introduced by Leopold Auenbrugger (1722–1809) in 1761. It was also difficult to apply successfully in a number of cases, including this one. Here, the obesity of the patient prevented Laënnec from getting the chest to produce adequate sounds. Laënnec thought of using another examination technique first suggested in the Hippocratic literature, which he knew well. It was used by one of his colleagues, Gaspard Bayle (1774–1816) and involved placing an ear directly on the patient's chest to glean, from the sounds heard, the nature of the disease within. However, Laënnec dismissed this technique as 'inadmissible' by the age and sex of the patient.[3] He then recalled the well-known acoustic phenomenon: that sound was augmented when it travelled through solid bodies, as when a scratch noise made at one end of a piece of wood can be heard at the other end. As he wrote:

Immediately, on this suggestion, I rolled a square of paper into a sort of cylinder and applied one end of it to the region of the heart and the other to my ear, and was not a little surprised and pleased, to find that I could thereby perceive the action of the heart in a manner much more clear and distinct than I had ever been able to do by the immediate application of the ear.[4]

Laënnec thereupon grasped that through this innovation, the sounds of the organs in the chest might be disclosed for medical analysis, leading to the evolution of a new set of signs to diagnose chest diseases. He also envisioned that the instrument through which these findings would pass, the cylinder or stethoscope as he would alternatively call it, would provide information as direct as 'the indications furnished to a surgeon'[5] placing a finger or probe into the body. This description reveals that Laënnec thought of the new set of diagnostics he was proposing as akin to a living anatomization of the patient. Further as he investigated the application of the stethoscope and the new technique of mediate auscultation (that is, auscultation mediated by an instrument), the association of the sounds from within the patient and the lesions discovered after death was the principal method he used to confirm diagnostic signs. Anatomical thinking, hence, was pervasive in working out the use of the stethoscope and other instruments of physical diagnosis that would be discovered as the nineteenth century wore on.

The discoverer of a new diagnostic technique must discuss not only its significant technical features, but comment too on techniques already in use. The main technique used at that time, as noted, was inquiry into symptoms of the illness as experienced and reported by the patient. Case reports consisted mainly of patients' accounts, and observations made visually by the doctor of the appearance of the body: the doctor was thus a biographer, the patient a narrator. These stories of illness gave rise to misgivings among doctors. For example, the American physician Benjamin Rush (1746–1813) in a lecture to his students in the 1790s advised:

Physicians by reviewing the history of complaints from their patients will often have them exaggerated but by frequent visits you cannot be deceived.... Endeavor to get the history of the disease from the patient himself and do not interrupt him till he has finished as he will always give the best symptoms tho' he may give the worst causes. Begin to interrogate your patient. By how long he has been sick? When attacked and in what manner? What are the probable causes, former habits and dress; likewise the diet, etc., for a week before especially in acute diseases.... In chronic diseases enquire their complaints far back and the habits of life.... Pay attention to the phraseology of your patients, for the same ideas are frequently conveyed in different words. A pain in the precordia is called by an Englishman a pain in his stomach, by a Scotchman in his breasts, an Irishman in his heart and by a Southern man mighty poorly. Enquire of your patients the diseases of their ancestors, the age to which they lived and the remedies which relieved them. It is of consequence because there is a hereditary idiosyncracies in some families. Patients often conceal the cause of their disease – therefore interrogate them particularly when you suspect intemperance as the cause of disease.[6]

Laënnec, too, was troubled by the inaccuracy of the patient by account, and the large role that subjective symptoms played in diagnosis. For example, he described the symptoms common to all heart diseases: habitually short and difficult respiration, palpitations, and a feeling of oppression produced by exciting emotions, frightful dreams, disturbed sleep, paleness, swelling of the body, constrictive feeling in the region of the heart, and pain or numbness in the arm. But for all of these symptoms, most being subjective reports of sensations the patient experiences, 'none', said Laënnec, 'suffice to character-ize disease of the heart . . . for a certain diagnosis we must recur to mediate auscultation'.[7] When Laënnec did, here is the result, as epitomized in one of his case reports:

> Phthisis Pulmonalis – Tuberculous excavation producing the metallick tinkling. A woman, aged 40, came into the Hospital 29th January, having been affected with cough for five months, and which had increased since her confinement, three months ago. At this time the respiration was short and quick, and difficult; the chest resounded pretty well in the back and left side before, – but better on the right side; there was distinct pectoriloquism near the junction of the sternum and left clavicle, and the same phenomenon, but less distinct, on the same side where the arm joined the chest; the sound of the ventricles was dull, and the heart gave hardly any impulse. Two days after, by means of the cylinder, we distinguished a sound resembling fluctuation, in the left side, when the patient coughed, and the metallick tinkling when she spoke. Succussion of the trunk did not produce the sound of fluctuation. From these results the following diagnostic was given: very large tuberculous excavation in the middle of the left lung, containing a small quantity of very liquid tuberculous matter. The patient died five days after this.
>
> Dissection twenty-four hours after death. In the right lung, through its whole extent, there were innumerable tubercles of a yellowish white colour, and varying in size from that of a hemp-seed to a cherry-stone, and even a large filbert. These last were evidently formed by the reunion of several smaller ones, and, for the most part, were more or less softened. . . . The left lung adhered closely to the pleura of the ribs and pericardium. On its anterior and lateral part it contained, near its surface, three cavities, one above the other, and communicating by two large openings. The upper, of the size of a pigeon's egg, occupied the top of the lung, and corresponded to the junction of the clavicle and sternum; the second might have contained a pullet's egg, and the lowest, which reached within an inch of the base of the lung, was the size of a walnut.[8]

We learn in the first line of this case the patient's age, that she had a continuous cough, and was confined for three months. After that we lose touch with her as a person. Instead, we are brought rapidly into the cavity of the chest; the patient is anatomized through auscultation; the diagnosis given in anatomical language; and the subsequent autopsy tells us how accurate the diagnosis was.

Laënnec's discovery, which began a new age in diagnosis that would extend for a century, had several significant influences. First, on diagnosis itself, the stethoscope challenged older methods through an ability to convey signs characteristic and hence diagnostic of a particular disease. For example, once while examining with the stethoscope a woman who recently contracted a cough, Laënnec found in an area confined to the space of about one square inch on the chest, a phenomenon in which her voice seemed transmitted to the examiner's ear directly from the chest. He proceeded to examine other patients in the hospital, looking for this unique sound and found it in about twenty, most of whom were in advanced stages of tuberculosis, or suspected of having it. But several, like the woman who started this investigation, had no symptoms of the disease, and in fact their robustness seemed to confirm its absence. Laënnec systematically autopsied all patients who exhibited this sign, which he called pectoriloquism, and found the characteristic lesions of tuberculosis. He thus wrote:

> I have detected pectoriloquism in subjects in whom, at the time, no other characteristic symptom of phthisis was present; as was, indeed, the case with the first patient in whom I recognized it. In cases of this sort, whose progress I have been enabled to trace, I have observed the gradual development of phthisical symptoms until they reached that point when their nature could be understood by no one. From all this, I think we are entitled to conclude, that pectoriloquism is a true pathognomonic sign of phthisis, and that it announces the presence of this disease sometimes in an unequivocal manner, long before any other symptom leads us to suspect its existence. I may add, that it is the only sign that can be regarded as certain.[9]

A second basic influence of the stethoscope was on physicians, in whom it encouraged an independent and self-reliant attitude. Before, the doctor depended on patients and families to provide crucial evidence to establish diagnoses. The stethoscope provided doctors with a means to seek for themselves the signs of disease and to evaluate their saliency in deciding what was wrong. Walled off from the external environment, connected to the world of sound in the chest of the patient, stethoscopists made their own judgements. Thoughts of the patients were replaced by sounds from the patient. The basic data of illness were judged and experienced in the diagnostic process not by the patient but the doctor. (➤ Ch. 34 The history of the doctor–patient relationship)

A third essential influence of the stethoscope was on the patient. To many who were first examined with it, the stethoscope was at the same time threatening and magical. Unaccustomed to being examined with instruments, and fearing that the appearance of one in the hands of a doctor meant that a surgical procedure was imminent, patients needed reassurance that the instrument's use would cause no pain. Yet the process of being examined physically required getting used to. The stethoscope was made in varied forms to accommodate this discomfort. One stethoscope was constructed as a tube several feet long, so that the examining end could be held in place on the body by the patient, while the earpiece end was grasped by the doctor standing in another room. This somewhat extreme need for privacy was, fortunately, not required by most patients. Apart from the embarrassment and threat to privacy and dignity that physical examination posed to patients, many were awed at the powers of the stethoscope, which in its original form developed by Laënnec was a simple wooden tube, one foot long, and hollowed out down the centre with a narrow bore to enhance the conduction of sound. Patients could not understand how this tube provided doctors with such dependable evidence about their complaints. What the doctor heard, after all, was not generally discernible to the patient.

Finally, the stethoscope had an influence on the organization of medicine. To learn the sounds of disease and their association with anatomical lesions required access to a large number of patients, the presence of colleagues who could teach auscultation, and autopsy facilities to check bedside judgements. All of these could be found in a hospital. Techniques of physical diagnosis helped establish the significance of the hospital as a place of medical learning. As Laënnec wrote: 'It is only in a hospital that we can acquire, completely and certainly, the practice and habit of this new art of observation.'[10] (➤ Ch. 49 The hospital; Ch. 11 Clinical research)

In sum, the success of the stethoscope was attributable to two basic circumstances. First, it allowed physicians to examine the patient's body without being in direct physical contact with it, permitting the social convention against such contact to be overcome. Second, it provided the doctor with access to a new range of physical events within the body that produced significant knowledge, made authentic and dependable by being detected and evaluated directly by doctors themselves. (see, for example, Figure 1).

The achievements in diagnostic evaluation of the chest made possible with the stethoscope, and the growing orientation of medicine toward an anatomical view of disease, created a climate in which doctors sought technologies that would extend their senses to other organs of the body. This resulted in a spate of innovations, basically developed in the second half of the nineteenth century. Chief among them was the ophthalmoscope (1850), the laryngoscope (1857), and visual scopes developed in the 1860s that permitted the examination of the bladder, stomach, rectum, and vagina. This last examination was criticised as a threat to decency. In a demonstration of how basic physical diagnosis had become to medicine, the American gynaecologist J. Marion Sims (1813–1883) responded to these views in 1868: 'There can be no indecency, and no sacrifice of self-respect in making any necessary physical

19. The following figures give an idea of some of the common forms of the instrument. *Fig.* 5 is copied from a stethoscope in my possession originally owned and used by Laennec. It is divided into two parts united by a screw (*fig.* 6), for the purpose of shortening it if necessary, and has a plug at its lower extremity. This last was thought necessary for the examination of the heart and of the sound of the voice. The instrument is wholly obsolete, being altogether too heavy and unwieldy.

20. *Figs.* 7, 8, 9, & 10, contain Piorry's stethoscope. *Fig.* 7 shows it prepared for auscultation. *Figs.* 8 & 9 represent its various parts separated; *fig.* 8 being the shaft of the instrument; *fig.* 9, *a*, being an ivory ear-piece, pierced with a screw to fasten it to the upper part of the shaft; *b*, a plessimeter (see plessimeters) which can be screwed to the bottom of the same; *c*, the plug to be used as in Laennec's instrument. *Fig.* 10 represents it in a portable form, the ear-piece being screwed upon the bottom of the plessimeter. This is a convenient form, but the ivory edge at the bottom of the shaft is apt to hurt the person who is ausculted. The plug likewise is found to be unnecessary.

20 a. One of the best instruments for conducting delicate shades of sound, is that proposed by Dr. C. J. B. Williams of London.

Fig. 11 represents the instrument prepared for use. It is made of soft sycamore wood. It is hollow; has thin parietes, and a trumpet-shaped mouth. *a* is a movable ear-piece, which can be introduced into the other end of the tube, as represented in *fig.* 12, to make the instrument more portable and less liable to receive injury in the pocket; or it may be placed on the chest, while the ear may be applied to the trumpet-mouth of the instrument, when we wish to examine the voice. To do this the stethoscope should be arranged as in *fig.* 11.

21. *Figs.* 13, 14, & 15 present a very convenient form proposed by Dr. Bigelow, of this city. *Fig.* 13 shows the instrument. It is wholly of soft wood. The ear-piece is broad, so that its side may be pressed on the chest and used as a plessimeter. *Fig.* 14 is a worsted ball, covered with velvet, through which a slender but firm handle of ebony passes. This is used as a precursor, instead of the tip of the finger, in order to avoid the click of the nails, which sometimes causes a confusion of sounds. *Fig.* 15 represents the instrument in its portable condition. This stethoscope is very convenient for auscultation. As an instrument for percussion, I use it, at times, behind the clavicle, but even there I prefer a piece of caoutchouc, or my fore-finger.

22. *Fig.* 16 is the flexible stethoscope used by Dr. Pennock, of Philadelphia, for the sounds of the heart. It is an elegant instrument, about two feet long. I have not used it much; but if Dr. Hope's rule is of importance, viz. that, while ausculting the heart, we ought to have one hand upon the pulse, it would evidently be impossible to use it, for it requires the use of both hands of the auscultator. A similar one is used by Dr. Golding Bird, of London.

23. *Figs.* 17 & 18. These plates are intended to represent the solid stethoscopes used by Drs. Cammann and Clark, in Auscultatory Percussion (386). They are made of soft wood. *Fig.* 17 is a cylinder, about six inches by three-quarters of an inch; the other (*fig.* 18) is like a cylinder of the same dimensions, made wedge-like, in order that the narrow part may be placed on the soft parts between the ribs.

Figure 1 Stethoscopes invented in the first half of the nineteenth century, with comments on them by Bowditch.

Source: H. I. Bowditch, *The Young Stethoscopist; or, the Student's Aid to Auscultation*, New York, Samuel S. & William Wood, *1848*, pp. *25–8*.

examination whatever, if it be done with a proper sense of delicacy, and with a dignified, earnest, and conscientious determination to arrive at the truth.'[11]

THE SCIENCE OF DIAGNOSIS – THE NUMBER AND GRAPH

By the end of the nineteenth century, doctors exulted in their power and prestige as finders and analysts of physical evidence. Indeed, the quintessential modern detective, Sherlock Holmes, created by a doctor, Arthur Conan Doyle (1859–1930) in the 1890s, was modelled on one of Doyle's teachers, Joseph Bell (1837–1911), who had great skill in physical diagnosis. (➤ Ch. 65 Medicine and literature) However, elsewhere in medicine, other technologies were being developed that ultimately would challange physical signs as the central features of diagnosis. The instrument that would initiate this transition was in shape like the stethoscope, and in its early forms quite as long: it was the thermometer. Like the stethoscope, the thermometer was catalysed into prominence by a single individual, and by a book that summarized and extended the possibilities of the technology: in 1868, the German physician Carl Wunderlich (1815–77) published *On the Temperature in Diseases: a Manual of Medical Thermometry.*[12] The work contains the insights of thousands of cases in which thermometric observations were made, and thermometer readings taken by himself and others. From these cases and readings, Wunderlich developed views on the physiological movements of body temperature in health, the variations in temperature produced by different diseases, and the meaning of temperature changes in diagnosis, prognosis, therapy, and disease prevention. He further provided a detailed account of the capabilities and limitations of thermometers, and instruction on their appropriate use to medical personnel and the public. While the earliest thermometer had been invented by Galileo (1564–1642) between 1593 and 1597, the absence of a detailed analysis of its application, such as Wunderlich provided, had limited its use in medical practice.

Early in his book, Wunderlich established two basic principles upon which the foundation of medical thermometry rests: first in healthy persons the temperature is constant (98.6–99.5 °F) and so an index of a sound constitution; and second it undergoes variations in, and is thus an important index of, disease. His research demonstrated that the particular course of these variations were hallmarks of particular diseases (Figure 2). Continual observations of the temperature, taken several times each day, not only permitted correct diagnosis, but also provided evidence of the progress and severity of the disease, the effectiveness of therapy, and the prospect for recovery or death. Thus, Wunderlich elaborated a new measure of the course and duration of diseases and the control of therapies for them, based not on a meticulous analysis of symptoms reported by patients or physical signs discovered by doctors, but on numerical results recorded by an instrument. (➤ Ch. 19 Fevers)

Wunderlich compared the nature of thermometric evidence with the physical signs of illness such as those produced in percussion and auscultation, which then held sway. He argued that thermometry had an advantage over acoustic-based investigations of disease in that it gave results that could be expressed in numbers. It thus produced diagnoses he believed were 'incon-

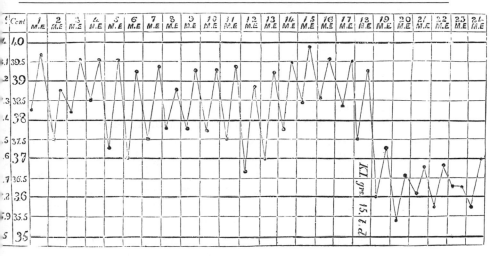

Figure 2 A graph drawn by Wunderlich of the general course of the temperature in lues. The following is Wunderlich's analysis of these observations, which provides the typical thermometric case history of lues:

> In luetic [syphilitic] cases, elevated temperatures are most commonly met with at the time when the first extensive hyperaemic papular or pustular skin eruptions are developed. The fever which accompanies the luetic [syphilitic] eruptions of the early periods may be very severe, and the maximal temperature may reach nearly 41 degrees C. [105.8°F]. The course of the temperature is markedly remittent [pseudointermittent], with a daily downfall which descends quite to normal, or very nearly so. The alternation of these deep morning remissions with the high evening exacerbations is tolerably regular, but in spite of the rapid rise of the evening temperature rigors only accompany it in exceptional cases. It is also equally exceptional for a day quite free from fever to intervene between the days of fever, or for the fever subsequently to display a tertian type, or for greater and more moderate exacerbations to prevail alternately from day to day. The duration of the fastigium is indefinite, sometimes it is short, occupying a few days only, but it may last over a fortnight [and even longer than this – Trans.]. The fever subsides by the evening, exacerbations gradually becoming less severe, in a manner which corresponds pretty closely with the behaviour of the temperature in advanced periods of convalescence from abdominal typhus.

Source: C. A. Wunderlich, *On the Temperature in Diseases: a Manual of Medical Thermometry*, trans. from the 2nd German edn by W. B. Woodman, London, New Sydenham Society, 1871, pp. 406–7.

testable and indubitable, which are independent of the opinion or the amount of practice or the sagacity of the observer. . . . Amongst all the phenomena of disease there is scarcely another which admits of such accuracy or is so reliable as the temperature.'[13]

This was not the only advantage claimed for thermometry over acoustic and other methods of physical diagnosis. While physical diagnosis generally detected permanent changes or slowly changing disease phenomena, thermometry provided insight into moment-to-moment disease perturbations. Further, while the other methods focused on site-specific alterations in the body, the thermometer measured the response of the whole body to illness, and thus was a more dependable index of the patient's prognosis.

The possibilities for benefit that thermometry promised could not be fulfilled unless its agents applied it properly. Wunderlich took great pains to educate his audience on what he called 'the art of medical thermometry'. He realized particularly that for ordinary practice, as opposed to research, absolute or 'painful' accuracy, as he called it, was not necessary to attempt, or aspire to. Making excessive demands on practitioners would have discouraged use. Moreover, as long as a disease followed its usual course, 'approximately accurate observations', frequently repeated, sufficed. Even in obscure or difficult cases where greater accuracy was called for, small errors of observation (one- to two-tenths of a degree) generally did not matter. 'We must not require impossibilities', he wrote, 'and in thermometry, as in all other affairs of life, we must be content with possibilities.'[14]

The thermometer recommended by Wunderlich was filled with mercury, 1/10–¼ inch in diameter, 4¾ inches long, and evaluated for accuracy by the user with periodic testing of its readings in a water-bath having a correctly marked thermometer. Although the part of the body in which the thermometer was placed depended on the circumstances, introducing it into the well-closed axilla was recommended for most cases. Physicians needed several instruments, each marked with a number. The same thermometer was to be used on a given patient so that observations could be corrected if errors were discovered in the instrument's readings. In private practice, physicians were to leave thermometers for patients who required repeated observations of temperature.

This raised the issue of who should take the temperature. Wunderlich recognized that to require the physician to make the observation involved too much time, and would thus limit use if more than one or two observations a day were required. He emphasized that a reasonably intelligent person, such as a nurse or relative, could be taught to use the thermometer. He distinguished between the tasks of observer and analyst: 'The role of the surgeon is not merely taking observations, but the superintendence, control, and right interpretation of them. The mere reading of thermometer degrees helps diagnosis no more than dispensing does therapeusis.'[15] Only confidence in the self-registering process by which the thermometer worked allowed Wunderlich to recommend the delegation of thermometric observation to non-physicians.

The distinctions that Wunderlich made between the character of the evidence produced by thermometry and that of the techniques of physical examination such as auscultation was elaborated on by others, including Edward Seguin (1843–98), an American physician who wrote on thermometry. In the 1870s, he classified the techniques of diagnosis into two divisions: those of physical diagnosis such as the stethoscope and ophthalmoscope, which were accessories to and extended the senses, but also reflected the impressionistic aspect of sensory data; and those of positive diagnosis, such as the thermometer and sphygmograph, which were substitutes for the senses, gave automatic results, and mathematically perceived and depicted phenomena unreachable by the senses, and unchangeable by the mind. He believed the results of these instruments literally to be 'given out by the instrument itself. . . . What all the instruments of positive diagnosis "indicate" are unchallengeable "indications" which it remains only to read and interpret correctly: what the thermometer says no man can "contradict".'[16]

The sphygmograph, which Seguin highly praised, was the most significant of a number of instruments developed in the nineteenth century, which converted the motions of internal organs into graphic form. These instruments basically linked the movements of a lever connected to the body at one end, and to a stylus at the other, which, in turn, continuously transcribed the motions into a revolving cylinder. The sphygmograph, developed in 1860 by E. J. Marey (1830–1904) to monitor the movement of the circulatory system, was the forerunner of twentieth-century electronic devices, such as the electrocardiograph (ECG).

Marey, Seguin, and Wunderlich each had an interest in the form best suited to the scientific notation of technological medical data. This became a significant issue in the second half of the nineteenth century. As self-registering instruments began to produce increasing amounts of data, attention turned to how best to display this without sacrificing accuracy. Wunderlich believed it was important that the results of the numeric thermometric observations be recorded sequentially. This was best done by describing them on a chart as a continuous oscillating line. He recommended that notations of the temperature be accompanied by a similar depiction of the frequency of the pulse and respirations. Other important pieces of data, such as remedies given, might also be incorporated on this chart. Thus, the whole course of the disease, with all of its turns, changes, and therapies, could be taken in by an observer in a single glance at this medical map. No memory could provide 'so "speaking" a likeness of the course of the disease as such a chart',[17] he observed.

In addition, a bringing-together of the charts of various patients allowed the general course of a given disease to be depicted, and thus to further scientific learning. Critically, Wunderlich believed the graphic, not the cipher, was the best way of integrating facts to form generalizations. He wrote: 'In order to extract the general facts from separate observations, we must look less to the *numbers* than to the *form*, that is, to the varied outline of the wave-systems which each separate curve furnishes us.'[18]

In this view, Wunderlich approximated the views of Marey, who saw in the graphic a key to medical diagnosis and other aspects of knowledge. However, Marey's graphic was different from Wunderlich's. Marey's was a transcription into curvilinear form of continuous, real-time, biological motions, such as the beating of a heart. Wunderlich's graphic was based on discontinuous recordings of biological events, taken at temporally spaced intervals. For Marey, the curve based on such real-time recording was the best expression of the changes of a medical phenomenon, and thus any physiological action that could be converted into such a form was well represented. Such curves also were readily and instantaneously comparable, and produced more rapid and clear views of difference and similarity. By comparison, columns of numbers were tedious and fatiguing to read. Marey wrote:

> To render accessible . . . all the phenomena of life – movements which are so light and fleeting, changes of form so slow or so rapid, that they escape the senses – an objective form must be given to them. . . . The graphic curve of a movement furnishes us with the double notion of time and space; it characterizes completely the act which it represents.[19]

For Seguin, a continuous representation of temperature readings equivalent to the curve produced by Marey's sphygmograph would have been ideal. Indeed, he praised Marey's thermograph, an instrument that sought to provide continuous temperature readings but never achieved success. Lacking such an instrument to measure body heat, he argued that Wunderlich's system of recording temperature did not portray its true movement. The lines connecting temperature observations merely filled in the gaps between them: 'the isolated points are true, the connecting lines are fictitious.'[20] Such graphics showed the movement, not the mathematics of a case, portrayed only the general course of the illness (and thus had been valuable to Wunderlich and others in demonstrating the basic temperature curves associated with disease), but none the less they failed to illustrate patient-specific temperature variants.

Seguin argued that mathematical charts in which the numbers represented the exact measures of temperature were superior to temperature graphics. They could provide a view of the relation of any temperature reading to other readings, the time of day, the period and complications of the disease, therapies, and life circumstances having prognostic significance (Figure 3).

For Wunderlich, Marey, Seguin, and others who would follow, giving medical findings an objective format was a means to create a scientific medicine. Like a physical scientist, Wunderlich spoke of discovering 'laws

NAME, GRACE G......	AGE, 10.	SEX, FEM.		DISEASE, SCARLATINA.				SEPTENARY NO. 2.		
Norme of Temperature, .2.		Of Pulse, 84.		Of Respiration, 26.						
872. MONTH, DECEMBER.	23	24	25	26	27	28	29	Maximum day, the 12th...	2.6	
DAYS OF DISEASE.	VIII.	IX.	X.	XI.	XII.	XIII.	XIV.	Minimum day, the 13th....	.1	
HOURS OF OBSERVATION.	M ⌇⌇ E	M ⌇⌇ E	M ⌇⌇ E	M ⌇⌇ E	M ⌇⌇ E	M ⌇⌇ E	M ⌇⌇ E	Total of morn. temp..	6.35 : 7 = .0
								Total of even. temp.......	9.35 : 7 = 1.3
Fever............	1.9 2.2	1.25 1.5	.9	.5 .5	1.4 .1	2.6 .1	" .7 "	Total up..................	15.35	
Zero Health....... } 0								Zeros............	"	
Depression........	⌇⌇	⌇⌇	⌇⌇	⌇⌇	⌇⌇	⌇⌇	⌇⌇	Total down..............	"	
Daily average..........	1.55	1.37	.7	.95	1.8	.1	.7	Average of temp..........	7.17 : 7 = 1.2	
Daily difference........	.3	.25	.4	.9	1.6	"	"	Id. of difference............	3.45 : 5 = .7	
ulse......................	86 106	102 104	100 "	96 "	102 "	100 "	100 "	Id. of pulse................	992 : 9 = 110	
espiration..................	30 36	34 32	28 "	28 "	31 "	27 "	28 "	Id. of breathing............	247 : 9 = 30	

* The other signs and symptoms, as well as the treatment—which happily was of the simplest nursery kind—have been omitted, to not ostruct the mathematical course of the case.

Figure 3 Seguin's chart for recording clinical data numerically.
Source: E. Seguin, *Medical Thermometry and Human Temperature*, New York, William Wood, 1876, p. 406.

that regulate the cause of disease'.[21] Seguin saw such data as making physicians 'nearer physicists and further from metaphysicians than they now are', and having medicine reclaim 'its place among the Natural Sciences'.[22] Marey looked to the possibility of bringing physiology and medicine nearer to the 'exact sciences' by describing biological events through curves, which epitomized their successive changes.[23]

However, at almost the end of the nineteenth century, a discovery was made that focused the medical world on a new form of diagnostic data.

THE SCIENCE OF DIAGNOSIS – THE IMAGE

Perhaps no innovation in medicine ever created the drama and astonishment of the X-ray. It came out of nowhere, for its discovery, like the stethoscope, was not a result of a long search, but of a chance event and prescient observation. Wilhelm Roentgen (1845–1923), a physicist, was in his laboratory on 8 November 1895 studying the properties of the energy produced by the cathode-ray tube, then a common laboratory device. As he discharged it, he noted that a screen coated with a fluorescent material, by chance placed about a yard from the tube, responded to the discharge by displaying a faint glow. This surprised Roentgen, for ample studies had proved that cathode rays could not travel more than several centimetres in air. He discharged the tube repeatedly, placing the screen at increasing distances from it, and was met with the same effect. This led him to conclude that he was not dealing with cathode rays, but some new form of energy which, since unknown, he labelled as X-rays. In the days that followed, he subjected a number of objects to the rays to test their ability to penetrate them. He found it was possible to produce photographic effects through a variety of opaque materials of low density, like wood, pages of a book, and flesh. However, denser materials such as lead or bone were not penetrated by the rays. He sent his findings to the Physico-Medical Society of Würzburg on 28 December 1895, for publication in its *Proceedings*, and he privately circulated some reprints on 1 January 1896.[24]

Word of his discovery spread swiftly in the scientific community. 'Probably never before has the entire scientific world been simultaneously aroused to such a pitch of excitement as that caused by the recent remarkable discovery of Professor Roentgen', wrote a professor of physics.[25] 'Roentgen's weird and wonderful discovery is destined to enrich medicine with possibly the most valuable diagnostic process which recent years have witnessed', commented a professor of pathology.[26] The public joined in the enthusiasm. At one bazaar at which X-ray apparatus was set up to demonstrate its effects, one of the assistants told of two elderly women who 'entered the small room, and solemnly seating themselves, requested me to close and fasten the door. Upon my complying they said they wished ' "To see each other's bones, but I was not to expose them below the waist-line".'[27] Another request was made by a woman to 'look through her young man unbeknown to him while he gazed at the pictures to see if he was quite healthy in his internals'.[28]

The diffusion of this technology was accelerated by a number of factors, in addition to its novel effects. Cathode-ray tubes were common in scientific laboratories and thus claims made for the technology could be readily tested. The X-ray picture could be captured on ordinary photographic plates, making use easy. Also, the cost of a basic set of apparatus did not exceed US $50. Rapidly, scientists and physicians tested X-rays on different medical conditions. Because bone and other dense objects were not penetrated by the rays and flesh was, the technology was most quickly adopted to locating foreign bodies and fractures (Figure 4). Physicians also used X-rays to evaluate arthritis, bony deformities, kidney- and gall-stones, bullet wounds, and gout, among other conditions. Two years after its discovery, a professor of surgery wrote: 'Proper surgery cannot be done in a certain variety of diseases without first using the X-ray. . . . It is to the surgeon what the microscope is to the pathologist.'[29] (➤ Ch. 42 Surgery (modern))

At this time, the technique was already standard practice, which made its use an increasing necessity not only on medical, but also legal, grounds. Doctors were warned that 'every doubtful case upon which the X-rays can throw any light, *must be made clear* before proceeding with treatment, or the surgeon will be liable for damages if he meets with bad results.'[30] (➤ Ch. 69 Medicine and the law) Some thought the urgency to have rapid resort to the X-

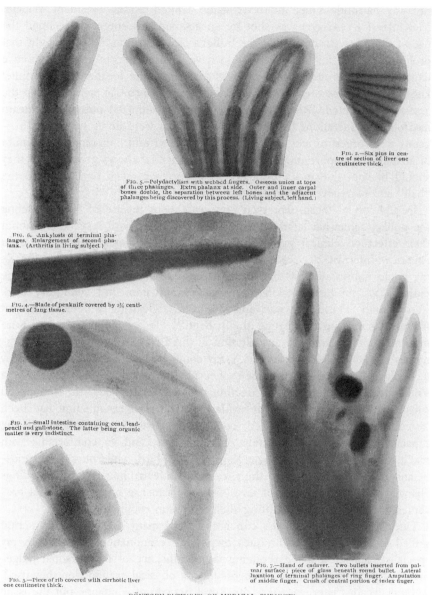

FIG. 2.—Six pins in centre of section of liver one centimetre thick.

FIG. 5.—Polydactylism with webbed fingers. Osseous union at tops of three phalanges. Extra phalanx at side. Outer and inner carpal bones double, the separation between left bones and the adjacent phalanges being discovered by this process. (Living subject, left hand.)

FIG. 6. Ankylosis of terminal phalanges. Enlargement of second phalanx. (Arthritis in living subject.)

FIG. 4.—Blade of penknife covered by 2¾ centimetres of lung tissue.

FIG. 1.—Small intestine containing cent, lead-pencil and gall-stone. The latter being organic matter is very indistinct.

FIG. 7.—Hand of cadaver. Two bullets inserted from palmar surface; piece of glass beneath round bullet. Lateral luxation of terminal phalanges of ring finger. Amputation of middle finger. Crush of central portion of index finger.

FIG. 3.—Piece of rib covered with cirrhotic liver one centimetre thick.

RÖNTGEN-PICTURES OF MEDICAL SUBJECTS,
Taken by HENRY W. CATTELL, M.D., in the Physical Laboratory of the University of Pennsylvania, with the kind permission of PROF. ARTHUR W. GOODSPEED.

For THE MEDICAL NEWS, New York, Feb. 15, 1896.

Figure 4   Early X-rays by pioneers in American radiology.

Source: H. W. Catell, 'Roentgen's discovery – its application in medicine', *Medical News*, 1896, 68: 169.

ray was harmful. Thus in 1901, when United States President William McKinley (1834–1901) was shot by an assassin, his surgeons declined the use of the X-ray to determine the bullet's exact location. They thought that prolonged search for the bullet would have exposed him to greater operative danger, and that once the X-ray was taken and the location of the bullet known, public pressure to extract it would have grown. As one report on the assassination noted: 'Roentgen rays are not an unmixed blessing, as death has followed operations for encysted bullets that were doing no harm.' Surgeons were urged to take care not to be coerced into operating 'on account of anxiety and importunings of patient and friends, always greater than they should be, but due to an exaggerated importance given by laymen to the "ball" and its recovery.'[31]

In addition to these expressed concerns about misuse of X-rays among the public, somewhat later physicians also began to have reservations about their effect on clinical practice. In 1921, George Dock (1860–1951), an American internist, declared that the many doctors who believed that the X-ray could abbreviate the diagnostic process and allow them to avoid 'the tedious task' of history-taking, physical examination, and laboratory work were wrong: 'The dream was, and still is, to endeavour to detect and treat the disease instead of treating the patient.'[32] He argued that X-rays were inferior to percussion and auscultation in three ways. First, unlike the techniques of physical diagnosis, the X-ray could be significantly influenced by technological failures of machinery. Second, the X-ray developed in an era when the rate of autopsy was declining, and thus it lacked the anatomical substantiation against which the evidence of physical examination had been tested. How then, Dock argued, could radiologists be so confident in the capacity of X-rays to accurately depict lesions, and so comfortable with making a diagnosis from a single X-ray plate? Third, while physical diagnosticians could readily follow their cases and learn how physical findings changed during the course of an illness, the expense of taking X-rays prevented radiologists from adapting such follow-up routinely.[33]

Dock's critique reflects the concerns felt by many doctors of this period skilled in applying the techniques of physical examination. The new X-ray specialists appeared to be reducing the significance of the personal judgements of the physician and the techniques of physical examination they used. Several decades later, in 1945, the Royal Society of Medicine put the issue to a test. A debate was held with the title, 'Stethoscope versus X-rays'. The views expressed showed that in the half-century since its discovery, the X-ray had assumed many of the diagnostic burdens the stethoscope had carried. Among the debaters, few made a spirited defence of the stethoscope as pre-eminent in evaluating chest diseases. At best, arguments in its favour were posed as using its findings in conjunction with radiological, historical, and other forms of evidence. Comments about the stethoscope had almost an elegiac tone to them. One doctor said he 'would be very sorry to see the physical signs and stethoscope abandoned'. On the whole, the discussion confirmed that medicine was in the age of the X-ray. 'In a hundred years', commented a doctor, 'the stethoscope had not altered fundamentally; it had reached its limits, and those limits, even in skilled hands was so narrow that radiography was indispensable.' Called to choose between the stethoscope and X-ray, 'it would be the X-rays every time,' said another. The stethoscope's significance 'still lingered in the imagination of the patient and medical men', declared a participant. 'It was difficult to avoid going through the gesture – it was not much more than that – of trying to hear vague mysterious sounds, when something quite definite could be seen on the X-ray film.'[34]

The victor in this debate was not merely the X-ray, but the form of evidence for which it stood – the picture. Photography had been invented in 1839, over half a century before the discovery of the X-ray. During this period, the belief had emerged that the photograph was a true depiction, if not the equal, of reality itself. A central reason for the rapid acceptance of the X-ray was a perception of it as a particular kind of photograph and thus vested with its reality-capturing properties. Shortly after their discovery, X-rays were called 'Roentgen photographs';[35] a number of early radiologists began as photographers. It seemed X-rays could easily capture the way things were. One medical observer wrote of these beginnings:

> The throat mirror needed the practiced eye, the stethoscope an acute ear, and the scalpel trained fingers but [in the early days] this new affair, these X-rays, their very name a confession of inexactitude, could be managed by any hospital photographer, ward orderly or nurse. The one thing needful . . . was a hand to start the machine and then to stop it. I heard it said . . . that any high-school boy, given a smattering of knowledge of human anatomy, should be able to 'take X-ray pictures,' to borrow the expression used.[36]

These photographs could bridge the opaque layers of the skin to reveal the organs beneath. They were viewed as the most dramatic extension of the senses into the body's interior ever facilitated by a technology, the equivalent of an autospy. Thus, the belief that photographic images were depictions of reality enormously furthered the acceptance of the X-ray, and helped it to triumph over other forms of diagnostic evaluation, such as those based on sound or touch.

Little more than two decades after the 1945 Royal Society of Medicine debate, A. M. Cormack (b. 1924), a physicist, and G. Hounsfield (b. 1919), an engineer, working separately in the mid-1960s, built the first computerized tomography (CT) scanning machines. In 1971, it was used clinically at the Atkinson Morley Hospital in England; and in 1973, the Mayo Clinic received the first commercial model.[37] This technology was revolutionary from several perspectives. It put together the X-ray and the computer in a way that allowed multiple, narrowly separated cross-section images of the body to be taken rapidly. By eliminating several problems of conventional X-rays – the overlap of organs and difficulty of distinguishing adjacent structures of similar density – great improvement in diagnosis was achieved, particularly in the less-dense aspects of the body such as the brain. It was also the most expensive diagnostic technology ever introduced into medicine: early scanners cost over US $300,000.[38] (➤ Ch. 57 Health economics)

Although the X-ray was already an established feature of diagnosis, the introduction of the CT scanner catapulted radiology, or imaging as it began to be called, to the pinnacle of diagnostic prominence. At this time, a variety of techniques of producing pictures of the internal structures of the body using energy other than that of the X-ray were being introduced. By the mid-1970s, the images produced by ultrasound technology were finding increasing use in medical practice, particularly in obstetrics, where the hazards of radiation to the foetus had limited the use of X-rays. The low biological danger of ultrasound, its modest cost, and ease of use (the examination took minutes and required no special preparation of the patient) made it an increasingly popular device.

In the 1980s, magnetic resonance imaging (MRI), a technique investigated for several decades in laboratories using magnetic fields and radio-frequency waves to obtain images of tissues, became clinically developed and was in wide use by the decade's end. Like the CT scanner, it produced cross-section images, but without the presence of ionizing radiation. Not only was the MRI safer for patients, but it was more sensitive than the CT scanner in a number of areas, such as the finding of brain tumours or lesions of the spinal cord. Its cost, even greater than the CT scanner, could run upwards of US $2 million. Other technologies just as costly as MRI have begun to be evaluated for clinical use in the 1990s, such as the positron emission tomography (PET) machine. It can produce images of actual biochemical activites in organs such as the brain and heart, as opposed to revealing structural changes that the other imaging processes now expose.

The organization of imaging technologies, our premier diagnostic instruments, and the role of the specialists who direct them have become daunting challenges in modern medicine. Increasingly, each of these major technologies is placed in a separate unit. Requests by clinicians for a particular test is referred to that unit, where the test is performed, interpreted, and the findings sent back to the clinicians. Given the growing array of alternative imaging examinations and the difficulties of choosing those most appropriate to evaluate a given patient, and having the test results comparatively interpreted, a strong warrant exists for imaging specialists to have a greater exchange with clinicians. At the Massachusetts General Hospital in the 1910s, Richard Cabot (1868–1939), a professor of medicine, encouraged pathologists, chemists, and physiologists to make ward rounds with him, to come out of their specialized enclaves detached from patient care and engage in dialogue about clinical choices. Increasingly, the need for better diagnostic management requires modern technological specialists to think of doing the same. (➤ Ch. 55 The emergence of para-medical professions)

Most of the new imaging technologies depend on the computer to integrate into readable images the data their sensors acquire. In this and in other aspects of medicine the computer's introduction heralded another fundamental change in the process of diagnosis.

THE SCIENCE OF DIAGNOSIS – THE PRINTOUT

Marey had extolled the virtues of the sphygmograph's depiction of physiological phenomena because it recorded faithfully the almost-infinite inflections of the organ whose movements it measured. The attraction of the computer to doctors, as it was introduced into medicine at the start of the 1960s, was a similar ability to store and analyse an almost unlimited amount of evidence. The computer was to the analysis of data what the sphygmograph was to its detection.

As the 1960s began, doctors were sorely in need of rescue from the torrent of diagnostic evidence pouring down upon them from the ever-increasing array of data-generating technologies, and the growing numbers of journals and books that discussed their value and meaning. By this time, the simplification, enhanced power, and cost reduction realized through the invention of the transistor made the computer a potent target of research among clinicians and scientists. The computer had the capability to store prodigious loads of data, and to sift through and analyse them. As one comparison of the machine and a person put it: 'Any computer will do in less than an hour what a man will do in a year with a pen and paper.'[39]

Specifically, computers were thought capable of solving the problem of medical record-keeping, diagnosis, physiological monitoring, and the processing and retrieval of administrative and clinical data (Figure 5). Medical records posed a particular dilemma. As described in the mid-1960s:

> Many millions of pieces of paper are added to medical records yearly; many thousands of record clerks, quite apart from doctors and nurses, are employed in maintaining these records, fetching them, carrying them and filing them; they occupy hundreds of thousands of square feet of floor space, and yet despite all this enormous effort and cost the utilization of this data, other than as an aide-mémoire, is very small indeed.[40]

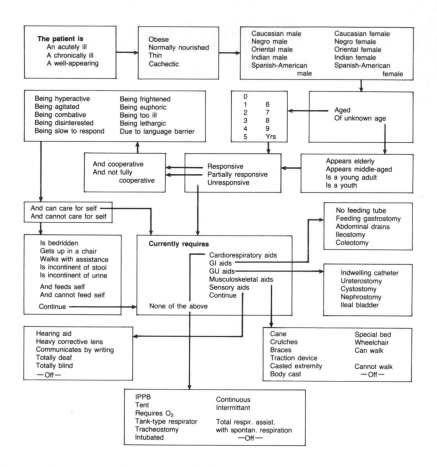

Figure 5 Recording and structuring findings of physical examinations through the computer by the American physician, Lawrence Weed. The following are his comments on the meaning and use of the computer program:

This figure represents the 'General Appearance' section of the physical examination. Each 'box' is a single TV terminal display. The series begins at #1 in the upper left corner and ends with #12. In order to write a description of this patient, the physician simply touches the TV-tube terminal at the point of appropriate selection. The machine responds by changing from one display to the next so rapidly that one is barely aware of the change of frames on the screen. Note that the sequence which the machine will follow depends entirely upon the choice of statements. Thus a choice of 'unresponsive' at #7 leads directly to #12. The 'General Appearance' section follows the vital signs, and once it is completed the physician touches either 'none of the above' or 'continue,' both of which are on display #12. He will immediately continue with the skin examination at this point. The title for the first display is recorded automatically, along with the modifying statement selected by the physician. Thus a touch of the finger would write, 'the patient is chronically ill.' The material is printed in final form as a complete sentence. Example: 'The patient is an acutely ill, obese, Caucasian male, aged 54 years. Responsive, not fully cooperative, being too ill, and can care for self. Currently requires GI aids, colostomy.' A 29-word statement is thus generated by touching the terminal only 13 times, faster than the material can be written with a pen.

Source: L. L. Weed, *Medical Records, Medical Education, and Patient Care*, Cleveland, OH, Press of Case Western Reserve University, 1971, pp. 232–3.

846

A 1966 study indicated that over 25 per cent of hospital budgets were consumed in information handling.[41] What an opportunity to prove its worth the information quagmire seemed to offer the computer!

Diagnostic analysis was another central theatre of operations for the strength of the computer. The sifting of pertinent from irrelevant data, and developing hypotheses from present but incomplete data, seemed tailor-made for a machine with its information-processing capabilities. In the 1960s, continuous monitoring of the major body systems, such as the renal, cardio-vascular, and respiratory systems, had become a regular feature of the newly developed intensive-care units that were springing up in all major hospitals. The computer became an essential tool in this process, for the data streaming out of these monitors ran at so rapid a rate that only automated tracking of its findings enabled use of the data to detect crises, measure therapeutic progress, and watch trends for prognoses.

Finally, there was great hope that computers would make possible Hospital Information Systems (HIS) to help deal with the flood of data generated by the hospital and its diagnostic and therapeutic-care work: the reports, scheduling data, requisitions for supplies, and patient bills.

By the end of the 1960s, virtually none of these hopes had been realized. Computer experts had been too optimistic about their ability to develop systems of logic and programming to lead the computer's data-analysing capacity to appropriate outputs. Engineers, physicists, mathematicians, and medically qualified computer experts did not do enough to allay the anxiety their machine stirred in doctors that one day it might take over their most prized capability: clinical judgement. The introduction of computers into patient-management activities was considered 'as a repugnant interference in what were essentially human activities quite unsuited to any form of mechanization'.[42] And the costs of introducing and using the machines in clinical settings had far exceeded estimates. As one computer expert wrote: 'There is a keen appreciation of the wide gap separating a demonstration project, however impressive, and an operational service system in daily use.'[43] There was harder work ahead for the promise of the computer to match its performance.

By the 1990s, computers had become ubiquitous in medicine, particularly in four areas. First, in the real-time monitoring of physiological functions during ordinary or critical patient care. Monitored signals include those of arterial and venous pressure measured from indwelling catheters, and blood chemistries of all kinds. A second use was the analysis of electric signals from machines such as the ECG and the electro-encephalograph (EEG). In 1970, about 1 per cent of all ECG analysis in the United States was done through the computer. By 1982, the figure had risen to 10 per cent, and it has been increasing. A third growth area (see pp. 843–45), noted previously, was in imaging systems, which depended on the computer to piece together an image from the data they produced. Finally, computers became widely used in the precise control of delicate interventions, such as drug infusions or therapy.[44]

However, while computer programs have been developed and used to deal with diagnosis in narrow areas of medical specialization, as yet no general diagnostic program has emerged and taken a regular place in practice, although research programs for this exist.[45] Even in the area of ECG diagnosis, where use is becoming widespread, one expert noted: 'Few observers would prefer any of the available computerized systems to an experienced, expert EKG [ECG] interpreter when confronted with a representative small sample of patient EKGs.'[46] It had been hoped that once a diagnostic ECG program had been developed and worked well, it could be gradually improved until it was better than the human expert, but since disagreement still exists among experts in the interpretation of a large percentage of ECGs, tuning the system has proved difficult. Computerized ECG analysis thus remains confined to use essentially as a screening tool to evaluate large populations where few complications are anticipated, and in rural sites where cardiologists are less available and practitioners can receive at least a rapid opinion. The difficulties of achieving success, even in this narrow area of medical diagnosis, illustrates the problems ahead in computer diagnosis.

Further, even in recent times, some three decades after its introduction in medicine, one still reads in the medical literature of the need to calm anxiety about the computer. For example, a 1987 essay by a physician and computer expert stated that physicians worried more than other professionals 'about computers "taking over".' Why? Because physicians 'take pride in the amount of factual knowledge they possess. They are, therefore, threatened by a machine that is superior to man in memorizing facts and retrieving them on command, and now it even aspires to emulate "human" intelligence.'[47]

At least a part of this anxiety is generational. Most physicians now in practice did not experience the computer as a regular feature of growing up. As computers become a routine part of childhood education, and as more adults become familiar with their function, their reach and limitations will be more evident and thus their use in fields like medicine less intimidating. As this familiarity grows, computers probably will be treated like other diagnostic technologies, as helpful extensions of a human capability – judgement in this case. Indeed, future application of computers may mirror that of many innovative diagnostic technologies that formerly caused trouble: not auspicious under-use, but unreflective over-use.

Like the diagnostic technologies preceding the computer, its adoption will not only be shaped by technological qualities. It will depend, too, on the technology's influence on the user's self-image, human relationships, and social standing. The technologies of diagnosis serve not only as extensions of the users' physical and intellectual selves, but of their personalities as well. Narratives about the adoption and use of these technologies ultimately are narratives about ourselves. (➤ Ch. 68 Medical technologies: social contexts and consequences)

ACKNOWLEDGEMENTS

I gratefully acknowledge the permission of the Historical Research Center of the Houston Academy of Medicine – Texas Medical Center Library to reproduce from volumes in their collection the material in Figures 1–4. I acknowledge also Mosby-Year Book, Inc., for permission to reproduce the material in Figure 5.

NOTES

1   J. N. Corvisart, *An Essay on the Organic Diseases and Lesions of the Heart and Great Vessels*, trans. by Jacob Gates, New York, Hafner Press, 1962, p. 17.

2   Ibid, pp. 15–18.

3   R. T. H. Laënnec, *A Treatise on the Diseases of the Chest*, trans. by John Forbes, New York, Hafner Press, 1961, p. 284.

4   Ibid., p. 285.

5   Laënnec, op. cit. (n. 3), p. 285.

6   B. Rush, 'A course of lectures on the theory and practice of medicine', MS student notes taken by an unidentified hand at Philadelphia: University of Pennsylvania Medical School, [c.1790] In the Francis H. Countway Library of Medicine, Boston, MA.

7   Laënnec, op. cit. (n. 3), p. 370.

8   Laënnec, op. cit. (n. 3), pp. 392–3.

9   Laënnec, op. cit. (n. 3), pp. 302–3.

10 Laënnec, op. cit. (n. 3), p. 288.

11 J. Marion Sims, 'On the microscope, as an aid in the diagnosis and treatment of sterility', *New York Medical Journal*, 1869, 8: 397.

12 C. A. Wunderlich, *On the Temperature in Diseases: a Manual of Medical Thermometry*, trans. from the 2nd German edn by W. B. Woodman, London, New Sydenham Society, 1871.

13 G. B. Morgagni, *The Seats and Causes of Diseases Investigated by Anatomy*, trans. by B. Alexander, 3 vols, London, Millar & Cadell, 1769; orig. pub. as De Sedibus et Causis Morborum per Anatomen Indagatis, Venice, Remondini, 1761.

14 Wunderlich, op. cit. (n. 12), p. 60.

15 Wunderlich, op. cit. (n. 12), p. 75.

16 E. Seguin, 'Suggestions on Thermometry and Human Temperature', in C. A. Wunderlich and Seguin, *Medical Thermometry and Human Temperature*, New York, William Wood, 1871, p. 243.

17 Wunderlich, op. cit. (n. 12), p. 79.

18 Wunderlich, op. cit. (n. 12), p. 289.
19 E. J. Marey, 'Lectures on the graphic method in the experimental sciences, and on its special application to medicine', *British Medical Journal*, 1876, 1: 1.
20 E. Seguin, *Medical Thermometry and Human Temperature*, New York, William Wood, 1876, p. 289.
21 Wunderlich, op. cit. (n. 12), p. 52.
22 Seguin, op. cit. (n. 20), p. 250.
23 Marey, op. cit. (n. 19), p. 1.
24 W. C. Röntgen, 'On a new kind of rays', *Nature*, 1896, 53: 274–6.
25 A. W. Goodspeed, 'Roentgen's discovery', *Medical News*, 1896, 68: 168.
26 H. W. Cattell, 'Roentgen's discovery – its application in medicine', *Medical News*, 1896, 68: 168.
27 B. Hunter, 'X-ray extravagances', *Lancet*, 1896, 1: 1203.
28 Ibid.
29 J. T. Dunn, 'Diagnostic value of the X-rays', *International Journal of Surgery*, 11 November 1898: 294.
30 Ibid.
31 Editorial, 'The wounds of Presidents Garfield and McKinley', *Journal of the American Medical Association*, 21 September 1901: 781.
32 G. Dock, 'X-ray work from the viewpoint of an internist', *American Journal of Roentgenology*, 1921, 8: 323.
33 Ibid.
34 Reports of Societies, 'Stethoscope versus X-rays', *British Medical Journal*, 15 December 1945, 2: 856–7.
35 Editorial, 'Roentgen photographs and some interesting features of the discovery', *Medical News*, 1896, 68: 171.
36 Ruth and Edward Brecher, *The Rays: a History of Radiology in the United States and Canada*, Baltimore, MD, Williams & Wilkins, 1969, p. 103.
37 D. Banta, 'Embracing or rejecting innovations: clinical diffusion of health care technology', in S. J. Reiser and M. Anbar (eds), *The Machine at the Bedside: Strategies for Using Technology in Patient Care*, New York, Cambridge University Press, 1984, p. 69.
38 Ibid., p. 74.
39 L. C. Payne, *An Introductin to Medical Automation*, Philadelphia, PA, J. B. Lippincott, 1966, p. 93.
40 Ibid., p. 14.
41 G. O. Barnett, 'Computers in patient care', *New England Journal of Medicine*, 1968, 279: 1321.
42 L. C. Payne and P. T. S. Brown, *An Introduction to Medical Automation*, 2nd edn, Philadelphia, PA, J. B. Lippincott, 1975, p. vii.
43 Barnett, op. cit. (n. 41), p. 1326.
44 F. D. Scott, 'The computer at the bedside: current use of dedicated systems in patient care', in M. Anbar (ed.) *Computers in Medicine*, Rockville, Computer Science Press, 1987, pp. 151–73.
45 A. H. Woods, 'Internal medicine', in D. Levinson (ed.), *Computer Applications in Clinical Practice: an Overview*, New York, Macmillan, 1985, pp. 103–9.
46 Scott, op. cit. (n. 44), p. 159.

47 M. Anbar and F. M. Snell, 'Artificial intelligence and its impact in medicine –
can the computer replace the doctor?', in Anbar, op. cit. (n. 44), p. 298.

FURTHER READING

Auenbrugger, L., *Nouvelle méthode pour reconnâitre les maladies internes de la pointrine par la percussion de cette cavité*, trans. by J. N. Corvisart, Paris, Migneret, 1808.

Davis, A. B., *Medicine and its Technology: an Introduction to the History of Medical Instrumentation*, Arlington, Printers' Devil, 1981.

Fox, D. M. and Lawrence, C., *Photographing Medicine: Images and Power in Britain and America since 1840*, New York, Greenwood Press, 1988.

Herrick, J. B., *A Short History of Cardiology*, Springfield, IL, C. C. Thomas, 1942.

Keele, K. D., *The Evolution of Clinical Methods in Medicine*, Springfield, IL, C. C. Thomas, 1963.

Mackenzie, J., *Symptoms and their Interpretation*, London, Shaw, 1920.

Marey, E. J., *Researches sur les pouls au moyen d'un nouvel appareil enregistrauer, de sphygmographe*, Paris, E. Thunot, 1860.

Mitchell, S. W., *The Early History of Medical Instrumental Precision in Medicine*, New York, Tuttle, Morehouse & Taylor, 1892.

Reiser, S. J., *Medicine and the Reign of Technology*, New York, Cambridge University Press, 1978.

Shryock, R. H., 'The history of quantification in medical science', *Isis*, 1961, 52: 215–37.

37

THE HISTORY OF MEDICAL ETHICS

Robert Baker

For the best and worst of reasons, there has been little primary research on the history of medical ethics. Among the more elevated reasons for the paucity of scholarship are beliefs about the nature of ethics itself. The subject is sometimes conceptualized in terms of ahistoric universal principles, insusceptible to change, and hence lacking a history – except in the realm of interpretation. Other scholars view history from the perspective of social science and tend to envision ethics as a mere epiphenomenon of more fundamental socio-economic forces. These theoretical considerations effectively discourage serious historical scholarship. The predilection for ahistoricism is reinforced for the history of medical ethics by the myth of the Hippocratic Footnote, that is, the view that Western medical ethics was established in ancient Greece by the Hippocratic Oath and for the subsequent two millennia amounted to little more than footnotes interpreting this foundational commitment. The myth is cultivated by physicians looking to ancient authority to legitimate their opinions, as well as by critics of medicine, who find the Oath a convenient focus for their critique. Complicating matters further, fundamental changes in moral conceptualization in different historical periods tend to trivialize earlier conceptions of morality in the eyes of later ethicists. Thomas Percival (1740–1804), for example, was universally regarded as the founder of modern medical ethics in the nineteenth century, but was summarily dismissed in the twentieth as fabricator of an obsolete medical etiquette.[1] Even the Hippocratic Oath itself is not immune to this phenomenon – Robert Veatch, a founder of contemporary bioethics, once remarked that calling the Oath ethical 'so stretches the meaning of the term *ethics* that one wonders if it has not simply been misused'.[2]

Despite these conceptual barriers, there is a limited scholarly literature on medical ethics that focuses one-dimensionally on codes, oaths, and other formalizations, ignoring standards of medical propriety stated or implied in the law, in regulatory statutes, in the diaries and letters of practitioners and patients, in the columns of journalists, and in the lyrics of poets and playwrights. Summaries are necessarily circumscribed by the limitations of the summarized, so this survey will also ignore these sources. Moreover, since the extant literature focuses on three eras – ancient Greece and Rome, the professionalization of medical morality in the English-speaking world during the eighteenth and nineteenth centuries, and the bioethical revolution of the second half of the twentieth century – I too follow this pattern, although it is recognized that a history of medical ethics that ignores the Islamic world and continental Europe is, at best, only partial. (➤ Ch. 31 Arab-Islamic medicine)

ANCIENT MEDICAL MORALITY: THE OATH

The Hippocratic Oath established the Western paradigm of a profession (etymologically, one who professes, or swears an oath) as a morally self-regulating discipline – where 'discipline' is defined in terms of those sharing esoteric knowledge and committed to using that knowledge to benefit others. Authorship of the Oath is sometimes attributed to Hippocrates of Cos (c.450–370 BC), but the document itself dates from anywhere between the fifth and third century BC. Scholars usually divide it into four sections:[3]

1   a *preamble*, invoking various gods as witnesses and stating the performatives of oath-swearing ('I swear by Apollo, Physician');
2   a *covenant*, stating the swearer's duties to the profession (that is, to the teacher, the teacher's family, and other oath-swearers), including the duty to 'teach them this art, if they want to learn it ... but to [teach] nobody else';
3   a *code*, stating the duties of the swearer to the patients;
4   a *peroration*, in which the swearer affirms the belief that reputation is dependent upon the faithful execution of the oath.

The *code* is formulated in terms of two basic injunctions: one delineating the nature of morally acceptable treatment, the other directing appropriate conduct towards patients. Both principles are supplemented by specific interpretations (numbered T1, C1, etc., below).

Injunction on treatment: 'I will use treatment to benefit the sick according to my ability and judgment, but never with a view to injury or wrong-doing.'

T1   'Neither will I administer a poison to anyone when asked to do so, nor will I suggest such a course.'
T2   'Similarly I will not give to a woman a pessary [i.e. a vaginal suppository] to cause an abortion.'

T3 'I will not use the knife, not even, verily, on sufferers from stone, but I will give place to such as are craftsmen therein.'

Injunction on conduct: 'Into whatsoever houses I enter I will enter to help the sick, and I will abstain from all intentional wrong-doing and harm.'

C1 '... especially from abusing the bodies of man or woman, bond or free.'
C2 'And whatsoever I shall see or hear in the course of my profession ... if it be what should not be published abroad, I will never indulge, holding such things to be holy secrets.'

The Oath's *code, covenant, preamble,* and *peroration* define a *deontological* (that is, an obligation or duty-based) role ethic, in which physicians are accepted into the profession only if (by swearing the Oath) they undertake to accept and enforce certain special obligations towards each other and towards their patients. The performative, 'I swear', in the *preamble* sets the moral stage for the rest of the Oath. As Edelstein noted,[4] the *preamble* and other passages in the *code* (for example, 'I will keep pure and holy both my life and my art') suggest that the Oath was modelled after priestly vows, effectively elevating medicine above such mundane activities as trade (and thereby establishing the idea of transcendent commitment as central to the Western ideal of professionalism). The *covenant* defines the community of physicians in terms of those who know 'the art' and have sworn the Oath (widening the cleavage between profession and trade by insisting that knowledge of the art be shared within that community, in a manner befitting priest-scholars, rather than being hoarded, or 'patented', as trade secrets used for financial gain). In the *peroration* (which some believe echoes the Athenian juror's oath[5]), censure (or ostracism or expulsion) are acknowledged as enforcement mechanisms (again, suggesting the idea of a self-regulating discipline).

The most substantive section of the Oath is the *code*. The presupposition underlying it is that the medical art is sacred and not to be profaned by: (T3) performing surgery; or (T2) performing abortions or prescribing abortifacients; or (T1) prescribing or administering poisons (even to assist suicide, a form of 'euthanasia'). The most fundamental obligation of the Oath-sworn physician is to help the sick and refrain from all wrong-doing and harm – including taking sexual advantage of patients, even slaves (C1), or violating patient 'confidentiality' (C2).

THE INFLUENCE OF THE OATH

Little is known about the Oath. We do not know who drafted it, nor for what purpose, nor even if it was sworn as an oath of apprenticeship. We do know of a tradition of oath-swearing, associated with the medical schools of ancient Alexandria, which continued through the Middle Ages, but we do not know if these oaths were Hippocratic in nature.[6] A clearer line of influence is the tradition of referring to and commenting on the Oath in medical writings such as those of the first century AD physician Scribonius Largus by Sarapion (*fl.* 339–59) (who recast the parts of the Oath as a poem[7]), and by the second-century physician, Galen (AD 129-*c*.200/210).[8] What is clear, however, is that as the West converted to Christianity, so did the Oath. (➤ Ch. 61 Religion and medicine)

In the Christianized Oath,[9] the swearer called on Christ as witness, the words were sometimes displayed on the page in cruciform array, and Christianity altered its substance to accommodate Christian conceptions of charity, as is evident from 1586 English translation of Thomas Newton (*c*.1542–1607).

> That I shal not be squeamish to bestow my skill in this Arte upon the poore and needie, freely, without either fee or other covenant certainly agreed upon.[10]

THE IMPORTANCE OF THE OATH IN ANCIENT GREECE AND ROME

It is unlikely that the Oath set the standards of propriety for most medical practitioners in the ancient world. Edelstein has argued persuasively that the Oath was *not* a strong influence on standards of medical morality until the Christian era; thus, he pointed out that the sanctity accorded human life in the Oath (T2, T3) is an anomaly in ancient secular moral thought and practice.[11] Abortion and exposure (that is leaving a child exposed in the open, where it would die if no one adopted it) were common practices in Greece and Rome,[12] condoned by such leading moral philosophers as Plato (*c*.427–347 BC)[13] and Aristotle (384–322 BC).[14]

Turning from the foetus and the infant to the adult, the following passage from the Roman stoic Seneca (*c*.4 BC–AD 65) is more representative of secular views on the 'sanctity of life' – it is especially informative because it suggests that physicians/surgeons assisted suicides (in direct contravention of T1 and T2).

> Must I await the cruelty of disease? . . . Live, if you so desire; if not, you may return to the place whence you came. You have often been cupped in order to relieve headaches. You have veins cut for the purpose of reducing your weight. If you would pierce your heart, a gaping wound is not necessary; a lancet will open the way to that great freedom, and tranquility can be purchased at the cost of a pin-prick. (Seneca, *Epistle LXX*, 14–18)[15]

Moreover, the Oath is inconsistent with known facts about Hippocratic medical practices, especially T3, the prohibition of surgery. We know that Hippocratics practised surgery from a number of texts (*Surgery*, *On Fractures*, and *On Joints*)[16] dealing with the subject. The Oath's characterization of medical knowledge as esoteric and 'holy' is also at odds with ancient practice, as Edelstein observed: 'Everybody was familiar with medicine ... physicians wrote books for the general public ... medical knowledge was perhaps diffused more widely in Greek and Roman times than in any other period of history.'[17]

ANCIENT VIRTUE ETHICS OF MEDICINE

If the Oath did not provide a standard of moral propriety, was there another source of secular medical morality? Morality, of course, is less an invention of philosophers than of peoples: philosophers critique and formalize conceptions that are essentially artifacts of culture. 'Ethics', a term that derives from the Greek for 'character', is no more the invention of the teacher student team of Socrates (*c*.470–399 BC), Plato, and Aristotle than 'rights' (a linguistic artifact of Anglo-Saxon resistance to the Norman conquest) are the invention of Thomas Hobbes (1588–1679), John Locke (1632–1704), and Jean Jacques Rousseau (1712–78). Standards of moral propriety may exist, therefore, without philosophers' idealized formalizations. This would appear to be the case with the dominant medical ethic of the ancient world – although at least one ancient philosopher, Plato, indirectly formalized the prevalent conception of medicine as an art governed by the ethics of *aretê*.

For Plato, *aretê*, or 'virtue', was the primary concept of moral appraisal – as it was for most ancient Greeks. MacIntyre tried to put the Socratic–Platonic–Aristotelian commentaries on *aretê* into perspective by noting that there was 'a received set of virtue-words in fifth-century Greek and, in that sense, a received set of virtues: friendship, courage, self-restraint, wisdom, justice'.[18] The problem facing the Greek and Roman philosophers was to reformulate the common conceptual coin of their culture into a coherent system – a task Plato undertook for the virtue of justice in the *Republic*. In Book I, as part of this analysis, Plato described a conception of medicine, which he seemed to expect his fourth century BC Greek audience to accept as obvious:

> the human body ... has weaknesses and defects, and its condition is not all it might be. That is precisely why the art of medicine was invented: it was designed to help the body and provide for its interests. ...
>
> ... the art of medicine does not study its own interest, but the needs of the body itself, just as a groom shows his skill by caring for horses, not for the art of grooming.
>
> So the physician, as such, studies only the patient's interest, not his own. For as we agreed, that business of the physician, in the strict sense, is not to

make money for himself, but to exercise his power over the patient's body. . . .
All that he says and does will be said and done with a view to what is good
and proper for the subject for whom he practises his art.[19]

In these passages, Plato presupposes that his audience will accept as truisms
that every activity aims at some good, and that the virtue of an art/craft or
an artisan/craftsperson is a function of its/their ability to attain this good.
Acts or character-traits that lead towards the attainment of the good are
virtues, or virtuous; those that lead away from the good are vices, or vicious.
These truisms lay the foundation for Plato's argument that the aim of the
groom and the physician is not to make money, but to attain the goal òf the
activity: in the case of medicine, to assist the body to deal with its flaws and
defects. Good medicine is thus medicine that attains this end; good physicians
are those who cultivate the skills and character traits (virtues) enabling them
to attain it.

This virtue conception of the good physician differs profoundly from the
ideal of the good physician in the Oath. The art of the Oath was esoteric
and holy, demanding a sacred commitment from practitioners, who could be
entrusted with the art only if they swore to undertake a special role. The
Oath thus presumes a 'fact-value' distinction: that is, it presupposes the
possibility that knowledge can be abused for unholy ends. Plato's medical
art, in contrast, is secular (like grooming). For Plato, activity, not role,
determines morality: anyone engaged in the activity (grooming a horse, healing
a sick person) partakes in the ethic generated by the goal of the activity (the
telos), in the sense that knowing the aim of the art determines what ought to
be done. On this view, empirical facts are inextricably interconnected with
what we would today characterize as 'values'. Thus immorality, for Plato,
was less a matter of intent than of ignorance; for no one who really knows
how to practise medicine will intentionally practise poor medicine.[20]

Perhaps the most profound difference between the two ethics is that the
Oath is *deontological*: that is, it is an ethic of duties created by, and set forth
in, the text of the Oath. Plato's virtue ethic, in contrast, is *teleological*: that
is, good medical practice, including the determination of obligation, is determined by an empirical assessment of which actions and which character-
traits best achieve the aim of the art (the *telos*). These apparently abstruse
differences have practical consequences. Consider the patient who asks a
physician to use a 'lancet' to 'open the way to that great freedom'; that is,
to bleed him to death. A physician whose conscience is dictated by the Oath
determines the propriety of such an act by consulting the text of the Oath.
Since T_1 and T_3 prohibit euthanasia by bleeding, whatever the consequences
to physician, patient, or society, the Oath-sworn physician cannot comply
with the patient's request.

Consequences, however, are relevant in teleological ethics. Just as questions about the best methods of grooming are to be answered empirically, in terms of consequences, so too are questions about the precise duties of the physician. Insofar as the aim of the medical art is to relieve bodily suffering, euthanasia (whether by bleeding or any other means), becomes a possible remedy – unless it conflicts with another aim of medicine. For, in virtue ethics, moral controversy also focuses on the aims of the medical art itself. Thus moral disputes in a virtue ethic will often take the form of arguments over the *aim* of the medical art.

Plato provides us with an example in Book III (405–410) of the *Republic*. In Book I, he indicated that it is generally held that the aim of the art of medicine was to serve the interests of the body; in Book III, he uses the literary convention of reinterpreting the myth of Asclepius, the mythological father of medicine, to argue that the 'proper' aim of medicine is to correct weaknesses of the mind, as well as the body, as long as life is meaningful.

> Herodicus . . . combined training and doctoring in such a way as to become a plague to himself first and foremost and to many others after him . . . [b]y lingering out his death. He had a mortal disease, and he spent all his life at its beck and call, with no hope of a cure and no time for anything but doctoring himself. Every departure from a fixed regimen was a torment; and his skill only allowed him to reach old age in a prolonged death struggle. . . . [Herodicus] never understood that Asclepius did not reveal these valetudinarian arts to his descendants . . . because he realized that in every well-ordered community each man has his appointed task which he must perform; no one has leisure to spend all his life in being ill and doctoring himself. . . . [H]e either regains his health and lives to go about his proper business, or, if his body is not equal to the strain, gets rid of all his troubles by dying. . . .
>
> Asclepius recognized this and revealed the art of medicine for the benefit of people of sound constitution who normally led a healthy life, but had contracted some definite ailment[.] He would rid them of this disorder by means of drugs or the knife and tell them to go on living as usual so as not to impair their usefulness as citizens. But where the body was diseased through and through, he was not to try, by nicely calculated evacuations and doses, to prolong a miserable existence and let his patient beget children who were likely to be as sickly as himself. Treatment, he thought, would be wasted on a man who could not live in his ordinary round of duties and was consequently useless to himself and society. . . . if a man had a sickly constitution and intemperate habits, his life was worth nothing to himself or anyone else; medicine was not meant for such people and they should not be treated, though they be richer than Midas. . . .
>
> The physically unfit [physicians] will leave to die and they will actually put to death those who are incurably corrupt in mind.[21]

Plato's alternative to conventional fifth-century medicine would widen its aim to encompass mind as well as body, and would focus the aim of medical interventions on preserving life *only* insofar as life was meaningful. Meaningless lives, those in which individuals can do nothing but nurse their own diseases 'and consequently is useless to [themselves] and society', are not worth living and should not enjoy fruits of the medical art. Good medical practice would have allowed, perhaps even (depending on one's reading of the last line) encouraged, Herodicus's death.

It might be supposed that Plato's indifference to Herodicus's patent desire to live is also a departure from standard fifth-century secular medical practice. In the ancient world, however, secular morality was primarily a matter of duty and virtue; wishes and desires were always suspect as potentially subversive to these fundamental aspects of morality. Thus Plato insists that, in spite of Herodicus's patent desires to live, insofar as his life 'was worth nothing to himself or anyone else', he 'should not be treated, though [he] be richer than Midas'. Both the virtuous physician and the Oath-sworn physician are morally obligated to ignore the patient's wishes (to be treated, to be given a poison or an abortifacient, etc.) and to resist the patient's 'bribes'. Wishes and desires would not, and could not, become morally relevant until they were conceptually metamorphosed into something quite different: that is, into 'values'. Before that transformation, the idea that it is morally proper for patients to participate in medical decision-making, and the correlative ideas of patient autonomy and medical paternalism, were inconceivable, if not meaningless.

TEXTUAL EVIDENCE OF A VIRTUE ETHIC IN THE HIPPOCRATIC CORPUS

From the historiographer's perspective, it is a singular virtue of the Oath that it has a physical text that has been revised: leaving tracks in the historical record. Outside of the passages cited in Plato, the textual evidence for a virtue ethic of medicine consists of statements interspersed throughout technical writings in the Hippocratic Corpus evaluating activities and character-traits in terms of their ability to achieve the aim of the art. Thus technical writings on bone surgery often contain discussions of improper treatments (*apodidaxia*) and malpractices (*mathemata*) characterized in terms of the aim of the art: that is, impropriety in these practical medical texts is characterized in terms of a virtue ethic of medicine.[22]

The better-known Hippocratic texts, *The Art*, *Epidemics*, and *Precepts*, also contain passages in which one can discern disagreements over the aim of the art and hence over medical ethics. It is possible, for example, to detect a debate between science-based technologists and medical humanists in such passages as *Precept V*, where the physician is enjoined to be a technician and hence to 'disregard' (but 'not to punish') patient requests for 'what is out of the way and doubtful'. In *Epidemics* (I, 11), however, the physician is encouraged to 'make a habit of two things to help, or at least to do no harm' because: 'The art has three factors, the disease, the patient, and the physician. The physician is the servant of the art. The patient must cooperate with the physician in combating the disease.' Thus, in this classical statement of medical humanism, the physician is exhorted not to be a technician, but to pay attention to the patient's wishes – even, presumably, when they request 'what is out of the way and doubtful' – because the patient is as much a factor in illness as the disease. The servant of the art, therefore, cannot disregard the patient's requests, as recommended in *Precept V*, but must secure the co-operation of the patient, because co-operation achieves the aim of the art: that is, it 'combat[s] the disease'.

Other moral disputes are also discernible in the Hippocratic Corpus. In *The Art*, the author characterizes the art's aim as: 'to do away with the sufferings of the sick, to lessen the violence of their diseases, and to refuse to treat those who are overmastered by their diseases, realizing that in such cases medicine is powerless'. Refusing 'to treat those who are overmastered by their diseases', however, was as controversial in ancient times as it is today.

> VII. Some there are who blame medicine because of those who refuse to undertake desperate cases and say that while physicians undertake cases which would cure themselves, they do not touch those where great help is necessary; whereas if the art existed, it ought to cure all alike ... if a man demand from an art what does not belong to the art.... his ignorance is more allied to madness than to lack of knowledge. For in cases in which we have mastery through a means afforded by a natural constitution, or by art, there we may be craftsmen, but nowhere else.

A seemingly direct critique of this position is found in *On Joints*.

> Now someone might say that conditions fall outside the medical art for, after all, why is it necessary to ponder further about diseases which have become incurable? It is, however, quite wrong to think that this were the case: surely it is obvious that one should be an expert in these as well, for it is not possible to separate the one from the other. For one has to apply one's art to the curable [morbid conditions] lest they become incurable, and this is done by knowing the best way to preventing them from advancing to incurability. But one has to be familiar with incurable conditions in order to avoid needless torments. Brilliant and conclusive predictions [are derived from] recognition of the trend, of the manner, and time, when each [morbid state] will come to an end, and whether it will take the turn to the curable or incurable.[23]

Thus, while acknowledging the obligation of avoiding 'useless torments', it is asserted that treating 'incurable' patients has a 'use': that is, enabling physicians to perfect 'the art' by developing diagnostic, prognostic, and therapeutic skill.

MEDICAL ETHICS IN THE MEDIEVAL AND RENAISSANCE PERIODS

For present purposes I shall ignore the evolution of the ethics of the Art and the Oath from the fall of Rome through the Enlightenment. The omission is slightly less criminal than the span of years suggests for two reasons: the paucity of primary scholarship and the apparent continuity of ancient, medieval, and early modern medical thought and practice. Sixteenth- and seventeenth-century translations of the Hippocratic Oath, a variety of apprenticeship manuals, and other medical writings, although Christianized, use language and employ conceptions of medical practice, decorum, etiquette, and moral propriety that would be readily understood by ancient Greek or Roman practitioners (and were often written in the same language: Latin).[24]

JOHN GREGORY AND THE INVENTION OF MODERN MEDICAL ETHICS

Evidence of a fundamental reconceptualization of medical morality first appears in the English-language literature with the publication in 1772 of *Lectures on the Duties and Qualifications of a Physician*, by John Gregory (1725–73).[25] Gregory (1725–73) was educated in Aberdeen and Leiden; in 1766, he became Professor of Practice of Physic at Edinburgh and gave a series of lectures on the duties of physicians. It seems probable that, in doing so, he was following the practice of his professors at Leiden – the *alma mater* of many eighteenth-century medical ethicists, including Thomas Percival.

The opening words of Lecture One place Gregory in the tradition of classical virtue ethics, the ethics of 'the Art': '[By] the *practice of medicine* ... I understand, the art of preserving health, of prolonging life, and of curing diseases.' Indeed, Gregory's first two lectures read like commentaries on the ethics of the Hippocratic Corpus. In Lecture Two, for example, he takes a position on treating patients 'overmastered' by disease, remarking that: 'It is as much the business of a physician to alleviate pain, and to smooth the avenues of death, when unavoidable, as to cure diseases.'[26] (➤ Ch. 67 Pain and suffering)

Yet, as Gregory appreciated, any attempt to teach traditional virtue ethics, that is, teleological ethics, to an eighteenth-century scientific audience was problematic because the very 'modernity' of modern science lies in its presupposition of a mechanistic conception of causation – a conception incompatible with the idea of a *telos* (an aim or purpose). The problem was delineated by

Thomas Hobbes in *Leviathan* (1651), a work that extended Galileo's picture of a non-teleological universe into human society, reducing all human interests to self-interest, and portraying competition as the force motivating all social activity. In such a world, Hobbes argues, the only rationally justifiable virtue is justice; 'arts' have no purposes (no aim) except the self-interests of those engaged in them. Hobbes's portrait of social relations dissolving in the acid of self-interest was especially vivid for eighteenth-century intellectuals because it aptly portrayed the psychological impact of capitalism on society.[27]

Revising or refuting Hobbes was thus tantamount to the project of developing an ethic for a competitive capitalist society in the context of a mechanistic scientific culture. Three such projects dominated eighteenth-century thought: John Locke's theory of natural rights grounded in a social contract; the subjugation of self-interest of Jeremy Bentham (1742–1832) through the calculus of utility, which postulated universal happiness as the end sought by everyone (thereby reasserting teleology); and the theory of moral sense or sentiments. The latter was the philosophy of the Scottish Enlightenment, developed by Francis Hutcheson (1694–1746), David Hume (1711–76), and Adam Smith (1723–90). For these Scottish philosophers, the moral sentiments, particularly 'humanity' and 'sympathy', offset the antisocial proclivities inherent in a competitive world motivated solely by rational self-interest, thereby providing a basis for morality.

In his lectures, Gregory (a friend of Hume) turned to the language and logic of the Scottish philosophers to address not only the problem of reasserting a traditional teleological medical ethic (of 'the Art') in the face of an antiteleological scientific culture, but also the interrelated problems of distinguishing etiquette from decorum (typically conflated in eighteenth-century medical manuals),[28] and of preventing medical practice from devolving into 'the sick trade': that is, a trade dominated by a market-place mentality in which the only ethic was *caveat emptor*.[29] More specifically, Gregory reinterpreted classical medical humanism in terms of the theory of moral sentiments, asserting that the virtues of the physician include 'humanity, patience, attention, discretion, secrecy and honour' as well as 'temperance and sobriety', 'candor', and, above all else, 'sympathy'. Gregory defined 'sympathy' as 'that sensibility of heart which makes us feel for the distresses of our fellow creatures, and which of a consequence, incites us to relieve them'.[30]

Gregory now had an answer to the basic moral problems confronting medicine in the eighteenth century. As he argued to his students, an ethic based on sympathy transformed medicine from a trade into an 'art' in which the classic ethic of the art remained meaningful:

medicine may be considered either as an art the most beneficial and important to mankind, or as a trade by which a considerable body of men gain their subsistence. . . . I shall endeavour to set this matter in such a light as may shew that this system of conduct in a physician, which tends most to the advancement of his art, is such as will most effectually maintain the true dignity and honour of the profession, and even promote the private interest of . . . its members.[31]

How can medicine, practised as an art, promote the 'private interests of its members'? Because, by displaying sympathy, the practitioner of the art 'naturally engages the affections and confidence of a patient', making the patient more amenable to cure – and a more satisfied customer. Thus sympathy, 'an attention which money can never purchase',[32] offers practitioners of the art a decisive competitive advantage over their trade-minded competitors. (➤ Ch. 34 History of the doctor–patient relationship)

Medical humanism founded on sympathy, moreover, provides a basis for distinguishing between real (or 'natural') moral propriety and etiquette.

> Decorum, decency and propriety, are words very indeterminate in their application, for this reason, that the ideas fixed to them are partly founded in nature and common sense; partly in caprice, fashion, and the customs of particular nations. In [natural propriety] the obligation is immutable, the same in all ages and nations. In the latter, it is fluctuating and less binding.[33]

For Gregory 'natural propriety' involves immutable obligations such as 'the principal duties a physician owes his patients' which he enumerates in terms of the sentiments of humanity, patience, attention, discretion, secrecy, honour, candour, sympathy, and temperance. Everything else is mere etiquette or decorum.

> There is no natural propriety in a physician's wearing one dress in preference to another . . . indeed . . . external formalities have been often used as snares to impose on the weakness and credulity of mankind; that, in general they have been most scrupulously adhered to by the most ignorant and forward of the profession.

By applying moral sense theory to medical ethics, Gregory not only formulated the first modern theory of medical ethics, he also created the ideal, still very much alive, of the humanistic physician whose effectiveness derives as much from an empathic understanding of illness as from medical science. Some scholars are tempted to treat Gregory as a precursor of the twentieth-century bioethicist. He might better be regarded as the inventor of medical paternalism. For Gregory's objective was that of classic medical humanism: that is, to use sympathy to 'manage [patients] properly'; and when humane management required, he even permitted physicians 'a deviation from the truth'.[34]

THOMAS PERCIVAL AND THE CODIFICATION OF MEDICAL ETHICS

Despite the enduring influence of Gregory's vision of the humanistic physician, a different physician-ethicist, Thomas Percival, laid the foundations for professional medical ethics in the nineteenth and twentieth centuries. Like Gregory, Percival was educated at Edinburgh (but not during Gregory's tenure) and Leiden, and was an acquaintance of David Hume. Instead of seeking an academic appointment, however, Percival settled into a successful private practice in Manchester, where he was a leader of the dissenting community[35] – in part, because of his renown as author of *A Father's Tales*,[36] a collection of parables for the moral education of children.

For most of his life, Percival's reformist inclinations involved him in what might be called 'biomedical politics' (or 'biopolitics' or 'medical politics') rather than 'biomedical ethics' (or 'bioethics' or 'medical ethics'). This distinction is important, not only for understanding Percival, but for the history of medical ethics in the last two centuries. Political action, insofar as it is successful, culminates in regulations and laws enforceable through state sanction. Ethical norms, in contrast, are enforceable through private sanction. For example, acts of wilful deception are generally considered wrong: when the only sanctions against these acts are conscience, censure, loss of status, ostracism, etc., the wrong is treated as ethical. If, however, government holds the wrongdoer liable for civil or criminal sanctions, the wrong is considered illegal as well. The same is also true of reforms which right wrongs: thus a figure like Edwin Chadwick (1800–90), who looked to government (that is, to regulations and laws) to right the wrongs of medicine, can be said to be engaged in biomedical politics, while someone seeking to remedy precisely the same wrongs by appeals to conscience and peer sanctions is engaged in biomedical ethics. In a country like the United States, which has an extensive private sphere and limited government, bioethics is often the dominant mode of moral reform in medicine. In countries where government plays a stronger role in health care, biomedical politics tends to dominate. (➤ Ch. 50 Medical institutions and the state)

Percival was an accomplished biomedical politician. As early as 1711, he was writing about the need for municipal regulation of hospitals. He conducted a census of Manchester in 1773, and from 1778 held an appointment at the Manchester Infirmary, then one of the largest hospitals in England. As physician-adviser to the Infirmary, he worked with the trustees to establish the Manchester Board of Health and to institute a House of Recovery (a contagious-disease section) at the Infirmary, both in 1796. What transformed Percival from a biomedical politician into a biomedical ethicist was a request from the trustees to draft a code of ethics, a request that had arisen in the wake of a dispute that threatened to destroy the Infirmary. In 1792, Percival completed this code, which he revised and published as *Medical Jurisprudence* in 1794. He circulated this edition to eminent physicians, theologians, and lawyers, who urged him to change the title to *Medical Ethics*.[37] An expanded and renamed work was published in 1803.

Medical Ethics was immediately treated as authoritative, especially by the Americans. Two of Gregory's students, Samuel Bard (1742–1821), a founder of New York's Columbia Presbyterian Hospital, and Benjamin Rush (1745–1813), cofounder of a number of Philadelphia medical institutions, had heralded the importance of medical ethics for the American medical profession. It was thus natural for a committee of physicians charged to draft a code of conduct for the newly formed Boston medical organization to turn to the medical-ethics literature for guidance. The code they produced, the 1808 *Boston Medical Police* – the first official code of ethics issued by a modern medical organization – borrowed extensively from Percival's *Medical Ethics*. Between 1817 and 1842, thirteen American medical societies adopted codes based on the Boston *Police*, while the Baltimore and the New York State societies adopted codes based directly on Percival.[38] In 1847, the newly formed American Medical Association (AMA) drafted a code modelled on Percival,[39] to such an extent that many passages were taken directly from *Medical Ethics*.[40]

What accounts for the extraordinary influence of *Medical Ethics*? Syncretism: Percival drafted the 1792 code to develop regulations preventing intrapractitioner disputes, a common problem for eighteenth-century medicine.[41] (➤ Ch. 47 History of the medical profession) Since practicality rather than originality was at a premium, Percival felt free to draw on the works of others. He openly acknowledged using the recommendations of a committee of Manchester practitioners which collected regulations and codes from various British hospitals. He also drew extensively on two contemporary treatises on medical ethics, John Gregory's *Lectures*, and *An Enquiry into the Duties of Men in the Professions* by Reverend Thomas Gisborne (1758–1846).[42] In addition, he revised *Medical Ethics* to accommodate the comments and criticisms of two dozen lawyers, physicians, and theologians to whom he had sent *Medical Jurisprudence*. *Medical Ethics* is thus an essentially syncretic work, which capitalized on practical experience as well as legal, medical, philosophical, and theological reflection, synthesizing them in one grand but concise amalgam.

Percival's treatment of Gregory is a case in point. After noting (Ch. 2, Art. I) that 'The *moral rules of conduct*, prescribed towards hospital patients, should be fully adopted in private or general practice', Percival recapitulates Gregory's list of virtues peculiar to the physician: 'Every case, committed to the charge of a physician or surgeon, should be treated with attention, steadiness and humanity'. The passage is entirely representative, reflecting the singular attraction of *Medical Ethics* for nineteenth-century practitioners – it summarized the moral insights of an era in the 'aphoristic form of a code'.

Chapter 1, article I, opens with another basic insight of the turn of the century, this time from Thomas Gisborne.

> 1. HOSPITAL PHYSICIANS and SURGEONS should minister to the sick, with due impressions of the importance of their office; reflecting that the ease, the health, and the lives of those committed to their charge depend on their skill, attention and fidelity.

The key word here is 'office'. The duties of the hospital practitioners are derived neither from their contract with trustees, nor from their relationship with patients; rather they derive from the 'office' of being a physician or surgeon. As Percival later explains (ch. 4, art. I), this 'office' confers obligations as well as privileges; indeed, acceptance of the privileges of 'office' constitutes a tacit social contract to exercise the duties of office. Consequently, practitioners incapable of performing their duties are obligated to resign their office (ch. 2, art. XXXII):

> when it becomes incumbent on a physician to decline the offices of his profession, it is not easy to ascertain.... [but] Let both the physician and surgeon never forget, that their professions are public trusts, properly rendered lucrative whilst they fulfil them; but which they are bound, by honour and probity, to relinquish, as soon as they find themselves unequal to their adequate and faithful exercise.

Gisborne's notion of 'office' also provides a basis for asserting practitioner independence of patrons; for, as 'public servants', practitioners are no one's private servant. Their 'office' even obligates them to challenge their patrons. Thus, in ch. 2, art. XXI, Percival calls on practitioners to 'discourage' private patients from using '*quack medicines* ... as ... injurious to health, and often destructive even of life'. A similar challenge is to be made by hospital practitioners if trustees attempt to economize by prescribing substandard medications (ch. 11, art. VIII), or by overcrowding wards (art. XV).

For Percival, hospital practitioners were also obligated by their office to challenge their own class prejudices. Percival accepts Gregory's moral sense version of medical humanism and concludes that the practitioners' obligation to promote 'the ease, health, and life of those in their charge' creates a correlative obligation to attend to patients' emotions. To quote ch. 1, art. II, since 'personal confidence is no less important to the comfort and relief of the sick poor than of the rich under similar circumstances', the wishes of the hospital patients too deserve to be indulged (to the extent that the practicalities of institutional life permit). The sick poor thus have an entitlement to humane empathy from their physicians and surgeons who, as Percival states in art. I, must: 'study... in their deportment, so to unite *tenderness* with *steadiness* and *condescension* with *authority* so to inspire the minds of their patients with gratitude, respect, and confidence'.

This statement may be misread because the meaning of 'condescension' has inverted over time. Contemporary society presupposes egalitarianism. Hence to 'condescend' is to presume to an elevated status to which one has no entitlement. In the openly hierarchical eighteenth century, however, social practices were predicated upon a presupposition of inequality. 'Condescension' was thus a measure of temporary egalitarianism; to condescend was to treat someone of lower social status as if they were one's equals. Which is why, as Percival remarks in art. XXVI, 'greater *condescension* will be found requisite in domestic attendance on the poor': that is, the greater the social distance between practitioner and patient, the harder the practitioner should strive to treat the patient as a social equal.

Percival's extension of Gregory's version of medical humanism to the sick poor derives from the traditional medical humanist concern to incorporate the patients' emotions in the treatment of the disease, not from any concern for patients' 'rights' to participate in decisions affecting their course of treatment. In ch. 1, art. IV, Percival asserts that patients are to play no role in discussions of their condition, since 'misapprehension may magnify real evils'. In ch. 2, he displays a parallel concern to protect private patients from unsettling knowledge.

> III... the physician should be the minister of hope and comfort to the sick; that by such cordials to the drooping spirit, he may smooth the bed of death; revive expiring life; and counteract the depressing influence of those maladies which rob the philosopher of fortitude, and the Christian of consolation.

In one of the first modern debates over medical ethics, Thomas Gisborne (a Lockean social contract theorist, who held veracity to be a fundamental duty) took Percival to task on this point. (Percival had sent Gisborne a copy of *Medical Jurisprudence*; Gisborne responded by publicly admonishing him on subject in the 1794 edition of his book, *An Enquiry Concerning the Duties of Men in the Professions*.)

> [T]he welfare of the sick man commonly require[s] that his drooping spirits be revived by every encouragement and hope, which can honestly be suggested to him. But truth and conscience forbid the physician to cheer [the patient] by giving promises, or raising expectations, which are known, or intended to be, delusive. The physician... is at liberty to say little; but let that little be true. St. Paul's direction, *not to do evil, that good may come*, is clear, positive, and universal.[43]

The debate between Gisborne and Percival anticipates a pattern familiar to any reader of the recent bioethical literature. Gisborne premisses his moral analysis on 'clear, positive, and universal' moral principles, which, by dint of their universality, apply just as surely to medical practitioners as to anyone else – overriding any specific obligations practitioners acquire through their office. In his reponse to Gisborne, Percival cites Francis Hutcheson, founder of Scottish moral sense theory,[44] but ultimately appeals to experience to prove his point, citing the following case as one in which deception is 'self-evidently' proper.

> Lady Russel's only son ... died of the small-pox in May 1711. ... To this affliction succeeded, in Nov. 1711 ... her daughter ... who died in child-bed. Lady Russel, after seeing her in the coffin, went to her other daughter ... from whom it was necessary to conceal her grief, she being at the time in child-bed likewise; therefore she assumed a chearful [sic] air, and with astonishing resolution agreeable to truth, answered her anxious daughters enquiries with these words: 'I have seen your sister out of bed to-day.'[45]

THE NINETEENTH CENTURY CODIFICATION OF MEDICAL ETHICS

The appropriation of Percival by Americans, Australians, Canadians,[46] and others in the English-speaking world was not simply a matter of copying articles out of *Medical Ethics*. Percival addressed his code to an eighteenth-century British context in which distinctions of social class permeated a medical division of labour formally segmented between university-educated physicians, hospital-trained surgeons, and appenticeship-trained apothecaries. (➤ Ch. 48 Medical education) These distinctions failed to take root in Britain's colonies. So, where Percival addressed his code to three categories of practitioner (physician, surgeon, and apothecary) and a variety of patients (private, hospital, dispensary, lock hospital, insane asylum), the non-British codes addressed all medical practitioners as 'physicians' and their charges as 'patients' – simplifying Percival's complex ethic into a single unified code for physician–patient, physician–physician, and physician–societal relationships. In the 1847 AMA code, these relationships were formulated as reciprocal obligations, in effect a tripartite social contract (making explicit Percival's presumption of a tacit social contract). Such a formulation was a natural outgrowth of the Americans' Lockean intellectual heritage and had been proposed as early as 1794 by Benjamin Rush – himself a signer of that quintessentially Lockean document, the Declaration of Independence.[47]

Chapter 1 of the 1847 AMA Code[48] specifies the duties of 'Physicians to their patients' and the reciprocal 'Obligations of patients to their physicians':

> 1. A physician should not only be ever ready to obey the calls of the sick, but his mind ought also [to] be imbued with the greatness of his mission, and the responsibilities he habitually incurs in its discharge. ... Physicians should,

therefore, minister to the sick with due impressions of the importance of their office; reflecting that the ease, the health, and the lives of those committed to their charge depend on their skill, attention and fidelity. They should study, also, in their deportment so to unite tenderness with firmness, and condescension with authority, as to inspire the minds of their patients with gratitude, respect, and confidence.[48]

The reciprocal obligations of patients towards physicians are stated in art. 2:

2. The first duty of a patient is, to select as his medical advisor one who has received a regular professional education. . . .

4. Patients should faithfully and unreservedly communicate to their physician the supposed cause of their disease. . . . A patient should never be afraid . . . a medical man is under the strongest obligations of secrecy. . . . However commendable a modest reserve may be in the common occurrrences of life . . . in medicine [it] is often attended with the most serious consequences, and a patient may sink under a loathsome disease, which might have been readily prevented had timely intimation been given to the physician.

6. The obedience of a patient to the prescriptions of his physician should be prompt. . . . He should never permit his own crude opinions as to their fitness, to influence his attention to them.

Chapter 2 of the Code deals with the reciprocal obligations of professionals to each other and to the profession, for the most part recapitulating Percival's complex regulations about professional consultation and the adjudication of disputes. In the third chapter, the profession states its contractual relationship to the public.

1 . . . it is the duty of physicians to be ever vigilant for the welfare of the community . . . and when pestilence prevails, it is their duty to face the danger, and to continue their labours for the alleviation of the suffering, even at the jeopardy of their own lives.

The same chapter delineates the public's reciprocal obligation to the profession.

1 . . . physicians are justly entitled to the utmost consideration and respect from the community. The public ought likewise to entertain a just appreciation of medical qualifications.

In sum, the 1847 Code committed the American medical profession to a contractual obligation to accept Gregory's empathic medical humanism and Percival's conception of the physician's office as a public trust – going beyond Percival in accepting a duty to serve the public in the face of epidemics, 'even at the jeopardy of their own lives'. In exchange, the AMA asked of patients and the community what they took to be justice: that is, respect and obedience from the former, and licensure from the latter.

The 1847 Code provoked controversy: some practitioners found it too constraining; others endorsed it, but objected to specific provisions. Among the latter was Worthington Hooker (1806–67), who, in his 1849 book, *Physician and Patient*,[49] took the AMA to task for accepting Percival's ideal of the physician as a 'minister of hope' and asserting a 'sacred duty to . . . avoid all things which have a tendency to discourage the patient or to depress his spirits' (ch. 1, art. I.4). Hooker rehearsed Gisborne's objections to Percival on the subject of veracity, and argued that if the AMA's policy be adopted by the community as a common rule:

> [it] will be self-defeating, because deception succeeds . . . because the patient supposes that all who have intercourse with him deal with him truthfully. . . . And if [deception] should become a settled policy . . . the result would be general distrust . . . defeating deception at every point.[50]

As Hooker's critique illustrates, the formalization of medical ethics in codes provided a vehicle, not only for articulating ideals of propriety, but also for debating them.[51] The codes were also instrumental in shaping the biomedical politics of the era: for example, the drive for educational standards and licensure. More often than not, however, biomedical politics held centre stage, even in America. In continental Europe, biopolitics appears to have completely dominated bioethics. Thus, where Percival urged the human treatment of the insane as a matter of egalitarian ethics in Britain, Philippe Pinel (1745–1826) unchained the insane at Bicêtre as a matter of egalitarian politics; Dominique Jean Larrey (1766–1842), Napoleon's Surgeon-General, replicated Percival's medical egalitarianism when he decreed:

> those who are dangerously wounded must be tended first, entirely without regard to rank or distinction. Those less severely injured must wait until the gravely wounded have been operated on and dressed.[52]

Ironically, Larrey's biopolitical policy, triage, was later to be converted to an ethical principle by American bioethicists.[53]

MEDICAL ETHICS IN THE TWENTIETH CENTURY

In the first half of the twentieth century, biomedical politics dominated discourse about standards of medical propriety in Europe, and even in America. Moreover, the modern rejection of teleology had become so entrenched that twentieth-century scholars routinely perused the history of medicine without perceiving any ethics, other than the Oath. The discussions of 'the art', of 'mission', or of 'office', which fill the Hippocratic Corpus, as well as eighteenth- and nineteenth-century codes, were read as ornamental rhetoric. Percival's code, and the codifications predicated upon it, were thus dismissed as mere etiquettes whose real function was to serve as fig-leaves disguising professional privilege,[54] and/or the politics of monopolization.[55] Although the bioethicists of the 1970s sometimes noted that the language of everyday clinical ethics is the language of 'appropriateness' and 'acceptability', and is adamantly teleological, they generally treated this fact as evidence of medical practitioners' misconceptions about the nature of morality.[56]

THE NUREMBERG CODE ON EXPERIMENTING ON HUMANS

The Nuremberg Warcrimes Tribunal raised new moral questions for medical professionals. During the Second World War, German physicians conducted destructive, often lethal, medical experiments on unconsenting captive populations. (➤ Ch. 66 War and modern medicine) In their defence, these physicians claimed that their experiments were not only lawful, but indistinguishable from those published in leading medical journals.[57] Moreover, although they admitted that their methods of conducting non-therapeutic research on humans violated some moral standards for research on humans[58, 59] – particularly the principle of Claude Bernard (1813–78) of 'never performing on man an experiment that might be harmful to him to any extent, even though the result might be highly advantageous to science, i.e. to the health of others'[60] – they pointed out that other eminent researchers also conducted non-therapeutic experiments that violated Bernard's principle.

Non-therapeutic research on humans had, in fact, been justified by a variety of expedients: auto-experimentation,[61] the 'voluntary consent' of subjects,[62] paying subjects (compensating extra for injury, or death),[63] and choosing as subjects only those exposed to the disease in the natural course of events.[64, 65] In justifying their experiments, the Germans asserted what they took to be an equally valid principle: the interests of the state in time of war. They argued that in the absence of any universally accepted standard, their justification was as good as any other. (➤ Ch. 69 Medicine and the law)

The German defence seemed airtight: in the absence of standards of propriety, there can be no impropriety; in the absence of law, no crime. None the less, the Warcrimes Tribunal (drawing on the same moral tradition as Gregory and Gisborne) found them guilty of violating universal principles of 'natural propriety':

> All agree . . . that certain basic principles must be observed in order to satisfy moral, ethical, and legal concepts:
> 1. The voluntary consent of the human subject is absolutely essential. . . .
> 2. The experiment should be such as to yield fruitful results for the good of society, unprocurable by other methods or means of study, and not random or unnecessary in nature.

3. The experiments should be so designed as to be based on animal experimentation and ... that the anticipated results will justify the performance of the experiment.

4. The experiment should be so conducted as to avoid all unnecessary physical and mental suffering and injury.

5. No experiment should be conducted where there is an *a priori* reason to believe that death or disabling injury will occur; except, perhaps, where the experimental physicians also serve as subjects.

6. The degree of risk taken should never exceed that determined by the humanitarian importance of the problem. . . .

7. [Adequate facilities should be used, and precautions taken] to protect the experimental subject against even remote possibilities of injury, disability or death.

8. . . . [E]xperiments should be conducted only by scientifically qualified persons. . . .

9. . . . [The] subject should be at liberty to bring the experiment to an end . . .

10. [The] experiment . . . must be . . . terminate[d] . . . [if] continuation is likely to result in injury, disability, or death to the experimental subject.

These ten principles, now known as the Nuremberg Code, eventually provided the basis for a universally accepted ethic for experimentation on humans.

THE PHYSICIAN'S OATH (GENEVA, 1948)

Many physicians were profoundly disturbed by the role German physicians had played during the Second World War – not only experimenting on unconsenting humans, but also participating in involuntary euthanasia, eugenic sterilization, and 'eugenic-euthanasia' (more commonly known as genocide – physicians presided over the gas-chambers and other killing mechanisms at all concentration camps).[66] At the Second General Assembly of the World Medical Association (WMA), representatives of the medical community attempted to reassert the claims of professional morality by issuing a new Physician's Oath.

Now being admitted to the profession of medicine I solemnly pledge to consecrate my life to the service of humanity. I will give respect and gratitude to my deserving teachers. I will practice medicine with conscience and dignity. The health and life of my patient will be my first consideration. I will hold in confidence all that my patient confides in me. I will honor the noble traditions of the medical profession. My colleagues will be as my brothers. I will not permit considerations of race, religion, nationality, party politics, or social standing to intervene between my duty and my patient. I will maintain the utmost respect for human life from the time of its conception. Even under threat, I will not use my knowledge contrary to the laws of humanity. These promises I make freely and upon my honor.[67]

The Physician's Oath ingeniously preserves not only the formal structure and deontological logic of the Hippocratic Oath (preamble, covenant, code, and peroration), but also the sense of the profession as sacred office in a secular setting. Yet it modernizes the content of the oath by eliminating the therapeutic injunctions (T1–T3) and by attempting to clarify a transcendental, transnational commitment that race, religion, etc., will not 'intervene between my duty and my patient', and that 'Even under threat I will not use my knowledge contrary to the laws of humanity.' Gregory had earlier predicated modern medical teleological morality on natural law; the penultimate line of the Physician's Oath grounds medical deontological ethics in the same tradition, but for a different purpose: to assert that professional morality overrides the laws proclaimed by national states. (➤ Ch. 59 Internationalism in medicine and public health)

INFORMED CONSENT TO THERAPEUTIC EXPERIMENTATION

Although the WMA issued an International Code of Medical Ethics predicated on the Golden Rule ('As ye would that men should do unto you, do ye even so to them') at their 1949 London meeting,[68] it did not specifically address experiments on humans until 1954, when it issued 'Principles for those in research and experimentation'. These principles clarified the Nuremberg Code and modified it to make it applicable to 'normal' hospital research. Specifically: they establish a clear distinction between therapeutic experiments, designed to test new cures on sick patients, and non-therapeutic experiments; they assert that written consent by a subject '*informed* of the nature of, the reason for, and the risk of the proposed experiment' should be the basis of all ethical experimentation; and they recognize the propriety of surrogate consent for incompetent patients.[69] In the following year, the Catholic Hospital Association of the US and Canada (CHA) endorsed consent as the ethical basis for experimenting on humans;[70] and the Public Health Council of the Netherlands (PHCN) transformed the WMA Code into practical guidelines by, among other things, recommending that they be interpreted by a 'permanent advisory committee of men experienced in human experimentation': the Dutch thus invented Institutional Review Boards or 'IRBs' (to use a later American acronym), fulfilling Percival's vision (*Medical Ethics*, ch. 1, art. 12) of subjecting proposed experiments to peer review.[71]

While medical societies and regulatory bodies around the world accepted the Nuremberg principles for non-therapeutic experimentation – and while, in 1957, the AMA abandoned the Percivalian model of a 'contract' for a WMA model code based on 'principles'[72] – few organizations followed the WMA by applying the requirement of informed consent to therapeutic experiments.[73] The 1962 US Army Regulations, for example, explicitly exempted therapeutic research from the informed consent requirement,[74] as did separate 1963 statements by the British Medical Association (BMA)[75] and the Medical Research Council (MRC), which stated:

> Provided . . . the medical attendant is satisfied . . . that a particular new procedure will contribute to the benefit of that particular patient . . . he may *assume* the patient's consent to the same extent as he would were the procedure entirely established practice.[76]

In its 1964 Declaration of Helsinki,[77] however, the WMA reiterated that explicit, rather than assumed, consent is the proper basis for ethical research on humans. In the end, the WMA's view prevailed, in large measure because of the efforts of two physicians, Henry Beecher (1904–76) in the US and M. H. Pappworth in the UK,[78] who alerted the public to the abuse of patients used as subjects in purportedly therapeutic research. Beecher reported his findings at a professional meeting in March 1965 and in a *New England Journal of Medicine (NEJM)* article, which focused on twenty-two papers published in such leading medical journals as *Circulation, JAMA, Journal of Clinical Investigation*, and *NEJM* between 1948 and 1965. The papers were written by eminent researchers at the Harvard Medical School, the National Institutes of Health (NIH), Sloan-Kettering, etc., reporting research sponsored by the NIH, the Surgeon-General's Office, the US Armed Forces, and the US Public Health Service, as well as by Merck, Parke-Davis, and other leading pharmaceutical companies; all of the papers involved morally questionable activities (for example, injecting live cancer implants into patients without their knowledge).[79] Propelled to action, the AMA endorsed the principles of the Declaration of Helsinki in 1966,[80] as did the Food and Drug Administration,[81] NIH,[82] and the US Public Health Service.[83] (➤ Ch. 11 Clinical research)

The worldwide reform of experimentation on human subjects set the paradigm for the bioethics movement. Appeals to universal moral principles had a demonstrable power to reform medical practice, and so the locus of debate shifted from the political to the ethical arena – to basic moral principles which were interpreted as conferring both responsibilities and rights. The particular right that was to occupy the limelight was the right to withhold consent and hence to refuse treatment.

PATIENTS' RIGHTS TO REFUSE TREATMENT: THE QUINLAN CASE

As early as 1973 the American Hospital Association affirmed in its 'Patient's Bill of Rights' that 'The patient has a right to refuse treatment to the extent permitted by the law.'[84] The legal status of this right was tested two years later by a case in New Jersey, Robert Morse, a young attending physician, and Joseph Quinlan, the father of a twenty-one-year-old woman, Karen. Karen Quinlan was in an irreversible vegetative state for several months when Joseph Quinlan and his family asked Dr Morse to turn off the MA-1 ventilator keeping her alive. The Quinlans were guided by their parish priest, who acted after consulting Pope Pius XII's 1958 pronouncement:[85]

> The doctor . . . can take action only if the patient . . . gives him permission. The technique of resuscitation [is one which] the patient if he were capable . . . could . . . give the doctor permission to use . . . [but] since these forms of treatment go beyond an ordinary means to which one is bound, it cannot be held that there is an obligation to use them. . . .
>
> The rights and duties of the family depend . . . upon the presumed will of the unconscious patient . . . they [too] are bound only to the use of ordinary means.
>
> Consequently, if it appears that the attempt at resuscitation constitutes in reality such a burden for the family that one cannot in all conscience impose it upon them, they can lawfully insist that the doctor should discontinue these attempts, and the doctor can lawfully comply.[86]

The Quinlans' priest evidently believed the burden Karen placed on her family was so 'extraordinary' that they could lawfully ask Dr Morse to disconnect the ventilator. Dr Morse, however, was more concerned with medical precedent and the laws of New Jersey than with Catholic doctrine, and declined. In the resulting case, the New Jersey Supreme Court 'affirm[ed] Karen's independent right of choice', or 'self-determination', as a constitutional 'right to privacy' and ruled that her family could exercise this right on her behalf, if 'the responsible attending physician concludes that there is no reasonable possibility of Karen's ever emerging from her present comatose condition', provided that an 'Ethics Committee' concur with this decision.[87]

THE BIOETHICAL CRITIQUE OF CONVENTIONAL MEDICAL ETHICS

The Quinlan decision set a moral and legal precedent for patients' right to refuse life-sustaining treatment. More subtly, it seemed to validate the bioethical critique of conventional medical ethics. Leading bioethical theoreticians of the day – Tom Beauchamp and Robert Veatch – were arguing that although physicians could properly claim expertise about the 'facts' of medical science, they lacked expertise in moral principles or 'values'.[88, 89] Traditional medicine was vulnerable to this critique because – from the Hippocratic Corpus, to Percival, to Beecher (who looked to Percival)[90] – its sense of moral propriety derived from a teleological understanding of the aim of the art (morally 'appropriate' practices were simply those that furthered this aim). Bioethicists, however, argued that rhetoric about the 'aim of the art', or what was 'medically indicated', or 'acceptable', or 'appropriate', begged the central moral question: 'Whose values decide?' To bioethicists, there is but one justifiable answer: 'the patient's'. To answer otherwise is to illicitly extend scientific expertise, committing the moral error of 'paternalism'.

The principles and rhetoric of patients' rights became extremely popular in America in the 1970s and 1980s,[91] as middle-class patients and their lawyers rejected the 'paternalistic' protections of an older teleological medical ethics (originally introduced to protect sick-poor hospital patients), opting instead to assert the bioethical principle of 'self-determination', and such authoritative voices as the American Hospital Association and the President's Commission for the Study of Ethical problems in Medicine publicly endorsed this principle.[92] By the 1980s, the ideals of bioethics were also embraced by European reformers such as Ian Kennedy and Peter Singer, who strove not only to empower patients, but also to criticize the biopolitical decisions of national health services.

MEDICAL TECHNOLOGY, MEDICAL HUMANISM, AND THE BIOETHICAL REVOLUTION

The dominant role of the bioethics movement since the 1970s is also an artifact of medical humanism's abdication of its traditional role as defender of the patient. Conventional wisdom has it that physicians opened the doors of the clinic to ethicists because they were overwhelmed by moral problems caused by scientific advances in medical technology. Historians of medical technology, most notably Michel Foucault and Stanley Reiser,[93, 94] tell a more complex tale. Two traditions of teleological morality are indigenous to medicine: the ethic of *techne*, propounded in *Precept V*, which identifies good physicians as those proficient at restoring health and preventing disease; and the humanism propounded in *Epidemics*, in which the patient (and, post-Gregory, the patient's feelings) are considered integral to the curative process. (➤ Ch. 36 The science of diagnosis: diagnostic techologies; Ch. 68 Medical technologies: social contexts and consequences)

Medical humanism claimed superiority to an ethic of *techne* because it recognized, as the technologists did not, the significant role patients play in the diagnosis and cure of their own illnesses. This claim was undercut by the scientific revolution in clinical medicine. Modern diagnostic techniques

– from auscultation, to stethoscopy, to radiology, to magnetic resonance imaging (MRI) – seemingly eliminate any need to rely on patients and their reported symptoms to access 'the disease', replacing them with the 'clinical gaze' (to use Foucault's terminology): that is, the perception of the living body and its pathologies as a set of scientifically detected signs. Advances in anaesthesia, antisepsis, and antibiotics also seemed to undercut the role of the patient in curative medicine. The humanistic preoccupation with the patient was thus seen to be irrelevant, if not retrograde. To quote Foucault: 'Our contemporaries [seeking] the establishment of a "unique dialogue", the most concentrated formulation of an old medical humanism, as old as man's compassion. . . . Miracles are not so easy to come by.'[95]

BRAIN DEATH AND THE FAILURE OF MEDICAL HUMANISM

As Foucault warned, the clinical revolution challenged traditional medical humanism, not only because the new sciences de-emphasized the significance of the patient, but also because they breathed life into areas that were traditionally problematic for humanism. Consider the 1968 report of the Ad Hoc Committee of the Harvard Medical School to Examine the Issue of Brain Death, 'A definition of irreversible coma'.[96] The committee was chaired by none other than Henry Beecher, and stated its purposes as twofold: to resolve the problems of resuscitating and providing life-support for patients in irreversible vegetative states; and to eliminate 'Obsolete criteria in the definition of death which can lead to controversy on obtaining organs for transplantation'. The Committee's solution to these problems was to offer a new definition of death, 'brain death', which legitimated treating as dead unresponsive comatose patients who lacked reflexes and had a 'flat' EEG. This redefinition of 'death' successfully pre-empted moral controversy over discontinuing life support for patients with flat EEGs, thereby permitting the appropriation of their organs for use by others.

Notice that, although 'brain death' is an ultra-modern concept, the Committee's strategy was entirely traditional: in redefining death, they resorted to a teleological technique for dealing with moral issues – redefining the 'aim of the art'. To paraphrase Gregory, the 'aim of the art' is to preserve health, cure disease, and prolong life. If irreversibly comatose patients with flat EEGs are 'alive', therefore, traditional medical ethics would obligate physicians to prolong their lives. By declaring these patients to be 'dead', the Harvard Committee obviated the traditional obligation to prolong their 'lives', providing an apparently definitive resolution to the problem of withdrawing life support from irreversibly comatose patients.

In reality, 'brain death' did *not* entirely obviate the traditional aim of prolonging life in the case of irreversibly comatose patients, for, as experience soon revealed, some of these patients had EEG activity. Karen Quinlan is the classic case of an irreversibly comatose patient who had a minimally active brain. Disconnecting her ventilator was morally problematic for physicians because she could not be defined as 'dead' by the Harvard criterion. Consequently, Karen Quinlan fell into the traditionally vexing category of patients 'overmastered by their diseases' for whom 'medicine is powerless' to effect a cure (to use the language of *The Art*). Teleological medical ethics had been unable to come to a consensus about terminating treatment in such cases from Plato's time to the present day – and, not unexpectedly, it failed to provide the New Jersey courts with clear moral advice. As an alternative, the court looked to Catholic moral theology (that is, the 'ordinary/extra-ordinary' distinction), to the collective wisdom of an ethics committee, and to the personal decision of Karen's parents. In doing so, they broke the monopoloy of the medical community on medical ethics, legitimating not only the patient's right to self-determination, but also the practice of looking to ethical traditions outside of medicine to resolve moral quandaries arising in medical practice.

THE BIOETHICAL TURN

The bioethical turn to a variety of religious and secular ethical traditions assumes especial importance, when, as in the Quinlan case, traditional appeals to the 'aim of the art' are controversial or meaningless. Thus, bioethics was particularly relevant to the abortion controversy (where appeals to the life-preserving aim of the art begs the question of the status of the foetus as human life), to the anti-psychiatry controversy (in which Thomas Szasz and others challenged the interpretation of madness as illness),[97] and to the human genome project (which involves a new realm of inquiry rather than a mode of intervention).

BIOETHICS AS A SOURCE OF MORAL CONSENSUS: THE WARNOCK REPORT ON *IN VITRO* FERTILIZATION

The emerging role of bioethics as social arbiter of biomedical controversies – especially in areas where traditional appeals to the aim of the art are feckless – is perhaps best illustrated by the work of the Warnock Committee (headed by the philosopher Mary Warnock). The committee was convened in July 1982 by the UK Department of Health and Social Security to deal with the problems arising from *in vitro* fertilization (IVF).[98] The controversy was triggered on 25 July 1978, when a 5 lb 12 oz baby girl, Louise Joy, was born to an infertile Manchester couple, John and Lesley Brown. To circumvent Lesley's infertility, Patrick Steptoe and Robert Edwards removed one of her eggs and placed it in a Petri dish, where it was fertilized by one of John's sperm. The extra-uterine embryo was then reintroduced into Lesley's uterus; the embryo's brief extra-uterine existence led the popular press to dub Louise a 'test-tube baby'.

Louise Joy Brown's birth was condemned by voices as diverse as Nobel Laureate James Watson and the Vatican; it continued to be condemned in later years by feminist philosophers (for example, Mary Ann Warren[99]) and, again, by the Vatican.[100] What sparked the controversy was the foetus's brief extra-uterine existence, which raised such questions as: did every extra-uterine embryo have a right to be implanted? Could unwanted extra-uterine embryos be destroyed? Could they be used for research? If so, was ectogenesis (that is, their growth in an artificial environment) permissible? IVF (along with such less spectacular technologies as artificial insemination by husband (AIH) or by donor (AID) also resurrected troublesome questions about surrogate motherhood (which date back to *Genesis* verses 16 and 30, when Sarah's infertility led Abraham to have a child by her servant, Hagar).

The Warnock Committee opted for a narrow focus, and ultimately recommended that IVF be considered a legitimate medical option for infertile women. It also limited the extra-uterine maintenance of an embryo to fourteen days after fertilization, during which time experimentation is permissible, and after which it is illicit. Additionally, it recommended against the implantation of embryos used as research subjects in humans or in other species. These recommendations became the focal point for a worldwide consensus legitimating IVF.

The Warnock Committee's function as a catalyst for consensus is highlighted by the absence of a comparable consensus on the question of surrogate motherhood, which the Committee opted not to address. Although a New Jersey Supreme Court decision outlawed surrogate motherhood contracts by 7–0 in the infamous Baby M case of 1988,[101] in the absence of a catalyst like the Warnock report, there is no consensus on the legitimacy of surrogate motherhood in the US or elsewhere.

BIOETHICS AS A FOCAL POINT FOR MORAL CONTROVERSY: ANIMAL RIGHTS

Despite the consensus-generating role often played by bioethicists and bioethical committees, the turn away from traditional medical ethics is also a significant source of discord. As bioethicists have been quick to point out, traditional medical teleology is problematic in contexts in which physicians and patients disagree about the 'aims of the art'. What often passes unnoticed is that, in the overwhelming majority of cases, there is consensus about the 'aims of the art', and so traditional medical morality functions unproblematically – it also insulates medical morality from more – general moral and political concerns. Bioethics, precisely because it is based on a morality external to medicine, tends to lack these virtues.

Consider the issue of animal experimentation. The use of animal precursors to human experimentation is explicitly required in the 1948 Nuremberg Code, the 1964 Declaration of Helsinki (and its reaffirmations in 1975 and 1983), and by the Council for International Organizations of Medical Sciences 1985, *International Guiding Principles of Biomedical Research Involving Animals*.[102] The use for animals is consistent with the narrow conception of the 'aim of the art' in traditional teleological medical ethics: to promote human life and health. Jeremy Bentham's utilitarianism, however, envisioned a broader teleological aim that of maximizing happiness. As many twentieth-century utilitarians (most notably Tom Regan and Peter Singer) fully appreciate,[103, 104] however, there is no a priori reason for favouring the happiness of humans over that of other sentient creatures. To quote Bentham:

> The French have already discovered that the blackness of the skin is no reason why a human being should be abandoned without redress to the caprice of the tormentor. It may come one day to be recognized that the number of the legs ... are reasons equally insufficient for abandoning a sensitive creature to the same fate ... a full grown horse or dog is beyond comparison a more rational, as well as a more conversable animal, than an infant of a day, or a week, or even a month, old. But suppose the case were otherwise, what would it avail? The question is not, Can they reason? nor, Can they talk, but, Can they suffer?[105]

As this passage from Bentham illustrates, opening biomedical ethical questions to moral frameworks external to medicine has the inexorable destabilizing effect of reopening matters long considered morally unproblematic within the medical community.

MERCY KILLING AND THE RESURGENCE OF MEDICAL HUMANISM

It is too early to write the epitaph for traditional teleological medical ethics. This ethic provides a generally unproblematic moral framework for both physicians and patients in most areas of medicine and generates ideals of professionalism and humanism capable of inspiring physician-led moral reforms. Mercy-killing is a case in point. In 1971, Geertruida Postma, a Dutch physician, killed her mother with a lethal injection of morphine and curare. When the case went to trial, the judge found Dr Postma guilty, but gave her only a one-week suspended sentence, stating that under certain circumstances mercy killing may be legitimate.

In 1973, the Royal Dutch Medical Association issued guidelines legitimating mercy killing if: (1) it is implemented by a physician, for (2) a competent patient experiencing (3) unbearable pain or suffering, whose requests for relief are (4) unambiguous, repeated, well-documented, and (5) clearly voluntary, provided that (6) there is consultation with another physician, and (7) it is found that there are no alternative measures, acceptable to the patient, for alleviating the pain or suffering.[106] The Postma case and the ensuing Dutch guidelines set the framework for discussions of mercy killing in both Europe and America.[107] They are particularly interesting because they suggest the possibility of a *rapprochement* between traditional teleological ethics and the ideology of patients' rights: that is, a teleological ethic that allows the patient the prerogative of selecting the appropriate 'aim of the art' in those few areas where the aims are either unclear, or in conflict with the patient's own aims. (➤ Ch. 46 Geriatrics)

CONCLUDING COMMENT

The history of medical ethics is one of continuity and change, of a resilient and dominant teleological paradigm torn internally by a long-standing conflict between technologists and humanists, and sometimes challenged, appropriated, or eclipsed by alternative paradigms offered by the deontological ethics of oaths, by contractarian ethics (of Gisborne and, more recently, Veatch), by principled ethics based on natural law, and by a bioethics predicated on patients' rights and the principle of patient autonomy. Although it is difficult to hazard a prediction about the future of medical ethics, its history suggests that ethics will remain integral to medicine, and will continue to be subject to change. (➤ Ch. 4 Medical care; Ch. 12 The concepts of health, illness, and disease)

NOTES

1   Ivan Waddington. 'The development of medical ethics – a sociological analysis', *Medical History*, 1975, 19: 36–51.
2   Robert Veatch, *A Theory of Medical Ethics*, New York, Basic Books, 1981, p. 94.
3   W. H. S. Jones (trans.), *Hippocrates, Works*, Cambridge, MA, Loeb Classical Library, Harvard University Press, 1923. The Jones translation is used because it appears to be the most universally acceptable rendering of the text. Except where otherwise indicated, all references and quotations from the Hippocratic Corpus are from the Jones translations in the Loeb Classical Library editions.
4   Ludwig Edelstein, *Ancient Medicine: Selected Papers of Ludwig Edelstein*, ed. by Owsei Temkin and C. Lilian Temkin, Baltimore, MD, Johns Hopkins Press, 1967.
5   Fridolf Kudlien, 'Medical ethics and popular ethics in Greece and Rome', *Clio Medica*, 1970, 5: 91–121.
6   Vivian Nutton, 'Healers in the medical market place: towards a social history

of Graeco-Roman medicine', in Andrew Wear (ed.), *Medicine in Society: Historical Essays*, Cambridge, Cambridge University Press, 1992, pp. 15–58.

7   James H. Oliver, 'An ancient poem on the duties of a physician', in Chester Burns (ed.), *Legacies in Ethics and Medicine*, New York, Science History Publications, 1977.

8   F. Rosenthal, 'An ancient commentary on the Hippocratic Oath', *Bulletin of the History of Medicine*, 1956, 30: 52–87.

9   W. H. S. Jones, *The Doctor's Oath*, Cambridge, Cambridge University Press, 1924.

10   Sanford V. Larkey, 'The Hippocratic Oath in Elizabethan England', *Bulletin of the History of Medicine*, 1936, 4: 201–19; reprinted in Burns, op. cit. (n. 7), p. 220; see also Paul Kirbe, 'Hippocratic writings in the Middle Ages', *Bulletin of the History of Medicine*, 1945, 18: 317–412; Martin Levey, 'Medical deontology in ninth century Islam', in Burns, op. cit. (n. 7), pp. 129–44.

11   Edelstein, op. cit. (n. 4), Part 1.

12   William Langer, 'Infanticide: a historical survey', *History of Childhood Quarterly: Journal of Psychohistory*, 1974, 1: 353–65. Perhaps the best collection of citations on this subject is to be found in two venerable but still informative works: William Lecky, *History of European Morals: from Augustus to Charlemagne*, London, Longmans, Green, 1905, esp. Vol. II, ch. 4, pp. 19–37; Edward Westermark, *The Origin and Development of the Moral Ideas*, 2nd edn, London, Macmillan, 1912, esp. Vol. I, ch. 17, pp. 383–417.

13   Plato, *Republic* V, 460–1.

14   Aristotle, *Politics*, Book VII, 1335b 20.

15   Seneca, *Ad Lucilium Epistulae Morales*, trans. by Richard Gummere, 3 vols, Cambridge, MA, Harvard University Press, 1962, Vol. II, p. 65.

16   There is evidence that the Hippocratics, like other ancient physicians, engaged in the practice. Some scholars try to reconcile T3 with the Hippocratic texts describing surgery by interpreting T3 as prohibiting castration. The consensus of scholarly opinion, however, endorses Edelstein's view that the prohibition is against shedding blood.

17   Edelstein, 'The relation of ancient philosophy to medicine', op. cit. (n. 4), p. 361.

18   Alasdair MacIntyre, *After Virtue*, London, Duckworth, 1982, p. 114. See also MacIntyre, *A Short History of Ethics*, New York, Macmillan, 1966, ch. 2.

19   Plato, *Republic*, Book I, 341–43, trans. by F. M. Cornford, New York, Oxford University Press, 1945, pp. 22–4.

20   Hence the famous Socratic dictum, *arete* is *episteme*, virtue is knowledge – if one knows how to achieve virtue, one will be virtuous: if one understands the virtues of living, one will live well: that is, one will live the good life.

21   Plato, op. cit. (n. 19), Book III, ch. 9, pp. 405–10, pp. 95–100. This position seems at odds with the position Plato ascribes to Socrates in the *Crito*, and at *Phaedo* 6b-c, where Socrates seems to accept the Pythagorean prohibition against suicide. Something of this attitude appears to be echoed in Plato's later work *Laws* at 873c-e.

22   Markwart Michler, 'Medical ethics in Hippocratic bone surgery', in Burns, op. cit. (n. 7), pp. 105–19.

23   Ibid., p. 107.
24   Sanford V. Larkey, 'The Hippocratic Oath in Elizabethan England', *Bulletin of the History of Medicine*, 1936, 4: 201–19; reprinted in Burns, op. cit. (n. 7), p. 220; see also Kirbe, op. cit. (n. 10); and Levy, op. cit. (n. 10).
25   John Gregory, *Lectures on the Duties and Qualifications of a Physician*, London, 1772; all references are to the American edition published by M. Carey, Philadelphia, PA, 1817.
26   Ibid., p. 37.
27   C. B. Macpherson, *The Political Theory of Possessive Individualism: Hobbes to Locke*, London, Oxford University Press, 1962.
28   Mary Fissell, 'Innocent and honourable bribes: medical manners in eighteenth century Britain', in Robert Baker, Dorothy Porter and Roy Porter (eds), *The Codification of Medical Morality: Historical and Philosophical Studies of the Formation of Medical Morality*, Vol I: *The Eighteenth Century*, Dordrecht, Kluwer Academic, 1992.
29   Dorothy Porter and Roy Porter, *Patient's Progress: Doctors and Doctoring in Eighteenth-Century England*, Cambridge, Polity Press, 1989.
30   Ibid., p. 15.
31   Porter and Porter, op. cit. (n. 29), p. 13.
32   Gregory, op. cit. (n. 25), p. 22.
33   Gregory, op. cit. (n. 25), p. 34.
34   Gregory, op. cit. (n. 25), p. 36.
35   Edmund Percival, *Memoirs of the Life and Writings of Thomas Percival*, London, J. Johnson, 1807.
36   Thomas Percival, *A Father's Tales*, in Percival, *The Works, Literary, Moral and Medical of Thomas Percival*, London, J. Johnson, 1807.
37   Thomas Percival, *Medical Ethics or a Code of Institutes and Precepts Adapted to the Professional Conduct of Physicians and Surgeons*, Manchester and London, J. Johnson & R. Bickerstaff, 1803.
38   Chester Burns, 'Reciprocity in the development of Anglo-American medical ethics, 1765–1865', in Burns, op. cit. (n. 7), pp. 300–7.
39   Morris Fishbein, *A History of the American Medical Association, 1847–1947*, Philadelphia, PA, W. B. Saunders, 1947.
40   Donald Konold, *A History of American Medical Ethics, 1847–1912*, Madison, WI, State Historical Society of Wisconsin, 1962.
41   Lester S. King, *The Medical World of the Eighteenth Century*, Chicago, IL, University of Chicago Press, 1958, pp. 227–62.
42   Thomas Gisborne, *An Enquiry into the Duties of Men in the Higher and Middle Classes of Society in Great Britain Resulting from their Respective Stations, Professions and Employment*, London, B. & J. White, 1794.
43   Thomas Gisborne, cited in Percival, op. cit. (n. 37), p. 158.
44   Ibid., p. 162.
45   Percival, op. cit. (n. 37), pp. 167–8.
46   Chester Burns, 'Medical ethics, history of: North America: seventeenth to nineteenth century', in Warren Reich (ed.), *Encyclopedia of Bioethics*, 4 vols, New York, Free Press, 1978, Vol. III, pp. 963–5.

47 Benjamin Rush, 'Duties of a physician', *Medical Inquiries and Observations*, Philadelphia, PA, 1794, Vol. I, Appendix.

48 'Code of Medical Ethics', *Proceedings of the National Medical Conventions held in New York, May 1846, and in Philadelphia, May 1847*, Philadelphia, PA, 1847.

49 Worthington Hooker: *Physician and Patient: or a Practical View of the Mutual Duties, Relations and Interests of the Medical Profession and the Community*, New York, Baker & Scribner, 1849.

50 Ibid.

51 See, for example, Austin Flint, *Medical Ethics and Medical Etiquette: the Code of Ethics Adopted by the American Medical Association, with Commentaries*, New York, D. Appleton, 1883.

52 Dominique J. Larrey, *Surgical Memoirs of the Campaign in Russia*, trans. by J. Mercer, Philadelphia, PA, Cowey & Lea, 1832, p. 109.

53 Gerald Winslow, *Triage and Justice*, Berkeley, University of California Press, 1982.

54 Chauncey Leake, *Percival's Medical Ethics*, Baltimore, MD, Williams & Wilkins, 1927; esp. noteworthy is Leake's introductory essay, which inspired Ivan Waddington's claim (cited in n. 1) that medical ethics is merely medical etiquette.

55 Jeffery Berlant, *Profession and Monopoly; a Study of Medicine in the United States and Great Britain*, Berkeley, University of California Press, 1975.

56 For a non-teleological and a teleological view of clinical ethics, see the Baker–Veatch debate in Barry Hoffmaster, Benjamin Freedman and Gwen Fraser, *Clinical Ethics: Theory and Practice*, Clifton, NJ, Humana Press, 1989, pp. 7–57.

57 *United States v Karl Brandt, Trials of War Criminals before the Nuremberg Military Tribunals, Vols I and II: The Medical Case*, Washington, DC, US Government Printing Office, 1948, in Jay Katz (ed.), *Experimentation with Human Beings*, New York, Russell sage Foundation, 1972.

58 Gisborne, op. cit. (n. 42), p. 407.

59 Percival, op. cit. (n. 37), ch. 1, art. 12.

60 Claude Bernard, *Introduction à l'étude de la médecine expérimentale (1865)*, pub. as *An Introduction to the Study of Experimental Medicine*, trans. by Henry Green, New York, Dover, 1957, p. 101.

61 In 1885, Daniel Carrion died from a self-administered inoculation when he used himself as a subject for research on verruga peruana. In 1929, Werner Forsmann was able to demonstrate the safety and efficacy of cardiac catheterization using himself as a subject; Forsmann lived and went on to receive the Nobel prize in 1956. For further information on auto-experimentation and the need felt by researchers to challenge Bernard's principle, see Katz, op. cit. (n. 57), pp. 136–42.

62 William Beaumont signed a contract with his experimental subject, Alexis St Martin (*c.*1806–*c.*1884), permitting him to study the subject's gastric juices, as Henry Beecher observed in *Research and the Individual: Human Studies*, Boston, MA, Little, Brown, 1970, p. 219. The US Committee on Medical Research (CMR) used informed consent for experiments using conscientious objectors during the Second World War; see David J. Rothman, *Strangers at the Bedside*, New York, Basic Books, 1991, pp. 41–7.

63 Rothman, op. cit. (n. 62).

64 CMR policy for prisoners and asylum inmates; Rothman, op. cit. (n. 62), pp. 41–40.

65 US Army surgeon Walter Reed (1851–1902) employed all these expedients in experimenting on yellow fever; see Rothman, op. cit. (n. 62), pp. 25–7.

66 Robert Jay Lifton, *The Nazi Doctors: Medical Killing and the Psychology of Genocide*, New York, Basic Books, 1986.

67 World Medical Association, *Declaration of Geneva 1948*, in Beecher, op. cit. (n. 62), p. 235.

68 General Assembly of the World Medical Association, *International Code of Medical Ethics* (London, 1949), in Beecher, op. cit. (n. 62), p. 237.

69 General Assembly of the World Medical Association, 'Principles for those in research and experimentation', in Beecher, op. cit. (n. 62), p. 240.

70 The Catholic Hospital Association of the United States and Canada, 'Ethical and religious directives for Catholic hospitals' (1955), in Beecher, op. cit. (n. 62), p. 245.

71 Public Health Council of the Netherlands, 'Report on human experimentation' (1955), published in the *World Medical Journal*, 1957; in Beecher, op. cit. (n. 62), pp. 241–4, quote on p. 244.

72 American Medical Association, *Principles of Medical Ethics*, reprinted in Stanley Reiser, Arthur Dyck and William Curran, *Ethics in Medicine*, Cambridge, MA, MIT Press, 1977, p. 39.

73 'Harvard University Health Services Code' (1963), in Beecher, op. cit. (n. 62), pp. 272–5.

74 Ibid., p. 252.

75 'Harvard University Health Service Code' in Beecher, op. cit. (n. 62), p. 268.

76 'Harvard University Health Service Code' in Beecher, op. cit. (n. 62), pp. 262–7, quote on p. 263, emphasis added; also reprinted in Reiser, Dyck and Curran, op. cit. (n. 72).

77 Ibid., pp. 277–8.

78 M. H. Pappworth, *Human Guinea Pigs. Experimentation on Man*, London, Routledge & Kegan Paul, 1967.

79 Henry Beecher, 'Ethics and clinical research', *New England Journal of Medicine*, 1966, 274: 1354–60. The cancer implant case is presented in detail in Katz, op. cit. (n. 57), pp. 9–65.

80 AMA, (1966), in Beecher, op. cit. (n. 62), pp. 222–3.

81 Ibid., p. 299.

82 AMA (1966), in Beecher, op. cit. (n. 62), p. 285.

83 AMA (1966), in Beecher, op. cit. (n. 62), pp. 293–8.

84 American Hospital Association, 'Patient's Bill of Rights', *Hospitals*, 1973, 47: 41.

85 Joseph Quinlan and Julia Quinlan, with Phyliss Battelle, *Karen Ann: the Quinlans Tell Their Story*, New York, Doubleday Anchor, 1977.

86 *The Pope Speaks*, 4: 1958, 393–8; also in Reiser, Dyck and Curran, op. cit. (n. 72), pp. 501–3.

87 *In the Matter of Karen Quinlan: an Alleged Incompetent*, 137 NJ Superior Court (1975); *In re Quinlan*, 70 NJ 10, 355 A2d 647, 429 US 922 (1976). The transcripts are available in *In the Matter of Karen Quinlan: the Complete Legal*

Briefs. Court Proceedings and Decisions of the Superior Court of New Jersey, Vols I and II, Frederick, MD, University Publications of America, 1982.

88 Tom Beauchamp and James Childress, *Principles of Bioethics*, New York and Oxford, Oxford University Press, 1979; Beauchamp and LeRoy Walters, *Contemporary Issues in Bioethics*, Belmont, CA, Wadsworth, 1978, 1982.

89 Veatch, op. cit. (n. 2).

90 Beecher, op. cit. (n. 62), p. 218, cites Percival, ch. 1, art. 12, as the earliest code of research ethics.

91 George Annas, *The Rights of Hospital Patients: the Basic ACLU Guide to Patient's Rights*, Carbondale, IL, Southern Illinois University Press, p. 199.

92 President's Commission for the Study of Ethical Problems in Medicine and Biomedical and Behavioral Research, *Deciding to Forego Life-Sustaining Treatment: Ethical and Legal Issues in Treatment Decisions*, Washington, DC, US Government Printing Office, March 1983.

93 Michel Foucault, *Naissance de la clinique*, Paris, Presses Universitaires de France, 1963; pub. as *The Birth of the Clinic: an Archaeology of Medical Knowledge*, trans. by A. M. Sheridan Smith, London, Tavistock and New York, Random House, 1973; reprinted New York, Vintage Books, 1975.

94 Stanley Reiser, *Medicine and the Reign of Technology*, Cambridge, Cambridge University Press, 1978.

95 Foucault, op. cit. (n. 93), pp. xiv, xv.

96 'A definition of irreversible coma: report of the Harvard Medical School to examine the definition of brain death', *Journal of the American Medical Association*, 1968, 205: 337–40.

97 Thomas Szasz, *The Myth of Mental Illness*, New York, Harper & Row, 1960, 1973.

98 Department of Health and Social Security, *Report of the Committee of Inquiry into Human Fertilisation and Embryology*, London, HMSO, 1984.

99 Mary Ann Warren, 'IVF and women's interests: an analysis of feminist concerns', *Bioethics*, 1988, 2: 37–57.

100 'Text of the Vatican's statement on human reproduction', *New York Times*, 11 March 1987, pp. 10 ff.

101 *In The Matter of Baby M*, New Jersey Supreme Court, *Atlantic Reporter*, 537 A.2d 1227, (NJ, 1988).

102 Council for International Organizations of Medical Sciences, *International Guiding Principles for Biomedical Research Involving Animals*, Geneva, CIOMS, 1985.

103 Tom Regan, *The Case for Animal Rights*, Berkeley and Los Angeles, University of California Press, 1983.

104 Peter Singer, *Animal Liberation*, New York, Avon Books, 1975.

105 Jeremy Bentham, *Introduction to the Principles of Morals and Legislation*, London, 1789, ch. 17, section 1.

106 George E. Pence, *Classic Cases in Medical Ethics*, New York, McGraw Hill, 1990, pp. 51–2.

107 Ibid., p. 54. 1987 Statement of Dr Peter Admiraal. For a US example of physician-led reform, see T. E. Quill, 'Death and dignity – a case of individual decision making', *New England Journal of Medicine*, 1991, 324: 691.

FURTHER READING

There are no general histories of medical ethics as such. Interested readers might peruse the works cited here, which are either specialized histories and/or edited collections.

Baker, Robert, Porter, Dorothy and Porter, Roy (eds), *The Codification of Medical Morality: Historical and Philosophical Studies of the Formalization of Medical Morality*, Vol. I: *The Eighteenth Century*; Vol. II: *The Nineteenth Century*, Dordrecht, Kluwer Academic Vol. I, 1993, Vol II, 1994).

Beecher, Henry, *Research and the Individual: Human Studies*, Boston, MA, Little, Brown, 1970; Beecher's appendices are especially noteworthy.

Burns, Chester (ed.), *Legacies in Ethics and Medicine*, New York, Science History Publications, 1977.

Edelstein, Ludwig, *Ancient Medicine: Selected Papers of Ludwig Edelstein*, ed. by Owsei Temkin and C. Lilian Temkin, Baltimore, MD, Johns Hopkins Press, 1967; esp. Parts 1 and 3.

Katz, Jay (ed.), *Experimentation with Human Beings*, New York, Russell Sage Foundation, 1972.

Konold, Donald, *A History of American Medical Ethics, 1847–1912*, Madison, State Historical Society of Wisconsin, 1962.

Pence, George E., *Classic Cases in Medical Ethics*, New York, McGraw Hill, 1990.

Reich, Warren (ed.), *The Encyclopedia of Bioethics*, 4 vols, New York, Free Press, 1978. Esp. noteworthy are the excellent articles by Chester Burns, Donald Konold, and Lawrence McCullough.

Reiser, Stanley, Dyck, Arthur and Curran, William (eds), *Ethics in Medicine: Historical Perspectives and Contemporary Concerns*, Cambridge, MA, and London, MIT Press, 1977.

Rothman, David J., *Strangers at the Bedside: a History of How Law and Bioethics Transformed Medical Decision Making*, New York, Basic Books, 1991.

38

WOMEN AND MEDICINE

Johanna Geyer-Kordesch

The discussion of gender invariably introduces a different system of co-ordinates when looking at the balances and imbalances of history. For one thing, gender is a recently introduced concept focusing on socially produced behaviour as it refers to men and women. Thus the negligible genitalia, usually decently hidden, have become profoundly significant by what they imply. No one can escape the fact that the pattern of what they do or appear to be refers to a set of assumptions based on sex.

These assumptions change, and indeed have had change forced upon them, as grievances and inequalities have found a political voice. The politics of sex were actually never private, as the varied heritage of poetry, plays, epics, and novels on wedding and bedding, languishing, pining away, and occasionally, successfully departing, either alone or together, attests. Even in the most idealized of literary works, such as Friedrich Schiller's plays about liberty and freedom, women are present as allegories of men's favourite political and moral ideas.[1]

Although women may be rarefied as allegories, the archetypal imagery of gender harks back to the old myths, those of the regeneration of the land by the sexual union of the earth goddess and her sacrificial son.[2] The modern sociological view of gender, the analysis of the social place of women and what is ascribed to them, cannot really detach this shadow, the deep-seated archetypal accompaniment that reflects the forces men and women are caught up in: sexuality, the giving of life, creativity and work, suffering, illness and death. The mythologizing of sexuality has to do with its power; the politicizing of gender roles has to do with social purposes, not least of them the dignity and autonomy of individuals.

The political and moral purposes of the women's rights movement, a creation of the nineteenth century, moved the social claims of womanhood on to national and international agendas. The underworld of sexual tension remained. Some issues connected with it, especially those dealing with morality and health, entered the arenas of public discussion. Others remain ideologically intact, predicating what gender means today, but the deep-rooted anarchy of sexual relations continues to guarantee turmoils in whatever enlightenment has come to pass.

This basic ambivalence between civilizing behaviour and the shifting sands of the 'natural', or nature's perversity, must be understood at the outset if a theme such as women and medicine is to have any descriptive validity. 'Women and medicine' thus includes more than just the obvious extension of female biology into obstetrics or gynaecology, or the invention of 'women's diseases', or the place of women in the health professions. It touches on the basic question of why belonging to one gender creates different conditions, for women on the one hand and men on the other.

Historians must do more than unearth women's past lives. The point is not that of investigating a separate sphere, but whether historical analysis has not been altogether ill-judged by ignoring the fundamental importance of disparate chances, separately ascribed roles, and constructed mentalities based on gender. For example, when historiography abandons the idea that witch-hunting is equivalent to woman-hunting, the analysis of bewitching, sorcery, and magic becomes a much more complex subject including the relative values of maintaining crops, domestic animals, and home life as they are part of what *women* did in a peasant economy.[3] Healing or causing harm is then related to the power of women *and* the economy they control. Again, we might consider the question of why perfectly capable women who pursued scientific work and wished to continue their research within prestigious bodies like the Prussian Royal Academy of Sciences (as in the case of Maria Winckelmann-Kirch (1670–1720), the astronomer) were *actively* dismissed.[4] Here, we have an insight into the scientific community creating 'the women's sphere' by debarring women.

Or, for instance, while food production, low income, and ill health have been variously linked, no one sees the homemaker as the substantial arbiter of what is bought, at what price, and how the customs of cooking relate to nourishment. After all, the family and the household controlled diet, the day-to-day nursing care of the sick, and expenditure for food in all the centuries before our own, and this is certainly crucial for health problems even today. The economic input and the public impact of women in philanthropy in the nineteenth century was also pivotal for social hygiene and public health, yet historians never seem to discuss the skills women learned in home management, as opposed to their organizational skills outside the home.[5] (➤ Ch. 63 Medical philanthropy after 1850)

WOMEN AND HEALING: THE MIDDLE AGES TO THE SEVENTEENTH CENTURY

Women healers have a continuous history outside the Hippocratic–Galenic tradition.[6] Medical education, where it was tied to universities, from which women were largely excluded, was not an option for women, although this does not mean there were no outstanding female scholars in the Renaissance. Where medical history concentrates on the legacy of antiquity or on textbook medicine, it misses the popular forms of healing, run by women. Before hospital medicine was linked to professionalized doctors seeking the exact aetiology of diseases, health care was based on different premises. These included attending the sick (nursing care), providing infirmaries for the chronically ill (such as lepers), almshouses for the poor and aged, knowledge about folk remedies, good housekeeping, and providing the right kind of nutrition for all and sundry, including patients in the home. Minor surgery and pharmaceutical skills were also outside the learned élite's practice. In all these areas, from the Middle Ages to the eighteenth century, the evidence for women practising is legion.

The case may thus be made that women were responsible for general health care from the Middle Ages to the eighteenth century, when medical men began to dominate hospital medical science. (➤ Ch. 49 The hospital) The exclusion of women from professionalized medical incorporations must then also be seen in relation to their being disadvantaged as western European society intensified its patriarchal structures through urban regulation of work.

Before the Reformation, the independent power of women to effect charitable works lay with the authority of powerful abbesses or the high nobility. The great abbesses of the Holy Roman Empire, such as Hildegard von Bingen (1098–1178), Mechthild of Magdeburg (1212–82), or Gertrude of Helfta (d. 1311), not only administered their communities and were great mystics, but founded and supervised infirmaries for the sick.[7] In these charitable works, virtues were not practised at arm's length. Medicines and foods were cooked under the guiding hand of the founder. This was part of her wisdom and knowledge, not so far removed from the office of the village wise-women in more circumscribed practice. (➤ Ch. 62 Charity before c.1850)

Women of the high aristocracy could also be independently effective.[8] Lady Margaret Beaufort (1443–1509), Countess of Richmond and Derby, was singularly active, and certainly not unrepresentative, in providing for education and health. She founded two Cambridge colleges (Christ's in 1506 and St John's in 1511, on the site of one of the first charitable hospitals in Cambridge) and an Oxford college, as well as hospitals and almshouses. She personally attended the sick in her hospital in Westminster. Across Europe, these same activities were characteristic of pious and strong-minded women.

In the fifteenth century, titled ladies founded private hospitals, many of them exemplary for their time, such as that in Santiago (Isabella of Spain) or Ewelme, England (Duchess of Suffolk).

The many women who can be named in connection with health care throughout Europe point to a seriously undervalued activity: whether in charge of a monastery or landed estates, their money and energy was used to establish a whole network of personally supervised private hospitals in the public interest. In effect, that was equivalent to health care, the other sectors of healing being the private practice of learned physicians (very small in number) or of barber-surgeons and apothecaries. Women were certainly numbered amongst the latter practitioners. However, only one group of women medical practitioners remained exclusively female: the midwives.

All told, no one can maintain that women were not actively skilled and frequently dominant in health-care provisions in a European society that saw caring for the sick as one of the great works of mercy to which all should aspire. Curing was a professional matter where it pertained to surgery and dispensing of medicines, but on a par with it was the supernatural, where saints and magic were both invoked, especially in a period in which the macrocosm and microcosm were seen to be intimately related. One might point to the great saints of the Middle Ages, amongst them St Elizabeth of Hungary (1207–30), St Bridget of Sweden (1304–73), St Catherine of Siena (1347–80), and St Teresa of Avila (1515–82), all of whom attended the sick and worked curative miracles. In this connection it may not be amiss to mention the great curative power of supplication to the saints and the Virgin Mary, the efficacy of which is amply documented for periods even extending into the nineteenth century in the dedicatory paintings and votive offerings in the churches of, for example, southern Germany and the old Austro-Hungarian Empire.[9] (➤ Ch. 61 Religion and medicine)

But women healers were steadily marginalized through male professional organizations and the sex-related persecution of magical practices in the sixteenth and seventeenth centuries. The seventeenth century saw a severe curtailment of their freedom to practise. The regulation of medical practice through the need to obtain licences was discriminatory in regard to sex.[10] For a woman in England, no matter what her skills, being a woman debarred her in 1614 from practising surgery, and in 1617 from becoming an apothecary or pharmacist. After 1642, a midwife had to be examined before six surgeons and six midwives to obtain a licence; and after 1662, had to pay a fee for a licence. In London in 1634, leading midwives petitioned for an act of incorporation for midwives, but it was not passed. A year later in Paris, the midwives unsuccessfully petitioned the Crown to allow Louise Bourgeois (1563–1638), the most accomplished French midwife of her time, to lecture them in public on obstetrics. (➤ Ch. 47 History of the medical profession)

It cannot be said that women were unwilling to update and reform the only area of legitimate medical practice left to them. In London, Mrs Elizabeth Cellier (*fl.* 1680), an accomplished, well-educated and well-to-do midwife, addressed plans to King James II in 1687 for a royal hospital to care for mothers, educate nurses, and provide for illegitimate babies. She also compiled statistics on the unnecessarily high mortality rate amongst women and infants. (➤ Ch. 45 Childhood) She was a Catholic at a time when this was a political disqualification, and therefore doubly disadvantaged. To her credit, it seems she was immensely angry when the promise of a hospital and the incorporation for midwives did not materialize. Her public anger earned her the pillory and the burning of her books before her eyes.

Jane Sharp (*fl.* 1670) (midwife in England), Louise Bourgeois, and Justina Dietrich (in Prussia) had international reputations and publishing successes. Treatises on chemistry, physic, pharmacy, cookery, and remedies were published by the female intelligentsia of the period, which saw a number of significant female heads of state: Elizabeth I of England (1533–1603), Christina of Sweden (1626–89), Catherine the Great of Russia (*c.*1729–96), and Maria Theresa of Austria (1717–80).

No one has comprehensively traced the books, the lives, or the work of the women who were the backbone of health care. The fault lies with a historiography that concentrates on family history or guild or institutional and corporate histories, leaving out the characteristic trait of female work: that is, their double careers in the household *and* skilled work outside. The writer of popular medical books, the widow who carried on craft skills in surgery or pharmacy, the wise-woman and the midwife, all of whom were engaged in healing, acquired expertise *within her surroundings* and worked from there. This is an entirely different story of 'practitioner–client' relationships than the one told through civic or professional perspectives. (➤ Ch. 34 History of the doctor-patient relationship)

TRANSITIONS? THE SEVENTEENTH AND EIGHTEENTH CENTURIES

Medical knowledge about women certainly changed as the medical disciplines of anatomy and physiology turned to a more graphic and precise description of the organs of reproduction and probed the mechanisms of procreation and generation. (➤ Ch. 5 The anatomical tradition; Ch. 7 The physiological tradition) The knowledge available through the work of Ambroise Paré (1510–90) and William Harvey (1578–1657) took a great deal of time to filter into medical teaching and literature (learned medical practice was highly dependent on written dissemination of knowledge in this period).[12] In the mid-eighteenth century in Prussia, for example, in medico-legal cases, conception, gestation, and parturition were still debated in medical terms among the experts, in particular for cases involving separation, divorce, inheritance, and infanticide.[13] It seems that for childbirth and gynaecology, still fields dominated by midwives and wise-women, the links with 'science' were not well established. (➤ Ch. 44 Childbirth) On the one hand, childbirth was not a purely technical event, but was much more encompassing because it was suffused with ritual and custom,[14] so that scientific medical knowledge may not have been seen as beneficial; on the other hand, by the seventeenth century, the question of competition and male predominance had become acute in these fields. The secret of the Chamberlain family, the obstetrical forceps, helped to establish the ascendency of the man-midwife,[15] but safe delivery in the hands of competent midwives was by no means superseded. Rivalry may not have been the order of the day everywhere: for example, Georg Ernst Stahl (1659–1734), first physician to Frederick William I of Brandenburg-Prussia, attended the Queen, Sophie Dorothea, together with her midwife. Indeed, William Hunter (1718–83) was left waiting outside the bedchamber and lost his fee while Mrs Draper delivered the future George IV in 1762 (although Hunter attended later royal deliveries). Women did not lose their strong role in attending childbirth, although they were gradually controlled and displaced not by male predominance as such, but by the gradual monopoly powers (regulations of licences, access to medical corporations, and medical education) of hospital doctors and surgeons.

Healing, if seen in the wider context of society – that is, not as the special expertise of doctors – probably remained an open and equally distributed, very diverse enterprise. If witchcraft gives an indication of magical healing practices, its demonological aspects declined in Holland, Italy, and Spain after 1620.[16] That indicates nothing, however, about beliefs on curing, and these were certainly culturally entwined with astrology and alchemical ideas on the transformation of substances. The idea that Nature was inherently unified and that thus sympathy (the correspondence of outward appearances with invisible forces, such as the sympathy cures between rubies and blood disorders) and symbolic actions (laying-on of hands, for example) were effective, involved much of general curative practice. (➤ Ch. 30 Folk medicine) Books written by women in this period, such as those by Eleonora, Duchess of Troppau and Jaegerndorff (Troppau was then in Silesia), or Margaret Cavendish, Duchess of Newcastle (c.1624–1674), or Elizabeth, Countess of Kent, or Ann Woolley of London, whose *Pharmacopolinum Muliebris Sexus* of 1674 was reprinted and translated into German and French, reflect the commonplace mixture of beliefs and remedies of the seventeenth century.[17] Only the aristocratic birth that enabled these women to receive an education separates them from the male doctors and empirics who wrote much the same kind of thing.

Where women came to prominence in a more unusual way was amongst the Nonconformist and separatist sects of a century filled with religious controversy. Here, amongst the Quakers, Covenanters, early Pietist radicals, and communities such as those led by Jane Leade (1623–1704) or Eleonora Peterson (née von Merlau), the power of prayer and prophetic gifts were female advantages.[18] Nonconformity, although puritan in some of its leanings, proved to be a bonus for courageous women. They could actively engage the promptings of their conscience, as did Elizabeth Fry (1780–1859), a Quaker, who started her life work after bringing up her family.[19] At the age of 40, Fry began to reform prison conditions, in particular for women. Her work in training nurses for better hospital care was one of the first among these endeavours (the training school for Protestant Sisters of Charity, who trained at Guy's Hospital). Most health-related Christian reform had international connections. For example, Fry went on a tour to Germany to press for prison reform. There she met Pastor Theodor Fliedner (1800–64) of Kaisersworth (near Düsseldorf), whose pioneer training of deaconesses for the care of the ill had repercussions for Great Britain, notably through the study visit there of Florence Nightingale (1820–1910). (➤ Ch. 54 A general history of nursing 1800–1900)

Strong religious belief, its democratic tendencies where women were concerned, and the high purpose and courage it engendered were crucial to women's high profile in public battles for reform, both for the suffering poor and their health, and for the educational and professional rights of women. Distinct religious motivation carried Josephine Butler (1828–1900) into campaigns against prostitution, Sophia Jex-Blake (1840–1912) into medical education, Florence Nightingale into nursing reform, and Elizabeth Blackwell (1821–1910) to her doctorate of medicine (1849).

But Puritan and strict Protestant morality also had severe consequences for women in other areas, particularly where sexual morality was involved. In the 1690s, the Scottish law made concealment of pregnancy a capital offence.[20] The same is true of Prussia in the early eighteenth century, where sexual offences were severely punished and medical expertise helped to convict.[21] In these legal cases, one can graphically perceive the plight of women seduced and abandoned when social mores identified the loss of sexual honour in terms of criminal law. Infanticide and illegitimate births are a consistent barometer of what happens in health, legal, and medical terms to women, but not men, as institutions and governments are predicated on male ideas of right and wrong. What eventually turned the tide for women's rights were ideas on natural law and democracy that also fed into the great revolutions: those of America (1776) and France (1789), and the belated and aborted European revolutions of 1848. (➤ Ch. 69 Medicine and the law; Ch. 37 Medical ethics)

WOMEN DOCTORS

Although women had been scholars and healers for centuries, the medical doctorates granted in the nineteenth century pushed open the doors of the universities and of an established profession for women. When the first handful of women won their degrees, domestic ideology was dented beyond repair. This ideological impact, rather than their small number, gives them an undeniable historical significance. The first women doctors have been diminished because they have been portrayed as superior girl-guides. But at issue was something far larger than medical practice itself: the rights of women to have jobs, earn degrees, and be paid.[22] What stood in their way was an array of strongly held views, particularly by doctors, that women's place was in the home, that women earning professional fees would demean the place of the (male) breadwinner, that professional work (no one seemed to care about agricultural or domestic labour) would make female bodies unfit for bearing children, that medical knowledge would defile their natural purity, and that intellectual work would end in neurosis. These opinions were so well documented in public pronouncements, the press, and scholarly and medical journals that it should once more be impressed on the historical mind that it was an *ideology*, not a passing aberration lately corrected, that stood its sexist ground for at least a century against women doctors.[23] The professions, the universities, governments, and public opinion changed exceedingly slowly and only under pressure. If this history is denied, it makes a doll's house out of a campaign that spanned western Europe and North America and illustrates an amazing autodidactic (the universities were closed to women) ability to produce cogent arguments in the face of no mean opposition. (➤ Ch. 48 Medical education)

A short prelude to the international campaigns of the nineteenth century for education and degrees took place in the small Prussian town of Quedlinburg. In 1740 Dorothea Christiane Erxleben-Leporin (1715–62) petitioned Frederick the Great to let her attend the University of Halle.[24] She was the daughter of the local doctor, who was an advocate of the educational reforms of the Enlightenment and therefore saw nothing amiss in teaching his medical skills to a female. Well-prepared as she was, Erxleben-Leporin's professional hopes succumbed to the circuitous route of marriage and a family – she married a clergyman, a widower with four children, and had five of her own – before she asserted her claim to be a physician on a par with male colleagues. These had forced her hand in 1753 by formally accusing her of quackery, which, after the state regulation of medical practice in Prussia in 1725, would have confined her to household duties. Sure of her own worth and her principles – she had written a book on the subject of why women were kept from studying, published in Berlin in 1742 – she submitted her doctoral dissertation and was examined on her medical knowledge in 1754. The degree was granted that year. Unfortunately, she remained a unique example of Prussian liberal thinking when the equalitarian tendencies of radical evangelicalism (Pietism) could still be counted upon.

While German Romanticism saw an important contribution to intellectual life through the salons and publications of women like Rahel Varnhagen (1771–1833), Bettina von Arnim (1785–1859) (née von Brentano), Henriette Hertz, and others, their influence was personal rather than public.[25] Their social sensibilities and arguments, like Rahel Varnhagen's against the limitations of being Jewish and female, or Bettina von Arnim's against social injustice (the Silesian weaver's plight) could only be expressed in letters or books rather than direct political action.

The early nineteenth century saw a good number of middle- and upper-class women who were educated through university attendance, but barred, ironically, from regular study and degrees. Two members of the same family, Regina von Siebold and her daughter Charlotte (1761–1859), both midwives, received degrees in obstetrics from the University of Giessen (an honorary degree in 1815 for Regina and a full degree in 1817 for Charlotte). Charlotte von Siebold wrote her thesis on 'Extra-uterine pregnancy'. As an acknowledged expert in obstetrics, she was engaged to come to England to deliver the future Queen Victoria.[26] But, yet again, these notable exceptions brought about no broad structural or ideological changes for educational or professional advance.

Another push for women's rights was seen in 1848, but on the European continent, the Metternich era restored *Biedermeier* domesticity or the frippery of love affairs. Women outside the moneyed safety of well-arranged marriages were disadvantaged by the industrial revolution or by the ghetto of their usual employment as domestic servants. Legally, crimes involving women, such as infanticide, suicide, and murder were dealt with leniently,[27] but they indicate the continued gender conflicts of the nineteenth century. Prostitution was policed on the Continent, and was on the rise.

One of the indications of the continual inability to grant women financial independence and education (the means to practise a profession, especially in view of state and university regulation of qualifications) revealed itself after German Unification (1871), when the Reichstag delayed in committee for some thirty years the repeated petitions to admit women to higher education. The barriers did not fall in the German Reich until 1908.[28]

Although Dorothea Christiane Erxleben-Leporin's doctorate in medicine became an isolated case, it was indicative of fundamental patterns that can be traced through European and North American attempts to establish educational and professional rights for women. As has been mentioned, Enlightenment ideology championed rationality, usefulness, and education. Erxleben-

Leporin tried to fit these ideals to the very real difference in women's obligations (the double burden of career and home, in modern usage). Her legacy was unconsciously taken up by Elizabeth Blackwell, the first woman in an English-speaking country to receive her medical doctorate.[29] Blackwell's Nonconformist family (in striking parallel to Erxleben-Leporin's) equipped her for self-confidence in her abilities (although not credited as such, she was a fine intellectual, albeit self-taught) and motivated her toward ideals of social usefulness. She could not, however, be a 'woman' as it was then understood, when she pursued her medical education. Henry Blackwell, her brother, called her an 'intrepid biped' because he knew about her complete ostracism by both men and women in Geneva, in New York State (she was not greeted, let alone invited to social gatherings), as she pursued her medical studies. Unlike Erxleben-Leporin, however, Blackwell could look to political support. Among her friends and acquaintances were Harriet Beecher Stowe (1811–96), author of *Uncle Tom's Cabin* and keen human-rights apologist; William Lloyd Garrison (1805–79), the abolitionist; Lucy Stone (1818–93), who was her sister-in-law (Henry's wife) and a prominent feminist; and Antoinette Brown (1825–1921), the first woman preacher in the USA and Samuel Blackwell's wife. Lucy Stone and Antoinette Brown were amongst the first graduates of Oberlin College, Ohio, founded in 1833, the first institution of higher education to admit women and blacks. The coupling of educational and economic outcasts such as women and blacks was symptomatic: in the 1847 refusal of Harvard University to admit 'women and Negroes', the reason given was that both would devalue the Harvard degree. But in 1849, Blackwell received her doctorate. Not far from Geneva, New York State, in Seneca Falls, the first women's rights convention was held in 1848. It is no accident that the Seneca Falls convention, which grew from the articulate involvement of women in the anti-slavery movement, was close in time and place to their first medical doctorate.[30] Women's entry into medicine was first a political act and then one of 'opening a profession'.

Blackwell's sister, Emily (1826–1910), and a Polish-German emigrant, Marie Zakrzewska (1829–1902),[31] whom the Blackwells befriended (Elizabeth spoke German, Marie no English, the latter ordering beefsteak in a boarding-house because she could not think of 'breakfast'), received their degrees in 1854 and 1856, respectively, from another liberal land-grant college, Western Reserve, Ohio. Marie Zakrzewska was Chief-of-Staff in maternity in the Berlin Charité, the most eminent teaching hospital of its day, and would have been the first female member of the obstetrics faculty had she not been driven out by a smear campaign.

The pre-Civil War period of evangelism and abolitionism corresponded well with pre-1848 radical thinking in Europe. The failure of the revolutions of 1848 in Germany and Austria were beneficial to medical women in several ways: those men fleeing political persecution, now scattered elsewhere, proved to be reliable on women's rights issues. Abraham Jacobi (1830–1919), often accorded the title of Father of American Paediatrics, and an accomplished doctor, was a pre-1848 Communist fleeing the crime of *lèse majesté* in Germany. He was not afraid to marry one of the first woman physicians, Mary Putnam (1842–1906), and was part of the Blackwells' circle of friends in New York. Mary Putnam, of the renowned American publishing family, was the first woman to receive a medical doctorate from the University of Paris, in 1868.[32] She was the first scientist of that pioneer generation, doing work on brain tumours. Other German medical men who fled after 1848 went to Zurich and Berne, Switzerland, where, as medical professors, they were instrumental in letting women study medicine. The first woman graduate in Zurich was Nadezhda Suslowa (1843–1918), a Russian, in 1867; she was followed by many others (Zurich was truly liberal), among them the first German national to receive her doctorate, Franziska Tiburtius (1843–1927).[33] In Berne, Rosalie Somanowitch graduated first (in 1874), and there, after losing the battle with the Medical Faculty of Edinburgh, Sophia Jex-Blake won her degree in 1877.[34]

Elizabeth Garrett Anderson (1836–1917) graduated in Paris in 1870.[35] Her road to the medical doctorate drew its direction from the British initiative for women's education headed by Emily Davies (1830–1921), her girlhood friend.[36] Garrett Anderson had been able to enter the medical register of Great Britain in 1866, the first woman after Blackwell to do so, because she qualified as a licentiate of the Society of Apothecaries. This, however, was not intentional on the society's part; they had inadvertently failed to include a sex clause. It may be noted that the medical colleges of Geneva and of Western Reserve University changed their admission rules to debar woman after their first laudable liberalism.

If one follows the careers of the pioneer generation of women doctors, it becomes clear that success was due to Nonconformist Protestantism, international links in the anti-slavery coalition and the women's rights movement, the liberalism of 1848 and its rebirth in Switzerland and Paris, and the broad network of social reform in which women were engaged. Medicine, and not theology or law as academic and professional disciplines, stood women in good stead (even though the majority of doctors were against them) because it was an eminently practical field linked decisively with the reform issues of the day.

The legislative side of the British regulation of medicine, on the other hand, was a retarding factor. The Medical Act of 1858 stipulated that no foreign degree would qualify anyone for the medical register. Until the 1870s, all the medical doctorates won by women were foreign. Only in 1876, with the Russell Gurney Enabling Act, were women assured of medical legitimacy.

This was the Act of Parliament that enabled all medical corporations to examine women, notwithstanding any restrictions to be found in their charters. The King and Queen's College of Physicians, Dublin, was the first to do so. The first seven women, amongst them Sophia Jex-Blake, presented themselves for examination, were successful, and joined the British medical register.

The list of hard-won medical doctorates deserve augmentation by the élite list of those who decisively discouraged women: besides Harvard, outright refusals were given at London in 1858; St Andrews in 1858/9; Cambridge and Oxford (without formal refusal, Jex-Blake being told: 'Even the most sanguine of reformers would advise against it' (that is, women attempting medical studies));[37] and all of the German and all of the Austrian universities until the end of the nineteenth century (because these were subject to government legislation which was not forthcoming).

Degrees are not everything, even though the pioneer generation of women doctors received the best medical education available (Paris, Zurich, Berne) and all of them graduated with honours or near the top of their classes. The most momentous hurdle was actual medical practice. Some women – it may even have been a not insignificant number, but no one has taken the trouble, even in these demographically interested times, to study available class lists for continental European universities – had attended lectures and paid fees in medicine and other subjects. Male animosity was select: when it came to earning money and the independence connected with a good job, the line was drawn. But not overtly, of course. As Abraham Jacobi publicly reminded his male colleagues, women were not trying to become another Virchow, Descartes, or Leibniz, they were merely attempting to ply a trade and be paid for it.[38] This reminder of 1896 fell on deaf ears, as the substantial outpourings against women doctors in the medical press in every European country attest. The arguments against women practising medicine were highly sexually discriminating;[39] medical men sadly proffered gender-specific, biological arguments, such as: mental and physical incapacity due to menstruation; lack of physical strength when compared to men; childbearing and lactation; mental inferiority due to smaller brain size; and the usual outcry that medical work desexed women. Biological determinism was, of course, not out of temper with an age attuned to eugenic thinking. Julius Pagel (1851–1912), a very prominent member of the medical faculty in Berlin, in his public lectures on medicine in 1905/6, pronounced that women doctors were only fit for one thing: to help in the hospital kitchens. By that time, the evidence must have been considerably against him, had he taken any trouble over empirical data: women doctors had been running successful dispensaries and clinics since 1857.

Prejudice was so keen, from New York to Berlin, that it was indeed a miracle of faith in the principles of human rights that women doctors came to practise medicine at all. None of them, in compliance with then current sexual taboos, treated male patients. But human rights radicalism had its sure allies. First the Quaker women in New York came to Elizabeth Blackwell's dispensary, the New York Infirmary for Women and Children, founded in 1857, and then those in dire need of help: the urban poor. Marie Zakrzewska emphasized that the poor are no less discriminating than the wealthy. The few pennies they have will be spent with more thought than by those for whom money is no object. Success confirmed this. In 1865, the Blackwell sisters were able to augment their now thriving dispensary and hospital through the medical college of the New York Infirmary for Women and Children, which trained that score and more of women doctors who carried the work outward to other, similar institutions. Philadelphia with its radical Quaker legacy established the Women's Medical College of Pennsylvania in 1861, attached to its own hospital of thirty-five beds. Zakrzewska built up the ever-expanding and very successful New England Hospital for Women and Children with forty-six beds and twelve maternity beds in Boston in 1862. Even though this was not a college, it afforded some of the best training available for women. In London in 1866, Garrett Anderson opened St Mary's Dispensary for Women, also a success story, which became the New Hospital for Women in 1872. In 1877, the London School of Medicine for Women opened under the organizing efforts of Jex-Blake and Garrett Anderson.

Sophia Jex-Blake was a woman of great conviction who had nearly won the battle for women's medical education at the University of Edinburgh in 1869; in 1894, she was present when the university finally decided to admit women. With the usual uphill battle for financing and approval, she established a dispensary and then the Edinburgh Hospital for Women and Children, which would also provide clinical study for women. Leith Hospital took over this function in 1886. But the hospital had a difficult existence between 1879 and its slow decline, especially after the founding of the medical side of Queen Margaret's College in Glasgow in 1890. None the less, Jex-Blake's activities were auspicious in a way she could not have known: by 1990, over 50 per cent of the medical students at the University of Glasgow were women.[40]

In Berlin in 1877, Franziska Tiburtius and Emilie Lehmus (both graduates of Zurich) encountered the dead hand of bureaucracy when first seeking to practise privately and later when setting up their small polyclinic. Denunciations and court injunctions by male doctors forced the police repeatedly to take down the brass plate advertising their practice (eventually everyone tired of this farce). The polyclinic was successful, and pioneered health care for women and children in Berlin. They were financially supported by women's groups. Eventually, Berlin became one of the largest centres for women physicians.

In Switzerland the opposition from bureaucracy was less unforgiving. Here Marie Heim-Voegtlin (1845–1916), the first Swiss woman doctor, managed to challenge all the prevalent prejudice: she became an excellent doctor, carried on a wide private practice, married and had several children, and was deeply involved in social-reform programmes.[41]

The hospitals for women and children and the attached colleges were the backbone of the success of the women doctors. By the early twentieth century, however, the pioneer generation of women doctors insisted that there should be no separate medical education for women. It must be equal, and they had proved that women were up to it. The future they envisioned, however, was, in the event, not open-minded enough: American medical schools that admitted women on 'equal' terms with men practised a hidden system of quotas against women and Jews.[42] And in Nazi Germany after 1933, women were forced out of higher education and back to the most vulgar ideas of reproduction. Numbers and opportunities have not been equal in western Europe or North America in the twentieth century, although the tide now seems to be turning.

NURSING AND SANITARY CAMPAIGNS

Florence Nightingale once wrote that she didn't wish women to become doctors at all, because they would become like their male colleagues.[43] Nightingale's objectives were breathtakingly broad.[44] She wanted no less than a medical reform so thorough in prevention and care that doctors might become redundant. She certainly thought little of the then current sanitary and military practices; instead, she pushed forward modern arguments for reform based on statistics and structural planning. She is hard to assess historically precisely because she had a steely brain rather than womanly tact. She was persistent, probably a formidable snob, and an antidote to the faint-hearted. Her genius was in planning and administration, as well as in that rare form of intemperate courage that attempts change out of high moral conviction, disregarding the interplay of plurality of interest or other points of view. She has been heavily criticized of late in nursing histories as unoriginal, and as ineffective because of being often divisive.[45] Given her objectives, she could not very well fit the development in nursing that was to supersede her ideas.[46] This progress, realized only in the early twentieth century, was to secularize nursing. The nursing tradition is a very old one and it was wedded to philanthropic and religious ideals, not to those of a profession (qualifications, regulated hours, salaries).

The Christian tradition always included ministering to the sick; one need only think of the Beguines, the mendicant orders, the orders founded in the Counter-Reformation (for example, the Sisters of St Vincent de Paul), the Protestant sisterhoods (for example, the Sisters' Institute of Nursing founded by Elizabeth Fry), or the deaconesses founded in the 1830s and taught by the wife of Pastor Theodore Fliedner in Kaiserswerth, near Düsseldorf, who, as mentioned on p. 894, inspired both Fry and Nightingale.[47] Beyond Protestant Great Britain and before the French Revolution, caring for the sick and the education of girls was a major part of the work of the religious orders of women.

A great many lay women also tended the sick, the 'handywomen', as they are termed in one nursing history. They were not gentrified and cared for people in the Poor Law infirmaries.[48] This was paid nursing, but on a par with domestic service rather than a profession. Unnamed legions of unmarried women attended family members and relatives when doctors were scarce, as well as expensive, and illness was a matter of home care rather than the hospital (that is, prior to the twentieth century). These could also be included as 'nurses', albeit here in the pattern of unpaid and amateur use of labour. In a book about the abortive careers of women painters of the *fin de siècle*, one of the prime reasons given for failure to realize a career in the arts is the long spells of home nursing required of female relatives.[49]

The uneven and often divisive path to professional nursing, which took as long as women's entry to medical practice, from the 1850s to after the First World War, cannot be exclusively seen as an institutional or a professional history. In contrast to the paradigm of men's organization of their work, to which the professionalized aspect of women's qualified work eventually accommodated itself, women's talents and women's work straddled the ambiguities of the private *and* the public, usually without the defining roles of administrative posts, public office, or a place in the professions (law, theology, medicine). The crippling effect of the closure of higher education with its concomitant laicizing of female work was unfortunately one of the best means of enforcing domestic roles.

Social and domestic (non-) qualifications, however, carried the day for women in quite another way. They were the basis of womanly effectiveness, as the various campaigns of Josephine Butler, Nightingale, Frances Power-Cobbe (1822–1904), Jex-Blake, and many others show. The sure organizational talent for criticizing the *status quo* of bad hygiene, nutritional deficiency, inadequate pay, and bad housing came from running large households. The professionalized (and paid) work of nurses and women physicians grew from women's traditions of voluntary organizational involvement with sanitary work and philanthropy. The Ladies National Association for the Diffusion of Sanitary Knowledge (founded 1858) was the first sanitary society to have national scope. Its aims were health education within the new concerns of the public-health movement.[50] All of the prominent women connected with these and other campaigns in education, antivivisection, nursing, the repeal of the Contagious Diseases Acts, prostitution, penal reform, anti-alcoholism, and better employment for women were aware, connected with, and well-versed in sanitary work and philanthropy. Before engaging in the lobbying, committee testimonials, and fund-raising connected with these enterprises (an extensive feat in itself), the women had seen and experienced the squalor, filth, and crime giving rise to public-health reform. All the biographies make this practical point, and also show the deep moral and religious component of sanitary reform. (➤ Ch. 51 Public health; ➤ Ch. 53 History of personal hygiene)

Even though women were usually on the receiving end of sermons and confined by conventional habit and dress, they took good housekeeping to mean the nation and the relief of the victims of *laissez-faire* capitalism. The original scope of sanitary reform was not narrowly medical (that is, curative or remedial) but was aimed at prevention. Good food, clean water, fresh air, non-restrictive and warm clothing, sanitation, maternity, and childcare were issues in which active lay women, newly autonomous women writers (Harriet Martineau (1802–76), Frances Power-Cobbe), political campaigners (Josephine Butler, Florence Nightingale), and the new women doctors (especially Elizabeth Blackwell) were unanimously engaged. Until medicine and nursing became scientific and offered women careers (after the 1890s), they were a means to another end: the reform of social evils. In this sense, therefore, one can conjecture that the professional opportunties women fought for and won against an unsympathetic and conservative alliance (this is well documented elsewhere) sprang from an active female tradition of voluntary service and public concern. The string that fashioned Diana's bow ran from anti-slavery campaigns, through women's rights, through sanitary reform, to abolishing the double standard, to being a medical professional.

MIDWIFERY

Midwifery remains the prime example of how an established field of expertise practised for centuries by women was changed into a medical speciality practised in hospital, mainly by men.[51] In tracing this shift, an aspect of medicalization comes to the fore that many find disconcerting. A good study comparing the traditional practice of childbirth (both historically and in today's traditional societies) with modern improvements shows how the best techniques in normal childbirth can share common benefits for the mother from all these approaches.[52] The delivery of babies, when seen in this dia-chronic perspective rather than in the usual chronological fashion, centres on an expertise common to observation and experience, and not on scientific or laboratory discoveries with their fragmented picture of technologically mediated physiology. Ethnographic and historical comparisons indicate that traditional techniques used psychological support from women and men throughout pregnancy, birth, and postnatal care, and helped the woman use positions (kneeling, squatting, etc.) that maximized her own muscle strength. Women were also encouraged to tone their bodies and control their diets. This particular study shows how practical empirical knowledge was replaced by male obstetricians, who concentrated on technical solutions, including refinements to the obstetrical chair. It is indeed revealing that the eventual supine position in childbirth coincided with progressive restrictions on midwifery as practised by women.

Midwifery schools on the European continent were founded by university-trained doctors, who taught supposedly backward women medicine.[53] (Göttingen's Hebammenschule, the first of its kind, was founded in 1751.) As the regulation of medicine through the state increased, medical acts, and also medical societies, curtailed the independent and autonomous practice of midwifery by women. The renaissance of a plurality of methods in giving birth today is probably the result of books criticizing modern childbirth, and the return of a measure of authority to women.[54] Although the high mortality rates in childbirth have declined because of better medical care, today's almost obligatory hospitalization does not seem entirely satisfactory. In this sense, midwifery and its decline is not solely the story of a profession and deserves a new approach, including questions on why the role of women became largely passive. (➤ Ch. 72 Medicine, mortality, and morbidity)

WOMEN: OUR BODIES, OURSELVES

The nineteenth-century climb into the professions – due to their own agitation – by middle-class women did not solve the more trenchant dilemmas posed by cultural habits of thinking, namely those assumptions that determine so much of projected and ascribed behaviour. There has been little reconciliation between the so-called scientific evaluation of disease and research into mental constructs of illness. However, both these approaches must be looked at in an area in which the problem of gender roles becomes significant.[55] The scientific orientation of medicine has largely precluded paying attention to questions of this kind. This is largely understandable, because the rationalities involved in abstracting a model of disease for science deal in measurable reactions and their prognostic patterns, which almost axiomatically select out cultural assumptions. Only within the scientific system of predictability does one have the power to diagnose disease in its current definition: that is, as a distinct set of symptoms. Medical therapies, in this system, also require scientific predictability, namely the controlled elimination of manifest symptoms. The efficacy of modern medical science rests on recognizable knowledge of this kind. In effect, medical science is necessarily loath to introduce variables whose cause and effect are based on social indications.[56] In medical science, as in the long tradition of fixing true anatomical knowledge, women often appear only as a structural variation of an abstracted whole, 'the body', albeit with a chapter to themselves on reproductive organs and hormonal functions. But these specialist areas are seldom amenable to approaches that render the scientific methodology out of place. Modern physiological discoveries, such as those on hormones, have caused some debate on sexual differentiation, but this, too, tends to be either scientific or quantitative, or (in a more speculative vein) seen to establish links between hormonal production and behaviour patterns. The latter equations belong to the contentious field of sociobiology.[57]

Modern medical science has developed a somatic model of disease in which health is largely negatively defined by the absence of those patterns recognized as belonging to pathological breakdowns of bodily systems. Although immensely sophisticated, this model functions within the imagery of maintenance and repair. Established scientific medicine has been criticized for its lack of incorporation of social determinants for some time, but only recently has it been pointed out that gender, rather than male or female bodily dysfunction, patterns how and why people become ill, and how differently they are judged – and judge themselves – in these processes.[58] Modern statistics show that women are ill more often, swallow more psychosomatic drugs, and (paradoxically) live longer than men.[59] Explanations for these numeric findings have opened the way for linking gender–role expectations with patterns of illness, both as to the inception of illness and the type of diseases developed. This is particularly true of general disorders, but also of specific diseases such as coronary ailments.

The more diffuse types of psychosomatic disability (headaches, sleeplessness, anxiety) are seen to be more prevalent amongst women, and it has been suggested that they correlate with cultural tendencies to define women as passive, easily influenced, and inclined to avoid conflict by somaticizing it. In Germany, recent data for the consumption of psychopharmaceutical drugs show that on average doctors prescribe over twice as many of these drugs for women than for men.[60] (On the other hand, statistics for illnesses related to men show a high prevalence for, in particular, heart disease and alcoholism.) This has led to the suggestion that a correlation between disease syndromes and images of masculinity and femininity are worth consideration. Statistics on disease and death among men point to cultural assumptions, namely that the assertiveness and denial of suffering or emotion required of men lead them to disregard symptoms. Heart attacks, in particular, have been seen as an end-result of the culturally enforced masculine inability to acknowledge suffering. (➤ Ch. 21 Mental diseases; Ch. 56 Psychiatry)

Women, on the other hand, are tainted with the assumption of feminine susceptibility to illness due to lack of such qualities as toughness, stamina, self-control, and repression of minor pain. It has been suggested that this image today indicates women's newly ambivalent situation, namely that femininity decrees susceptibility and weakness, while health and achievement (in the masculine mode) are based on the denial of behaviour indicating uncertainty, hesitation, caution, fear, and intuitive alarm.[61] These characteristics are certainly culturally 'unmasculine' and lead to cultural assumptions of unfitness for leadership roles, as, for example, any war film indicates.

Such gender-related readings of health and illness should at least disquiet the process of a quick suppression of these issues in supposed normalcy, in effect the re–assertion of cultural clichés. Indeed, cultural assumptions have a long history in medicine's brief of 'overcoming' illness. Recent books and articles on the history of hysteria and psychiatry suggest that there might be such an entity as *die Krankheit Frau*,[62] meaning that to be a woman is equivalent to illness. Lest this be thought of as far-fetched, the book so entitled traces ideas ascribed to persons harbouring a uterus (Gr. *hystera*, the womb) that leave little doubt as to the localization of imbalance, suffering, and unpredictable waywardness in that organ and ascribed to women. Being a woman was often equivalent to the imagery connected with the female body. If pre-modern times were sexist on this scale, the nineteenth century did not alleviate the problem by a change of these dominant beliefs, namely defining women as inherently healthy, strong, and given to self-confidence. One merely has to look at the long train of wreckage, often self-inflicted in psychological and bodily terms, by women, who were caught in the quandary of losing their femininity when they became active in public campaigns. They were censured for not conforming to the role of passive womanhood, and of contravening their 'proper' spheres. The result of this ideologically imposed ambivalence is clearly discernible in the 'tiredness' and 'illness' thematic in prominent biographies (Florence Nightingale being the best example).

The suggestion has been made that the ideology of 'separate' spheres developed with the division of labour in early industrialization (Great Britain) and proto-industrialization (Germany).[63] This ideological separation seems to pertain to cultural images rather than work, since most women always worked. However, work done in the home and in the drawing-rooms and salons of Europe (being a society hostess was certainly work) was taken out of paid labour and merged with the idea of the private household. With the division of labour (men in the factory, women at home), women were forced to move within a limited space. This development produced further taboos of where they could 'safely' go, and that they must be chaperoned. Such social constraints were particularly strong in the moral realm, where women were punished culturally if they were not seen to be 'pure' or did not conform to the stereotype of sexual ignorance, physical limitation, mental frivolity, and the passivity inherent in the prerogative of the male (father, husband, government) acting and judging on their behalf.

Much of male 'romantic' literature reinforced these distinctly morbid qualities of limitation, weakness, and agoraphobia by asserting that the proper woman pines away or dies when she is abandoned (for example, in *Anna Karenina*, *La Traviata*, *Effie Briest*, or Arthur Schnitzler's very revealing *Liebelei*).[64] These objects of male erotic romanticism are hardly ever robust, backtalking survivors. the tales of Sigmund Freud (1856–1939) of sexual and social neurosis fit well with the enervating atmosphere of women confined to erotic intrigue where males have it both ways:[65] married women socially coded to uphold strictures while at the same time prey to the love affair. (➤ Ch. 43 Psychotherapy) Somatic illness and neurosis are easily inferred in conflicts of morality and erotic codes. This also indicates how women came to carry the stigma of patterns of illness: emotional instability, indecisiveness, enervation, lack of physical stamina, irrationality, and physical debility. Even their sexuality was severely damaged by investing it with a demonic component: that is, the idea of 'succumbing' to 'baser' instincts, or sexual corruptibility. (Frank Wedekind's *Lulu* is the unleashed projection of the male sexual drive. Lulu shoots her lover in the finale, another revealing male fantasy of how it should end.)[66]

In the *Sadian Woman*, Angela Carter has important things to say about the extreme passivity of the heroine of the Marquis de Sade's novel *Justine*.[67] As Carter points out, Justine can be seen as morally outstanding because she never lifts a finger to liberate herself from where fate has put her. The other side of this Sadian psychopathology projected on to women resides in a Viennese grave, the writer Sacher-Masoch (after whom Masochism is named). If there is no female Shakespeare, there is also no female Marquis de Sade. (➤ Ch. 65 Medicine and literature)

By the late nineteenth century, gender stigmatization had refined the idea of *die Krankheit Frau* to a subtle morass of physical weakness and erotically significant psychopathology. The Viennese turn-of-the-century pornographic classic *Josephine Muetzenbacher*, while not denying women sexual fulfilment, clearly tends toward child abuse, male predatory behaviour, and the indiscriminate availability of women for men's sexual demands.[68] Pornographic thought plays the same Sadian role as in *Justine*, a debasement of women in which a male fantasy seeks nothing more than the compliance of what it has fabricated. Different cultural assumptions led, at least, to more robust fantasies, for example *Fanny Hill*, whose cavortings show a sense of enjoyment and that she had a choice.[69]

Prostitution is not an illness, but there is no denying that it can lead to disease. (➤ Ch. 26 Sexually transmitted diseases) This was the epidemiological aspect of nineteenth-century sexual mores that led to a functional solution completely oblivious to gender issues until faced with the campaign of Josephine Butler and her Ladies' National Association against the Contagious Diseases Acts (1864, 1866, and 1869).[70] A purely medical solution was shortreined when its obvious sexual discrimination was pilloried on human-rights issues (police regulation and custodial hospitals); the double standard (no measures against philandering men); victimization (the economic plight of women); and ethical grounds (the bodies of women sold for the sexual gratification of men, and the abuse of minors). The subsequent purity campaigns turned on health issues (venereal disease and alcoholism) and had an international scope. These campaigns should be evaluated as the first political manifestations of protesting women discussing their own sexuality and indignant about issues threatening their own dignity and way of life: conjugal sexual violence (ensconced in law); the fight for the legal barrier against sexual abuse of minors: the so-called 'age of consent'; the violence and economic threats connected with alcoholism; sexual transmission of disease through infected husbands; the right to birth control; the right for medical abortion (rather than backstreet or amateur disasters). Public-health issues, such as better housing and hygiene, were also addressed. Through historiographical selectivity, the issue of women's right to vote has seemed to mirror the advance of the women's movement, but this seems far from the full truth, because, in practical terms, women were fighting for basic social changes specific to their needs. It is therefore vastly irritating to see issues crucial to women represented as marginal (when highlighting only the administrative side of health care) or oddly moralistic (the purity campaigns are often represented as the moral visions of unworldly spinsters).[71]

CONCLUSION

One develops a great sympathy for the polemics of feminist writings when they challenge the insidious disappearance of women from history. The fact is that history does have to be rewritten,[72] and what stands in the way is the very pervasiveness of the seemingly 'objective' approach: the invisible hand of economics, health care, medical theory, epidemiology, and so forth. What is wanted is a bit more of a healthy emotional and mental breakdown in the writing of medical history, because in that unstructured state, gender issues might not be disqualified and their originality taken seriously.

NOTES

1   Friedrich Schiller, *Maria Stuart*, Tübingen, Cotta, 1801; *Die Jungfrau von Orleans*, Berlin, Johann Friedrich Unger, 1802. On the meaning of female imagery, see Marina Warner, *Monuments and Maidens. The Allegory of the Female Form*, London, Weidenfeld & Nicolson, 1985.

2   Robert Graves, *The White Goddess*, London, Faber & Faber, 1975; Heide Göttner-Abendroth, *Die Gottin und ihr Heros, Die matriarchalen Religionen in Mythos, Märchen und Dichtung*, Munich, Frauenoffensive, 1980 (1988); Ursula K. Le Guin, *Dancing at the Edge of the World. Thoughts on Words, Women, Places*, London, Gollancz, 1989.

3   Marijke Gijswijt-Hofstra, 'Witchcraft in the Northern Netherlands', in Arina Angerman, Geerte Binnema, Annemieke Keunen, Vefic Poels and Jacqueline Zirkzee, *Current Issues in Woman's History*, London, Routledge, 1989, pp. 75–92.

4   Linda Schiebinger, 'Maria Winkelmann: the clash between guild traditions and professional science', in ibid., pp. 21–38.

5   The excellent monograph by F. K. Prochaska, *Women and Philanthropy in Nineteenth-Century England*, Oxford, Clarendon Press, 1980, op. cit. (n. 3) discusses 'The power of the purse' and 'The power of the Cross', but never looks at the power of the household!

6   Kate Campbeall Hurd-Mead, *A History of Women in Medicine*, Haddam, KS, Haddam Press, 1938. This is still the most encompassing overview. Also a classic: Sophia Jex-Blake, *Medical Women. A Thesis and a History*, Edinburgh, 1886.

7   See Hurd-Mead, op. cit. (n. 6), pp. 183 ff. 223 ff.

8   Hurd-Mead, op. cit. (n. 6), pp. 320 ff., for the following information.

9   See literature given in Norbert Stefenelli, 'Ärzte, Krankheitspatrone, heilige Fürbitter und Nothelfer', in *Kunst des Heilens*, Exhibition Katalog, Niederösterreichische Landesausstellung, Kartause Gaming, 1991, pp. 438–49.

10 See for a summary history, Jean Donnison, *Midwives and Medical Men*, London, Heinemann, 1977.

11 Hurd-Mead, op. cit. (n. 6), pp. 395 ff.

12 Audrey Eccles, *Obstetrics and Gynaecology in Tudor and Stuart England*, London, Croom Helm, 1982.

13 Esther Fischer-Homberger, *Medizin vor Gericht, Gerichtsmedizin von der Renaissance bis zur Aufklärung*, Berne, Hans Huber, 1983.

14 Jacques Gélis, *History of Childbirth: Fertility, Pregnancy and Birth in Early Modern Europe*, Cambridge, Polity Press, 1991.

15 Adrian Wilson, 'William Hunter and the varieties of man-midwifery', in W. F. Bynum and Roy Porter (eds), *William Hunter and the Eighteenth-Century Medical World*, Cambridge, Cambridge University Press, 1985, pp. 343–70.

16 Short bibliography on European witchcraft in Gijswijt-Hofstra, op. cit. (n. 3), pp. 91 ff.; Richard van Dulmen (ed.), *Hexenwelten. Magie und Imagination vom 16–20 Jahrhundert*, Frankfurt, Fischer Taschenbuch Verlag, 1990.

17 Hurd-Mead, op. cit. (n. 6), pp. 359, 401 ff. Hurd-Mead is instructive as a source on the vast variety of medical publications by women (not a theme taken up since!), but her interpretation reveals a scientific bias not always in sympathy with the view or needs of a period.

18 Keith L. Sprunger, 'God's powerful army of the weak: Anabaptist women of the radical reformation', and R. Greaves, 'Foundation builders: the role of women in early English nonconformity', in Richard Greaves (ed.), *Triumph over Silence: Women in Protestant History*, Westport, CT, and London, Greenwood Press, 1985; Phyllis Mack 'Feminine behaviour and radical action: Franciscans, Quakers and the followers of Gandhi', *Signs*, 1986, 11: 457–77; Melvin B. Endy Jr, *William Penn and Early Quakerism*, Princeton, NJ, Princeton University Press, 1973; Margaret Hope Bacon, *Mothers of Feminism: the Story of Quaker Women in America*, San Francisco, CA, Harper & Row, 1986.

19 June Rose, *Elizabeth Fry*, London, Macmillan, 1980.

20 Lionel Rose, *The Massacre of the Innocents, Infanticide in Britain 1800–1939*, London, Routledge & Kegan Paul, 1986, p. 2; Rosalind Mitchison and Leah Leneman, *Sexuality and Social Control, Scotland 1660–1780*, Oxford, Basil Blackwell, 1989.

21 Johanna Geyer-Kordesch, 'Infanticide and medico-legal ethics in eighteenth-century Prussia', in A. Wear, R. French and J. Geyer-Kordesch (eds), *A History of Medical Ethics*, Rodopi.

22 The older histories and biographies are exemplary on fighting prejudice; see Josephine Butler, *The Education and Employment of Women*, London, Macmillan, 1868; Sophia Jex-Blake, *A Visit to Some American Schools and Colleges*, London, Macmillan, 1867; E. Moberly-Bell, *Storming the Citadel: the Rise of the Woman Doctor*, London, Constable, 1953.

23 Mary Roth Walsh, *Doctors Wanted: No Woman Need Apply. Sexual Barriers in the Medical Profession 1835–1975*, New Haven, CT, Yale University Press, 1977; Johanna Geyer-Kordesch, 'Geschlecht und Gesellschaft. Die Ersten Ärztinnen und sozialpolitische Vorurteile', *Berichte zur Wissenschaftsgeschichte*, 1987, 10 (4): 195–205.

24 Heinz Bohm, *Dorothea Christiane Erxleben. Ihr Leben und Wirken*, Quedlinburg, 1965.

25 Hannah Arendt, *Rahel Varnhagen. Lebensgeschichte einer deutschen Jüdin aus der Romantik*, Munich, Piper, 1981 (orig. pub. 1959); Ingeborg Drewitz, *Bettina von Arnim*, Düsseldorf, 1969; Christa Wolff, *Lesen und Schreiben*, Darmstadt, Luchterhand, 1980 (essays on Bettina von Arnim and Karoline von Günderrode on pp. 225–318. These essays are especially valuable for understanding the problems of talented women in the Romantic period.)

26 Hurd-Mead, op. cit. (n. 6). pp. 475, 503 ff.

27 Rose, op. cit. (n. 20).

28 For a polemical overview (not good on the *Reichstag* debate) with bibliography, see Margrit Twellmann, *Die deutsche Frauenbewegung. Ihre Anfänge und erste Entwicklung 1843–1889*, Kronberg, Athenäum Verlag, 1976; Richard Evans, *The Feminist Movement in Germany, 1894–1933*, London, Sage, 1976.

29 Elizabeth Blackwell, *Opening the Medical Profession to Women*, reprinted, New York, 1977; Ishbel Ross, *Child of Destiny. The Life Story of the First Woman Doctor*, London, Gollancz, 1950; J. Geyer-Kordesch, 'Vorkämpferinnen im Ärzteberuf. Der Einstieg der angelsachsischen Frauen in die professionalisierte Medizin des 19. Jahrhunderts', *Feministische Studien*, 1983/2, 24–45.

30 For the interrelationship of medical reform, the anti-slavery movement (human

rights), and women's rights, see J. Geyer-Kordesche, 'Sozialhygiene und Sexual-reform. Die Kritik der "Feministinnen" in England im 19. Jahrhundert', in J. Reulecke and Adelheid Gräfin von Castell Rudenhausen (eds), *Stadt und Gesund-eit*, Stuttgart, Franz Steiner Verlag, 1991, pp. 257–70; Blanche Glassman Hersch, *The Slavery of Sex. Feminist-Abolitionists in America*, Chicago, University of Illinois Press, 1978; Ellen Dubois, 'Women's rights and abolition: the nature of the connection', and Blanche Glassman Hersch, 'Am I not a woman and a sister? Abolitionist beginnings of nineteenth-century feminism', in Lewis Perry and Michael Fellman (eds), *Antislavery Reconsidered: New Perspectives on the Abolitionists*, Baton Rouge, Louisiana State University Press, 1979, pp. 238–51 and 252–86, respectively.

31 Agnes Vietor, *A Woman's Quest. The Life of Marie Zakrzewska*, London, 1924.

32 Mary Putnam-Jacobi, *Mary Putnam Jacobi, MD, A Pathfinder in Medicine. With Selections from Her Writings and a Complete Bibliography*, New York, Women's Medical Association of New York City, 1925; Rhoda Truax, *The Doctors Jacobi*, Boston, MA, Little & Brown, 1952.

33 Christa Lange-Mehnert, 'Marie Heim-Vögtlin und Franziska Tiburtius: Erste Ärztinnnen im Zeitalter der naturwissentschaftlichen Medizin. Motive, Hintergründe und Folgen ihrer Berufswahl', unpublished medical dissertation, University of Munster, 1988.

34 Margaret Todd, *Life of Sophia Jex-Blake*, Lauda Macmillan, 1918.

35 Jo Manton, *Elizabeth Garrett Anderson*, London, Methuen, 1965.

36 Daphne Bennett, *Emily Davies and the Liberation of Women 1830–1921*, London, Andre Deutsch, 1990.

37 See the interesting correspondence, reproduced in Todd, op. cit. (n. 34), pp. 218–31.

38 Johanna Geyer-Kordesch, 'Geschlecht und Gesellschaft', *Berichte zur Wissenschaftsgeschichte*, 1987, 10 (4): 195–205.

39 See ibid for substantiation of the following facts.

40 Wendy Alexander, *First Ladies of Medicine. The Origins, Education and Destination of Early Women Graduates of Glasgow University*, Glasgow, Wellcome Unit for the History of Medicine, 1987.

41 For F. Tiburtius and Marie Heim-Vögtlin, see Lange-Mehnert, op. cit. (n. 33).

42 Walsh, 'Moving backward', op. cit. (n. 23), pp. 178–206.

43 Quoted in Brian Harrison, 'Women's health and the women's movement in Britain: 1840–1940', paper given at the Roots of Sociobiology Conference held by the Past and Present Society in conjunction with the British Society for the History of Science, September 1978, p. 11; published as 'Women's health and the women's movement in Britain 1840–1940', in Charles Webster (ed.), *Biology, Medicine and Society*, Cambridge, Cambridge University Press, 1981, pp. 15–71.

44 Edward Cook, *The Life of Florence Nightingale*, 2 vols, London, Macmillan, 1913; Brian Abel-Smith, *A History of the Nursing Profession*, London, Heinemann Educational Books, 1960; Celia Davies (ed.), *Rewriting Nursing History*, London, Croom Helm, 1982; Judith Moore, *A Zeal for Responsibility. The Struggle for Professional Nursing in Victorian England*, Athens, University of Georgia Press, 1988.

45 Anne Summers, *Angels and Citizens, British Women as Military Nurses 1854–1914*, London, Routledge & Kegan Paul, 1988.

46 Ibid.; and Robert Dingwall, Anne Marie Rafferty and Charles Webster, *An Introduction to the Social History of Nursing*, London, Routledge, 1988.

47 On church communities and deaconesses, see Martha Vicinus, *Independent Women. Work and Community for Simple Women, 1850–1920*, London, Virago, 1985.

48 Dingwall, Rafferty and Webster, op. cit. (n. 46).

49 Renate Berger, *Malerinnen auf dem Weg ins 20. Jahrhundert. Kunstgeschichte als Sozialgeschichte*, Cologne, Du Mont, 1982.

50 Perry Williams, 'The laws of health: women, medicine and sanitary reform 1850–1990', in Marina Benjamin (ed.), *Science and Sensibility: Gender and Scientific Enquiry 1780–1945*, Oxford, Basil Blackwell, 1991.

51 Donnison, op. cit. (n. 10).

52 Liselotte Kuntner, *Die Gebärhaltung der Frau, Schwangerschaft und Geburt aus geschichtlicher, volkerkündlicher und medizinischer Sicht*, Munich, Hans Marseille Verlag, 1985.

53 A comprehensive article on midwifery in the Netherlands: M. J. van Lieburg and Hilary Marland, 'Midwife regulation, education, and practice in the Netherlands during the nineteenth century', *Medical History*, 1989, 33: 296–317.

54 Adrienne Rich, *Of Woman Born. Motherhood as Experience and Institution*, London, Virago, 1977; Ann Oakley, *Women Confined: Towards a Sociology of Childbirth*, Oxford, Martin Robertson, 1980.

55 Irmgard Vogt, 'Medizinsoziologie und weibliche Leidensweisen', in K. Hausen and H. Nowotny (eds), *Wie Männlich ist die Wissenschaft?*, Frankfurt, Suhrkamp, 1986, pp. 179–98: this work looks at somatic illnesses and their potential origins in gender-related behaviour. Most books deal with psychiatric illness or with illnesses traditionally associated with women. Elaine Showalter, *The Female Malady: Women, Madness and English Culture, 1830–1980*, New yorak, Pantheon Books, 1985; Regina Schaps, *Hysterie und Weiblichkeit: Wissenschaftsmythen über die Frau*, Frankfurt, Campus Verlag, 1983; Mark Micale, 'Hysteria and its historiography: the future perspective', *History of Psychiatry*, 1990, 1: 22–124; Micale, 'Hysteria male/hysteria female: reflections on comparative gender construction in nineteenth-century France and Britain', in Marina Benjamin (ed.), *Science and Sensibility 1780–1948*, Oxford, Basil Blackwell, 1991, pp. 200–42; Charles Bernheimer and Claire Kahane (eds), *In Dora's Case: Freud-Hysteria-Feminism*, New York, Columbia University Press, 1985; I. S. L. Loudon, 'Chlorosis, anaemia and anorexia nervosa', *British Medical Journal*, 1980, 281: 1669–75; Irmgard Vogt, *Für Alle Leiden gibt es eine Pille*, Wiesbaden, Westdeutscher Verlag, 1985; Brenda Parry-Jones, 'Historical terminology of eating disorders', *Psychological Medicine*, 1991, 21: 21–8.

56 Ruth Hubbard, Mary Sue Henifin, Barbara Fried (with the collaboration of Vicki Dross and Susan Leigh Star) (eds), *Women Look at Biology Looking at Women: a Collection of Feminist Critiques*, Boston, G. K. Hall, 1979; Brighton Women and Science Group, *Alice through the Microscope: the Power of Science over Women's Lives*, London, Virago, 1980; Sandra Harding, *The Science Question in Feminism*,

Ithica, Cornell University Press, 1986; Evelyn Fox Keller, *Reflections on Gender and Science*, New Haven, CT, Yale University Press, 1985.

57 Ruth Bleier, *Science and Gender. A Critique of Biology and its Theories of Women*, Oxford, Oxford University Press, 1984; Sandra Harding and Merrill Hintikka (eds), *Discovering Reality: Feminist Perspectives on Epistomology, Methodology and Philosophy of Science*, Dordrecht, Reidel, 1983; Anne Fausto-Sterling, *Mythos of Gender. Biological Theories about Women and Men*, New York, Basic Books, 1985.

58 H. E. Richter, 'Konflikte und Krankheiten der Frau', in D. Claessens and P. Milhoffer (eds), *Familiensoziologie*, Frankfurt, Athenäum Verlag, 1973, pp. 293–308.

59 Ibid.

60 Vogt, op. cit. (n. 55).

61 Vogt, op. cit. (n. 55).

62 Esther Fischer-Homburger, *Krankheit Frau, zur Geschichte der Einbildungen*, Darmstadt, Luchterhand, 1984.

63 Karin Hausen, 'Die Polarisierung der Geschlechtscharaktere – eine Spiegelung der Dissoziation von Erwerbs- und Familienleben', in W. Conze (ed.), *Sozialgeschichte der Familie in der Neuzeit Europas, Neue Forschungen*, Stuttgart, Klett-Cotta Verlag, 1977, pp. 363–93.

64 Alexander Tolstoy, *Anna Karenina*, 1877; Giuseppe Verdi, *La Traviata*, 1853; Theodor Fontane, *Effie Briest*, 1895; Arthur Schnitzler, *Liebelei*, 1895.

65 The extremely interesting book *In Dora's Case* (Kahane, op. cit. (n. 55)) shows the inherent prejudice based on male sexual perogatives in psychoanalytical interpretations.

66 Frank Wedekind, *Lulu*, in several parts, the whole entitled *Die Büchse der Pandora*, written 1892–94.

67 Angela Carter, *The Sadian Woman. An Exercise in Cultural History*, London, Virago, 1979.

68 Roland Pinson (ed.), *Josephine Muetzenbacher, Geschichte einer Wiener Dirne*, Brigitte Verlag, 1982.

69 John Cleland, *Memoirs of a Woman of Pleasure*, ed. by Peter Sabor, New York, Oxford University Press, 1985.

70 Judith Walkowitz, *Prostitution and Victorian Society, Women, Class and the State*, Cambridge, Cambridge University Press, 1980; Glen Petrie, *A Singular Iniquity: the Campaigns of Josephine Butler*, New York, Viking Press, 1973; Johanna Geyer-Kordesch and Annette Kuhn (eds), *Frauenkörper, Medizin, Sexualität*, Düsseldorf, Schwann, 1986.

71 Sheila Jeffreys, *The Spinster and Her Enemies, Feminism and Sexuality, 1880–1930*, London Pandora, 1985, takes issue with this interpretation.

72 The polemic classic is Sheila Rowbotham, *Hidden from History. Rediscovering Women in History from the Seventeenth Century to the Present*, New York, Vintage Books, 1976; Adrienne Rich, *On Lies, Secrets and Silence, Selected Prose 1966–1978*, New York, W. W. Norton, 1979; M. McNeil, (ed.), *Gender and Experience*, London, Free Association Books, 1987.

FURTHER READING

Bell, E. Moberly, *Storming the Citadel. The Rise of the Woman Doctor*, London, Constable, 1953.

Blackwell, Elizabeth, *Opening the Medical Profession to Women*, London, Longmans, Green, 1895.

Bonner, Thomas N., *To the Ends of the Earth*, Cambridge, MA, Harvard University Press, 1992.

Brighton Women and Science Group, *Alice through the Microscope: the Power of Science over Women's Lives*, London, Virago, 1980.

Cook, E. T., *The Life of Florence Nightingale*, 2 vols, London, Macmillan, 1913.

Donnison, Jean, *Midwives and Medical Men*, London, Heinemann, 1977.

Harding, Sandra, *The Science Question in Feminism*, Ithaca, NY, Cornell University Press, 1986.

—— and Hintikka, Merrill B. (eds), *Discovering Reality. Feminist Perspectives on Epistemology, Metaphysics, Methodology and Philosophy of Science*, London, Reidel, 1983.

Hubbard, Ruth *et al.* (eds), *Women Look at Biology Looking at Women: a Collection of Feminist Critiques*, Boston, MA, G. K. Hall, 1979.

Hurd-Mead, Kate Campbell, *A History of Women in Medicine*, Haddam, KS, Haddam Press, 1938.

Jeffreys, Sheila, *The Spinster and Her Enemies: Feminism and Sexuality, 1880–1930*, London, Pandora, 1985.

Morantz-Sanchez, Regina M., *Sympathy and Science: Women Physicians in American Medicine*, New York, Oxford University Press, 1985.

Moscucci, Ornella, *The Science of Woman*, Cambridge, Cambridge University Press, 1990.

Pinchbeck, Ivy, *Women Workers and the Industrial Revolution, 1750–1850*, London, Virago, 1981;orig. pub. 1930.

Prochaska, F. K. *Women and Philanthropy in Nineteenth-Century England*, Oxford, Clarendon Press, 1980.

Sapiro, Virginia (ed.), *Women, Biology and Public Policy*, London, Sage, 1985.

Showalter, Elaine, *The Female Malady. Women, Madness and Culture, 1830–1980*, London, Virago, 1987.

Todd, Margaret, *The Life of Sophia Jex-Blake*, London, Macmillan, 1918.

Vicinus, Martha (ed.), *A Widening Sphere: Changing Roles of Victorian Women*, Bloomington, Indiana University Press, 1977.

——, *Independent Women. Work and Community for Single Women, 1850–1920*, London, Virago, 1985.

39

DRUG THERAPIES

Miles Weatherall

DRUGS IN ANTIQUITY

The use of drugs to treat ill health is as old as recorded history. The practice appears at first to have been based on appeals to magic, and any result of medication was attributed not only to the natural properties of the remedy but also to the favour of the gods and their approval of the ceremonies associated with its use. The Greek word *pharmakon* referred to a drug or a charm, whether beneficial or noxious.[1] It gave the derived words 'pharmacy', meaning knowledge of drugs or a place where drugs are kept; and 'pharmacology', the science of drugs or medicines. That there could be an essentially physiological explanation of the action of drugs appears in the writings of Hippocrates of Cos (*c*.450–370 BC), accompanied by a view of medical practice based on observation and experience instead of appeals to the gods.[2]

In the following centuries, in the civilizations that existed around the Mediterranean, many plants were tried and found to have, or appear to have, medicinal properties. Most of them can be identified more or less accurately, and a certain amount learned about the diseases for which they were used. Galen (AD 129–200/210) wrote extensively on medical knowledge as it then existed, and, for many centuries, the use of drugs in Western society was dominated by his authority.

Other parts of the world were developing independently, especially China and Arabic-speaking countries. Chinese medicine had little impact on European knowledge and practice, but contact between the Middle East and other countries around the Mediterranean allowed the passage of medical ideas and medicines. The encyclopedia of the Persian physician Avicenna (980–1037) was added to the standard authority of Galen. (➤ Ch. 31 Arab-Islamic medicine; Ch. 32 Chinese medicine)

THE RENAISSANCE AND THE ENLIGHTENMENT

In the early sixteenth century, Paracelsus (1493–1541), who for a short time held the position of town physician and university professor in Basle, began to rebel against the respect for authority as a source of information. He made extensive chemical experiments, and recommended the use of minerals as well as plants in medicine. He may have introduced mercury for the treatment of syphilis. He made much of a secret remedy, which he named laudanum. Opium was probably the main constituent, used in preparations still called laudanum until well into the twentieth century. He also had an elaborate mystical philosophy, which justified rejection of traditional authorities and possibly encouraged experiments in therapeutics to discover what really worked. He was one of the first doctors to separate completely the material treatment of patients from attention to their beliefs and feelings, a separation that continues to be a source of problems in therapeutics.[3]

New ideas of therapeutics had more chance of flourishing and many new remedies were adopted in the following century. Some arose from the products of alchemy and the more rational chemistry that followed it, and others from an increasing awareness of the possibilities of plants, and sometimes portions of animals, as medicaments. Knowledge of these medicaments spread as society in western Europe became more organized. Colleges and academies concerned with the practice of medicine slowly became established, and, among other activities, sponsored pharmacopoeias, books of recipes for the preparation of medicines, essential for any physician, apothecary, or druggist who wished to provide medicines that conformed with the standards of the time. The Ricettaria Fiorentino of 1497 was influential in northern Europe through the sixteenth century, and was followed by the Dispensatorium Pharmacopoearum of Lyons in 1546.[4] In England, the Royal College of Physicians issued its first pharmacopoeia, containing nearly 2,000 recipes, in 1618. Subsequent editions reflect changing fashions in therapeutics for two hundred years. Herbals also contained much information about medicinal uses of plants, but less about standards for preparing drugs.

In the seventeenth and eighteenth centuries, medicines were used freely. There is little evidence that they did much good, and many reasons for thinking that they were often harmful. Until knowledge of physiology was advanced by animal experiments, and that of pathology by post mortem examinations, reasons for choosing particular substances as drugs continued to be based on casual clinical observations and on the beliefs and hopes of the times.[5] For instance, according to the doctrine of signs, the yellow colour of saffron showed that it was good for jaundice, the red colour of rust or wine that they relieved anaemia, and the leaves of the plant lungwort, which had some resemblance to the appearance of the lungs, announced that the plant alleviated lung diseases. (➤ Ch. 30 Folk medicine)

The old humoral theory still had much influence and justified physical methods of treatment, such as bleeding, cupping, and the application of leeches, to achieve the removal of unwanted humours. (➤ Ch. 14 Humoralism; Ch. 40 Physical methods) Purgation was another way of getting material out of the body, and the extensive use of cathartic medicinal plants and of salts of mercury became notorious. Strong purgatives caused colic, which could be relieved by the leaves of deadly nightshade, *Atropa belladonna*. So there were grounds for using two drugs at once, and extended reasoning of this sort led to complicated prescriptions containing many supposedly active drugs. Most of them were probably innocuous. Nightshade was not, and caused mental confusion and death if too much was used. Opium or laudanum gave comfort, sometimes more desirable than prolongation of life. (➤ Ch. 67 Pain and suffering) Scepticism about the value of remedies and doctors was often expressed, from Petrarch to Molière, and scientifically respectable observations were too rare to have much influence on the chaotic state of therapeutics.

The range of materia medica was increased by plants brought from far away by growing numbers of explorers. Peruvian bark, the source of quinine, was brought to Europe c.1630–40, probably by Jesuit missionaries.[6] It was specific for the easily recognized fever that recurred every third or fourth day and which is now called malaria. (➤ Ch. 19 Fevers) It was widespread in Europe until large tracts of marshland were drained in the nineteenth century. (➤ Ch. 15 Environment and miasmata) The demand for Jesuit's bark had important consequences in promoting new exploration, and in starting new cultivation in different lands. (➤ Ch. 58 Medicine and colonialism; Ch. 18 The ecology of disease) Ipecacuanha ('the little plant which grows by the wayside and causes vomiting') also came from South America. It cured one kind of dysentery, and was used indiscriminately for a long time. It was necessary to discover more, both about dysentery and about the drug, before proper use could be made of it. Other novel important plants that contained drugs were used socially rather than medicinally. Tobacco was brought to England by Sir Walter Raleigh (1552–1618) at the end of the sixteenth century, and tea and coffee came from the East Indies in the seventeenth.

Among plants indigenous to England, the bark of the willow was reported to the Royal Society of London in 1763 to be successful in curing ague. Willow bark did not work as well as the Peruvian material, but, a century later, salicylates were isolated from it and became useful in another 'ague', rheumatic fever. Twenty years later, William Withering (1741–99) of Birmingham, wrote *An Account of the Foxglove and Some of its Medical Uses etc. with Practical Remarks on Dropsy and Other Diseases*. From his carefully recorded clinical experience, he recognized that digitalis increased the flow of urine

917

and reduced dropsy, and had a powerful action on the heart. But his analysis was handicapped by the general lack of knowledge of bodily mechanisms at this time. The circulation of the blood was known, but its role in transporting water was not yet understood, nor was dropsy due to heart failure distinguished from dropsy due to disease of the kidneys.[7] (➤ Ch. 7 The physiological tradition; Ch. 9 The pathological tradition)

A SCIENTIFIC BASIS FOR THE USE OF DRUGS

The necessary advances in understanding normal physiology could be made only by experiments in animals, such as those in France towards the end of the eighteenth century. In measuring and accounting for the heat production of animals, Antoine Lavoisier (1743–94) developed ideas of the living body as an elegant piece of chemical machinery and provided an essential foundation for a science of drug action. Another basis was given by the experiments in physiology of Xavier Bichat (1771–1802) and his post-mortem dissections to discover the immediate causes of death. His successor, François Magendie (1783–1855), often regarded as the founder of modern experimental physiology, was perhaps the first to recognize that poisons were invaluable tools in the armoury of a physiological investigator.

The growing scepticism of the period bore heavily on the practice of medicine, and began a much-needed questioning of the value of remedies and the best ways of judging their efficacy. The importance of observation, measurement, and counting received its strongest support from Pierre Charles Alexandre Louis (1787–1872), who insisted on the 'numerical method' and was one of the earliest physicians to require what would now be called statistical evidence of the outcome of alternative treatments.[8]

Medicine was further influenced by the emergence of the profession of pharmacy, combining the skills of apothecaries, botanists, and chemists in advancing knowledge of drugs. Magendie, most clear-sightedly, saw that the drugs used by him as tools were most reliable when they were purest. He collaborated with the pharmacist Pierre Joseph Pelletier (1788–1842) in studies of poisonous plants. The substance in ipecacuanha that caused vomiting was isolated and named emetine; and from the seeds of the small Indian tree *Strychnos nux-vomica* a convulsant poison, strychnine, was prepared. It became a cornerstone in Magendie's analysis of reflex activity of the spinal cord, and for over a century was a popular ingredient of 'tonic' medicines.

Pelletier and his colleague, Joseph Bienaimé Caventou (1793–1877), also developed the discovery of 'morphium' (morphine), a substance first isolated from opium in Westphalia by an apothecary's assistant, Friedrich Sertürner (1783–1841), who showed by experiments on himself and his friends that he had isolated a powerful sedative or narcotic. His material was much more potent than anything that had previously been isolated from opium, and he nearly killed himself with an excessive dose. He is generally credited with first making known the existence of drugs which, like inorganic alkalis, formed salts with acids, and so were called alkaloids.

Pelletier and Caventou adapted Sertürner's methods and, between 1817 and 1821, isolated a remarkable range of alkaloids. They included a close relative of strychnine, which was named brucine; the febrifuge and antimalarial quinine; caffeine from coffee beans; and a drug from hellebore, veratrine, which has complex physiological effects and limited medicinal use. Isolation of active principles from any therapeutically active material became an established basic procedure. It required collaboration between chemist and physiologist in order to show that the substances had the same actions as the parent material. This required trials in humans, such as Sertürner had rashly conducted, or, less hazardously, experiments on animals, in which analysis of the mode and site of action was also possible. (➤ Ch. 8 The biochemical tradition)

The study of poisons was extended by the Majorca-born physician Joseph Orfila (1787–1853), who went to Paris and published a famous textbook, *Traité des Poisons*, in 1814. He does not appear to have been a great experimentalist himself, but his encyclopedic work was an obvious source-book for scientists as well as for physicians and lawyers. It became increasingly clear that poisons were distinguished from potent therapeutic drugs only in the matter of dosage, and the investigation of poisons, or toxicology, developed inseparably with experimental physiology, and with pharmacology when the subject became more explicitly recognized.

Magendie was succeeded by Claude Bernard (1813–78), who made some of the earliest experiments which showed that drugs act as specific sites in the body and not in some diffuse way all over the system. He showed that the paralysis caused by curare was due not to an effect on either nerves or muscles, but to an action on the specialized tissue called the neuromuscular junction. Such a specific site was a new idea, and it started a search for similar sites. This was the beginning of a new and rewarding approach to physiology and pharmacology. (➤ Ch. 11 Clinical research)

THE BEGINNING OF PHARMACOLOGY

Bernard had few followers and did not found a school of physiology and pharmacology. The impetus passed to Germany, where the new knowledge of physiology was systematized and propagated, experimental physiology was advanced, and the aim was pursued of 'reducing' the science of life to a description purely in terms of physics and chemistry. The study of drugs received its greatest impetus at the University of Dorpat (now Tartu) in

Table 1 Potent drugs known before the nineteenth century

Drug	Plant	Recognition	Active principle
wine	*Vitis vinifera*	Ancient Greece	ethyl alcohol
opium	*Papaver somniferum*	Ancient Greece	morphine, etc.
hemlock	*Conium maculatum*	Ancient Greece	coniine
mandragora	*Mandragora officinatum*	Ancient Greece	hyoscine
ma huang	*Ephedra* spp.	Ancient China	ephedrine
belladonna	*Atropa belladonna*	Middle Ages	atropine
ergot	*Claviceps purpurea*	Middle Ages	ergotamine, etc.
ipecacuanha	*Cephaelis ipecacuanha*	Brazil *c.*1600	emetine
Jesuit's bark	*Cinchona* spp.	Peru *c.*1630	quinine
coca leaves	*Erythroxylon coca*	Bolivia and Peru *c.*1688	cocaine
foxglove	*Digitalis purpurea*	England, 1775–85	digitoxin, etc.

Estonia. Dorpat had strong German connections and attracted many outstanding individuals in science and medicine. A chair of pharmacology was established, the first under that name in Europe and probably in the world. It was filled by Rudolf Buchheim (1820–79), a graduate of Leipzig, who had learned much of his subject by translating an important new English textbook on drugs written by Jonathan Pereira (1804–53), physician and chemist in London. Buchheim studied the effects of the familiar drugs of the time – metals, purgatives, alkaloids, and alcohol, among others – and, when a pharmacological institute was built, he trained younger men as pharmacologists.[9]

Buchheim made no great discovery, but did much to establish the science as a distinct discipline. One of his pupils, Oswald Schmiedeberg (1838–1921), succeeded him at Dorpat and in 1872 moved to Strassburg (Strasbourg), where the university was being made a showplace of German culture in the province of Alsace, newly acquired after the Franco-Prussian war. Here, Schmiedeberg created a great centre for the development of experimental pharmacology.

The work of the Strassburg laboratory marks a great advance in the understanding of drugs. Medicines in common use were investigated to discover how they acted on bodily tissues, and their supposed therapeutic benefits were related, if possible, to observable physiological facts. Chloroform and other anaesthetics and narcotics, drugs such as nicotine and muscarine with actions related to the autonomic nervous system, digitalis, and heavy metals were all studied, with varying success. More importantly, the principle was established that this kind of investigation was valuable, indeed essential, as a background to the clinical use of drugs and as a means for finding better drugs.

The pharmacologists trained by Schmiedeberg went elsewhere in Germany and further afield, and created departments of pharmacology where there had been only those of materia medica (the study of the plants and minerals from which medicines were prepared), or none at all. By the time Schmiedeberg retired in 1918, over a hundred pupils had been trained in his laboratory and had gone to many parts of the world to establish the new science.[10]

The science of pharmacology developed strongly also in Edinburgh, where it evolved from long-established courses in materia medica. Toxicology was included with pharmacology, as well as in the teaching of forensic medicine. Robert Christison (1797–1882), who had studied in Paris under Magendie and Orfila, investigated the poisonous seeds of the tropical plant *Physostigma venenosum*, partly by self-medication. His successor, Thomas Fraser (1841–1920), isolated the alkaloid eserine or physostigmine from the plant, though he was not the first person to do so, and made the important discovery that another alkaloid, atropine, blocked some of the actions of eserine. Eserine continued to play a key part in many investigations in the next eighty years.[11]

Interaction between two drugs had not been carefully analysed before, and invited studies of their chemistry. Fraser collaborated with the organic chemist Alexander Crum Brown (1838–1922) in studying the antagonism between drugs and how chemical structure affected the ways drugs acted. At this time, the approximate atomic composition of various alkaloids was known, but almost identical formulae, in terms of the number of atoms present, did not correspond to similar pharmacological actions. Crum Brown modified various alkaloids, including strychnine, codeine, morphine, and atropine, by attaching an additional methyl group to the nitrogen atom which each of them contained. Fraser showed that this change had striking pharmacological results. The original alkaloids differed widely in their actions: strychnine was convulsant, morphine soporific, and atropine relieved colic (among many other actions). All the new compounds had a new action, like that of curare, in causing paralysis. Sometimes, they also lost their own typical actions. The presence of the ammonium-like structure, later known as an onium compound, consistently conferred curare-like action on any drugs to which it could be introduced. Crum Brown and Fraser were less successful than they had hoped in applying their discoveries to the invention of useful drugs: Curare and curare-like drugs did not come into medicinal use for another seventy or eighty years, but their experiments were fundamentally important as the first clear demonstration of a connection between chemical structure and pharmacological action.[12]

CHEMISTRY APPLIED TO MEDICINE

A quite different aspect of the study of drugs began in 1841 when the English physician Alexander Ure treated gouty patients with benzoic acid and noted that the urine contained crystals of hippuric acid.[13] Hippuric acid results when benzoic acid combines with glycine, but the reaction does not ordinarily take place when the components are put together at body temperature. Evidently, chemical combination, of a kind that did not happen spontaneously, had occurred in the living organism. The results were confirmed in other laboratories, and the mechanism was investigated further under Schmiedeberg's aegis. The conversion was an example of what would now be called 'biotransformation' of drugs. Very few drugs pass through the body unchanged, and study of the chemical changes which they undergo has gradually become increasingly important in interpreting their actions and the time for which they act. Changes of this kind, which make drugs less active or inactive, became known as detoxication.

Biotransformations with the opposite effect were also recognized. A possibility was envisaged both by Buchheim at Dorpat and by Oscar Liebreich (1839–1908) in Berlin. The substance chloral hydrate had been prepared by Justus von Liebig (1803–73) in 1832, about the same time as chloroform had been first made. The fairly close resemblance between the two substances suggested that the body might convert chloral to chloroform and release the anaesthetic gradually but effectively. Buchheim and Liebreich each tried the idea, and found that chloral hydrate produced sleep. Liebreich published an account of his discovery in 1869, and chloral hydrate became established as a useful drug. The reason for the experiment was right in principle, but not in detail. It was shown many years later that chloral undergoes 'biotransformation' not to chloroform but to trichlorethanol, which is the active agent in producing sleep.[14]

It has now become common practice to devise drugs that are transformed before acting, sometimes called 'pro-drugs'. The active substance is released gradually, without the dangers of a single large dose acting all at once, or the inconvenience of continuous infusion of the agent. Biotransformation is not necessarily beneficial: the transformed material is sometimes more dangerous than the parent substance (for example, fluorocitrate from the rat poison fluoroacetate) and may have lethal consequences.[15]

With the rise of synthetic chemistry, substances previously unknown came into existence. There was no reason to expect them to have any effects on humans, though chemists no doubt treated them with respect. Volatile substances were not easily avoided, and the stupefying powers of nitrous oxide and of ether were known for thirty or more years before their practical application as general anaesthetics was shown between 1842 and 1846. (➤ Ch. 41 Surgery (traditional)) Another novel volatile substance, chloroform, was used on animals by M. J. P. Flourens (1794–1867), a colleague of Magendie, in 1847; and in humans, after adventurous self-experimentation by J. Y. Simpson (1811–70) in Edinburgh in the same year. In spite of some opposition, the use of nitrous oxide, ether, and chloroform extended widely, and a search has continued ever since, sometimes fruitfully, for safer and more effective agents. Other volatile substances had quite different effects. The vasodilator properties of amyl nitrite and of glyceryl trinitrate were recognized by the chemists who made them. They were later investigated by experimentally minded physicians, and seen to be useful for the treatment of angina pectoris.

When previously unknown substances made in a laboratory were found to have medicinal properties, it became both attractive and necessary to make them on a large scale. The existing suppliers of drugs and medicines – druggists, apothecaries, pharmacists – were familiar with botanical and inorganic materials, but were not experienced in more elaborate organic chemistry. To meet this difficulty, some wholesale businesses, notably Merck of Darmstadt, sent employees to laboratories where technical knowledge could be obtained, and embarked on the isolation of alkaloids that could be marketed as pure and more reliable medicines than cruder preparations from plants.

At the same time, innovative organic chemists, especially Liebig in Germany, were promoting the industrial applications of their subject, including the extraction from raw materials of reactive ingredients and the synthesis of novel compounds with innumerable possible uses. The crystallization of pure plant alkaloids was a tiny and highly specialized part of such work. Chemical analysis of the new alkaloids suggested that they might be prepared synthetically, and so avoid all the problems of collecting or cultivating medicinal plants and extracting the required drugs, often in quite unpredictable yields.

An attempt in 1856 by the English chemist W. H. Perkin (1838–1907) to synthesize quinine failed in its objective: the complexity of the quinine molecule was far beyond anyone's chemical knowledge at that time, and its synthesis was not achieved until the 1940s. But Perkin's synthesis gave a coloured compound, and led him to synthesize the dyestuff mauvein, which he exploited commercially: thus began the foundation of the synthetic dyestuffs industry. Good dyestuffs were valuable, and organic chemistry advanced as ways were sought of making new ones. Other uses for new compounds were examined, and, in time, the dyestuffs industry became an industry of fine chemicals, including medicinal substances among its products. So Perkin's attempt to synthesize quinine had much greater consequences for medicine than the artificial preparation of a single drug.

Other alkaloids were less troublesome. Once organic chemistry had advanced sufficiently to give a clear picture of the structure of at least the simpler alkaloids, synthesis became possible and was achieved for coniine in 1886. The more complex substances, atropine, cocaine, and nicotine, were all synthesized soon after 1900. The way was open for studying the relation of chemical structure to pharmacological activity, denied to Brown and Fraser forty years earlier, and for inventing new compounds which were simplified imitations of natural alkaloids.

The earliest major group of compounds produced by the new chemical industry and found to have medicinal properties were the antipyretic analgesics derived from coal tar. They included phenacetin, paracetamol, and several others later discarded because they were too toxic. Other early synthetic drugs including several hypnotics, notably the barbiturates, and various volatile anaesthetics. Sometimes, compounds produced either in industry or in university laboratories were found to be useful drugs only after many years. Aspirin was synthesized in 1852, but its medicinal properties were not recognized until 1899; and sulphanilamide lay on the shelves of organic chemists from 1908 until the mid-1930s, while childbed fever and other diseases which it could cure remained unchecked. (➤ Ch. 44 Childbirth)

The ingenuity of organic chemists had further scope when they synthesized compounds modelled on existing drugs, usually alkaloids, in the hope of finding materials easier to make and equally or more effective and safe. The earliest, and one of the greatest, successes came with local anaesthetics that resembled cocaine. 'Novocain' or procaine appeared in 1899: it was effective, much simpler chemically, avoided most of the hazardous properties of cocaine, and was the forerunner of a range of drugs adapted to special kinds of local anaesthesia.

So the nineteenth century saw the introduction of partially purified drugs, some active principles (especially pure alkaloids), and a number of synthetic drugs of undoubted potency. Their discovery had been empirical: none of the original compounds had been made in the first place with a medicinal purpose in mind. But they were the harbingers of an incoming tide of new remedies, increasingly purpose-designed, and not seriously checked during the next eighty years.

CHEMOTHERAPY

While the chemical industry was growing and producing new remedies, advances in biology gave a second foundation from which new therapeutic substances were developed. The discovery of microbes which caused particular illnesses, the germ theory of disease, and the investigation of immunity are dealt with elsewhere in this encyclopedia. (➤ Ch. 16 Contagion/germ theory/specificity; Ch. 10 The immunological tradition) Here, we need note only the consequence that medicaments for preventing certain diseases were becoming possible. Immunization against smallpox by vaccination had indeed an ancient history, but by the end of the nineteenth century, vaccines were being devised for protecting against cholera, typhoid fever, and other diseases. Also, a novel kind of remedy appeared, prepared from the blood serum of immunized animals and containing antitoxins which saved the lives of patients with diphtheria or tetanus.

Such remedies of biological origin are not usually classed as drugs. The distinction is more practical than fundamental, and, historically, ideas of antibacterial drugs are rooted in research related to vaccines and antitoxins. Indeed, it is reasonable to suggest that all modern concepts of the mode of action of drugs spring from studies of antibacterial agents, and particularly from the work of the German physician and scientist Paul Ehrlich (1854–1915).

Ehrlich's earliest observations dealt with the staining of tissues for microscopic examination, and so with the processes by which particular dyestuffs combined with and were fixed to specific components of the tissues. (➤ Ch. 6 The microscopical tradition) Ehrlich supposed that the action of drugs on bodily organs was likely to involve similar fixation, and throughout his life he followed the principle '*Corpora non agunt nisi fixata*' (substances do not act unless they are fixed). As an early test of this thesis, he treated a small number of malarial patients with the dye methylene blue, which was known to stain (that is, be fixed by) the malaria parasite, and he showed that it had a modest therapeutic effect. An important example of fixation was seen when bacterial toxins combined with cells, or with antitoxins. The question that followed was: 'What substances in the tissues or what part of the antitoxin produced by the tissues combines with or fixes the dye or toxin?'

Ehrlich called the unidentified material a 'receptor'. The term was used in a similar sense, at about the same time, by the English physiologist J. N. Langley (1852–1925) for the material which 'received' nicotine and curare in the motor end plates of skeletal muscle. Knowledge of the chemical structure of tissues was inadequate for either Ehrlich or Langley to isolate and identify the actual receptors, but the concept was a fundamental advance. Much basic pharmacology evolved from attempts to identify receptor substances or structures, and to account for the quantitative aspects of drug action in terms of theoretical receptors.

The early part of Ehrlich's career was concerned with the new biological remedies, and he made major contributions both to the practical problems of standardizing the remedies and to theories of their mode of action. He abandoned antitoxins and studied simpler substances, essentially products of chemical laboratories, both as drugs and as a basis for advancing knowledge of receptors. He recognized that microbes could fix small molecules – that is, they had receptors for them – because they were stained selectively by dyes. The last quarter of Ehrlich's life was spent in the study that he called chemotherapy, the attempt to cure microbial diseases with substances of known chemical composition.

Many compounds were examined for antiprotozoal and antibacterial activity. The known antibacterial substances, such as phenol, were too poisonous to be tolerated if administered as medicines. Substances such as quinine, active against certain protozoa, were tolerated but were not effective against bacteria. Ehrlich had some success against experimental infections with trypanosomes, protozoa of the family that cause sleeping sickness, in rodents. Malaria was not a satisfactory topic, because patients were uncommon in northern Europe, and no means of producing the infection in animals was then known. In the light of clinical reports that organic arsenical compounds were effective against trypanosomes, Ehrlich pursued the chemistry and anti-microbial actions of such compounds. (➤ Ch. 24 Tropical diseases)

The organism that causes syphilis, the spirochaete *Treponema pallidum*, had recently been identified and offered another target, especially after the discovery that rabbits could be infected successfully with it. A Japanese scientist, Sahachiro Hata (1873–1938), who came from a laboratory in Tokyo with some German affiliations, brought the technique to Ehrlich, and together they found effective antisyphilitic organic arsenicals, of which the one numbered '606' appeared most promising. Ehrlich arranged for it to be made on a larger scale and for samples to be sent to colleagues for testing in patients, both in Germany and elsewhere. Early clinical trials of '606' were satisfactory, and Ehrlich announced publicly the discovery of the new remedy at the Congress for Internal Medicine held at Wiesbaden in April 1910. (➤ Ch. 26 Sexually-transmitted diseases)

However, '606', later named 'salvarsan' and arsphenamine, was unstable and the potency of successive batches varied. It was effective only by intravenous injection. Treatment required many months, and a substantial proportion of patients suffered from toxic effects on the liver, bone marrow, or skin. A better compound, '914' or neoarsphenamine, was introduced shortly before Ehrlich's death, and for twenty years became the principal drug for the treatment of syphilis.[16]

The principle of chemotherapy was established, and remained as a guiding light to those who sought new antibacterial agents. But advance in this field was, until the late 1930s, largely confined to the discovery of antimalarial drugs that could be used instead of quinine. They attracted little attention outside the tropics, and most experts in bacteriology and medicine in the 1920s regarded chemotherapy as an impractical dream. Before describing the overthrow of such scepticism, however, the progress up to 1935 in other fields of pharmacology will be reviewed.

PHYSIOLOGICAL AGENTS AS DRUGS

In the later part of the nineteenth century, physiologists began to postulate and sometimes demonstrate the existence of substances which were released by specific cells or organs and which had specific effects on other cells. These substances were of two kinds. One kind, later named hormones, was released into the bloodstream from certain ductless glands and acted on distant organs. The other kind was released at nerve endings and stimulated or inhibited other nerve cells, muscles, or glands. Their action was strictly localized, and they were known as humoral transmitters. Later, the simple name local hormone was used.[17]

Experiments on the effects of removing certain ductless glands, especially the thyroid or the adrenals, from animals supported and supplemented clinical observations of patients with diseases of these glands, and suggested that the glands contained valuable therapeutic principles. (➤ Ch. 23 Endocrine disorders) Extracts of thyroid gland were used to relieve myxoedema in 1891; and adrenal extracts were shown in 1894 to raise the blood pressure of experimental animals. An active principle, adrenaline, was isolated from the adrenal gland in several laboratories, notably by John J. Abel (1857–1938) at Johns Hopkins University in Baltimore, and its chemical identity was established and confirmed by synthesis. Testicular extracts were claimed in 1890 to have rejuvenating powers, and the ovaries were recognized as a source of internal secretion from about 1900, though more than thirty years passed before active principles were identified and their properties established. The word 'hormone' was adopted by E. H. Starling (1866–1927) in connection with his observations on gastro-intestinal chemical regulators in 1905.

From these beginnings, the complex science of endocrinology emerged. Hormones became important as drugs:

a to replace a deficiency of the natural secretion, due to disease or to traumatic or excessive surgical removal of individual glands;
b to modify immune responses and check unwanted inflammatory reactions (cortisone and its congeners); and
c to modify healthy bodily functions, notably the reproductive cycle of women as a means of contraception.[18]

In addition, new drugs were developed which either acted like the natural hormones (for example, the synthetic oestrogen, stilboestrol) or stimulated the release of hormone (for example, certain antidiabetic drugs), or prevented the release of hormone and so were valuable in glandular overactivity (for example, thiouracil and related antithyroid drugs).

The treatment of myxoedema with preparations of thyroid gland was effective, but a long sequence of investigations of the thyroid hormone continued. Thyroxine was isolated by E. C. Kendall (1886–1972) at the Mayo Clinic in 1915. C. R. Harington (1897–1972) established its correct structure, and synthetic thyroxine was shown to be as efficacious as the biological product. Further research, much under Harington's aegis, identified tri-iodothyronine as a second thyroid hormone, and revealed unsuspected complexities of the physiological system.

The discovery of adrenaline did not help the treatment of Addison's disease (adrenal insufficiency): adrenaline comes from the adrenal medulla, and the life-preserving agent that was lacking in Addison's disease originates in the cortical part of the gland. Adrenal extracts that alleviated the consequences of adrenal deficiency were not discovered until about 1930, and the identity of their active principles began to be established in the following decade.

A historic achievement in 1922 was the isolation from the pancreas of material that prevented the fatal outcome of diabetes mellitus. The importance of the pancreas in preventing diabetes was recognized before the end of the nineteenth century, and at least four attempts had been made to isolate an antidiabetic principle before the experiments of Frederick Banting (1891–1941) and Charles Best (1899–1978) in Toronto. The problem centred round the nature of insulin, which is a protein, a much more complex substance than either the thyroid or the adrenal hormones. As it is subject to digestion in the alimentary canal, it is not effective by mouth, and as the digestive enzymes originate in the pancreas, it seemed likely to be destroyed before it could be isolated from the gland. These problems were overcome, but the resources of a university laboratory were in no way equal to the task of providing insulin for all those who needed it. Practical application of the Toronto discovery depended much on the resources of the Connaught laboratories in Toronto and of Eli Lilly in Indianapolis, and thereafter on judicious licensing of production to manufacturers in every part of the world. Then sufferers from diabetes no longer awaited a distressing death within months, and could expect to live for a normal span of life.[19] The outcome was one of the first spectacular triumphs of science applied to medicine, and depended entirely on the conduct of experiments in animals, mostly dogs. The structure of insulin was not fully determined until the 1950s: it was too large to be made by chemical synthesis, and could be obtained only from the pancreas of recently killed animals until the genes that controlled synthesis were successfully transferred to microbes in the 1970s.

Further developments in endocrinology included identification of the sex and pituitary hormones and the synthesis of related drugs, a growing understanding of the functions of the pituitary gland as a regulator of all endocrine activity, and clarification of the functions of the parathyroid glands.

Another branch of physiological research was concerned with the transmission of messages from nerve cells to other nerve cells and to muscles and glands on which nerves acted.[20] For nearly a century, controversy centred on the mechanism of transmission – was it by electrical impulses or by pulses of chemically identifiable substances? The similarity of the actions of adrenaline to those of the sympathetic nerves suggested that adrenaline might be a transmitter. The resemblance of the actions of muscarine to those of the vagus and other parasympathetic nerves invited the question of whether muscarine was a transmitter. Although neither supposition was correct, ideas were developing on the right lines. O. Loewi (1873–1961) showed that the transmitter at vagal endings was likely to be acetylcholine. The extensive work of H. H. Dale (1875–1968) and his colleagues, and of U. S. von Euler (1905–83) and others, identified the principal transmitters as noradrenaline at sympathetic endings and acetylcholine at most other sites. It was then possible to draw a comprehensive picture of the actions of atropine (blocking muscarine-like actions of acetylcholine), eserine (delaying the destruction of acetylcholine and so imitating and enhancing its actions), curare (blocking non-muscarine-like actions of acetylcholine), ergotoxine (blocking certain actions of adrenaline), and a number of other drugs.

The immediate benefit of these advances to therapeutics was small. Some new drugs related to acetylcholine were useful for postoperative retention of urine, and the drug ephedrine, long known in Chinese medicine, was shown to resemble adrenaline, both chemically and pharmacologically, and to be beneficial in asthma. But the fundamental knowledge provided a background without which many advances after the Second World War would have been impossible.

ESTABLISHMENT OF A SCIENCE OF DRUGS

Advances in chemistry, in chemotherapy, in endocrinology, and in physiology all contributed to knowledge about drugs, and made their use more complicated, but pharmacology as a science in its own right progressed haltingly. As already recorded (see pp. 919–21), the science was established in Germany, both academically and industrially, during the nineteenth century, and flourished until the First World War. In the 1930s, it was ravaged by Nazi persecutions, and one outstanding pharmacologist after another was driven to seek refuge in Britain, the United States, or elsewhere.

In England between 1880 and 1930, research on drugs flourished in physiological laboratories and in the state-supported National Institute for Medical Research, but academic facilities were scanty and teaching about the use of drugs was usually in the hands of clinicians with no scientific training or interests. A national society to oversee all the interests of British pharmacologists was not founded until 1932, after which the subject gradually received wider recognition.[21] The British pharmaceutical industry was less oriented to research than that in Germany, but one firm, Burroughs Wellcome, supported substantial research laboratories, interestingly named 'chemical' and 'physiological', from the beginning of the century.

In the eastern United States, as in Scotland, experimental pharmacology replaced the old curricula in materia medica. The west was still being opened up, and developments came later. Early drug firms in America acquired a bad reputation for their commercial practices, and the industry was held in such low esteem that the American Society for Experimental Pharmacology and Therapeutics, founded and dominated by Abel, excluded industrial pharmacologists from its membership. The prohibition was repealed in 1941, by which time it had become an evident source of weakness.[22]

Elsewhere, research on drugs was increasing. International physiological congresses provided a meeting-ground for pharmacologists, who did not have an international meeting of their own until 1961. (➤ Ch. 59 Internationalism in medicine and public health)

A number of scientific problems were specific to pharmacology. The most fundamental related to the mode of action of drugs. By the beginning of the twentieth century, it was generally accepted that drugs act at specific sites and not diffusely throughout the body. These sites were described as receptors, but their identity was obscure. The ways in which drugs combined with and were removed from receptors, and how combination of a drug with a receptor produced some physiological effect, had yet to be discovered. Arthur Cushny (1866–1926), a pupil of Schmiedeberg and later successor to Fraser in Edinburgh, best known for his work on digitalis, studied the relation of optical activity to potency of drugs and elucidated the geometrical properties of drug receptors. His successor in the Edinburgh Chair, A. J. Clark (1885–1941), wrote two classic monographs about drug receptors and the mode of action of drugs.[23] He discussed ways in which drugs might block the actions of other drugs by competing for the same receptors, and laid the foundation for discoveries made after the Second World War.

An immediately practical activity specific to pharmacology was the use of living tissues to detect, identify, and measure minute quantities of drugs. In the nineteenth century, biological tests for organic poisons began to be used for legal purposes. A means of detecting digitalis and similar poisons was required, because chemical tests were too insensitive to identify potentially lethal quantities of digitalis. Biological tests were not only sensitive but could be made very specific, such as in distinguishing digitalis from other drugs that acted on the heart. Biological tests, developed to give estimates of the quantities of drug present, were necessary also for quality control of manufactured products: at first, antitoxins; and later, potent drugs of plant origin, such as digitalis or curare; as well as hormones and vitamins. The principles of good assays were laid down by Ehrlich, and their refinement by suitable statistical methods owed much to J. W. Trevan (1887–1956) at the Wellcome Laboratories, and J. H. Gaddum (1900–65) at the National Institute.

However, the major activity of most pharmacologists was the investigation of familiar medicines and the search for improvements. Especially when there were chemists eager to collaborate, or when chemists found pharmacologists willing to undertake tests for them, a pattern of research developed which was and still is a standard approach to finding new drugs. Once a drug was known to have a particular action, and its chemical structure was known, new compounds resembling the original substance were made, tested by whatever biological experiment seemed appropriate, and were investigated further if they had promise. This operation of synthesis and screening became the principal activity of industrial pharmacological research. It was applied to important alkaloids, including cocaine as a local anaesthetic, eserine as an anticholinesterase, and atropine as a spasmolytic, and to physiological agents such as adrenaline and acetylcholine. Synthetic substances that had shown interesting physiological activity also served as starting-points, such as substituted ammonium compounds, which blocked autonomic ganglia and showed the way to a long sequence of hypotensive agents.

The weakest aspect of pharmacology, especially in Britain, lay in its separation from clinical medicine. An aspect of this weakness can be seen in the history of attempts to identify the active principle of ergot, which made the womb contract and so was useful for controlling bleeding after childbirth. Ergotoxine, active in laboratory experiments, was discovered in 1906, and for many years was regarded as 'the' active principle. Clinical experience preferred the well-known watery extract of ergot, and confusion existed for nearly thirty years, not diminished by the discovery of another uterus-contracting alkaloid, ergotamine. The problem was not resolved until clinical studies were undertaken in collaboration with laboratory scientists in 1933–5, and the clinically active principle of the watery extract was shown to be yet another alkaloid, ergometrine or ergonovine.

The important advances in therapeutics between the First and Second World Wars came from physiological and biochemical laboratories, and were developed by clinical scientists. Vitamins were discovered, mainly by biochemists and chemically oriented nutritionists, and hormones came into clinical use. Physiological studies of the value of liver in some kinds of anaemia led to trials in treatment of the hitherto fatal disease, pernicious or Addisonian anaemia. The liver treatment was successful, and represented the next important therapeutic advance after the introduction of insulin. Potent extracts of liver became a new life-saving medicine, and their further purification led, in the mid-1940s, to the identification of vitamin B_{12}. (➤ Ch. 22 Nutritional diseases)

CHEMOTHERAPY REVIVED

The success of salvarsan showed that microbes could be destroyed in patients by synthetic drugs, but the search for other chemotherapeutic drugs did not prosper greatly. There was little light to guide the search, and discoveries were made empirically. An acridine dye that inhibited trypanosomes was named 'trypaflavine': related acridines were found to be active against bacteria and were adopted as antiseptics, but they were too toxic for systemic use. In the laboratories of the Bayer Company, compounds were discovered that attacked protozoa and were sufficiently harmless to humans. The work was conducted in secrecy and even the chemical identity of the first important compound, 'Bayer 205' or germanin for sleeping sickness, was not divulged at first. Two important antimalarials, Plasmaquin (pamaquine) and Atebrin (mepacrine in England and quinacrine in America) were also discovered. None of these advances contributed to *antibacterial* chemotherapy, and eminent authorities in Britain and America continued to dismiss the subject as an unrealizable dream.

However, Gerhard Domagk (1895–1964), who came to the Bayer laboratories in 1927, pursued potential antibacterial drugs, including a red dye later named 'Prontosil'. In 1935 Domagk reported an experiment in which it saved the lives of mice infected with haemolytic streptococci. Clinical trials were widespread and the drug became well known.

Later in the same year, J. Tréfouël (1897–1777) and his colleagues at the Pasteur Institute in Paris showed that a simpler compound was equally effective. This compound, chemically named *p*-aminobenzenesulphonamide or, more conveniently, sulphanilamide, was part of the whole molecule of Prontosil, and, as appeared soon afterwards, was liberated from Prontosil *in vivo*. Sulphanilamide provided a model for new compounds, of which several thousand were described in the next decade, some useful against other microbes, some less toxic, and some which acted for longer after each dose than did sulphanilamide.[24]

During the 1920s and 1930s, the biochemistry of microbes was studied on a rapidly increasing scale, and had so advanced that the mode of action of sulphanilamide could be explained within a few years of the discovery of its therapeutic power. A growth-promoting substance in yeast extracts resembled sulphanilamide in its chemical properties. Known compounds were tested, and *p*-aminobenzoic acid (PABA) was found, like the yeast material, to support the growth of various kinds of microbe and also strongly to counteract the effects of sulphanilamide. The species of microbe that depended on a supply of PABA were the same as those that were sensitive to sulphanilamide.

Competitive antagonism between chemically allied compounds as substrates for an enzyme system had been recognized in earlier biochemical studies, but was now seen to be of great practical importance for inventing new drugs. The discovery could be applied by identifying some metabolite essential to a pathogenic microbe and without an important role in human physiology. Analogues could be synthesized and tested for competitive blocking activity, and the most effective could be developed for medical purposes. The principle was sound. The practical difficulties became more obvious as time progressed, but a substantial number of new drugs have been discovered in this way, useful not only against bacterial and protozoal infections, but also for cancer chemotherapy. (➤ Ch. 25 Cancer)

ANTIBIOTICS

The next advance in the control of microbial infections came from a quite different approach. A phenomenon known as antibiosis – that is, the prevention of growth or actual destruction of one species of micro-organism by substances produced by another species – was known to bacteriologists from the time of Pasteur (1822–95). Certain moulds had this property: the antibacterial effects of some species of *Penicillium* were observed in the 1870s, and a crude preparation was used by Joseph Lister (1827–1912) in Edinburgh to treat an infected wound. From time to time, various extracts of moulds and bacteria were tried. A preparation named pyocyanase, from *Pseudomonas pyocyanea*, was available commercially about 1910, but gradually lost its reputation and was abandoned. Alexander Fleming (1881–1955) used the name penicillin to refer to the antibacterial matter produced by the mould that fell on his plate, but did not succeed in isolating the very unstable active principle. The chemical problems were overcome in Oxford early in the Second World War by E. B. Chain (1906–79), working with H. W. Florey (1898–1968), as part of a broad study of antibiotics. By a remarkable feat of organization, enough crude penicillin was produced in an academic laboratory to show that it was innocuous and to treat a small number of patients successfully, and so justify attempts at large-scale production. British resources were fully committed to wartime needs, and the development of penicillin depended on the brilliant work of American laboratories and manufacturers.[25]

It was soon found that there was more than one penicillin, but the chemistry was unexpectedly difficult, and no large-scale synthesis has been achieved. Manufacture still depends on fermentation processes. The original penicillins attacked many organisms which were insensitive to sulphonamides, but the penicillins decomposed in the acid contents of the stomach and were effective only when injected. They were rapidly excreted, and so frequent doses were required, typically every three hours, to maintain adequate antibacterial activity throughout a course of treatment. In time, modified penicillins were made, partly by fermentation and partly by synthesis, that were active by mouth and less rapidly excreted. Some were not destroyed by bacterial penicillinases, and so were effective against strains that produced this enzyme.

Another fungal product, streptomycin, was reported by S. A. Waksman (1888–1973) and others at Rutgers University, New Jersey, in 1943 to be active against tubercle bacilli and other organisms. The clinical efficacy of streptomycin against tuberculosis was established by W. H. Feldman (b.

1892) and H. C. Hinshaw (b. 1902) at the Mayo Clinic, but resistant bacilli appeared with discouraging rapidity. American and Swedish studies in competitive antagonism led to the drug *p*-aminosalicylic acid (PAS), which was less potent than streptomycin, but very effective when combined with it for preventing resistance. In Britain, a series of trials organized by the Medical Research Council established the clinical importance of these facts quickly and clearly; the shortage of streptomycin, which made it impossible to treat all eligible patients, greatly simplified the ethical difficulty in withholding a treatment from some patients, who served as controls in evaluating the drugs. (➤ Ch. 37 History of medical ethics)

The success of penicillin and streptomycin stimulated a search for other antibiotics, and vast programmes were undertaken which yielded many new antibiotics active against various organisms, and sometimes also against tumours. Few were as innocuous as penicillin, and their main merits were their activity against a wider range of organisms (so making exact bacteriological diagnosis less critical), or against unfamiliar organisms or strains resistant to first-choice antibiotics.

THE AGE OF THE PURE DRUG

Not only antibiotics, but new drugs of all kinds, appeared after the Second World War. Human thirst for medicine was unquenched, and the pharmaceutical industry, greatly strenghthened by advances in the sciences of chemistry, pharmacology, and all other subjects related to the manufacture and use of drugs, did its best to meet the demand. The principle of competitive antagonism gave a reasoned basis for seeking new drugs, and advances in the biochemistry of infectious organisms, of cancer, and other pathological processes showed enzymes worthy of attack and new models for chemists to modify. Pure, stable substances were more reliable and easier to store and use than tinctures and dried extracts, so that nearly all traditional and widely used remedies were gradually displaced. (See Table 2.)

The design of clinical trials was greatly improved, particularly under the influence of A. Bradford Hill (1897–1991) and the authority of the Medical Research Council in Britain. Few drugs came into use without trials of some sort, and some drugs, especially against tuberculosis, were exceptionally well evaluated as soon as they became widely available. However, it did not follow that all the new remedies were of lasting benefit. Many were superseded within a few years of introduction by more recent discoveries that had some clear advantage, or were free from some obviously undesirable property. Other drugs were discredited after a brief period of enthusiasm, when unsuspected toxic effects appeared, or when evidence accumulated that their use was no more beneficial than their omission.

Table 2 The introduction of some purified or synthetic drugs

Drug	Purpose or use	Decade
nitrous oxide	general anaesthetic	1840
ether	general anaesthetic	1840
chloroform	general anaesthetic	1840
amyl nitrite	angina pectoris	1860
trinitrin	angina pectoris	1860
phenacetin	analgesic	1880
Novocain etc.	local anesthetic	1900
Veronal etc.	hypnotic	1900
insulin	diabetes mellitus	1920
liver extract	pernicious, Addisonian anaemia	1920
steroid hormones	Addison's disease	1930
	disorders of reproduction	
mepacrine	malaria	1930
Prontosil, sulphonamides	streptococcal infections	1930
penicillin	Gram-positive infections	1940
streptomycin	tuberculous	1940
chloroquine	malaria	1940
nitrogen mustard	blood-cell cancers	1940
antifolates	blood-cell cancers	1940
cortisone	anti-inflammatory	1940
methoniums	hypertension	1940
chlorpromazine	anxiety, schizophrenia	1950
isoniazid	tuberculosis	1950
chlorothiazide	diuretic	1950
progestogen and oestrogen	contraceptive (oral)	1950
monoamine oxidase inhibitors	antidepressant	1950
Imipramine	antidepressant	1950
propranolol	angina, hypertension	1960
diazepoxides	anxiety	1960
allopurinol	gout	1960
cimetidine	peptic ulcers	1960
acyclovir	herpes virus infections	1980

Source: M. Weatherall, *In Search of a Cure*, Oxford, Oxford University Press, 1990.

With the introduction of many new substances as drugs and their production and distribution on a wider scale, ill effects were observed from time to time and were, perhaps, an unavoidable price to pay for therapeutic successes. Drugs did not come into clinical use until they had been extensively assessed in animals, and many potential disasters were prevented in this way. However, tragedies occurred. Some were a consequence of ignorance on the part of manufacturers: for example, when a manufacturer of an elixir of sulphanilamide used ethylene glycol as a sweetening agent and over seventy deaths resulted before the sale of the medicine was stopped. Others arose when drugs had ill effects of a kind not previously recognized, notably the injury to the developing foetus caused by thalidomide.

After the thalidomide tragedy, the toxicity of drugs was tested much more extensively in animals. The tests delayed the introduction of new drugs, especially in the United States (the so-called 'drug lag'): numerous drugs were not sanctioned there for months or years after they were freely in use in other parts of the world, despite available evidence of the life-saving value of some of them. The elaboration of formalized toxicity testing in animals diverted resources from more useful ways of assessing toxicity, and the protracted poisoning of groups of animals probably contributed to the growth of protests, some more reasonable than others, against experiments of any kind on animals, and a consequent check to innovation. Nor did elaborate ritual testing in animals prevent further tragedies, for example, with practolol and benoxaprofen.

Therapeutics has always suffered swings of fashion. The heroic treatments widely used in the eighteenth and early nineteenth century led to disillusion and a phase of therapeutic nihilism, which was well justified by discoveries of the extent of tissue damage in advanced disease and of the lack of real activity of most of the remedies in use. A crescendo of scientific discoveries, from antitoxins and early chemotherapy to penicillin and the drugs of the post-war era, brought the age of the pure drug and of 'a pill for every ill'. Once again, optimism was excessive and a sure foundation for new disillusion. Public understanding is not well equipped to distinguish drugs that do more good than harm from inappropriate, ineffective, or misused drugs, and it is becoming fashionable to take refuge in hopes for 'natural' remedies: that is, unpurified materials of uncertain potency and uncertain toxicity, and in systems of therapy such as homoeopathy, which contradict the most elementary scientific knowledge. (➤ Ch. 28 Unorthodox medical theories) There is ample historical evidence for the value of belief in a remedy as an aid to therapeutics, but belief in a remedy is no proof of its efficacy, and the history of drugs shows that the chemical identity of the remedy is fundamental to its curative powers. (➤ Ch. 4 Medical care)

NOTES

1 Homer, *Odyssey*, iv, 230 ff.
2 O. Temkin, 'Historical aspects of drug therapy', in P. Talalay (ed.), *Drugs in Our Society*, Baltimore, MD, Johns Hopkins University Press, and London, Oxford University Press, 1964.
3 W. Pagel, *Paracelsus. An Introduction to Philosophical Medicine in the Era of the Renaissance*, 2nd rev. edn, Basle, Karger, 1982.
4 G. B. M. Bettolo, 'The evolution of the pharmacopoeias in Europe', *Pharmaceutical Journal*, 1966, 197: 535–8.
5 M. P. Earles, 'Early theories of the mode of action of drugs and poisons', *Annals of Science*, 1961, 17: 97–110.
6 A. W. Haggis, 'Fundamental errors in the early history of cinchona', *Bulletin of the History of Medicine*, 1941, 10: 417–59, 568–92.

7   J. K. Aronson, *An Account of the Foxglove and its Medical Uses 1785–1985*, Oxford, Oxford University Press, 1985.

8   A. M. Lilienfeld, '*Ceteris paribus:* the evolution of the clinical trial', *Bulletin of the History of Medicine*, 1982, 56: 1–18.

9   G. Kuschinsky, 'The influence of Dorpat on the emergence of pharmacology as a distinct discipline', *Journal of the History of Medicine*, 1968, 23: 258–71.

10   J. Koch-Weser and P. J. Schechter, 'Schmiedeberg in Strassburg 1872–1918: the making of modern pharmacology', *Life Sciences*, 1978, 22: 1361–72.

11   J. H. Gaddum, 'The development of materia medica in Edinburgh', *Edinburgh Medical Journal*, 1942, 49: 721–35.

12   W. F. Bynum, 'Chemical structure and pharmacological action. A chapter in the history of nineteenth-century molecular pharmacology', *Bulletin of the History of Medicine*, 1970, 44: 518–38.

13   A. Ure, 'On hippuric acid and its tests', *Provincial Medical and Surgical Journal, London*, 1841, 2: 317–18.

14   T. C. Butler, 'The introduction of chloral hydrate into medical practice', *Bulletin of the History of Medicine*, 1970, 44: 168–72.

15   R. A. Peters, 'Lethal synthesis', *Proceedings of the Royal Society*, 1952, (series B), 139: 143–70.

16   The collected papers of P. Ehrlich have been republished, with English translations of the most important, as follows: *The Collected Papers of Paul Ehrlich*, Vol I: *Histology, Biochemistry and Pathology*, Vol. II: Immunology and Cancer Research; Vol. III: *Chemotherapy*, ed. by H. H. Dale, F. Himmelweit and M. Marquardt, London, Pergamon Press, 1956–61.

17   J. H. Burn, 'A discussion on the action of local hormones', *Proceedings of the Royal Society*, 1950 (Series B), 137: 281.

18   G. Pincus, *The Control of Fertility*, New York, Academic Press, 1965.

19   M. Bliss, *The Discovery of Insulin*, Toronto, McClelland & Stewart, 1982.

20   Z. M. Bacq, *Chemical Transmission of Nerve Impulses. A Historical Sketch*, Oxford, Pergamon Press, 1975.

21   W. F. Bynum, *An Early History of the British Pharmacological Society*, British Pharmacological Society, 1981.

22   K. K. Chen, *The American Society for Pharmacology and Therapeutics Inc. The First Sixty Years 1908–1969*, Bethesda, MD, American Society for Pharmacology and Experimental Therapeutics, 1969.

23   A. J. Clark, *The Mode of Action of Drugs on Cells*, London, Edward Arnold, 1933; Clark, 'General pharmacology', in W. Heubner and J. Schüller (eds), *Handbuch der experimentelle Pharmakologie*, Vol. IV. Berlin, Springer, 1937.

24   E. H. Northey, *The Sulfonamides and Allied Compounds*, New York, Rheinhold, 1948.

25   G. Macfarlane, *Howard Florey. The Making of a Great Scientist*, Oxford, Oxford University Press, 1979; Macfarlane, *Alexander Fleming. The Man and the Myth*, London, Chatto & Windus/Hogarth Press, 1984.

937

FURTHER READING

Binden, J. S. and Ledniger, D. (eds), *Chronicles of Drug Discovery*, New York, Wiley, 1982.

Fluckinger, F. A. and Hanbury, D., *Pharmacographia. A History of the Principal Drugs of Vegetable Origin Met with in Great Britain and British India*, London, Macmillan, 1879.

Leake, C. D., *An Historical Account of Pharmacology to the Twentieth Century*, Springfield, IL, Thomas, 1975.

Lesch, J. E., *Science and Medicine in France. The Emergence of Experimental Physiology, 1790–1855*, Cambridge, MA, Harvard University Press, 1984.

Liebenau, J., *Medical Science and Medical Industry. The Formation of the American Pharmaceutical Industry*, Basingstoke, Macmillan, 1987.

Mann, R. D., *Modern Drug Use: an Enquiry on Historical Principles*, Lancaster, MTP Press, 1984.

Manske, R. H. F. and Holmes, H. L. (eds), *The Alkaloids. Chemistry and Physiology*, New York, Academic Press, 1958. 35 vols pub. by 1989, ed. by A. Brossi).

Matthews, L. G., *History of Pharmacy in Britain*, Edinburgh, Livingstone, 1962.

Moberg, C. J. and Cohn, Z. A. (eds), *Launching the antibiotic era: personal accounts of the discovery and use of the first antibiotics*, New York, The Rockefeller University Press, 1990.

Parascandola, J., *The development of American pharmacology: John J. Abel and the shaping of a discipline*, Baltimore and London, Johns Hopkins University Press, 1992.

Parascandola, J. and Kenney, E., *Sources in the History of American Pharmacology*, Madison, WI, American Institute of the History of Pharmacy, 1983.

Parish, H. J., *A History of Immunization*, Edinburgh, Livingstone, 1965.

Paton, W. D. M., 'The early days of pharmacology', in F. N. L. Poynter (ed.), *Chemistry in the Service of Medicine*, London, Pitman, 1961.

Sneader, W., *Drug Discovery: the Evolution of Modern Medicines*, Chichester, Wiley, 1985.

Swann, J. P., *Academic Scientists and the Pharmaceutical Industry*, Baltimore, MD, and London, Johns Hopkins University Press, 1988.

Weatherall, M., *In Search of a Cure*, Oxford, Oxford University Press, 1990.

Wootton, A. C., *Chronicles of Pharmacy*, 2 vols, London, Macmillan, 1910.

40

PHYSICAL METHODS

Harold J. Cook

Physical methods might be loosely defined as therapeutic methods for relieving somatic ills without surgical intervention or the administration of medicines. Such methods of treatment have been among the most important ways of relieving bodily pains, especially before the most recent historical epoch. Physical methods have been used not only for the relief of ills, but also for their prevention. The person who underwent the use of physical methods need not be sick at all.

But there are many problems with even so general a definition. The most basic problem stems from deciding where to draw the lines between physical methods and surgical and medicinal therapies. For instance, while bloodletting (also known as phlebotomy or venesection) will be considered below (pp. 940 ff.), it might also be considered a surgical method, since it required the use of a knife. Equally, when patients 'took the waters', they sometimes drank them for their medicinal properties as well as bathed in them. Then too, it would be wrong to ignore the often non-'scientific' reasons for using physical methods: bathing might be done to purify a person's being as much as to wash the body; while rubbing and stroking to drive out pains might be performed by someone who was assumed to have inherent healing powers rather than merely understanding the techniques of massage. Clearly, the range of the human experience of the body and the variety of the ways people have tried to achieve a state of well-being cannot be readily made to fit a neat set of intellectual categories.

Nevertheless, despite these problems of definition and the almost endless range of physical methods, several major and many minor topics need consideration and explanation. The major topics include dietetics and regimen, and bloodletting. Among the other topics are bathing, gymnastics, touching, stroking, and massage. Many of these methods had ritualistic and religious as well as medical or scientific origins and explanations. It can be said, though, that those who engaged in such methods ordinarily assumed to a greater or lesser degree that the body needs to be kept 'in tune', 'in harmony', or 'in balance'. It might help to pursue one or more of these physical methods to stay in balance and so prevent disease; once diseased, a person might seek physical treatment in order to be returned to a state of balance. In short, while physical methods might be interventionist or manipulative, they did not try to change the nature of a person or attack a disease entity so much as to maintain someone in or restore someone to a state of harmony.

DIETETICS AND BLOODLETTING

Long before the ancient Greeks, and throughout the world, various kinds of physical methods were used. Two of the most important have been dietetics and bloodletting. Bloodletting is reported as a practice among many people still. (➤ Ch. 60 Medicine and anthropology) As the stuff of life, blood often had (and has) ritualistic associations such as the sealing of an association of 'blood-brothers', blood sacrifice of animals or other people, and Faust's pact with the devil written in his own blood. Controlling the special properties of the 'life-blood' itself, including letting some of it out of the body, has appealed to many people as an important way of ordering one's harmony with the world. Equally, rules of diet have concerned almost every group. What a person raised in one culture understands as good and even tasty nourishment may be seen by someone raised in another group as bad or unwholesome. Some of these attitudes toward food and drink are taken in from the society in which people are raised, others may be explicitly set down (like those in Leviticus), others may be self-consciously adopted for reasons of personal conviction (such as modern vegetarianism), and still others may be practised during special periods (such as fasting before certain ceremonies). It would be wrong to divide clearly the 'medical' from what one can only call the religious purposes of such rules. (➤ Ch. 61 Religion and medicine) As with bloodletting, regulating the diet may be thought to be even more important for prophylaxis than for therapeutics. But the Greeks meant more by 'diet' than simply the kind of food and drink taken in: the Greek word *diatia* meant a way of life. Dietetics therefore concerned not only food and drink, but exercise and other matters of daily life that could be regulated. For many Greeks, living according to a 'diet' or regimen appropriate to each person meant to maintain or restore balance (*krasis*), the foundation of health.

THE ANCIENT GREEKS AND ROMANS

Several physical methods are described in the oldest Greek medical texts, most of which were written between about 430 and 330 BC. These are the Hippocratic works, ascribed to the renowned physician Hippocrates (*c.*450–370 BC). Among many of them, dietetic regimen takes a very prominent place. One of the longest Hippocratic texts is now simply entitled *Regimen*, and it includes practical advice on how to live according to one's geography, climate, foods and drinks, baths, emetics, sleep, and exercise, arguing that eating and exercising are the two most important matters that need to be kept in balance. (➤ Ch. 14 Humoralism) Its concluding sentence emphasizes the preventative as well as curative nature of regimen: 'By following the instructions I have given [on regimen], one may live a healthy life.' Another important Hippocratic text, *Regimen in Acute Diseases*, explains the use of regimen – especially food and drink – to treat pleurisy, pneumonia, brain-fever, and continual fever; and one of the strongest statements in ancient medicine about the importance of dietetics is the Hippocratic treatise *Ancient Medicine*. Clearly, the ancient Greeks considered *diatia* or regimen to be the foundation-stone for the maintenance of health, and one of the primary instruments for its restoration.

Even the strangest of diseases could be treated by regimen. The well-known Hippocratic work *Sacred Disease* (which deals with a condition that may have been epilepsy) argues that the disease could be prevented by controlling the regimen of the affected person. It describes the cause of the disease not in terms of mysterious or divine antecedents, but in terms of blocked physiological functions of the body. The motions of phlegm, in particular, were of concern to the author. The treatise concludes:

> This so-called 'sacred disease' is due to the same causes as all other diseases, to the things we see come and go, the cold and sun too, the changing and inconstant winds. . . . A man with the knowledge of how to produce by means of a regimen dryness and moisture, cold and heat in the human body, could cure this disease too provided that he could distinguish the right moment for the application of remedies. He would not need to resort to purifications and magic spells.[1]

The author's faith that the causes of this most mysterious of diseases could be understood through a knowledge of nature rather than the supernatural is remarkable. But just as remarkable is the faith in regimen as a way of regulating a sufferer's constitution in order to prevent the disease from recurring. By altering the four qualities (hot, cold, wet, and dry) at just the right moment, a person who knew about nature could prevent the disease.

By discussing the qualities, the author of the *Sacred Disease* touched on a set of ideas becoming increasingly popular in the Hellenic world. The general principles of physiological theory were not the same in all the Hippocratic treatises, and indeed, the author of *Ancient Medicine* argued against the easy adoption of them. But as people codified them later, they were simple enough, although the details involved difficult philosophical niceties. The elements of nature were four: earth, air, fire, and water; and each of these consisted of a combination of two of the four qualities: hot, cold, wet, and dry. Accordingly, everyone's temperament or constitution could be analysed in terms of how it combined the four humours (blood, phlegm, black bile, and yellow bile), each of which also combined two of the four qualities. Phlegm was cold and wet. Since excess phlegm generated in the brain and blocked from running off to lower parts of the body caused the symptoms of epilepsy, using regimen to dry and warm the body at the appropriate moment would prevent the formation of excess phlegm and so the disease. (➤ Ch. 7 The physiological tradition)

If necessary, other physical methods could be employed to remove the causes of disease. Among them were steps to restore humoural balance by removing excesses. One of the main methods for removing excess was to remove blood – one of the four humours, but a medium that also contained the other humours. Letting blood could therefore be used both to remove a general surplus (*plethora*) and to lower the amount of the humour, blood. Like regimen, phlebotomy could be used prophylactically as well as therapeutically. Bloodletting was known to the ancient Egyptians and Mesopotamians (and other peoples throughout the world) as well as to the Hippocratics. But while the Hippocratic texts mention bloodletting on several occasions, there seems to have been no widespread urge to use it extensively, nor to prefer it to other methods.

While the Hippocratic authors did not systematically develop physiological theories to promote physical methods over other means of prophylaxis or treatment, several authors of the Hellenistic period (after the rise of Alexander the Great, *c.*330 BC) did. Many of the ancient medical systematists continued to stress physical methods as the best means of preserving health and treating disease, to the extent that some people even felt compelled to defend the use of drugs at all (that is, non-physical methods).[2] Among the most important authors of this period were Erasistratus (*c.*325–*c.*250 BC) and Herophilus (*c.*335–*c.* 250 BC), both associated with Alexandria (although Erasistratus may have been at Antioch). Each of these noted rationalists developed a rich system of rational physiology that underpinned their use of physical methods.

Erasistratus began to develop physiological theories based upon a growing knowledge of anatomy, theories that supported his main interest: medical practice. (➤ Ch. 5 The anatomical tradition) One of the most important principles of regimen that he, like his predecessors, stressed, was habit. People should follow the ways of life and diets to which they had become accustomed. The remaining fragments of Erasistratus's writings so stress the use of regimen to prevent and treat diseases that Galen (AD 129–*c.*200/210) later held him not to have used bloodletting at all.[3] For Erasistratus, many diseases had their causes in plethoras, or an overabundance of nourishment in the blood. If the nutriment is not digested according to how each person is accustomed, or if matter is not excreted as appropriate, then the vessels of the body would become too full and cease being capable of fulfilling their functions. He preferred to reduce a plethora of blood by moderately increased exercise, sweats, drying in a vapour-bath, reducing the amount of food, eating foods that could easily be excreted, and vomiting. Herophilus, however, advocated bloodletting. This excellent anatomist also advocated physical methods such as regulating exercise, food and drink for both prophylaxis and treatment, but he also used phlebotomy. He thought the removal of blood from the body could be more efficacious than a lowered diet in the treatment of plethoras.[4]

The use of both regimen and bloodletting became a major feature of Hellenistic and then Roman medicine. Debates about the efficacy of each continued. The growing use among the Greeks of phlebotomy in many illnesses meant that one of the first Greek physicians to practise in Rome, Archagathus (*c.*220 BC) acquired a quite bloodthirsty reputation. Other physicians voiced their concern that in phlebotomy, removing a therapeutically useful amount of blood would be too close to a dangerous amount of blood. But both regimen and phlebotomy gained great support from the great medical systematizer, Galen. For Galen, anatomy, physiology, and treatment went together in a rational system, which he developed so well (despite some internal contradictions) that it became the foundation for rational medicine for 1,500 years.

Galen's views are complicated, set out in numerous and voluminous works, and not always consistent. To simplify, however, he strongly advocated the view that for health one needed to be in balance, having an appropriate mixture of four humours just right for each person. Like most other philosophers, he believed in an active and purposeful nature, which operated in the body through various 'faculties' or powers (*dynameis*). The main philosophical questions pertaining to living organisms had to do with how beings come into existence, how they grow, and how they maintain life. For ordinary physiology, answers to the latter problem – that of nutrition – provided the focus of rational and investigative inquiry. The living, working body needed its parts replenished, just as a fire needs continuous fuel; and it needed ways to get rid of the residue. Intake and output therefore came in for close attention. Food was concocted (cooked) into chyle in the stomach; the chyle was further concocted and imbued with the nutritive faculty in the liver to become raw (venous) blood, which provided the main source of nutrition. Some of the venous blood reached the heart, where it became further digested and imbued with vital faculty to become arterial blood, which provided the animal spirits supplying heat and the ability to respond to reason. Some of the arterial blood was yet further concocted and imbued with the rational faculty in the brain to become nervous fluid (or psychic *pneuma*), providing sensation, voluntary motion, and all the aspects of thought. The body also had various eliminative faculties. Problems might occur when the digestive tracts became blocked, when superfluous matter was not properly evacuated, when foods containing qualities not proper for the person's temperament had been ingested, when organs ceased to function properly, and so on. Because Galen's physiology centred upon a theory of progressive stages of digestion, it placed much emphasis on food and drink, exercise, the evacuations of the body, the perturbations of mind, and, in general, the way of life.[5] Like other contemporaries, then, Galen advocated the use of prophylactic and therapeutic regimen to maintain or restore balance.

Among the physical methods Galen used, however, he may be best known for his use of reasoned arguments in favour of bloodletting. He wrote that 'the most accurate and balanced evacuation of humours is effected by venesection. Next ranges incising of the skin near the ankles, exercises, friction [massage], bathing and fasting.' Because he thought many diseases (especially fevers) were caused by a general plethora or an over-abundance of a single humour (*cacochymia*), he thought that they could be prevented or treated by removing blood. (➤ Ch. 19 Fevers) Blood might be let from the arteries (arteriotomy), which relieved the overheated blood coming directly from the heart; or, more commonly, it could be let from the veins (venesection). Arteriotomy needed to be done very cautiously, but venesection could be done more readily and copiously. Galen also gave further explanation to the two major techniques of 'revulsion' and 'derivation'. The first drew blood from a place away from the part of the body most affected, the second drew blood from nearby.[6] (➤ Ch. 41 Surgery (traditional))

To understand Galen's rationales and techniques, an analogy common among the ancients is helpful. Ignoring the other parts of Galen's physiological system and concentrating on the crucial issue of nutriment flowing into the veins, one can picture a water-source flowing into a set of interconnected ditches. The water flows into the ditches, drawn on by the absorbent power of the earth. When more water flows into the system than is being absorbed, however, a general plethora occurs, threatening to swamp the whole area. To relieve such a situation, breaking a ditch at one place that can be quickly repaired (cutting a vein) is most useful to draw off the excess fluid; reducing the flow of fluid into the system (a lowered diet) or heightening the absorptive need of the earth (a higher rate of exercise) will remedy the situation more slowly but perhaps avoid a catastrophic failure. If the ground is saturated in one place alone, making a breech nearby (using derivation) is most sensible;

on the other hand, if too much water is flowing toward one part, making a breech on the other side of the system (using revulsion) will draw off the fluid to that other area. Moreover, in the Galenic system, various arteries and veins were connected to different organs, so that drawing blood from them would draw it away from the organ they fed. For liver problems, for example, the vein in the right hand would be let; for the spleen, the vein in the left hand.[7]

Galen thought that the more serious the illness, the more blood needed to be let, and that in general complaints like fevers, copious amounts might be called for. However, blood should never be let during a crisis (a turning-point in a disease), and the amount taken needed to be closely regulated according to the season, climate, age and gender, and other indications. In some cases, as when the peripheral veins were clogged by heavy humours, venesection proved inadequate, and other physical methods such as scarification, cupping, blistering, purging, vomiting, and sweating were called for. Nevertheless, Galen's reasoned arguments in favour of bloodletting in many kinds of illness and in large amounts made bloodletting a sign of Galenic medicine for many centuries to come. His general views indicate how much importance he placed on maintaining or restoring a physiological balance using a rational analysis of the functions of the parts of the body to determine treatment properly.

THE ANCIENT LEGACY

The wide popularity of phlebotomy in the late antique world is attested by the adoption of rules on bloodletting among many people of the Empire, often in conjunction with numerological or astrological assumptions. For instance, the Jewish Talmud (AD c.200–500) spelled out a series of rules to govern bloodletting. According to the Talmud, Sundays, Wednesdays, and Fridays were favourable days for bloodletting, with Mondays, Tuesdays, and Thursdays unfavourable (and the Sabbath was out). Moreover, Wednesdays that were the fourth, fourteenth, or twenty-fourth days of the month, or too late in the month to be followed by four more days, were dangerous, while bloodletting on the first and second days of the month caused weakness. Taking blood from someone on the third day of the month or on the eve of Shavuot (Christian Pentecost) and all religious festivals would bring danger; and phlebotomy should not be performed on cloudy days or days when the south wind blew.[8] Similar rules on venesection, often with detailed astrological signs or, for Christians, lists of appropriate saints' days, could be found among many people of the Mediterranean region.

The greatest rationalists and systematists of classical medicine, the Islamic authors, also continued to advocate the use of bloodletting and dietetics.

945

(➤ Ch. 31 Arab-Islamic medicine) They extracted from a variety of ancient authors a general theory of physiology and, related to it, a general theory of medicine that placed great weight on physical methods. The scholastic medicine developed by the Islamic authors and adapted by the Latin West placed special emphasis on regulating the non-naturals. These were six (occasionally seven) in number: air, food and drink, exercise and rest, states of sleep and wakefulness, evacuations and retentions (of such things as semen, menstrual blood, urine, and faeces), and affections of the mind. The faith in the ability of learned persons to offer reasoned advice on how each of these non-naturals should be regulated so as to maintain a humoural balance became the foundation-stone of learned medicine.

For instance, the great theorist Avicenna (980–1037) believed that even medical practice was a rational science (that is, it held certainty) because it was rooted in an understanding of the principles of nature.

> The practice of medicine is *not the work* which the physician carries out, *but is* that branch of *medical knowledge* which, when acquired, enables one to form an opinion upon which to base the proper plan of treatment. . . . Once the purpose of each aspect of medicine is understood, you can become skilled in both theoretical and applied knowledge, even though there should never come a call for you to exercise your knowledge.[9]

The practice of physic, then, concerned the ability to move intellectually from certain knowledge to opinion based upon an understanding of how nature operated: to associate the universal and the particular. The physician ideally did this based upon skill in philosophy rather than upon clinical experience, so that no patient needed to be seen in order to practise. Keeping someone in harmony with nature through advice on regimen rooted in natural philosophy was the epitome of rational medicine.

Yet another aspect of Islamic rational medicine was the continued use of bloodletting, especially in fevers, through revulsion and in conservative quantities. While physicians prescribed phlebotomy and sometimes carried it out, the practice was so popular that a group of professional venesectors also came into being.[10]

When Islamic theories became known in the Latin-speaking lands of Europe, some of the first medical works to gain popularity were works of regimen and phlebotomy. Among the former, the *Regimen Sanitatis* of Salerno became one of the best-known medical works of the medieval and early modern periods, going through many manuscript versions and printed editions. Salerno, a cosmopolitan town in southern Italy, became known as a centre of medical teaching in the eleventh and twelfth centuries. The poem giving advice on regimen probably had its origin in the twelfth century, a period when many Islamic medical works were being translated into Latin.

Its main purpose was to instruct the auditor on how to live an orderly and thus a healthy life, with most of the advice centred on diet: when to eat or not to eat certain things according to season and constitution, based upon a rational account of physiology and the non-naturals. For instance, in the early seventeenth-century English translation of Sir John Harington (1561–1612):

> Although you may drink often while you dine,
> Yet after dinner touch not once the cup,. . . .
> To close your stomach well, this order suits,
> Cheese after flesh, Nuts after fish or fruits.

The poem also offers advice on treatment of illness, again stressing physical methods:

> As diet, drink, hot baths, whence sweat is growing,
> With purging, vomiting, and letting blood:
> Which taken in due time, not overflowing,
> Each malady's infection is withstood.
> The last of these is best, if skill and reason,
> Respect age, strength, quantity, and season.
> Of seventy from seventeen, if blood abound,
> The opening of a vein is healthful found.[11]

The poem continues with an account of the various benefits of venesection, before giving explicit instructions on how to do it, and what days to avoid. Similar rules on the use of diet and phlebotomy became widespread in Europe after the eleventh century, as the rational medicine of the Islamic physicians was taken up among the Latins.

The high science of regimen in the Latin-speaking West is best exemplified in the practice of granting *consilia*. A learned physician might write a *consilium* (an often lengthy piece of written dietetic and medical advice) for a particular person. It took into account all the details of someone's constitution and social and physical surroundings, and then gave written recommendations on the non-naturals so as to preserve or restore health. It sometimes went on to recommend some medicinal treatment. Some of the most learned physicians, like Ugo Benzi (1376–1439), had their *consilia* collected together as manuscript works on medicine. The written form not only made a physician's learning available to other consultants and the client, it also gave the physician the opportunity to study books in order to bring to bear all the wisdom of the most respected learned writers.

Learned physicians in Europe also continued to recommend phlebotomy, although they sometimes complained that the actual cutting of veins had become something performed by the barbers rather than the physicians. The learned Latins also tended to follow the learned Arabic-speaking physicians in being moderate in their use of bloodletting and in adopting Islamic ideas about how and when to prescribe it. Good and bad days for venesection were sometimes chosen according to saints' days, astrological assumptions, the constitution of the patient, his or her state of health, or learned physiology. A detailed lore about which vein to open for various purposes also existed, with some verses being composed to aid memory.[12] For instance, one learned treatise explained that for an ephemeral fever, the cephalic vein in the right arm should be let in the summer, the same vein in the left arm in the winter.[13] By the later medieval period, too, many manuscripts contained illustrations pointing out the veins and which ones to open in which conditions, detailing how to diagnose according to the colour and consistency of the blood taken, and so forth.[14] It became common for many people to have regular lettings of blood (especially in the spring and autumn) in order to prevent disease.

The tradition of giving prophylactic and therapeutic regimen and phlebotomy continued from the late Middle Ages into the early modern period, but was expanded through the new medium of printing to widen the advice for all. Many medical works printed in vernacular languages as well as in Latin gave instructions about bloodletting. Even the cheap little almanacs intended for a popular audience frequently contained woodcuts of the 'vein man' showing the sites from which to let blood, alongside astrological instructions on timing. Many books containing medical advice made regimen and dietetics based upon the non-naturals central to their instruction. Most of these medical works amounted to something like *consilia*, with this difference: readers had to make their own judgements about their constitutions before going on to see what advice would therefore be appropriate to them. For instance, early in the sixteenth century, Andrewe Boorde (b. 1490), a physician and former monk, offered his *Compendyous Regyment or a Dyetary of Healthe* (1547) as a testament to the Duke of Norfolk, but also as a general set of rules that might benefit many well-to-do readers. The rules began with where to situate a house, how to plan and construct it, how to organize a household, what to eat and drink and what to avoid, and what exercise to take, before moving on to more detailed physical methods of preserving and restoring health.

THE DECLINE AND RISE OF DIETETICS AND BLOODLETTING

The use of both regimen and phlebotomy suffered serious intellectual blows in the sixteenth and seventeenth centuries, however. On the one hand, the recovery of many ancient medical texts by the humanists made it clear that the 'Arab' medicine adapted by the Latins differed in some ways from Galen's recommendations. Pierre Brissot (1478–1522), working in Paris, took up what he considered to be Galen's methods in an epidemic of pleurisy in 1514, bleeding patients copiously and without regard to left or right. This caused a stir, which was excited still further when Brissot took his methods to Portugal, and in 1518 again had success with his treatments, provoking a polemical attack from one of the royal physicians. When Brissot's reply gained posthumous publication in 1525, the issue was joined, dividing the classical physicians from the 'arabists'.[15]

Moreover, intellectual attacks from several directions undermined the rationale for many physical methods. Since physical methods like bloodletting and regimen were rationally defended in terms of certain principles of nature and physiological theories (such as the four elements and active faculties), attacks on those theories caused the prophylactic and therapeutic uses of the methods to be called into question. Moreover, the discovery of the circulation of the blood by William Harvey (1578–1657) undercut accepted Galenic ideas of nutrition. While Harvey remained convinced that many problems could be caused by plethoras, so that phlebotomy was useful, and while he himself never attacked regimen, the larger implications of his theory were to call into doubt the intellectual principles behind both.[16] Perhaps even more importantly, those who adopted the non-academic theories of medical chemistry often rejected bloodletting and other physical methods wholesale in favour of treating disease through the use of chemical medicines. (➤ Ch. 40 Drug therapies) For example, Joan Baptista van Helmont (1577–1644) rejected the idea that a plethora of blood could cause disease, since he equated blood with the vital strength itself: according to his view, someone with a large quantity of blood would be stronger than someone with less.[17]

Dietetics therefore underwent significant changes in the later seventeenth century. The essence of regimen and dietetics – advice tailored for one person's constitution, which might not be good advice for anyone else – gradually disappeared, to be replaced by universal advice, good for anyone. Manuals of popular medicine continued to stress prophylactic and therapeutic regimen. But such handbooks increasingly offered rules of life for anyone to follow, rather than those tailored for particular constitutions. A science of medicine rooted in universalities rather than individual differences came to mark Western medicine. The practice of changing location to take advantage of the climate best suited for particular conditions continues to be popular, general exercise has reappeared as a prophylactic against various ills, and the science of nutrition has developed apace. But all these practices are built upon general rules, and so differ from the learned art of individualistic dietetics. (➤ Ch. 15 Environment and miasmata; Ch. 18 The ecology of disease)

In regions of Europe where iatrochemistry flourished – in the north, especially – people also tended to abandon bloodletting. The English physician Walter Harris (1647–1732) commented of the Dutch that they let blood so little and so infrequently, that they had 'an extremity of bleeding little'.[18] In England, the seventeenth century saw some notorious quarrels over the efficacy of bloodletting; and during the eighteenth century, the practice gradually declined, until early in the nineteenth century, when it was revived because of its efficacy in treating tropical fevers. Benjamin Rush (1745–1813) became notorious in the United States for advocating copious bloodletting, probably based on the same experience of tropical fevers.[19] (➤ Ch. 24 Tropical diseases) Venesection also became the focus of a vigorous debate in Edinburgh in the middle of the nineteenth century.[20]

In France, the physicians of court and university continued to let blood often and in large amounts. When the West German aristocrat Liselotte von der Pfalz (1652–1722), married into the French dynasty in the later seventeenth century, she was shocked by the frequent and copious phlebotomy of the Parisian court physicians.[21] At the beginning of the nineteenth century, François Joseph Victor Broussais (1772–1838), a military physician and leading figure of the Paris school, argued that all diseases took their origin from inflammation, and that bloodletting served as the best anti-inflammatory: he was said to have used 100,000 leeches per year in his hospital practice. One of his students, however, Pierre Louis (1781–1872), did statistical studies on hospital patients (published as *Recherches sur les Effets de la Saignée*, 1835) to show that phlebotomy was not beneficial in all diseases.

By the later nineteenth century, because of new physiological and pathological theories, the practice of phlebotomy seemed to be discarded throughout Western medicine. But it underwent another brief resurgence at the turn of the twentieth century,[22] and is even indicated in the 1990s in certain illnesses.[23] Advice about regimen grew to be increasingly focused on food. In a period marked by the great wealth and great poverty of the nineteenth and early twentieth centuries, great multi-course meals and the bodily bulk that came from them signified high status and good health. The development of a science of nutrition and metabolism at the same time focused on how the absence of certain kinds of food could cause disease. During the 1880s, various researches showed that small quantities of certain foods could prevent physiological problems; by 1911, the term 'vitamin' had been coined to denote the missing factor in certain foods that brought on diseases like beriberi: vitamins A, B, and C were isolated or postulated in 1913; cod-liver oil became a popular supplement to diets, and from it vitamin D was identified. (➤ Ch. 22 Nutritional diseases) Medical advice on eating mixed diets of carbohydrates, proteins, and vegetables undoubtedly promoted good health in many people. Since the mid-twentieth century, however, nutritional advice has increasingly concentrated on eliminating from diet unwanted substances. As wealth has come to be signified in slim and trim bodies, dangers to health have been identified in fatty foods leading to excess of certain cholesterols, possibly leading to heart attacks; in too much salt, and so high blood pressure; in sugar and consequent frantic behaviours or dangerous blood-sugar levels; in chemicals that may promote cancers; and so on. The sciences of nutrition, physiology, and oncology have made the choices about what to eat (among those with sufficient disposable incomes) sometimes difficult. But this modern focus on diet as limiting food intake is far from ancient ideas about dietetics as a healthy way of life.

WATER-BATHING

The use of water-bathing shows a history similar to those of phlebotomy and dietetics: late antique medical theory placed a firm foundation under a practice already in use; it was continued through the early modern period; the new learning and iatrochemistry of the sixteenth and seventeenth centuries challenged various rationales for it; and it then underwent important transformations in the last two hundred years as medical theories and popular views put down new roots. (➤ Ch. 28 Unorthodox medical theories)

Water has a long tradition of use in rites of religious purification as well as in personal hygiene. Water is not only essential for life; it is associated with life-threatening storms and the mysteries of travel by water. Where it emerges from the ground in springs, it has associations with the chthonic. The Jewish bath cleansed people after certain occasions, such as giving birth, before they could be readmitted to the community; Christian baptism by water signified spiritual purification. Many Greek cults, too – like that of the healing god, Asclepius – urged not only the offering of sacrifices but bathing in water before approaching the god.[24] The Greeks and Romans therefore often built large baths into their temple complexes. (➤ Ch. 53 History of personal hygiene)

PUBLIC BATHS

The Greeks and Romans, especially the latter, also built public baths for hygienic reasons. Together with the application of oils, the use of water in warm or cold baths became a frequent feature of bodily care after exercise. Wherever the Romans built a town, they built a bath, often taking over the site of a spring used for religious purposes by the previous occupants. By the first century BC, they were building baths of great complexity for the use of the urban population. The bath at Pompeii, for instance, had a series of large rooms for men, and some smaller rooms for women. The bather entered into a room to undress, and then proceeded to a warm room. After a while, the visitor entered a hot and steamy room. In this sauna bath, people used metal strigils to scrape off the sweat and grime. The men then had access to a large water-bath in which they could immerse themselves. At the bath, Romans would exercise and socialize, and get medical and dietetic advice, manicures, and massages. Aristocrats built villas in the neighbourhood of rural baths and spas. The specific qualities of the waters of various sites gained reputations for being especially helpful in certain kinds of diseases. Bathing in warm or cold waters could help balance the cold, hot, wet, and dry qualities, or soften or strengthen the constitution. The latter idea made bathing particularly important among the sect of methodist physicians. Cold water might also be recommended as a medicinal drink in certain regimens. As the best summary of the use of waters among the Greeks and Romans concludes: 'water was frequently, widely, and enduringly used in classical medicine'.[25]

After the fall of Rome, many Roman public baths fell into disrepair, but the Middle Ages was hardly the 'thousand years without a bath' that some have claimed. The rules of life for monks included bathing in cold or occasionally warm water several times a year (together with tonsuring). A few municipal baths continued to be used by other people after Roman occupation, while holy wells and springs drew the faithful desiring relief from physical suffering. Many towns formerly settled by Romans kept up or built public baths where whole families might go to soak and play. These medieval baths offered hot water and steam rather than cold water or medicinal water to drink. Bath-houses also sometimes acquired a reputation for lewdness, since men and women were not always kept apart. As issues of public morality became increasingly sensitive during the Reformation and Counter-Reformation, many town leaders felt compelled to close the public baths, although in places like London proposals were put forward in the seventeenth century to rebuild them.

At the same time, however, the revival of ancient medical doctrines emphasized that the ancients had recommended bathing as the best treatment for certain kinds of illnesses. Many learned people in the sixteenth century therefore began to seek out medicinal baths supplied by springs: Michel de Montaigne (1533–92), for instance, travelled to Italy to seek relief in the baths for the pains of his bladder-stone. While he encountered few baths and spas ready to accommodate the traveller in comfort, within a few decades many places throughout Europe began to restore the ancient foundations and to construct new facilities for the well-to-do visitors.[26] The building activity around spring-fed baths became so great that the main character in the seventeenth-century novel *Simplicissimus* discovers a spring and immediately imagines the riches he could acquire by attracting people to it for its health-giving benefits.[27] By the eighteenth century, many spas had become fashionable resorts; it was at Bath in England that the first casino came into being. Public baths also reappeared in many cities later in the seventeenth century, although they were operated by private proprietors, and often became notorious as places of licentious behaviour.

In the later sixteenth and the seventeenth centuries, however, the development of iatrochemistry gave new meaning to 'taking the waters'. Increasing weight came to be placed on imbibing the waters, as an accompaniment to immersion – or even as an alternative. As iatrochemical practitioners increasingly turned their attentions to specific diseases and specific treatments, they tended to investigate the special medicinal properties thought to be contained in certain waters rather than their general physical benefits. That is, the waters of many baths and spas (the tastes and smells of which clearly differed from one another) contained therapeutic properties which, if drunk, could fight certain conditions even better than by immersion. ($\blacktriangleright$ Ch. 8 The biochemical tradition) From the late sixteenth century, many waters came in for chemical analysis, as the proponents of one place promoted its benefits over those of all others. Some people began to bottle and market special waters; others, like Nehemiah Grew (1641–1712), used the latest techniques to extract the special medicinal substance from the waters in order to sell the 'salts'.[28] Many people remain of the opinion that drinking certain mineral waters is medicinally beneficial.

By the middle of the nineteenth century, the steam railroad and steamship made the great baths and spas easier to get to and so more popular than ever. Places like Bath, Baden-Baden, Aix-les-Bains, Bad Ischl, Karlsbad, and Hot Springs remained popular among the well-to-do until the early twentieth century: or rather, they used to be popular among the English-speakers, and today remain a well-respected part of the medical armamentarium elsewhere. But as each special water developed its own proponents arguing for its unique properties, and as each place developed its own special (and sometimes unseemly) social atmosphere, attempts to use plain cold-water treatments in universally beneficial physical therapies began to come to light. Among the most popular was the system developed by Vincent Priessnitz (1799–1851), born in Austrian Silesia. His system forbade the use of drugs, urging instead exercise, coarse diet, and the use of cold water inside and out, on the premise that water purifies the blood. He advocated an elaborate system of wrapping the patient in wet sheets, giving injections of water, shower-baths, and other physical therapies. When in 1838 the imperial court sent Baron Turkheim to inspect his practice, it received a very favourable report, which brought Priessnitz's hydrotherapy into widespread use throughout Europe. Variants on hydropathy, like kneipping, developed by Father Sebastian Kneipp (1821–97), spread widely. In England, James Wilson (1807–67) and James Gully (1808–81) established a fashionable treatment centre at Malvern that specialized in hydrotherapy, where people including Darwin, Tennyson, and Carlyle took cures.[29]

PRIVATE BATHING

The use of the small bath is also very old, reaching back to the Minoans. The Greeks and Romans preferred public to private baths, although wealthy people might luxuriate in their own private warm-water bath – a practice sometimes condemned by moralists. Medieval people, too, sometimes bathed the body in hot water (as well as washing their hands in cold water before each meal, daily washing of their teeth and face, and somewhat less often their hair and feet). When doing so, they often put herbs or flower petals in the water to make it more pleasant and sometimes to increase its medicinal effects. It is said that King John of England (r. 1199–1216) bathed his body every three weeks.[30] When royalty, aristocrats, or the upper classes bathed, they often invited guests to share the tub – a sense of privacy about the body has been acquired in the West only recently. But without many servants to warm and carry the water, and to bail it out afterwards, the inconvenience of bathing was great. Moreover, by the seventeenth century, medical advice tended to condemn the warm-water bath: it was thought to weaken the constitution, as well as to open the pores wide, letting noxious airs into the body. At the same time, however, some physicians argued for the medical usefulness of the cold-water bath in many illnesses. By the later seventeenth century, too, princes began to install large baths for their own use in their palaces, sometimes with piped water heated by coal, and with drainage outlets.

The fashion for the private warm-water bath increased in the eighteenth century as notions of privacy and luxury became more allowable. Moreover, the improving supply of piped water and heating facilities brought into being a whole host of kinds of private baths in the early to mid-nineteenth century: the bidet, the steam-bath, the shower-bath, the sponge-bath, the hip-bath, the sitz-bath and, what we recognize today as 'the' bath, the lounge bath. Gas-fired boilers to supply warm water to private baths came into being in the mid-nineteenth century, as did the bathroom attached to increasing numbers of middle-class bedrooms. At the same time, baths came to be used not so much for helping to regulate the bodily humours, but to make the body clean: it was the early nineteenth century that popularized the phrase 'cleanliness is next to godliness', and saw the use of soap in the bath increase (formerly, people had rubbed the body with the hands or sponges). With the coming of the germ theory and general improvements in the supply of water to individual dwellings in the later nineteenth century, regular bathing as an important part of hygiene became common – so much so that at the present, personal hygiene has become almost synonymous with cleanliness rather than a healthy constitution.[31]

There have been important variants on water-bathing. Benjamin Franklin (1706–90) advocated fresh-air bathing, sitting unclothed in front of an open window each morning for a period of time, rubbing himself all over (just as people rubbed themselves in water-baths before the use of soap). An English contemporary, James Graham (1745–94), advocated sitting for long periods in earth or mud to restore the vital properties of the body. And by the middle of the eighteenth century, too, sea-bathing at Brighton had begun, on the assumption that salt water had good preservative properties against various ills. In bathing as in other treatments, then, as the intellectual foundations of classical physiology disappeared, a hodge-podge of other systems developed, with almost every practitioner proclaiming a special treatment.

RUBBING, MASSAGE, AND GYMNASTICS

Other physical methods have been many, and like bloodletting, dietetics, and bathing, have had both enduring popularity among orthodox healers and a long association with ritual. For instance, Galen mentioned rubbing (or friction) in conjunction with other physical methods to treat fevers. The art of massage and physical manipulation of the body had long been used before him for prophylaxis and treatment. Medical flagellation (therapeutic beating) gained increased attention in the seventeenth and eighteenth centuries, and long remained a therapy for the mentally ill. (➤ Ch. 21 Mental diseases) Bonesetters plied the countryside, not only setting bones, but exercising their art of physical manipulation.[32] With the development of the modern hospital, medical massage gained greater attention as a necessary nursing practice for keeping skin and muscle healthy during long periods in bed. (➤ Ch. 49 The hospital) These practices became the foundation for the modern science of physical therapy. Another group of medical practitioners who believed that physical manipulation held the key to maintaining and restoring health have developed into modern chiropractors.

In addition to people who artfully or aggressively rubbed, stroked, manipulated, and pummelled the body were those who possessed special spiritual properties that could cure the ill by touching or stroking. Even a faithful touch of Jesus's garment was said to heal, and thereafter the faithful sometimes sought somatic as well as spiritual relief in the Christian sacraments. On the other hand, it was believed that the touch of a dead person's hand or the rope with which one had been hanged might cure, too. Moreover, until the end of the seventeenth century, the French and English kings who maintained their sacerdotal claims to power touched those suffering from the king's evil (scrofula) in the hope of performing miraculous cures.[33] Not only God, saints, and kings could heal by their touch, so too could seventh sons and a host of other strokers. Perhaps the most famous of the strokers was the mid-seventeenth-century English-Irish gentleman Valentine Greatrakes

(1629–83), whose powers attracted the attention of the likes of Robert Boyle (1627–91).[34] But the healing touch remains important.

Gymnastics (or exercise) figures as an important part of ancient regimen. For the Greeks and Romans, a healthy body meant a body fit for use, and their statuary makes plain how they idealized the athletic body. Daily training in the gymnasium was common for males: the Greek gymnasium became a major place of resort for all sorts of activities, not least among them the education of the mind as well as the body. As an accepted part of regimen, exercise long remained an important preventive measure, and through late antiquity and the Middle Ages, moderate exercises like walking and riding were ordinarily suggested: immoderate exercise might be dangerous. Dancing and the exercise of arms called for more rigorous training to acquire skill and strengthen the body. But the notion that moderate exercise was essential to everyone's good health remained a commonplace through to the nineteenth century.

The modern development of medical gymnastics is usually associated with the 'Swedish gymnastics' of Pehr Henrik Ling (1776–1839) who, by the patronage of Charles XIII (r. 1809–18), opened the Central Institute of Gymnastics in Stockholm in 1813. Ling taught a theory of muscles, in which the motion produced by groups of agonist muscles were moderated by antagonist groups. Based on this theory, he developed a system of exercises in which a gymnast provided resistance for the exerciser, the resistance being designed to strengthen the body, as well as to make it healthier. But the idea of therapeutic exercise was developed most by another Swede, Jonas Gustaf Wilhelm Zander (1835–1920), who introduced 'mechanotherapy' in 1864, in which assistance and resistance could be provided through machines. The Zander machines were used to remedy physical ills, and the Zander institutes employed physicians. Physical therapy and rehabilitation gradually developed into medical specialities.[35] (➤ Ch. 55 The emergence of para-medical professions)

The Romantic movements of the nineteenth century also emphasized individuality and moral and physical fortitude, and Swedish exercise proliferated and diversified, with branches of physical theory like kinesitherapy taking root in the 1840s onwards. In an age of industry, mass warfare, and colonial adventures, Western national governments also wished to promote the physical fitness of their citizens. By the later nineteenth century, physical exercises were being promoted for both genders in school; outside the governmental system, private groups like the Boy Scouts and Young Men's Christian Association (YMCA) urged their programmes of muscular Christianity upon the world, while competitive sports began to develop professional leagues in which outstanding athletes stood as popular heroes and models of virtue worthy of emulation. The need for fit draftees in two world wars also focused governmental attention on the physical health of the public. During the Cold

War, in the USA a Presidential Commission on physical fitness again promoted bodily strength for the nation, but that was soon coupled with the voices of a few advocates of running and other vigorous exercises as health promoting. The 'jogging craze' soon spread widely, and has received a qualified blessing from medical researchers, who increasingly see exercise as helpful for many conditions, including the prevention of heart trouble. Whether the tyranny of the 'body beautiful', which is inducing millions to enter upon courses of rigorous physical training, will be so medically advantageous is questionable – but only time will tell. (➤ Ch. 4 Medical care)

CONCLUSION

Physical methods, then, have always been an important part of medical practice, for the prevention as well as treatment of illnesses. Various ritual practices and cultural attitudes have been at least as influential as medical theory for sustaining their use, but classical physiological theory, with its emphasis on health as the maintenance of balance and harmony with nature, provided a firm rationale for the prophylactic and therapeutic uses of dietetics, bloodletting, bathing, rubbing, exercise, and many other physical methods. As that theory came under attack from the sixteenth through nineteenth centuries, the use of physical methods continued, but became more centred upon general rules, good for anyone, rather than advice tailored for each person. As medicine in the nineteenth century became ever more focused on laboratory research, examining specific causes for specific diseases, many physical methods – which always had prevention even more than therapy as their goal – declined. For better or worse, the rise of holistic thinking in the later twentieth century may be the cause of a growing return to physical methods, but since the strong individualism of classical physical treatments, based upon humoralism, is unlikely to flourish in the foreseeable future, how the theory of prevention and treatment comes to be worked out with regard to physical methods will be a subject of much concern.

NOTES

1 'The sacred disease', in G. E. R. Lloyd (ed.), *Hippocratic Writings*, Harmondsworth, Pelican Classics, 1978, p. 251.
2 For example, see J. S. Hamilton, 'Scribonious Largus on the medical profession', *Bulletin of the History of Medicine*, 1986, 60: 209–16.
3 Wesley D. Smith, 'Erasistratus's dietetic medicine', *Bulleatin of the History of Medicine*, 1982, 56: 402–4; Peter Brain, 'Galen's book on venesection against the Erasistrateans in Rome', in Brain, *Galen on Bloodletting: a Study of the Origins, Development and Validity of his Opinions, with a Translation of the Three Works*, Cambridge, Cambridge University Press, 1986, pp. 38–66.

4   Heinrich von Staden, *Herophilus: the Art of Medicine in Early Alexandria: Edition, Translation and Essays*, Cambridge, Cambridge University Press, 1989, pp. 397–426.

5   For more information, see Owsei Temkin, *Galenism: Rise and Decline of a Medical Philosophy*, Ithaca, NY, Cornell University Press, 1973, pp. 10–50; Brain, op. cit. (n. 3), pp. 1–14; and Ch. 14: 'Humoralism' in this *Encyclopedia*.

6   Rudolph E. Siegel, 'Galen's concept of bloodletting in relation to his ideas on pulmonary blood flow and blood formation', in Allen G. Debus (ed.), *Science, Medicine and Society in the Renaissance: Essays to Honor Walter Pagel*, New York, Science History Publications, 1972, Vol. I, pp. 243–75, See p. 258.

7   Brain, op. cit. (n. 3), pp. 122–44; Joseph Bauer, *Geschichte der Aderlässe*, Munich, Werner Fritasch, 1666, pp. 68–76.

8   David L. Cowen, 'A late medieval Yiddish manuscript on bloodletting', *Clio Medica*, 1975, 10: 267–76.

9   Avicenna, *Canon*, trans. by O. Cameron Grüner, modified by Michael McVaugh, in Edward Grant (ed.), *A Source Book in Medieval Science*, Cambridge, MA, Harvard University Press, 1974, p. 716, emphasis added.

10 Bauer, op. cit. (n. 7), pp. 95–109; Ghada Karmi, 'State control of the physician in the Middle Ages: an Islamic model', in Andrew Russell (ed.), *The Town and State Physician in Europe from the Middle Ages to the Enlightenment*, Wolfenbüttel, Herzog August Bibliothek, 1981, p. 74.

11 John Harington, *The School of Salernum: Regimen Sanitatis Salernitanum*, Salerno, Ente Provinciale per il Turismo, [1966], pp. 40, 83.

12 For example, Charles F. Mayer, 'A medical leechbook and its fourteenth-century poem on bloodletting', *Bulletin of the History of Medicine*, 1939, 7: 381–9.

13 Linda Voigts and Michael R. McVaugh (eds), *A Latin Technical Phlebotomy and its Middle English Translation, Transaction of the American Philosophical Society*, 1984, Vol. LXXII Part 2, 1984, p. 41; see also pp. 1–7 for a fine brief summary of medieval phlebotomy.

14 Peter Murray Jones, *Medieval Medical Miniatures*, London, British Museum, 1984, pp. 119–24.

15 John B. de C. M. Saunders and Charles Donald O'Malley (eds), *Andreas Vesalius Bruxellensis: the Bloodletting Letter of 1539: an Annotated Translation and Study of the Evolution of Vesalius's Scientific Development*, New York, Henry Schuman, 1947.

16 See esp. Jerome J. Bylebyl, 'Nutrition, quantification and circulation', *Bulletin of the History of Medicine*, 1977, 51: 369–85; Bylebyl, 'The medical side of Harvey's discovery: the normal and the abnormal', in Bylebyl (ed.), *William Harvey and his Age*, Baltimore, MD, Johns Hopkins University Press, 1979.

17 Peter H. Niebyl, 'Galen, Van Helmont, and blood-letting', in Debus, op. cit. (n. 6), Vol. II, pp. 14–15.

18 Walter Harris, *A Description of the King's Royal Palace and Gardens at Loo*, London, R. Roberts, 1699, p. 68

19 Peter Niebyl, 'The English bloodletting revolution, or modern medicine before 1850', *Bulletin of the History of Medicine*, 1977, 51: 464–83

20 John H. Warner, 'Therapeutic explanation and the Edinburgh bloodletting controversy: two perspectives on the medical meaning of science in the mid-nineteenth century', *Medical History*, 1980, 24: 241–58.

21 Elborg Forster, 'From the patient's point of view: illness and health in the letters of Liselotte von der Pfalz (1652–1722)', *Bulletin of the History of Medicine*, 1986, 60: 297–320.

22 Gunter B. Risse, 'The Renaissance of bloodletting: a chapter in modern therapeutics', *Journal of the History of Medicine*, 1979, 34: 3–22.

23 Delavan V. Holman, 'Venesection, before Harvey and after', *Bulletin of the New York Academy of Medicine*, 1955, 31: 661–70; Lawrence K. Altman, 'Iron in diet is poison for a million Americans', *New York Times*, 27 November 1990, p. B8.

24 Emma J. Edelstein and Ludwig Edelstein, *Asclepius: a Collection and Interpretation of the Testimonies*, Baltimore, MD, Johns Hopkins University Press, 1945, p. 149.

25 Ralph Jackson, 'Waters and spas in the classical world', in Roy Porter (ed.), *The Medical History of Waters and Spas, Medical History* (Supp)., 10), London, Wellcome Institute for the History of Medicine, 1990; 1–13.

26 L. W. B. Brockliss, 'Taking the waters in early modern France: some thoughts on a commercial racket', *Society for the Social History of Medicine, Bulletin*, 1987, 40: 74–7; Brockliss, 'The development of the spa in seventeenth-century France', in Porter op. cit. (n. 25): 23–47; Phyllis Hembry, *The English Spa 1560–1815: a Social History*, London, Athlone Press, 1990, pp. 4–38.

27 H. J. C. von Grimmelshausen, *The Adventurous Simplicissimus: Being the Description of the Life of a Strange Vagabond named Melchoir Sternfels von Fuchshaim*, trans. by A. T. S. Goodrick, Lincoln, University of Nebraska Press, 1962, pp. 338–9 (also see p. 333).

28 Alex Sakula, 'Doctor Nehemiah Grew (1641–1712) and the Epsom salts', *Clio Medica*, 1984, 19: 1–21.

29 Robin Price, 'Hydrotherapy in England 1840–70' *Medical History*, 1981, 25: 269–80; Janet Browne, 'Spas and sensibilities: Darwin at Malvern', in Porter op. cit. (n. 25) pp. 102–13.

30 Lawrence Wright, *Clean and Decent: the Fascinating History of the Bathroom and the Water-Closet*, New York, Viking, 1960, p. 39.

31 Georges Vigarello, *Concepts of Cleanliness: Changing Attitudes in France since the Middle Ages*, trans. by Jean Birrell, Cambridge University Press, 1988; Jean-Pierre; Goubert, *The Conquest of Water: the Advent of Health in the Medical Industrial Age*, trans. by Andrew Wilson, Princeton, NJ, Princeton University Press, 1989; Wright, op. cit. (n. 30).

32 Roger Cooter, 'Bones of contention? Orthodox medicine and the mystery of the bone-setter's craft', in W. F. Bynum and Roy Porter (eds), *Medical Fringe and Medical Orthodoxy 1750–1850*, London, Croom Helm, 1987, pp. 158–73.

33 Marc Bloch, *The Royal Touch*, trans. by J. E. Anderson, London, Routledge & Kegan Paul, 1973; Frank Barlow, 'The king's evil', *English Historical Review*, 1980, 95: 3–27.

34 James R. Jacob, *Robert Boyle and the English Revolution: a Study in Social and Intellectual Change*, New York, Burt Franklin, 1977, pp. 159–76; Eamon Duffy, 'Valentine Greatrakes, the Irish stroker: miracle, science, and orthodoxy in Restoration England', *Studies in Church History*, 1981, 17: 251–73; Nicholas Steneck, 'Greatrakes the stroker: the interpretations of historians', *Isis*, 1982, 73: 161–77; Barbara Kaplan, 'Greatrakes the stroker: the interpretations of his contemporaries', *isis*, 1982, 73: 178–85.

35   Sidney Licht, 'History', in Licht (ed.), *Therapeutic Exercise*, 2nd edn., New Haven, CT, Elizabeth Licht, 1961, pp. 426–71.

FURTHER READING

Bauer, Joseph, *Geschichte der Aderlässe*, Munich, Werner Fritsch, 1966.

Brain, Peter, *Galen on Bloodletting: a Study of the Origins, Development and Validity of his Opinions, with a Translation of the Three Works*, Cambridge, Cambridge University Press, 1986.

Goubert, Jean-Pierre, *The Conquest of Water: the Advent of Health in the Industrial Age*, trans. by Andrew Wilson, Princeton, NJ, Princeton University Press, 1989.

Niebyl, Peter H., 'The English bloodletting revolution, or modern medicine before 1850', *Bulletin of the History of Medicine*, 1977, 51: 464–83.

Porter, Roy (ed.), *The Medical History of Waters and Spas*, Medical History (Suppl. no. 10), London, Wellcome Institute for the History of Medicine, 1990.

Price, Robin, 'Hydrotherapy in England 1840–70', *Medical History*, 1981, 25: 269–80.

Risse, Guenter B., 'The renaissance of bloodletting: a chapter in modern therapeutics', *Journal of the History of Medicine*, 1979, 34: 3–22.

Smith, Virginia, 'Prescribing the rules of health: self-help and advice in the late eighteenth century', in Roy Porter (ed.), *Patients and Practitioners: Lay Perceptions of Medicine in Pre-industrial Society*, Cambridge, Cambridge University Press, 1985, pp. 249–82.

——, 'Physical puritanism and sanitary science: material and immaterial beliefs in popular physiology, 1650–1840', in W. F. Bynum and R. Porter (eds), *Medical Fringe and Medical Orthodoxy 1750–1850*, London, Croom Helm, 1987, pp. 174–97.

Smith, Wesley D., 'The development of classical dietetic theory', in M. D. Grmek (ed.), *Hippocratica: Actes du Colloque Hippocratique de Paris, 4–9 Septembre 1978*, Paris, CNRS, 1980, pp. 439–48.

Vigarello, Georges, *Concepts of Cleanliness: Changing Attitudes in France since the Middle Ages*, trans. by Jean Birrell, Cambridge, Cambridge University Press, 1988.

Voigts, Linda, and McVaugh, Michael R. (eds), *A Latin Technical Phlebotomy and its Middle English Translation*, Transactions of the American Philosophical Society, Vol. LXXII, Part 2, 1984, p. 41.

Warner, John H., 'Therapeutic explanation and the Edinburgh bloodletting controversy: two perspectives on the medical meaning of science in the mid-nineteenth century', *Medical History*, 1980, 24: 241–58.

41

SURGERY (TRADITIONAL)

Ghislaine Lawrence

INTRODUCTION

An ideal history of surgery has been described as having three parts: the history of the surgical profession, surgical pathology, and surgical technique.[1] To these could be added the history of everyday practice and of patients' experience. The task of writing such a history is not helped by the profound separation of surgery and medicine that occurred in the West and elsewhere from the late Middle Ages until the eighteenth century. Throughout this period in most of Europe, practical surgery was a craft, learned by apprenticeship and controlled by trade guilds, its practitioners of much lower social standing than literate, Latinate, university-trained physicians. (➤ Ch. 48 Medical education) Written sources are not necessarily revealing of craft practices. Most surgical authors from whom, perforce, we reconstruct the history of the subject were atypical practitioners – if only because they had the ability to commit themselves lucidly to paper. In general, surgical authors seem to constitute an élite group, often doubly qualified as physicians. Prior to about 1500, many of them came from the rather separate, southern-European tradition of academic surgery, which flourished particularly in Italy, where it retained a place in university curricula. Here, the emphasis was on surgical theory and anatomy, taught by physicians.

When it comes to practice, surgical authors, at least prior to the eighteenth century, often described operations that they admitted they had never performed, and perhaps never seen performed. Even for well-known surgeons, it seems likely that everyday practice was more conservative than has been suggested by some histories of operative surgery. And for the average practitioner, surgery must largely have entailed wound treatment, bandaging, and bleeding, combined most often with barbering but sometimes with another trade, such as inn-keeping, to make a living. We should guard against using the written sources to construct only a history of modern surgery, for which operations are constitutive. Prior to the nineteenth century, operative intervention was rare and practitioners performed functions we would consider 'non-surgical', such as the treatment of skin complaints or venereal disease. The operations that were performed were those of dire necessity. The accidents and injuries of daily life, including those of warfare or judicial punishment, demanded treatment. Other conditions, such as urinary stone or hernia, which were so debilitating as to persuade the sufferer to undergo surgery without anaesthesia, might also be treated operatively. However, these risky procedures were often shunned by the whole spectrum of licensed practitioners and left to travelling empirics.

Fundamental changes in the organization of surgery took place in the eighteenth century, most notably the severing of links with trade guilds and the commencement of academic teaching and regulation of practitioners, whose status rose markedly between 1700 and 1800. Such changes presaged the successful and scientific surgery of the nineteenth and twentieth centuries, often attributed to the replacement of empiricism with rationally based practice. However, the role of empiricism in surgery has been hotly debated both by practitioners and later commentators and has been applauded or derided in different contexts.

ANCIENT AND CLASSICAL SURGERY

To those for whom the history of surgery is the history of operations, it has seemed logical to locate its origins in the prehistoric period, following the sporadic discovery from the late seventeenth century onwards of neolithic trephined skulls in Europe, and later in the Americas and Oceania. These skulls bear one or more roughly circular defect, the bone margins of which show evidence of healing. During the late nineteenth and early twentieth centuries, some medical historians experimented with flint scrapers and primitive drills to demonstrate the feasibility of prehistoric skull trephining. Much conjectural history was subsequently written about the origins of this technique, which was certainly later an established and long-standing part of the surgical repertoire. It was frequently suggested that trephining was performed to release demons or evil spirits responsible for ill health. This was entirely supposition, extrapolated from studies of 'primitive' societies still in existence; the anthropological realm has also been tapped by historians seeking the origins of surgery. Study of non-literate societies in the 1900s revealed practices such as the suturing of wounds and the splinting of fractured limbs with hide or bark, and these have been taken as indicative of what may have constituted prehistoric surgery. (➤ Ch. 60 Medicine and anthropology)

Fragmentary written evidence on surgical practice in the ancient civilizations of Egypt and Mesopotamia is available. The Edwin Smith papyrus (c.1600 BC) was translated and published in 1922. It is a large fragment of a book on wounds and lists, from head to foot, various injuries, their prognosis and, if applicable, their treatment. This papyrus first indicated an empirico-rational content for ancient Egyptian medicine, which, like Mesopotamian medicine, historians had previously considered entirely magico-religious in character. Cuneiform inscriptions on the stele of Hammurabi (King of Babylon c.1792–c.1750 BC), dating from the second millennium BC and preserved in the Louvre in Paris, include laws relating to manual operations by doctors in Mesopotamia. From it we learn the fees chargeable for successful treatment of broken bones, eyes, and internal organs, and the penalties for failed operations. Of actual practice, however, we know very little.[2]

In the study of the ancient Greek authors, we first encounter detailed instructions for surgical procedures together with a theoretical context for surgery. However, in both the Hippocratic Corpus (fifth-third centuries BC) and in later Hellenistic works, subjects we would now regard as surgical are in general not treated separately from 'medical' ones. This is consistent with what we know of physicians in the Greek and Roman period; peripatetic practitioners with both medical and surgical skills were apparently the norm. The Hippocratic Corpus contains much material which would now be regarded as surgical, including a treatise on wounds (*De Ulceribus*) and one on head injuries (*De Capitis Vulneribus*). Discussion of head injuries, of which five types were recognized, was considerable, and included indications for trepanation. Fractures were treated by reduction and immobilization with bandages and later splints. In the management of dislocation, there is a description of the extension apparatus subsequently referred to by Galen (AD 129–c.200/210) as the Hippocratic bench. The knife was used for excising nasal polyps and ulcerated tonsils and for draining empyema, and for the cautery for treating haemorrhoids, but, in general, a very conservative picture emerges. Amputation as a last resort was carried out through gangrenous tissue. Catheterization, never lithotomy (operative removal), was advocated for bladder stone, the latter being left to 'such as are craftsmen therein'. Vascular ligature was apparently unknown to the ancient Greeks. The suturing of wounds, although metioned, was either too familiar or too infrequent to merit further explanation. In the Hippocratic treatment of wounds, we encounter theory that was to prove influential for centuries to come. Some degree of suppuration was considered essential to healing, the pus deriving from changed and heated vitiated blood. In general, wounds should be kept dry.

The eight books of *De Medicina*, written in the first century AD by the Roman encyclopedist Aulus Cornelius Celsus (25 BC–AD 50) are an important source for classical Greek medicine. The seventh book deals with 'the third part of the Art of Medicine' after dietetics and the use of dressings, namely 'that which cures by the hand'. It is devoted to surgical matters. Scarcely referred to throughout the Byzantine and medieval periods, though apparently available in some centres, *De Medicina* was nevertheless one of the earliest medical works to appear in print in 1478. Thereafter, it enjoyed great success, with new editions appearing even in the nineteenth century. Many of its subjects are also those of Hippocrates, but Celsus expands on hernia repair, fractures, and dislocations, and couching for cataract. In amputation, he used a saw as well as a knife, and made the incision through healthy tissue. Lithotomy had apparently entered the legitimate practice of a surgeon since Hippocrates's time, and Celsus provides detailed instructions. Book five of *De Medicina* concerns the treatment of injuries. Celsus describes the vascular ligature in a discussion of haemostasis, and also wound closure, by suture or the 'fibula', a pin passed through the wound edges with a thread twisted around it in figure-of-eight configuration.

The prolific works of Galen, practising in Rome in the second century AD, contain specifically surgical matters largely in the *Methodus Medendi*. The influence of Hippocrates is marked. Of wounds, Galen wrote that primary healing was best (that is, without the formation of any other matter). Closure was achieved by bandaging, suture, or a fibula. Haemostasis was attained by torsion of the blood vessels or their ligation with yarn or silk (the latter was not mentioned by Hippocrates). Eight varieties of head injury were recognized, and for depressed skull fracture trephining was indicated. In penetrating abdominal wounds, the large intestine might be sutured successfully, the ileum occasionally, but the jejunum not at all. Closure of the abdomen was achieved by two alternative kinds of running suture. Galen's actual experience as a surgeon is a subject of debate. The specific surgical content of his work is perhaps less important for the history of surgery than his entire system of medicine, which encompassed what we would now refer to as anatomy, physiology, pathology and therapeutics. The Galenic system based on humoralism became the established orthodoxy for Western medicine, unchallenged until the sixteenth century, remaining influential to some degree until the nineteenth. (➤ Ch. 14 Humoralism) This had important consequences for surgery. Surgical matters which were not purely empirical came to rest on Galenic assumptions about the body in health and disease. Academic, theoretical surgery explained pathology in terms of humoral imbalance in the individual concerned, rather than the localized changes which the practising surgeon was perforce obliged to diagnose and treat. On a practical level, the bloodletting advocated by Galen in the correction of humoral imbalance became, from Hellenistic times onward, an important therapy. (➤ Ch. 40

Physical methods) Because of its practical nature, it was left to surgeons to perform and became a staple part of their work.

MEDIEVAL AND ARABIC SURGERY

The fall of the Western Roman Empire from the fourth century AD, and the Arab conquests of the seventh century, led to the destruction of north-west Europe's trade links, an increased importance for agriculture, and a corresponding decline in city life. Learned works, including medical texts, survived only in monasteries. There is evidence of some medical practice by monks, especially Benedictines. Anecdotal accounts indicate that monks may have undertaken surgery, as perhaps did some lay practitioners, but, apart from brief tracts on phlebotomy and cautery, there is little mention of surgery in the medical literature of the Latin West from the sixth to the eleventh centuries. In surgical matters, as in other fields of learning, Arabic authors had a key role in preserving and adding to classical teaching during this period. Initially compilers and editors of earlier Indian, Persian, and, in particular, ancient Greek texts, medical authors writing in Arabic drew particularly on the *Epitome* of the Greek physician, Paul of Aegina (*c.*625–90). The seven books of the *Epitome*, translated into Arabic in the ninth century, were largely taken from the compilatory works of Oribasius (325–403) who, in turn, drew heavily on Galen. The sixth book of Paul's *Epitome* informed much of what the Arab authors wrote on operative surgery. (➤ Ch. 31 Arab-Islamic medicine) (Apparently available in the West by the fourteenth century, Paul's operative surgery, written in late antiquity, was to form a staple part of the surgical 'revival' of the late Middle Ages and Renaissance.)

Those dealing with surgical matters include Rhazes (d. 925) in the seventh book of his *Liber Medicinalis ad Almansorem*, Haly Abbas (930–94) in the ninth book of the *Practica* of his *Libri Pantechni*, and the greatest Arabic medical scholar, Avicenna (980–1037), whose *Canon Medicinae* was enormously influential in the West throughout the Middle Ages. Avicenna's *Canon* provided a complete, largely Galenic, system of medicine. Material on surgery and external diseases is contained in the third book, and is mainly derived from Paul of Aegina. Our most important Arabic source for surgery is the author known in the West as Albucasis (936–1013), of Cordoba, whose thirty surgical treatises appeared in Latin translation in the twelfth century as the *Liber Alzaharavii de Chirugia*. This was subsequently widely referred to in the West, perhaps because of its practical nature and copious illustrations of surgical instruments. Its content draws, once again, on the classical authors, especially Paul.

The impression we obtain of Arabic surgery from the authors mentioned above is that the use of the knife definitely took second place to other therapies such as pharmacy, bloodletting, and cupping. When operative surgery was practised, lamented Albucasis, the standard was low, the art having fallen into disrepute. Nevertheless, his work illustrates an impressive armamentarium of instruments, some of which, such as the tonsil guillotine and a concealed knife and case for opening abscesses, appear to be innovative. There are also detailed accounts of the use of the cautery, treatment of wounds, fractures, and bone diseases. Cauterization appears to have had a central role in Arabic surgical practice, being used to open abscesses, burn skin tumours and haemorrhoids, stop arterial bleeding, or produce intentional scarring to limit mobility of the parts in, for example, recurrent dislocation of the shoulder. Cauterization, like bloodletting, was also performed in the treatment of internal diseases, in line with humoral theory. Apart from Albucasis and possibly Avenzoar (c. 1092–1162), it is unlikely that the Arabic surgical authors known to us ever practised surgery themselves. We should therefore be aware of the limitations of these, our only sources, as an indication of everyday practice.

In the medieval West, there was a striking rise in the production of technical surgical literature from the twelfth to fifteenth centuries, in both Latin and, later, the vernacular. In part, this was initiated by the translation of Arabic authors into Latin, which provided the West with a considerable amount of surgical writing, much of it deriving ultimately from Hippocrates. Italy, less isolated than the rest of Europe, saw the founding of the first universities in the early twelfth century, and theoretical surgery was revived there and flourished first at Salerno, a centre of medical practice since the mid-900s. The earliest medieval surgical work in the West originated from Salerno in the second quarter of the twelfth century: an anonymous compilation of earlier authors known as the Bamberg surgery (after the city where the oldest surviving manuscript resides). This was certainly not a specialist work, but new Latin textbooks of surgery did soon appear, perhaps because the translated ancient and Arabic material was by no means easy to use. One of the earliest of the new Latin texts was that of Roger Frugard, practising in Parma c.1170. Roger's *Practica Chirurgiae* dealt with the treatment of injuries in a head-to-toe arrangement and spawned a large derivative literature, including an expanded version by his pupil, Rolando, who took Roger's teaching to Bologna in the early thirteenth century. Roger's work formed the basis of Latin instruction in surgery at Salerno, at the northern Italian universities, and at Montpellier until the late thirteenth century, when it was to some extent supplanted by direct study of Galen and the Arabic authors as translations became available. Vernacular surgical treatises also began to be produced from this period onwards.

The focus for medical studies moved in the thirteenth century to the northern Italian universities of Bologna, Padua, and Verona. Surgical authors from Bologna, including Bruno Longoburgo, Teodorico Borgognoni (c.1205–98) and William of Salicet (1201–77) continued the Latinate tradition. All these authors show indebtedness to Galen and, to a varying degree, the Arabs. It was at Bologna in 1302 that the first human dissection since the Alexandrian period appears to have taken place. (➤ Ch. 5 The anatomical tradition) This was conducted for legal purposes, but subsequently (1315) a limited amount of anatomy teaching using human dissections was begun by Mondino de' Luzzi (c.1275–1326), whose influential book of human anatomy, eventually printed in 1478, was wholly Galenic in character. It should be noted that these dissections were not intended to teach practical anatomy to surgeons, but were rather expositions of a rational basis for medicine, by and for physicians.

Italian academic surgery spread during the fourteenth century to France by both personal and geographical connections. The surgeon Lanfranc (d. c.1315) fled from Guelph and Ghibelin feuding in Milan to Paris, where he established a flourishing school from 1295. His *Chirugia Magna*, completed a year later, was disseminated throughout the West. In turn, Lanfranc's pupil, Jan Yperman (d. c.1330) took northern Italian techniques and teaching, together with those of the Paris school, to Flanders and Germany. At Montpellier, geographically close to the Italian schools, Henri de Mondeville, (c.1260–c.1320), a former pupil of Teodorico Borgognoni, wrote his unfinished, five-part work. The only major operation discussed is amputation. Much attention is paid to wound treatment, a notably controversial subject in medieval surgical writing. De Mondeville supported the method of Teodorico, and Teodorico's father Hugo, who advocated simple cleansing of wounds with wine and immediate closure, followed by dry dressings for fresh wounds with no great loss of flesh or skin. By this means, healing without the formation of pus was promoted. This view encountered considerable opposition from supporters of the more traditional use of wound salves, plasters, and powders designed to promote, amongst other things, a degree of suppuration. Certain types of pus were regarded as beneficial, and both ancient and Islamic sources, and the Salernitan school, advocated keeping wounds open to allow for suppuration and healing by second intention (from the bottom of the wound up). Advocates of both methods defended their practice in humoral terms, contesting the relative claims of the dry and the moist in wound healing. De Mondeville's anatomy was drawn from Avicenna. He stated that anatomical knowledge is essential to surgeons, as is a general pathology, which he derived from Galen. His works contain numerous asides on topics such as the professional bearing of a surgeon, his relations with physicians (apparently poor) and the difficulty of obtaining fees.

The major surgical author of the late Middle Ages was Guy de Chauliac (1298–1368), a physician and surgeon apparently educated, like De Mondeville, at Montpellier and Bologna. His *Inventorium sive Collectorium artis Chirurgicalis Medicinae*, or *Chirugia Magna*, was to be translated many times and quoted in European surgical literature until the eighteenth century.

The French and Italian authors of the late Middle Ages – de Chauliac, de Mondeville, and their predecessors – seem to have come from a small, élite group of university-trained men, some of whom were also physicians and all of whom were active in literate, Latin circles. They both wrote about and practised surgery, though they made it clear that they had never performed certain of the procedures they described. Undoubtedly, this is partly due to the compilatory nature of technical surgical writing, which characterized the Latinate tradition extending from Roger Frugard to Guy de Chauliac. The works were often innovative in arrangement, content, and scope, but the details of operative technique, and the range of operations described, do not differ radically from the ancients. These works are not a reliable guide to what surgical proceduers were actually performed or how they were carried out in practice. The Salernitan manuscripts contain some of the earliest surviving illustrations of surgical procedures (as opposed to instruments) but, as one commentator puts it, in medieval illustrations the surgeon and patient 'seem often to be engaged in a swaying dance', the patient making anatomically impossible gestures, the faces always impassive.[3] Likewise, the stylized portrayals of operations in the woodcuts of later vernacular works convey little of what actual practice must have been like. We do know that literate, Latinate surgeons had difficult relationships with physicians, with whom they competed for patients, and that they tried hard to distinguish themselves from other types of surgical practitioners who were, according to Bruno Longoburgo, 'for the most part ignorant and stupid peasants'. Undoubtedly, there was a very broad spectrum of practitioners, with much everyday practice by now in the hands of barber-surgeons (see below), regulated by guilds. To a lesser extent, from the tenth century, there is also evidence of travelling specialists – cataract couchers, hernia 'specialists', and the like – prepared to undertake high-risk procedures shunned by licensed practitioners of all kinds.

THE DIVISION BETWEEN MEDICINE AND SURGERY: THE BARBER-SURGEON

In most of western Europe by the time of the Renaissance, until the eighteenth century, surgery and medicine were the province of separate groups of practitioners.[4] The licensing of physicians, first recorded in the West in 1140, was in the hands of the universities. Surgeons, however, were regulated by the trade guilds and had their closest occupational links with the barbers. It became usual, though not inevitable, for the two trades to be carried on by a single practitioner, the barber-surgeon. Guilds of barber-surgeons are recorded in Europe from the thirteenth century. Training was by apprenticeship, and it seems possible that many surgeons were illiterate. They enjoyed considerably lower status than the physicians, who continued to be university-educated men versed in Latin. In Italy, the continuing tradition of university surgery mitigated against the separation between medical and surgical practice, but in northern Europe this was profound, perhaps at its height from the fifteenth to the seventeenth centuries. Historians have ascribed the origins of this division to Christian teaching in the early Middle Ages, which proscribed the shedding of blood by clerics, who often provided some form of medical care. (➤ Ch. 61 Religion and medicine) However, there is little evidence to suggest that surgical knowledge or practice was separated to any degree until the late Middle Ages. As we have noted, the Graeco-Roman physician was expected to be competent in surgery, and such source material that is available on the largely clerical medical practitioners of the early Middle Ages in western Europe suggests that they too carried out surgery on occasion. A very early reference to surgery being performed by a barber is found in Gratian (fl. 1140), but this was before the advent of medical licensing in the West, when any individual could practise medicine or surgery. Rather, it has been suggested that an influential revision of the medieval schematic literature in the twelfth century threatened medicine in general with relegation to the mechanical arts, rather than the place it formerly occupied as a division of physics. In late schematic works, medicine is restored to its former place but surgery is separated and demoted to the mechanical arts. This has been seen as a strategy of the medical professors, at a time of socio-economic growth and increased professional consciousness generally, to preserve the status of medical knowledge.[5] (➤ Ch. 47 History of the medical profession)

The rigid organization of trades into guilds, which also began at this period, may have contributed to the separation. Guilds served several social and economic purposes, and full members or freemen had many incentives to enforce their regulations. These controlled numbers entering a given trade and ensured a basic level of competence through apprenticeship, which also brought in revenue to freemen. Small guilds and corporations of surgeons who were not barbers maintained a precarious existence in some countries, many being engulfed by the larger barbers' corporations during the sixteenth century. The small Fellowship of Surgeons in London was united with the Barber-Surgeons' Company by Act of Parliament in 1540. The Act distinguished between the two crafts, largely proscribing the practice of surgery by barbers, and vice versa. Barber-surgeons considerably outnumbered physicians and had an important role in what would now be regarded as primary medical care, especially in metropolitan areas. It seems clear that many engaged in 'physic' as well as strictly surgical procedures. For example, they treated skin complaints and venereal diseases, sometimes with the internal remedies which were officially the province of the physician. A study of the London Barber-Surgeons (already by 1537 the strongest City company, with 185 freemen) suggests they were well placed, both because of the location of their premises near centres of 'low life' and because of the personal nature of the services they offered, to treat the syphilis which raged in early six-teenth-century England.[6] (➤ Ch. 26 Sexually transmitted diseases) These 'craftsmen shopkeepers' perhaps more readily took economic advantage of the new chemical drugs, especially mercury, than physicians who clung to galenicals. One of the earliest (1579) English vernacular treatises on a single disease – syphilis – was by the surgeon William Clowes (1544–1603). Elsewhere in Europe, barber-surgeons had already contributed to a growing vernacular literature on surgery. Many, like Clowes, drew on areas of experience not available to physicians, namely military and naval service. Barber-surgeons' companies often administered tests for ships' surgeons' licences, which were simpler than the regular examinations for guild membership. The latter usually involved displays of practical skills such as bandaging, together with theoretical questions from a panel of guild officials. In several European countries, the demand for naval surgeons was high and the posts lucrative. Perforce, ships' surgeons gained experience in medical as well as surgical matters.

After the introduction of gunpowder into warfare in the fifteenth century, the number and variety of injuries presenting to field surgeons increased substantially. Vernacular surgical handbooks, such as the *Buch der Wund-Artzney* (1497) of Hieronymus Brunschwig (1450–1533) and the *Feltbuch der Wundartzney* (1517) of Hans von Gersdorff, both of Strasburg, were based on their authors' practical experience in the field – in this case in campaigns against Charles the Bold (1433–77; Duke of Burgundy 1467–77). Brunsch-wig's book was the first printed book on surgery to appear in English (1525). It also contains the earliest printed illustrations of surgical instruments, but, in general, these and other Renaissance surgical authors, such as Giovanni da Vigo (1450–1525) of Rome or the Spaniard Francisco Arceo (1493–1571), display a conservative stance when it comes to practice, preferring salves and plasters, or cautery, to the knife, and sometimes employing magical cures and weapon-salves. A combination of extreme conservatism and a reliance on mystical elements is to be found in what Paracelsus (1493–1541), who accompanied military campaigns in the Netherlands, Denmark, and Italy, wrote on surgical matters.

There was a move towards more active surgical intervention in the works of Ambroise Paré (1510–90), a barber-surgeon with the French armies who developed new forms of wound treatment and new techniques for amputation. Paré abandoned the pouring of boiling oil into gunshot wounds, which were generally held to be poisoned by the gunpowder, but did advocate the use of traditional suppurative agents. In amputation, he operated through healthy tissues and attempted a form of vascular ligature rather than cautery to arrest haemorrhage. His great surgical work, forty books in length, was written in the vernacular, but displayed familiarity with the ancient classical and Arabic authors. Hippocrates informed much of his treatment of fractures and dislocations. Paré's wound treatment was, in general, traditional, using cooling and drying medicaments in line with the clasical Galenic pathology, which he presented in his introduction. His anatomy, however, comprising four books, was Vesalian (see below). Paré appears to many historians a transitional figure in the history of surgery and is lauded for his combination of empiricism – careful observation and operative innovation – with scholarship. Less attention has been paid to other areas of his published work: for example, on reproduction and on monsters, a favourite Renaissance topic. The trend in Paré's work towards more-active surgical intervention is also present in the writings of the Provençal surgeon Pierre Franco (c.1500–61), and the Italian Mariano Santo (1498–after 1550), both of whom give detailed directions for procedures such as hernia repair and lithotomy, which were formerly left to empirics.

Santo was also a doctor of medicine, a product of the flourishing Italian tradition of university surgery whose centres, particularly Padua, became a focus for foreign students in the seventeenth century. It was in these universities that the controversy over Vesalian anatomy had raged, following the publication of *De Humani Corporis Fabrica* in 1543, while Vesalius (1514–64) was lecturing in surgery at Padua. Post-Vesalian anatomists included surgeons such as Marcus Aurelius Severinus (1580–1656), whose *De Recondita Abscessuum Natura* of 1632 is considered by some to be the first textbook of surgical pathology. The relationship of the new anatomy to surgical practice is hard to decipher, however, particularly elsewhere in Europe. Here, during the seventeenth century, anatomical teaching did begin to have a more prominent place in both the university curricula for physicians and in the training of surgeons, which was still governed by guild regulations. The well-known anatomy theatre of Leiden was completed by the university in 1593, a professor from the medical faculty having been detailed to lecture on anatomy to the medical students since 1587. During the seventeenth century, the town's surgeons and their apprentices were also admitted to these (Latin) demonstrations, although they obtained their own dissecting room in 1636. Elsewhere in the Netherlands and in other European countries, anatomical demonstrations in the vernacular specifically for surgeons, and sometimes also midwives, were provided at municipal or guild expense.

Other seventeenth-century discoveries and innovations, often included as part of the history of surgery, had little connection with, or application in, the surgical practice of the period. The announcement by William Harvey (1578–1657) of the circulation of the blood in 1628 was the work of a professed disciple of Aristotle and an exposition of the latter's teleological and vitalist philosophy. Animal experimentation pursued in several European countries during the seventeenth century was, in general, concerned with philosophical debate. It was in this context that Richard Lower (1631–91), an English member of the 'invisible college', the precursor of the Royal Society, experimented with direct blood transfusions between animals and, in one case, a man. Attempts at therapeutic blood transfusion were made by the Parisian physician Jean-Baptiste Denis (c.1625–1704), who reported on them in 1667. A fatal outcome prevented further experimentation. (➤ Ch. 7 The physiological tradition)

Such activities can hardly have touched the everyday world of practising seventeenth-century surgeons. A few accounts, drawn from day-books, guild records, and the like, are now available of the activities of some of these men who, like the great majority of their colleagues, left no published record. Records from the barber-surgeons' guild in Cologne have enabled the practice of one member to be reconstructed.[7] In 1634–5, this master-surgeon saw some two hundred patients. The majority of his serious cases were men, and there is evidence to suggest that he specialized to some extent in the treatment of severe injuries. These, whether accidental or the result of deliberate wounding, might be expected to be more prevalent amongst males. Another study records the London practice of Joseph Binns (d. 1664), who left a written case-book covering the years 1633–63.[8] The author finds Binns's actual therapeutic interventions rather more conservative than those advocated by Richard Wiseman (1622–76), the foremost English surgeon of the period, in his *Several Chirurgical Treatises* (1676).

MEDICINE AND SURGERY REALIGNED

During the course of the eighteenth century, the practice of surgery became dissociated from barbering and from trade links generally in most of northern Europe. Increasingly, centres of academic training were established for surgeons. These changes first began in late seventeenth-century France. In Paris, the College of Saint Côme, founded in 1210, had enjoyed a precarious existence as a centre of academic surgery until 1655, when its members were finally forced to merge with the guild of barbers, thus making all surgeons officially barber-surgeons. Within a few decades, however, royal patronage allowed the surgeons to begin a rapid process of emancipation. In 1672, the leading French surgeon Pierre Dionis (c.1650–1718) secured an appointment to lecture in anatomy and surgery at the Jardin du Roi. In 1687, the celebrated case of Louis XIV's anal fistula, successfully operated on by C. F. Félix

(1650–1703), added to surgery's growing prestige. Teaching demonstrations were held in the new amphitheatre built at Saint Côme in 1694 at what became, in effect, a school of surgery. Courses in anatomy, osteology, and operative surgery were available there at the beginning of the eighteenth century. These changes marked the beginning of the end of surgical training by apprenticeship, finally abolished in France in 1768. The status of Paris surgeons had continued to rise as, during the first half of the eighteenth century, they engaged in so-called 'pamphlet wars' with the physicians. The strategy of these surgeons, amongst whom were Georges Mareschal (1658–1736) and François de la Peyronie (1678–1747), was to stress the importance of a separate, surgical theory. Empiricism was everywhere condemned.[9] In 1731, permission was granted to establish the Académie Royale de Chirurgie, and in 1743, a declaration was issued by Louis XV ending the union of the surgeons and barbers. These changes contributed to the pre-eminent position in surgery that France occupied for at least the first half of the eighteenth century. French surgeons were of international repute and drew students and observers from all over Europe. Depending on their status, these observers were admitted to ward rounds and operations – in other words to an increasingly hospital-based training where clinical instruction played an important role. (➤ Ch. 49 The hospital)

In London, the Company of Surgeons split from the barbers in 1745; and here, another important new form of surgical education was to flourish: the private anatomy school. (During this period, hospital-based training was also 'private' in that, in France and elsewhere, it generally involved the payment of fees directly to the surgeons involved.) Private anatomy schools taught a good deal more than anatomy. Perhaps the most famous, that established in 1770 in London's Great Windmill Street by William Hunter (1718–83), also offered instruction in surgery, physiology, pathology, midwifery, and diseases of women and children. Teaching was by means of an extensive number of anatomical models and human material for dissection.

The private schools flourished particularly in London, a capital city without a university, because of wide changes in the 'medical market-place' of the eighteenth century. A growing and increasingly socially stratified populace demanded new and more sophisticated forms of medical care, which the traditional 'primary carer', the barber-surgeon, was not well placed to provide. Thus, a new type of general practitioner arose – the surgeon-apothecary – who, in turn, demanded new forms of education. In northern Europe generally, several years' apprenticeship for surgeons remained compulsory, but this was increasingly supplemented by subsequent attendance at private anatomy schools, hospitals, and public lectures. This represented a considerable departure from the earlier situation where the experience of an apprentice barber-surgeon was limited to that provided by a single master. Aspiring surgeons were able, if they had the means, to pick and choose from courses, some of which were on traditionally 'medical' subjects. They could and did travel internationally to gain wider experience, with Paris, Edinburgh, and London, in turn, being the most popular cities for aspiring medical practitioners of all persuasions. By the end of the eighteenth century, the surgeon-apothecary was a representative of a new and, especially in provincial towns, relatively prosperous form of general practitioner, whose employment possibilities had expanded with the increasing commercialism of health care, together with, in England, changes attendant on the Industrial Revolution. Surgeons were engaged by parishes, dispensaries, gaols, workhouses, and private mad-houses. They were involved in the examination of factory apprentices and army recruits. Increasingly, they gained resident and consulting appointments to hospitals. (➤ Ch. 4 Medical care)

In several countries, the late seventeenth century saw the establishment of small surgical élites, whose members sometimes possessed university degrees in medicine or had the means to avail themselves of the high-quality private medical and surgical tuition available. It is from this surgical élite, rather than from rank-and-file practitioners, that much of our knowledge of eighteenth-century surgery is drawn. Those to the fore in teaching and publishing on surgical matters were now also skilful and relatively frequent operators. In France, J. L. Petit (1674–1750) dominated surgery for the first half of the century, attracting numerous foreign students, among them Lorenz Heister (1683–1758), who was to become pre-eminent in German surgery. Heister's *Chirurgie* (1718), translated into English as *A General System of Surgery* (1743), was regarded by late eighteenth-century surgeons as the first complete and systematic treatment of the *science* of surgery.

By the late eighteenth century, however, the greatest living exponent of scientific surgery was considered by many in Britain to be the Scot John Hunter (1728–93). The younger brother of William Hunter, in whose anatomy school he worked on first coming to London, John rapidly became a skilful and prolific dissector and preparer of both human and animal material, eventually setting up his own school. In contrast to William, who became a successful society practitioner specializing in midwifery and possessed of a considerable fortune, John devoted almost all his energies and income to his research work. Broadly, this concerned comparative studies on the relationship of structure to function throughout the animal kingdom. It also encompassed observation and experimentation on more specifically surgical topics such as inflammation, shock, disorders of the vascular system, and venereal disease. His four treatises, *Natural History of the Human Teeth* (1771), *On Venereal Disease* (1786), *Observations on Certain Parts of the Animal Oeconomy* (1786), and *Treatise on the Blood Inflammation and Gunshot Wounds* (1794), are regarded as the most important of his writings. He amassed a huge collection of anatomical, pathological, and embryological specimens which was subsequently given to the newly established Royal College of Surgeons.[10] He was made a member of the Royal Society in 1767, and remained pre-eminent among London surgeons, with an appointment at St George's Hospital and a considerable private practice, until his death.

The subsequent adulation given to John Hunter by his former surgical colleagues (though not by his first biographer, Jesse Foot (1744–1826)) can be related in large part to their professional aspirations, particularly those of a small élite.[11] At the turn of the nineteenth century, London surgeons strove for equal status with physicians. Like that of the Paris surgeons before them, their strategy lay in emphasizing that surgery was no longer an empirical craft, but a science resting on a secure body of theoretical knowledge. John Hunter's work, with its stress on studying the normal as well as the pathological, and the relationship of structure to function as an essential prelude to surgery, served its purpose well. Furthermore, his studies of comparative anatomy were akin to the pursuits of gentleman scholars, and did indeed attract an aristocratic audience. Hunter's ideas found rather little application in practical surgery until the late nineteenth century, his usefulness to his immediate successors lying elsewhere.

John Hunter's vitalist perspective, which led him to stress the role of the blood as bearer of a vital principle, has sometimes been seen as a form of humoralism and somewhat at variance with the solidist physiologies of, for example, Albrecht von Haller (1709–77) and, later, Xavier Bichat (1771–1802). The Solidist physiologi were to have an integral role in one of the most striking developments in both medicine and surgery in the eighteenth century: the emphasis on the anatomical localization of disease. This is conventionally recognized as having one of its most important expressions in the 1761 publication of Giovanni Battista Morgagni (1682–1771), *Seats and Causes of Disease*, which correlated clinical symptoms with autopsy findings in some seven hundred patients. (➤ Ch. 9 The pathological tradition) This approach to disease by surgeons was eventually to make internal intervention a plausible therapeutic approach. In France, this view of disease, sometimes called 'anatomico-localist' or 'anatomico-clinical' to distinguish it from the physicians' stress on balancing individual systems, was integral to the internal medicine practised in the hospitals of post-Revolutionary Paris, where the radical reorganization of medical education imposed by the Revolutionary Council in 1794 had caused both medicine and surgery to be taught to all medical students. Also in Paris, the tissue pathology developed by Bichat in the 1790s was later to be used as the general pathological basis of what was seen as a new scientific surgery. From France, too, came new diagnostic instruments, such as the stethoscope, which were used to localize disease in the living patient. After death, these findings, along with other clinical observations, were systematically correlated with post-mortem appearances. The Paris hospital system, with an estimated 20,000 inmates in 1790, provided the huge numbers of (poor) patients necessary to this approach, which was far removed from the 'client-centred' concern with patients' symptoms still prevailing in circles where physicians depended on patronage. (➤ Ch. 34 History of doctor patient relationships) So radical was this change that it has been claimed that a complete ideological rupture occurred during the creation of what became, in effect, modern clinical medicine. Other commentators have suggested that the growing influence of surgical thinking and factors in the institutional organization and teaching of surgery during the preceding century can explain this seemingly abrupt change. It was noted on p. 973 that the private anatomy schools taught surgical and 'medical' subjects to both medical and surgical students. At the Edinburgh medical school, a mecca for aspiring medical men by the mid-eighteenth century, Alexander Monro *primus* (1697–1767), first incumbent of the Chair of Anatomy and Surgery, taught a theoretical course, but also the operations of surgery to medical students, as well as surgical apprentices, in English. Both were thus 'exposed to the most up-to-date medical theory, capped by a surgical, natural historical account of disease'.[12]

The new 'Paris' medicine was hospital based, and it is clear that the career structures of surgeons had, during the century, come to be more closely tied to hospitals than those of physicians. Surgeons had made more systematic use of hospitals for teaching apprentices, dressers, and pupils. The surgeon P. J. Desault (1744–95), at the Hôtel Dieu in Paris, had introduced the bedside teaching integral to the new form of clinical medicine. House-surgeons were resident at some London hospitals by the early 1760s. Many of the managing bodies of hospitals, originally lay but increasingly medicalized, had surgeons as members. In France, it was recognized by contemporaries that the organization of the new *écoles de santé* owed a great deal to the practice and organization of Paris surgeons.

OPERATIVE SURGERY TO 1800

It is a measure of the somewhat underdeveloped state of scholarship in the history of surgery that surveys of operative techniques are often, like the brief outline that follows, not fully integrated into more general accounts of the social, cultural, and cognitive issues attendant on practice. Much work remains to be done in relating changes in technique to these wider issues. As has been noted, until the very end of the period under review, the only operations performed with any regularity were those of dire necessity. As far as can be judged from the sources available, many techniques remained, in the eighteenth century, much as they had been in antiquity. In other cases, such as trepanation, the indications for surgical intervention had changed, but the techniques remained largely unaltered. In a few areas, for example in operating for stone in the bladder, innovative changes were made, largely during the eighteenth-century expansion of surgery. By 1800, channels existed and were used to communicate new techniques to other surgical practitioners. During the eighteenth century, surgeons wishing to publish in learned journals had used the magazines of their local literary and philosophical societies or organs such as the *Philosophical Transactions* of the Royal Society in Britain, or the *Ephemerides* of the German Academia Naturae Curiosorum. In both types of publication, surgical papers were mixed with others on widely varying, often literary, subjects. In contrast, the *Mémoires de l'Académie Royale de Chirurgie*, appearing between 1743 and 1773, was a specialist publication. A separate surgical journal, the *Chirurgische Bibliothek*, was published in Germany from 1771 to 1796 at the instigation of A. G. Richter (1742–1812). In earlier periods, some of the procedures outlined below were the particular province of itinerant specialists, who took pains to guard their trade secrets. The operations characteristically associated with this type of unlicensed practitioner, such as cataract couching and hernia repair, were not usually attempted by guild surgeons, presumably in fear of an unfavourable outcome. There is also evidence that only certain licensed surgical practitioners undertook major operations at all, with barber-surgeons unable or unwilling to perform, for example, amputations. Only the roughest estimates of the incidence of the disorders submitted to surgical treatment can be made, using case reports and so forth. Similarly, the success of surgical intervention can be judged only from rare individual case series or registers of operations, such as that kept by the city of Amsterdam for lithotomies performed there from 1700 to 1821. Excluding the years 1704–24, which are missing, 363 operations are recorded with an overall operative mortality of about 20 per cent.[13]

Some of the conditions in which, from antiquity, surgical management had had an established role are discussed below.

Head injuries and broken or dislocated bones were usually considered to require treatment, whether or not a flesh wound was also involved. In injuries to the head, operative treatment by means of trephination was known to Hippocrates, and the indications rather than the procedure were varied by later surgeons. In the sixteenth and seventeenth centuries, it appears to have been one of the few operations both described and performed frequently. Indications came to include, for some eighteenth-century surgeons such as Percival Pott (1714–88), all cases of depressed fracture. Others, including Pierre Dionis, had taken unconsciousness following a blow to the head as enough indication. Multiple trepannings were not uncommon. By the late eighteenth century, a much more conservative approach had supervened. The treatment of fractures, from the Hippocratic period onwards, consisted in reduction and fixation, sometimes by unqualified bone-setters.

Gangrene or serious injury to the extremities was always the principal indication for the amputation of whole or parts of limbs. Amputation above the knee was rarely performed prior to the sixteenth century. In the actual severing of the limb, progressive attempts were made to remove more bone and less soft tissue, thus allowing the latter to heal over the bone and form a usable stump. Paré's technique, in use throughout the seventeenth century, involved pulling skin and muscles as high as possible above the amputation site and securing them there with a tight cord before severing the soft tissues in one cut. Subsequent two-stage procedures approximated to the double circular procedure of J. L. Petit, which became standard after its description in 1736. In it, skin, muscles, and bone were sectioned separately at progressively higher levels. Management of the amputation stump involved all the problems and controversies attendant on wound treatment generally. The actual cautery continued in regular use to arrest haemorrhage until the mideighteenth century. Styptics and compression bandaging persisted as popular alternatives. Paré's method of vascular ligature (in reality a form of undersewing of the vessels) only slowly gained ground as more-refined versions of his artery forceps were developed during the eighteenth century. In closure of the wound as well, Paré's use of suturing was less popular than tight bandaging or adhesive strapping. Other controversial elements included the level of amputation, the fitting of prostheses (devised by Paré and others and, by the eighteenth century, extremely well crafted), and the indications for operations.

The question of whether compound fracture (where the bone fragments punctured the skin's surface) warranted immediate amputation gave rise to what was perhaps the first major international dispute in surgery, in the mideighteenth century. For the first time also, statistical evidence of operative results was presented in this debate. The widely differing views of the participants were perhaps related to the very different circumstances attendant on military and civil practice. Soldiers were often better able to seek shelter without their damaged limb. Many historians of surgery have commented on the role of the battlefield as an age-old 'school for surgery', but it is perhaps worth stressing that warfare presented not only new forms of injury but large numbers of serious cases at any one time. In this situation, quite different from civilian practice, military surgeons had often drawn conclusions about the relative merits of various therapies based, however impressionistically, on large numbers of cases. In practical matters, military surgeons were to the fore in organizing systems of transportation for large numbers of injured. The subsequent nursing of many recently wounded or postoperative patients in close confines had few equivalents in civilian life before the nineteenth century (with the possible exception of lying-in wards), and it was hardly surprising that army surgeons penned many of the descriptions of wound sequelae, such as hospital gangrene, tetanus, and erysipelas, which fuelled debates on contagionism during the late eighteenth and early nineteenth centuries. (➤ Ch. 16 Contagion/germ theory/specificity; Ch. 66 War and modern medicine)

Renal stone was prevalent throughout western Europe until the nineteenth century, particularly in country areas and in children. Calculi formed in the urinary tract became impacted and obstructed flow. Until the early sixteenth century, operative treatment, if resorted to, was by the method Celsus described in the first century AD: the stone was cut down on and removed, a finger in the rectum making it bulge into the perineum. This technique, requiring few instruments, became known as the 'apparatus minor'. Early in the sixteenth century, the method of Mariano Santo of Barletta, described in 1522, was widely adopted. It involved dilating and incising the urethra just anterior to the bladder neck to allow the introduction of various instruments to extract the stone. Known as the 'apparatus major', the method avoided damage to the prostate gland and seminal vesicles, which frequently led to haemorrhage and incontinence after the Celsan operation. At the end of the seventeenth century, lateral cystotomy was introduced, apparently by the itinerant, unlicensed practitioner Jacques de Beaulieu (or Frère Jacques; 1651–1719). It involved an incision in the perineum to one side of the midline and the opening up of both bladder and bladder neck. The established surgeons Johannes Rau (1688–1719), in Amsterdam, and William Cheselden (1688–1752), in London, took up the method with considerable success and it became widely used throughout Europe during the eighteenth century, many surgeons developing their own variations and instrumentation. The almost exclusive province of unlicensed practitioners in the sixteenth century, lithotomy had gradually been appropriated into the repertoire of qualified surgeons by the eighteenth.

Surgical treatment of hernia was one of the operations that remained longest in the hands of travelling empirics, with licensed surgeons unwilling to perform operative repair with the almost inevitable castration that accompanied it. Itinerant 'hernia masters' were active in Europe until the early eighteenth century, when their demise seems to have been as much due to an improvement in truss-making as to any greater inclination of surgeons to operate on unobstructed hernias. Strangulated hernias, on the other hand, had always required attention, with local poultices, compresses, purging or bleeding (to produce relaxation by syncope) the first line of attack. Failing these measures, manual reduction was indicated. Operative intervention was a last resort. This consisted in surgically enlarging the orifice through which the intestines had prolapsed in order to replace them in the abdominal cavity. Cutting into a nearby blood vessel was a frequent hazard.

The procedures outlined above, together with a few others such as emergency surgery for aneurysms (abnormal dilatations of the blood vessels), the removal of superficial tumours, and, occasionally, Caesarean section, made up the bulk of operative surgery. This remained the situation during the opening decades of the nineteenth century. Even for the more-complex procedures, a relatively small number of fairly unspecialized surgical instruments sufficed. These were generally owned by the surgeon, although in some countries, such as the Netherlands, eighteenth-century guilds are known to have held loan collections from which surgeons could borrow expensive or infrequently used items. From Graeco-Roman times, the surgical armamentarium consisted of knives, forceps, probes, cauteries, and needles of various types.[14] Some ancient bronze instruments, including a trivalve vaginal speculum from the ruins of Pompeii, still exist. Few medieval instruments have survived, since they were generally of iron or steel, but authors such as Paré and Fabricius of Aquapendente (1537–1619) provide plentiful woodcut illustrations. Evidence of actual everyday usage is harder to obtain.[15] Originally crudely made by blacksmiths and armourers, surgical tools were produced by cutlers and other artisans during the seventeenth century. Pewterers, engravers, mathematical instrument-makers, and gold- and silversmiths became involved as instruments became more precise and more decorative. By the late eighteenth century, specialist instrument-makers were in existence, often working closely with surgeons in the design of new instruments. Until the late nineteenth century, a typical general set comprised instruments for amputation, lithotomy, and trepanation, put up in a velvet-lined, polished wood box. Instrument handles were of decoratively cut ebony or ivory, and carbon steel was used for knife blades until mid-century, with silver for cannulae and probes. Not until the last decades of the nineteenth century did all-metal instruments, devoid of decoration, begin to be used as aseptic techniques were adopted. Easier to clean and sterilize, these instruments also served to distinguish surgeons' tools from those of the physician, which continued to be made of materials such as wood and ivory.

THE EARLY NINETEENTH CENTURY

During the early decades of the nineteenth century, surgeons were prominent among the medical élite of both France and England, with Paris and London attracting many foreign students, including Americans. The 'eye-witness' accounts of these students and the lecture notes they made provide additional insight into a mode of operating where, in the absence of anaesthesia, speed remained at a premium. In Paris, Alexis Boyer (1757–1833) at the Charité and, above all, Guillaume Dupuytren (1777–1835) at the Hôtel Dieu, attracted numerous foreign observers. In London, Robert Liston (1794–1847) at University College Hospital and Astley Cooper (1768–1841) at Guy's and

St Thomas's Hospitals, held pre-eminent positions. The Bell brothers, John (1763–1820) and Charles (1774–1842), were leading representatives from the still-flourishing Edinburgh school. Surgical mortality remained very high, but in all these centres the numbers and types of operations attempted increased as the techniques of a more-conservative surgery were established. Leading surgeons were careful to stress the dependence of surgical practice on suitable theory. In France, the highly organized and institutionalized surgical profession based its theory on the tissue pathology of Bichat, who had taught Dupuytren. The more-individualistic tradition of British surgery took John Hunter's principles as its guide. His pupils included Astley Cooper, John Abernethy (1764–1831), Henry Cline (1750–1827), William Blizard (1743–1835), and other luminaries of the London surgical scene. The increasing demand by surgeons and anatomists for corpses during this period resulted in the resurrectionist scandals and, ultimately, the Anatomy Act of 1832 in Britain, which extended the circumstances in which human dissection might legally be performed.

The experiences in London, Edinburgh, and Paris of Americans such as John Collins Warren (1778–1856), Professor of Anatomy and Surgery at Harvard, contributed to the development of surgery in the United States. With Philip Syng Physick (1768–1837) at Pennsylvania, Warren led an essentially practical tradition of American surgery. Despite the influence of French surgical teaching on many Americans, their surgery remained, until later in the century, less concerned with theoretical matters than its European counterparts. It was in this context that Ephraim McDowell (1771–1830), a country practitioner from Kentucky, performed a number of successful ovariotomies from 1809 onwards. His cases became known through reports addressed to John Bell in Edinburgh, whose courses McDowell had attended in the 1790s. They were met with scepticism. Elective operations within the abdominal cavity were not yet widely accepted in European surgical practice.

In the German-speaking countries, expansion in both academic and theoretical surgery came rather later than in France and Great Britain. This was characterized in the 1820s and 1830s by the rebuttal of French influence and a corresponding interest in English surgical literature. C. J. M. Langenbeck (1776–1851) led the profession in Göttingen. At Vienna, Vincenz von Kern (1760–1829) founded a school of surgery in 1806. There was a surgical clinic at the University of Berlin from its foundation in 1810. Its professors were Carl Ferdinand von Graefe (1787–1840), and then J. F. Dieffenbach (1792–1847). A slightly anomalous situation existed in the Netherlands, where medical education continued on an eighteenth-century pattern well into the nineteenth. Continuing allegiance to Hermann Boerhaave (1668–1738) and the small size of the university hospitals did not favour the adoption of 'Paris medicine'. A broad spectrum of practitioners, including barber-surgeons, persisted, and it was possible to pursue a non-academic training in surgery until the 1860s.

The middle of the nineteenth century is usually regarded as a cut-off point in the history of surgery, dividing the pre- and post-anaesthetic eras. Historians have rightly seen successful anaesthesia (1840s) and also (from the 1880s) the adoption of antiseptic, then aseptic, techniques as changing the character of operative surgery virtually beyond recognition. Increasingly, intricate procedures in the innermost parts of the body were attempted successfully in the longer operating times and calmer conditions allowed by anaesthesia. It became accepted that gentle operative technique with meticulous attention to controlling haemorrhage and conserving body tissues gave better postoperative results. However, the radical changes in the surgical profession itself, and in the perception of the body and its pathology, had begun nearly a century earlier. By the 1850s, there was, in Europe and North America, an institutionalized surgical profession with an established body of theoretical knowledge in which the innovations of the second half of the century were generated, appraised, and disseminated. These earlier changes were a prerequisite for the subsequent technical success of surgeons. (➤ Ch. 42 Surgery (modern))

NOTES

1   O. Temkin, 'Review of Richard A. Leonardo *History of Surgery*, New York, Froben Press, 1943', *Bulletin of the History of Medicine*, 1944, 15: 430–2.

2   P. B. Adamson, 'Surgery in ancient Mesopotamia', *Medical History*, 1991, 35: 428–35.

3   Peter Murray Jones, *Medieval Medical Miniatures*, London, British Library Board, 1984, p. 105.

4   T. Clifford Allbutt, *The Historical Relations of Medicine and Surgery to the End of the Sixteenth Century*, London, Macmillan, 1905.

5   Darrel W. Amundsen, 'Medicine and surgery as art or craft: the role of schematic literature in the separation of medicine and surgery in the late Middle Ages', *Transactions and Studies of the College of Physicians of Philadelphia*, 1979, (Series 5, I (I): 43–57.

6   Margaret Pelling, 'Appearance and reality: barber-surgeons, the body and disease', in A. L. Beier and Roger Findlay (eds), *London 1500–1700: the Making of the Metropolis*, London, Longman, 1985, pp. 82–112.

7   Robert Jütte, 'A seventeenth-century German barber-surgeon and his patients', *Medical History*, 1989, 33: 184–98.

8   L. Beier, 'Seventeenth-century English surgery: the casebook of Joseph Binns', in C. J. Lawrence (ed.), *Medical Theory, Surgical Practice*, London, Routledge, 1992.

9   Toby Gelfand, 'Empiricism, and eighteenth century French surgery', *Bulletin of the History of Medicine*, 1969, 43: 40–53, see p. 41.

10 J. Dobson, 'The place of Hunter's Museum', *Annals of the Royal College of Surgeons* 1963, 33: 32–40.

11 L. S. Jacyna, 'Images of John Hunter in the nineteenth century', *History of Science*, 1983: 85–108.

12 C. J. Lawrence, 'Ornate physicians and learned artisans', in W. F. Bynum and R. S. Porter (eds) *William Hunter and the Eighteenth-Century Medical World*, Cambridge, Cambridge University Press, 1985, pp. 153–76, see p. 159.

13 Daniel De Moulin, *A History of Surgery*, Dordrecht, Martins Nijhoff, p. 245.

14 J. Kirkup, 'The history and evolution of surgical instruments', *Annals of the Royal College of Surgeons of England*, 1981, 63: 279–85; 1982, 64: 125–32; 1983, 65: 269–73; 1985, 67: 54–60; 1986, 68: 29–33.

15 G. Lawrence, 'The ambiguous artifact: surgical instruments and the surgical past', in Lawrence, op. cit. (n. 8), pp. 295–314.

FURTHER READING

De Moulin, Daniel, *A History of Surgery*, Dordrecht, Martinus Nijhoff, 1988.

Gelfand, Toby, *Professionalizing Modern Medicine: Paris Surgeons and Medical Science and Institutions in the Eighteenth Century*, Westport, CT, Greenwood Press, 1980.

Manjo, Guido, *The Healing Hand: Man and Wound in the Ancient World*, Cambridge, MA, Harvard University Press, 1991.

Nutton, Vivian, 'Humanist surgery', in A. Wear, R. K. French and I. M. Lonie (eds), *The Medical Renaissance of the Sixteenth Century*, Cambridge, Cambridge University Press, 1985, pp. 75–99.

Siraisi, Nancy G., *Medieval and Early Renaissance Medicine*, Chicago, IL, University of Chicago Press, 1990, Ch. 6.

Wangensteen, Owen H. and Wangensteen, Sarah D., *The Rise of Surgery*, Minneapolis, University of Minnesota Press, 1978.

42

SURGERY (MODERN)

Ulrich Tröhler

INTRODUCTION

Modern surgery, that is surgery after the introduction of antiseptic/aseptic wound management in the late 1860s, can be divided into three periods, namely. the localistic or anatomical period from 1860 until the First World War; the functional or physiological period up to the 1950s; and the systemic period of the decades since.

During the first period, surgery was revolutionized, but the First World War in many ways marked a change in outlook. By 1900, those giants born around 1840, who had known the old, dirty surgery leading to hospital gangrene and had contributed to or accepted its aseptic conversion, were just about to leave. The principles of avoiding germs were self-evident to the generation of their successors, who were ready to tackle new issues with new methods, some being prompted by the First World War. The influence of para-surgical methods on surgery grew, and the combined advances of surgical and para-surgical knowledge continued yet at an increasing pace from the 1950s, particularly with respect to technology, leading in many fields to a clear break with the past.

The localistic period dominated by the triumvirate of anaesthesia, asepsis, and pathological anatomy was characterized by *resection* in order to cure tumours, inflammations, injuries, or anomalies. The functional period, in addition, emphasized surgical (patho)physiology and pharmacology, and developed methods respecting functions and procedures of *restoration* of impaired or endangered function. The third era can be characterized by the term '*replacement*'. First, while fostering function by the novelty of artificial or biological organ or tissue replacement, necessitating an unprecedented degree of technology as well as biochemical and immunological knowledge, it featured an increasingly systemic approach to diagnostics, treatment, risk, and outcome assessment, often blurring the traditional frontiers between surgery and other disciplines, medical and beyond. (➤ Ch. 8 The biochemical tradition; Ch. 10 The immunological tradition) Second, this was also the era when surgery was being replaced by other therapies based on metabolic rather than localistic understanding of disease. And finally, it is the time when a good deal of what remained from the first period in terms of surgical technique is, in a second revolution, seemingly being replaced by entirely novel procedures.

While features of each of the periods persisted and were subsequently improved, these periods nevertheless were distinct from each other and were perceived as such by their contemporaries. Furthermore, each of them is characterized by a change and differentiation of surgically treatable disorders. Therefore the dates of the three periods might vary according to a specific field, so that a survey is appropriately sectional rather than chronological.

This article thus describes in a first part each period from the point of view of general surgery: that is, management of pain and wounds, handling of the risks and consequences of operations (for example, haemorrhage and shock), and general surgical technique (instruments, sutures), as well as general theories of inflammation and tumours. It is concluded by a brief section on evaluation of surgical therapy and the place of the surgeon in society. This chapter then illustrates surgery's evolution, using examples from special fields. Specialization in, as well as institutionalization and professionalization of surgery are phenomena increasingly observable throughout the last 120 years. They are issues on their own, only marginally hinted at in this chapter, which had to focus, albeit not exclusively, on information on ideas, concepts and – important for surgery – on technical developments. This information is presented in the form of a periodization model derived from empirical data. Other historically relevant questions such as the reasons for the very existence and the kind of development (and decline) surgery took cannot be addressed to the desirable extent. Nor can national peculiarities be dealt with.

THE SURGICAL REVOLUTION OF THE NINETEENTH CENTURY

THE DEVELOPMENT OF GENERAL PRECONDITIONS
1846–1900

Anaesthesia

The breakthrough of ether anaesthesia in 1846 can be seen as a heroic landmark in the history of modern surgery. The rapidity with which the news of the obliteration of pain during a surgical operation spread to Europe shows the impact of this first great American contribution to medicine. On 16 October 1846, the Boston surgeon J. C. Warren (1778–1856) operated on a neck tumour under ether inhalation administered by W. T. G. Morton (1819–68), and the resulting publication was read at a meeting on 3 and 9 November. The London surgeon R. Liston (1794–1847) performed the first leg amputation on 21 December of the same year. The next day, ether anaesthesia was tried in Paris; on 23 January 1847 in Berne; 28 January in Vienna; 6 February in Berlin; 8 March in The Hague, etc.[1] (➤ Ch. 67 Pain and suffering)

Remarkably, some doctors learned about this sensation from the New World through the lay press, which had, a few years earlier, reported the effects of mesmeric 'anaesthesia'. Inhalation anaesthesia was quickly seen as a welcome tool to foster a powerful surgical (and obstetrical) community within established university medicine. Surgery, still considered a mere craft by many physicians and patients, had already achieved this in some places. Legal prescriptions helped. They were introduced against criminal abuse of anaesthetics as early as the spring of 1847, for example, in Germany and Switzerland: henceforth, only qualified doctors were allowed to administer anaesthetics. (➤ Ch. 4 Medical care)

On 19 January 1847, barely four weeks after the first painless operation in London, J. Y. Simpson (1811–70) of Edinburgh first used chloroform to ease childbirth. Soon afterwards, this was also tried on the European continent, and in the same year, the dentist, H. Wells (1818–97) of Hartford, Connecticut, published his work on nitrous oxide. Thus, within a few months, three general anaesthetics became known, a true revolution causing an extraordinary amount of debate in professional and lay circles on medical and ethical aspects of pain control. It led to research on animals and on patients, and self-experimentation by doctors, to elucidate the various mechanisms of action, to describe the stages of this artificially induced sleep and analgesia, and to establish dosage. Until the First World War, the pros and cons of ether, chloroform, or other gases, or the 'right' mixture or sequence, were discussed. This research set standards of accurate reporting of successes and failures. Thus in many ways, anaesthesia established the relation between the surgeon as practitioner and as clinical or physiological researcher. (➤ Ch. 11 Clinical research)

Several significant discoveries followed, such as the introduction of new agents for inhalation anaesthesia, and of techniques for local infiltration, spinal application, and blocking of nerve trunks. Local anaesthesia, for example, with cocaine in ophthalmology, according to C. Koller (1857–1944) of Vienna, made minor operations easier for both patient and surgeon. However, bigger ones, like thyroid extirpations or trepanations, where local anaesthesia was applied for safety reasons, often remained distressing for the patient. From the 1870s, intratracheal insufflation for total anaesthesia was tried in Scotland, France, and Germany, where F. Kuhn (1866–1929) experimented c.1900 with positive-and negative-pressure insufflation. This was developed by S. J. Meltzer (1851–1920) and J. Auer (1875–1948) of the Rockefeller Institute, New York, in 1909.

Theory of disease

Turning back to the late 1840s, it becomes clear from hospital reports – which were then rather novel – and from archival sources, that the introduction of painless operating, although hailed by patients, did not influence the success of surgical interventions. Surgical mortality was still very high due to blood loss and postoperative infection. Furthermore, a theoretical precondition for more invasive surgery than was necessary for the customary amputations, subperiostal resections, fistulas, superficial tumours, abscesses – that is, for mainly 'external diseases' – was not present as long as humoralism prevailed. (➤ Ch. 14 Humoralism) A new localistic theory was advanced in the work by R. Virchow (1821–1902), *Cellularpathologie, in ihrer Begründung auf physiologische und pathologische Gewebelehre* (1858), and soon gained wide acceptance. The book was translated into English in 1860 and became a cornerstone of mainstream medical theory for decades. It finally did away with humoralism, which had been anti-surgical for centuries.[2]

The therapeutic implementation of cellular pathology was, in fact, the surgical removal of the pathologically altered tissues, from which diseases were understood to take their origin. (➤ Ch. 9 The pathological tradition)

Germ theory of wound infection, antisepsis, and asepsis

At the same time, successes in the fight against acute infections were reported. I. P. Semmelweis (1818–65) first showed in Vienna in 1848/9 that puerperal fever was a contagious septicaemia that could largely be prevented by scrubbing the hands with soap and water, using a fingernail brush, followed by a similar scrub in chlorine water before internal examination of lying-in women. This, and his later book-length contribution, being entirely empirical and with no theoretical foundation, were only partially recognized by the academic community. (➤ Ch. 16 Contagion/germ theory/specificity)

In parallel and independently, a school of 'cleanliness and cold water surgery' established itself in London around T. S. Wells (1818–97). From 1860, Wells washed with cold water and used fresh towels when operating, used metallic thread, and admitted only those spectators who testified in writing that they had not been in an autopsy room for seven days.

This procedure – as Semmelweis's physical examination – can with hindsight be called 'aseptic': that is, all parts in intimate contact with the patient (hands, instruments, dressings) were relatively germ-free. Neither Semmelweis nor Wells was aware of the pathogenicity of germs as we understand it. Such micro-organisms were then often regarded as microscopical artefacts or as results of chemical processes. (➤ Ch. 6 The microscopical tradition) Bacteriology had not become established. Rather, Semmelweis's and Wells's practice stemmed from chance observations, influenced by a very strong public-health movement, which was effective in reducing infections by cleanliness and hygiene. (➤ Ch. 51 Public health) The theoretical background, as established in the eighteenth century (but, in fact, much older) was that infections were caused either by miasmata (emanations given off by non-human sources) and/or by contagions (emanations from humans suffering from a disease). (➤ Ch. 15 Environment and miasmata) All kinds of emanations were transmitted by air, and this dogma therefore emphasized ventilation and control of overcrowding as preventive measures. There was a kind of dialectical relationship between the patient and the environment, which explained disease; the treatment of surgical patients derived from this old theoretical principle. In 1862, J. Paget (1814–99) held that:

> The cleanliness should, however, include more than it commonly does, such as the use of . . . baths, and of the frequent change, not only of dressings . . . and of bed-linen, but of beds . . . the best plan is to let patient be as ready as possible in the ordinary mode of prudent life . . . to observe all rules of personal cleanliness, to provide abundant fresh air, and a sufficient or liberal mixed diet.[3]

Hygiene encompassed bodily and moral constitution alike. (➤ Ch. 53 History of personal hygiene) In London and other European cities, it was a hotly debated issue, on statistical grounds, whether large hospitals with their filthy, crowded wards constituted a real danger to patients. For surgery, this meant, among other things, the so-called open treatment of wounds: ventilation and fresh air favoured the natural process of healing, of which infection was still seen as a normal stage. (➤ Ch. 49 The hospital)

Into this debate came J. Lister (1827–1912), Professor of Surgery at Glasgow, who in 1867 published a series of three articles in the *Lancet*, starting with 'On a new method of treating compound fractures, abscesses etc.' and ending with 'Illustrations of the antiseptic system of treatment in surgery'. Antisepsis was the destruction or suppression of agents of wound infection by disinfectants. Lister's practice depended on two entirely new theoretical points concerning infection: first, that germs, which were ubiquitous, were the causative agents of infections; and second, that infection was not a normal stage in the wound-healing process. They were in complete opposition to the above-described concept, which, besides its age, had the proven efficacy of public-health measures on its side: Lister's new view derived from the work of Louis Pasteur (1822–95) on fermentation and putrefaction, phenomena which he interpreted as biological processes due to the action of bacteria and/or yeasts both in the presence and absence of air (1859–63), and from his observations on the spoiling of wine by micro-organisms (1868). The analogy to wound infections, however, was not yet experimentally demonstrated.

Thus Lister's method could convince only by its results. He presented them as a statistical comparison of the mortality rates of compound fractures before and after the introduction of dressings soaked with carbolic acid (phenol). Its disinfectant or, rather, deodorizing properties (directed against the 'emanations') had already been described by F. J. Lemaire (1814–86) in France in 1860. In fact, Lister had chosen phenol amongst other substances known for their deodorizing action. Although it is possible that he presented 'selected' statistics, as a modern analysis of the case records suggests, the difference between the mortalities as shown by the method of historical controls impressed many a practitioner. This was particularly true for empiri-cally minded doctors, who cared for results rather than for theoretical justifi-cations: in 1864 and 1866, sixteen of his thirty-five patients undergoing amputation (46 per cent) died, whereas in 1867–9 it was only six out of forty (15 per cent).[4]

However, the new wound dressing had its drawbacks. It was costly, compli-cated and, as we know from the diaries of a few patients, as long-lasting and disagreeable to them and doctors alike as traditional treatment.[5] Furthermore, the implication of antisepsis (that is, the germ theory of infection) placed the responsibility for the outcome of a treatment no longer on the patient's susceptibility to infection, nor on the environment, but on the surgeon. Thus, there were good reasons for the long-lasting opposition to antisepsis on theoretical (or from the absence of 'proven' theoretical) and administrative grounds, as well as for subjective and social motives, that made it unlikely to appeal to a professionalizing group as surgeons were at that time. Ethical considerations also played an important role, at least in Germany.[6] In fact, the high death rate of amputations in Glasgow at the time of Lister was neither ubiquitous nor constant, but rather new, possibly due to the mid-century social crisis caused by the Industrial Revolution. Since the incidence of postoperative infections was not suddenly reduced when carbolic acid was introduced, it may from hindsight be suggested that the decreasing mortality rate was also due to better resistance to infection as a consequence of better nutrition, and of fresh water supply and sewage systems being introduced – at least in Lister's Glasgow – at the same time as antiseptic methods.[7] This interpretation would agree with the fact that Lister continued to perfect his method through the 1870s and 1880s. It ultimately resulted in the disinfection of operative and accidental wounds, surgical instruments, and the surgeon's hands, and for a time even the air, using a spray.

In parallel, the Semmelweis and Wells prophylactic approach was being adopted in England and Germany. This meant the prevention of putrefaction by securing the absence of infective agents as opposed to their destruction by antiseptic chemicals. In this view, the surgeon was not equated with pollution, but rather became the mediator between a potentially dangerous environment and the patient's susceptibility. Aseptic means were completely in accordance with the notions of cleanliness in matters both moral and medical, so typical for Victorian times, at least in Protestant countries. This notion was also basic to the successful public-health approach, and to the improvement of hospital cleanliness: for example, by ventilation and avoidance of cross-infections by prophylactic measures such as the pavilion system of hospital architecture. (➤ Ch. 64 Medicine and architecture) It is a fact that the aseptic ritual of sterilized gowns – which were not necessary according to Lister, and not used by him – masks, and gloves was introduced gradually from the early 1870s without much opposition and discussion, as it connected popular ideas of cleanliness with the notion of surgical sterility.

Nevertheless, the scientific work that established this old dialectic interplay between the patient and the environment on a new basis must be stressed as the important factor. This work was mostly done in the late 1870s in Germany by people such as R. Koch (1843–1910). It furnished, first, the hitherto-lacking experimental basis for the germ theory of specific wound infection by showing the possibility of culturing and identifying bacteria and by the transfer of pure cultures into animals, thereby producing specific types of wound infections. Second, bacteriology also furnished objective criteria for evaluating the efficacy of the measures taken to prevent or to fight surgical infection. Thus measures and agents of the aseptic ritual could be tested as to whether they effectively diminished the number of pathogenic germs. The bacteriologists' experimental work on wound infection left no doubt that infection could not occur without a certain number of bacteria: the culture of smears taken from the skin of doctors and patients, as well as from wounds, dressings, and instruments, relentlessly revealed whether or not a significant number of bacteria was present. Evaluation even included the hygiene of hospital and private laundries, and the bacteriostatic action of soaps.

By 1874, Pasteur suggested immersing the instruments in boiling water and passing them through a flame, and by the end of the decade advocated these methods to replace chemical antiseptics, as did Koch in 1881. The earliest steam-sterilizers were built by these same microbiologists for laboratory use. Gradually, heat superseded chemical methods.

A few leading scientifically oriented surgeons in Germany and Switzerland, such as E. von Bergmann (1836–1907), T. Kocher (1841–1917), and J. von Mikulicz-Radecki (1850–1905), set up bacteriological laboratories in the 1880s within their clinics. The laboratories were staffed by specialists, and contributed markedly to modern standards of preparation for aseptic operations. Each elaborated his own controlled system of wound management. This is subject to modification even today, yet still according to the same criteria of evaluation.

Bergmann propagated antisepsis with sublimate ($HgCl_{12}$), before his assistant, K. Schimmelbusch (1860–91), proved in the 1880s that streaming steam outdid phenol in its bactericidal effect, and had the drums which still bear his name constructed. Kocher, an even quicker adept of Lister, observed the toxicity and sometimes the inefficacy of phenol, and also tested various other antiseptics. He started boiling his instruments in 1886. Together with the bacteriologist E. Tavel (1858–1912), he later introduced the quicker method of pressure steam-sterilization. The two Swiss also showed the rationale for Kocher's gentle handling of tissues, starting with the skin incisions parallel to the fissure lines of the skin and his refined haemostasis (Kocher's clamp). These lay in the phenomena of 'lesion-infection' and 'haematoma-infection', terms coined by them (1895/1909). Kocher warned that antisepsis and asepsis gave no reason to neglect anatomical and physiological features of the natural healing process. Von Mikulicz-Radecki, an equally early advocate of boiling and washing, together with his microbiologist colleague C. Flügge (1847–1923), showed that speaking during operations enhanced droplet infection – a term coined by him – and that this risk could be markedly diminished by wearing face-masks, except when the surgeon was bearded.

Cotton and silk gloves were in use before the Europe-trained American surgeon, William S. Halsted (1852–1922), of Johns Hopkins Hospital, introduced rubber gloves in 1890. He did so to protect the hands of his operating-room nurse (his fiancée), whose skin was allergic to the antiseptic in use then. There was much opposition to rubber gloves, for they were expensive and allegedly reduced the delicacy of touch. Von Mikulicz-Radecki described cotton gloves in 1897 which could be boiled and used up to twelve times and which he changed up to three times during a long operation.

Extensive experiments on the problems of sterility of surgeons' hands were conducted, particularly in Germany. The finding that it was impossible to achieve absolute sterility finally persuaded most surgeons to wear rubber gloves, although it was decades before this became routine for the whole operating team.

However, in the final years of the nineteenth century, pre-operative prophylactic antiseptic and aseptic methods were adopted in one combination or another by all surgeons. Gone were the days when a surgeon operated in an eternal black frock caked with blood, the patient lying on a wooden dining table in a barely lit room, the floor of which was covered with sawdust. (➤ Ch. 41 Surgery (traditional)) As one of them recalled in 1927:

> Operating theatres which resembled a shambles in 1860 are replaced by rooms of spotless purity containing scintillating metal furniture and ingenious electric lights. All concerned in the operation are clothed from nose-tip to toe-tip in sterilised linen gowns, and their hands covered with sterilised rubber gloves.[8]

Operating techniques

In general, operating before 1900 was quick, a relict of the pre-anaesthetic and -antiseptic era. Techniques, above all, had to ease the surgeon's work. An enormous number of new, individualized – and potentially prestigious – instruments were devised. Surgery was centred on the intuition, perseverance, and technical brilliance of the individual master. Only a few operations eventually became internationally standardized. Yet with diagnostic and post operative control taking new dimensions after the introduction of X-rays in 1896, some of the idiosyncratic procedures, for instance of fracture treatment, became rapidly obsolete.[9]

If operative surgery was dominated by the idea of resection and extirpation in connection with the Virchowian concept of disease, this also implied the finding of reliable methods of closing an injury. For example, intestinal suture opened up the whole new territory of gastro-intestinal surgery. In all tubular structures of the body, this involves closing a partial injury created by the doctor or even reuniting two completely transected ends. Anaesthesia and asepsis enabled crude suture techniques to be systematically elaborated and refined. The principle of the inverting suture, in which the insides of a tubular wall are turned slightly inward on both sides of the lesion, which is then sutured together using their outside surfaces without entering the lumen of the organ, was proposed in 1826, first successfully performed by J. F. Dieffenbach (1792–1847) in an accidental case in 1836, and became the basis of almost all suture techniques. Kocher, in 1888, replaced the customary catgut by more sterilizable fine silk thread, even for lasting sutures.

From the 1820s, a great deal of animal experimentation was devoted to finding mechanical devices as aids to intestinal suture by compression of linear bowel lacerations. Individual chips and needle-armed anastomosing blocks were tried. The best known was (and still is) the metal device based more or less on the principle of the snap fastener, the 'Murphy button', introduced clinically in 1892 by the Chicago surgeon J. B. Murphy (1857–1916).

THE CONQUERING SURGICAL PRACTICE 1870–1910

The complete statistics that T. Billroth (1829–94) published on his work as chief of the surgical clinics of Zurich (1860–7) and Vienna (1867–8) universities, reveal that most of his 700-odd in-patients per annum suffered from acute and chronic infections (frequently tuberculosis and syphilis), and tumours and injuries of the lower extremities; followed by the upper extremities, face, mouth, thorax, and neck, sexual organs, pelvis, head, and spine. The category that Billroth termed 'varia' included plastic operations for cleft palate and tenotomies for club-foot as already introduced in the first half of the century by the German surgeons Dieffenbach and B. von Langenbeck (1810–87), and G. F. L. Stromeyer (1804–76). The overall mortality in both Zurich and Vienna varied around 10 per cent. In most cases, the surgeon dealt with these conditions in either a conservative way – that is, by punctures, injections of iodine, orthopaedic fixation, and rest – or, rarely, in a radical way by amputation and/or resection of the diseased part. This held also for tumours and cysts, of which only superficial ones were reported. There was no carcinoma of an abdominal, intrathoracic or endocranial organ, but a few goitres, skin tumours (atheromas, lipomas, angiomas), osteosarcomas, carcinomas of mouth and pharynx, and lymphomas were operated on, besides breast tumours, which were relatively frequent. Two out of six cases of rectal cancer were deemed too extended to be extirpated: three of the four patients operated on died. Anorectal fistulas or prolapsed haemorrhoids could be treated successfully.[11]

Thus Billroth dealt, above all, with superficially localized disorders often complicated by infections. His methods were 'conservative'. Only as a last resort would he choose a 'radical' measure: amputation or resection with a high risk of death by infection or circulatory problems.

Twenty years later, the first German edition of a classic textbook of operative surgery, T. Kocher's *Chirurgische Operationslehre* (1892), was 200 pages long; its fifth German edition (1907) comprised nearly 1,100 pages. Old procedures such as ligatures of arteries (for syphilitic aneurysms) and veins, amputations, and bone resections alone now took over 250 pages. There was an entire 100-page section on pre- and postoperative care, and nearly half of the book treated the new fields of abdominal and thoracic surgery and that of the nervous system including brain and spinal cord. Surgeons had, in their own terms, 'conquered' all body cavities and organs.

Paradigmatic operations were the excision (rather than the earlier puncturing) of sometimes enormous ovarian cysts and goitres by so-called ovariotomy and resection, respectively. The former, transgressing the hitherto absolute barrier of the peritoneum, preluded abdominal surgery in the 1860s already, and was therefore debated through the world medical press.[12] Wells performed his thousandth ovariotomy in 1880 with a lethality of 11 per cent in the last 100. In the hands of Kocher, thyroid resection for endemic goitre, much feared hitherto because of haemmorrhage and infection, became safe. In 1895 he had performed his first thousand; in 1909 his fourth thousand resections, with lethalities decreasing from 14 per cent to 1.1 per cent and finally to 0.7 per cent, respectively, in the last thousand.

The expansion of surgical practice and research is also reflected in the increasing number of papers delivered at the meetings of newly founded surgical societies. Their contents afford particularly rich illustrations of the wealth of innovation as well as of its practical rationale. In the German series, for example, which started in 1872, cancer was an important subject. It was selected five times as a main congress topic (1883, 1895, 1900, 1902, and 1905). There was a constant flow of papers on cancer, averaging about 20 per cent of all communications: 52 organs or organ systems were concerned, the most frequent being the gastro-intestinal tract (26.5 per cent), followed by thyroid (18 per cent), breast (16.2 per cent), and bone (12.9 per cent). Total 'eradication' was aimed at, which ended up sometimes in mutilating interventions. Other main topics continued to be the surgery of infections, both acute (for example, appendicitis, cholecystitis) and chronic (extrapulmonary tuberculosis, osteomyelitis). Fracture treatment, on the other hand, was a kind of Cinderella. At the first four meetings after the Franco-German war, 18.4 per cent of all papers dealt with fractures; afterwards, the rate fell to below 10 per cent.[13] This held also, albiet to a lesser extent, for what was then called 'war surgery': that is, the management of battle-wounds, characterized by discussion of the pros and cons of debridement.

Often, both tumours and infections led to obstruction or stenosis, above all in the digestive, respiratory, and urogenital tracts. These could be – if only temporarily – cured by fissuring or extirpation, which made the surgeon the 'saviour' of patients. Obvious examples were safe tracheotomy for tuberculosis or cancer of the larynx, and relief of intestinal obstruction caused by cancer or strangulation. With relatively safe procedures, operative surgery entered its 'golden age' when it was unquestionably the most therapeutically active branch of somatic medicine.

INSTITUTIONALIZATION AND PROFESSIONALIZATION OF SURGERY

In this unprecedented revolution, which occurred within one generation, the German-speaking countries gained a leading position in the nineteenth century. Clinical practice, teaching, and research were united in the surgical departments of twenty-seven medical faculties in Austria, Germany, and Switzerland. These university departments with their clear hierarchical organization set the example for other countries, such as the United States (Johns Hopkins) or the Netherlands (where Austrian and Swiss-trained chiefs became professors). There were also great surgeons in the other European countries and the United States, yet the environment (including the relatively later adoption of asepsis) and the 'school-type' organization of medical studies made achievements more difficult than in the 'faculty-type' in central Europe.[14] (➤ Ch. 47 History of the medical profession)

The scientific expansion in Germany is reflected in the foundation of four journals devoted exclusively to surgery: *Archiv für klinische Chirurgie* (1861), *Deutsche Zeitschrift für Chirurgie* (1872), *Centralblatt für Chirurgie* (1874), and *Beiträge zur klinischen Chirurgie* (1886). Travel was about to become faster and easier. Many national surgical societies were founded, the first being in Germany (1872), reflecting the fact that German-speaking Europe had by then become the world's centre of medical science in general. The American Surgical Association, the first of many American ones, soon followed in 1880. It published *Annals of Surgery*, the first modern non-German surgical journal, from 1885. The second and third American periodicals followed in 1888 and 1905, respectively. In Britain and France, however, surgical work continued to be published in the general medical press. The *British Journal of Surgery* was started only in 1913. The Italian and French surgical associations were founded in 1882 and 1884, respectively, and the Dutch and Swiss ones in 1902 and 1913. The Société Internationale de Chirurgie held the first three of its triennial meetings as from 1905 in Brussels.[15] Thus surgery had become fully professionalized.

X-ray diagnostics and aseptic therapeutic procedures could be safely performed only in special premises: that is, in a clinic equipped with the necessary technical infrastructure and built according to the new and controllable standards of hygiene. Surgical clinics were no longer reserved for lower-class patients, although special facilities guaranteed the privacy and comfort the well-to-do were accustomed to and ready to pay for.

But a spirit of optimism for the future of surgery also arose within the profession and in hospital administrations, governments, and patients around the turn of the century. Two surgeons were honoured with an early Nobel Prize (first bestowed in 1901). These were Kocher in 1909 for his work on physiology, pathology, and surgery of the thyroid gland; and the Franco-American A. Carrel (1873–1944) in 1911 for his development of the suturing of blood vessels and his work on transplantation. Throughout the Western world, old premises were completely renovated or, more often, entirely new operating suites and surgical clinics were built and equipped, particularly in university towns. The favoured plan was still the pavilion system championed for half a century by Florence Nightingale (1820–1910).

Nightingale also pioneered professional nursing, a further precondition for the success of modern hospital-based medicine, particularly of surgery with its increasingly demanding pre- and postoperative care. Antisepsis, and particularly asepsis, required a strict set of rules, and became instrumental in transforming surgery to a form of teamwork. The first trained nurses exclusively employed in the operating theatre appeared in the early twentieth century. (➤ Ch. 54 A general history of nursing 1800–1900)

SUMMARY AND OUTLOOK

Up to the First World War, surgery principally based on anaesthesia, asepsis, and pathological anatomy was extremely rich in ideas and the creation of new operative procedures, the lethality of which progressively decreased. Many operations on the gastro-intestinal tract, nervous system, thyroid, mammary glands, bones, and blood vessels were included by the turn of century in 'systems of [safe] surgery'.[16] E. von Küster (1839–1930) of Marburg, who had done the first successful plastic operation for the relief of hydronephrosis in 1892, concluded in his state-of-the-art lecture on urological surgery: 'It is impossible not to have the impression that the main work has been done and that for our successors there only remain scanty gleanings.'[17]

Thus the years preceding the First World War can be seen as the first heyday of surgery in the traditional narrow sense of the term: there was the operative 'conquest' of all cavities and organs of the body. Even difficult procedures on brain, lung, and heart were performed. Yet such great work, albeit based on valuable ideas and technical brilliance, remained chancy or isolated, since it required theoretical concepts and/or material resources which were increasingly felt to be lacking. How was one to understand graft rejection after a technically successful kidney transplantation, or to find material for osteosynthesis and joint replacement biologically better tolerated than the iron or ivory at hand?

Although the disputes between surgeons and physicians on operative versus conservative treatment of some acute conditions such as appendicitis had been decided in favour of early operation, there remained the subsidiary problem of social acceptance of surgery by physicians, general practitioners, and patients, particularly for chronic diseases. Immediate complications of operations such as embolism or blood loss were feared, as were delayed consequences and relapses: one even spoke of stigmatizing scars. Patients were sometimes more afraid of the nightmare induction of inhalation anaesthesia than of the operation itself. Nor was the psychological problem of abandoning one's consciousness to a doctor negligible. In addition, new therapeutic alternatives were coming up, such as X-rays, and radiotherapy for cancer and high-alpine heliotherapy for extrapulmonary tuberculosis. Often, the decision to operate for chronic diseases depended on social rather than medical motives, since in the absence of public-health insurance long-lasting conservative treatment was accessible for the well-to-do only.[18]

The lack of success of even total extirpation of the larynx by 1888 (only 8 of 138 cases were successful[19]) shows the problem surgery in this 'golden age' still encountered in terms of accurate and, above all, early diagnosis. Despite X-rays and the optical devices developed in the second part of the nineteenth century, allowing the visual examination of ear, nose, throat, larynx, oesophagus, stomach, rectum, abdominal cavity, urinary bladder, and vagina, inspection was often treacherous. It was not yet possible to take pre-operative biopsies from the stomach or urinary bladder, and even for the other organs, parts of tumours containing characteristic elements might some-times not be accessible through the existing instruments. Thus the pre-operative diagnosis had to rely, above all, on clinical findings. The misman-agement of the 'laryngeal swellings' (carcinoma) of Frederick III of Germany in 1887/8, involving top doctors like the British laryngologist M. Mackenzie (1853–1925), the German surgeon von Bergmann, and the pathologist Vir-chow, tragically illustrated these difficulties.[20] In fact, histological examinations were mostly done in postoperative preparations. And many doctors renounced even these, since operations were often carried out only in advanced stages with seemingly clear clinical diagnoses. This lack of precise diagnostic criteria as well as of statistical insight hindered the comparison of results, but, together withever changing techniques, made it easy to explain results not in agreement with theoretical expectations.

Leading surgeons felt these challenges and feared that surgery *per se*, having in many ways become a technically safe routine, was in danger of reverting to the mere handicraft of the old stone-cutters and bone-setters, if its theoretical concepts and their clinical application and evaluation were not continually revised and researched. For this reason, von Mikulicz-Radecki and the physician B. von Naunyn (1839–1925) founded the interdisciplinary periodical *Mitteilungen aus den Grenzgebieten der Medizin und Chirurgie* in 1896. Kocher commented: 'Operative therapy at the culmination of its quickest progresses was entirely based on the direct elimination of the cause of disease by its mechanistic means without greatly considering other factors.'[21] He knew what he was talking about, for in his thyroid resections he had passed over more and more to total extirpation of the gland, which prevented relapses, until by discovering the ensuing 'cachexy' (myxoedema) in 1883 (see p. 1010) he realized a functional limit of the idea of localization and extirpation of disease. Modern thyroid research, and indeed endocrine research, starting immediately thereafter became an important guideline for a new scientific outlook of surgery in the twentieth century. It lead to one of the rare Nobel Prizes ever bestowed upon a surgeon (Kocher, 1909). And G. Crile (1864–1943) of Cleveland, Ohio, who pioneered the experimental study of shock, concluded at a meeting in London in 1910: 'It would seem, that this era of the great triumvirate of anaesthesia, asepsis and pathological anatomy is nearing its zenith. . . . Are we not on the threshold of the era of physiology, the interpretation of the laws of life itself?'[22]

Thus the advances and the challenge of surgery generated the need for interdisciplinary research both in the laboratory and in the clinic. Part of this programme was hampered, and in part stimulated, by the First World War, and was greatly influenced by American authors. Indeed, in 1914, The Société Internationale de Chirurgie held its fourth congress in New York.

FACING NEW CHALLENGES WITH PHYSIOLOGY AND PHARMACOLOGY 1914–60

PHYSIOLOGICAL SURGERY

Two features characterize the progress of surgery in the period up to the 1950s. First, while the limits of technical feasibility were still extended (see new radical operations elaborated, for instance, in gastro-intestinal and gynae-cological oncology and psychosurgery), previous heroic procedures and even already standardized ones were gradually altered in the sense that an inter-vention had to be comfortable for the patient, not for the surgeon, even if this meant it lasted longer. Gentle procedures, already introduced by Kocher in Europe and Halsted in the USA by the turn of the century, were adopted gradually by some of their younger colleagues such as von Mikulicz-Radecki (Breslau); E. Payr (1871–1946) (Leipzig); the American leader of physiologi-cal surgery, Crile; or the Frenchman R. Leriche (1879–1955); who, in turn, trained others. These surgeons were as much concerned to increase the resistance of the tissues against infection as to carry out barely successful germ-free extirpation. This holds for specific surgical techniques as well as para-surgical methods, such as for the pre- and intra-operative consideration of physiological factors regulating blood circulation (particularly of the brain), in order to prevent surgical shock, a frequent complication of more extensive surgical interventions. Care for the position of the patient during the oper-ation, heated operating tables, control of blood pressure, use of body-warm isotonic saline for infusion and cleansing, differentiated techniques of anaes-thesia and haemostasis all contributed to prevent or ameliorate dangerous side-effects of surgery.[23] Intravenous feeding and gastro-intestinal decom-pression by continuous suction were further methods introduced between the wars, which revolutionized abdominal surgery.

But second, the trend was doubly on physiological lines since the results of surgery had no longer to be anatomically but also functionally satisfying. (➤ Ch. 7 The physiological tradition) This meant that surgeons had to develop an interest in patho-physiology beyond traditional mechanical conceptions. Examples are the artificial hand of F. Sauerbruch (1875–1959), with its mechanical yet physiological prehensile functions (1915–17), or of anatomically *and* functionally oriented system of fracture treatment F. de Quervain (1868–1940). This whole outlook was epitomized in the book by F. Rost, (1884–1935), *Die Pathophysiologie des Chirurgen*, with three editions between 1920 and 1925 and an English translation. Elucidating patho-physiological alterations by assessing, for example, heart, lung, kidney, or endocrine function by laboratory tests requiring biological, pharmacological, and statistical knowledge and technological procedures, have since continuously completed and even replaced traditional clinical diagnosis. This implied more precise criteria for indications to operate and for intra- and postoperative control, and – as far as radiology was concerned – also direct guidelines for operations. However, with the exception of some leading personalities, the main interest of surgical research was still the improvement of technique.

Wounds

During the First World War, debates over the proper method of treating wounds predominated. In particular, infected wounds, by then rare in civilian practice, became a topic of fervent discussion. It was soon realized that neither the aseptic techniques used in civilian circumstances nor the experiences of recent wars had much bearing on the conditions encountered in the trenches of the Western front. In fact, since the Industrial Revolution, weaponry changed in every war, confronting surgeons with new types of wounds. Thus, experimental hospitals emerged, such as that run by Carrel near Paris, which pioneered the Carrel–Dakin treatment. It consisted in cleansing the wound, irrigating it with a specific antiseptic (hypochloride in Dakin's formula) until it was bacteriologically sterile, and then closing it by suturing or lacing. Despite serious – and justified – criticism by English and American doctors from both scientific and practical points of view, this method came to prevail in both military and civilian practice up to The Second World War.[24] (➤ Ch. 66 War and modern medicine)

In parallel, the management of compound fractures, wound infection, and plastic surgery was technically improved. The availability of sulphonamides and, later, penicillin further changed former local treatment to a general one. Finally, the instillation of antiseptics into wounds was abandoned, as it was realized that they failed to sterilize already contaminated ones and might impede the natural reparative process, just as debridement proved useless once infection was well established. Thus, the role of the surgeon in wound management, which for centuries had been that of local pus evacuator, gave way to more general treatment. (➤ Ch. 39 Drug therapies)

Shock

Two early examples of the interplay of (patho)physiology and surgery were the management of surgical shock and endocrine research. Prevention and management of shock were still poorly understood, although the importance of blood loss and/or distribution in its genesis had been experimentally shown by Crile before The first World War. However, until the work of A. Blalock (1899–1964) established it firmly after 1930, a toxic factor was still debated. Treatment consisted in the administration of cardiotonics and, occasionally, since the late 1880s, in the intravenous infusion of saline or glucose solutions, although it had already been shown by a British–American research committee appointed during The First World War that macromolecular (gum acacia) solutions should be preferred.[25] In 1944, Swedish researchers recommended dextrane. The ideal solution is not yet found. Despite the discovery of the blood groups by K. Landsteiner (1864–1943) and other Viennese workers in 1900–2, blood transfusion played hardly any role up to the eve of The Second World War. Blood was still transfused directly from donor to recipient, and the procedure was deemed dangerous and time consuming. In the Spanish Civil War (1938), it was shown that blood which had been kept for several days could be indirectly transfused from the bottle to the patient. A first blood bank was established in the United States at the Mayo Clinic in Rochester in 1935.[26]

Endocrine glands

The Mayo Clinic was also a centre of endocrine research. Founded in 1889 as a predominantly surgical institution, it now set the example of clinical and theoretical scientists co-operating more closely than was customary in the compartmentalized central European structures. Through this work, within some twenty-five years, surgery for toxic goitre became safer, adreno-cortical tumours were successfully removed, and two hormones, thyroxine and cortisone, were isolated there by E. C. Kendall (1886–1972) in 1914 and 1936, respectively.[27] Cortisone became a most important therapeutic agent in many fields of medicine and surgery; it rendered adrenalectomy and hypophysectomy safe. Surgery of endocrine organs became a factor in the treatment of other diseases, such as cancer of the breast and the prostate, or of renal stones due to hyperparathyroidism, illustrating a metabolic rather than localistic concept of disease. (➤ Ch. 23 Endocrine disorders)

Such an interdisciplinary approach became common in central Europe only gradually. This was partly due to the post-war economic difficulties during the 1920s, and the ideological isolation of Germany in the 1930s after the

Nazi government had taken over, leading to the emigration of Jews. Also, German doctors were not yet accustomed to reading foreign literature.

ANAESTHESIOLOGY[28]

There were, however, major para-surgical advances during this period. Between 1923 and 1935, four new narcotic gases were introduced, followed in 1956 and 1974 by two more. They were mostly applied by endotracheal intubation, which is still considered the safest means to maintain undisturbed aeration of the lung. Although known in France and in Britain and extensively treated in a monograph by F. Kuhn of Berlin in 1911, the technique was rarely used in central Europe until after 1945. American army surgeons used it extensively during The Second World War as a consequence of the experimental work of Meltzer and Auer (see p. 987). A small technical modification, the use of an inflatable cuff to fit the tube gas-tight with the trachea (proposed by F. Trendelenburg (1849–1924) in the nineteenth century) was crucial: it enabled the anaesthetist to 'breathe' the patient, and allowed operations without time constraint, notably on the thoracic organs.

A series of soluble narcotic compounds found in Germany and the United States between 1929 and 1934 led to a further differentiation of anaesthesia by intravenous and intramuscular application. J. S. Lundy (1894–1973) of the Mayo Clinic, who contributed three of them, is sometimes called the 'father' of intravenous anaesthesia. This allowed short operations in total unconsciousness by a method easy to handle; above all, it was used to control induction of a lengthy inhalation anaesthesia, eliminating the patient's subjective stress without the dangers of rectal application. These substances were widely used until, in the 1960s, barbiturate-free ketamines and diazepam (also known as a tranquillizer in psychiatry and psychosomatic medicine) became popular.

Muscle relaxation via Crile's 'anoci-association' (ether inhalation completed with regional procaine) in 1915 marked a further surgically relevant pharmacological innovation. A next step was the first clinical use of curare, the Indian arrow-poison, by the Americans H. R. Griffith (1894–1985) and G. E. Johnson in 1942. The curare-like substances of the Swiss Nobel Prize winner D. Bovet (1907–92) and coworkers (1946), who also discovered succinyl-choline (1949), and the methonium compounds found by the British pharmacologist W. D. M. Paton (b. 1917) in 1948, further transformed intra-abdominal operations.

In consequence, in this period anaesthesiology, in turn, became a professionalized discipline with periodicals and societies. The first periodical was the *American Yearbook of Anesthesia and Analgesia* (1915) (*Current Researches in Anaesthesia and Analgesia* from 1922). Periodicals in Britain, Germany, France,

Italy, and Argentina began to appear before The Second World War. After the war, journals followed in Asia (Japan, India), Mexico, Scandinavia, and in other European countries. The World Federation of Societies of Anaesthesiology was founded in 1955. Training courses and specialized examinations were introduced first in the Anglo-Saxon countries. H. Beecher (1904–76), the world's first Professor of Anaesthesiology (at Harvard University, 1941), wrote *The Physiology of Anesthesia* (1938). The first American textbook was *The Art of Anesthesia* (1916) by P. J. Flagg (1886–1970). Works such as *Chemistry of Anesthesia* and *Physics for the Anaesthetist*, both published in the USA in 1946, as well as *Pediatric Anesthesia* and *The Pharmacology of Anesthetic Drugs*, published there in 1948 and 1952, respectively, illustrate the development of anaesthesiology as a speciality based on respiratory and circulatory physiology, pharmacology, and medical technology. Further developments included the introduction (again in the USA) of such complicated measures as artificial hypothermia, controlled lowering of blood pressure to diminish blood loss, and extracorporeal circulation by the heart–lung machine (see p.1020). The mass spectrograph, developed between 1950 and 1952 in Minnesota, marked a new stage of monitoring narcosis.[29]

EXTENDING AND DIFFERENTIATING SURGICAL PRACTICE

By the mid-1950s, these para-surgical and general surgical procedures had greatly increased the possibilities of operability, both with respect to the age of patients and to the underlying disorder. This held also for cases hitherto deemed too risky because of imminent danger of infection, for example, for certain interventions in the lung, which is always in contact with the microorganisms of the air. These patients could now be treated pre- and/or post operatively with sulphonamides and/or antibiotics.

Thus the spectra of both surgically treatable disorders and of surgical methods were further widened but also differentiated, as is reflected in the development of surgery of the urogenital tract, orthopaedics, neurosurgery, and thoracic surgery as specialized branches, sometimes with their own university chairs.

With increasing feasibility and safety, however, the temptation to operate became sometimes irresistible. Appendectomy for so-called 'chronic' appendicitis was fashionable in the 1920s and 1930s, as were operations devised to fix an abdominal organ found by X-ray examination to be misplaced (that is, in a position considered to be anatomically incorrect) in order to treat chronic functional disorders. Similarly, tonsillectomies in children with sore throats became increasingly routine.[30] Total gastrectomy and radical pneumonectomy with excision of the mediastinal lymph nodules were recommended, in the early 1950s, for every stomach and lung cancer, respectively, as was ultra-radical mastectomy for breast cancer a decade later. These variants of possible therapeutic approaches called for comparative evaluation of results with proper statistical methods.

THE IMPACT OF TECHNOLOGY AND OF ASSESSMENT OF RESULTS SINCE THE 1960s

During the first period up to The First World War, operability had depended primarily on the surgeon's experience, intuition, and the brilliance and technical spectrum of his skills. While this may still be the case in emergencies, it has become much less so in elective surgery where still-growing precision in diagnostics, operating techniques, pre-operative treatment and postoperative and intensive care have come to influence indication and management. Specific clinical, physical, and laboratory parameters are considered in checklists according to the planned intervention, in order to estimate the risks, which sometimes also depend on psycho-social preparation. Whereas curability was a further important factor for the determination of operability in the first period, and respect of and restoration of function since the second, this third period is characterized by the new possibility of organ replacement due to new technologies. On the other hand, it features the replacement of surgery alone by other forms of treatment, and the replacement of by-now conventional techniques by radically new ones, phenomena to which more widespread attempts to assess therapeutic outcome by the methods of the controlled clinical trial, including the quality of life, are linked.

DIAGNOSTICS

Visual diagnostics gained precision with the introduction of the computerized tomograph (CT) by G. N. Hounsfield (b. 1919) of Great Britain in 1972, and of nuclear magnetic resonance (NMR) a decade later, both especially useful for neurosurgery (see p. 1018). More-recent methods include position emission tomography (PET). Sonography (visualization by ultra sound) was developed clinically in Sweden and the USA from around 1955, and soon became relevant for cardiac surgery. Nuclear medicine, using radioactive isotopes with a short half-life for quantitative determination of hormones and their metabolites in the laboratory as well as for clinically localizing tumours and metastasis by scintigraphy, became increasingly important in assessing the function of endocrine organs, lung, and kidney. Various catheterizations allowed the measurement of heart and liver functions. They can also be used therapeutically for mechanical dilating or local application of drugs. Finally, clinical neurophysiology elaborated many diagnostic approaches to assess the function of brain and nerves, as well as of the sense organs. (➤ Ch. 36 The science of diagnosis: diagnostic technologies)

THE SECOND REVOLUTION OF SURGICAL PRACTICE

Operating techniques

In 'traditional' surgery, operating techniques greatly changed due to new instruments and materials. As in the nineteenth century, new suturing techniques opened new territories, passing through a new experimental phase from the 1950s. The Moscow Scientific Institute for Experimental Surgical Apparatus and Instruments (with Gudov and Androsov) developed stapling apparatus for every conceivable surgical application, and stimulated research elsewhere.[31] Stapling was one of the preconditions for the deep resection of the rectum via the abdomen, allowing extirpation of a cancer while maintaining a functional sphincter ani: that is, faecal continence.

Vascular suture, thanks also to the introduction of anticoagulants, now became established. The possibilities of vascular anastomoses, in turn, stimulated the precise diagnosis of congenital and acquired heart disease, and the development of open-heart and transplantation surgery (see pp. 1020–21, 1022–24, respectively). Microsurgical techniques played a great role in this process of specialization. These procedures have been applied increasingly since the 1960s, particularly in plastic, neuro- and ophthalmic surgery, and in operations on the urogenital tract and the ear. They allow, on the one hand, precise destruction and excision of tissues (for example, by electro- or cryo-coagulation or lasers); on the other hand, they allow correction of malformations, reconstructions, and the implantations and transplantations typical of this period of replacement surgery.

Even in the traditional field of cancer surgery, ultra-radical procedures have mostly been abandoned whereas radical operations are seldom the sole treatment. They are complemented – not anatagonized – by radio- and/or chemotherapy (so that one even speaks of 'radiosurgery' and 'chemosurgery'), by hormones, by psycho-social support, and by rehabilitation, reflecting the interdisciplinary approach of the late twentieth century. (➤ Ch. 25 Cancer) In yet other fields, such as gastro-intestinal ulcer or endocrine disorders, where the disturbances can now justifiably be seen from a metabolic rather than a merely local point of view, traditional surgery has been increasingly replaced or complemented by other forms of standard treatment since the 1960s.

Intensive care

The differentiation of anaesthesiology continued, with the aim of contributing to each major intervention a specific procedure for the individual patient; correction of cardiac malformations in very small babies necessitating extra-corporeal circulation, as well as total hip replacement in 90-year-old diabetics are thus possible. For both these interventions, the risk of thrombosis and embolism was markedly diminished from the early 1970s by prophylactic prescription of small doses of anticoagulants such as heparin, which was purified in 1929 by C. Best (1899–1978) of Toronto, and was first used in Sweden and the USA in high doses.

The possibilities of controlling, re-establishing, and maintaining cardiac, respiratory, and kidney function, fluid and electrolyte balance using complex technologies, and of intravenous feeding, widened the field of medicine as a whole. Anaesthesiology was particularly concerned. It gradually evolved further into rescue and intensive medicine, fields that naturally overlap with operative surgery. Thus, the intensive-care units increasingly installed in many hospitals from the 1960s are often run by interdisciplinary teams.

The new endoscopes

A new generation of endoscopes made of flexible fibreglass was developed in the 1960s. They were not only used for diagnostics – making biopsies much easier – but soon had also therapeutic implications. Traditional abdominal operations, such as for isolated gallstones in the biliary ducts, appendectomies, and herniotomies could be performed through a laparoscope. Most recently, laparoscopic cholecystectomy and hysterectomy are being inaugurated and quickly spreading worldwide. Even a perforated gastro-intestinal ulcer can be treated by the laparoscopic route. Thus abdominal surgery, so important in changing surgery from a craft to a scientific discipline in the nineteenth century, is about to open the new era of video-mediated surgery.

Surgical pathology

Around 1910, herniotomies and appendectomies, each averaging about 15 per cent of all operations, were the most frequent operations. Together with other gastro-intestinal interventions, they amounted to some 40 per cent in Kocher's clinic at Berne, which covered the whole of surgery except treatment of eye, ear, nose, and throat diseases.[32] These rates were still true in the mid-1950s and justified the existence of 'general surgeons' with a broad spectrum of competence, ranging from subdural haematoma via lung tumours, diseases of endocrine organs, of the abdominal viscera and the vessels, as well as orthopaedic, urological, and accident surgery.

In the early 1990s, herniotomies and gastro-intestinal operations total only 10 per cent of the interventions in the same university surgical centre, while operations on the nervous system, rare at the beginning of the century, constitute the specialized field of neurosurgery. This holds also for urogenital, thoracic, and orthopaedic surgery.[33] The latter sometimes includes the operative treatment of fractures, which have become much more frequent due to the increased mobility and the sports activities of the population. The rapid decline of tuberculosis and other chronic infections in the antibiotic era is another example of the changed spectrum of surgical pathology: bone and joint resections and amputations for infectious diseases are seldom done in the Western world. Yet the operative access to the bones and joints developed a hundred years ago has proved useful for osteosynthesis and implanting artificial joints.

The first implantation of an artifical apparatus concerned the heart pacemaker constructed by R. Elmquist and performed by A. Senning (b. 1915) in Sweden in 1959. In the 1990s the spectrum includes, in addition, eyelenses, middle-ear ossicles, cochlear implants, vascular prostheses, heart valves, and pneumatic penile prostheses. Organ and tissue transplantations are routine. In a word, most of today's operations were not known in the early 1900s, and those standardized by then are – with a few exceptions – relatively rarely performed now.

Despite today's sophisticated possibilities, duration of hospital stay in Berne, for instance, decreased from an average of more than three weeks c. 1910 to below ten days in 1990, and it will tend further to diminish with ambulatory surgery. Provided that bed occupation is constant, this means that the number of operations per hospital bed will rise considerably, necessitating an enormously increased staff. The number of surgeons per bed has increased about sixfold, and that of nursing staff even more. These figures do not take into account anaesthetists and intensive-care staff.

SURGICAL ASSESSMENT

The success of rationally indicated and devised operations was customarily expressed in terms of (peri)operative complication rate and/or mortality. Technical changes were nearly always said to reduce both. Since the nineteenth century, such data were sometimes completed with reports about the post-hospital course of the patient, first obtained from the patient, his or her family doctor, or a relative upon written request. In the twentieth century, easier communications enabled this information to be obtained by re-examination. This method, although yielding somewhat fortuitous results, was deemed sufficient.[34]

Such unilateral assessment was important in its time for the self-regulation of surgery, as well as for winning the confidence of other doctors and patients alike. It has been systematically elaborated since then. However, it allows no conclusion of the value of any particular procedure as compared to another. The Swiss F. de Quervain published the first long-term follow-up comparing various forms of breast-cancer therapy, with the help of a professional statistician in 1920 and 1930.[35] The methodology of the prospective randomized comparison was introduced first in England: in 1957 H. J. B. Atkins and coworkers published such a trial comparing hypophysectomy and adrenalectomy for advanced cancer of the breast. Not all technical 'improvements' have, by this new standard, proved themselves as such. The comparison of two surgical procedures raises, however, specific methodical and ethical issues since the (double-)blind approach is obviously not applicable and since surgeons tend to have individual technical preferences. The world's first working group for clinical trials in surgery was instituted within the German Surgical Society in 1980.[36]

Therapeutic evaluation is just one example illustrating the enormous extent to which methodological standards for the originality and morality of scientific statements have increased since the 1950s. They require the consideration and integration of a much greater spectrum of information from various clinical and theoretical disciplines (including psychiatry, nursing, physio- and ergotherapy, statistics, psychology, sociology, history, philosophy, theology, and politics) from home and abroad, than had been the case in the preceding periods of one-sided statistical returns and animal experiments.

This meant a transformation of the prestigious autonomous surgeon, assisted by a nurse and a junior resident, customary by 1900, to a surgical team and, more recently, to the multidisciplinary group of professionals, assisted sometimes by an ethics committee progressively blurring the traditional distinctions between (academic) fields and entailing a change of the surgeon's place within medicine and society as a whole. (➤ Ch. 72 Medicine, mortality, and morbidity)

Emphasis on assessment as a form of quality control is one thing, but this process has opened broader questions about the efficacy of surgery and its unintended consequences for some patients. It has by now become evident (if not so earlier for everyone) that surgery cannot be considered (also not historically) as an isolated, autonomous discipline.[12]

SPECIALIZATION IN SURGERY

Abdominal and endocrine surgery are examples of a first type of specialization (that is, the development of fields in which practice has mostly remained with the 'general surgeon'), although there are specific scientific societies and departments here and there. A second type concerns fields which – both in terms of professionalization and institutionalization – were already more or less ubiquitously constituted in the nineteenth century (for example, ophthalmology and otorhinolaryngology), later (for example, gynaecology, urology, neurosurgery and thoracic surgery), or are about to become so (transplantation surgery). In between are, for example, orthopaedic surgery and its subspecialities, since the general surgeon is still traditionally expected to be competent in first-stage traumatology and fracture treatment.

ABDOMINAL SURGERY

Gastro-intestinal surgery was really founded by T. Billroth and his school. He pioneered, albeit unsuccessfully, partial and total extirpation of the larynx in 1870 and 1873 for tuberculosis and cancer, respectively, and undertook the first partial resection of the oesophagus in 1872. In 1881, he performed the first successful gastric resection (actually pylorectomy) for cancer. The feasibility of all these operations had been previously studied over years in dogs (in which pylorectomy had been successfully carried out in 1810 by the German army surgeon O. C. T. Merrem (1790–1859)).[37] In fact, two colleagues in France and Germany, who had tried without such careful preparation, had lost their stomach patients from suture leakage. By 1890, forty-one gastric resections had been performed at Billroth's Vienna clinic with nineteen operative successes.[38] Billroth, who was a fine teacher and generous man, had his co-workers take their own part in realizing his ideas. Thus it was also in his clinic that anterior and posterior gastroenterostomies for stomach cancer and ulcer were developed from 1881; and von Mikulicz-Radecki pioneered the electric oesophagoscope in the same year. Later, von Mikulicz-Radecki was the first to make a plastic reconstruction of the oesophagus after its partial resection for carcinoma (1886).

Although by no means the first, Billroth became the leading advocate in continental Europe for surgical account-keeping and complete reporting of his cases, successes and failures alike. This method of evaluation spread as his pupils occupied chairs in Austria, Belgium, Germany, Italy, the Netherlands, Switzerland, and the United States, but it concerned mostly the operated cases. Billroth's basic training in pathological anatomy, including microscopy, was characteristic of many surgeons of the period. This holds also for his self-taught interest in microbiology. Very special, however, was his friendship with the composer J. Brahms (1833–97), and his love for music and wide cultural interests.[39]

From the 1880s, methods to extirpate cancer of the rectum, to treat hernias, acute and chronic cholecystopathy, and acute appendicitis were developed. The latter, first conservatively treated as 'perityphilitis' by physicians by procrastination, had better surgical results when operated on earlier. The names of R. M. Fitz (1843–1943) from Harvard Medical School, who coined the pathogenetically correct term 'appendicitis'; C. McBurney (1845–1913), and J. B. Murphy (1857–1916) in the USA; and the Swiss C. Krafft (1863–1921) were particularly linked with the introduction of this strategy.[40] Its superiority in terms of lethality and cost (shorter hospital stay, no relapses) were conclusively shown in an elegant comparative study by de Quervain in 1913.[41] The domination of the hitherto often-dramatic course of acute appendicitis was an important stage for the social acceptance of modern surgery.

The 'Murphy button' (see p. 992) was a safe device for intestinal anastomosis, which permitted easier resections of cancer of the colon, rectum, and the small intestine. Pre-operative diagnosis was eased by radio-opaque contrast media first containing bismuth (H. Rieder (1858–1932) of Munich in 1904), then the less-toxic barium (P. Krause (1871–1934) of Bonn c. 1910), allowing visualization of form, position, and movements of the alimentary tract.

This held also for biliary surgery by the introduction of cholecystography by E. A. Graham (1883–1953) and W. H. Cole (b. 1898) in 1923.[42] Cholecystectomy had outweighed dietary measures as standard treatment of chronic cholecystopathy for patients of all social classes by 1960. In the 1990s, it is in competition again, namely with litholytic drugs and shock-wave lithotrity (see p. 1016).

Around 1960, functional operations such as (selective) vagotomies became popular in the treatment of gastro-duodenal ulcers, replacing the traditional approach of local resection and short-circuiting operations. From the 1980s, they were, in turn, replaced as primary therapy by modern drugs. Surgery became mostly reserved for complicated cases; but in the 1990s even perforated ulcers can be operated on by the laparascopic route (see p. 1005).

One of the typically difficult operations of the second period, pancreatico-duodenectomy for carcinoma of the pancreas was introduced in 1935 by A. O. Whipple (1881–1963) of Columbia University, New York. It is still performed in the 1990s. Whipple also pioneered operation of insulinomas (tumours of the endocrine pancreas).

Abdominal surgeons meet in international associations, such as the Collegium Internationale Chirurgiae Digestivae (1969) and the International Hepatobiliary and Pancreatic Association (1978), at congresses held partly independently, and partly in connection with those of the still-existing Société Internationale de Chirurgie, as in the case of the International Association of Endocrine Surgeons (1979). (➤ Ch. 59 Internationalism in medicine and public health)

ENDOCRINE SURGERY[43]

The door to the practical-clinical concept of endocrine disease was definitely opened by unforeseen – and long unlooked for – consequences of ever-better thyroid surgery in humans. Its uncontested leader was Kocher (see p. 995).[44] During the first two years of his professorship in Berne (1872–3), he operated on thirteen goitres – nearly as many as his two predecessors had done in forty-two years. Thanks to anatomical studies, he systematized the operative technique, insisting on very careful haemostasis (Kocher's clamp). At the time of his death, he had performed the operation over 5,000 times. On a hint from J. L. Reverdin (1842–1921), he accidentally discovered the 'cachexy' (myxoedema) following total thyroidectomy in 1883. This led to worldwide in-depth study of thyroid function, hitherto explained only speculatively by both surgeons and physiologists, and to the understanding of the already well-described clinical conditions of myxoedema and cretinism, and Graves's (Basedow's) disease as hypo- and hyperthyroidism, respectively. From 1883, Kocher tried to cure the myxoedema he had caused by homografts of thyroid tissue, with only transitional success.

A world leader in a period that brought forth these typical master-surgeons, he made outstanding contributions to abdominal surgery (Kocher's manœuvre), neurotopographical diagnosis, and neurosurgery. Characteristically enough for the time, he was engaged in not a few priority quarrels, particularly with Reverdin of Geneva over thyroid function, in which his pretensions were actually not justified.

Thyroid surgery was epidemiologically important because of the high prevalence of goitre, particularly in regions remote from the sea. But it also showed the biological limits of the idea of localization and extirpation of disease, and thereby became an important guideline for the new functional outlook of surgery in the twentieth century. Thyroidectomy, oriented according to a 'function test' quantifying the degree of hyperthyroidism or, alternatively, thyroid replacements in the case of hypothyroidism, were introduced as 'physiological therapy' by Kocher. Thyroidectomy became safer by preoperative iodine treatment after The First World War. At the same time, the occurrence of endemic goitre started to decrease in certain areas when iodinized table salt was introduced. Since the late 1960s, nuclear medicine has increasingly replaced surgery in the treatment of other specific forms of goitre.

Today, endocrinology is recognized as a specialized clinical and research field, although it deals with organs in many areas of the body. For precisely that reason, surgical practice is often in the hands of the generalist or of various specialists, depending on local arrangements.

OPTHALMOLOGY AND OTORHINOLARYNGOLOGY

Fragmentation of surgery into specialized branches originated when new fields took shape from within both surgery and internal medicine around new diagnostic instruments, such as the ophthalmoscope introduced by H. Helmholtz (1821–94) in 1851, the otoscope by A. T. von Troeltsch (1829–90) in 1860, and the laryngoscope by M. Garcia (1805–1906) in 1854/5.

The founder of ophthalmology and creator of modern eye surgery was Albrecht Graefe (1828–70) of Berlin.[45] He introduced, among other things, iridectomy for glaucoma, and linear extraction of cataract. By 1880, all twenty-seven faculties of the German-speaking lands except Jena had full chairs of ophthalmology, and ophthalmic surgery was also segregated as a special branch elsewhere.

The full institutionalization of otorhinolaryngology was slower:[46] by the 1950s, chairs existed in only 80 per cent of the German-language universities, although by 1880 there were already extraordinary professors in two-thirds of them. The field developed in Germany and Austria around von Troeltsch of Würzburg and A. Politzer (1835–1920) of Vienna. Hundreds of American doctors travelled to Vienna in the 1900s to learn endoscopic and ophthalmo-scopic techniques.[47] Von Troeltsch invented the modern otoscope and in 1861 devised the operation for mastoiditis, which was first performed in England in 1868 by J. Hinton (1827–75). Politzer's contributions included a method of effecting permeability of the Eustachian tube (1863) and the first report of otosclerosis as a separate clinical entity (1893). The standard oper-ation to restore hearing by fenestration of the external semicircular canal described in 1937/8 by M. L. J. Sourdille (1885–1961) and J. Lempert (b. 1890) was replaced in 1952 devised the elegant functional intervention of mobilization of the stapes by S. Rosen (b. 1897). Microsurgical approaches then took the lead in the field, by construction of an artifical tympanic membrane for example.

ORTHOPAEDICS[48]

Orthopaedics, concerned at first with congenital osseous deformities, became orthopaedic surgery when it extended its territory to developmental anomalies and to disabilities due to age, infections, or injuries of the locomotor appar-atus. The Italian *Archivio di Ortopedia* (from 1884) shows the starting-point and reflects the development: there were the traditional tenotomies for club-foot (see p. 993), the conservative management of pes equiro-varus, genua valga, congenital hip dislocation, kyphosis, arthrosis, and closed fractures. Treatment was characterized by an array of metal appliances, plaster-of-Paris casts, splints, and bandages: that is, by methods necessitating long periods of bed-rest, or – in the case of open injures – by resections and amputations. From the 1870s, some of the above conditions were increasingly being operated on, the procedures involving osteotomies, reconstruction of spinal column and extremities by bone-grafting and tendon-transplantation. Skin-grafting also became important (see p. 1022). The motor bone-saw of the American, F. H. Albee (1876–1945) led from 1909 to a new era in bone-grafting methods.

There were pioneers of these new approaches in every European country; the first nationally affiliated group of orthopaedic surgeons was the American Orthopaedic Association, founded in 1887. A first British society followed in 1894, its German counterpart in 1901, and an international society was planned for 1914 (delayed until 1929 because of the First World War). Since 1935, it has been called Société Internationale de Chirurgie Orthopédique et de Traumatologie.

The history of implants[49] – as well as of transplantation – illustrate that it is always possible to have the right ideas at the wrong time.[49] Thus, the empirical methods of internal fixation of femoral neck fractures and of total knee-joint replacement using metal and ivory, respectively, published in Germany (for example, by T. Gluck (1853–1942) in 1890), were supported by neither current technology (metallurgy, biomechanics, biocompatibility) nor by knowledge of bone physiology. The first treatise on internal fixation of fractures by cerclage, suturing, or impaction of spikes by the French naval surgeon L. Bérenger-Féraud (1832–1900) suffered from the same drawback in 1870 as did – nearly forty years later – those by A. Lane (1856–1938) of London and A. Lambotte (1866–1955) of Brussels, describing the use of plates and screws and introducing the term 'osteosynthesis' (Lambotte, 1907). Ingenious empiricism prevailed until the 1960s.

The first animal experiments to grasp the metallurgical and mechanical requirements for implants were performed in the USA and Britain before the First World War, and continued thereafter alongside the newly developed techniques of tissue culture. In the 1920s, bone was slowly being understood as a living tissue, and its diseases were studied from a metabolic point of view. Anatomists, physiologists, and surgeons started investigating it in an interdisciplinary way; for example, the group of R. Leriche (1879–1955) and, A. Policard of (1881–1972) in Lyons. A decade later, vitamin D allowed the prevention and cure of rickets without orthopaedics. (➤ Ch. 22 Nutritional diseases) This approach was also the key to modern scientifically founded osteosynthesis, built on the empirical clinical observation by R. Danis (1880–1962) of Brussels that fractures could heal without visible callus when rigidly fixed by osteosynthesis. This was achieved on an experimentally defined scientific basis by the Swiss Arbeitsgemeinschaft für Osteosynthesefragen, founded in 1958. This interdisciplinary group also developed standard techniques. As asepsis had done away with the 'normality' of wound healing via suppuration, the possibility of rigid fixation by compression now identified fracture-healing via the callus as a detour.[50] Intramedullary nails advocated by G. Küntscher (1900–72) of Kiel are still a competitive technique in certain cases.

The removal and replacement of the femoral head and the hip-joint were attempted early in modern surgery because of frequent arthritic degeneration, chronic infections, and the often precarious blood supply after an injury with ensuing necrosis. By 1954, an American research committee reported on nearly forty types of femoral endoprostheses, suggesting that none was really satisfactory. As was the case with internal fixation of fractures, the many problems of materials, biomechanics, and fixation linked with permanent endoprostheses were systematically tackled from the 1950s, illustrating again the onset of the second surgical revolution during this decade. Plastics came into play – but which plastics? A new era was opened in 1961, when John Charnley (1911–82), of Manchester, published his epochal paper on low-friction arthroplasty using a metal femoral head, neck, and stem and a plastic acetabular cup: total hip replacement has since been performed all over the world according to his basic principles. Its success led to their application to the knee, ankle, and other joints.

GYNAECOLOGICAL SURGERY[51]

Around 1850, a few surgeons in America and Britain, at the price of human experimentation, ended up dealing successfully with vesico-vaginal fistula (J. M. Sims, 1813–83) and sometimes excised enormous ovarian cysts by the so-called ovariotomy (T. S. Wells), stimulating worldwide medical debates (see pp. 993–94).

By 1880, Caesarean section was recommended for specific intrauterine foetal positions and pelvic deformities. Several methods – classical transverse uterotomy (M. Sänger, 1853–1903), vaginal operation, suprasymphyseal section, and the extraperitoneal approach – were developed between 1882 and the First World War. The mortality remained high during the nineteenth century, as the operation was considered only after difficult labour for days – similar to the case of delay in acute appendicitis (see p. 1009). Today, mortality in planned Caesarean sections is so low that there is discussion on its merits as an alternative to normal childbirth. (➤ Ch. 44 Childbirth) This holds also for hysterectomy to prevent dysmenorrhoea and uterine cancer. Certainly, diffeent incidences of disease do not explain most of the highly variable rates for this and other operations, from one population to another.[52]

From the late 1870s, in accordance with the trend to extirpate, the cancerous uterus was also removed by the vaginal and abdominal routes, yet initially with appalling lethalities of around 75 per cent. These operations were worked out in Germany, and by the Billroth school in Austria. By 1900 the more radical operation of E. Wertheim (1864–1920), including the additional removal of the pelvic lymph-nodes and of part of the vagina, and by 1950 the possible benefit of exenteration of the pelvic organs in patients with advanced pelvic cancer pioneered by A. Brunschwig (1901–69) of New York, were described. The extirpation of the ovaries, however, developed particularly in the USA in the 1870s and 1880s, was highly contested in Europe. This, and other radical operations, brought about professional disputes between surgeons and obstetrical physicians over the performance of gynaecological interventions, leading gradually to the organization of a speciality uniting gynaecology with obstetrics.[53]

The treatment of mammary cancer was greatly influenced by Halsted's method of radical mastectomy (1890/4). He continued the work of his teacher, Billroth, who, in 1878, had already published the results of 170 operations for this disorder. Halsted was the first Professor of Surgery at Johns Hopkins Medical School. His work on cocaine was important for the discovery of conduction and lumbar anaesthesia, and he was the first to use rubber gloves. His experimental approach made him one of the leading American surgeons and teachers, and his pupils included neurosurgeons H. Cushing (1869–1939) and W. Dandy (1886–1946) (see p. 1017).

Treatment of breast cancer went through the typical developments corresponding to the three periods of modern surgery outlined in the outset of this article: that is, from Halsted's radical extirpation via supraradical mastectomy including lymph nodes, local muscle and bone (despite de Quervain's statistical evidence (see pp. 1007), but according to the prevalent theory of formation of metastases), back to quadrantectomy, and finally reduced to lumpectomy (1980s). In addition, radiotherapy and chemotherapy were introduced first as alternatives and more recently as complements in various combinations. Furthermore, by 1900, removal of the ovaries was recommended as the second-stage operation in cases of relapse. In the 1940s adrenalectomy and ablation of the pituitary were the next logical steps in an endocrine conception of mammary cancer (see p. 1000). This type of hormone-elimination by surgery has now been superseded by drug therapy.

UROLOGY[54]

Urology grew independent of surgery in the nineteenth century, mostly outside the traditional university network. The old tradition of unorthodox, itinerant lithotomists even reflected on some of the early nineteenth-century pioneers of modern lithotrity, such as J. Civiale (1792–1867) and C. L. S. Heurteloup (1793–1863), who put the crushing of stones inside the bladder on a firm basis.

As a modern speciality, however, urology developed around general surgery and new diagnostic possibilities. After G. von Simon (1824–76) had performed the first nephrectomy in 1869, the leading general surgeons of the first generation who concentrated on the urogenital tract were H. Thompson (1820–1904) in London, who worked on bladder tumours (1884); F. Guyon (1831–1920) in Paris; J. Israel (1848–1926) in Berlin; and L. von Dittel (1815–98) in Vienna. It was at the latter's great polyclinic that M. Nitze (1848–1906) developed an electrically lighted cystoscope (1879), which rendered possible great improvements in bladder surgery, including the excision of tumours *in situ*. Israel inaugurated the operative treatment of stenosis of the ureters, due to the still-frequent calculi, and he decreased the morbidity of nephrectomy to below 10 per cent (1893).

Diagnostic improvements included catheterization of the ureters, first introduced at Johns Hopkins Hospital in 1893. In the year after the discovery of X-rays, calculi could already be visualized. In 1905/6, the first retrograde cysto- and pyelograms were obtained by F. Voelker (1872–1955) and A. von Lichtenberg (1880–1948), respectively. Voelker also described one of the various kidney function tests (1903) developed from 1895 in the form of cryoscopy of the urine. Although retrograde urography was a pioneer achievement of local diagnostics, it was an unphysiological method, often leading to pyelonephritic infections. A great change occurred when intravenous urography using an iodine substance was introduced in 1929, again by von Lichtenberg.

Various procedures for treating hypertrophy of the prostate by extirpation were acomplished from the 1890s in Italy (E. Bottini, 1837–1903), England (suprapubic and vesical prostatectomy by E. Fuller, 1858–1930), and the United States (perineal prostatectomy by F. S. Watson, 1853–1942). Although still crude by present-day standards, this operation interrupted the miserable vicious circle of prostatic enlargement, infection, and bladder stones, which had dominated the surgery of middle-aged men for centuries. Another American specialist, H. Young (1870–1945), performed the first radical operation for carcinoma of the prostate (1905). These procedures, as well as nephrectomy for unilateral tuberculosis of the kidney, were typical examples of the pathological-anatomical period of surgery.

In urology particularly, the shift through the second period, which lay more stress on functional aspects although often only mechanically understood, was well marked by the introduction of intravenous pyelography. This allowed a systemic and functional diagnosis of the kidney and the descending urinary tract. It led to systemically oriented and conservative operative procedures. While nephrectomies were previously performed in 80 per cent of unilateral kidney diseases, today the figure is 20 per cent. The first plastic operations were tried to normalize urinary flux in cases of stenosis. At the same time, extirpation of the bladder for carcinoma was completed by R. C. Coffey (1869–1933) by conducting the ureters into the large bowel in 1911, and after the Second World War, by utilizing isolated parts of the intestine with a cutaneous opening (stoma) to replace the bladder (for example, the ileal pouch of E. M. Bricker (b. 1908) in the United States, and of Seifert in Germany). In the 1990s in male patients, functional bladders can be reconstructed using parts of the intestine sewn on to the urethra. Clearly, the field profited from the possibility of local (paravertebral) conduction anaesthesia, from the possibilities of visual control, and finally from the institutionalization of urology in the universities after the Second World War.

Urology is also an excellent example to illustrate the shift of surgery into the third period. It was one of the first fields in which the extirpation of malignant tumours was challenged by radiotherapy: in 1906, the American A. L. Gray (1873–1932) introduced it for carcinoma of the bladder, and it was soon also used to treat carcinoma of the prostate. This tumour was one of the first successfully treated with hormones (1941): for his work on hormone-dependent tumours, C.B. Huggins (b. 1901) of Chicago shared a Nobel Prize in 1966. This development was helped by early diagnosis by needle biopsy, developed in Sweden.

Operative urology had further been transformed by yet another diagnostic technology developed from 1955 in Sweden: compound sonography. It marked a change analogous to that from retrograde to intravenous urography in the 1920s. Sonography is easily handled, needs relatively simple equipment, and avoids radiation damage. It provides precise operative guidelines, allowing differentiation of the structure of tumours, cysts, and urinary calculi. It also permits puncturing of the kidney and the urinary tract under direct visual control so that stones can be removed or crushed with special endoscopes. Such new optical systems mark the perfecting of endoscopic urology, which started with Nitze and which has also led to the transurethral resection of the prostate. This elegant operation was developed in the United States in the 1970s, and has now largely replaced traditional open-prostate surgery.

In 1980, the experimental surgeon W. Brendel (b. 1922) and the urologist E. Schmiedt (b. 1920) of Munich published their first clinical results with shock-wave lithotrity. Since then, yet another traditional urological field, extraction of calculi, has been transformed and operations have dramatically decreased. At the same time, another bloodless approach, the pharmacological dissolution of stones, had its first successes in the (rare) pure urea stones by alkalization of the urine. Hormone treatment of tumours and chemical methods for dissolving stones illustrate the third, systemic period that urology has entered in the last decades, which includes biochemical aspects in the consideration of urological diseases, allowing also dietary prevention of certain stone diseases. This development holds for all operative disciplines when patients are suffering from metabolic disorders. An early example was the prevention of endemic goitre (see p. 1010); a recent one was the treatment of certain gallstones.

NEUROSURGERY

Surgery of the nervous system is another field that developed as a speciality in parallel with improved diagnostic techniques.[55] Prior to the First World War, certain surgeons took a special interest in it, such as W. Macewen (1848–1924) and V. Horsley (1857–1916) in Britain; von Bergman, Kocher, and F. Krause (1856–1937) in German-speaking Europe; A. Chipault (b.1833) in France; and L. M. Puusepp (1875–1942) in Russia. But the major problem was topical diagnosis, which had to rely on clinical symptoms, and the still rather imprecise localization of functional centres in the cortex. By 1890, so-called craniocerebral topographies with corresponding 'craniometers' were established to localize such centres in individual patients.[56] But mostly, the operator depended on the diagnosis of a neurologist.

This changed when direct visualization of the ventricles and the brain became possible with the introduction of air-ventriculography and pneumoencephalography by W. Dandy in 1918 and 1919, respectively. X-ray examination of the spinal cord (myelography) in 1921, and cerebral radiology using iodinated compounds in 1921 (J. A. Sicard (1872–1929), and in 1929) J. Forestier (b. 1890), in Paris), followed, as well as cerebral angiography in 1927 (A. C. de Egas Moniz (1874–1955), in Lisbon): the surgeon could diagnose and localize the disease much more precisely.

The first to practise neurosurgery almost exclusively before the First World War was H. Cushing of Baltimore and Boston. He was also an accomplished neuropathologist. He was the first to collect a large series of cerebral tumours, which he was able to classify in the 1920s. His further research interests concerned the hypophysis and hypothalamus. This specialist approach transformed neurosurgery, which had hitherto been limited to the evacuation of pus or blood and the elevation of depressed skull fractures. Brain and spinal tumours as well as vascular lesions became accessible for systematic operations. Cushing developed electro-surgery, providing cutting and coagulating currents, and introduced the silver clips for haemostasis as well as intra-operative monitoring of blood pressure (1903). He was an excellent teacher and trained many second-generation international neurosurgeons.

Through the work of Cushing and others of his generation, such as Dandy of Baltimore, C. Elsberg (1871–1948) of New York, and C. Frazier (1870–1936) of Philadelphia, the USA dominated the field. In 1920, the Society of Neurological Surgeons was founded there, and in 1944 publication the *Journal of Neurosurgery* was begun.

In Europe, the distinguished neurologist O. Foerster (1873–1941) of Bres-lau deserves mention. He started operating at the age of 40 because he was dissatisfied with the execution of his advice by surgeons. This illustrates the institutional delay in Germany, where the first full chair of neurosurgery was created only in 1937.

The most original French contribution was the surgery of the autonomic (sympathetic) nervous system by M. Jaboulay (1860–1913) and R. Leriche of Lyons, Strasburg, and Paris for many conditions (for example Raynaud's disease, causalgia, senile arteriosclerosis, and hypertension) which have been accessible to pharmacotherapy since the 1960s.

Continuous improvement of diagnostic apparatus after the Second World War allowed pre-operative diagnosis of vascular alterations and of the charac-ter of tumours. Around 1980, fine catheters could be placed in definite areas of the brain and the spinal cord. Yet even these procedures have been largely replaced by non-invasive methods: computerized tomography (CT) and nuclear magnetic resonance (NMR) are not only harmless and painless, they can be used in ambulatory practice, and have an even greater power of resolution.

On the operative side, the greatest progress in neurosurgery stemmed from the developments of anaesthesiology and microsurgery mentioned above, (pp. 1001, 1005). Artificial hypothermia and hypotension rendered certain operations easier and more successful.

On the other hand, 'psychosurgery' (for instance leucotomy for chronic schizophrenia (1936), for which the Portuguese Egas-Moniz shared a Nobel Prize in 1949), was a widening of surgical indications typical of the second period due to greater safety of operations on the brain. Its success was doubtful and it is now, in the third period, practically obsolete.

THORACIC SURGERY[57]

While some heroic operations were attempted in the nineteenth century to eradicate cancer of the oesophagus and lung or to treat an injury of the heart, chest surgery really originated as a treatment for pulmonary tuberculosis. Quantitively, this dominated the field until the 1950s, when the decrease of lung tuberculosis coupled with an increase of cardiovascular morbidity made surgery of the heart and the great vessels more important.

Mechanistic patho-physiology had its bearing on thoraic surgery from the early 1900s. Theoretically, the development of the negative pressure chamber by Sauerbruch in Breslau (1904) was justified, but it never became functional in humans. It was the much less complicated endotracheal tube completed by an inflatable cuff towards the end of the First World War that paved the way for thoracic surgery as a speciality, as it also allowed controlled artificial respiration (see 997 above). This first took place predominantly in the United States.

Lung surgery

The surgical approaches to pulmonary tuberculosis started with the collapsing therapies designed to put the infected lung at rest. Artificial pneumothorax by puncturing the interpleural space was inaugurated in 1888 by C. Forlanini (1847–1918) of Torino. Other approaches followed, such as thoracoplasty, an invasive procedure comprising the section of many ribs, developed largely by German surgeons, as was phrenicotomy. The latter was soon abandoned because of its negative impact on respiratory function, whereas drainage of tuberculous caverns and of chronic empyemas, other typical operations of the localistic period, kept their place.

Because of the problem of negative intrapleural pressure, lung surgery entered the period of extirpation somewhat later than abdominal surgery. Except for a few isolated earlier cases, pulmonary resections (including 'dissection lobectomy') were pioneered in the early 1920s by A. T. Edwards (1890–1946) at London's Brompton Hospital, inspiring a British School of chest surgeons. In Germany and America, total pneumonectomies were performed in 1931–3 by rather crude methods using mass ligatures of the hilus of the lung in two stages: for accident by R. Nissen (1896–1981), for bronchiectasis by C. Haight (1901–70), and for cancer by E. Graham (1883–1957), respectively. From 1933, one-stage operations with individual dissection and ligature of specific bronchi were also developed by American surgeons, and a school of thoracic surgery was established at the Massachusetts General Hospital. Limited resections of tuberculous foci tended to replace the collapsing operations.

After the Second World War, surgery of tracheo-bronchial reconstruction was developed in the United States and in France, for both tuberculosis and lung cancer. The morbidity of the latter increased, whilst tuberculosis virtually disappeared after the introduction of chemotherapy. Thanks to antibiotics, tracheo-bronchial anastomosis also became safe, which allowed conservative resections and reparative surgery to maintain or re-establish pulmonary functions. This was the case for pulmonary transplantation, which began to be performed in 1963.

Heart surgery

Three phases can be distinguished in this field: that is, those of extracardiac, blind intracardiac (closed-heart), and eye-controlled intracardiac (open-heart) surgery.

During the extracardiac pioneer phase, drainage of the pericardial space was performed, and occasionally an injury of the heart was successfully sutured: for example, in 1896 by L. Rehn (1849–1930). The first successful pericardectomy for constrictive pericarditis was performed in 1921 by V. Schmeiden (1874–1945). The surgical correction of vascular abnormalities in humans, however, originated in Boston, where in 1939 R. E. Gross (1905–89) and J. P. Hubbard (b. 1903) performed the first successful ligature of a patent ductus arteriosus. In 1945, Blalock and H. Taussig (1898–1986) of the Johns Hopkins Hospital succeeded in the palliative correction of pulmonary stenosis by creating an artificial ductus arteriosus. In the same year, C. Crawfoord (1899–1984) of Stockholm resected congenital coarctation (stenosis) of the aorta, and in 1951 C. Dubost (b. 1914) of Paris an aneurysm of the terminal aorta with replacement using homologous venous tissue.

The period of blind intracardiac surgery on the closed heart was opened prior to the First World War by the first dilatation of an aortic vascular stenosis by T. Tuffier's (1857–1929) in 1912; this was a success, as was the commissurotomy for stenosis of the mitral valve performed by H. Souttar (1875–1964) in London (1925). Whle other operations done in Boston between 1923 and 1928 were not functionally successful, because they transformed stenosis into insufficiency, the new procedures of H. G. Smithy (1914–48), C. P. Bailey (b. 1910) of Philadelphia, and D. E. Harken (b. 1910) of Boston, all in 1948, succeeded. This was also the case for valvulotomies for pulmonary stenosis performed in 1947/8 by T. Holmes-Sellors (1902–87) and R. Brock (1903–80) in London, and two years later, for aortic stenosis, again by Bailey.

It was at the Rockefeller Institute in New York that Tuffier and Carrel had already performed experimental open-heart surgery in animals before the First World War. Afterwards, together with the famous pilot C. Lindbergh (1902–74), Carrel first developed a 'pump' for extracorporeal circulation, that functioned in animals (1938). Three developments enabled open-heart surgery: the design of the heart–lung machine maintaining artificial circulation through the great vessels while the heart is bypassed; the use of hypothermia to reduce the oxygen need of the tissues (1950); and the discovery that the deeply cooled and bypassed heart can be stopped for up to an hour and started again without suffering damage (1959).

After Carrel, research on extracorporeal circulation continued in the United States. In 1953, results applicable in humans were achieved by J. H. Gibbon (1903–73), who was supported by IBM's technological department but whose apparatus failed because he thought he had to deal with the whole blood volume. When it was discovered that the patient can survive with only 10 to 20 per cent of the normal total blood volume, the problem was finally solved. Other great names in this development were J. Kirklin (b. 1917) of the Mayo Clinic and C. W. Lillehei (b. 1918) of Minneapolis. The latter succeeded first in cross-circulation between father and son, and in 1955 had a break-through with the bubble-oxygenator. These achievements relied on the pre-vention of blood coagulation by heparin (see p. 1005).

Open-heart surgery started in 1952 with the implantation of valvular pro-stheses, first by the American C. Hufnagel (1917–89). The Starr–Edwards model of Portland, Oregon, became the most popular: by 1962, 18,00 oper-ations had been performed. Valvular reconstruction and repair surgery, as well as the implantation of biological valves needing no anticoagulation, have become important since the late 1960s, particularly influenced by the Paris school of C. Dubost and A. Carpentier.

The possibility of open-heart surgery also permitted procedures for coro-nary revascularization. After F. M. Sones Jr (1918–85) had introduced coro-nary arteriography at the Cleveland Clinic, Ohio, in 1958, precise local diagnosis of coronary occlusions became possible, and various procedures of bypass using autologous venous grafts were tried successfully from 1964 by M. E. de Bakey (b. 1908) in the USA and V. Kolesov (b. 1904) in Russia. F. C. Spencer and co-workers, taking up the technique of bypass using the internal mammary artery successfully realized on dogs by Carrel in 1914, introduced it on a large scale in 1968; 4,600 patients were treated in Cleve-land up to 1972, with a lethality below 1 per cent and a patency around 80 per cent. From 1988, endoluminal interventions using inflatable balloon catheters, lasers, and endoprostheses, as well as local application of throm-bolytic drugs by catheters, are in international evaluation and, in part, replace invasive surgery.

While the chief indications for open-heart surgery had been, until the end of the 1960s, congenital or acquired heart defects and valvular diseases, coronary operations have increased since, partly due to changes in the popu-lation structure, and in the attitude of referring physicians: in 1970, 170 open-heart operations were performed per million inhabitants in the Federal Republic of Germany, and ten years later the number had trebled.

TRANSPLANTATION[58]

Transplantation of both non-vital and living tissues and organs was begun in the nineteenth century. Successful skin-grafts were described in 1869 by J. L. Reverdin (1842–1929) of Geneva and systematized by C. Tiersch (1822–95) in Leipzig (1872). These were autografts (transplantations of tissues within the same patient). They were soon applied in the treatment of ulcers, severe burns, and to repair skin defects resulting from extirpation of underlying tissues. Skin-grafting marked the onset of plastic and reconstructive surgery.[59]

Homografts (tissues from donors) were tried in the late 1880s, using also skins of cadavers or of amputated limbs. However, the results were disappointing, although some authors reported 'good success' even after heterografting frog-skin. Even so, it was realized that such transplantations could serve as a kind of 'pacemaker'. This was also the case for implanted decalcified bone, as reported by Gluck in Berlin in 1890. He also used nerve autotransplantation in humans. E. Ullmann (1861–1937) of Vienna experimented on autotransplantation of parts of the intestine in heterotopic sites (1901). This marked the beginning of living organ transplantation.[60]

Venous autografting was first used clinically by J. G. Capdevila (1876–1964) in Madrid (1906), and by E. Lexer (1867–1937) at Königsberg (1907). Lexer was to become a pioneer of plastic surgery during the First World War. After a reliable method of vascular suture had been obtained particularly by Carrel (1902), who later also showed that explanted vessels could be kept alive for days in defined laboratory conditions, the transplantation of vessels and consequently of organs became an important field of experimental research. Indeed, the technique of renal transplantation was perfected in animals in Vienna, Berlin, Lyons, and New York. Jaboulay (see p. 1018), a great pioneer of vascular surgery, and E. Unger (1875–1938) of Berlin even performed clinical transplantations in 1906 and 1910, respectively. The latter tried a heterograft using a kidney of a monkey. This was also tried with pancreas as early as 1894.[61] But because of graft rejection, organ transplantation fell into disuse until after the Second World War.

During this war, transplantation of non-vital or non-vitally conserved tissue had become urgent for 'pacemaker' support in regeneration of connective tissues after severe injuries. Since the 1960s, a rapid development of transplantation of vital and vitally conserved tissues has occurred, with bone marrow and endocrine tissue being particularly successful. Autotransplantation of tissue gained before the onset of aggressive chemotherapy or radiotherapy for cancer was also introduced.

At this point, a new wave of interest in organ transplantation was led by the invention of the so-called 'artificial kidney', the extracorporeal haemodialysis machine invented by the Dutch internist W. Kolff (b. 1911) during the Second World War. It allowed reversibly damaged kidneys (for example, due to shock) to recover, and chronic renal failure to be compensated over a long time. Chronically ill patients were, however, tied to this initially huge machine for the rest of their lives, which motivated an entirely new approach to kidney transplantation. The first longer-lasting successes were obtained by transplantations among close relatives, particularly twins (for example, J. Murray *et al.* of Boston) from the early 1950s.[62]

Meantime, the concept of the immunological nature of homograft organ rejection, formulated before the First World War, had been substantiated, particularly by the experiments of M. Burnet (1899–1985) of Melbourne and P. B. Medawar (1915–87) of London. In 1953, Medawar and his collaborators described the possibility of 'actively acquired tolerance', but the first kidney homo- and heterografts performed in American and French centres mostly failed, even if they were done after whole-body irradiation with X-rays or under cortisone treatment to suppress immune response by analogy to cancer treatment. Around 1960, by the same analogy, the first immunosuppressive drugs blocking the production of antibodies without producing susceptibility to every kind of infection were introduced (6-mercaptopurine, azathioprine). Because of their high toxicity and side-effects, the search for more specific compounds went on, leading to the clinical introduction of cyclosporine in 1980. This drug greatly improved the management of immunological problems of transplantation. At the same time, solutions and conditions for preserving cadaver kidneys were defined so that they could be transported. On a European level, Eurotransplant, an organization in Leiden, is in charge of the optimal distribution of transplantable organs according to their immunological compatibility with the receiver, for kidney homografting has now become the treatment of choice.

The first to breach the considerable moral barrier against transplanting the heart was C. Barnard (b. 1922) of Cape Town in December 1967. The technique had been ready for some time, and hearts were soon being transplanted at centres all over the world: by 1971, a total of 180 operations had been performed by 56 teams. Most of them abandoned the procedure since survival was mostly short, due to graft rejection. N. Shumway (b. 1923) of Stanford, however, methodologically developed the conditions to be met for successful heart transplantation. By 1990/1 it had a high success rate for narrowly defined indications, and some 14,500 transplantations had been performed worldwide.

This holds also for liver transplantation, for which T.E. Starzl (b. 1926) of Denver established the first successful programme in 1967/8. He also introduced clinical histocompatibility testing. This work greatly stimulated traditional liver surgery, such as resection of tumours and metastasis. The history of pulmonary transplantation began also in the 1960s with isolated successes. The systematic work of J. Cooper of Toronto, culminating in his successful series between 1977 and 1982, showed the method's potentiality for strictly defined indications. Intestinal and pancreatic transplantations are now being tried, whereas bone-marrow transplantation has achieved the stage of a clinical treatment; and cornea, middle ear ossicles, cartilage, bone, and heart valves are transplanted very frequently.

Organ transplantations are just one illustration of replacement surgery characterizing the last three decades. Many kinds of prostheses (see p. 1006), have become routine treatments, whereas the artificial heart (both orthotropic and heterotropic) is still in an experimental stage. These artificial replacements particularly illustrate the interdisciplinary nature of surgery of this third period, necessitating the collaboration not only with traditional experimental sciences, but also with the electronics, metal, and plastics industries, to the benefit of all concerned. (➤ Ch. 68 Medical technologies: social contexts and consequences)

The field of organ transplantation was accompanied by serious deliberations of concomitant general medical, moral, and legal issues: the definition of brain death of potential organ donors replacing the century-old heart death, as well as rules for explantation, had to be elaborated and accepted by both doctors and the lay public. The humane questions of patients waiting for organ transplantation and the ethical issue of criteria for justice in the distribution of too-few available organs, and of resource allocation, were and still are repeatedly addressed.[63] Transplantation marks the tip of the iceberg of the kind of issues facing progressing surgery and medicine as a whole: their medical and social functions are being seen by health professionals, the public, and historians as being problematic rather than self-evident. Finally, the history of transplantion is just one illustration of the old psychological and/or social motives for doctors insisting on actually rare but conceptionally interesting problems. (➤ Ch. 37 History of medical ethics; Ch. 69. Medicine and the law)

NOTES

1   H. A. Walser, *Zur Einführung der Äthernarkose im deutschen Sprachgebeit im Jahre 1847*, Aarau, Sauerländer, 1973; A. Winter, 'Ethereal epidemic and the introduction of inhalation anaesthesia in early Victorian London', *Social History of Medicine*, 4: 1–28.

2   E. H. Ackerknecht, *Rudolf Virchow: Doctor, Statesman, Anthropologist*, Madison, University of Wisconsin Press, 1953.

3   N. Fox, 'Scientific theory choice and social structure: the case of Lister's antisepsis, humoral theory and asepsis', *History of Science*, 1988, 26: 367–97, see p. 371–2.

4   J. Lister, 'On the effects of the antiseptic system of treatment upon the salubrity of a surgical hospital', *Lancet*, 1870, 1: 4–6, 40–2.

5   M. Goldman, *Lister Ward*, Bristol and Boston, MA, Hilger, 1987.

6   B. Elkeles, 'Der moralische Diskurs über das medizinische Menschenexperiment zwischen 1835 und dem ersten Weltkrieg', Med. Habilitationsschrfit, University of Hanover, 1991, pp. 168–83.

7   D. Hamilton, 'The nineteenth-century surgical revolution – antisepsis or better nutrition?', *Bulletin of the History of Medicine*, 1982, 56: 30–40.

8   Fox, op. cit. (n. 3), p. 388.

9   U. Tröhler and A.-H. Maehle, *Die Knochenbrüche – Wege zur modernen Behandlung*, Basle, Pharma-Information, 1991.

10 F. M. Steichen and M. M. Ravitch, *Stapling in Surgery*, Chicago, IL, and London, Year Book Medical Publishers, 1984, pp. 1–77.

11 T. Billroth, 'Chirurgische Klinik Zürich 1860–1867', *Archiv für klinische Chirurgie*, 1868, 10: 1–194, 421–654, 749–893; *Chirurgische Klinik Wien 1868*, Berlin, Hirschwald, 1870.

12 A. Dally, *Women under the Knife. A History of Surgery*, London, Hutchinson Radius, 1991, pp. 135–41.

13 S.-S. Krudup, 'Das Krebsproblem in den 'Verhandlungen der Deutschen Gesellschaft für Chirurgie' von 1872–1914 mit besond. Berücksichtigung der Magen-Darm-Tumoren', unpublished MD thesis, University of Göttingen, 1990, pp. 41–2; L. Linnemann, 'Die Frakturbehandlung von 1872–1914, dargestellt anhand der Verhandlungen der Deutschen Gesellschaft für Chirurgie', unpublished MD thesis, University of Göttingen, 1985.

14 E. H. Ackerknecht, 'Typen der medizinischen Ausbildung im 19. Jahrhundert', *Schweizerisch medizinische Wochenschrift*, 1957, 87: 1361–6.

15 U. Tröhler, *Der Schweizer Chirurg J. F. de Quervain (1868–1949) Wegbereiter neuer internationaler Beziehungen in der Wissenschaft der Zwischenkriegszeit*, Aarau, Sauerländer, 1973.

16 W. W. Keen (ed.), *Surgery, its Principles and Practices*, Philadelphia, PA, and London, Saunders, 8 vols, 1907–21; F. Pitha and T. Billroth (eds), *Handbuch der allgemeinen und speziellen Chirurgie*, Stuttgart, Enke, Vols I–IV, 1865–8.

17 E. Küster, 'Die Nieren-Chirurgie im 19. Jahrhundert. Ein Rück- und Ausblick', *Verhandlungen der Deutschen Gesellschaft für Chirurgie*, 1901, 30: 420–39, see p. 438.

18 U. Tröhler, ' "To operate or not to operate? Scientific and extraneous factors in therapeutic controversies within the Swiss Society of Surgery 1913–1988', *Clio Medica*, 1991, 22: 89–113.

19 O. H. Wangensteen and S. D. Wangensteen, *The Rise of Surgery*, Folkestone, Dawson, 1978, p. 183.

20 Ibid., pp. 180–4.

21 U. Tröhler, *Der Nobelpreisträger Theodor Kocher 1841–1917. Auf dem Weg zur physiolgischen Chirurgie*, Basle, Boston, MA, and Stuttgart, Birkhäuser, 1984.

22 P. C. English, *Shock, Physiological Surgery, and George Washington Crile*. Westport, CT, Greenwood Press, 1980, pp. 167–8.

23 U. Tröhler, 'Die Wechselwirkung von Anatomie, Physiologie und Chirurgie im

Werk Theodor Kochers und einiger Zeitgenossen', in U. Boschung (ed.), *Theodor Kocher 1841–1917*, Bern, Stuttgart, and Toronto, Huber, 1991, pp. 53–71.

24 T. I. Malinin, *Surgery and Life. The Extraordinary Career of Alexis Carrel*, New York, Harcourt Brace Jovanovich, 1979, pp. 66–93.

25 English, op. cit. (n. 22), pp. 198–206.

26 N. S. R. Maluf, 'History of blood transfusion', *Journal of the History of Medicine*, 1954, 9: 59–107.

27 A. E. Nourse, *Inside the Mayo Clinic*, New York, St Louis and San Francisco, McGraw-Hill, 1979; O. T. Clagett, *General Surgery at the Mayo Clinic 1900–1970*, Rochester, MN, [n.p.], 1980.

28 R. B. Knapp, *The Gift of Surgery to Mankind. A History of Modern Anaesthesiology*, Springfield, IL, Thomas, 1983.

29 T. E. Keys, *Die Geschichte der chirurgischen Anaesthesie*, Heidelberg, Springer, 1968.

30 D. de Moulin, *A History of Surgery*, Dordrecht, Nijhoff, 1988, p. 333.

31 Steichen and Ravitch, op. cit. (n. 10).

32 [Inselspital Bern], *Jahresbericht der Inselkorporation pro 1916*, Berne, Büchler, 1917.

33 [Inselspital Bern], *Tätigkeitsbericht d. Chirurg. Universitätskliniken 1990*, Berne, 1991.

34 Tröhler, op. cit. (n. 21), pp. 82–120.

35 U. Heusser, 'F. de Quervain 1868–1940 als Weberbereiter der kontrollierten Studie in der Klinischen Chirurgie', unpublished MD thesis, University of Basle, 1990.

36 H. J. B. Atkins *et al.*, 'Adrenalectomy and hypophysectomy for advanced cancer of the breast', *Lancet*, 1957, 1: 489–96; K. L. J. Bonchek, 'The role of the randomized clinical trial in the evaluation of new operations', *Surg. Clin. North America*, 1982, 62: 761–9; W. Lorenz and H. Rohde, 'Prospektive, kontrollierte Studien in der Chirurgie. Kontroverse Standpunkte zur Motivierung und Durchführung', *Klinische Wochenschrift*, 1979, 57: 301–10.

37 O. Temkin, 'Merrem's youthful dream. The early history of experimental pylorectomy', *Bulletin of the History of Medicine*, 1957, 31: 29–32.

38 Wangensteen and Wangensteen, op. cit. (n. 19), p. 149.

39 K. B. Absolon, *The Surgeon's Surgeon. Theodor Billroth 1829–1894*, 3 vols, Kansas, Coronado Press, 1979–87.

40 P. Gasser, *Charles Krafft (1863–1921). Ein Pionier der Appendektomie und der Krankenpflege in Europa*, Basle and Stuttgart, Schwabe, 1977; G. R. William, 'Presidential address: a history of appendicitis', *Annals of Surgery*, 1983, 197: 495–506.

41 Tröhler, op. cit. (n. 18).

42 G. Altmeier, *Von der Wahrsagekunst zur modernen Chirurgie der Gallenwege*, Herzogenrath, Murken-Altrogge (Studien zur Medizin-, Kunst- und Literaturgeschichte, Vol. XV), 1987.

43 R. B. Welbourn, *The History of Endocrine Surgery*, New York, Praeger, 1990.

44 Tröhler, op. cit. (n. 21).

45 H. E. Henkes and Cl. Zrenner (eds), *History of Ophthalmology 1–3, sub auspiciis*

Academiae Ophthalmologicae Internationalis, Dordrecht and Boston, MA, Kluwer Academic, 1988–90.

46 N. Weir, *Otolaryngology: an Illustrated History*, London and Boston, MA, Butterworth, 1990.

47 T. N. Bonner, *American Doctors and German Universities*, Lincoln, University of Nebraska Press, 1963.

48 D. Le Vay, *The History of Orthopaedics*, Basle, Editiones Roche, 1990.

49 L. F. Peltier, *Fractures. A History and Iconography of their Treatment*, San Francisco, CA, Norman, 1990, pp. 114–67.

50 Tröhler and Maehle, op. cit. (n. 9), pp. 39, 57, 61–2.

51 Wangensteen and Wangensteen, op. cit. (n. 19), pp. 209–45; Dally, op. cit. (n. 12).

52 J. Wennberg, 'Which rate is right?', *New England Journal of Medicine*, 1986, 314: 310–11.

53 O. Moscucci, *The Science of Women. Gynaecology and Gender in England, 1800–1929*, Cambridge, Cambridge University Press, 1990, pp. 157–64.

54 L. P. Wershub, *Urology from Antiquity to the Twentieth Century*, St Louis, MO, Warren H. Green, 1970.

55 E. H. Ackerknecht, 'Aus den Anfängen der Neurochirurgie', *Schweizer Archiv für Neurologie, Neurochirurgie und Psychiatrie*, 1975, 116: 233–9.

56 U. Tröhler, ' "Why grope in the dark in the light of precision?" Theodor Kocher and neurotopographical diagnosis around 1900', *Cogito* 1992, 1: 75–8 (supplement to *Italian Journal of Neurological Sciences*).

57 A. L. Naef, *The Story of Thoracic Surgery*, Toronto, Hogrefe & Huber, 1990.

58 Francis D. Moore, *Give and Take. The Development of Tissue Transplantation*, Philadelphia, PA, Saunders, 1964.

59 H. J. Klasen, *History of Free Skin Grafting*, Berlin, Springer, 1981; A. F. Wallace, *The Progress of Plastic Surgery: an Introductory History*, Oxford, Meeuws, 1982.

60 J. M. Oppenheimer, 'Taking things apart and putting them together again', *Bulletin of the History of Medicine*, 1978, 52: 149–61.

61 H. P. Schmiedebach, R. Winau and R. Häring (eds), *Erste Operationen Berliner Chirurgen 1817–1931*, Berlin and New York, de Gruyter, 1990, p. 209; T. Schlich, 'Vom physiologischen Experiment zur Therapie: die Pankreastransplantation', *Medizinhistorisches Journal*, 1993.

62 D. M. Hume, 'Early experiences in organ homotransplantation in man and the unexpected sequelae thereof', *American Journal of Surgery*, 1979, 137: 152–61.

63 W. Land and J. B. Dossetor (eds), *Organ Replacement Therapy. Ethics, Justice and Commerce*, Berlin, Springer, 1991.

FURTHER READING

Cartwright, F. F., *The Development of Modern Surgery*, London, Arthur Barker, 1967.

De Moulin, D., *A History of Surgery with Emphasis on the Netherlands*, Dordrecht, Boston, MA, and Lancaster, Nijhoff, 1988, p. 333.

Friedmann, S. G., *A History of Vascular Surgery*, Mount Kisco, NY, Futura, 1989.

Goerke, H., *Medizin und Technik – 3000 Jahre ärztliche Hilfsmittel für Diagnostik und Therapie*, Munich, Callwey, 1988.

Gorin, G., *History of Ophthalmology*, Wilmington, DE, Publish or Perish, 1982.

Haeger, K., *The Illustrated History of Surgery*, New York, Bell, 1988.

Lawrence, C. (ed.), *Medical Theory, Surgical Practice: Studies in the History of Surgery*, London and New York, Routledge, 1992.

Meade, R. H. (ed.), *An Introduction to the History of General Surgery*, Philadelphia, London and Toronto, Saunders, 1968.

Ogilvie, W.H., 'History of surgery', *Encyclopaedia Britannica*, Chicago, 1967, Vol. XV, pp. 92–106.

Pernick, M. S., *A Calculus of Suffering. Pain, Professionalism and Anaesthesia in Nineteenth-Century America*, New York, Columbia University Press, 1985.

Ravitch, M. M., *A Century of Surgery. The History of the American Surgical Association*, Vols I and II, Philadelphia, PA, Lippincott, 1982.

Ruprecht, J., *et al.* (eds), *Anaesthesia. Essays on its History*, Berlin, Springer, 1985.

Schreiber, H. W., and Carstensen, G. (eds), *Chirurgie im Wandel der Zeit 1945–1983*, Berlin, Springer, 1983.

Wangensteen, O. H. and Wangensteen, S. D., *The Rise of Surgery. From Empiric Craft to Scientific Discipline*, Folkestone, Dawson, 1978.

43

PSYCHOTHERAPY

Sander Gilman

Psychotherapy is the non-invasive treatment of those mental or emotional states understood by the patient and the therapist as pathological or maladaptive. It may be used independently of or in addition to somatic procedures and psychopharmacology (somatotherapy). (The 'therapist' may or may not be a physician; the 'patient' may nor may not manifest the symptoms that are defined as 'mental illness' in the various standard nosological handbooks such as the *Diagnostic and Statistical Manual of the American Psychiatric Association*.)

Psychotherapy presupposes a specific relationship between therapist and patient and more or less clearly defined roles for both; it is undertaken in a physical space labelled as a therapeutic context; it presumes that therapy can be effective, and so sets an optimistic prognosis; it is so structured that both therapist and patient have specific, assigned tasks that permit the therapist's interventions.[1]

While the term psychotherapy was recorded in English as early as 1853, it came into common medical use only in the late 1880s through French-language publications.[2] The tradition of an interpersonal, physically non-invasive psychotherapy, however, has long roots in Western culture.[3] It is possible to speak of the sacrament of confession within the Catholic church as a model for the overall practice of psychotherapy.[4] Present within the rhetoric of the Gospels is the image of 'Christ as the physician'. The church, using this biblical metaphor of healing, saw confession (the verbal articulation of sins by the parishioner to the priest within the confessional, and the priest's absolution through the assignment of specific ritual tasks) as healing the soul of those ailments that caused both physical and psychic distress. In addition to the confessional, 'healing miracles' such as those experienced by the Jansenists in the seventeenth and early eighteenth centuries, like other forms of faith-healing, led to cures of both somatic and psychological disorders. Such successes were believed to be the result of the intervention of the divinity through the action of saints represented by relics. But it is clear, if the Jansenist accounts are read, that such cures took place through the active intervention of the clergy and the participation through assigned roles of those undertaking to be healed. In both cases, the roles of patient and therapist, the place of healing, and the potential for intervention were present. (➤ Ch. 61 Religion and medicine)

THE EIGHTEENTH CENTURY

With the medicalization of specific practices of psychotherapy in the course of the late eighteenth century, a secular definition of psychotherapy evolved. Given its secular nature, the roots of this new psychotherapy were within – but often combated by – the traditional medical establishment of the late Enlightenment. The European asylum tradition of the eighteenth century had established a specific model for treating those mental and emotional states that rendered an individual unable to function within the increasingly urbanized and industrial society of Europe. (➤ Ch. 27 Diseases of civilization) Using the traditional pharmacopoeia, diet, baths (especially popular in the latter half of the nineteenth century), and other forms of somatic intervention, physicians attempted to treat debilitating emotional or psychological states with greater or lesser success. (➤ Ch. 40 Physical methods) With the medicalization of animal magnetism or what came to be called 'mesmeric treatment', the path to a psychological procedure which seemed overtly different enough from both conventional medicine and religious tradition was introduced. It was in the theory and practice of the Viennese physician Franz Anton Mesmer (1734–1815), but even more in the work of his disciple, Armand-Marie-Jacques de Chastenet, Marquis de Puységur (1751–1825), that the theory of animal magnetism was applied as a healing tool. They both used the rhetoric of the high science of the eighteenth century, such as chemistry and physiology, to provide a 'scientific' veneer for their treatment.[5] The very name, 'animal magnetism', reflects the Enlightenment interest in concrete forms of physical science, such as electricity and magnetism. The procedure was one of suggestion, but its outward trappings were those of physical science. The use of a *baquet*, the object which was to gather the body 'fluid' to be magnetized by the physician and thus cure the patient, was a clear replica of one of the most avant-garde pieces of scientific instrumentation of the day, the Leyden jar. (One of the more accepted forms of treatment for a wide range of psychological and emotional disorders during the nineteenth century was low-voltage electrolization.) The magnetizer's power over the patients did not rely solely on these scientific substitutes for religious relics.[6]

Rather, Mesmer stressed that the power of healing lay solely with the magnetizer and the special relationship, the 'rapport', with the patient. While individual treatment soon gave way to mass treatment, the relationship between the magnetizer and the patient was a personalized one of trust and belief. (➤ Ch. 28 Unorthodox medical theories)

Mesmer's patients were often suffering from what seemed to be physical symptoms and yet were healed by his non-invasive procedures. Such a blanket claim for the efficacy of mesmerism placed it in direct competition with all forms of institutionalized medicine. The scientific establishment quickly came to view animal magnetism, both in its theoretical as well as its applied form, as bad science and dangerous quackery. The pre-eminent commission appointment by Louis XVI of France in 1784 (the astronomer Jean Bailly (1736–93), the chemist Antoine Lavoisier (1743–94), the physician Joseph Guillotin (1738–1814) and the American ambassador to France, Benjamin Franklin (1706–90)) to examine Mesmer's approach to healing totally rejected the existence of any fluid that could explain animal magnetism. But it also pointed out the dangers that might lie in the sexual exploitation of the suggestible subject through the special rapport, which was evidently generated through the act of mesmeric healing. There is a tension between the tradition of psychotherapy as practised by marginalized physicians such as Mesmer and the mainstream practice of a medicine which defined itself in terms of the high science of its time.

In the German Enlightenment, pre-Romantic writers and thinkers such as Karl Philip Moritz (1756–93) concerned themselves with the social and cultural context of aberrant emotional states, their relationship to physical ailments, and to language and its use as a means of therapy. In practice, the treatments for such states were often through mesmerism or suggestion. Academic physicians in Germany, such as Dietrich Georg Kieser (1779–1862), continued to stand in this tradition in their treatment of the mentally ill, and the poet-physician Justinius Kerner (1786–1862) used a *baquet* in his treatment of psychological, emotional, and physical disorders well into the 1850s. Because of the rapport between therapist and patient, such an approach was understood to be more humane than alternative treatments. Exponents of what came to be called 'moral treatment' of the mentally ill elsewhere in Europe, such as the Quaker reformer of the British asylum, William Tuke (1732–1822), while advocating very different approaches to psychotherapy adapted the close, personal sense of rapport which marked the tradition of mesmerism without the overt use of mesmeric treatment. Like the German Romantic therapists, they spoke and interacted with their charges in terms of accepted social convention, had specific places where treatment took place, and assigned specific tasks for both therapist and patient in the course of the treatment.

THE NINETEENTH CENTURY

With the medicalization of the treatment of the mentally ill in the mid-nineteenth century, certain modes of therapy, such as mesmerism, came to be understood as having some basis in the science of that time. In the 1850s, the work of James Braid (1795–1860) had restored mesmerism as an accepted form of therapy through his realization that pure suggestion rather than instruments such as the *baquet* could be used to place patients in a trance. Braid relabelled 'mesmerism' with the more 'scientific' and less pejorative name, neuro-hypnotism or hypnotism. However, he did this in the context of his interest in phrenology, another 'new' science of the mind in the mid-nineteenth century, as he discussed in his principal work, *Neurypnology, or the Rationale of Nervous Sleep, Considered in Relation with Animal Magnetism* (1843). Braid's interest in phrenology and hypnotism was branded as unscientific by the materialists of his day, such as Wilhelm Griesinger (1817–68) who reduced 'mind illness to brain illness'. This epiphenomonalism made the study of the psyche as an independent or dominant phenomenon impossible for those 'mainstream' physicians who dealt with the mentally and emotionally ill. Dominated by this view during the latter half of the nineteenth century, the study of human physiology and anatomy came to be the sole manner of exploring all those mental and emotional states which were labelled as pathological. (➤ Ch. 7 The physiological tradition)

Thus it was only within the new scientific rhetoric of brain localization, the search for the place within the structure of the brain where the lesions that caused specific forms of mental or emotional illness were to be located, that psychotherapy was able to reappear within mainstream medicine. Given the search for the material basis for the mind, access to the mind (and therefore to the brain) through its psychological manifestations, such as the hypnotic state, again became of interest. Auguste Ambroise Liébeault (1823–1904) in Nancy began, like Mesmer, to treat all the ills of the poor through hypnosis. Liébeault, in his *Concerning Sleep and Analogous States, Considered from the Angle of the Mind-Body Relationship* (1866), explained hypnotism to be a natural state, analogous to normal sleep, but induced in the subject by the suggestion of the physician. For Liébeault, this accounted for the special relationship between the patient and the hypnotizer. Liébeault's work influenced Hippolyte Bernheim (1840–1919), the Professor of Internal Medicine at the new University of Nancy. Bernheim's work was based on a broad application of the implications of his findings concerning hypnotism. In his *Suggestive Therapeutics: a Treatise on the Nature and Uses of Hypnotism* (1886) he suggested that everyone – both the 'ill' and the 'normal' – has the potential to be hypnotized and that this universal aspect of the psyche permitted not only a therapeutics (of negative as well as positive suggestion), but also a research agenda concerning the normal structure of the psyche independent of any material structures within the brain.

Bernheim's furtherance of Liébeault's work was in the light of the dominance of French neurology by Jean Martin Charcot (1825–93), the first Professor of Clinical Diseases of the Nervous System (from 1882) at the University of Paris. (Psychiatry was not yet an independent speciality, as all aberrant psychological phenomena were understood to be physical and therefore 'nervous' diseases.) Charcot, too, employed hypnotism or 'Braidism' to treat the seemingly organic problems of one category of mental illness, hysteria. He understood his ability to place these subjects into a trance as a further symptom of their illness. For Charcot, suggestibility was itself a symptom of the functional deficit of the hysteric. (➤ Ch. 21 Mental diseases)

The conflict between the Parisian and the Nancy schools could be summarized in their self-definition of the efficacy of therapy. Charcot's work became more and more rooted in his understanding of the physiological state, which he saw mirrored in the symptoms of his hysterics. He understood this state as the direct result of some physically traumatic shock on the nervous system. His lack of long-term success in treating the symptoms of his hysterical patients through hypnotism became a further proof of the constitutional nature of their disease. Bernheim, on the other hand, came more and more to abandon hypnosis as the primary mode of therapeutic treatment, relying on direct suggestion. This mode of treatment came to be labelled as 'psychotherapy', a term employed by Bernheim in the title of his *Hypnotism, Suggestion, Psychotherapy* (1891).

FREUD AND HIS FOLLOWERS: THE PSYCHOANALYTIC MOVEMENT

In the midst of this debate between Bernheim and Charcot concerning the treatment of specific forms of mental illness, the Viennese neurologist Sigmund Freud (1856–1929) went to Paris (1885–6), where he attended Charcot's lectures and through them became interested in hysteria.[7] He subsequently visited Bernheim in 1889, in order to further his facility in hypnotism. Freud eventually translated works by both Charcot and Bernheim into German. His personal exposure to both schools, as well as his biological training in the laboratories of the University of Vienna, led him to evolve a three-pronged approach, which he came to call 'psychoanalysis': a therapeutics of psychopathology initially based on hypnosis but quickly evolving to the use of Bernheim's suggestive psychotherapy; a theory of the mind employing the model of hidden or subconscious levels taken from German Romantic psychiatry and philosophy; and a research agenda concerning the impact of history on the mind and of the mind on history which reflected the importance of anthropological models as well as biological models to *fin-de-siècle* medicine.[8] Freud's initial work in the area of the therapeutics of hysteria was undertaken with his somewhat older and more established Viennese colleague, Josef Breuer (1842–1925).[9] Their jointly authored *Studies in Hysteria* (1895) was the initial statement of both the theoretical basis of their approach as well as their therapeutic innovations. These essays and case studies outlined three areas of investigation in terms of vocabularies of science taken from other fields. The 'economic' aspect described the quantity of excitation of the nervous system which, in the normal state, was released in order to create pleasure. In the hysteric, it was dammed up and created symptoms. This 'dynamic' aspect was evoked to explain the creation of specific symptom by specific emotionally charged experience. They argued that all hysterical symptoms were the product of the memory of real events forgotten by the conscious mind but retained elsewhere in the psyche. For Freud, these were recent events of a sexual nature which evoked memories of early sexual experiences of seduction. The 'topographic' aspect of the theory locates where these events took place: the unconscious, a powerful area of the mind not directly accessible to the conscious mind. Later, Freud refined this aspect of his theory. Between the conscious and the unconscious mind stood the preconscious, the screen situated between the conscious and the unconscious. It was here that neuroses arose as preconscious material was repressed into the unconscious.

Freudian theory evolved during the first decade of the twentieth century, but its contours followed these initial categories. Initially, Freud and Breuer (as had Bernheim) substituted a form of suggestion for the hypnotic trance when they found that their patients' experiences were not sufficiently resolved through posthypnotic suggestion. Their therapy for hysterical neurosis, free association, was developed in concert with their patients, especially the patient whom Breuer called 'Anna O.', Bertha Pappenheim (1859–1936). (She later in life became one of the founders of modern German social work.) She evolved a system of what she labelled as 'chimney sweeping'. In discussing with Breuer the meaning and origin of each symptom, the underlying cause of the symptom was articulated and the symptom vanished. Anna O., like many of Freud's and Breuer's patients, was middle class and well educated.[10] These patients entered into the therapeutic situation with a sense of having or needing some control over the therapeutic situation not offered through traditional medicine. Indeed, Freud's own record of those patients who terminated treatment abruptly is a sign of the overall sense of autonomy granted to the patient within the psychoanalytic milieu as opposed to that of establishment psychiatry at the *fin de siècle*. (➤ Ch. 56 Psychiatry)

The centrality of human sexuality, while clear to Freud in his initial work with Breuer in the 1890s, was most clearly expressed in his work at the *fin de siècle.* The force repressed in the hysteric, the experiences which were shaped by the fantasy over the first few years of life, was sexual – the underlying driving-force of human instincts (libido). Freud's model for the id was male sexuality. While he recognized the existence of models of male and female sexuality, reflecting cognitive as well as anatomical difference, he departed from an explicit model of aggressive male sexuality. The Oedipus complex was a clear expression of this male model: it was the successful or unsuccessful renunciation of the attraction to the mother and the concomitant fear of punishment through castration by the father that determined the psychological health or pathology of the male child. The female child must not only abandon her attraction to the mother but must also deal with the sudden awareness of her own physical incompleteness, her envy of the penis. Freud's discussion of the fantasies of female anatomy reflected a male fantasy of castration rather than potential female fantasies of fecundity and childbirth. Likewise, Freud's use of the categories of 'active' and 'passive' to represent the male and female character reflected his presumption about the definition of gender.

By 1897, Freud transcended his initial view that all neuroses were the results of real events and came to understand that the origins of neurosis were in universal psychological drives and the fantasies of sexually arousing events. And the source for all of these fantasies was the nature of the unconscious. The unconscious was the space where all of the basic libidinal drives were housed. This would include the sexual drive, but also those such as hatred and shame. It is the place within the psyche that the repressed incestuous desires of the child were hidden. Freud in no way excluded the possibility that real disturbing events, in the form of childhood sexual experience, could exist. To examine the underlying processes which structure human fantasy in the unconscious, Freud turned to universal experiences which he saw as revealing unconscious processes: dreaming, slips of the tongue, errors of memory, and jokes. In *The Interpretation of Dreams* (1900), he set out a model for interpreting the underlying structure of the unconscious 'dream work'. His primary source for his work in this period was his analysis of own experiences and dreams. He illustrated how the manifest content of the dream (its overt story) employed aspects of daily experience to both mask and expose the underlying sexual fantasies of early childhood. He thus saw the analysis of dreams by the psychoanalyst and the analysand as a central means of psychotherapy.

The analysis of all aspects of the analysand's mental life – dreams, memories, thoughts, preoccupations – presented the key to the underlying tension between the social demands of the world (represented in the psyche as the superego) and the immediate demands of libidinous instincts (the id). It is in the ego, the realm of reason and balance, that there is an attempt to resolve these conflicts. What occurs in therapy is transference, an intense rapport (which may take the positive form of love, but may also take the negative form of hate) with the neutral figure of the analyst, who comes to replace that 'object' (parent, authority figure). The means of therapy is the free association of ideas, thoughts, images and feelings. (➤ Ch. 34 History of the doctor–patient relationship)

The rapport that Mesmer had described between the subject and the magnetizer, the suggestion which Bernheim (and unconsciously Charcot) had seen between the patient and the physician, evolved within the psychoanalytic model as the transference between the analyst and the analysand. The therapeutic dimension thus rested on the relationship between the analyst and the analysand as well as on the roles that they accepted as part of the therapy. The 'talking cure' was not merely the secular confession of failings. The analysand was to tell the analyst:

> what he knows and conceals from other people; he is to tell us too what he does not know. . . . He is to tell us not only what he can say intentionally and willingly, what will give him relief like a confession, but everything else that his self-observation yields him.[11]

Freud's central therapeutic approach, which impacted either positively or negatively on virtually all forms of psychotherapy, arose to no little degree out of the social milieu in which he and Breuer found themselves. They were not psychiatrists dealing with the institutionalized mentally ill. As neurologists, they dealt with what was perceived as somatic illnesses. They thus spoke with their patients, asking them about their experience as well as their symptoms. As physicians with a mainly middle- and upper-middle-class, educated clientele, there were few problems in finding a common language about more or less common experiences. And as Jews treating a mainly Jewish patient population, they could lay claim to an immediate rapport between themselves and their patients, as all found themselves in an extremely hostile environment. They themselves bore the stigma of difference while being part of the select world of medical power.

In 1905, Freud published his descriptive study on the theory of sexuality (*Three Essays on the Theory of Sexuality*). He evolved a model of phases of psychosexual development. The infant's early experiences revolved about its oral activity with its focus on the mouth; then the anal stage, which evolved with the appearance of teeth; then the phallic stage (from three to seven), with the Oedipus phase for males and the Electra phase for women (the attraction to the opposite-sex parent and fear of the same-sex parent); a latency stage (with a strong identification with the same-sex parent); and finally, the genital stage. Here in the greatest detail Freud laid out the relationship beyond psychosexual development and neurotic symbol formation.

Freud also applied the development model taken from nineteenth-century biology to the study of 'primitive' societies. In a series of anthropological works from *Totem and Taboo* (1913) to his final work *Moses and Monotheism* (1938), he used the mythic embryological model of 'ontogeny recapitulating phylogeny' (the development of the species repeating in the development of the individual) to trace the historical impact of the model of psychosexual development he evolved. He returned to a model of trauma, but a model of historical trauma, in which he saw an earlier act – the murder of the 'primitive' father by the sons or the murder of Moses by the Jews – as historical realities which came to be implanted in the memory of the group or race and which provided a model for human action. Freud's debt to nineteenth-century anthropology for the materials and approaches to these questions were certainly as great as his debt to nineteenth-century neurology for the talking cure, and to nineteenth-century biology for his underlying views of the structures of the psyche. (➤ Ch. 60 Medicine and anthropology)

Belonging to the mainstream of Freudian theory and practice, from the *fin de siècle* to the present, meant following the general therapeutic milieu of the talking cure, holding to the centrality of the sexual origin of neurosis, and seeing a parallel between development and historical or cultural manifestations of the psyche. The orthodoxy of psychoanalysis was challenged by many of those who had been Freud's closest followers during the beginnings of the organization of the psychoanalytic movement. A major role in mainstream Freudian psychotherapy during the very beginnings of the movement was played by the Hungarian-Jewish psychoanalyst Sándor Ferenczi (1873–1933), whose innovations both in theory and therapy altered the primary Freudian model of the neutral stance of the psychoanalyst. Initially, Ferenczi was much more rigid than Freud in terms of forbidding any release of the analysand's libido, hoping that the damming of libidinous drives would be released within the therapeutic setting. He came to reject this position and evolved an intensive interactive therapy based on his view that the analysand's neurosis was the result of not having had enough love as a child. Frued's neutral analyst was substituted by Ferenczi with a therapist who replaced the parent and provided this lost love. Likewise, Otto Rank (1884–1939), whose cultural history of incest, *The Incest Motif in Poetry and Legend* (1912), was the prototype of all later psychoanalytic approaches to cultural artefacts, broke with Freud over the question of the length of therapy, among other reasons. He advocated a specific, pre-set time limit rather than an open-ended therapy. Rank's theoretical emphasis was on the manner by which each person separated from the mother and became a 'self-realized' individual. This was initially seen through his focus on 'birth trauma'. For

Rank, the anxiety of the birth trauma became a means of understanding all the later developments of the adult, considering separation necessary for the individual fully to mature. Thus Rank's planning of the length of therapy was a means of introducing the anxiety of separation as part of the psychotherapeutic method.

Without a doubt the most orthodox follower of the second generation of psychoanalysts was Freud's youngest child, Anna Freud (1895–1982).[12] Her work on child analysis, begun with a paper in 1926, developed the ego psychology outlined by her father. Especially in *The Ego and the Mechanisms of Defence* (1936), she outlined the means (repression and projection) by which the ego protected itself from unpleasant ideas and emotions. She escaped with her father from Nazi-occupied Vienna in 1938, and settled in England where she founded the Hampstead nurseries for wartime children.[13] Out of that experience came a series of studies of the mental lives of children in institutional settings.

Anna Freud's great opponent within the London psychoanalytic community was Melanie Klein (1882–1960), an analysand of Ferenczi, who had come to London from Vienna in 1926.[14] Like Anna Freud, her initial interest lay in the area of child development. Her focus on the meaning of play in the mental world of the child and its symbolic language was best outlined in *The Psychoanalysis of Children* (1932). She expanded Freud's discussion of the formation of the ego and focused on the internalization of the representation of those objects in the world, such as the mother, that the child first understands as different from itself. She described introjection, the process by which internal representations of good and evil, of control or lack of control, are generated by the developing psyche of the child.

The number of psychoanalytic schismatics is extensive. The primary figures who came to found independent psychoanalytic schools were also the first major disciples of Freud who were seen by him as his potential successors within the psychoanalytic movement: Alfred Adler (1870–1937) and Carl Gustav Jung (1875–1961). Both broke with Freud over the question of the centrality of sexuality in the structure and treatment of the human psyche. Adler stressed the physical nature of the individual as the source of mental illness.[15] As early as his 1907 *Study of Organ Inferiority and its Psychical Compensation*, Adler emphasized the attempts of children to compensate for their physical inferiority by producing specific pathological character structures which led to specific 'life-styles'. He expressly rejected Freud's sexual theory in *The Neurotic Constitution* (1912), and was the first of Freud's major followers to break with him (in 1911). Adler's creation of 'individual psychology' emphasized the fictions through which the individual created and achieved life goals. The central tenet of Adlerian psychotherapy reflected the individual's creation of socially meaningful, personal goals. This was to be achieved through the analysis of early memories as the source of an understanding of the patient's social maladaptation. Adler's approach became the primary model for psychotherapy among psychotherapeutic social workers in the 1920s and 1930s.

Jung, the first important non-Jewish follower of Freud, was trained in Switzerland as well as in Paris. He was a colleague of the Swiss academic psychiatrist Eugen Bleuler (1857–1939), the first major figure in academic psychiatry to accept and apply Freud's therapeutic methods. Basing his work on the mental-association methods of Wilhelm Wundt (1832–1920), Jung developed a word-association test, which was initially employed to explore the unconscious, following Freud's model. Through the analysis of the test results, Jung was able to describe the 'complexes' of the individual. For Jung, however, the unconscious which was to be so explored came more and more to be a historical rather than a sexual unconscious. What for Frued was sexual libido became for Jung 'life force'. Jung, who broke with Freud in 1912, stressed the inheritance of psychological models of the world, archetypes. He saw these as inherent and motivating, rather than (as did Freud) the articulation of the repression of instinct. Sexuality was thus relegated to a minor feature within Jung's system. Central to his therapeutics was the image of 'coming to selfhood' or 'self-realization'. This was the integration of the various 'persona', of social and individual personalities, into a whole. Where Freud departed from the pathological in order to present an understanding of the human psyche, for Jung normal psychic development stood at the centre of his system.

Jung's archetypes were not bound by time and space: they were truly universal. He generated a series of images, restructuring the Freudian vocabulary of sexuality into a vocabulary of archetypes. Thus the Freudian image of bisexuality (the view that all individuals contained the potential for 'masculine' as well as 'feminine' qualities) became the syzygy, the anima, the feminine quality of the male; and the animus, the male quality of the female. These became asexual driving forces, Jung's libido, existing as part of the collective unconscious. This is the origin of all creativity, but also all mental illness. It is the balance between psychic forces within the collective unconscious that structured the human being's manner of relating to world. The domination of one pole created the 'introvert'; of the other, the 'extrovert.'

THE NEO-FREUDIANS

Adler had set a social agenda only peripheral to Freud's own interest; how does the experience of the self in society structure the psyche? The question of the social context of the individual and its role in creating circumstances that could be labelled as pathogenic became the agenda of the neo-Freudian or culturally oriented psychoanalysts in the 1930s and 1940s. For Erich Fromm (1900–80), the organization of society provided the structure for definition of the self. He visualized a political choice for the individual, which also shaped and gave form to the psyche: either the productive use of freedom to fulfil the individual, or the flight from individual freedom into the control of totalitarianism. His categories of ego formation (relatedness, transcendence, rootedness, identity, and orientation) all stressed the social factor in the shaping of the psyche.

It is in the work of the neo-Freudian psychoanalyst, Karen Horney (1885–1952), that Freud's analysis of feminine psychology had its first and most intensive critique.[16] While some female followers of Freud had supported his male-oriented model of sexuality, Horney challenged Freud over this question.[17] Beginning in a series of papers in 1924 (on the 'Dissolution of the Oedipus complex'), she saw feminine psychology as a process parallel to but different from the development of male sexuality. Rather than being robbed of the penis, she argued in a 1926 paper ('The flight from womanhood'), the woman's fecundity became an object of envy for men – the ability to conceive and bear. Horney's neo-Freudian work extended into her American experience after she went to the University of Chicago from Berlin in 1932. Her interest in the question of feminine psychology gave way to broader questions about the cultural context of neurosis. In the late 1930s she broke with orthodox Freudian theory over the primacy of Freud's libido theory. Her most important work of the American period was *The Neurotic Personality of Our Time* (1937). For her, the origin of neurosis was not the articulation of the Oedipus complex, but basic existential anxiety common to all human beings. Other psychoanalysts who dealt with the question of the psychology of women and their therapy, Edith Jacobson (1897–1978) and Melanie Klein, were of central importance during this period in drawing attention to the social as well as the biological specificity of the female experience.[18]

In the United States, Freudian theory and therapy had had a powerful beginning in the first decade of the twentieth century. The attraction and support of established psychologists, such as William James (1842–1910) of Harvard University and G. Stanley Hall (1844–1924) of Clark University, for psychoanalysis opened the doors for the wide dissemination of this therapy after Freud's visit to the United States in 1909. Of all the American reinterpreters of Freud, none was more influential than Harry Stack Sullivan (1892–1949), who, like Horney, stressed the central role of anxiety in the shaping of maladaptive behaviour. Sullivan carried on Ferenczi's interests in anxiety. Ferenczi's work had been brought to the United States by his analysand, Clara Thompson (1893–1958), with whom Sullivan, in turn, worked.[19] For Sullivan, this anxiety is transferred empathetically from mother to child. Psychotherapy is the interpersonal process of alleviating the psychic tension which is the result of this anxiety, and, if successful, it results in equilibrium. Sullivan's therapeutic model was widely influential in the 1940s and 1950s. But it was not only within the Americanization of the 'talking cure' that psychotherapy found its therapeutic tools. It was also in the United States that hypnosis was reintroduced after the Second World War within mainstream psychology by Milton H. Erickson (1901–80).[20]

In France, following the Second World War, it was in the work of Jacques Lacan (1901–81) that Freudian theory had its most controversial representative.[21] Lacan, like the Freudo-Marxist Herbert Marcuse (1898–1979) in the United States, placed psychoanalysis at the centre of political change during the 1960s and 1970s. He laid claim to the revolutionary history of psychoanalysis and saw it as a force of eventual social change. Central to Lacan's views was a developmental model in which the process of acquiring language and the internalization of symbols shaped the inner structure of the psyche. Lacan argued for the universality of transference into all spheres of social interaction. Lacanian psychoanalysis came to structure and focus French (and to a limited extent Anglo-American) cultural life during this period. But Lacan also developed a strikingly innovative mode of psychotherapy. His introduction of very short session therapy, with its intense moment of transference, related to certain developments by Ferenczi in the field of brief (short-term) psychotherapy.[22] In the United States and western Europe, the open-ended therapeutic model of traditional psychoanalysis came to be restructured into the needs of a more mobile patient population, the cost of whose therapy was no longer borne personally, but by third parties (such as the state or private insurance).

In Great Britain, psychoanalysis acquired a place in the traditional medical establishment through the work of Ernest Jones (1879–1958), the founder of the British Psychoanalytic Society (1919).[23] Jones had invited Melanie Klein to England, and was helpful in relocating both Sigmund and Anna Freud there in 1938. He was also able to maintain a working relationship between the dominant groups within British psychoanalysis during the 1940s and 1950s. This was quite unlike the experience in the United States, where schism after schism fragmented the various organized Freudian groups. In Britain, the conflict between Melanie Klein and Anna Freud reflected itself in the therapeutic milieu as well as in the protagonists' theoretical positions. Both groups were concerned with child therapy. The Kleinians, however, were quite willing to intercede earlier and more rigorously in the child's treatment than the Freudians, and employed free-association play therapy with very young children rather than those verbal methods that could only be effective with slightly older children. Anna Freud's impact on the wider culture in the United States and western Europe came with her collaboration in the 1950s and 1960s in a series of studies that defined the legal framework for societies' treatment of children. (➤ Ch. 45 Childhood; Ch. 69 Medicine and the law)

The impact of Melanie Klein was felt within psychotherapy with the rise of object-relationship theory, the theory of how the developing child related to the earliest and most intense relationship with the care-giver or mother.[24] This work departed from Freud's 1914 paper 'On Narcissism', in which he described how the infant differentiated itself from the world in which it found itself. The continuation of Freud's interest in ego psychology in the United States was furthered by Margaret Mahler (1897–1985), who had come from Vienna to New York in 1938.[25] Her interest, best expressed in *On Human Symbiosis* (1968), focused on the problems of the process of individuation in severely mentally disturbed infants as well as in normal development. Donald Woods Winnicott (1896–1971) in Great Britain, Hans Kohut (1913–81) at the University of Chicago, and Otto Kernberg (b. 1928) at Cornell University all contributed to the discussion of how the child differentiates itself from the world and constructs an ego and superego.[26] The reflection of this view in therapy surfaced with the renewed emphasis on very early childhood, pre-Oedipal development at the core of the formation of psychopathology, such as the 'borderline' or 'narcissistic' personality.

OTHER PSYCHOTHERAPIES

The psychotherapists who radically departed from Freudian theory and evolved their own models of psychotherapy range widely across the therapeutic field. The Freudo-Marxist Wilhelm Reich (1897–1951), who had begun as a traditional, if politically radical, follower of Freud in the 1920s, evolved a theory of mass neurosis and its origin in sexual repression.[27] Reich stressed the meaning of body position and contact. Out of this theoretical view came the 'orgone box', a device developed by him in the 1940s to harness psychic energy as a treatment for neurosis, as well as 'vegetotherapy'. Parallel devices for psychological (and physical) healing were developed in the 1950s by the Scientologists. Such devices were the exception within mainstream psychotherapy, but they harked back to the tradition of Mesmer's *baquet*. Reich's work assumed that psychological maladaptation reflected itself in the structure of the body. He saw the development of a 'character armour' which was mirrored in the very musculature of the body. His followers evolved various therapies out of his basic views.

Similar claims were made for the impact of the body on the psyche in the work of F. Matthias Alexander (1869–1955) and Moshé Feldenkrais (b. 1904).[28] These approaches were purely somatic ones, stressing the question of body alignment and physical self-awareness. Yet they were also psychotherapies in that they treated emotional and mental states as well as physical ailments. The entire development of the biofeedback method of psycho-therapy during the 1960s and 1970s was a more-sophisticated form of self-suggestion using an apparatus.[29] During the late 1960s, it was reported that subjects could control their EEGs (brain-wave measurements) while watching them on a screen. The explosion of interest in biofeedback therapy made use of various traditional medical-monitoring devices and trained patients to alter their emotional levels. The line between somatic therapies and psycho-logical therapies remained very fine.

Alternative therapies such as the re-enactment of lived experience, 'psycho-drama', in groups rather than in individual sessions with a therapist had been developed in the 1920s. Jacob Levy Moreno (1892–1974) evolved a role-playing structure in which aspects of the patient's life were re-enacted in order to come to a clinical resolution.[30] Moreno introduced the term 'group therapy' in 1932. A standard feature of his therapy was 'role reversal', in which the patients reversed their antagonistic social roles, each playing the others. Such group treatments had begun with patients suffering from pul-monary tuberculosis at the turn of the century. Frederick Perls (1894–1970) developed 'Gestalt therapy' as a means of allowing patients to make creative adjustments to their present situations.[31] The patient constructed a dialogue by which the warring aspects of the personality were reunited into a single Gestalt or structure. Through Perls's institute at Esalen, California, Gestalt therapy had a disproportionate influence on the anti-psychoanalytic views of the 1960s. Family therapy arose after the Second World War with the attempt to treat the entire family unit rather than only the patient through psychotherapy. The Wisconsin psychiatrist Christian Fredrick Midelfort (b. 1906) developed the view that there were compensatory and opposing psycho-pathologies within every family, which might well only manifest themselves overtly with any given member. Treating the family unit was necessary in treating the individual.

Ronald David Laing (1927–89) also postulated a re-enactment of childhood and a retraining of the mentally ill individual in his therapeutic community at Philadelphia House, London.[32] Alexander Wolf (b. 1907) evolved a means of treatment for large groups, and group therapy spread widely in specific environments (such as public hospitals) during the 1950s.[33] The psychologist Carl Ransom Rogers (1902–87) evolved a variation of the group: the encoun-ter group, which is a client-centred therapy based on existentialist philo-sophy.[34] Related to this were the 'T-groups', which evolved from the work of Kurt Lewin (1890–1947). There, the rules of the group demanded com-plete self-disclosure. These groups had the quasi-religious parallel in the twelve-step movement of group psychotherapy, initially developed by William G. Wilson (1895–1971), known as 'Bill W.', for the treatment of alcoholism (Alcoholics Anonymous) but evolving during the 1960s and 1970s to cover a wide range of addictive or assumed-addictive behaviours (including food-related disorders, co-dependency, tobacco addiction, as well as the impact of addictive behaviour on family members (Al-Anon).[35] These movements were all extensions of the idea of a total therapy to combat a total illness. Their models were shaped by religious models (such as the Protestant tradition of bearing testimony) rather than strictly medical ones, but they have come to be a major adjunct to the treatment of various addictions, tendencies, and habits. The stress in these movements, as in the 'Mental Hygiene Movement' begun in the 1920s, by Clifford Beers (1876–1943), is on patient self-identification and self-help.[36]

Various American popular psychotherapeutic movements, such as the transactional analysis of Eric Berne (1910–70),[37] EST devised by Hans Werner Erhard (b. 1935), or the Primal Therapy of Arthur Janov's, evolved variant forms of treatment for neurosis.[38] All combined psychodynamic therapies with various notions of the unconscious and all achieved a broad popular success for a relatively short period of time in the 1960s and 1970s. Indeed, the quick development and often quicker demise of such popular psychotherapies during the twentieth century reflects more the increased level of communication and the power of modern advertising than the need for ever newer and different approaches to the treatment of psychopathologies.

While there was a lowering of the prestige of traditional psychoanalysis in the United States and western Europe with the introduction of psychoactive drugs, such as lithium for the treatment of manic-depressive psychosis, during the 1960s, psychoanalysis retained its importance in certain areas such as feminist therapy. The continuation and abridgement of traditional psychotherapy through the feminist model can be best seen in the 1970s in the work of the British psychoanalytic theorist, Juliet Mitchell (b. 1940).[39] Mitchell's work synthesized streams coming from France (Lacan) and Britain (Winnicott). She stressed the underlying unconscious forces depicted in Freud's theory and his rejection of biologically based instinct theories. Her reading of Freud's work as a more abstract and symbolic system made Freudian psychoanalysis not only a central feature of feminist theory of the 1970s and 1980s, but also provided the intellectual background for the development of a feminist psychotherapy. Parallel trends can be seen in the work of Helene Cixous (b. 1937) in France and Margarete Mitscherlich-Nielsen (b. 1917) in Germany.[40]

Another major tradition of late nineteenth-century mental science, the developments of clinical psychology, especially as evolved in the laboratory of Wundt, were translated into a psychotherapeutic approach during the first decades of the twentieth century. In Switzerland, Jung had used Wundt's model of word association in describing the creation of 'complexes' within early psychoanalytic theory. At about the same time, a quite different appropriation of Wundt's psychological theory was being undertaken in Russia. Central to these were the behavioural psychotherapies which evolved out of the work of Ivan Petrovitch Pavlov (1849–1936), a student of Wundt. Pavlov's description of 'conditioned reflexes' set the stage for a redefinition of 'consciousness' as purely instinctual and learned responses, and for the denial of the existence of the unconscious. For Pavlov, the assumption was that the only 'unconscious' processes that existed were simple reflexes which could be conditioned to affect behavioural change. Pavlov found that he could condition dogs to respond in specific ways to specific, set stimuli. He could also generate what he labelled as 'experimental neurosis' by providing what would have been perceived by the dog as contradictory or overly fine distinctions between stimuli. Pavlov's work on experimental neurosis had a major impact on American psychology and psychotherapeutics through the work of Howard S. Lidell (1895–1962) at Cornell University. (➤ Ch. 11 Clinical research)

The central difference between the behavioural model and the psychoanalytic model was one of level of treatment. Freudian psychotherapy assumed that the treatment of the symptom without addressing its underlying, interpsychic cause would not be effective. Indeed, this was Freud's own critique of Charcot's treatment of hysterics through hypnosis. Behaviourists assumed that the therapist could directly treat and eliminate the symptom, which was making the person maladaptive or ill. The British psychologist Hans J. Eysenck (b. 1916) provided a detailed critique of psychoanalytic psychotherapy in an essay in 1952, which encouraged behavioural therapies as a more effective manner of treating emotional and psychological problems.[41]

By the 1950s, there was a long tradition of successful treatment of various forms of emotional or psychological maladaptation through behavioural therapy. John Broadus Watson (1878–1958), whose treatment of phobic conditions in children and adults was through direct conditioning, provided a set of clinical case studies. Patients were exposed, under a strict regime, to the source of their anxiety. They gradually became desensitized and demonstrated fewer negative responses as their exposure was increased. In Boston during the 1920s, Douglas A. Thom (1887–1951) set up a 'habit clinic' to treat pre-school children. The development by Burrhus Frederick Skinner (1904–90) of 'operant conditioning' as a basic approach to behaviour modification presented a means of controlling the development of positive behaviours (rather than the elimination of negative behaviours) based on the controlled responses to specific reward stimuli. Skinner applied his views to child-rearing (developing the Skinner box, which had a controlled environment) and undertook the treatment of psychopathologies. During the early 1950s, Skinner and his colleagues applied the principle of operant behaviour to the treatment of severely mentally ill patients, using a larger version of the Skinner box, a 6 ft by 6 ft room in which therapeutic tasks performed were directly rewarded by small gifts such as cigarettes or candy.[42]

By the 1980s, psychotherapy had become so complex and fragmented that no single approach could be understood as primary.[43] With the rise of psychopharmacological treatments for psychosis, neurosis, as well as behavioural problems, beginning in the 1960s, many of the forms of psychotherapy were adapted as supportive psychotherapy both within and beyond the clinical setting. (➤ Ch. 39 Drug therapies) Indeed, one of the ironies is that Freudian psychotherapy, stripped of its theoretical basis, comes by the 1970s and 1980s to be a substantial addition to the chemotherapy of emotional and psychic illness as 'supportive psychotherapy'. Psychotherapy from the 1980s onwards has been extraordinarily diverse and holds an important position within both medical and non-medical aspects of culture.

NOTES

1 This definition is based on the discussion of Jerome Frank, *Persuasion and Healing, a Comparative Study of Psychotherapy*, Baltimore, MD, Johns Hopkins University Press, 1961.

2 Walter Cooper Dendy, 'Psychotherapeia, or the remedial influence of mind', *Journal of Psychological Medicine and Mental Pathology*, 1853, 3: 268. The first modern use of the term seems to be in the work of A. W. van Renterghem and F. van Eeden, *Clinique de psychothérapie suggestive fondée à Amsterdam le 15 août 1887*, Brussels, A. Manceaux, 1889. See I. N. Bulhof, 'From psychotherapy to psychoanalysis: Frederik van Eeden and Albert Willem van Renterghem', *Journal of the History of the Behavioural Sciences*, 1981, 17: 209–21; D. Pivnicki, 'The beginnings of psychotherapy', *Journal of the History of the Behavioural Sciences*, 1969, 5: 238–47; and E. Harms, 'Historical background of psychotherapy as a new scientific field', *Diseases of the Nervous System*, 1970, 31: 116–18.

3 On classical ideas of psychotherapy see C. Gill, 'Ancient psychotherapy', *Journal of the History of Ideas*, 1985, 46: 307–25; and on a case of psychotherapy which would meet our definition during the Middle Ages see J. P. Williman and R. G. Kvarnes, 'A medieval example of psychotherapy', *Psychiatry*, 1984, 47: 93–5.

4 Hanna Wolff, *Jesus als Psychotherapeut: Jesu Menschenbehandlung als Modell moderner Psychotherapie*, Stuttgart, Radius, 1986; P. W. Sharkey (ed.), *Philosophy, Religion and Psychotherapy: Essays in the Philosophical Foundations of Psychotherapy*, Washington, University Press of America.

5 Robert Darnton, *Mesmerism and the End of the Enlightenment in France*, Cambridge, MA, Harvard University Press, 1968; Leon Chertok and Raymond de Saussure, *The Therapeutic Revolution, from Mesmer to Freud*, New York, Brunner Mazel, 1979.

6 As, for example, in the Jansenist healings. See Louis Basile Carré de Montgeron, *La Verité des miracles operés par l'intercession de M. de Pâris et autres appellans*

demontrée contre M. L'Archevêque de Sens, 3 vols., Cologne, Chez les libraires de la Campagnie, 1745–7.

7 Peter Gay, *Sigmund Freud: a Life for Our Time*, New York, Norton, 1988.

8 Edwin Wallace IV, *Freud and Anthropology: a History and Reappraisal*, New York, International Universities Press, 1983.

9 Albrecht Hirschmüller, *The Life and Work of Josef Breuer: Physiology and Psychoanalysis*, New York, New York University Press, 1989.

10 E. Jones, 'Social class and psychotherapy: a critical review of research', *Psychiatry*, 1974, 37: 307–20.

11 Sigmund Freud, *Standard Edition of the Complete Psychological Works of Sigmund Freud*, ed. and trans. by J. Strachey, A. Freud, A. Strachey and A. Tyson, 24 vols, London, Hogarth, 1955–74, Vol. XXIII, p. 174.

12 Elisabeth Young-Bruehl, *Anna Freud: a Biography*, New York, Summit Books, 1988.

13 On the tradition of psychotherapy under the Nazis, see Geoffrey Cocks, *Psychotherapy in the Third Reich: the Göring Institute*, New York, Oxford University Press, 1985.

14 Phyllis Grosskurth, *Melanie Klein: Her World and Her Work*, New York, Knopf, 1986.

15 Paul E. Stepansky, *In Freud's shadow: Adler in Context*, Hillsdale, NJ, Analytic Press, 1983; B. Handlbauer, *Die Entstehungsgeschichte der Individualpsychologie Alfred Adlers*, Vienna, Geyer-Edition, 1984.

16 Susan Quinn, *A Mind of Her Own: the Life of Karen Horney*, New York, Summit Books, 1987.

17 Nellie Louise Buckley, 'Women psychoanalysts and the theory of feminine development: a study of Karen Horney, Helene Deutsch, and Marie Bonaparte', unpublished dissertation, University of California at Los Angeles, 1982; Janet Sayers, *Mothers of Psychoanalysis: Helene Deutsch, Karen Horney, Anna Freud, and Melanie Klein*, New York, W. W. Norton, 1991.

18 Otto Kernberg, 'The contributions of Edith Jacobson: an overview', *Journal of the American Psychoanalytic Association*, 1979, 27: 793–819.

19 R. Moulton, 'Clara Thompson, M.D.: unassuming leader', in L. J. Dickstein and C. C. Nadelson (eds), *Women Physicians in Leadership Roles*, Washington, DC, American Psychiatric Press, 1986, pp. 87–93; H. S. Perry, 'Clara Mabel Thompson', *Notable American Women: the Modern Period*, Cambridge, MA, Belknap-Harvard University Press, 1980.

20 J. D. Beahrs, 'The hypnotic psychotherapy of Milton H. Erickson', *American Journal of Clinical Hypnosis*, 1971, 14: 73–90.

21 Sherry Turkle, *Psychoanalytic Politics: Freud's French Revolution*, Cambridge, MA, MIT Press, 1981; Michael Clark, *Jacques Lacan: an Annotated Bibliography*, New York, Garland, 1988; Shoshana Felman, *Jacques Lacan and the Adventure of Insight: Psychoanalysis in Contemporary Culture*, Cambridge, MA, Harvard University Press, 1987.

22 P. E. Sifneos, 'Short-term dynamic psychotherapy: its history, its impact and its future', *Psychotherapy and Psychosomatic Medicine*, 1981, 35: 224–9.

23 Gregorio Kohon (ed.), *The British School of Psychoanalysis: the Independent Tradition*, London, Free Association Books, 1986.

24 Jay R. Greenberg and Stephen A. Mitchell, *Object Relations in Psychoanalytic Theory*, Cambridge, MA, Harvard University Press, 1983.

25 In general on the relationship between Viennese and American psychoanalysis, see A. Schick, 'Psychotherapy in Old Vienna and New York: cultural comparisons', *Psychoanalytic Review*, 1973, 60: 111–26. On Mahler, see J. R. Smith, 'Margaret S. Mahler, M.D.: original thinker, exceptional woman', in Dickstein and Nadelson, op. cit. (n. 19), pp. 109–19.

26 A. Phillips, *Winnicott*, Cambridge, MA, Harvard University Press, 1989; F. R. Rodman, *The Spontaneous Gesture: Selected Letters of D. W. Winnicott*, Cambridge, MA, Harvard University Press, 1987.

27 M. Sharaf, *Fury on Earth. A Biography of Wilhelm Reich*, New York, St Martin's Press/Marek, 1983; Erwin H. Ackerknecht, 'Wilhelm Reich (1897–1957)', in K. Ganzinger, *et al.* (eds), *Festschrift für Erna Lesky zum 70. Geburtstag*, Vienna, Bruder Hollinek, 1981, pp. 5–12; Paul A. Robinson, *The Freudian Left: Wilhelm Reich, Geza Roheim, Herbert Marcuse*, Ithaca, NY, Cornell University Press, 1990.

28 F. Matthias Alexander, *The Resurrection of the Body*, ed. by Edward Maisel, Boston, MA, Shambala, 1986; Moshé Feldenkrais, *Body and Mature Behavior: a Study of Anxiety, Sex, Gravitation and Learning*, New York, International Universities Press, 1949; Feldenkrais, *The Case of Nora: Body Awareness as Healing Therapy*, New York, Harper & Row, 1977.

29 John V. Basmajian, *Biofeedback: Principles and Practice for Clinicians*, Baltimore, MD, Williams & Wilkins, 1987.

30 Jacob Levy Moreno, 'Psychodrama', in Silvano Arieti (ed.), *American Handbook of Psychiatry*, New York, Basic Books, 1959, pp. 1375–96.

31 Martin Shepard, *Fritz*, New York, Saturday Review Press, 1975.

32 A. Collier, *R. D. Laing: the Philosophy and Politics of Psychotherapy*, New York, Pantheon, 1977; and Richard I. Evans, *R. D. Laing: the Man and His Ideas*, New York, Dutton, 1976.

33 M. F. Ettin, ' "Come on, Jack, tell us about yourself": the growth spurt of group psychotherapy', *International Journal of Group Psychotherapy*, 1989, 39: 35–57; Ettin, ' "By the crowd they have been broken, by the crowd they shall be healed": the advent of group psychotherapy', *International Journal of Group Psychotherapy*, 1988, 38: 139–67. See also H. Papanek, 'Adler's psychology and group psychotherapy', *American Journal of Psychiatry*, 970, 127: 783–6.

34 Richard I. Evans, *Carl Rogers: the Man and His Ideas*, New York, Dutton, 1975.

35 Bill W., *Twelve Steps and Twelve Traditions*, New York, Alcoholics Anonymous, 1953. See also Robert Thomsen, *Bill W.*, New York, Harper & Row, 1975; H. M. Trice and W. J. Staudenmeier, 'A sociocultural history of Alcoholics Anonymous', *Recent Developments in Alcoholism*, 1989, 7: 11–35.

36 Norman, Dain, *Clifford W. Beers: Advocate for the Insane*, Pittsburgh, PA, University of Pittsburg Press, 1980.

37 E. W. Jorgensen and H. I. Jorgensen, *Eric Berne, Master Gamesman: a Transactional Biography*, New York, Grove Press, 1984.

38 See R. D. Rosen, *Psychobabble: Fast Talk and Quick Cure in the Era of Feeling*, New York, Atheneum, 1979.

39 Juliet Mitchell, *Psychoanalysis and Feminism*, New York, Pantheon Books, 1974. See also Hannah Lerman and Natalie Porter (eds), *Feminist Ethics in Psycho-*

therapy, New York, Springer, 1990; Toni Ann Laidlaw, Cheryl Malmo and associates, *Healing Voices: Feminist Approaches to Therapy with Women*, San Francisco, Jossey-Bass, 1990.

40 Elaine Marks and Isabelle de Courtivron (eds), *New French Feminisms: an Anthology*, New York, Schocken Books, 1981; Edith Hoshino Altbach *et al.*, (eds), *German Feminism: Readings in Politics and Literature*, Albany, NY, SUNY Press, 1984.

41 Hans J. Eysenck, 'The effects of psychotherapy: an evaluation', *Journal of Consulting Psychology*, 1952, 16: 319–24.

42 Ogden R. Lindsley 'Operant conditioning applied to research in chronic schizophrenia', *Psychiatric Research Reports*, 1956, 5: 118–39.

43 Yehuda Fried and Joseph Agassi, *Psychiatry as Medicine: Contemporary Psychotherapies*, The Hague and Boston, MA, Nijhoff, 1983.

FURTHER READING

Chessick, Richard D., *Great Ideas in Psychotherapy*, New York, Jason Aronson, 1977.

Ehrenwald, Jan (ed.), *The History of Psychotherapy: from Healing Magic to Encounter*, New York, Jason Aronson, 1976.

Ellenberger, Henri F., *The Discovery of the Unconscious: the History and Evolution of Dynamic Psychiatry*, New York, Basic Books, 1970.

Fine, Reuben, *A History of Psychoanalysis*, New York, Columbia University Press, 1979.

Gilman, Sander L. (ed.), *Introducing Psychoanalytic Theory*, New York, Brunner/Mazel, 1982.

Harper, Robert A., *Psychoanalysis and Psychotherapy: 36 Systems*, New York, Jason Aronson, 1974.

Healy, David, *The Suspended Revolution: Psychiatry and Psychotherapy Re-examined*, London, Faber & Faber, 1990.

Hilgard, Ernest R., *Psychology in America: a Historical Survey*, San Diego, CA, Harcourt Brace Jovanovich, 1987.

Hothersall, David, *History of Psychology*, Philadelphia, PA, Temple University Press, 1984.

Jones, Wilfrid Llewelyn, *Ministering to Minds Diseased: a History of Psychiatric Treatment*, London, William Heinemann, 1983.

Kazdin, Alan E., *History of Behavior Modification: Experimental Foundations of Contemporary Research*, Baltimore, MD, University Park Press, 1978.

Kurzweil, Edith, *The Freudians: a Comparative Perspective*, New Haven, CT, Yale University Press, 1990.

Malan, D. H., *A Study of Brief Psychotherapy*, New York, Plenum, 1963.

Sahakian, William S., *History and Systems of Psychology*, New York, John Wiley, 1975.

44

CHILDBIRTH

Irvine S. L. Loudon

Today, when childbirth in Western countries has become almost wholly a surgical speciality conducted in hospitals, it is easy to forget how recently this has occurred. In England and Wales only fifty years ago, less than half of all deliveries took place in hospital, and a hundred years ago only about 3.5 per cent. Indeed, in historical times, obstetrics is a very recent addition to medical practice. It is the purpose of this essay to outline some of the ways in which childbirth, and its management, has changed over the last 250 years.

Until the early years of the eighteenth century in Britain and the late seventeenth century on the European continent, childbirth was a social rather than a medical event. It was confined exclusively to women, and men were rigorously excluded. Expectant mothers invited a carefully chosen group of friends, the 'gossips', to keep them company in labour and lying-in. Midwives, whose role was part-servant or employee and part-expert, delivered the babies.

Midwives did not offend female modesty or disturb the all-female milieu of childbirth, and some of them developed considerable skills in dealing with complications. (➤ Ch. 38 Women and medicine) But if major complications arose and all else failed, a surgeon was called in. Knowing little, if anything, about normal labour and certainly less than a midwife, he was necessarily unskilled. Armed only with the crudest of destructive instruments, his job was usually confined to dealing with obstructed labours in mothers already close to death. Calling a surgeon was very much a last resort, largely because 'the fear of being indecent, the fear of being seen in the throes of suffering – these great ageless concerns were at the core of the debate over the indecency of having men deliver women'.[1] (➤ Ch. 34 History of the doctor–patient relationship)

MATERNAL CARE IN THE EIGHTEENTH CENTURY

All this changed during the eighteenth century, which is where we begin. I should make two things clear. Throughout this essay I shall be talking about England and Wales unless other countries are specified; and I shall use the terms 'midwifery' and 'obstetrics' interchangeably, as they were always so used in the past, and not to indicate deliveries by midwives and doctors, respectively. Why the regular employment of medical practitioners as the attendants, not only at abnormal labours but also at normal ones, was rare in 1700 but common in 1750 is hard to explain. The canard that it was a forcible takeover by forceps-wielding doctors, greedy for money and power over women, is nonsense. The notion that the introduction of forceps delivery was the bait that tempted women away from midwives is certainly false; and the idea that medical men founded lying-in hospitals and received so much publicity by so doing that women flocked to them as the new experts in childbirth has nothing to commend it. Lying-in hospitals were small institutions of minor importance strictly for the poor; in any case, the large-scale employment of men-midwives took place in areas where lying-in hospitals were unknown.

It was the public, the women themselves, who in substantial numbers deliberately chose to engage a medical practitioner when there were plenty of skilled and capable midwives of high reputation to choose from. Their choice must have had something to do with the rise in the status of the medical practitioner. In an age which, according to some historians, saw the birth of the consumer society, orthodox medical care was seen as something worth buying, and medical practitioners thrived as a consequence. (➤ Ch. 4 Medical care) At all events, the employment of medical men for normal childbirth occurred quite suddenly. Numerous reports confirm the story of the very capable and experienced midwife, Sarah Stone: following in the footsteps of her mother, she practised in Bridgewater and Taunton in the early eighteenth century. When she began her career, men-midwives were unknown. When she moved to Bristol in 1730, however, she found that 'every young MAN who hath served his apprenticeship to a Barber-Surgeon, immediately sets up for a man-midwife, although as ignorant, or indeed much ignoranter than the meanest woman of the Profession'.[2] What Sarah Stone reported was occurring, then or soon after, all over the country.

What is so remarkable about the eighteenth century is not just the birth of man-midwifery but the speed with which midwifery advanced, and since there are feminist historians who deplore the intervention of medical men in childbirth, I must emphasize that I mean advances in knowledge, not necessarily in the effectiveness or satisfactoriness of maternal care. By the end of the century, the anatomy of the gravid uterus, the physiological mechanism of normal labour and the nature and management of the major complications had all been described. So had the three stages of labour. The correct management of the dangerous third stage of labour, which depended on understanding the normal process of placental separation, was accurately described, and *accouchement forcée* (forcible dilatation of the cervix in order to speed up labour) rightly condemned. Almost none of this was known in 1700. The forceps were introduced around 1730 (having remained a secret of the Chamberlen family for more than a hundred years) and, most important, the indications for their use had been refined until, by the end of the century, obstetric practice had become judicious, conservative, and non-interventionist. By mid-century, the centre for the publication of treatises on midwifery had moved from Paris to London. The works of men such as William Smellie (1697–1763), William Hunter (1718–83), John Leake (1729–92), William Osborne (1736–1808), Alexander Gordon (1752–99) of Aberdeen, and especially Thomas Denman (1733–1815), excite our admiration today. For originality and clarity they were seldom equalled by anything published on obstetrics in England during the nineteenth century.

Medical men in the eighteenth century regarded obstetrics as a new and important addition to the field of orthodox medical practice, undertaken with the expressed aim of saving as many mothers and babies as possible from death due to complications. By the end of the century, most surgeon-apothecaries, as well as some physicians and surgeons, were regularly delivering babies and finding there was no surer way of building a practice and establishing a reputation. Of course, the penalty if a mother or a succession of mothers died, was severe. Whether it was bad management or sheer bad luck, mothers who distrusted 'unlucky' practitioners promptly went elsewhere.

Apart from their role in home deliveries, doctors joined with philanthropically minded lay people in the eighteenth century to establish lying-in hospitals and out-patient lying-in charities, almost all in London. These provided care for women too poor to pay a practitioner, as well as serving as teaching centres for young medical practitioners and midwives. (➤ Ch. 62 Charity before *c*.1850)

The involvement of medical men in childbirth was bitterly opposed by some midwives. A few practitioners, joined by some lay people, took their side, asserting that men-midwives undertook midwifery solely for perverse erotic satisfaction. They formed a sort of anti-man-midwife brigade whose importance has often been exaggerated. Since the brigade poked fun at the sexually ambivalent term 'man-midwife', many physicians and surgeons adopted the fancy French name of 'accoucheurs' and justified the addition of midwifery to medical practice on the grounds of their knowledge of anatomy and the mechanisms of normal and abnormal labour. It would be wrong, however, to suppose that these accoucheurs were intent on abolishing the midwife. They knew midwives would continue to contribute to maternal care and meet the needs of women too poor to pay a doctor, and they sought to improve midwives by instructing them in the principles of midwifery. To take just one example, when Alexander Gordon arrived back in Aberdeen in 1785, as almost the only practitioner with any obstetric training, he saw it as one of his first duties to institute courses of instruction for the midwives of the town.

MATERNAL CARE IN THE NINETEENTH CENTURY

The man-midwife, accoucheur, or obstetrician, call him what you will, was firmly established by the end of the eighteenth century. From the viewpoint of 1800, there seemed every reason to believe obstetrics would forge ahead, building on the strengths of eighteenth-century knowledge. Instead, it entered a phase of stagnation, at least until the 1880s. The prime reason was the rejection of obstetrics by the medical establishment. The first half of the nineteenth century, the period of medical reform, was characterized by the growth of medical education, registration, and the hardening of divisions between practitioners. All this was accompanied by intra-professional strife in which the Royal Colleges of Physicians and Surgeons sought to affirm their supremacy. The College of Physicians considered delivering babies an ungentlemanly occupation. The College of Surgeons, intent on creating an élite who devoted their lives to 'pure' surgery, refused to have anything to do with childbirth. The Society of Apothecaries was primarily concerned with pharmacy, although after the Apothecaries Act of 1815, they were required to examine candidates in the practice of physic, but not midwifery. These three institutions called the tune as far as medical education was concerned. Obstetrics was pushed to one side to such an extent that an accoucheur protested:

> Here in a department of the medical profession, the practice of which involves at the same time the existence of two individuals, that practice is left without any control whatsoever and there are no means of ascertaining the qualifications of the persons who take it in charge.[3]

Even when the Medical Act of 1858 was introduced, medical students could qualify as doctors in total ignorance of midwifery. This was remedied only by the introduction of the Medical Act Amendment Act of 1886; but even then, training in midwifery was often derisory. (➤ Ch. 47 History of the medical profession)

Rejected by all but a minority of physicians and surgeons, obstetrics throughout the nineteenth century was much more a branch of general practice than a specialty. In the first half of the century, so few were the medical men who resembled consultants in anything like the modern sense and so concentrated were they in the metropolis, that if you took away London, you would be hard put to it to find twenty elsewhere. Take away Edinburgh, Glasgow, Dublin, and two or three other cities, and there would be scarcely enough to count on the fingers of one hand. In 1850 (and quite possibly in 1900), you could have travelled west from London through Reading, Oxford, Gloucester, Bath, Bristol, and Exeter to Plymouth without finding a single physician- or surgeon-accoucheur of the standing of such London practitioners as Francis Ramsbotham (1801–68), Sam Merriman (1771–1852), John Lever (1811–58), and Robert Lee (1793–1877). You would, however, have met hundreds of general practitioners all busily engaged in the practice of midwifery.

To the general practitioners, midwifery was essential to build and keep a practice, but it had grave disadvantages. It was time-consuming, badly paid, hard, tiring, and worrying work. As one general practitioner put it:

> I have no hestiation in saying, after more than thirty years' experience as student and practitioner that midwifery is the most anxious and trying of all medical work, and to be successfully practised calls for more skill, care, and presence of mind on the part of the medical man than any other branch of medicine.[4]

But deliveries by doctors were only half the picture. What about the midwives? We know a good deal about the number and distribution of nineteenth-century medical practitioners, but very little about the midwives who, with rare exceptions, were untrained in the formal sense and unregistered. The census returns are unreliable. In 1841, just over 700 women put their occupation as midwives; in 1851, 2,204. This apparent increase was certainly spurious. Confusion arose because many women practised occasionally, attending only one or two cases a year, while others made a regular living by it. For some, delivering babies was a sideline to other occupations, such as nursing or field-labour. Even those who were a cut above manual labour were usually known by their neighbours not as 'the midwife', but as 'the woman who goes about nursing'. Such would have been more likely to have put down 'nurse' or some other occupation than 'midwife' as their occupation. The 1871 census showed 3,349 midwives and 31,180 nurses; there is a strong likelihood that many of the latter acted as midwives. (➤ Ch. 54 A general history of nursing 1800–1900)

An investigation in the 1860s revealed that deliveries by midwife were very common in villages. In small non-manufacturing towns with a population of between 6,000 and 10,000, midwife deliveries formed a much smaller proportion. In large manufacturing towns such as Birmingham, Leeds, or Shef-field, the majority (often the large majority) of deliveries were by midwives. In Coventry, they amounted to 90 per cent. In Wakefield (population 23,000), midwife delivery was the rule amongst the Irish, but the English were almost all attended by medical men. London showed a clear division between the East End where 30–50 per cent of the deliveries were attended by midwives, and the West End and suburbs where midwife deliveries seldom exceeded 5 per cent.

That there was a division between doctor deliveries and midwife deliveries in terms of social class seems certain. We tend to assume that the landed gentry and the rich employed obstetricians; the middle classes, general prac-titioners; and the working classes, midwives. The first two of these assump-tions may largely be true; but the third is a pitfall of potential errors. It is now recognized that the 'working classes' were an intensely diverse group, going far beyond such simple divisions as skilled and unskilled labourers.

Within this diversity, was the choice of birth-attendant influenced by the hierarchies between and within occupational groups? Among railway workers, for instance, did the wives of the 'carriage finishers and upholsterers . . . a class in themselves' and the wives of the footplatemen and signalmen, the 'aristocrats' of railway workers, choose a doctor to deliver them, while the wives of the 'porters, shunters, cleaners, loaders, carters and the like who were unskilled' chose a midwife?[5] Did printers, piano-makers, engine-fitters and lathe-operators routinely employ doctors while the wives of the multitude of pick-wielders, barrow-pushers and sweeper-uppers employed midwives? It would not be surprising if they did, for it is certain that general practitioners delivered large numbers of working-class women, and the choice of doctor or midwife must have been determined by some internal logic, however complex. What evidence we have suggests that the choice of birth-attendant was often determined by geographical location; sometimes by occupational status; sometimes by ethnic origin, like the Irish women in Wakefield; often, probably, by the local reputations of midwives and doctors; sometimes by membership of sick clubs and friendly societies, and very often by available income. There must have been a complex interaction of all these factors in different regions. This, however, is only guesswork. The truth is we know very little, although these are among the most interesting of the many questions concerning childbirth in the nineteenth century.

What of hospital deliveries? In general, they were a disaster throughout the Western world. In lying-in hospitals in London, Edinburgh, Paris, Vienna, Copenhagen, Boston, New York, and Sydney, there were dreadful recurrent epidemics of puerperal fever in which the risk of the mothers dying in hospital was five or even ten times higher than it was for the poorest women delivered in hovels or slum tenements by untrained midwives. The voluntary

Table 1 Average annual deliveries of women in England and Wales in the 1880s for the different places and types of delivery

Place/type of delivery	Average annual deliveries	
Deliveries in institutions	67,700	(7.5%)
In-patient deliveries	31,700	(3.5%)
Voluntary hospitals	2,700	(0.3%)
Workhouse infirmaries	29,000	(3.2%)
Out-patient deliveries	36,000	(4.0%)
Home deliveries	822,300	(92.5%)
Midwife deliveries (rough estimate)		(50.0%)
Doctor deliveries (rough estimate)		(42.5%)
Average annual number of live births	890,000	(100.0%)

Source: Report of the Select Committee on Midwives Registration, PP 1892 *XIV*, text and appendices.

hospitals were dangerous places to have a baby. In contrast, the records of out-patient lying-in charities were almost uniformly excellent. Institutional deliveries, however, formed only a very small proportion of the total, as Table 1 shows. (➤ Ch. 49 The hospital)

What was the situation in the nineteenth century in other countries? In the USA, midwifery was practised by a wide range of medical practitioners; full-time obstetricians were rare, as in England, and lying-in hospitals were broadly similar. Midwives were very diverse indeed, especially with European immigration at the end of the century, and there were far more neighbour deliveries in remote rural areas. By the end of the century, it was accepted policy in Britain that the midwife should be retained, but she must be trained and registered. In the USA, the medical profession was intent on abolishing the midwife and pursued this objective with almost total success into the twentieth century.

In most European countries, there were two major differences. First, obstetrics was not despised to the same extent as in England. It was an accepted and respected part of the medical curriculum in the early nineteenth century, if not in the eighteenth. Second, midwife training and state registration were introduced in the nineteenth century so that the standard and status of the midwife was much higher. Indeed, in France there were two classes of midwife, the first class independent and powerful (they ran the lying-in hospitals and taught students) and able to command high fees; the second class, closely supervised and controlled, were typical of rural areas. In Europe, and especially in Sweden, Denmark, and the Netherlands, a high proportion of home deliveries were conducted by midwives of much higher standards than those found in England; it was a feature that stood those countries in good stead in the early twentieth century.

Before moving into the twentieth century, however, it is worth considering the way the quality or effectiveness of maternal care in the past can be assessed.

EFFECTIVENESS OF CARE AND MATERNAL MORTALITY

If we need to compare the outcome of childbirth in different periods or countries or regions, or assess the effectiveness of various types of birth-attendants or obstetric institutions, we must have a recognized standard of comparison. Until very recently, that standard was the rate of maternal mortality, defined as the number of maternal deaths (deaths, that is, during pregnancy, labour, or the lying-in period) per 1,000, 10,000 or 100,000 births. The choice of the denominator is arbitrary, and I shall use 10,000. Although deaths related to childbirth were not the most common cause of death in women of childbearing age – that place was held by tuberculosis – they were, and always have been, a tragedy unlike other deaths, partly because of the devastating effect on the family, and partly because of the deeply held feeling that mothers should not die in the course of the normal process of reproduction. Recognizing the particular tragedy of a death following safe delivery (and the large majority of maternal deaths occurred after, not during, labour), an American obstetrician said in the 1850s, 'It is a sort of desecration for an *accouchée* to die'. From the practical point of view, the statistics of maternal mortality provided the means by which policies were determined and judged.

Maternal mortality therefore occupies a central position in the history of childbirth. Some historians, however, have looked at the statistics, judged them unreliable, and thrown them out of the window. This is absurd. No mortality statistics are wholly reliable, not even today. It is true that for various reasons the interpretation of maternal mortality rates presents special problems; however, it is the job of the historian not to reject statistical evidence, but to assess its worth and estimate the limits of accuracy. In practice, differences in maternal mortality were often so wide that they remain significant in spite of confounding factors. (➤ Ch. 71 Demography and medicine; Ch. 72 Medicine, mortality, and morbidity)

By the final years of the nineteenth century, maternal mortality began to become a matter of public concern, largely through the persistence of William Farr (1807–83), the Compiler of Abstracts at the General Register Office who, in the 1870s, returned time and again to the scandal of preventable deaths and the failure to reduce maternal mortality. The first major breakthrough came with the introduction of antisepsis and asepsis in the 1880s and the effect of these on the lying-in hospitals.

Before the 1880s, hospital mortality often reached quite unacceptable levels

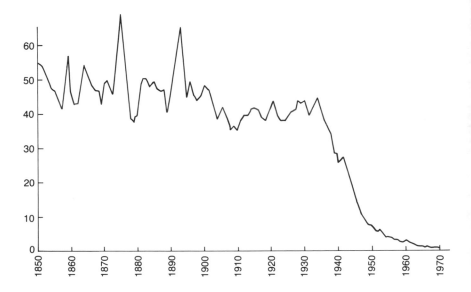

Figure 1   The trend in maternal mortality in England and Wales from 1850 to 1970. Maternal deaths per 10,000 births. Annual rates.

of 200 or more deaths per 10,000 births, while the level in England and Wales as a whole remained steady at around 40–50 per 10,000. The fall in maternal mortality in lying-in hospitals after the 1880s was dramatic, reaching levels of 20 or less by the end of the century. There seemed no reason why such levels should not be obtained in home deliveries. Antisepsis and asepsis were neither complex nor difficult to put into practice. As Figure 1 shows, however, no such fall occurred in England and Wales, where maternal mortality remained on a high plateau from the time vital registration began until 1934. Infant mortality, on the other hand, and a wide range of death rates from common infective diseases such as scarlet fever and tuberculosis, declined steadily from the beginning of this century. (➤ Ch. 45 Childhood) Thus maternal mortality was an anomaly, not only in its failure to decline, but also in its surprising relation to social-class. Whereas most death rates, such as infant mortality, showed a strong social class gradient, being highest in the labouring classes and substantially lower in the middle and upper classes, maternal mortality was the reverse. Was the trend in maternal mortality similar to or quite different from that seen in other countries? Figure 2 shows in diagrammatic form the broad trends in maternal mortality in various countries from the late nineteenth century to 1960.

In Scandinavia and the Netherlands, deaths from puerperal sepsis (see

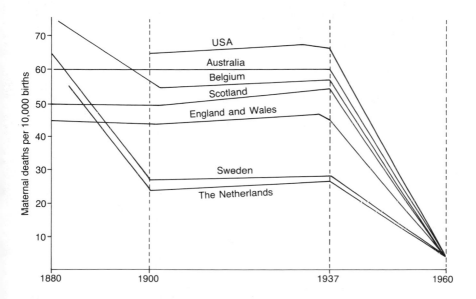

Figure 2 A schematic representation of the broad features of the trends in maternal mortality in certain countries between 1880 and 1960.

p. 1066) fell significantly after the introduction of antisepsis: in England, Wales, and Scotland, no such fall occurred (see Table 2). By 1910, however, in every Western country maternal mortality either remained on a level plateau or, more often, actually rose until the mid-1930s. Some authorities asserted that the plateau was an artefact; that an underlying fall in mortality was masked by an improvement in the accuracy of death registration, especially in the USA where the gradual expansion of the 'death registration area' – the group of states selected for the collection of national statistics – makes interpretation immensely difficult. But this was only true to a small extent, if at all. Another feature, the increase in deaths from septic abortion after the end of the war, contributed to rising maternal mortality; but even when this is allowed for, the underlying trend was still level rather than downwards throughout the civilized world. By the yardstick of maternal mortality, there was no improvement in the effectiveness of obstetric care between 1910 and the mid-1930s, and we come in due course to what happened after that.

The causes of maternal mortality appear to have been remarkably constant everywhere. Before the mid-1930s, puerperal fever (also known as 'childbed fever', 'metria', 'puerperal sepsis/septicaemia') was by far the most common cause. It is popularly associated with the name of I. P. Semmelweis (1818–65).

Table 2 Mortality due to puerperal sepsis before and after the introduction of antisepsis in the 1880s. The upper line for each country gives the maternal mortality rate due to puerperal sepsis (expressed as deaths per 10,000 births) and the lower line shows those values indexed to the first year for which values could be obtained, the first value being expressed as 100 to facilitate comparison.

Maternal mortality rate	1870	1875	1880	1885	1890	1895	1900	1905
England and Wales	18	28	18	26	22	20	21	18
1870=100	100	155	100	144	122	111	116	100
Scotland	17	30	14	29	26	19	17	18
1870=100	100	176	82	170	160	112	100	106
Ireland	23	31	26	31	23	29	22	18
1870=100	100	134	113	135	100	126	96	78
Norway	28	31	24	26	25	14	16	9
1870=100	100	111	104	93	89	50	57	32
Sweden	31	32	24	22	12	13	8	12
1870=100	100	103	77	71	39	42	26	39
The Netherlands	13	16	11	14	12	9	9	7
1870=100	100	123	85	107	92	69	69	54
Amsterdam	–	36	26	28	12	8	4	2
1875=100	–	100	72	77	33	22	11	5
Switzerland	–	–	41	52	31	25	20	26
1880=100	–	–	100	127	76	61	49	63

Sources: F. W. N. Haultain, 'A retrospect and comparison of the progress of midwifery and gynaecology', *Edinburgh Medical Journal* (NS), 1911, 6 (1): 17–37. *Amsterdam Statistical Bulletins.*

In fact, there were three major contributions to the understanding of puerperal fever before the advent of bacteriology. During an outbreak of puerperal fever in Aberdeen in 1789–92, Alexander Gordon provided proof for the first time that it was a contagious disorder spread by the birth-attendant from case to case, and also that it was closely associated with erysipelas. In 1843, Oliver Wendell Holmes (1809–94) published a famous paper based on a review of published reports of the disorder which confirmed Gordon's work. In 1847, Semmelweis, a Hungarian obstetrician in the Vienna maternity hospital who was not influenced by the work of Gordon or Holmes, demonstrated that doctors and students going straight from post-mortem examinations to the maternity wards were directly responsible for infecting women in labour with 'morbid matter', which he believed was the cause of puerperal fever. This explained why the mortality was very much higher on the wards attended by doctors than those attended by midwives. Further, he showed that washing hands in disinfectant could prevent the spread of puerperal fever in hospitals. (➤ Ch. 19 Fevers; Ch. 16 Contagion/germ theory/specificity)

The work of all three was unpopular because it indicted medical practitioners as the transmitters of this much-dreaded disease. It was therefore denied or ignored or forgotten, until a group of bacteriologists at the end of the nineteenth century (including Louis Pasteur (1822–95)) showed that a large majority of deaths from puerperal fever were due to one organism, *Streptococcus pyogenes* (later known as the ß-haemolytic streptococcus, Lancefield group A) which was also the cause of erysipelas and scarlet fever. Only in the 1930s was the last vital piece of information added, when it was recognized that this organism was a common inhabitant of the noses and throats of healthy people, including doctors and midwives: the 'asymptomatic carriers'. Many previously puzzling features of puerperal fever then became clear, and the importance of strict asepsis and the wearing of masks by birth-attendants was obvious.

The other common causes of maternal mortality were puerperal haemorrhage and toxaemia of pregnancy, now known as hypertensive disease in pregnancy. Each contributed about 15 per cent to total maternal mortality, while puerperal fever contributed 40–50 per cent, and septic abortion became an increasing problem in the inter-war period.

CHILDBIRTH IN THE TWENTIETH CENTURY: 1900–35

To understand the anxieties of this period, we must remember the sudden success of antisepsis in the lying-in hospitals. Here at last, it seemed, was the answer to maternal mortality, which, like so many medical advances, started in the hospitals and spread to general practice. The surge of optimism that this generated was dashed when maternal mortality in general, and deaths due to puerperal sepsis in particular, failed to decline. In a period that prided itself on scientific advance, the statistics of maternal mortality were a bitter reproach to all concerned with childbirth.

Whereas childbirth in the nineteenth century was a private domestic affair between mothers and those they chose to deliver them, apart from the smattering of charitable provision for the poor, the characteristic feature of the twentieth century was the increasing involvement of authorities, medical and lay, charitable and governmental, in the care of mothers and children. The politics of maternal care was indicated by such terms as 'maternal welfare' and 'maternal and child health'. High maternal and infant mortality were the spur to involvement at local and national levels. Internationally, the extent of government involvement varied widely, being, on the whole, most conspicuous (and oldest) on the European continent, least so in the USA, and in-between in Britain.

When the Ministry of Health was established in England and Wales in 1919, maternal and child health was one of its major concerns, not least because the recent slaughter in the trenches added to the anxieties of the declining birth rate and fears of depopulation. A team led by Dr Janet Campbell (1877–1954) produced a series of reports on maternal care and mortality in various areas. The Ministry also produced a report on maternal mortality and morbidity in 1932, and another and much better one in 1937, which was followed by similar reports on Wales (1937), Scotland (1942), and Northern Ireland (1943).

In the USA, an even larger series of reports on maternal and child health was published, reflecting national discomfort at the revelation that it had the highest recorded level of maternal mortality of any country in the civilized world. Some of the reports from the Children's Bureau of the Department of Labor in Washington were the most impressive ever published anywhere; and they were accompanied by many others from state departments, medical institutions, and other bodies concerned with maternal welfare.

Thus there was no shortage of detailed statistical analysis or policies. One of the recurrent themes, which preoccupies historians today as it concerned health authorities in the inter-war period, was the question of the relative importance of social and economic factors, on the one hand, and clinical factors on the other, as the major determinants of maternal and infant mortality. The practical importance of finding the answer was obvious. Where the health of mothers and infants was found wanting, how could it be improved? By better medical care or better living conditions? Better obstetrics or better housing? More medicines or more food?

The answers for maternal care and for child care were quite different, although, in general, it was believed that both factors (or rather, sets of factors) played a part. As far as maternal mortality was concerned, that a woman was more likely to die in childbirth if she was poor, undernourished, and worn-out seemed to be common sense; that she was also likely to die if her labour was grossly mishandled by an incompetent doctor or midwife was just as obvious; that the two were not mutually exclusive – that a woman may die because of poor clinical care combined with her chronic ill health – was also self-evident. It was therefore a question of the relative importance of the two distinct groups of determinants – poverty and malnutrition on the one hand, poor clinical care on the other. Elsewhere, I have presented evidence that has led me to the conclusion that when malnutrition is extreme and approaches, or reaches, levels of famine, there is little doubt it is the factor of overriding importance, but only then. Otherwise, the standard of clinical care was always the dominant factor, even in conditions of poverty such as those in the industrial slums of the nineteenth century and the depression of the late 1920s and early 1930s. (➤ Ch. 52 Public Health) This was shown by the low maternal mortality of mothers in the poorest areas of nineteenth-century London attended by the well-trained midwives of out-patient charities; the high mortality of the middle classes attended by incompetent doctors; and the ability of certain individuals to reduce very greatly the mortality of childbirth in poverty-stricken areas such as the mountains of Kentucky or the streets of Rochdale by the provision of a high standard of maternal care while the social and economic circumstances of the population remained unaltered.[6] In other words, maternal mortality seems to have been very sensitive to standards of care and surprisingly insensitive to the ill-effects of quite severe degrees of deprivation.

For the reduction of maternal mortality, prevention became the byword; prevention through antenatal care, better hospital provision, more clinics, better training of midwives and doctors, better provision of services, better publicity directed towards mothers. It became fashionable to say that obstetrics was, above all, a branch of preventive medicine. To formulate policies, however, is one thing; to put them into practice, quite another.

In retrospect, what was lacking was imaginative leadership from respected institutions. Some shining exceptions apart, men and women of the necessary energy and persuasiveness were rarely found in public-health departments or the corridors of the Ministry of Health, neither of which were highly regarded by the medical profession, least of all by general practitioners. In any case, the power of such authorities was limited. After the Midwives Act of 1902, probably the single most important reform in maternal care this century, midwives could be monitored, but doctors could not; nor could mothers. The authorities could only exhort and persuade. So, when maternal mortality failed to decline, the fault was laid at the door of careless general practitioners, foolish uncaring mothers, and the 'handywomen' who were still delivering some babies in deprived areas. (➤ Ch. 50 Medical institutions and the state)

Taking maternal care as a whole, leadership was not the forte of the Royal College of Obstetricians and Gynaecologists when it was established in 1929, this late date providing a telling contrast with the Royal College of Physicians (established in 1518) and the Company of Surgeons (1745), which became the Royal College of Surgeons in 1800. The College of Obstetricians endorsed the midwife and the general practitioner as the 'backbone' of British obstetrics and introduced a diploma in obstetrics for the latter. The energies of the College, however, were consumed by the need to create a cadre of high-quality consultants in hospitals, by which the College would claim a position alongside its sister-institutions, and the battle with the College of Surgeons, whose obstructive attitudes echoed the early nineteenth century. Maternal care in general, and the practice of general practitioners and midwives, was not their territory.

What, then, were the changes in maternal care compared with the nineteenth century? The obstetrician Victor Bonney (1872–1953) observed in 1919: 'Taking the conduct of labour in general not much more than a bowl of antiseptic stands between the practice of today and the practice of the [eighteen] sixties.'[7] He was right, at least in a limited sense. Most women were still delivered at home, institutional deliveries increasing slowly compared with the USA, Sweden, and New Zealand. The middle classes were generally delivered by general practitioners, at home or in nursing-homes of sometimes dubious quality. Midwives formed the backbone of hospital care, and care in the community. Since the 1890s, Caesarean section had become increasingly safe. Certain conditions such as placenta praevia were managed much better than they had been in the nineteenth century. Twilight sleep, invented in Germany in 1902, was a technique designed to avoid the risks of total anaesthesia. The idea was not to abolish pain, but the memory of pain, by administering injections of scopolamine and morphine in doses calculated to render the patient amnesic while retaining consciousness. (➤ Ch. 67 Pain and Suffering) When it worked, the mother, though conscious throughout, could remember nothing of her labour. In practice, however, it often produced a disorientated and restless mother, unable to co-operate and extremely difficult to manage, who needed constant attention throughout labour. This, and the unpredictable response of individuals to the drugs, made childbirth under twilight sleep so difficult that it was virtually abandoned soon after the end of the First World War and was referred to as the 'twilight sleep fiasco'. It was replaced by an increasing use of drugs to produce analgesia, if not total anaesthesia, increasing the need for instrumental delivery or Caesarean section. (➤ Ch. 42 Surgery (modern))

In the first two-thirds of the nineteenth century, inactivity and patience were seen as the greatest virtues in the management of all but a small minority of seriously complicated labours. Students were constantly urged to trust to 'nature' and avoid interference, whenever possible. Some obstetricians turned against instrumental delivery to such an extent that they boasted their forceps had become rusty from disuse. There is little doubt they erred on the side of excessive caution, and it was perhaps inevitable that there would be a swing to a greater degree of intervention. By the 1870s, obstetricians were beginning to say they had been too conservative in the past when they had powerful instruments that could ease the sufferings of parturient women.

The argument put forward to justify the change in the management of labour was a theory, not new, but rediscovered and widely proclaimed in the late nineteenth and early twentieth centuries. It was held that women had become so weakened by the vitiating effects of modern civilization that they could not withstand the pain of normal labour or be expected to deliver themselves without assistance. For evidence, anthropologists and doctors contrasted the slow, painful, and complicated labours of modern civilized women with the supposedly quick, easy, painless, and uncomplicated labours of 'savage, uncivilized' peoples such as the Eskimo, the Hottentot, and those North American Indians still unspoilt by contact with white people. How much they really knew about the deliveries of these peoples was never revealed, but the story of their easy labours was soon accepted as common knowledge. (➤ Ch. 60 Medicine and anthropology)

As a result, in Britain and even more in the USA, the application of forceps and the extensive use of anaesthesia in normal deliveries increased steadily from the 1870s to the 1920s. One of the most influential obstetricians in the USA, Joseph Bolivar DeLee (1869–1942) of Chicago, described his 'prophylactic forceps operation' in 1920. He believed that, ideally, every woman in labour should be fully anaesthetized at the end of the first stage and delivered by forceps, followed by a manual removal of the placenta.[8]

By this time, most obstetricians (partly through the influence of gynaecology) had become more surgically minded. 'Midwifery', said Bonney in 1919, 'is a purely surgical art.' The baby was a 'neoplasm'; labour, a process accompanied by self-inflicted wounds; the puerperium, a period of surgical healing. Ideally, he said, patients should never be delivered at home. 'There should be large lying-in hospitals all over the country.'[9] In the USA, unnecessary interference in labour ran riot during the inter-war period. It did so in Britain to a lesser extent, but such excesses were unknown in the Netherlands and Scandinavia.

The excessively surgical approach was by no means unopposed. In the USA, J. Whitridge Williams (1866–1931) of Philadelphia bitterly opposed DeLee's philosophy (the two were described as the 'giants' of obstetrics in their day) and consistently preached the need for a quiet, patient, conservative approach to normal labours. The work of Grantley Dick Read (1890–1959), the advocate of natural childbirth, was a more extreme but still direct reaction against the surgical approach to labour. His book *Natural Childbirth* was published in 1933, followed by *Childbirth without Fear*. He stressed the 'psychosomatic' as opposed to the 'mechanistic' approach, believing that too little attention had been paid to the psychology of childbirth and that careful psychological preparation and relaxation could abolish the pain of normal childbirth without recourse to drugs. He had many ardent followers on both sides of the Atlantic.

A high rate of surgical intervention was only one of a series of factors that sustained the high level of maternal mortality. In England and Wales, the desultory nature of maternal care was revealed by surveys carried out by the Ministry of Health in the late 1920s and early 1930s. They found that some counties (for instance, Gloucestershire in 1932) had no consultant obstetricians at all, and maternity beds were scattered haphazardly through various general and cottage hospitals. Other counties, Lancashire for example, had ample maternity departments and many consultants. In some counties, there were too few midwives; in others, too many. Some areas relied on midwives working for voluntary organizations; others used midwives employed by county councils; and in others again, most midwives were independent. Local administration of maternity services was often defective (but again, very patchy and sometimes excellent), and the degree of co-operation between midwives and general practitioners ranged from close and friendly to open warfare. Indeed, the provision of maternal care was so variable that generalizations about the country as a whole are very difficult. Part of the problem was that much of the relevant legislation was permissive; the amount of money and energy devoted to maternal care was often dependent on the political persuasions and priorities of local councils. In the provision of maternal care between 1900 and 1935, Britain was certainly not a shining example to other countries. For shining examples, one needed to look towards north-west Europe.

CHILDBIRTH IN THE TWENTIETH CENTURY: SINCE 1935

In 1935, Gerhard Domagk (1895–1964) in Germany found that if living streptococci were injected into the peritoneal cavity of mice, they all died; but if the streptococci were injured by heat or chemicals, some of the mice survived. He then tried the experiment of administering a series of chemicals to mice just after injecting them with live streptococci. In a list of chemicals selected almost at random, the only one that had any effect, and indeed led to 100 per cent recovery, was a red dye, prontosil rubrum. Prontosil was the first sulphonamide. In a little over two years, there were at least a dozen brands on the market. (➤ Ch. 39 Drug therapies)

By the end of 1935 on the European continent, and early 1936 in Britain, patients with severe puerperal fever were treated with sulphonamides. The rate of recovery was so high as to rule out chance or a decline in the virulence of the streptococcus as possible explanations. By the spring of 1937, when sulphonamides were generally available, maternal mortality began the steep fall shown in Figure 1. It had already fallen in 1935 and 1936, but no more than on many previous occasions. The fall became statistically significant for the first time in 1937.

Those who saw puerperal fever in the 1930s remember the sulphonamides as a 'miracle drug', for it must be remembered that previously none of the extremely large number of treatments for puerperal fever had been of any use whatsoever. The sulphonamides provided 'one of the rare situations which endorse the identification of an agency of major importance as contributory to a statistical trend'.[10]

Between 1937 and 1940, 80 per cent of the fall in maternal mortality consisted of a reduction in deaths due to puerperal fever. People have been puzzled, however, to note that a decline also occurred in the other non-infective categories of maternal mortality, although not so steeply as the decline in deaths due to puerperal fever. There were two reasons. First, many of the deaths before 1935 due to other causes were aggravated by puerperal sepsis. Faced with a case in which death was associated with haemorrhage and puerperal fever, many doctors would have put down haemorrhage as the primary cause of death because of the opprobrium surrounding puerperal infection; secondary causes of death do not appear in the statistics. Second, hard on the heels of the sulphonamides came a number of significant improvements in maternal care.

The Midwives Act of 1936, which made it obligatory for every county and county-borough to provide an adequate salaried domiciliary service, 'revolutionized the standard and practice of midwives'.[11] The Second World War led to an improvement in maternity services and a wider availability of consultant services. Through special rations, the war improved the diet of expectant mothers. Blood transfusion became widely available, and just at the end of the war, the introduction of penicillin into civilian practice pushed the still-useful sulphonamides backstage. Penicillin was not only highly effective in puerperal fever, but even more in septic abortion, in which the spectrum of organisms responsible for sepsis was quite different from those causing puerperal fever. From 1948, the National Health Service not only made obstetric care at all levels available to the whole of the population, but, by effectively removing the financial competitive element, it allowed for a greater degree of co-operation than ever before between midwives and general practitioners and hospital obstetricians. It also led to an increased provision of maternity beds and consultant obstetricians, and standards of teaching improved.

Thus no single cause, but a whole series of events, ensured that the fall in maternal mortality initiated by the sulphonamides continued at the same rate. In the mid-1940s, doctors and midwives who had been students in the 1920s and had witnessed the rise in maternal mortality to the peak of 1934 could hardly believe its decline would continue. Many expected it to level out at a minimum of unavoidable maternal deaths, probably in the region of 1 per 1000 births (10 per 10,000). In fact, that level was reached in the 1950s and the decline continued.

Table 3 is worth a moment's attention because it shows something quite extraordinary. Countries in which the national levels of maternal mortality

Table 3 Maternal mortality rates in the USA, England and Wales, and the Netherlands from 1920 to 1960. Rates expressed as maternal deaths per 10,000 births.

Year	USA	England and Wales	The Netherlands
1920	68.9	43.3	24.0
1930	63.6	44.0	33.3
1940	37.6	26.1	23.5
1950	8.3	8.7	10.5
1960	3.7	3.9	3.7

Source: The vital statistics of each of the three countries.

were widely different in 1920 and 1930 had converged by 1960 to almost identical levels, in spite of totally different histories. By 1960, the USA had gone down the path of private enterprise to nearly 100 per cent deliveries by specialists in hospitals. Britain, with its free National Health Service, retained the general practitioner obstetrician and the midwife, and used the hospitals for high-risk cases and an ever-increasing number of normal ones. By 1960, less than half of all deliveries took place at home, and the number was falling fast; by the 1980s, over 98 per cent of deliveries took place in hospitals. The Netherlands, where maternal care was part private, part health insurance, continued to have far more home deliveries than any other Western country. It still does. In 1960, about two-thirds of deliveries were at home, conducted largely by midwives of high status and a good deal of independence.

These international differences were not due to chance; they were due to deliberate policies based on different historical backgrounds. But each country was able to claim with equal justification that its policies were vindicated by the criterion of maternal mortality. This is a point well worth bearing in mind when faced with people intent on advocating a particular form of maternal care and decrying all others. By judicious selection, historical evidence is always available to support their cause.

It should also be remembered that systems of maternal care evolve within the historical, political, and geographical context of each country. Like trees or bushes that do well in some soils and badly in others, systems of maternal care appropriate for one country might be quite inappropriate if exported to another. In the Netherlands, the system works well because of the high tradition of midwives, and perhaps because it is a small non-industrial country with such excellent communications that everyone is within less than half-an-hour's distance from at least one of the large number of hospitals.[12] The Dutch system of maternal care might not be so successful in a country the size of the USA.

CONCLUSION

By this point in the story, somewhere around the 1960s, someone reading this short history who had never given a moment's thought to childbirth, a bachelor recluse perhaps, might conclude that dissension in obstetrics was a feature of the past. If so, he would be startled to learn that the more maternal and perinatal mortality has declined, the greater the number of lawsuits against obstetricians, and that the last few decades have seen obstetricians under constant attack for too much science, too much technology, and too little appreciation of the feelings of mothers. (➤ Ch. 69 Medicine and the law)

The expectations of women have changed. In the early years of this century, almost every mother knew of a member of her family, a friend, or a neighbour who had died in childbirth. It is only a slight exaggeration to say that in the past a successful delivery was one in which the mother survived, although one must not exaggerate the fear this may have caused, because people tend to adapt to the causes of death with which they have grown up. Today, when few of us have personal knowledge of a maternal death, most women expect not only to survive childbirth, but to do so in perfect health after a perfect and satisfying delivery of a perfect baby. The majority of obstetricians believe that if these expectations are to be satisfied for the largest possible number of women, they need to employ all the technology that has become available. In other words, they see a direct link between modern hospital delivery and low maternal and foetal mortality and morbidity. (➤ Ch. 68 Medical technologies: social contexts and consequences)

This is hotly denied by a small but vocal and mainly middle-class minority of women who question the importance of the whole apparatus of ultrasound, foetal monitoring, pH estimations, widespread induction of labour and increasing rates of Caesarean section. They believe the general standard of life and health is so much higher now than in the past that all but a few would do just as well, and would certainly achieve much greater satisfaction, by a home birth with a midwife and a supportive group of family and friends, like the mothers of the seventeenth century. Proponents of this view are vociferous, and the debate is highly emotional. So, for reasons that will appear, it is worth completing this essay with a short account of two modern North American religious groups, who live in separate communities apart from the rest of the population.

First are the Hutterites, who are healthy and prosperous farmers. They live a spartan communal life without such entertainments as radio or television. Except for business purposes, they do not mix with their non-Hutterite neighbours. They pray a lot, dress demurely, and spend little or nothing on modern comforts, although they buy the best of modern kitchen and farming equipment. Birth control is forbidden, and the fertility of the Hutterites is so high that it is used as a standard of comparison for other populations. The Hutterites do, however, believe in modern Western medicine. Previously, they were delivered by their own orthodoxly trained midwives; now they are delivered by local obstetric specialists in maternity hospitals. As one might expect, their maternal and perinatal mortality rates are the same as those in the general North American population.

The second group are the Faith Assembly in Indiana. They too are a religious group, in which prayer plays a central part in their lives. They are nearly all white, well fed and healthy. They differ from the Hutterites in two respects. They mix readily with the local community and work in a wide variety of occupations alongside the rest of the population; but they refuse all aspects of modern medical care. They employ neither doctors nor midwives in childbirth, but rely on prayer, faith, and the help of family and neighbours. They therefore provide a unique example of a healthy and prosperous late twentieth-century community that rejects every form of modern maternal care. Between 1975 and 1982, maternal mortality in this community was 87.2 per 10,000 birth compared with 0.9 in the state of Indiana as a whole, a relative risk of 92. The number of deaths was small, however, and the 95 per cent confidence limits of relative risk were 19 to 280. In short, the risk of a Faith Assembly mother dying in childbirth was at least 19 times as high as the risk for mothers statewide, and possibly as much as 280 times as high.[13] To find a national maternal mortality rate of 87.2 in England and Wales, one would have to go back to the beginning of the eighteenth century.

This is not to say that modern American-style 'high-tech' hospital childbirth is essential for all. Childbirth in the Netherlands proves otherwise. Indeed, the risks of childbirth have been transformed over the last fifty years in all Western countries. In Britain, maternal mortality today is only one-fiftieth of what it was in 1934. Without a comprehensive system of modern medical care, however, a healthy upbringing and healthy style of life – with or without prayer – is not enough to maintain, let alone improve, the present low level of maternal and perinatal mortality and morbidity.

NOTES

1 M. Laget, 'Childbirth in seventeenth- and eighteenth-century France: obstetrical practices and collective attitudes', in R. Fraser and O. Ranum, *Medicine and Society in France*, Baltimore, MD, Johns Hopkins University Press, 1980, pp. 137–76.

2 Sarah Stone, *A Complete Practice of Midwifery*, London, 1737.

3 A. B. Granville 'Political condition of midwifery in the metropolis', *Lancet*, 1830–1, 1: 301–2.

4 *Report of the Select Committee on Midwives Registration*, PP 1892 *XIV* Q. 1660. Evidence of Mr Brown MRCS LSA, general practitioner.

5 F. M. L. Thompson, *The Rise of Respectable Society. A Social History of Victorian Britain, 1830–1900*, London, Fontana, 1988, pp. 216–43.

6 Mary Breckinridge, *Wide Neighborhoods*, Lexington, University Press of Kentucky, 1981; A. Topping, 'Maternal mortality and public opinion', *Public Health*, 1936, 49: 342–9.

7 V. Bonney, 'The continued high mortality of childbearing', *Proceedings of the Royal Society of Medicine*, 1918–19, 12 (3): 75–107.

8 J. B. DeLee, 'The prophylactic forceps operation', *American Journal of Obstetrics and Gynecology*, 1920–1, 1: 34–44.

9 Bonney, op. cit. (n. 7).

10 W. Taylor and M. Dauncey, 'Changing pattern of mortality in England and

Wales: II. Maternal mortality', *British Journal of Preventive and Social Medicine*, 1954, 8: 172–5.

11 J. Towler and J. Bramall, *Midwives in History and Society*, London, Croom Helm, 1986, p. 226.

12 J. M. L. Phaff, 'The organisation and administration of perinatal services in The Netherlands', in Phaff (ed.), *Perinatal Health Services in Europe*, London, Croom Helm, 1986, pp. 117–127, see p. 118.

13 A. Kaunitz *et al.*, 'Perinatal and maternal mortality in religious groups avoiding obstetric care', *American Journal of Obstetrics and Gynecology*, 1984, 150: 826–31.

FURTHER READING

Aveling, J. H., *English Midwives, their History and Prospects*, ed. by J. L. Thornton, London, H. K. Elliot, 1967; orig. pub. London, 1872.

Garcia, J., Kilpatrick, R. and Richards, M., *The Politics of Maternity Care*, Oxford, Oxford University Press, 1990.

Glaister, J., *Dr. William Smellie and his Contemporaries: a Contribution to the History of Midwifery in the Eighteenth Century*, Glasgow, James Maclehose, 1894.

Gordon, Alexander, *A Treatise on the Epidemic Puerperal Fever of Aberdeen*, London, 1795.

Leavitt, J. W., *Brought to Bed: Childbearing in America, 1750 to 1950*, New York, Oxford University Press, 1986.

Lewis, J., *The Politics of Motherhood*, London, Croom Helm, 1980.

Loudon, I., Death in Childbirth: *An International Study of Maternal Care and Maternal Mortality*, Oxford, Clarendon Press, 1992.

Ministry of Health, *Report of an Investigation into Maternal Mortality*, Cmd. 5422, London, HMSO, 1937.

Moscucci, O., *The Science of Woman*, Cambridge, Cambridge University Press, 1990.

Report of the Select Committee on Midwives Registration, PP 1892 *XIV*.

Sandelowski, Margarete, *Pain and Pleasure in American Childbirth: from Twilight Sleep to the Read Method, 1914–1960*, Westport, CT, Greenwood Press, 1984.

Semmelweis, Ignaz, *The Etiology, Concept and Prophylaxis of Childbed Fever*, trans. by K. Codell Carter, Madison, University of Wisconsin Press, 1983; orig. pub. 1861.

Wertz, R. W. and Wertz, D. C., *Lying-in. A History of Childbirth in America*, New York, Free Press, 1977.

White, Charles, *A Treatise on the Management of Pregnant and Lying-in Women*, London, 1772; reprinted with introd. by L. D. Longo, Canton, MA, Science History Publications, 1987.

Williams, W., *Deaths in Childbed*, London, H. K. Lewis, 1904 (the Milroy Lectures delivered at the Royal College of Physicians of London, 1904).

45

CHILDHOOD

Debórah Dwork

In 1893, the physician Gaston Variot (1855–1930) opened an infant consultation service supported by private charity at the Belleville Dispensary, which was located in one of the poorest districts in Paris. He distributed sterilized milk free of charge or at a nominal sum to babies 'of the lowest and poorest classes' whose mothers were 'obliged to work in the manufactories or in the workshop'. Far from being an obscure event, Variot's work attracted the attention of intellectuals, artists, politicians, and reformers. An effective writer as well as an eminent paediatrician, Variot established and edited the journal *La Clinique infantile*, which publicized his own endeavours and those of others in the field. His consultation service was examined by a host of visitors, including the artist Jean Geoffroy, who painted 'The Philanthropic Society of the *Goutte de Lait de Belleville*', which was exhibited in the Salon of 1903 and subsequently acquired by the municipality of Paris.[1]

Variot's clinic, and the interest it aroused, was just one example of the way in which a specific ideology of childhood was translated into practical efforts to preserve the health of individual children. Throughout the industrialized West, children had captured the popular imagination, and child-rearing philosophies, child-protection policies, and child-saving programmes proliferated. From the second half of the nineteenth century, childhood was recognized, as never before, to be a special and discrete stage in the life cycle. Novelists and newspaper reporters, politicians and philanthropists, and physicians and educators were fascinated with the ideology, concept, and needs of children in the modern industrial age. Their interest was expressed variously, but the subtext was the same: the sanctity of childhood must be preserved by efforts to save, succour, and rescue children. Charles Dickens's *Nicholas Nickleby*, for example, publicized the plight of destitute orphaned children. Victor Hugo's *Les misérables* awoke interest in abandoned waifs.

J. M. Barrie's *Peter Pan* celebrated, through the character of Wendy, the fantasy of children; and through Peter, the epoch of childhood. Barrie's book did not address the pain children suffered and its need for alleviation, but the proceeds from its sale were donated to the Great Ormond Street Hospital for Sick Children. On the other side of the Atlantic, the journalist Jacob Riis (1849–1914) published photographs and stories concerning neglected and oppressed children in the New York City slums which stirred the public to demand rescue and relief operations for them. Works such as these encouraged the development of a wide variety of professional and philanthropic efforts to help children. It was at this time that juvenile court systems, child-labour laws, kindergartens, playgrounds, and universal public-education plans were introduced.

THE DEVELOPMENT OF PAEDIATRICS

While the establishment of special hospitals for children, the growth of paediatrics as a separate medical discipline, and the institution of child-care programmes can thus be seen as manifestations of a wider concern about the welfare of children, they also have their own history. Their development depended on the felicitous nexus of scientific, political, economic, and social factors – and on the way in which physicians, scientists, parents, and politicians perceived children and their needs.

The earliest paediatric hospitals date from the first half of the nineteenth century. The Hôpital des Enfants Malades in Paris, for example, was established in 1802. Others were opened on the European continent over the course of the next five decades (St Anne's Hospital in Vienna, 1837; Kaiser Franz Joseph Hospital in Prague, 1842; Elizabeth Hospital in Berlin, 1843; Ospedaletto di Santo Filomena in Turin, 1845; etc.), but it was not until the mid-1800s that, concomitant with the increased interest in children, hospitals for these youngest members of society were established in growing numbers. In London, the Hospital for Sick Children in Great Ormond Streeet began to function in 1852, and by 1910, seventeen in-patient facilities were opened. In the United States, the first paediatric hospital was the Children's Hospital of Philadelphia, which opened in 1855. By 1930, there were seventy such institutions that treated an estimated 10 per cent of all hospitalized children.[2] (➤ Ch. 49 The hospital)

The establishment of a speciality hospital was not at all unusual during this period. However, other medical specialities (such as ophthalmology) focus on a particular anatomical part or system; by contrast, paediatrics is based entirely on age, and encompasses all areas of clinical medicine. The parameters of the discipline are the physiology and normal development of young children and the specific diseases and ailments that affect them.

However unique the specialty of paediatrics may have been, it was just as profoundly affected by scientific developments as were the other branches of medicine. The germ theory of disease and the practice of asepsis led to the control of infection in hospitals and the admission of children with contagious diseases. Prior to these discoveries in bacteriology, the majority of paediatric patients had suffered from chronic ailments. After the identification of pathogenic microbes and the introduction of specific antitoxins, those suffering from acute conditions were hospitalized. (➤ Ch. 16 Contagion/germ theory/specificity)

Only a small percentage of sick children were admitted to hospitals. By and large, paediatrics was practised in the patients' homes, in the physicians' offices, and in ambulatory clinics. Hospitals were important in that they served as a training-ground for clinical practice and fostered research into the physiology and pathology of children. But they did not, in themselves, affect or even influence the gross morbidity or mortality rates of children as a whole. The prevention and treatment of disease among children depended on developments in bacteriology and the establishment of public-health programmes. It also depended on the recognition by politicians of children as an essential national resource, the demand by mothers for help, and the growth of a group of professional paediatricians. (➤ Ch. 50 Medical institutions and the state; Ch. 51 Public health)

POLITICS AND CHILD WELFARE: THE FRENCH INITIATIVES

In the late nineteenth and early twentieth centuries, politicians throughout the industrialized West began to be concerned about the health of their youngest citizens. It seemed to them, with some justification, that not only was the birth rate declining, but that the infant mortality and morbidity rates were increasing. The prospect of fewer and less-healthy children to attain adulthood and to take on the responsibilities of a premier nation made contemporary statesmen uneasy. That prospect also served as a convenient rhetorical tool. The mid-century message of the pristine childhood of yesteryear, both lost and regretted, was superseded by the image of the fecund and hearty population of yore debilitated by slums, factories, fecklessness, and vice. Where were the stalwart men for the army and the robust women to bear children? Where was the next generation of healthy miners, nimble factory hands, and able educators and administrators? (➤ Ch. 71 Demography and medicine; Ch. 72 Medicine, mortality, and morbidity)

The perceived problems of national degeneration and depopulation became an issue in France a generation earlier than in Britain or the United States. The profoundly demoralizing débâcle of the Franco-Prussian War (1870–1) gave rise to the fearful spectre of present and future French national impotence, and politicians began to pay increased attention to their population problems in response. They were deeply concerned that France would lag in the race for cultural and military supremacy. Physicians who dealt with children on a daily basis were sincerely committed to the reduction of disease and the alleviation of suffering, but they shared these nationalistic sentiments. The rhetoric of the time reverberated through the popular and medical press: France would become a second- or even third-rate nation.[3]

The single greatest cause of infant mortality in France was the diarrhoea of childhood called epidemic diarrhoea, and bottle-fed babies suffered disproportionately.[4] Bacteriologists in France, Germany, Britain, and the United States investigated the flora of the normal intestine as well as the specific pathological conditions found in affected infants, but were unable to identify or isolate the aetiologic agent.[5] French physicians therefore turned to pragmatic solutions. The first of these was the establishment in 1890 of the *Oeuvre de la maternité* at Nancy by François-Joseph Herrgott (1814–1907). The object of this charitable society was to educate and aid the mothers delivered at his clinic in the maternity hospital, and to encourage them to breast-feed.[6]

Much more influential, however, was the infant-welfare scheme of Pierre Budin (1846–1907), which he began when he was head of the Charité Hospital in Paris. In 1892, with the authorization of the director of the Assistance Publique of Paris, Budin organized the first formally structured *consultation de nourrissons* (suckling-infant clinic). The women who were delivered at the Charité (where they were admitted free of charge) were requested to attend an out-patient clinic (the *consultation*) established specifically for their infants every Friday morning. There, the child was weighed and examined. Records were kept of this information and particulars such as teething, illness, method of feeding and quantity of milk consumed, and general observations regarding growth and development were noted. These findings were discussed with the mothers to increase their interest in the health and growth of their infants. Budin's and the mothers' achievement, throughout the 1890s, in slashing the morbidity and mortality rates among the children attending the *consultation*, especially when compared with the statistics of the general infant population of Paris, were inspiring.[7] Indeed, the system promised so well that the following year Gaston Variot opened another *consultation*. The situation he faced differed from that of Budin. The Belleville Dispensary was not a maternity hospital and Variot did not have prenatal contact with the mothers, nor did he see the infants immediately or even shortly after birth. Infants who were failing to thrive, who were weak and ill, were brought to his *consultation*, often already 'deficient in weight by one-third and sometimes one-half of the normal'. Unlike Budin, Variot could not encourage breast-feeding. 'It is utterly impossible to resort to suckling to combat infantile mortality,' he declared, 'the mothers no longer have any milk.' Variot organized a system of milk distribution accompanied by medical examination of infants, who were weighed and examined, and at the Charité. The results of both physicians were remarkable.[8]

The number of *consultations de nourrissons* increased rapidly throughout the 1890s. By 1898, four of the twelve maternity services in Paris had established them. In addition, a number of physicians opened similar services at dispensaries and general hospitals. Due to the ardent advocacy of Paul Strauss (b. 1852), a politician (member of the Senate), philanthropist, and friend of Budin, the General Council of the Seine organized similar services in the municipal dispensaries and charities throughout Paris. By 1903, there were twenty-five *consultations* in the city, twelve funded by private charity and thirteen through municipal monies.[9]

INFANT WELFARE IN THE USA

Nathan Straus (1848–1931), a New York philanthropist, followed Variot's example, and in 1893 established a system of milk stations in Manhattan. Convinced of the prophylactic value of pasteurized milk in the reduction of infant and child morbidity and consequent mortality, Straus generously and enthusiastically championed the cause. The milk was modified according to formula, pasteurized, and dispensed in nursing-bottles. One milk depot distributed 34,400 bottles of milk to poor children in the first year of operation. Straus enlarged his scheme: in 1895, more than 500,000 bottles were supplied. Over the next decade, the figure continued to rise: in 1905, 2.5 million bottles and more than 1 million glasses of milk were sold from Straus booths in the city parks; and in 1906, seventeen Straus stations dispensed 3,140,252 bottles and 1,078,405 glasses of milk. The milk stations also had an educational function, and provided simple instruction about infant and child feeding.[10] (➤ Ch. 63 Medical philanthropy after 1850)

Straus was not alone in his attempts to alleviate disease among the children in New York. In the early years of the twentieth century, many philanthropists, politicians, and physicians in New York and other large American cities were deeply concerned about the high disease rates of the urban poor, especially among the multitude of immigrants who had recently settled in the slum districts of the metropolis. Unlike the French, the Americans were not concerned about a national degeneration due to a low birth rate and high infant and child morbidity and mortality rates. It was the poverty, disease, ignorance, and foreign cultures of the immigrants and the filthy conditions in which they lived that alarmed the reformers.[11] Provision of clean milk to mothers and children appeared to be an efficient way to effect change on a large scale. The results Variot had obtained and the impact of Straus's endeavours persuaded others to follow suit. The New York Association for Improving the Condition of the Poor, for example, established the New York Milk Committee in 1907, and set up milk depots in the immigrant neighbourhoods.[12]

It became clear that provision of milk was only a partial solution. Many immigrant women needed and, as it transpired, wanted instruction about infant and child care. These mothers were uprooted and decontextualized. Often, they were the first generation from their families to have gone to the United States, and they did not have their own mothers to help them. They did not speak English, and did not know how to get the help they required. And the exigencies of poverty complicated their situation further.

In 1908, S. Josephine Baker (1873–1945) (who would shortly become the Chief of the Division of Child Hygiene – the first anywhere in the world) was a child-health inspector for the New York City Health Department. While working in an Italian immigrant ward on the lower east side of New York in the early summer of that year, she evolved a system for providing care to infants and young children. The name and address of every newborn baby in the district was obtained from the Registrar of Records the day after birth. Baker detailed a public-health nurse to visit the mother and child. The mothers were helped to breast-feed, if their situation permitted it, and they were taught the rudiments of how to keep the baby well: the importance of ventilation, frequent bathing, thin summer clothes, and outdoor airings was explained. Finally, the baby was examined and given medical care, if necessary. Results tabulated at the end of the summer revealed that there had been 1,200 fewer deaths among infants in that ward than during the preceding summer, while elsewhere in the city the summer baby death rate remained as high as ever. When the Division of Child Hygiene was created in August, Baker instituted her system on a city-wide basis.

Baker was convinced of the value of education, in additon to the provision of milk and simple medical care. To reach the largest possible number of children she instituted a few avenues of access. First, she extended the milk-depot system. Milk depots were economically useful to mothers, and were also a means of teaching them basic health care and familiarizing them with the official health machinery. This contact with the mothers was crucial. Aided financially by Mrs J. Borden Harriman (1870–1967), Baker transformed the milk depots into Baby Health Stations. Mrs Harriman had raised the money to open and operate thirty stations for the summer months. When those resources were exhausted, the city officials were so pleased with the results that they provided the funds to maintain all those in existence and to open ten more.

Baker persistently sought new means to educate those who looked after small children. Recognizing that 'little mothers' were a reality of life for the working poor, the Division delivered a lecture on baby care in each public school in the city (1909). This was the beginning of a drive to start Little Mothers' Leagues. Membership was open to girls over twelve years old. The leagues met once a week, and after six meetings the girl received a silver badge. The children were taught by nurses and they learned to feed, clothe, and exercise a baby. Two years later, there were 239 leagues in New York City. Leaflets and folders about baby care were published in simple English, Yiddish, and Italian, and distributed by the hundreds of thousands in tenements. The Baby Health Stations remained the primary means of contact between the official health system and the population it sought to serve, and pocket cards with the locations of milk stations were given to everyone to circulate. Every policeman and park employee, for example, was expected to have several of these cards in his pocket when on duty. Baker also convinced the English, Yiddish, and Italian newspapers to print a series of twelve articles on baby care.[13]

THE BRITISH APPROACH TO CHILD WELFARE

Like the Americans, the English politicians, physicians, and reformers turned to the examples provided in France when they awoke at the turn of the century to their own national peril. Bismarck's merging of Germany (1866–71) and its subsequent military and industrial growth and colonial expansion aroused anxiety in Britain, as did the adoption of conscription throughout the European continent. Similarly, the Dual Alliance between France and Russia emphasized the potential weakness of Britain's naval power. Furthermore, as industrial production in France, Germany, Italy, and the United States increased, the importance of Britain as a commercial power declined.[14] The reverses suffered by the British Army during the Boer War (1899–1902) crystallized and emphasized the hitherto latent fears of national deterioration and depopulation. While the news from South Africa of military failures reflected the incompetence of the officers, the news at home of eager but unfit recruits reflected the physical debility and ill health of the would-be soldiers. Indeed, the statistic that three out of every five men were rejected by recruitment officers became an issue of imperial importance and reflected social conditions that were of national significance.[15]

Child welfare programmes based on the French experience appeared to be a possible remedy: they reduced mortality and morbidity, and the healthy children produced by these systems would become healthy adults. It was not, however, Variot's *consultation* that provided a model for the British (as it had for the Americans), but a plan instituted by Léon Dufour (1856–1928), a physician in Fécamp, Normandy. In 1894, Dufour opened an independent baby-welfare clinic, unattached to any hospital or dispensary and supported by private subscriptions. Dufour named his establishment the Goutte de Lait, and the term became popular. Its principles were to encourage and aid breast-feeding, to supply good-quality sterilized milk for those infants who required it, and to provide weekly medical care and supervision of the infants during their first one to two years of life. Dufour welcomed any and every infant. He asked no questions concerning legitimacy or the occupation of the mother. His results, like those of Budin and Variot, were excellent. The mortality from diarrhoea throughout the year 1895–6 was 6.80 per cent among the infants attending the Goutte de Lait, while it was 18.18 per cent among the entire infant population of Fécamp. By 1898–9, the figures had dropped to 1.28 and 9.67, respectively. With results like these, *guottes de lait*, like *consultations de nourrissons*, quickly became popular throughout the country, and the number of infants in attendance increased each year.[16]

A leader in the *Journal of State Medicine* of December 1898 enthusiastically describing Dufour's work caught the attention of F. Drew Harris, the Medical Officer of Health for St Helen's. After a visit to Fécamp, he opened the St Helen's milk depot on 8 August 1899. Although it was based on the French model, the two establishments differed greatly. Whereas the French provided medical care for the children during their first two years, which included child-hygiene instructions for the mothers and a proper milk supply if necessary, the St Helen's depot undertook only the latter function and charged prices their clients could not afford. Nevertheless, the depot was popular, at least initially, and Harris claimed a reasonable success. He certainly received a positive response from his colleagues, and perhaps he inspired them. In 1901, three municipalities established milk depots.[17] Despite the early enthusiasm, the infant milk depot idea never really got off the ground. By 1913, only thirteen depots in England and Wales had been opened, of which three had closed. Not all aspects of the milk-depot system had failed, however. While the provision of milk without supervision came to be seen as having only limited usefulness, health visitors were increasingly incorporated into the scheme to oversee the normal development of the babies and to teach the principles of child care to the mothers.

This educational component was developed in the early years of the twentieth century in Britain as in the United States. Health visitors in Britain and visiting nurses in the USA taught mothers in their own homes the principles of child hygiene and care. Many women welcomed them. Letters from working women collected by the Women's Co-operative Guild for a campaign for improved maternal- and child-health services revealed a widespread desire for and appreciation of education, maternity centres, and 'baby welcomes'. The mothers saw themselves as the key to child welfare. Lack of education was specifically mentioned repeatedly. They demanded instruction with regard to sex, contraception, hygiene, and child-rearing. 'I think ignorance has more to do with suffering than anything', one woman contended.[18] Health authorities originally intended to reach only working-class mothers, but by 1913 it was clear that the more affluent also wanted this help. In the majority of communities which had adopted the Notification of Births Act, over 75 per cent of all births were visited at least once, and in a significant number of towns 90 to 100 per cent were visited.[19] The mothers approved.

THE SCHOOL HEALTH MOVEMENT

Just as proper feeding in conjunction with hygiene instruction and medical supervision were understood to be the primary factors in maintaining the health of infants, adequate nourishment coupled with periodic medical examination and treatment were perceived to be the key to preserve and even ameliorate the mental as well as physical condition of schoolchildren. Food came first, and once again France provided a model for the USA and Britain to copy.

The compulsory-education legislation enacted in France in March 1882 required all communes to establish a *caisse des écoles* (school fund), to be funded by charitable donations and subventions given by the commune, department, or state. This Act also provided for free education and mandatory attendance; thus the school funds could be utilized to promote the physical health of the pupils so that they could take full advantage of their studies. All the communes began to provide one hot meal each day to children whose parents were in receipt of poor relief. By the time the British began to consider this sort of child-health programme, the establishment of *cantines scolaires* (school canteens), which provided a hot meal of soup, meat, and vegetables, had become universal in France. As a special report on the subject in the *Lancet* in 1904 remarked, 'Is there not in all this the making of a healthy people and a strong race? Can we in England afford to ignore the example here given? ... Without hesitation, if we would preserve the race, without the loss of a moment and without making a single exception, every hungry child must be fed.'[20]

A number of charitable organizations had begun to provide meals to schoolchildren after the passage of the 1870 Education Act. The *Referee* fund, for example, was started in 1874 by the head-teacher of the Orange Street School in Southwark. Publicized by George R. Sims (1847–1922) in his *Referee* articles on 'How the poor live', this charity funded dinners for children throughout the winter, and it was found that, contrary to prior experience, the pupils were healthier and attended school more regularly in winter than in summer. The correlation between increased attendance, improved academic performance, and the provision of a meal was corroborated by another philanthropist, Sir Henry Peek (1825–98) who, in the autumn of 1876, organized a system of penny dinners for the children attending the schools on his estate in Devonshire. But these were small-scale, local efforts which did not and could not answer the need of the estimated 13 per cent of schoolchildren who required nourishment.[21]

Educators, political theorists, philanthropists, and the public articulated their demands for state action and responsibility at the Guildhall Conference on Feeding School Children in January 1905. It was attended by approximately 250 delegates representing labour and other organizations with a total membership of about two million. All but thirteen of them adopted a proposal for the free maintenance of schoolchildren by the state, with national rather than local funds. A year later, in 1906, the Education (Provision of Meals) Bill was passed. The Act was permissive, and allowed 'a Local Education Authority [to] take such steps as they think fit for the provision of meals for children in attendance at any public elementary school in their area'. It authorized the creation of school-canteen committees and the use of public money to defray the cost of food.[22]

Bradford was one of the first communities to undertake the provision of meals to schoolchildren. Bradford had already acquired a reputation for remarkable school-health work. In 1893, the Bradford School Board had appointed James Kerr (1849–1911) as a full-time medical officer; he was the first elementary-school doctor with responsibilities for the health of the students and not simply the hygiene of the physical premises. After the passage of the Provision of Meals Act, the Bradford Education Authority instituted a pilot study. Forty children in schools in the poorest area of the city were chosen to receive breakfast and dinner five days a week for three months, except during the school holidays. The effect was judged by changes in general appearance and in weight. Improvement in appearance was 'more or less apparent in all, and very obvious in some of the children, who visibly filled out and brightened up. The reverse process was equally apparent when the children were seen after the summer holiday' when no meals had been provided. Weight gain was compared with a control group of sixty-nine children; it was found that those who received the meals gained approximately 1.2 kilograms, while the other children gained less than half a kilogram during the three months. On the basis of this study, and of the medical officer's examination of 1,840 children which revealed that about 11 per cent of the entire school enrolment were malnourished, the Bradford authorities instituted a general programme for the provision of meals. All children were encouraged to take them. Either the parents or the teacher could apply for free meals for a child. A poverty standard was fixed, but as such eligibility tests went, the Bradford standard was rather liberal; children of many working-class families qualified.[23]

Despite the example set by Bradford and the perceived need throughout the country, the provision of meals to schoolchildren was not made mandatory before the First World War. When the Provision of Meals Act was passed, there were 322 local education authorities in England and Wales; during the first fifteen months of its operation, only forty authorities had taken advantage of it. The next year, this figure more than doubled to eighty-five, but by 1912 only 131 of the 322 had instituted feeding programmes.[24] It is no coincidence that it was in June 1914 that a bill empowering the Board of Education to compel local authorities to feed malnourished pupils was enacted. It was an astute politician who said that programmes that sounded 'terribly like rank Socialism' were nothing more than 'first-class Imperialism'.[25]

The provision of meals was only one aspect of the school-health movement. Schools provided specific sites where the state's public-health arm could reach children, and physicians and reformers were anxious to take advantage of the opportunity. Medical inspection of approximately one-fifth of the population in each industrialized country could be instituted through the educational system, and treatment provided to those in need. It was the United States, with its enormous, newly arrived immigrant population requiring medical care, that took the lead in this area. The schools enabled health authorities and social workers to have contact with the immigrant population, and medical inspection systems, treatment clinics, and hygiene classes were organized. These programmes were a tool for Americanization and a means of social control, but they were also the products of a sincere desire to improve the health of these newest citizens. In a number of respects they were successful, most notably in the treatment of diphtheria and skin infections.

In September 1894, four years after two French bacteriologists Émile Roux (1853–1933) and Alexandre Yersin (1863–1943) had developed a diagnostic technique to demonstrate the diphtheria organism, and three years after diphtheria antitoxin was first used to treat a child in Berlin, Roux presented his work at the 8th International Congress of Hygiene and Demography in Budapest. William Hallock Park (1863–1939), head of the diagnostic laboratory at the New York City Health Department, took note and began to produce diphtheria antitoxin in New York. Massachusetts followed suit, and within a few years nearly every state and city in the USA had a diagnostic laboratory. At the same time as diphtheria antitoxin was first produced in his state, the Chairman of the Board of Health in Boston instituted the medical inspection of schoolchildren. An epidemic of diphtheria led the Board to appoint fifty physicians to examine the children. It was in New York, however, that plans for treatment were translated into direct care. Under the leadership of Hermann Biggs (1859–1923) and William Park, the New York City Health Department made practical use of antitoxin. A popular newspaper, the *New*

York Herald, supported the health authorities' efforts and established the *Herald* Antitoxin Fund for the use of antitoxin in the treatment of diphtheria. That year, the diphtheria death rate was reduced by 33 per cent. Previously, at least 45 per cent of all diphtheria cases had ended in death; by 1906, this had dropped to 13 per cent.[26]

Soon afterwards, New York, like Boston, Chicago, and Philadelphia, organized the medical inspection of its schoolchildren. In March 1897, 150 school medical inspectors were appointed to visit the public schools and examine children suspected of having communicable disease. This was a crude method to screen for the worst cases, and experience soon proved that it was not enough. Aside from diphtheria, measles, and scarlet fever, schoolchildren suffered from skin diseases such as pediculosis, scabies, ringworm, and impetigo; eye conditions such as trachoma; malnutrition; and physical defects.

It was not until a new administration came into office in 1902 that a real effort was made to institute effective school medical inspections. At the request of the Health Commissioner, the founder of the Henry Street settlement, Lillian Wald (1867–1940), loaned one of her best-qualified nurses, Lina Rogers (1870–1928), to carry on experimental work in a public school notorious for its incidence of disease. At that time, it was estimated that 80 per cent of the school children of New York were infected with head lice (pediculosis), and 20 per cent suffered from trachoma. Rogers quickly evolved an effective and educational approach to deal with these problems. She examined the children in school, having them pass by her in a line while she inspected their hands, teeth, throat, eyes, scalp, and general physical appearance. She provided protective treatments for skin infections to prevent them from spreading, and thereby allowed the child to remain in school. Children with ailments subsequently reported for daily treatment to a clinic established in each public school and supplied with simple remedies. Special classes were established for children with trachoma. Finally, Rogers also started a system of home care, teaching whole families how to prevent and cure minor contagious infections.[27] (➤ Ch. 54 A general history of nursing 1800–1900)

Rogers was the first full-time school nurse appointed in the USA, and within months the Health Department added seventeen nurses to her staff. By 1908, when the Division of Child Hygiene was established by the Health Department, there were about thirty school nurses; during the summer, they were detailed to infant-health work. The Chief of the Division, S. Josephine Baker, dramatically expanded the scope of the programme. She appointed a staff of 141 to conduct medical inspections of schoolchildren during the school year and to teach proper baby care at milk depots and in homes during the summer months when morbidity and mortality from epidemic diarrhoea was highest. During the school year 1908–9, 323,344 pupils were examined in school and 242,048 were found to be suffering from some non-contagious physical defect. Of this number, 203,488, or 84 per cent, were treated.[28]

School medical services were not new to European educators, physicians, and public-health officers. They had been instituted in Brussels in 1874, Sweden in 1878, Paris in 1879, and Lyons in 1880.[29] In Germany, between 1898 and 1903, a total of 676 school doctors were appointed in 234 towns and districts.[30] The New York City school-health programmes, however, were the most comprehensive and extensive, and they served as a model for future developments. For European reformers, as for their transatlantic colleagues, medical inspection was never the real issue: treatment for discovered ailments was their goal. Whether viewed as a patriotic measure to safeguard the nation's future, a medical measure to alleviate physical distress, or an educational measure to improve academic performance, medical examination followed by appropriate treatment was wanted. In France, the first such programme was instituted eight years after the Franco-Prussian War. In England, the national reaction to the Boer War recruitment statistics and to the Army's losses on the field demanded change, and school medical inspection was suggested as one remedy for the poor physical condition of the young. Reformers argued that such programmes would enable children to profit from their education; the nation would be saved the expense of trying to educate children who, due to physical ailments, could not learn; and this system had been undertaken successfully in other countries, which might bode ill for the Britain of the future. In other words, the claims of education, a profitable national economy, and apprehension about the future of the nation were the concerns that motivated child-health activity. School medical inspection was instituted in 1907, and the post of Chief Medical Officer of Health to the Board of Education was created. School clinics to treat the discovered ailments soon followed, as did systems for follow-up visiting in the children's own homes. According to a 1913 study, there were approximately 118 centres in England where treatment schemes or school clinics were in operation.[31]

COMPREHENSIVE WELFARE SYSTEMS

On the eve of the First World War, some form of infant-health service and school medical inspection and treatment scheme had been instituted in each of the industrialized nations of Europe and America. Not surprisingly, however, the First World War engendered a renewed sense of urgency among the hostile states for the establishment of a comprehensive infant- and child-welfare system. As Europe prepared for war again in 1939, S. Josephine Baker wrote:

It may seem like a cold-blooded thing to say, but someone ought to point out that the World War was a backhanded break for children. . . . As more and more thousands of men were slaughtered every day, the belligerent nations, on whatever side, began to see that new human lives, which could grow up to replace brutally extinguished adult lives, were extremely valuable national assets. [The children] took the spotlight as the hope of the nation. That is the handsomest way to put it. The ugliest way – and, I suspect, the truer, is to say flatly that it was the military usefulness of human life that wrought the change. When a nation is fighting a war or preparing for another . . . it must look to its future supplies of cannon fodder.[32]

Baker was a competent commentator. An innovative, imaginative, and indefatigable activist in child care, she had created and engendered support for child-health schemes for thirty years and she had found that in Europe and America enthusiasm for such programmes was much more easily aroused and maintained during hostile than in peaceful times.

In Britain, the quickened interest in infant health was reflected in the increase and in the number and variety of services that were made available. In 1914, local authorities employed 600 health visitors; by 1918, this figure had more than quadrupled to 2,577. Whereas 300 municipal and 350 voluntary maternity and child-welfare centres had been established by the beginning of the war, 700 of the former and 578 of the latter were in operation in 1918. The scope of activities carried on by the centres also expanded: more attention was paid to antenatal work; medical consultations were extended to include all pre-school children; milk and meals for toddlers as well as for pregnant and nursing women were more commonly offered; and dental care for mothers and children began to be provided at a number of clinics.[33] School health services also increased. In his report of 1917 George Newman (1870–1948), the Chief Medical Officer of Health to the Board of Education, noted with satisfaction that 'the School Medical Service is now a national system (it may be said as complete of its kind and more universal than elsewhere in the world) at work in all the 318 educational areas of England and Wales, [and] in all the 21,000 Public Elementary Schools.' Medical inspection and treatment for discovered ailments were provided to all students in the state schools, regardless of ability to pay or degree of physical distress. As Newman put it, 'the School Medical Service has recognized that the ordinary child is the key to the nation's health, and therefore it has exercised its duty to *all* children of school age.'[34] In August 1918, close to the end of the war, comprehensive legislation was passed which systematized and regulated the provision of welfare services for pregnant and nursing mothers and children up to school age. The welfare system explicitly and definitely structured by the 1918 Act remained essentially intact until it was superseded by the National Health Service in 1948.

The United States entered the war in April 1917. Much to the surprise and chagrin of politicians, physicians, and the public, 50 per cent of the men reporting to their draft boards were found to have physical defects. Analyses of draft-board figures revealed that only 65 per cent of inducted men aged 21 to 30 years were physically fit for military service.[35] This discovery, coupled with the extraordinary loss of life in the field, had the same effect in America as the Franco-Prussian War had had in France nearly half a century earlier and the Boer War had had in England some twenty years before: it stimulated interest in preserving the health of children. In the USA, newspapers and magazines began to report infant-mortality statistics as if they were news items, and ran lead articles on 'baby-saving campaigns'. (➤ Ch. 66 War and modern medicine)

The second year of American involvement in the war (1918) was named 'Children's Year' as part of a national campaign to emphasize the importance of the youngest members of society in a time of national peril. This message was promulgated and manifested in many ways, but one of the most effective techniques was designed by the newly formed Child Health Organization, whose goal was to improve health through education and nutrition, operating through the public-school system. The cartoon 'instructors', the Health Fairy, and Cho-Cho the Clown familiarized children with health principles and encouraged good health and hygiene habits like eating a balanced diet and brushing teeth.

Concern for the children culminated in the Sheppard-Towner Act (1921), which was the first measure undertaken in the USA to appropriate federal funds for health and social-welfare purposes. The Act provided for a range of health activities for children such as maternal-, infant-, and child-health centres, Little Mothers' leagues, and public-health physician and nurse services for rural populations. The legislation ran for seven years. In 1935, it was re-enacted on a more ambitious scale as Title V of the Social Security Act.

CONCLUSION

Who benefited from the ever-increasing interest in and concern for children, and the plethora of programmes, systems, and plans instituted to safeguard their health? Clearly, children profited. As the twentieth century wore on, infant- and child-mortality rates in the industrialized West declined, and a smaller percentage suffered from malnutrition and disease. Mothers also appear to have benefited. They wanted to know how to look after their children properly, and were delighted with their success. Both well-to-do and poor women in Europe continued to welcome the health visitor, and mothers in the USA took their children to paediatric clinics or offices. It is equally clear that the burgeoning field of child welfare and paediatrics was a boon to women seeking employment in this area and to physicians interested in the care of children. Traditional ideas about the special relation between women and children helped to create new opportunities for women as school physicians, school nurses, visiting nurses, health-centre personnel, and health visitors.[36] (➤ Ch. 38 Women and medicine) With the introduction of school lunch programmes, dieticians and cooks were in demand. And finally, the evolution of paediatrics into a distinct medical speciality was a means for the collective upward mobility of those in the field.[37]

The main party to have benefited, however, was the state. The rhetoric, so sanctimoniously intoned, that children were the 'hope of the nation' or, as the *British Medical Journal* called them, 'the true dreadnoughts of the nation'[38] was all too literally meant. Without power, financial resources, or the vote, children were, and still are, fundamentally the property of the state. 'Childhood' is a social construct, and it can be – and has been – manipulated for good and for ill. Politicians, physicians, and reformers may use the ideology of children as the hope of the nation to improve their health, but they may use it also for the political socialization of their youngest citizens. The Fascist regime under Mussolini, for example, saw young people as the hope for the future; indeed, their motto was, *'largo ai giovani'* ('make way for the young').[39] Young people held the same place in Hitler's National Socialism, receiving special attention and care; and after the 1 December 1936 Hitler Youth Law, they had to belong to their age-appropriate organization.[40] Children were the darlings of the fledgling Soviet state, with the Communist youth (the Komsomols) taking pride of place. And the newly established socialist states in eastern Europe after the Second World War adopted the same theoretical principles and rhetoric. Children in the German Democratic Republic, for example, were hailed as the most precious national asset, and extensive child-care systems were established.[41] They also participated in state youth organizations: the Young Pioneers became Thaelmann Pioneers, and then went on to become Free German Youth.

In the final analysis, the concept of childhood as it has been defined in the nineteenth and twentieth centuries and utilized by physicians and medical scientists must be understood to have a history that includes the German experimentation on children during the Second World War. These scientific endeavours were no mere aberration. The experiments of J. Mengele (1911–79) and K. Heissmeyer (1905–67) are as much a part of the construction of childhood in the industrialized West as are those of Koch (1843–1910), von Behring, and Ehrlich. It was in the interests of the state for Jewish children, especially twins, to be human subjects in lethal research which had as a goal the study of tuberculosis and, in the case of the latter, genetics.[42] They were indeed 'the hope of the nation' and 'the true dreadnoughts' of the state. (➤ Ch. 37 History of medical ethics; Ch. 44 Childbirth)

NOTES

1   Gaston Variot, 'L'élevage des enfants atrophiques par l'emploi méthodique du lait stérilisé', *Revue Scientifique*, 1902, 17: 225–35. See also Variot, 'Gouttes de lait', *British Medical Journal*, 14 May 1904: 1125–6; and 'Dr. Variot's goutte de lait', *Lancet*, 19 November 1904: 1458–9.

2   Arthur F. Abt and Fielding H. Garrison, *History of Pediatrics*, Philadelphia, PA, W. B. Saunders, 1965, pp. 120–1.

3   See, for example, Jacques Bertillon, *Élements de démographie*, Paris, Société d'Éditions Scientifiques, 1896; Bertillon, *La Dépopulation de la France*, Paris, Librairie Félix Alcan, 1911; Henri de Rothschild, *Dépopulation et protection de la première enfance*, Paris, Octave Doin, 1900.

4   Albert Balestre and A. Gilletta de Saint-Joseph, *Étude sur la mortalité de la première enfance dans la population urbaine de la France de 1892 à 1897*, Paris, Octave Doin, 1901.

5   Deborah Dwork, *War is Good for Babies and Other Young Children*, London, Tavistock, 1987, pp. 36–51.

6   Gaston Variot, 'La goutte de lait', *La Clinique infantile*, 1 November 1903; and in English, George Frederick McCleary, *The Early History of the English Welfare Movement*, London, H. K. Lewis, 1933, pp. 43–4.

7   Pierre Budin, 'La mortalité infantile', *L'Obstétrique*, 1903, 8: 1–44; Budin, *The Nursling*, London, Caxton, 1907; Budin, 'Sur le lait stérilisé', *Bulletin de l'Académie de Médecine*, 1897, 37: 685–7; Budin and Pierre Planchon, 'Note sur l'alimentation des enfants', *Bulletin de L'Académie de Médecine*, 1904, 51: 23–40.

8   Gaston Variot, 'Gouttes de lait', *British Medical Journal*, 14 May 1904: pp. 1125–6; see also Variot, 'L'élevage des enfants', op. cit. (n. 1).

9   Pierre Budin, 'Précis de *Consultations de nourrissons par Charles Maygrier*', *Bulletin de l'Académie de Médecine*, 1903, 50: 266; Charles Porak, 'Rapport au nom de la Commisson permanente de l'Hygiène de l'enfance, sur les mémoires et travaux envoyé a cette Commission en 1901', *Bulletin de l'Académie de Médecine*, 1901, 46: 668–769.

10 Deborah Dwork, *Biomedical Research and Infant and Maternal Health: a Chronology*, Washington, DC (written under contract to and property of the National Institutes of Health), 1979, p. 6.

11 See, for example, Annie S. Daniel, 'The wreck of the home', *Charities*, 1905, 14: 624–9; Harold M. Finley, 'The congestion of Manhattan', *Federation*, May 1908, 5: 10–18; and the entire issue of *Federation*, April 1906, 4; Arthur Henry, 'Among the immigrants', *Scribner's Magazine*, 1901 29: 301–11; Claude H. Miller, 'The menace of crowded cities', *World's Work*, 1908, 16: 10268–72; Jacob Riis, *How the Other Half Lives*, New York, Hill & Wang, 1957; Riis, *The Children of the Poor*, London, Sampson, Low, Marston, 1892; Riis, *The Peril and the Preservation of the Home*, Philadelphia, PA, George W. Jacobs, 1903; Riis, *A Ten Years' War*, Boston, MA, Houghton Mifflin, 1900; Anon., 'The moral side of the tenement problem', *Catholic World*, May 1885, 41: 160–4.

12 For a history of the New York Association for Improving the Condition of the Poor, see Roy Lubove, 'The New York Association for Improving the Condition of the Poor: the formative years', *New York Historical Quarterly*, 1959, 43: 307–29.

13 S. Josephine Baker, *The Bureau of Child Hygiene of the Department of New York*, monograph series 4, January 1915; Baker, *Fighting for Life*, New York, Macmillan, 1939; Baker, 'The reduction of infant mortality in New York City', *American Journal of Diseases of Childhood*, 1913, 5: 151–61.

14 For a contemporary discussion of the issue, see *inter alia*, Charles Wentworth Dilke, *Army Reform*, London, Service & Paton, 1898; Dilke, *The British Army*, London, Chapman & Hall, 1888; Dilke, *The British Empire*, London, Chatto & Windus, 1899; Dilke, *The Present Position of European Politics*, London, Chapman & Hall, 1887; T. H. Huxley, 'The struggle for existence: a programme', *Nineteenth Century*, 1888, 23: 169–80; George Bernard Shaw (ed.), *Fabianism and the Empire*, London, G. Richards, 1900; Ernest Edwin Williams, '*Made in Germany*', London, Heinemann, 1896. With regard to the secondary literature, see D. H. Aldcroft (ed.), *The Development of British Industry and Foreign Competition, 1875–1914*, London, Allen & Unwin, 1968; Eric John Hobsbawm, *Industry and Empire, an Economic History of Britain since 1750*, London, Weidenfeld & Nicolson, 1968; H. C. G. Matthew, *The Liberal Imperialists*, London, Oxford University Press, 1973; G. R. Searle, *Eugenics and Politics in Britain: 1900–1914*, Leiden, Nordhoff, 1976, Searle, *The Quest for National Efficiency*, Oxford, Blackwell, 1971; Bernard Semmel, *Imperialism and Social Reform*, London, Allen & Unwin, 1960; John Ecclesfield Tyler, *The Struggle for Imperial Unity, 1868–1895*, London, Longman, 1938.

15 'Miles' [pseud. of Frederick Maurice], 'Where to get men', *Contemporary Review*, 1902, 81: 78–86; 'Miles', 'The national health: a soldier's study', *Contemporary Review*, 1903, 83: 41–56; B. Seebohm Rowntree, *Poverty: a Study of Town Life*, London, Macmillan, 1901, pp. 216–21; Arnold White, 'Efficiency and empire', *Weekly Sun*, 28 July 1900, p. 5. See also, Aimée Watt Smyth, *Physical Deterioration, its Causes and its Cure*, London, John Murray, 1904; the wide coverage of the issue in the medical press: *British Medical Journal*, 11 July 1903: 99–100; 25 July 1903: 207–8; 8 August 1903: 345; 24 October 1903: 1101; 21 November 1903: 1339–40; 6 February 1904: 319–20; Arthur Newsholme, 'Alleged physical deterioration in towns', *Public Health*, 1905, 17: 292; and Dwork, op. cit. (n. 5), pp. 11–21.

16 Léon Dufour, 'L'oeuvre de la goutte de lait', *Bulletin de l'Académie de Médecine*, 1897, 38: 530–1; Porak, op. cit. (n. 9), 753–4; in English, see Budin, *The Nursling*, op. cit. (n. 7), p. 155; George Frederick McCleary, 'The infants' milk depot: its history and function', *Journal of Hygiene*, 1904, 4: 332, Leonard Robinson, 'Consultations for infants in France', *Practitioner*, October 1905: 485.

17 'La goutte de lait', *Journal of State Medicine*, 1898, 4: 612–14; F. Drew Harris, 'The supply of sterilized humanised milk for use of infants in St. Helens', *British Medical Journal*, 18 August 1900: 427–30.

18 Margaret Llewelyn Davies (ed.), *Maternity: Letters from Working Women*, London, Virago, 1978, p. 81; see also p. 147.

19 Arthur Newsholme, 'Second report on infant and child mortality', *42nd Annual Report of the Local Government Board* (suppl.), Cd 6909, London, HMSO, 1913.

20 'The feeding of school children', *Lancet*, 17 September 1904: 862.

21 Louise Stevens Bryant, *School Feeding*, Philadelphia, PA, J. B. Lippincott, 1913, pp. 14–22; M. E. Bulkley, *The Feeding of School Children*, London, G. Bell, 1914, pp. 1–49; Anon., *Prize Essays on Feeding School Children*, London, Sir Joseph Causton & Sons, 1890.

22 Bryant, op. cit. (n. 21), Appendix A, pp. 299–302.

23 Ralph H. Crowley, 'The provision of meals for school children', *Public Health*, 1908, 5: 325–35; Crowley, *The Hygiene of School Life*, London, Methuen, 1910, pp. 193–201.

24 Harry Beswick, 'Feeding the children', *Clarion*, 11 October 1912: 7.

25 T. J. Macnamara, 'Physical condition of working-class children', *Nineteenth Century*, August 1904: 311.

26 Diphtheria Prevention Commission, *Saving Children's Lives*, New York, Department of Health, 1932; William H. Park, M. C. Schroder and Abraham Zingher, 'The control of diphtheria', *American Journal of Public Health*, 1923, 13: 23–32; Zingher, 'Active immunization of infants against diphtheria', *American Journal of Diseases of Children*, 1918, 16: 83–102; Zingher, 'Preventive work in the public schools of New York City', *Archives of Pediatrics*, 1921, 38: 336–59.

27 Baker, *Fighting for Life*, op. cit. (n. 13), pp. 77–82. See also Lillian Wald, *The House on Henry Street*, New York, Henry Holt, 1915.

28 Dwork, op. cit. (n. 10), p. 33.

29 George Rosen, *A History of Public Health*, New York, MD Publications, 1958, p. 365.

30 'Medical inspection of school children', *British Medical Journal*, 16 July 1904: 137–8; see also William Harbutt Dawson, *School Doctors in Germany*, London, HMSO, 1906 (Board of Education, educational pamphlets, no. 4).

31 Lewis D. Cruickshank and W. Leslie MacKenzie, *School Clinics at Home and Abroad*, London, National League for Physical Education and Improvement, 1913, p. 111.

32 Baker, *Fighting for Life*, op. cit. (n. 13), p. 165.

33 William S. Craig, *Child and Adolescent Life*, Edinburgh, Livingstone, p. 164.

34 Board of Education, *Annual Report for 1917 of the Chief Medical Officer of the Board of Education*, Cd 9206, London, HMSO, 1918, pp. 162, 173.

35 Dwork, op. cit. (n. 10), p. 44.

36 Dwork, op. cit. (n. 5), pp. 125–9, 155–62, 198–205.

37 Sydney Halpern, *American Pediatrics: the Social Dynamics of Professionalism*, Berkeley, University of California Press, 1988.

38 'The war and the falling birth-rate', *British Medical Journal*, 30 October 1915: 649.

39 Tracy H. Koon, *Believe, Obey, Fight: Political Socialization of Youth in Fascist Italy, 1922–1943*, Chapel Hill, University of North Carolina Press, 1985.

40 Detlev J. K. Peukert, *Inside Nazi Germany: Conformity, Opposition, and Racism in Everyday Life*, New Haven, CT, Yale University Press, 1987, pp. 145–74.

41 Eva Schmidt-Kolmer, *Fruehe Kindheit*, Berlin, Volk und Wissen Volkseigener Verlag, 1984, sections 1.1, 2.3, and part 3.

42 Robert Jay Lifton, *The Nazi Doctors*, New York, Basic Books, 1986, pp. 347–60;

Guenther Schwarberg, *The Murders at the Bullenhuser Damm: the SS Doctor and the Children*, Bloomington, Indiana University Press, 1984.

FURTHER READING

Ariès, Philippe, *Centuries of Childhood*, London, Cape, 1962.

Beaven, Paul W. (ed.), *For the Welfare of Children*, Springfield, IL, American Academy of Pediatrics, 1955.

Crubellier, Maurice, *L'Enfance et la jeunesse dans la société française, 1800–1950*, Paris, Armand Colin, 1979.

Davin, Anna, 'Imperialism and the cult of motherhood', *History Workshop Journal*, 1978, spring: 9–65.

Fuchs, Rachel, *Abandoned Children: Foundlings and Child Welfare in Nineteenth Century France*, Albany, State University of New York Press, 1984.

Hirst, J. D., ' "A failure without parallel": the school medical service and the London County Council, 1907–12', *Medical History*, 1981, 25: 281–300.

Lewis, Jane, *The Politics of Motherhood: Child and Maternal Welfare in England, 1900–1939*, London, Croom Helm, 1980.

Lomax, Elizabeth M. R., Kagan, Jerome, and Rosenkrantz, Barbara G., *Science and Patterns of Child Care*, San Francisco, W. H. Freeman, 1978.

McCleary, George Frederick, *The Early History of the Infant Welfare Movement*, London, H. K. Lewis, 1933.

——, *The Development of British Maternity and Child Welfare Services*, London, National Association of Maternity and Child Welfare Centres and for the Prevention of Infant Mortality, 1945.

Newman, George, *Infant Mortality: a Social Problem*, London, Methuen, 1906.

——, *The Building of a Nation's Health*, London, Macmillan, 1939.

Newsholme, Arthur, *Fifty Years in Public Health*, London, Allen & Unwin, 1935.

Spargo, John, *The Bitter Cry of the Children*, New York, Macmillan, 1906.

Winter J. M., *The Great War and the British People*, London, Macmillan, 1985.

46

GERIATRICS

Pat Thane

EARLY HISTORY OF IDEAS ABOUT AGEING

Since classical times, there have been advocates of old age as an object of specialized study within medicine and other professional and intellectual disciplines, though they have never been numerous or powerful. Throughout this long history, there have been competing interpretations of the meaning of ageing: whether it is an unalterable natural condition or one susceptible to control or arrest by human agency; whether it is in itself a pathological or a natural condition; whether it is attended by pathological conditions peculiar to it or by diseases common to younger age-groups; a time of life to be dreaded or to be enjoyed; to be mocked or respected. In other words, whether or to what extent older people as such *should* be an object of specialist concern. Consideration of ageing has long put in focus the question of what constitutes health or disease, and the difficulty of answering it. Nuances have shifted back and forth over time, but the central themes and controversies have remained remarkably stable up to the present, with ancient and modern, 'scientific' and 'magical' perceptions of the management of ageing endlessly intertwined in no simple progressive pattern.

Cicero's *De Senectute*, written when he was 63, is a classic of consolation literature for older people, arguing that:

> he does not do those things that the young men do, but in truth he does much greater and better things . . . by talent, authority, judgement; of which faculties old age is usually so far from being deprived . . . the intellectual powers remain in the old, provided study and application be kept up.

Yet he also wrote 'Senectus ipsa morbus est' (old age is itself a disease).[1]

The latter view had been installed in the medical tradition by Hippocrates (*c*.460-*c*.370 BC), who differentiated and enumerated a catalogue of ailments peculiar to old people. His interpretation was fundamentally humoral: that the process of ageing was caused by a progressive loss of the body's store of heat. As people aged, they became colder and also moister compared with the warmth and dryness of the body's physical peak. This resulted in a depletion of vitality and increased susceptibility to disease.[2] (➤ Ch. 14 Humoralism)

Galen (AD 129–c.200/210) gave authority to a different tradition and, to the present, the two views have competed and been confused. He shared the humoral interpretation of the ageing process, but regarded this as natural rather than pathological or necessarily having pathological effects. Individuals could protect themselves against these effects by taking care of their bodies. He recommended suitable protective regimens for each phase of life, whilst recognizing that each individual aged somewhat differently. Humoral theory regarded the balance of humours in the body of any individual as affected by a number of independent variables, of which age was only one.[3] Galen installed another enduring approach: that due protection could enable a body to age more slowly.

However, the belief that human beings could prolong their lives was long at war in Western thinking with faith that nature or God organized things for the best and could not be tampered with. With Christianity emerged the conviction that people had been created in Eden without physical imperfections and destined for longevity, even immortality. This was forfeited at the Fall: sickness, degeneration, and death were among the punishments. However, God offered spiritual redemption through Christ, and Christianity held out to believers the hope that those who achieved a state of grace would also gain health and the prolongation of life. Biblical imagery was contradictory. Whilst stressing that the survival to great age and the wisdom of the Patriarchs was the reward for righteous living, the gloomy twelfth chapter of Ecclesiastes had a lasting influence, beginning: 'Remember now thy creator in the days of thy youth, while the evil days come not, nor the years draw nigh wherein thou shalt say, I have no pleasure in them.' (➤ Ch. 61 Religion and medicine) And the 90th Psalm fatalistically fixed the life-span at seventy years, conjoining with the mystical notion of the power of the number seven to encourage the popular division of life into seven ages; though scholars in the ancient and medieval worlds were more inclined to divide life into three, four, six, or twelve stages. Descriptions of ageing in ancient and early medieval times were embedded in cosmologies of growing complexity, but throughout these centuries, old age was defined as a distinct stage of life. The notion of human life as divided rather rigidly into stages, each with different health and behavioural characteristics, without clear phases of transition between them, remained powerful in Western thought until developmental lines of reasoning gained power from the eighteenth century.[4]

THE MIDDLE AGES AND RENAISSANCE

Nevertheless, an optimistic approach to ageing became embedded in popular culture, whilst in medical discourse it ebbed and flowed. From Hindu tradition, the notion that a 'fountain of youth' existed in some place or time, which could not merely prolong strength but could turn age back into youth, became absorbed into medieval Western imagery (for example, the *Fountain of Juventa* of Cranach the Elder). In medieval Western writing, the conviction recurs that there had once existed, and indeed existed still in remote places, the Golden Age or Place where youth is eternal and could be repossessed if only it or its secret could be discovered. Equally long-lived and widespread was the belief that the breath of youth, living and/or sleeping with young people, could restore warmth to the older body. Medieval alchemists in the West sought the elixir of life.[5] Yet such seeking after fantasy and hope coexisted in medieval Europe with a variety of other images, verbal and visual, which often distinguished active old age from final decline and attributed to the former almost every imaginable quality from good health and wisdom to boorish pettishness, with none clearly predominating.[6]

Among scholars, the belief that fitness and even life itself could be prolonged, and the more pathological conditions associated with ageing delayed or wholly averted, overrode belief in magical elixirs. Ancient ideas about ageing flowed into the Middle Ages through a multitude of channels. These further increased from the end of the eleventh century in the great age of translation of ancient Greek, Latin, and Arabic texts. These intensified the influence of humoralism, while introducing a new interpretation that old age was cold and dry, though in both versions loss of heat was the key characteristic. They also introduced from ancient sources regimens for the regulation of diet and behaviour, combining moral rules with practical advice for the prolongation of health and perhaps life. One of them, Galen's *On Maintaining Health* was translated into Latin in the twelfth century.[7]

Such regimens themselves experienced an active longevity. The late twelfth-century *Regimen Sanitatus* of the medical school of Salerno provided precise maxims for the maintenance of good health throughout life, emphasizing exercise, hygiene, diet, and moderation in all things, including sexual activity. It achieved 240 printed editions in Latin, Hebrew, Persian, and all European languages, and is the first known of a stream of health codes through the following 800 years.[8] It was, in fact, the only practical advice that could be given about ageing and the body throughout this time and for some time afterwards. Such influential scholars as Roger Bacon (1210–93), whose *Cure of Old Age and the Preservation of Youth* was much influenced by ancient texts, translated into English in 1683 and widely disseminated thereafter (demonstrating how little changed in this field in the intervening four centuries), believed that by these means human beings could reach 150 years and, in later generations, 300 to 500. He accepted the Christian belief that humans were naturally immortal and believed that even after the Fall human-kind had retained a residual capacity to live for 1,000 years.[9]

A conviction that the worst ills of old age could be alleviated or avoided implied that such ills existed in those who failed to follow the correct regimen. Hence it was consistent with a belief in the need to diagnose and treat the illnesses and weaknesses of older people. Bacon described such inventions as the use of glass to magnify and to assist weak eyes. The question was long left open and controversial whether such conditions were *solely* caused by intemperate life-styles or had other causes; and whether certain pathological conditions or syndromes were specific to older ages. The study of ageing in itself and the study of pathological conditions associated with old age, the disciplines that have become known in the twentieth century as, respectively, gerontology and geriatrics, were not, and have rarely been, wholly satisfactorily distinguished.

Not all of the medieval advocates of health regimens believed that they would or should produce supercentenarians; rather, that they could enable more people to attain old age and to experience it in comfort. Such an influential regimen as the *Discorsi della Vita sobria* of Luigi Cornaro (1464/6–1566), written at the age of perhaps 83, and translated into English in 1634, went through fifty editions in the eighteenth and nineteenth centuries. He believed that a temperate life enabled the body's supply of vital energy to last longer, until it ebbed peacefully away in a natural death between the ages of 100 and 120. (Cornaro was said to have practised what he preached and lived to around 100.)[10] There was some imprecision in claimed or ascribed ages at this and indeed at all times before the accurate recording of age became bureaucratic routine during the eighteenth century; recorded ages should be treated with caution.[11]

Advocates of health regimens among the *Gerontocomi* (Greek: *geron* – old man; *komeo* – to take care of it) of fifteenth-century Italy also made careful observations of the common pathological conditions that regimens were intended to avert. Gabriele de Zerbi (1445–1505), author of one of the first printed works on the care of old people in 1489, concluded that 'old age is inevitable . . . but its end uncertain', for if numerous conditions could be described and some prevented, they could not be cured.[12] This was part of a shift towards a more empirical approach to medicine, away from the more abstract Galenism.

The belief that old age virtually free of sickness was attainable was reinforced by the belief that many indeed attained it, sinking gradually into peaceful expiration. This appeared to be supported by results of the increasing practice of diagnosis through observation of the living and dissection of the dead. By this means, Leonardo da Vinci (1452–1519) concluded that the aged who enjoyed good health died through lack of nourishment due to the thickening of the walls of the veins and the closing up of capillaries.[13] This was 'natural' death.

THE SCIENTIFIC REVOLUTION

That healthy *super*longevity was attainable was also supported by the existence of apparently attested cases. That these were generally found among the rural poor was taken as proof that the immoderate life of modern, especially urban, society was the chief cause of 'premature' sickness and death. (➤ Ch. 27 Diseases of civilization) Thomas Parr for example, who was allegedly 153 when he died in London in 1635, aroused both élite and popular excitement. His death followed being brought as a curiosity to the Court. William Harvey (1578–1657) dissected him, and attributed his death to the sudden transition to the sulphurous air and rich living of London from the 'perfect purity' of air, meagre diet, and freedom from care of the rural labourer. Harvey did not question the longevity of 'Old Parr', which was probably attained by his, consciously or not, adopting his father's birth-date.[14]

The growing interest in pathology, dissection, and practical anatomy in Europe from the sixteenth century increased descriptive knowledge of the ageing body, and to some degree of the ageing neurological system. Harvey's discovery of the circulation triggered new explanatory models. With investigation of the chemical properties of inorganic substances and of the flora of the New World and of Europe, new horizons gradually opened up for pharmacology and nutrition.[15] (➤ Ch. 5 The anatomical tradition; Ch. 7 The physiological tradition)

André du Laurens (*c.*?1558–*c.*1609), Physician to Henri IV and Professor at the University of Montpellier, published in 1597 a book which was translated in 1599 as *Discourse of the Preservation of the Sight; of Melancholic Diseases; of Rheumes and of Old Age*. Written in French, it was translated many times into Latin, and ran to nine French and two Italian editions. Du Laurens recognized that different individuals aged at different rates, and that the causes were mental and occupational as well as physical: 'Nothing hastens old age more than idleness', 'Melancholie . . . is a dotage, not coupled with an ague, but with fear and sadness . . . old folks ordinarilie are fearfull.'[16]

One of his successors at Montpellier, François Ranchin (1560–1641), in 1627 published in his *Opuscula Medica* a plea that medicine should take the needs of older people more seriously, for:

> Not only physicians, but everybody else attending old people, being accustomed to their constant complaints and knowing their ill-tempered and difficult man-

ners, realize how noble and important, how serious and *difficult*, how *useful* and even *indispensable* is that part of practical Medicine called Gerocomica, which deals with the conservation of old people and the healing of their diseases. . . . [T]his science has been neglected by our forefathers and even by modern authors too. What has been written about the conservation of old people and the healing of the diseases of old age, is so bad and so unproductive that we get the impression not only that this noblest part of Medicine was not cultivated but even that, yes, it has been flatly suppressed and buried.

He described what were seen as the specific disorders of older people, both physical and neurological. He strongly emphasized the importance of diet and temperate living, but also that the 'conservation and duration of life depend partly on nature and partly on the medical art, the former through proper nourishment, the latter through chosen remedies'. He related particular types of diet to particular physical and mental ailments, insisting that even diseased elderly people could be cured.[17]

Arousing as it did such fundamental questions about human survival, the study of old age remained as much, and possibly more, a preoccupation of philosophers as of medical specialists. The great natural philosophers of the seventeenth century were attracted by the belief that human beings could control nature and prolong life. In *History Natural and Experimental of Life and Death* (1623), Francis Bacon (1561–1621) advocated the preservation of health, the cure of disease, and the prolongation of life through temperate living, combined with systematic collection of medical data through which physicians would come to a new understanding of the mechanisms of the body and the nature of disease.[18] In the concluding section of his *Discourse on Method* (1637), René Descartes (1596–1650) pledged his talent to finding ways of retarding or overcoming senescence: scientific knowledge could extend life and move beyond prevention to cure; though when torn by religious conflict, he favoured acceptance of the 'natural span'.

Yet for most of recorded time, neither philosophical nor medical comment on old age (a small proportion of the full range of medical discourse) touched the actual lives of most older people. They had little contact with formal medicine, due either to poverty or to a realistic assessment that it could not do them much good. This changed little before the 1920s, or, on a mass scale, the 1950s. Hence the continuing popularity of health and hygiene regimens and the preference for traditional remedies for the cure or alleviation of specific conditions in old and young alike. In the seventeenth century, 'knowledge of the virtues of plants and herbs was an essential part of a gentleman's education'.[19] There was an increasing flow of vernacular manuals spreading such knowledge: in Britain, those published by Nicholas Culpeper (1616–54), for example.[20]

THE EIGHTEENTH CENTURY

In more-orthodox medical circles, knowledge about bodily changes associated with ageing grew much faster than effective therapies. Through the seventeenth century, knowledge accumulated about, among other things, strokes and their effects, and arteriosclerotic changes. Johann Bernard von Fischer (1685–1772) in *De Senio eusque Gradibus et Morbis* (Erfurt 1754) described how by means of necropsy he explored the anatomy and physiology of old age, differentiating normal and pathological ageing. In Padua, Giovanni Battista Morgagni (1682–1771) in 1761 published *De Sedibus et Causis Morborum*, based on clinical and pathological reports of older people, and devoted some of his clinical lectures to old age. Still essentially a humoralist, he was especially celebrated for his contributions to cardiology. He commented accurately that many diseases experienced in old age, especially lung infections, ran a chronic, almost symptomless, course and might be more easily overlooked than in younger people: apparently disease-free 'natural ageing' might mask disease.[21] (➤ Ch. 9 The pathological tradition)

Gerard van Swieten (1700–72), Physician to Empress Maria Theresa from 1745, in 1763 gave at the University of Vienna an *Oratio de Senum Valetudine tuenda* (On protecting the health of the elderly), again emphasizing the efficacy of preventing serious conditions in old age through preserving the bodily fluids by means of lifelong temperance. But he believed that some symptoms of ageing could be alleviated. Bending and stretching could counteract stiffness of the limbs, as could the rubbing in of oils.[22]

Benjamin Rush (1745–1813), an immigrant from America who trained in Edinburgh, published in 1793 his *Account of the State of the Body and Mind in Old Age, with Observations on its Diseases and their Remedies*, based on personal observations of patients over the age of 50. He listed the factors favouring longevity as: descent from long-lived ancestors, temperate eating and drinking, matrimony, and equivocality of temper. He concluded that 'few persons appear to die of old age. Some one of the diseases . . . generally cuts the last thread of life.'[23]

Still the only practical advice that could be given to older people in most circumstances was to adopt a preventive regime, most influentially that of the physician Christian Wilhelm Hufeland (1762–1836), friend of Goethe (1749–1832) and Schiller (1759–1805), Professor in Jena and Berlin. His *Makrobiotik, oder die Kunst das menschliche Leben zu verlangen* (1796) (translated as *The Art of Prolonging Life*, (1797) aroused much enthusiasm and was translated into several languages. Essentially, it was yet another restatement of advice about means to conserve the vital energies in order to attain longevity, a tradition which remained the predominant approach to ageing in Germany throughout the nineteenth century.[24]

Enlightenment thinkers were attracted to the idea that free individuals could bring all bodily processes under rational control. William Godwin (1756–1836) believed that life would be lengthened by cultivating benevolent and optimistic attitudes and a clear, well-ordered state of mind until, ultimately, sleep, ageing, and death were banished.[25] Condorcet (1743–94) held that a little more human effort would be required to achieve this: improvement of the environment and a comprehensive programme of scientific research designed to improved the physical quality of the population.[26] Napoleon became one of a succession of powerful rulers to be convinced that a way would be found to prolong life indefinitely. *Essay on the Principle of Population* (1798) by Thomas Malthus (1766–1834) disparaged such hope and raised the spectre of overpopulation in a world of infinite longevity. (➤ Ch. 71 Demography and medicine)

THE NINETEENTH CENTURY

Such visions gradually thereafter became intellectually less respectable, though not necessarily less popular, and, periodically through the nineteenth century, rules for extending life were published and widely sold. William Thoms (1803–85) sought in 1873 in his *Longevity in Man: its Facts and Fiction* to knock superlongevity theorics on the head. He investigated all reported cases of survival beyond 100 years, and found them unsubstantiated. The controversy which his book aroused suggests the popularity of the aspiration for superlongevity. More effectively, the rise of social hygiene, the growth of the belief that health is the responsibility of the state, or at least of the community, rather than only that of the individual, and the development of rather more sophisticated aetiological concepts and therapeutic methods in the nineteenth century provided alternatives to individual preventive regimes. Humoral pathology was gradually superseded by the development of pathological anatomy and bacteriology, which revealed complex causes of disease on a microscopic level unknowable before. As medicine improved its capacity to diagnose and, much more gradually, to cure, it perhaps sought too enthusiastically to bury the more-sensible aspects of the preventive regimens. Yet still in the nineteenth century, progress in diagnosis and therapy was slow and both still had minimal impact on the lives and deaths of most old people.

In France between the mid-eighteenth and mid-nineteenth centuries, medical knowledge about ageing advanced particularly fast; *gérocomie* was a clearly defined medical specialism. By the 1830s, every major medical treatise for teaching purposes, in Paris at least, had a section on the special diseases of the old. Until the 1870s, research, along with pleas for a *médecine des vieillards*, came almost entirely from the great *hospices* designed for the indigent infirm and elderly, the Sâlpetrière for women and the Bicêtre for men, especially the former. The primary focus was pathological, through case studies and autopsies, with an overwhelming though selective organic emphasis. The lungs, brain, and vascular system, and to a lesser extent the liver, received a great amount of attention, leading to improvements in the description and classification of disorders afflicting them. The heart and kidneys were neglected because they were exempted from what was seen as the general rule of organic atrophy as a characteristic of ageing, since autopsies demonstrated that they did not generally atrophy. C. L. Durand-Fardel (1815–99) in his *Traité clinique et pratique des maladies des vieillards* (1854) claimed that heart problems were uncommon among the elderly, despite the cardiac weaknesses found in many who were said to have died of other disorders. The widely used *Traité des maladies des vieillards* (1909) of Louis Ranvier (1834–1922) still claimed that heart attacks were possible but rare. Understanding of heart disease in the elderly was to develop in the twentieth century through work in cardiology not specifically directed towards the aged. (➤ Ch. 11 Clinical research)

In consequence of the focus on vital organs, medical researchers largely ignored most of the conditions that killed older people: overwhelmingly, respiratory diseases, especially pneumonia; diseases of the nervous system; and cancer. But much was discovered about the distinctive physiology of older people. The influential lectures of J. M. Charcot (1825–93) at the Sâlpetrière between 1862 and 1870, published as *On Senile and Chronic Diseases*, encapsulated this work.

Diagnosis and symptomology received much less attention than pathology, but the precise observation that accompanied the pathological approach aided more precise diagnosis and usefully dispelled some long-held beliefs. The common ideas that a strong pulse in a stroke victim denoted a greater likelihood of a second attack, and that thin people were more prone to brain haemorrhage, were dispelled. Doctors were told how to use the stethoscope to distinguish between catarrh and emphysema. It was recognized by the end of the century that the elderly *could* suffer from tuberculosis, although symptoms presented more gradually than in younger people. (➤ Ch. 36 The science of diagnosis: diagnostic technology)

Treatment received least attention of all, and at best was relegated to a small final section in any geriatric treatise. Pathological observation did, however, produce a number of warnings against common therapeutic practices that were not helpful and might be harmful to the elderly: for example, bleeding following a stroke or brain haemorrhage, or use of strong emetics. This challenge to long-established and common practices was the most concrete contribution of geriatric research to the potential health of older people in the nineteenth century. But the fact that in France the traditional treatments were being urged as strongly in the 1850s as at the beginning of the century and still warned against at the end of the century, suggests that everyday practice was extremely slow to change, not least due to the lack of alternatives. Treatment in France differed little from other countries, though it may have relied more on bleeding. (➤ Ch. 40 Physical methods) Towards 1880 in France and elsewhere, surgery was applied to the elderly for the first time for cataracts and broken bones. By the end of the century, digitalis was increasingly used for heart problems.

In nineteenth-century France, as elsewhere in most times, the fact that old age was overwhelmingly a female condition could hardly be detected from the textbooks, which unswervingly presented the typical patient as male and gave more attention to problems of the prostate than to female afflictions. Indeed, in women, ageing had from the earliest times been seen as itself an adequate explanation of disease, since the menopause seemed to offer clear proof of humoralism. It brought old age earlier to women than to men, a critical time when disease emerged, due to the reflux of humours that could no longer escape through menstruation. There was long a conflict between the medical view of menopause as marking the onset of old age for women and social perceptions of women as acquiring a new independence and authority once they were emancipated from childbearing. Nineteenth-century doctors, at least in France, were puzzled that though women aged earlier than men and died of the same diseases, they died at later ages.[27] Relatively greater longevity of females is said to have characterized western Europe since at least the twelfth century.[28]

Alternatives existed even in France to the dominant Parisian pathological school, but they were much less influential. Some were variants of the preventive-regimen tradition, though with modern inputs. Leopold Turck (1797–1887) of Strasburg in *De la Vieillesse étudiée comme maladie* (1852) proposed a range of new therapies, ranging from restorative hibernation to electrical treatment to revive 'nervous fluids', restore hair colour, and tone up skin and body.

Parisian pathology had a certain influence upon German geriatrics, though this remained dominated throughout the nineteenth century by a version of vitalism, a transformation of the Galenic tradition, which saw ageing as the natural ebbing of the life-force. This was thought to be susceptible to a certain degree of human control, but it encouraged the belief that certain infirmities were exclusively associated with old age. This belief survived into the twentieth century, though challenged by adherents of the pathology school.[29]

Nineteenth-century geriatric researchers generally took little account of changes in other branches of medicine. They ignored the implications of biological advances, in contrast to such fields as obstetrics, where biological findings were taken up quickly at the research level. The experimental investigations in the field of internal secretions by Claude Bernard (1813–78), Professor of Experimental Medicine in the Collège de France, and by his successor, Charles Eduard Brown-Séquard (1817–94), provided a biomedical basis for the ancient belief that use of sexual substances could assist rejuvenation. In 1888, aged 72, Brown-Séquard claimed to have achieved rejuvenation by self-experimentation with extracts of animal testicles. Though derided by contemporary scientists, his work did increase interest in internal secretions and established a basis for modern endocrinology. (➤ Ch. 23 Endocrine disorders) He was not quite alone. The Russian biologist Elie Metchnikoff (1845–1916) considered toxicity induced by external factors to be the preventable cause of old age and death. In his widely read works, *The Nature of Man* and *The Prolongation of Life*, he advocated ingestion of sour milk for the destruction of putrefactive bacteria and the injection of stimulating hormonal sera. Hormone injections were still being dismissed in France in the 1900s, when they were being widely and successfully used in the USA, Germany, and elsewhere. Similarly, the relevance to the study of ageing of work on bone-grafts was not recognized in France.[30]

Fundamentally, in most countries, the field was still constrained by the belief that the elderly were incurable. The emphasis of French pathology on the decay of organs reinforced more strongly than in most countries the classical view of ageing as a time of unrelieved decay, a process of disease in itself. Durand-Fardel judged emphysema to be almost natural, the result of prolonged use of the lungs. The pathological school having been initially a force for progress in French geriatrics, at least on a research level, became increasingly limiting and sterile after the 1870s.

In Britain, George Day (1815–72), Professor of Medicine at St Andrews, published his *Practical Treatise on the Domestic Management and Most Important Diseases of Advanced Life* (1849), which gave some of the first surviving descriptions of the symptoms and some of the causes of senile dementia.[31] Daniel Maclachlan (1807–70), Physician to the Royal Hospital, Chelsea (for veteran servicemen) from 1840–63, where he achieved a creditably low death rate, published in 1863 his 718-page *Practical Treatise of the Disease and Infirmities of Advanced Age*. He pointed out – as did others at the time – the difficulty of diagnosis in the elderly since several diseases commonly coexisted. He stated that the most common causes of death were tuberculosis, and renal or lung failure. As regards therapy, he mentioned only some twenty drugs, the most potent of which were opium, digitalis, quinine, mercury, colchicum, potassium iodine, and the vegetable purgatives. His treatments can at best have produced delaying actions.[32]

John Milner Fothergill (1841–88) in his *Diseases of Sedentary and Advanced Life* (London, 1885) linked the socio-psychological and preventive interpretation of ageing with the findings of scientific medicine. In this and other publications, he emphasized that bad dietary and physical habits in early life contributed to the development of disease in the elderly, and also applied the contemporary physiological and chemical principles to the study of diabetes mellitus, renal disease, and gout. He suggested that ageing altered the connective-tissue content of organs (describing the process in biomedical rather than humoral terms) and thereby predisposed them to the irreversible disease states that occurred in old age, a view which was echoed in Germany.[33] (➤ Ch. 8 The biochemical tradition; Ch. 20 Constitutional and hereditary disorders)

THE TWENTIETH CENTURY

By 1914, there was no tidy separation between advocates of prevention and of medical therapy nor any clearly drawn distinction between normal and pathological features of ageing. There was recurrent lively debate about the latter. This was clear in the work of the very man who invented the term 'geriatrics', the Austrian-born émigré to the United States, Ignatz Nascher (1863–1945). Indeed, the main advances in medical understanding of old age in the early twentieth century came from the USA. Research grew in parallel with that in the life sciences, such as bacteriology, and the application of their findings to conditions found in older people. Research in neuropathology, such as that of Alois Alzheimer (1834–1915), further refined the classification of senile brain diseases. Emil Kraepelin (1856–1926) named one disease after Alzheimer, and did much to clarify the clinical concepts of pre-senile dementia. Among other things, neurosyphilis was distinguished from the senile dementias, which, in turn, were further divided into the senile psychoses and psychoses with cerebral arteriosclerosis. (➤ Ch. 21 Mental diseases)

It was Nascher, however, who did most to promote geriatrics as a speciality. A medical practitioner in New York, he first developed his ideas fully in *Longevity and Rejuvenescence* in 1909, proposing:

> Geriatrics, from *geras*, old age, and *iatrikos*, relating to the physician, is a term I would suggest as an addition to our vocabulary to cover the same field, in old age, that is covered by the term 'paediatrics' in childhood ... to emphasize the necessity of considering senility and its diseases apart from maturity and to assign to it a separate place in medicine.

Nascher described senility as 'a physiological entity, and its diseases not as diseases of maturity with senile complications, but as diseases of senility apart and distinct from maturity'. He did indeed appear to believe that a large number of disease processes were due to ageing, and his separation of diseases in the elderly from the ageing process itself was not always precise. However, his distinction between geriatrics and gerontology sharpened with his statement that 'disease in old age ... is ... a pathological process in a normally degenerating body'. He concluded: 'So little has been done in the field of geriatrics that until it receives the attention its importance deserves, and we know more about the metabolic changes in the period of decline, we must fall back upon empiricism in the treatment of diseases in senility.' He wrote further pleas for the study of geriatrics, and was invited to lecture on the subject at medical schools in Boston and Chicago, after pointing out that 'there is not a lecture given in any medical college on that branch of medicine dealing with senility and its diseases.' By 1914, he had published more than thirty articles on the subject, and written his text *Geriatrics: the Diseases of Old Age and their Treatment; including Physiological Old Age, Home and Institutional Care and Medico-legal Relations*, though he had difficulty in finding a publisher. A second edition appeared in 1916.

Nascher advocated the treatment of elderly patients as people with diseases. However, the three points he felt were of most importance in dealing with old-age problems were mental stimulation, food, and exercise. Geriatric medicine could still offer little more. By the 1920s, the main causes of death were hardly changed from the early nineteenth century, and for most of them nothing could be done. Of the major killers, geriatric researchers had investigated only strokes directly. Not surprisingly, preventive health regimes remained big sellers. Nascher's regular articles for the Sunday magazine of the *New York American* helped to spread his ideas, and from 1917, the *Medical Review of Reviews* added a section on geriatrics, to which he contributed regularly, helping to spread knowledge of geriatrics within the profession. It was the first medical magazine in the world to do so.

In 1929, Nascher retired as Chief Physician of the Department of Hospitals of the City of New York. Two years later, he asked to be put in charge of the 1,200 inmates of the New York City Farm Colony, many of whom were elderly. He aimed:

> to change the antiquated methods of dealing with aged public dependents and rehabilitate them as a far as possible physically and mentally... I tried to promote incentive to work, stimulated pride in appearance, tried to improve attitudes on life, created reading and games rooms, made workers' clubs, stimulated competition with private clubs, etc.

He used the inmates as research subjects to generate and test hypotheses about rehabilitation, ideas of motivation, persistence in purposeful activity, and attempts at maintaining ties between older people and the lives they had formerly led. He made careful, agonized notes on his wife's mental deterioration in her later years, which he summarized in his last paper, *The Aging Mind*, published one month before his death.

But for all Nascher's efforts, by the time of his death, geriatrics was still not a regular part of the curriculum of medical schools, though regular lectures were introduced in the New York Medical School in 1940. When, around this time, Nascher replied in answer to a questionnaire that his speciality was geriatrics, he was informed that this was not a recognized speciality.[34]

His work was carried on by his pupil and devoted admirer Malford W. Thewlis (1889–1956), who published in 1919 *Geriatrics: a Treatise on Senile Conditions*, which had an enlarged second edition in 1924. In 1941 and 1942, greatly enlarged and revised third and fourth editions appeared. The time-gap demarcated two major surges of interest in ageing, separated by a period of slow progress. The growing body of knowledge that these successive editions encompassed was rooted, as Nascher advised, in observation, including that derived from pathological anatomy, including autopsies. Such work developed fastest in the USA. From the 1920s, medicine acquired greater therapeutic capacity, although more slowly in geriatrics than in other specialities. Also from the 1920s, popular medical treatises and newspaper articles were written by medical practitioners for older people, such popularization having been rare through the preceding centuries in this branch of medicine, in contrast to others. In consequence of these changes, older people turned more frequently to doctors and, in turn, their rising expectations put more pressure upon the medical profession to attempt to meet their needs – though the pressure was less, and less effective, among old than young people.

Another important though slow change was the growth of psychotherapy and counselling for elderly people, also centred in the USA. Lillien J. Martin (1851–1943), a pioneering German-trained child psychiatrist (and suffragist) founded, in 1920, the first child-guidance clinic in the USA. (➤ Ch. 43 Psychotherapy) She discovered that disturbed behaviour in young people was often linked with the presence of a disturbed elderly person in the household. This led her to recognize that 'old age is a stress period to which too little attention has been paid and no help given except the offer of organized physical comfort'. 'When we have arrived at the place of looking at old age as a period of life rather than as a bodily condition, we shall give it the intelligent and careful study that we have applied to other such periods, infancy, childhood, adolescence etc. i.e. as a period with its own struggles, its aspirations and its accomplishments.' She occupied her own old age, from her retirement at 65 to her death at 92, to the Old Age Counselling Centre she founded in San Francisco. Her work was based on the principle that mental and physical decline are related, and that both can be retarded and even reversed through counselling designed to identify potential for fulfilment, leading to a regime of self-improvement, including exercise and diet, but above all the development of motivation and a sense of self-worth. As she described in *Salvaging Old Age* (1930), unhappiness and discontent were widespread among the elderly and had little to do with material or physical environments.

In the *Handbook for Old Age Counsellors* (1944), which she was revising on the day before her death, she wrote that counsellors must be free of the notion that old age implies only deterioration and decrepitude. The work 'involves the double task of breaking down a prevalent social misconception and of rebuilding a personality that has accepted that misconception and all the misery that goes with it.' But her approach has been slow to be accepted.[35]

In the inter-war years, both diagnosis and treatment of a number of conditions common in older people improved. The rise of biochemistry, physiology, and experimental medicine made the study of geriatrics less dependent upon pathological anatomy. It became clear that disease can be present even though the cellular structure might appear normal under the microscope. Diagnosis of heart problems, especially the use of the electrocardiogram, and medication for them improved, as also for hypertension. Diagnosis and the capacity to operate for various cancers improved, indeed the age of normally successful operability began slowly to rise. (➤ Ch. 42 Surgery (modern); Ch. 25 Cancer) Work on endocrinology in France and especially in the USA assisted, among other things, in the treatment of prematurely senile menopausal women and in the prevention of osteoporosis. Most of these medical improvements derived from research not primarily directed to the needs of older people.

More specifically directed to the needs of older people, in France, the Russian-born Serge Voronoff (1866–1951) worked on glandular grafts, aiming to provide more-durable treatment than the hormones then available. His injections into humans of extracts from monkey glands caught, via the popular press, the strand of the popular imagination which for centuries had longed for rejuvenation. Such work was regarded with disdain by the mainstream medical profession, in part no doubt because it *was* popular.[36]

In the USSR, dogmatic conviction of the power of humanity to control nature, and perhaps Stalin's own aspirations for immortality, brought encouragement of research into endocrinology and its geriatric applications (and more legends of supercentenarian peasants, this time in Georgia[37]). The first international gerontology conference was held in Kiev in 1938. In the USA, meanwhile, work was developing on plastic surgery and its application to older people. Yet still in 1937, in France and elsewhere, medical manuals recommended bleeding in apoplexy and cold baths for obese heart patients.

The study both of gerontology and of geriatric medicine, sometimes in close association, leaped forward in the later 1930s and 1940s, again with the USA in the lead. The growth in interest in all things associated with ageing at this time was directly due to the panic in all developed countries about the ageing of society due to the decline in the birth rate.[38] (➤ Ch. 45

Childhood) Also very important was the introduction of the sulphonomides and penicillin, and equally important, their rapid application in the more widely accessible and trusted medical services that simultaneously became available. (➤ Ch. 39 Drug therapies) This ensured that many more elderly people recovered from acute illnesses, above all pneumonia. They survived, however, only to succumb to other often chronic ailments which, becoming more commonplace, demanded greater medical attention. More widespread use of antibiotics after the Second World War heightened this effect.

The first medical journal devoted to geriatrics was published in Nazi Germany in 1936: by the 1950s, Germany had eight, Italy four, and France founded its first. In the USA, the early years of the Second World War, in particular, saw a growth of conferences and symposia on geriatrics and gerontology, and greater attention to geriatrics in medical schools. The emphasis was upon integrating biological, clinical, and socio-economic aspects of the study of ageing. From 1942, students at the Harvard Medical school were for the first time given regular lectures in geriatrics, though still in the USA in the 1950s there were bitter complaints from geriatricians about the unwillingness of general hospitals to admit older patients and about the few nursing specialists in the field.[39]

There were similar but rather slower developments in Europe. By the late 1940s, gerontological societies had appeared in at least seventeen countries. The International Association of Gerontology was formed in Liège in 1950. In most Western countries, geriatrics became established as a specialism, but nowhere with high prestige. In most of them, publicly funded medical care became dramatically more widely accessible and improved in quality. Yet a government report published in Britain in 1956 concluded that 'the old age group are currently receiving a lower standard of service than the main body of consumers and there are also substantial areas of unmet need among the elderly'.[40]

Britain from the mid-1930s established a lead in the physical rehabilitation of the sick elderly, beginning with the work of Marjorie Warren (1897–1960) at the West Middlesex Hospital. She found that old people were generally neglected, on the assumption that they were incurable and untreatable. They were placed in the care of general physicians, who gave their attention to younger 'remediable' patients. They were kept warm in bed and fed, though in depressing surroundings with minimal stimulus or incentive for activity, becoming apathetic, suffering bedsores, obesity, stiffness, and atrophy of the limbs.

Warren found that in more attractive and hopeful surroundings, and with therapy, many could be rehabilitated and leave hospital. She investigated the management of stroke victims, and evolved a series of exercises that enabled patients to become active. This work, and that of others, attracted special attention during the Second World War, when the Ministry of Health took control of most hospitals to meet the needs of war victims. Both the Ministry and the British Medical Association began to encourage best practice in geriatrics, drawing also on European and American experience.[41] The formation of the National Health Service in 1948, at a time when there was still concern about the ageing of society and the consequent costs of caring for the higher proportion of elderly people in the population, gave further organized stimulus, though change was slow.[42] (➤ Ch. 50 Medical institutions and the state) By 1953, there were three professors of geriatrics in the USA; in Britain, one lecturer and a few recognized clinical teachers. The first professor of geriatrics in Britain was appointed at Glasgow in 1964, though in Britain it remained controversial within the profession whether geriatrics should be a separate speciality.[43] In 1975, a leading British geriatrician could still comment that:

> There are few doctors with special knowledge of disease in the elderly; there are no nurses deliberately trained to care for the elderly. . . . Geriatrics is more a state of mind than a branch of medicine or a mode of treatment. It is a reaction against the belief that after 60 a patient is too old to be medically interesting or therapeutically rewarding. . . . The first stage of the Geriatric philosophy is the discovery that the ordinary methods of medicine and surgery can be applied successfully to elderly patients. Once diagnosed, pneumonia can respond to sulphonamides as well at 80 as at 18.[44]

A leading American geriatrician summed up the position in 1962:

> Our present concept [of old age] as an inherent property of living matter, manifested in man, by functional and structural changes which lead gradually by poorly understood intercellular and intracellular pathways to the development of associated superimposed diseases. The answer in any given situation to the question, aging process or disease, depends on interpretations which are subject to change on short notice. We have learned with difficulty to avoid the facile explanation of obscure conditions in the elderly as being due to 'old age'.[45]

In the post-war period, there was a clearer diagnosis of the medical conditions common among elderly people and real advances in treatment. There was increased awareness of the interplay between functional and psychological factors, and growing knowledge of psychopharmacology increased the capacity to cure. There were wider but still limited developments of specialized institutions for the treatment and care of older people, including those suffering from psychological and psychiatric problems. (➤ Ch. 56 Psychiatry) Conceptual and diagnostic refinement and the search for causes and cures has continued in these fields throughout the twentieth century, at different rates in different countries, developing into the distinctive specialism of psychogeriatrics. The growth and urgency of this research was especially noticeable from the 1980s, with the recognition of the increasing number of sufferers from dementia (about 20 per cent of people over 80, according to some UK estimates) and to fears that the ageing of populations, which was becoming evident at the same time, would bring about a further increase. The fears may be unduly pessimistic, but the problem remains that even in the early 1990s little is known about the epidemiology and aetiology, let alone prevention and treatment, of such major disorders as Alzheimer's disease. Perhaps more important than dramatic changes in medical knowledge, more older people than ever before received help with mundane but fundamentally disabling conditions affecting hearing, eyesight, teeth, and feet, again largely due to more widely available publicly funded services. And more have learned to seek treatment for such conditions rather than regard them as natural accompaniments of ageing to be endured rather than treated. (➤ Ch. 55 The emergence of the para-medical professions)

Compared with other forms of medicine, it was clearer that a strict line could not be drawn between the medical and social problems of patients. It was obvious that many older people could be kept out of institutions and could manage at home with the assistance of local social and health services: for example, in Britain, district nurses and home-helps. It was widely recognized that remaining integrated within the community enabled more people to retain maximum activity for longer.

This was perhaps just as well. Improvements in medical treatment remained slow. Studies in the USA in the 1960s and 1970s showed that medical students became *less* sympathetic to geriatric patients in the course of their training. This has been attributed to the conflict between the dominant paradigm in twentieth-century medical training – that each condition has a cause and a cure and the role of the medical practitioner is to cure – and the reality that geriatric patients generally suffer from multiple conditions, some of which might be palliated (though a growing problem was that drug therapies might have conflicting effects) but many of which could not be cured.[46] It has also been suggested that the development of geriatrics as a specialism has had ambiguous effects: in many respects, it has enhanced the quality of care of the elderly, but it has influenced some physicians to take less interest in them and to look to geriatricians excessively for their care.[47]

Works on geriatric medicine continued to be shot through with social and psychological assumptions, often of the kind the authors were allegedly seeking to dispel. For example, the fourth edition of a widely used British textbook, first published in 1960, opened by emphasizing the importance of promoting a positive image of elderly people, but was typical in proceeding to assume, among other negative stereotypes, that it was unnatural for different age-groups to mix socially, that elderly men disliked the company of elderly women, and that neither was sexually attractive.[48]

In 1975, a distinguished British geriatrician still felt the need to devote a prestigious annual medical lecture to an attempt to change attitudes to geriatrics within the medical profession:

> Today, the harder one tries to impress on one's colleagues from other medical specialties the reality of geriatric medicine – its clinical and educational role in medicine – the less they appear to believe it.

He sought to do by surveying the history of the speciality, concluding by crystallizing its central problem. History, he believed,

> demonstrated the importance of distinguishing the effects of disease from those of ageing; but it is just as important to realize that elderly ill patients will not become young well ones when treatment has been successful.[49]

Medical research made real breakthroughs in making cure possible, most notably the use of cardiac pacemakers from the 1960s, kidney dialysis from the late 1960s, coronary artery surgery from the 1970s, and hip- and organ-replacement surgery. Except for the birth-control pill, all of the major breakthroughs in medical technology since the late 1950s have had their most widespread impact on people who are past their fifties, and the further past their fifties, the greater the impact. The growth since the Second World War of various forms of state subsidy for health services in all Western countries has made these advances very widely available. However, in the late 1980s and the 1990s, economic recession in many countries, combined with increased demand due to increased client awareness and, above all, the potential growth in demand due to the growing proportion of elderly people in all Western populations, is creating a tendency towards age-based rationing of treatment: for example, in the British National Health Service, refusal of kidney dialysis to older patients. (➤ Ch. 57 Health economics) However, reductions in some causes of death in older age groups – above all, the unexpected drop in cardiovascular disorders since the late 1960s – appear to owe hardly anything to medical advance, but rather to popular and growing adoption of late twentieth-century regimens of exercise and diet. Similarly, hypertension has been shown to respond to low-cost techniques and sometimes very ancient therapies that induce relaxation and control over mind and body.

At the other extreme, developments in medical technology to a point at which people can be kept technically 'alive', but hardly meaningfully functioning, apparently indefinitely, seem to have delivered the long-desired superlongevity, in the least desirable of ways. In the 1990s, they pose medicine with its greatest ethical dilemma.[50] (➤ Ch. 37 History of medical ethics; Ch. 68 Medical technologies: social contexts and consequences)

Awareness has grown of the interaction of physical and mental illness with the environment: that poverty, bereavement, lack of status, and disability can lead to depression. Incontinence, for example, can be the result of social rejection rather than just a normal feature of ageing. Yet counselling for older people is not readily available. Both out-patient and institutional services for older people with psychiatric or neurological disorders, though less appalling than before the Second World War, remain in most countries markedly inferior to other health-care services, though it is one of the health-care sectors in which demand is growing fastest.[51] The issue of making survival to later ages worthwhile for the individual, and also for their kin and for the wider society, is raising new moral, as well as material, dilemmas for geriatrics in the 1990s. At the same time, cutting against a trend to integrate the medical care of the elderly with that of other age-groups (the term 'geriatric ward' officially no longer exists in the British National Health Service, 'medical ward for the elderly' having replaced it) is the continuing lack of certainty about which experiences and conditions are, or are not, peculiarly associated with the ageing process.

The outcome in the 1990s is the simultaneous emergence of the largest numbers of fit people in their sixties and seventies ever known, and the largest numbers of chronically ill elderly people ever known. For the first time in history, longevity has become a normal rather than a minority experience. Commonly, older people recover from acute medical problems which would have killed them in the past, only to succumb to sometimes complex sets of chronic non-lethal disorders for which relatively little can be done (for example, strokes and senile dementia) except to be kept alive with (not necessarily rapidly) diminishing functional capacity. For the major disabling conditions of old age, such as Alzheimer's disease, arthritis, and diabetes, despite continuing research, little can be done. The major diseases of the elderly from an epidemiological point of view are not specific lesions in particular organs. Overlapping, multi-system diseases predominate that are degenerative in nature and for which no single research breakthrough can bring the answer. These problems continue to be worsened by the slowness of some older people to consult doctors until their conditions are advanced, because they regard such ill health as a normal feature of ageing, as do their doctors, though such attitudes may decline as new age-cohorts more influenced by the health consciousness of the 1980s, and the many cautionary regimens it created, enter old age. Everywhere, there is great emphasis upon therapy and rehabilitation as means to maintain maximum function for as long as possible. Cost factors in populations in which the over-eighties are the fastest-growing age-cohort provide a constant stimulus for such approaches.[52]

It should also, however, be noted that research indicates that a majority of people surviving to their eighties and nineties do not suffer from acute illness and regard themselves as in good health and capable of a satisfactory degree of independent activity. For most, even at high ages, death is not preceded by a long period of invalid dependence. Also, even at these later ages, health experience is strongly influenced by class, gender, and ethnic background as well as by age in itself.[53]

The irony of modern medicine is that the least-valued medical specialism takes up most of general practitioners' time and fills most hospital beds (over-65s occupied over half the beds in Britain in the 1980s, though only 2.5 per cent of old people were in hospital at any time[54]). The central problem of geriatric medicine 'is that human beings are in fact mortal, we must die of some terminal event'.[55] It remains as it has been throughout its history, uncertain about how this event is to be approached or managed.

NOTES

1 Note Finley's warning that this text should not be read as accurately conveying the reality of Cicero's own old age or that of his time. Moses I. Finley, 'The elderly in classical antiquity', *Ageing and Society*, 1984, 4: 391–408; reprinted from *Greece and Rome*, October 1981, 28 (10).

2 Sona Rosa Burstein, 'The historical background of gerontology', part 1, *Geriatrics*, 1955, 10: 189–93, Part 1; Brian Livesley, 'Galen, George III and geriatrics', The Osler Lecture 1975, Worshipful Society of Apothecaries of London, 1975, p. 9.

3 J. A. Burrow, *The Ages of Man: A Study in Medieval Writing and Thought*, Oxford, Clarendon Press, 1988, pp. 12 ff.; Elizabeth Sears, *The Ages of Man. Medieval Interpretations of the Life-cycle*, Princeton, NJ, Princeton University Press, 1986, pp. 14 ff; Livesley, op. cit. (n. 2); Gerald G. Gruman, 'Longevity', in Philip P. Wiener (ed.), *Dictionary of the History of Ideas*, New York, Scribner's, 1973, Vol. III, pp. 89–90.

4 Burrow, op. cit. (n. 3), *passim*; Sears, op. cit. (n. 3), *passim*; H.-J. von Kondratowitz, 'The medicalization of old age: continuity and change in Germany from the late eighteenth to the early twentieth century', in M. Pelling and R. M. Smith (eds), *Life, Death and the Elderly. Historical Perspectives*, London, Routledge, 1991, pp. 134–64.

5 Gruman, op. cit. (n. 3); Burstein, op. cit. (n. 2): 536–40, Part 3.

6 Burrow, op. cit. (n. 3); Sears, op. cit. (n. 3), *passim*; Samuel C. Chew, *The Pilgrimage of Life (1485–1642)*, New Haven, CT, Yale University Press, 1962.

7 Burrow, op. cit. (n. 3), Sears, op. cit. (n. 3).

8 Burstein, op. cit. (n. 2): p. 328.

9 Charles Webster, *The Great Instauration. Science, Medicine and Reform, 1626–1660*, p. 246; Gruman, op. cit. (n. 3); Sona Rosa Burstein, 'The foundations of geriatrics', *Geriatrics*, 1957, 12: 494.

10 Gerald G. Gruman, 'The rise and fall of prolongevity hygiene, 1558–1873, *Bulletin of the History of Medicine*, 1961, 35: 221–5.

11 Creighton Gilbert, 'When did a man in the Renaissance grow old?', *Studies in the Renaissance*, 1967–8, 14: 7–32.

12 Livesley, op. cit. (n. 2), pp. 11–12.

13 J. O. Leibowitz 'Early accounts in geriatric pathology (Leonardo, Harvey, Keill)', *Koroth*, 1980, 7: ccliv-cclvi.

14 Gruman, op. cit. (n. 10), p. 225; Livesley op. cit. (n. 2), p. 15.

15 Webster, op. cit. (n. 9), pp. 247 ff.

16 Burstein, op. cit. (n. 9), p. 494.

17 J. T. Freeman, 'François Ranchin. Contributor of an early chapter in geriatrics', *Journal of the History of Medicine*, 1950, 5: 422–31.

18 Webster, op. cit. (n. 9), p. 249.

19 Webster, op. cit. (n. 9), p. 255.

20 Webster, op. cit. (n. 9), pp. 268 ff.

21 F. D. Zeman, 'Pathologic anatomy of old age. Notes on the development of our knowledge', *Archives of Pathology*, 1952, 73: 52.

22 J. Schouten 'Gerard van Swieten, a pioneer in the field of geriatrics', *Gerontologica Clinica*, 1974, 16: 231–5.

23 Livesley, op. cit. (n. 2), p. 17.

24 Gruman, op. cit. (n. 10), pp. 226–7; von Kondratowicz, op. cit. (n. 4).

25 William Godwin, *Enquiry Concerning Political Justice* (1793), quoted in Gruman, op. cit. (n. 3), p. 92.

26 M. J. de Condorcet, *History of the Progress of the Human Mind* (1793), quoted in Gruman, op. cit. (n. 3), p. 92.

27 P. Stearns, 'Old women: some historical observations', *Journal of Family History*, 1980, 5 (1): 46.

28 V. Bullough and C. Campbell, 'Female longevity and diet in the Middle Ages', *Speculum*, 1980, 55: 317–25.

29 Von Kondratowitz, op. cit. (n. 4).

30 Peter N. Stearns, *Old Age in European Society*, London, Croom Helm, 1977, pp. 80–118; Zeman, op. cit. (n. 21), pp. 131–2.

31 Livesley, op. cit. (n. 2), p. 54.

32 T. H. Howell, 'Geriatrics one hundred years ago', *Medical History*, 1973, 17: 199–203.

33 Livesley, op. cit. (n. 2), p. 26; von Kondratowitz, op. cit. (n. 4), p. 155.

34 J. T. Freeman, 'Nascher: excerpts from his life, letters and works', *Gerontologist*, 1961, 1: 17–26.

35 Sona Rosa Burstein, 'Lillien Jane Martin, pioneer in old age rehabilitation', *Medicine Illustrated*, 1950, 4 (2): 8290; 1950, 4 (3): 153–8.

36 Gruman, op. cit. (n. 3), p. 93.

37 As Hopkins has commented, in discounting claims of immense longevity in parts of the Roman Empire: 'The number of claimed centenarians in a population can often be considered a function of illiteracy rather than of longevity'; Keith Hopkins, 'On the probable age structure of the Roman population', *Population Studies*, 1966–7, 20: 247.

38 Pat Thane, 'The declining birth-rate in Britain: the "menace" of an ageing population, 1920s–1950s', *Continuity and Change*, 1990, 5: 283–305.

39 Sona Rosa Burstein, 'Gerontology: a modern science with a long history', *Postgraduate Medical Journal*, July 1946: 3–5.

40 Ministry of Health, *Report of the Committee of Enquiry into the Cost of the National Health Service*, Cmnd 9660, London, HMSO, 1956, p. 40.

41 T. H. Howell, *Our Advancing Years. An Essay on Modern Problems of Old Age*, London, Phoenix House, 1953, pp. 131–48.

42 Charles Webster, 'The elderly and the early National Health Service', in Pelling and Smith, op. cit. (n. 4), pp. 165–93.

43 Ivor Felstein, *Later Life: Geriatrics Today and Tomorrow*, Harmondsworth, Pelican, 1969, pp. 13–34.

44 T. H. Howell, *Old Age. Some Practical Points in Geriatrics*, 3rd edn, London, H. K. Lewis, 1975, p. 101.

45 Zeman, op. cit. (n. 21), p. 48.

46 J. L. Avorn, 'Medicine: the life and death of Oliver Shay', in A. Pifer and L. Bronte, *Our Aging Society*, London and New York, W. W. Norton, 1986, pp. 290–2.

47 Anthea Tinker, *The Elderly in Modern Society*, London, Longman, 1981, p. 74.

48 Kenneth Hazell (ed.), *Social and Medical Problems of the Elderly*, 4th edn, London, Hutchinson, 1976, pp. 12, 15, 40–1; 1st edn, 1960.

49 Livesley, op. cit. (n. 2), p. 29.

50 Avorn, op. cit. (n. 46), pp. 283–96.

51 Tinker, op. cit. (n. 47), pp. 58–79.

52 Avorn, op. cit. (n. 50).

53 C. Victor, 'Continuity or change? Inequalities in health in later life', *Ageing and Society*, 1991, 11 (1): 23–40; M. Bury and A. Holme, 'The challenge of the oldest old', in M. Bury and J. MacNicol (eds), *Aspects of Ageing*, Department of Social Policy and Social Science, Royal Holloway and Bedford New College, Social Policy papers, no. 3, 1990, pp. 129–52.

54 Tinker, op. cit. (n. 47), p. 74.

55 Avorn, op. cit. (n. 46), p. 295.

FURTHER READING

Burrow, J. A., *The Ages of Man. A Study in Medieval Writing and Thought*, Oxford, Clarendon Press, 1988.

Burstein, Sona Rosa, 'The historical background of gerontology', *Geriatrics*, 1955, 10: 189–93, Part 1; 1955, 10: 325–9, Part 2; 1955, 10: 536–40, Part 3.

Comfort, A., *The Process of Ageing*, London, Weidenfeld & Nicolson, 1965.

Grmek, M. D., *On Aging and Old Age*, The Hague, Vitgeveris Dr W. Junk, 1958.

Gruman, G. R., 'A history of ideas about the prolongation of life: the evolution of prolongevity hypotheses to 1800', *Transactions of the American Philosophical Society*, 1966: 3–102.

Jefferys, M. (ed.), *Growing Old in the Twentieth Century*, London, Routledge, 1989.

Laslett, P., *A Fresh Map of Life: the Emergence of the Third Age*, London, Weidenfeld & Nicolson, 1989.

Libow, L. S., 'From Nascher to now. 75 years of American geriatrics', *Journal of the American Geriatric Society*, 1990, 38 (1): 79–83.

Pelling, M. and Smith R. M., *Life, Death and the Elderly. Historical Perspectives*, London, Routledge, 1991.

Pifer, A. and Bronte, L., *Our Aging Society*, London and New York, W. W. Norton, 1986.

Sears, Elizabeth, *The Ages of Man. Medieval Interpretations of the Life Cycle*, Princeton, NJ, Princeton University Press, 1986.

Tinker, A., *The Elderly in Modern Society*, London, Longman, 1981.

Webster, C., *The Great Instauration. Science, Medicine and Reform, 1626–1660*, London, Duckworth, 1975; esp. Section IV, 'The prolongation of life'.

PART VI

MEDICINE IN SOCIETY

47

THE HISTORY OF THE MEDICAL PROFESSION

Toby Gelfand

The history of the medical profession, taken in its broadest sense, is virtually coterminous with the history of medicine. It comprises the cognitive component around which medical personnel define their profession; that is, the history of medical knowledge, the ethical component regulating relationships between practitioners and between practitioners and patients, and the various institutional arrangements, especially schools and societies, by which medicine propagates and perpetuates itself. One recurrent theme throughout the history of the medical profession has been the effort to define who is a member and who is not, on the basis of these three criteria of knowledge, ethics, and institutional organization.

ANTIQUITY: THE ORIGINS OF THE PROFESSION

Little need be said about the period of antiquity because of the ill-defined or, at any rate, historically obscure nature of professional organization. Greek medicine had an extensive knowledge base in the Hippocratic Corpus, which also included several treatises dealing with ethical issues, the best known of which is the *Oath*. There were putative 'schools' of medicine such as that on the island of Cos, the birthplace of Hippocrates (*c.*450–370 BC). Evidently, the better-trained physicians found posts as resident or 'public doctors' whose presence was retained by a community for a fee.[1] Later, Alexandria established a reputation as a leading medical centre. And in the centuries following the lifetime of Galen (AD 129–*c.*200/210), ancient and, eventually, medieval medical knowledge coalesced around the synthesis made possible by the voluminous writings of that author.[2]

But the status of medicine in Roman antiquity indicated its limitations as much as its successes in becoming a profession. Medical schools tended to be *ad hoc* arrangements loosely organized around the founding persona of a physician but lacking any secure institutional structure; nor, with the exception of the body established by the Emperor at Rome in AD 368 and concerned only with the selection of public doctors, were there provisions for licensing or regulation. In general, the educated laity held a rather low opinion of medical practitioners. At times considered a liberal art, the study of medicine became part of an educated man's general knowledge, while medical practice, particularly manual skills comprising surgery, were looked down upon and regulated to social subordinates such as foreigners or slaves.[3]

Professional fragmentation also stemmed from the various sects like the Dogmatists, Empiricists, and Methodists, each of which held philosophically distinct points of departure with radically different roles for anatomy in medical epistemology. The Methodist position, in particular, with its assumption that an adequate physician could be trained in a relatively brief tenure of six months, did little to enhance medicine's pretensions to be a learned profession. Although Galen rejected narrow sectarianism and in part overcame its divisiveness by asserting anatomical rationalism as the basis for a synthesis, the practice of medicine in antiquity remained open to secular and religious healers of all kinds. Galen himself was sympathetic to religious healing carried on in hundreds of temples of Asclepius throughout the ancient world. The Hippocratic Corpus, while resolutely naturalistic, reflected diverse authors and points of view without any consensus as to the distinguishing marks of a medical professional. The closest a Hippocratic author comes to this kind of category is in the treatise *On the Sacred Disease*, where pejorative reference is made to 'conjurors, purificators, mountebanks, and charlatans' who might, under the guise of religious healing, use incantations to compete with secular physicians in treating epilepsy as a sacred or divine disease.

THE MIDDLE AGES: THE INFLUENCE OF THE UNIVERSITIES

Medical knowledge found a home in the medieval monastery, beginning with the monastic schools of the Benedictine order at the end of the sixth century. Latin versions of works attributed to Hippocrates, Dioscorides (*c*.40–*c*.90 AD), Galen, and Caelius Aurelianus (fifth century AD) formed the basis of medical knowledge at the monasteries and early urban centres such as Ravenna and Bordeaux. Cathedral schools offering instruction in medicine emerged by the end of the ninth century at Rheims and especially at Chartres. Professional terminology from that time suggests the beginning of a distinction between physicians, surgeons, and apothecaries. The school at Salerno acquired an outstanding reputation, particularly following its assimilation of translations from Arabic medical authors in the eleventh century. During the ensuing centuries, prior to the founding of the universities, Salerno became renowned as the foremost centre for medical theory and practice; its 'masters' engaged in some form of organized instruction based on textual commentaries, animal dissection, and surgical interventions.[4]

Medicine became institutionalized within the medieval university during the twelfth and thirteenth centuries. Together with theology and the law, medicine took its place as one of the higher faculties in the corporate university structure constituted by the legal association of teachers and/or students. The now-familiar trappings of academia – a graded curriculum based on classic texts in Latin, a series of examinations, theses, fees, and ceremonies to mark advancement from bachelor, to licentiate, to doctorate or master – conferred a sense of professional identity within the framework of the Christian university. (➤ Ch. 48 Medical education) At Montpellier, Paris, Bologna, Oxford, Cambridge, and their successors throughout Europe, a reasonably uniform body of doctrine embraced knowledge of the diagnosis and treatment of disease, including such subjects and techniques as uroscopy, pulse lore, astrology, humoral theory, anatomy, bloodletting and other surgical procedures. Codes of etiquette governing relationships with patients and colleagues, versions of what became known as the Hippocratic Oath for graduating students, and other deontological conventions applying to autopsies, plagues, and the public responsibility of physicians strengthened the professional project.[5] (➤ Ch. 37 History of medical ethics)

The example of Bologna epitomizes the status of medicine as a learned profession within the medieval university. During the late thirteenth century, under the leadership of Taddeo Alderotti (c.1210–95), a man who had risen from humble social origins to become a learned and wealthy medical professor, a secular medical profession coalesced around innovative scholarship.[6] Going beyond the relatively elementary treatises which had up until then constituted the medical curriculum, the Bologna masters introduced sophisticated Aristotelian natural science and philosophy, new and more complex Galenic works, and the *Canon* of Avicenna (980–1037). These greatly expanded the domain of medical theory and debate. Taddeo and his pupils also included surgery in their teaching and practice (unlike the northern European universities) and introduced formal anatomical dissection of the human cadaver to the curriculum. (➤ Ch. 5 The anatomical tradition) Medical practice remained the ultimate goal of their interests, even though clinical experience does not seem to have been included in the requirements for the degree at Bologna as it was at Montpellier. Drawing upon their medical practice, the Bologna masters produced hundreds of *consilia* or written responses to individual patient requests for their professional advice. The *consilia* formed a basis for teaching by case example and probably derived from earlier analogous methods used by the law faculty at Bologna. Emerging secular professions of law and medicine also collaborated when it came to the determination of the cause of death by autopsy, and various public-health concerns such as the certification and status of lepers or the establishment of quarantine in the wake of the Black Death of the mid-fourteenth century. (➤ Ch. 51 Public health; Ch. 52 Epidemiology)

Learned medical professionals drew their clients from among the only members of society who could afford their fees, the narrow segment of upper classes. Indeed, it was royalty – the Norman king Roger in 1140 and the Holy Roman Emperor Frederick II (r. 1212–50) a century later – who promulgated early statutes for the examination and licensure of medical practitioners by the Salernitan masters. Within the medieval universities, religious authorities, ultimately representing the Pope, conferred the licence to practise. But the vast bulk of the population, constituted by the rural masses and urban poor, had little access to physicians. To the extent that they availed themselves of any professional medical services, they had recourse to barber-surgeons, apothecaries, midwives, and various empirics or 'specialists', including bone-setters, oculists, hernia experts, tooth-drawers, and so on. During the late medieval period, some of these practitioners organized themselves in craft guilds, at times in affiliation with other artisans. In principle, they were subordinate to medical faculties, but, in practice, they had a good deal of autonomy. At Florence, a single guild, that of doctors, apothecaries, and grocers, founded in 1293, encompassed diverse kinds of practitioners.[7]

The guilds too were largely an urban phenomenon, and they were to be the main professional source of ordinary healers down through the modern period. Their statutes dealt with apprenticeship, examinations to move up the hierarchy from journeyman to master, standards of licensing and practice for various levels of healers, the protection and security of families of guild members, all with the ultimate aim and hope of enforcing a shaky, if legal, claim to exclusive control over practice.

Women, with the exception of midwives, were mainly excluded from the healing guilds, as they were from the university medical faculties. Some evidence, however suggests professional recognition of women surgeons by the medieval Paris surgical guild, and a surgical manuscript by the British physician John of Arderne (1307–c.1390), depicts women engaged in a number of procedures. Women practised extralegally, but effectively enough to pose a threat to the medical faculties, as a suit brought against one Jacqueline Félicie by the Paris faculty in 1322 indicates.[8]

Although learned physicians at times achieved renown on an individual basis as surgeons – some, like Guy de Chauliac (d. 1368), were even clerics – the institutional cleavage between physicians and surgeons became more pronounced as each group developed its own professional structures. The church, under whose jurisdiction university medicine fell, formally prohibited its members to engage in procedures involving bloodshed or the risk of a fatal outcome. Until the mid-fifteenth century, ecclesiastical marriage prohibitions applied to physicians of the Paris medical faculty, even though few faculty doctors remained full-fledged clergy; until the end of the sixteenth century, 'bachelors' of the faculty had to swear an oath of celibacy.[9] (➤ Ch. 61 Religion and medicine)

Bloodletting, wound-dressing, major surgical procedures like amputations and anything else deemed part of 'external medicine', such as skin and venereal diseases and obstetrics, thus belonged largely to the practice of non-university-trained members of guilds. (➤ Ch. 40 Physical methods) Apart from small groups of surgeons with academic pretensions in the largest cities, like the so-called 'long-robe' surgeons of Paris whose confraternity of Saint-Côme originated in the early fourteenth century, professional surgery was in the hands of barber-surgeons' guilds, which emerged in both Paris and London in the early years of the fourteenth century. Guild healers, rather than the learned physicians, became familiar practitioners to the bulk of the population.[10] But even the most talented of the guild barber-surgeons tended to eschew certain major operations like lithotomy, which had a high mortality, leaving such work to travelling empirical 'specialists' down through the early modern period. (➤ Ch. 41 Surgery (traditional))

THE INFLUENCE OF THE RENAISSANCE

Renaissance medicine saw a renewal and expansion of the cognitive base upon which a learned profession could draw. The recovery of Galenic anatomy and physiology via the preparation of new texts translated directly from Greek into Latin, and the naturalist thrust of Renaissance art gave impetus to human dissection and led to the criticism and, ultimately, the undermining of the authority of ancient knowledge. Major scientific innovations epitomized by the publication of *De Humani Corporis Fabrica* (1543) by Andreas Vesalius (1514–64) and *De Motu Cordis* (1628) by William Harvey (1578–1657), although they constituted revolutions against Galenic anatomy and physiology, respectively, were the work of learned physicians thoroughly conversant with and respectful of the tradition they called in question. Each man also exemplified an elevated standing for experiential and, in the case of Harvey, fully experimental epistemology in the acquisition of medical knowledge. Thus it is not surprising that both deplored the division between head and hand that had become institutionalized in separate professions of medicine and surgery, and both urged physicians not to scorn manual functions by delegating them to subordinates. Finally, as royal physicians to the rulers of Spain and

England, respectively, Vesalius and Harvey also represented a new locus of medical professional patronage, around the early modern nation-state as opposed to the medieval church. (➤ Ch. 7 The physiological tradition)

The career of another Renaissance medical personage, Paracelsus (1493–1541), had even more radical implications for medical theory and professional structure. By his frontal attack upon humoral doctrine (➤ Ch. 14 Humoralism) and his categorical rejection of learned authority, he initiated a rift within medicine that bears comparison with the impact of his contemporary, Martin Luther (1483–1546), on the Roman Catholic church. Paracelsus's chemically based theory and practice of medicine provided an alternative to orthodox medicine's reliance on anatomy, humoral pathology, and an essentially botanical therapy. During the latter sixteenth and seventeenth centuries, the Paracelsian option gained a professional following among physicians and apothecaries dissatisfied with Galenism on intellectual and/or social grounds. Paracelsians, or chemical physicians, were particularly conspicuous in northern Europe and in England.[11]

THE EARLY MODERN PERIOD

The early modern period saw a growing association between organized medical practitioners and government at the central as well as municipal levels. In particular, royal patronage of the healing professions came to be significant. At first in Sicily and southern Italy, as early as the turn of the fourteenth century, and then in Spain, beginning in the fifteenth century, royal *protomedicato*, boards of medical men named by the crown, were entrusted with the examination, licensing, and policing of the entire spectrum of health professionals.[12]

Similarly, colleges of physicians, distinct from the university medical faculties and the guilds, and vested with licensing authority, emerged in the university towns of northern Italy, beginning with Pisa, Bologna, and Milan in the fourteenth century. By the early seventeenth century, there were fourteen such colleges. In general, the colleges consisted of a medical élite.[13] The one at Florence, established in 1560 by the Grand Duke of Tuscany, contained only twelve physicians, who were appointed for life. Its jurisdiction over examining and licensing of practitioners for the entire region superseded the traditional authority of the local healing guild; as well, the college served in an advisory capacity to the government, especially on matters of epidemics and public health.[14]

In part because of the extensive implantation of universities in the northern Italian states, their economic prosperity, and the abundance of public and private salaried posts, the density of learned physicians to the population in urban areas and even in the countryside appears to have been substantially higher here than elsewhere in Europe. The Italian cities of the early modern period often had between five and ten medical doctors per 10,000 inhabitants, and even rural areas in Tuscany contained university-trained doctors supported by public funds. By contrast, other European urban centres, such as Paris and London, possessed only two physicians per 10,000 inhabitants and virtually none in the countryside.[15]

THE MEDICAL PROFESSION IN LONDON

In 1518, Henry VIII chartered the London College of Physicians in response to a petition presented by several royal-court physicians and Cardinal Wolsey. The establishment of the college removed the great city from the anomalous position of lacking a medical corporation. Foreign precedents were cited in the founding charter, and it is likely that Henry's humanist physicians had in mind the Italian colleges. The college held examining, licensing, and police powers over medical practice in the City of London and environs. Public health also fell within its purview as a learned advisory body to the crown, and it was no coincidence that the year of its founding was a plague year.

Although the college gained exclusive licensing authority over medical practice in London (with the exception of Oxford and Cambridge degree-holders, who routinely became Fellows), it did not succeed, as did the Italian colleges and other European counterparts, in extending its jurisdiction to a wider region, much less the kingdom. According to the only prior parliamentary legislation (1511), medical professional regulation was the responsibility of bishops in each diocese, aided by medical and surgical examiners. It was thereby hoped that 'a great multitude of ignorant persons', including various artisans, women, and witches, might be deterred from medical practice.[16] Nor did the London college, despite its pretensions of professional dominance, have control over the licensing of subordinate practitioners, namely the surgeons and apothecaries. When royal patronage raised the status of these guilds, individual court physicians may have played key roles, but the new companies, particularly the barber-surgeons and eventually the apothecaries as well, were effectively independent of the college.

The chequered fortunes of the London College of Physicians during the seventeenth century provide a graphic illustration of the linkage between political history and that of the medical profession during what has been aptly termed the 'old medical regime'.[17] Patronage relationships based on socio-cultural values as opposed to collegial associations resting on scientific and technological training and expertise tended to result in a hierarchy of medical professions dominated by physicians rather than the unified, fairly homogeneous profession of modern times. Despite modest numbers (fewer than forty fellows for most of the century), the College of Physicians wielded considerable professional power, thanks to its royal patronage. For the same reason, however, it experienced serious crises during the two political revolutions against the Stuart monarchs in the seventeenth century. Thus the college's regulatory power, the vigour of which enabled the introduction of a malpractice concept into English law and prosecution of hundreds of illegal practitioners, dropped off precipitously during the decades of Civil War and parliamentary rule.[18] (➤ Ch. 69 Medicine and the law) In 1665, the Great Plague of London further compromised claims to monopoly by college physicians; the public perceived them to have fled the city, while chemical physicians and apothecaries remained, many dying with their patients.[19]

Deeper structural changes in Western society and culture were altering the traditional tripartite professional hierarchy in which learned physicians, in principle, presided over artisanal subordinates, the barber-surgeon and apothecary. To remain with the London example, the aspirations of the guilds, encouraged by royal support, resulted in new professional organizations: the Barber-Surgeons' Company, chartered in 1540, became the Royal Company of Surgeons in 1745, and the Royal College of Surgeons in 1800; while the apothecaries gained independence from the grocers in 1618. These 'new men' (the professional medical groups were exclusively male) had ambitious designs on the practice of medicine; apothecaries, in particular, not content merely to prepare and furnish drugs to physicians' prescriptions, provided increasing competition in diagnosing and treating disease during the course of the seventeenth century. In 1704, their existing status as medical practitioners received legal confirmation when the House of Lords found in favour of William Rose, an apothecary, against the College of Physicians. The Rose case virtually ended the physicians' efforts to regulate other healers.[20]

Expansion of the medical market-place, growth of a cash economy, and free competition encouraged under the economic liberalism characteristic of eighteenth-century Great Britain made physicians more vulnerable at the same time as the status of rival healers improved. A graphic illustration of the liberal medical economy in action was the acceleration, particularly from mid-century, of the demand for men-midwives. (➤ Ch. 44 Childbirth) Free competition between medical doctors and surgeons for a large lucrative market in middle-class clients enabled men with a professional surgical background to prevail, while traditional female midwives lost out.[21]

Intellectual developments also had professional consequences. While individual physicians contributed to the 'new science' of the seventeenth century and collectively sought to assimilate iatromechanism (medical theories derived from physical and chemical models), the College of Physicians remained identified, to its detriment, with Galenic medical theory.[22] On broader epistemological grounds, the resurgence of empiricism in the late seventeenth and eighteenth centuries militated against physicians' claims to comprehensive knowledge based essentially upon scholarship rather than experience. Utilitarian, technical, specialized skills increasingly took precedence over knowledge of the classics; the new ideal of a gentleman-physician became one whose 'wit' exceeded his learning.[23] As its power waned, the London College of Physicians conferred its licence upon a greater proportion of practitioners who never became Fellows. But these licentiates could none the less wield considerable professional power. One of them, Thomas Sydenham (1624–89), licensed by the College in 1663 and lacking the MD degree until he was 52 years old, was the most influential English physician of his age. Known as the 'English Hippocrates', Sydenham epitomized the turn toward empirical medical epistemology.

THE MEDICAL PROFESSION IN PARIS

What has been described for the early modern London profession was in some respects even more pronounced in a second important instance: Paris. As with the London College of Physicians, the Paris medical faculty controlled licensing and the regulation of medical practice in the capital. But the Paris medical guild also claimed wider jurisdiction over the entire kingdom, and even ubiquitous prerogatives for its graduates. The Paris faculty constituted a school with the power to determine the content and conditions of professional education in a way that the London college could not.

At least three centuries older than its London counterpart, the small élite of scholarly physicians constituting the Paris faculty maintained a consistently more conservative position regarding medical knowledge and control over guilds of subordinate practitioners.[24] Staunch defenders of Galenic doctrine, the leading Paris physicians refused to recognize the discovery of the circulation of the blood until near the end of the seventeenth century, just as they condemned therapeutic deviance in the form of chemical remedies.

The faculty's rigid adherence to traditional knowledge and practice seems almost worthy of the caricature to which it was subjected by the contemporary royal playwright, Molière. Public perception of the Paris physicians as pedants, coupled with the faculty's own commitment to institutional autonomy, deprived it of the kind of royal patronage the London physicians enjoyed and which the French crown extended to rival medical professionals.[25]

By favouring Montpellier graduates for its own court physicians, the Bourbon monarchy gave its support to a faculty whose reputation for Hippocratic empiricism, Paracelsian chemical doctrines and remedies, and a progressive attitude toward surgery contrasted with Paris.[26] The crown also encouraged surgeons directly. From the mid-seventeenth century, when the small company of Paris academic surgeons had joined the large prosperous guild of barber-surgeons, the king's premier surgeon began to dominate the unified corporation. Following the centralizing monarchical model, this officer asserted his jurisdiction over an extensive network of local communities of barber-surgeons. Royal patronage, via the agency of the premier surgeon and often accompanied by substantial financial support, resulted in new institutions that transformed the status of surgeons in the capital and provincial centres from craftsmen to liberal professionals: a royal college or school (1724) and an academy (1731) in Paris. In 1743, royal legislation terminated the union of Paris surgeons with barbers, required surgeons henceforth to pursue liberal studies, and recognized the effective independence of surgeons from the medical faculty. Paris apothecaries achieved similar, if less dramatic, professional gains later in the century.[27]

THE ENLIGHTENMENT

The London and Paris examples indicate several general phenomena of medical professionalization during the Enlightenment. Subordinate guilds of healers gained status and effective autonomy by means of state patronage. Philosophical empiricism legitimized these practitioners' claims to specialized knowledge and expertise based upon scientific training as well as craft skills even as it called into question the physician's traditional role and education. The Paris surgeons, for example, used empiricist strategies to good effect in their polemics against the medical faculty in the 1740s. Their leading spokesman, François Quesnay (1694–1774), drew upon Enlightenment philosophy and science to support surgical expertise.[28] In return, the *Encyclopédie* of Denis Diderot (1713–84), an epitome of Enlightenment culture, gave conspicuous attention to the achievements of surgeons. A glance at the group-portrait of the barber-surgeons' guild of Amsterdam painted by Rembrandt in 1632 reveals the mercantile success and scientific curiosity of new professional men. Careers such as those of the Hunter brothers, whose modest provincial Scottish origins did not prevent remarkable upward mobility in the medical world of eighteenth-century London, William (1718–83) as a man-midwife and John (1728–93) as a surgeon, illustrated novel opportunities in these fields.[29]

While physicians and surgeons realigned their corporative relationships according to a division of labour between internal and external medicine, the same process encouraged convergence of what had previously been separate professions. Quesnay himself followed an increasingly popular eighteenth-century pattern by adding a medical degree to his surgical mastership. In 1765 the proposal of John Morgan (1735–89) to introduce British corporative distinctions between physic and surgery to colonial Philadelphia met with indifference, but Morgan and his generation of educated physicians generally had training and some experience in surgery. They regarded the two branches of the healing art as partners, while pharmacy remained subordinate to each.[30]

Clinical training in the hospital setting became a more conspicuous part of medical education during the eighteenth century. (➤ Ch. 49 The hospital) Although precedents existed in Renaissance Padua, the clinical project achieved prominent stature only in 1714, when Hermann Boerhaave (1668–1738) used hospital beds for university teaching at Leiden, and his students diffused the practice throughout Europe, particularly to Vienna and Edinburgh.[31] Nevertheless, the formal status of the hospital clinic in professional education remained problematic and ultimately marginal, an option for élite students rather than a requirement. The eighteenth-century hospital had more intimate ties with the surgical profession. In exchange for their work in large urban hospitals, young French surgeons could satisfy guild training requirements, and a mechanism even existed whereby the surgical mastership could be earned by six years' residence and service in the hospital.[32]

Civil hospitals, along with service in the army and navy, afforded opportunities for medical training outside traditional corporate professional structures. Unlike the formal and local requirements of university and guild, the hospital and military provided informal but valuable professional experience on a large scale. Throughout the Austro-Hungarian and German realms, hospital medical officers in effect worked for and derived their legitimacy from central and municipal governments. In eighteenth-century France, as well, state bureaucrats gradually took over the administration of hospitals from the church, transforming them into secular instruments of training and healing.[33] (➤ Ch. 50 The medical institutions and the state) In England and its American colonies, the growth of the voluntary hospital movement resulted in the establishment via private subscriptions of numerous institutions in which clinical training took place. (➤ Ch. 62 Charity before c.1850)

The Englightenment thus saw a medical profession, or rather groups of medical professionals of various backgrounds and designations, whose training and practice were determined less by guild regulations and more by free-market forces. *Laissez-faire*, a doctrine of political economy first propounded in late Enlightenment France by the Physiocratic school, found an application to medical professionalization *avant la lettre*. In 1748, François Quesnay, surgeon-turned-physician and future founder of Physiocracy, argued that *laissez-faire* principles ought to govern whether one chose to practise primarily as a physician or surgeon. But patient demand, he held, determined what kinds of ordinary practitioners would be chosen by common people. On technical, economic, and social grounds, in town and countryside alike, barber-surgeon phlebotomists had captured this market.[34]

In matters of education, *laissez-faire* also overshadowed a prescribed course of professional studies. A proliferation of competing new medical schools in Scotland and on the European continent broke the monopoly of the medieval universities in granting degrees. The growing market in MD degrees, in many cases a venal business, provoked Adam Smith (1723–90), Quesnay's Scottish counterpart as a champion of free enterprise, to question the very principle of exclusive privilege implied by the degree.[35] In any case, superior education on which professional excellence and public reputation could be based had become something acquired outside of official schools, something purchased in the medical market-place in private courses. There, entrepreneurial teachers offered students who could afford their fees opportunities to learn anatomy, midwifery, and surgical operations by dissecting cadavers, and to gain clinical experience on hospital wards.[36]

Outside urban centres and for most of the population in cities as well, medical professionals remained, as they had been since medieval times, barber-surgeons, surgeon-apothecaries, and empirics. The latter, according to common practice in Old Regime France and elsewhere, might hold special 'privileges' or licences for particular procedures and remedies from police, judicial authorities, or even from the medical guilds. Such ordinary practitioners had to cope with competition from a host of non-professional practitioners – clergy, artisans, domestic and folk healers of both sexes – whom the professionals considered 'charlatans' but whose practice seldom met legal obstacles.[37]

Claims of medical corporations to license, regulate, or even define a profession thus became increasingly problematic during the Enlightenment. Central government and free enterprise, each intruding from opposite directions, undermined the power and autonomy of medical guilds. Physicians raised the spectre of 'medical anarchy' in complaining of the wholesale practice of internal medicine by surgeons, while they propounded codes of ethics that sought to reduce the tensions of intraprofessional competition.[38]

Despite substantial progress in empirical knowledge that contributed to as well as helped rationalize a new concept of specialization between doctors and surgeons (adhered to, in practice, only by a small surgical élite), medical knowledge in the eighteenth century did not serve as a basis for professional power. Medical institutions like the Royal College of Physicians of London, which functioned as centres of learning as well as professional regulatory bodies, lost their cognitive role to scientific academies like the Royal Society. In France, the Société Royale de Médecine, a Paris-centred but nationwide medical academy founded with royal funding in 1776, limited itself to the promotion and diffusion of knowledge and did not attempt to extend its authority to medical education or licensing. Numerous medical societies founded in late eighteenth-century London and colonial America – fourteen in New England alone after 1750 – tended to be oriented towards knowledge and self-improvement, and largely ineffectual with respect to professional regulation.[39]

In this professional context, patients enjoyed a number of advantages *vis-à-vis* medical practitioners. First, as had been the case since antiquity, patients tended to be equal or superior to their professional healers in social standing. At the upper levels of the social hierarchy, doctors importuned the patronage of wealthy, influential patients. Comparable economic and social constraints characterized more modest healing transactions as well. Dependency of practitioners on clients rather than collegial bonds between practitioners, was the general pattern. (➤ Ch. 34 The history of the doctor–patient relationship) Given this state of affairs, it is not surprising that professional knowledge too was responsive to patients' needs and expectations. Professional conceptions of disease in humoral, constitutional, or psychological categories were understandable in general terms to the educated public, just as diagnosis and therapy rested on symptoms, signs, and procedures visible to doctor and patient alike. (➤ Ch. 35 The art of diagnosis: medicine and the five senses) Medical knowledge remained, by and large, accessible to educated lay people; gentlemen and ladies of fashion attended public lectures in anatomy, and some pursued their medical interests at the private courses.[40]

THE INFLUENCE OF THE FRENCH REVOLUTION

The French Revolution (1789–99) had enormous consequences for medical professionalization. By abolishing medical institutions, along with the other guilds, universities, and scientific academies of the Old Regime, the Revolution removed obstacles to professional changes already under way. Thus, for a decade, *laissez-faire* medicine prevailed to an unparalleled extent, with practice open to all and no legal distinctions between professional and nonprofessional healers. Upon payment of a fee, virtually anyone could purchase a legal permit to practise. This extreme instance of deregulation or 'radical free field' has remained unmatched in modern Western medical history.[41]

At the same time, the Revolutionary French state introduced new institutions that brought medicine into much closer relationship with and control by government. In 1794, the National Convention decreed the establishment of a central 'school of health' in Paris (parallel, but smaller-scale, schools were formed at Montpellier and Strasburg) to recruit and train 'health officers'. Beyond the immediate medical needs generated by wartime crisis, the Paris school aimed to respond to progressive concepts of medical knowledge and education. Its curriculum embodied a radical empirical epistemology with an emphasis on learning by doing, translated into practical courses in anatomical dissection, laboratory work, and especially clinical courses. Just as the integration with hospitals fulfilled an eighteenth-century professional reform ideal, the common education provided to future physicians and surgeons in the 'health schools' accomplished in tangible and dramatic fashion the movement towards professional unification.[42]

Building upon its success in institutionalizing major reforms like the unification of medicine and surgery and the integration of the hospital clinic, the so-called Paris school became the world centre for medicine during the first half of the nineteenth century. Pathological anatomy, another innovation with eighteenth-century antecedents particularly within surgery, and heavily dependent on the large numbers of cadavers furnished by the state charity hospitals, emerged as the basis for a new science of disease.[43] (➤ Ch. 9 The pathological tradition)

These cognitive developments represented by the Paris school had dividends for medical professionals, especially for élite practitioners and, in that sense, ultimately for the status of the profession generally. Pathological anatomy, for example, broke definitively with the Hippocratic humoral tradition, which still informed professional and lay conceptions of illness and bedside practice. Although it had little, if any, immediate impact on therapy, pathological anatomy had a great deal of meaning for medicine as its first modern science. Disease, in this conception and in contrast with traditional medicine, was local, specific, anatomical, and hidden from view. Professional knowledge could thus claim an epistemological basis whose technical sophistication and instrumental needs excluded lay participation. The pathology of tissues (1800) described by M. F. X. Bichat (1771–1802) even at a gross anatomical level, to say nothing of microscopic anatomy, and the stethoscope (1819), designed by R. T. H. Laënnec (1781–1826) to hear the consequences of lesions of lungs and heart, presumed a new kind of special professional expertise. Doctors were putting themselves in position to know what was wrong with their patients better than the patients themselves. Hospital medicine furthered intellectually, as it always had socially, the power of professionals over patients. In that setting, traditional patient-centred knowledge and patronage became obsolescent.[44] (➤ Ch. 6 The microscopical tradition; Ch. 36 The science of diagnosis: diagnostic technology)

The Napoleonic regime reinstituted professional structure to the Revolutionary reforms in medical ideology and training. In 1803, national laws mandated direct state examination and licensing of two levels of medical practitioner. Doctors of medicine or surgery, who held degrees signifying at least four years of medical-school education, were qualified to practise anywhere in France, while health officers, the recipients of a more-limited practical training, were restricted to rural practice of routine procedures within the geographical locality where they had been examined and certified. In some respects, the health officers represented the successors of the guild barber-surgeons of the Old Regime (themselves tolerated by a 'grandfather' clause to remain in practice), but they differed by their formal training in general medicine and their clear regulation by both the French state and élite medical professionals.

Within little more than a decade, then, the medical profession in France had passed from freedom or absence of professional regulation to a strict, uniform national licensing system, thereby exemplifying models of opposite extremes, a 'Scylla and Charybdis between which most nineteenth-century legislators tried to steer a course'.[45] In those parts of Europe subjected to Napoleonic conquest, medical reforms and the new professional structure travelled with the Empire, to Italy, the Rhineland, and the Low Countries, where they sometimes remained after Waterloo. Within France, despite discontent with the two-tier system and other matters relating to education, medical professional structure remained until 1893 essentially as defined at the beginning of the century. Sharp legal distinctions between professionals and illegal practitioners were enforced by prosecution of the latter; special privileges to practise, characteristic of the Old Regime, were eliminated. The medical profession gained an effective monopoly over urban practice and penetrated the countryside, despite the persistence of traditional lay healers of both sexes. Even in mental disorders, the preserve of the church for centuries, medical specialists had by mid-century established their professional control.[46] (➤ Ch. 21 Mental diseases)

The medical profession in France thus emerged in the early nineteenth century substantially stronger than its Old Regime counterpart, a beneficiary both of unprecedented clinical experience afforded by the hospitals of the capital as well as the battlefields of Europe, and of direct linkage with the modern nation-state. Obviously, a great gap separated élite Paris physicians, who began academic careers by competing for hospital internships and displayed signs of nascent clinical sub-specialization, from humble provincial health officers. But if Charles Bovary, the literary creation of Gustave Flaubert 1821–80, accurately reflected the marginal status and technical limitations of the health officer, Balzac's *médecin de campagne* testified to a new prestige, moral as much as intellectual, of the medical practitioner even in the countryside. In real life, Flaubert knew from personal experience the stature that provincial medical men like his father and brother, both surgeons at the Rouen Hôtel-Dieu, could enjoy. Degree-holders in medicine and surgery never fell below half the profession in numerical terms; and by 1893, when the subordinate cadre of practitioner was legally revoked, health officers had dwindled to less than 10 per cent of the total.

THE PROFESSION IN NINETEENTH-CENTURY BRITAIN

In Great Britain, where no political revolution destroyed the institutional *status quo*, change within the medical professions followed a much more gradual evolutionary process. Unlike in Paris, London physicians and surgeons continued to be licensed by their respective distinct royal colleges. These élite corporations tended to resist professional-reform projects directed at their own antiquated educational and licensing requirements and the reorganization of rank-and-file practitioners nationwide. Until after the mid-nineteenth century, unchecked and uneven licensing authority resided in nearly twenty different institutions.

None the less, *de facto* unification of training had been taking place in private courses and in the seven London general hospitals since the middle of the previous century. With the termination of the Napoleonic Wars, the Paris clinical school became accessible to significant numbers of channel-crossing medical students.[47] 'General practitioner' emerged as a new term for a professional group consisting of surgeon-apothecaries, many of whom held dual licences from the Royal College of Surgeons and the Society of Apothecaries, and medical graduates of the Scottish universities. The aspirations of general practitioners, as reflected in the establishment of several early nineteenth-century professional associations, led to the passage of the Apothecaries' Act (1815), the first parliamentary effort to set standards of professional education throughout England and Wales. The Act has been interpreted as a backlash by the royal colleges against general practitioners, an effort to degrade them by emphasizing apprenticeship training and failing to protect them with effective prohibitions against irregular practitioners . On the other hand, acknowledgement of a role for scientific courses and clinical training signified official state endorsement of progressive modes of education which had long been available. The Act made compulsory what had previously been voluntary.[48]

British toleration of relatively unregulated medical practice, a 'modified free field' in which licensed practitioners, although privileged, did not enjoy a legal monopoly, made the profession particularly vulnerable economically, and lacking in social prestige. 'Overproduction' of general practitioners led to levels of medical density (10.7 per 10,000 inhabitants) in the 1840s for England and Wales nearly twice those that obtained in France, while competition from druggists, chemists, sectarians, and other irregulars was fierce.[49]

The Medical Act of 1858 introduced a single medical register for all legally qualified practitioners, thus reflecting further movement towards professional unification and standardization of training. But the General Medical Council, created to enforce the Act, remained dominated by representatives of the élite corporations. It failed to establish a single portal of entry into the profession, continued to accept a variety of licensing authorities for separate practice of medicine and surgery, and did not abolish unlicensed practice, merely making it illegal for a practitioner to misrepresent himself. The 1858 Act 'was a liberal victory in the sense that it abolished the last vestiges of corporate monopoly while instituting only the weakest form of bureaucratic regulation ... [it] stopped far short of the radical reforms of the French Revolution; where the French had slain the monster of privilege [the medical corporations], the English were content to draw its teeth'.[50]

Not until the 1880s did the British achieve professional unification with combined examinations by the royal colleges in medicine and surgery and certification of general practitioners in medicine, surgery, and midwifery. By then, medical density had fallen to 6.6 per 10,000 inhabitants of England and Wales (still twice the levels of France and Germany). Consultants, the élite physicians and surgeons, consolidated their position in hospitals by gaining control over medical matters formerly decided by lay administrators, ranging from clinical teaching to the appointment of personnel.[51]

None the less, the social prestige of medical men according to the British gentlemanly ideal remained inferior to other liberal professionals in law, the ministry, and the military.[52] General practitioners, as ever dependent on patronage-style relationships with middle-class clients, working-class sick clubs, and poor-law practice, often struggled to make a living. Despite marked stratification within the profession, the Medical Amendment Act (1886) evidenced unification. The practice of referral, by means of which patients could only gain access to a consultant via a general practitioner, became an accepted ethical principle in the late nineteenth century. This made for a unifying interdependence between the two levels of a profession in which 'the physician and surgeon retained the hospital but the general practitioner retained the patient'.[53]

The specific structure of the medical profession, its relationship with state authority, and its legal entitlement to monopoly varied with a given country's political culture. Thus France, under Napoleon and subsequent regimes, fostered a tightly regulated medical monopoly with legislation against illegal practice, whereas British commitment to liberal principles of political economy militated against legal prohibition of extraprofessional healers. The eighteenth-century medical liberalism of Adam Smith found a resounding echo in that of Herbert Spencer (1820–1903) in the 1840s; the possession of a medical degree and membership on the Royal Commission on the Medical Acts did not prevent Thomas Henry Huxley (1825–95) from declaring in the 1880s that, when it came to one's choice of a doctor, government should not interfere, but rather 'let everybody do as he likes'. In 1909,

Parliament passed a law which, in fact, did away with compulsory vaccination.[54]

INTERNATIONAL TRENDS IN THE
NINETEENTH CENTURY

The situation of the medical profession in Germany combined aspects of the French and British models. Prussia, the Austro-Hungarian Empire, and other German-speaking states inherited a tradition from the eighteenth century of centralized regulation with an extensive system of medical police or public-health officers. Medical practitioners, like young Robert Koch (1843–1910), were often civil servants living on government stipend. Illegal practice was forbidden by the penal code. On the other hand, in 1869 Prussia, and, shortly thereafter, a united Germany, adopted the free field. As in Britain, broader political and cultural values associated with freedom of trade, occupations, and opposition to state paternalism promoted freedom of healing (*Kurierfreiheit*). Social democrats, like the pathologist Rudolf Virchow (1821–1902), and conservatives like Chancellor Bismarck (1815–98) both opposed medical professional monopoly. Aided by their own aggressive political action, unlicensed healers practising parallel types of medicine flourished in Germany during the last two decades of the nineteenth century and had the state on their side until the Nazi period.[55]

Despite variations in professional structure from country to country related to political and cultural particularism, certain convergences on an international scale were evident by the time the international medical scientific congresses began to meet in the late 1860s. Most countries had a two-tier medical profession: an élite, at the summit of which were academics and hospital-based specialists; and a broad spectrum of practitioners of lesser training and status. But, in contrast to the diverse medical corporations of earlier centuries, professional training and organization had become increasingly standardized and unified under the control of the élite. This group set the standards for subordinate practitioners, gradually reduced their numbers, and ultimately abolished their legal status. Prussia eliminated second-class surgeons in 1852, when a single title joined physicians and surgeons; Great Britain legally unified its general practitioners in 1886, after their numbers had fallen by half relative to the population over the previous four decades; and France abolished the subordinate category of health officer in 1892, by which time most of them were already gone. In 1905, an international league against charlatanism came into being, and two decades later, a report including nearly 200 countries revealed that more than 90 per cent had legislation prohibiting unlicensed practice; among developed nations, there were only two (the

United Kingdom and Germany) that did not.[56] (➤ Ch. 59 Internationalism in medicine and public health)

During the course of the nineteenth century, national medical societies were established in most countries, with the conspicuous exception of Germany (in 1832, the Provincial Medical and Surgical Association, which became the British Medical Association in 1856; in 1847, the American Medical Association (AMA); in 1858, the Association Générale des Médecins de France; in 1867, the Canadian Medical Association). A sign of heightened professional consciousness and solidarity, the national societies explicitly sought, among other goals, to defend their interests against irregular healers. By the early twentieth century, they had established their authority in terms of numerical strength, being a majority of practitioners instead of the embattled minorities they had been at their origins, and as vehicles for reform under the banner of scientific medicine.

Even in Tsarist Russia, where the medical profession differed sharply from Western counterparts, doctors held particularly unenviable collective status as salaried servants of the state. Reforms after mid-century culminated in the foundation of the Pirogov Medical Society (1881). This national society commemorated and dedicated itself to the goals of N. I. Pirogov (1810–81), a professor of surgery who represented élite scientific medicine as well as social and humanitarian reform of practice based upon science. In *Uncle Vanya*, Anton Chekhov (1860–1904), himself a some-time government or *zemstvo* medical officer, testified to the enhanced scientific and social prestige of the Russian profession at the turn of the century.[57] (➤ Ch. 65 Medicine and literature)

If the economic and social circumstances of nineteenth-century medical professionals ran the gamut from the upward mobility of the *nouveau riche* to the continuing marginality of the mass of practitioners, the cultural authority of the profession attained unprecedented heights by the closing decades of the century. Bernard Shaw (1856–1950) exclaimed: 'Have we lost faith? "Certainly not; but we have transferred it from God to the General Medical Council" '.[58] Shaw posed the 'doctor's dilemma' in terms of moral choices over whose lives doctors should save, choices made possible by advances in medical science. His contemporaries, whether creative artists or professional leaders, satirical social critics or self-interested apologists, concurred that medical power was in the ascendancy and that its source, for better or for worse, derived from scientific progress.[59]

Universal human experiences as basic as birth and death, formerly mediated by folk and religious practices, shifted to a medical context. (➤ Ch. 30 Folk medicine) Public health, an arena for progressive lay-reform leadership during the first part of the century, became a field of applied medical science and technology. Civic action, as embodied in leagues against tuberculosis, alcoholism, and venereal disease, came increasingly under the auspices of professional medical men. Legislation dealing with prevention, diagnosis, and treatment of communicable diseases privileged community or state welfare over individual or private interests. In practice, class distinctions limited the application of such measures. But the extreme case, the coercive authority of professional medicine to 'inspect' and treat prostitutes in a campaign against venereal disease (a measure adopted in limited fashion for a time even in liberal Great Britain under the euphemism, Contagious Diseases Acts), showed the lengths to which professional intervention could go.[60] (➤ Ch. 26 Sexually transmitted diseases) In a more benign mode, new industries created opportunities for middle-class medical professionals to have an impact on the lives of working-class populations: the chief physician of a French railroad company, for example, estimated that a total of some 600,000 persons (workers and families) had access to approximately 1,500 physicians employed by that industry. Doctors, he concluded, fortified by scientific truth, served the nation by defending 'not only sanitary interests, but also social and political interests', and by exerting a favourable moral influence.[61]

SCIENCE AND THE MEDICAL PROFESSION: THE UNITED STATES EXPERIENCE

Substituting secular, material values for traditional spiritual ones, Western society embarked on what has been characterized as a process of medicalization in which the medical profession acted as agent and beneficiary of new cultural attitudes and practices.[62] For contemporaries, it seemed obvious that science was responsible for medicine's new stature. In retrospect, the connection between science and professionalization appears much more problematic. On the one hand, modern professional structures sometimes developed, as the example of France indicates, before the advent of modern laboratory medical sciences. On the other hand, the take-off in experimental physiology, pathology, and bacteriology after the middle of the nineteenth century had little direct or immediate impact on reducing mortality from disease. With the significant exception of antiseptic surgery, conceptual breakthroughs epitomized by the experimental physiology of Claude Bernard (1813–78), the cellular pathology of Rudolf Virchow, and the germ theory of Louis Pasteur (1822–95) and Robert Koch did not produce a revolution in medicine's ability to cure. Physicians did not possess the power over life and death often claimed by them and attributed to them by the public. Aside from a few ailments, like diphtheria and rabies, they remained helpless against most diseases. (➤ Ch. 42 Surgery (modern); Ch. 16 Contagion/germ theory/specificity; Ch. 11 Clinical research)

This is not meant to deny any relationship between science and professionalization, only that the relationship was complex, rather than one of straightforward cause and effect. Science did transform nineteenth-century medicine or, it might be better put, the medical profession incorporated and used science to transform itself. By the closing decades of the century, the profession and public shared an expectation of therapeutic power derived from science, if not the power itself. In this respect, and by providing a cogent causal explanatory framework, germ theory, in particular, yielded enormous dividends for the medical profession.[63] More generally, the profession availed itself of the cultural prestige of science; it appropriated scientific positivism and its optimistic faith in progress through materialist and reductionist approaches. Nowhere was this more graphically illustrated than in the rise of the specialties of psychiatry and neurology after mid-century. What had once been sins or troubles of the soul, the domain of theology, became pathology of the brain and nervous system, the province of physicians. In making good its claim to jurisdiction over emotional life, including defining milder neuroses like hysteria and neurasthenia, as well as frank insanity, the profession in effect reduced the mind to the body and extended its power considerably.[64] (➤ Ch. 56 Psychiatry)

The process of interaction between science and the medical profession may be fleshed out by reviewing developments in the United States, where a striking transformation occurred over a relatively brief period. Based upon eighteenth-century precedents, notably that set by New Jersey, many states vested licensing and regulatory powers in medical societies. But by the middle of the following century, such professional authority, fragile at best, had virtually disappeared. New states failed to enact licensing regulations, while legislation was repealed where it had formerly been in place, resulting in the least-regulated system in the Western world.[65]

The reasons for this situation were many and varied. In the first place, an effective licensing system for medical practitioners, apart from a relatively small élite in the eastern centres, had never really been workable. A mid-century survey of eastern Tennessee showed, for example, that only 17 per cent of 'physicians' were medical graduates, while about half of those practising medicine had received no instruction other than 'reading'.[66] Barbed criticism, as well as jokes at the expense of the low social and intellectual level of medical students, were commonplace. Second, medical degrees became recognized as equivalent to licensure, and thus legal certification shifted from societies to proliferating numbers of inferior private or proprietary schools, most of which lacked all but the most rudimentary facilities and standards.

Third, the growth of rival organised medical groups or sects with distinctive theoretical and therapeutic systems successfully challenged professional claims to exclusive legitimacy of doctrine and practice. The emergence of homoeopathy and Thomsonianism posed serious threats to all levels of regular practitioners: the homoeopaths' competition with urban élite physicians took the form of separate institutions and specialization. Regular medicine was now allopathy, simply another sect. Thomsonian herbal medicine appealed to a broad base of rural clientele.[67] Finally, the Thomsonians in particular, with effective marketing of do-it-yourself healing and political lobbying in a populist vein, tapped into the cultural ethos known as Jacksonian democracy. Individualist, anti-intellectual, antimonopolist ideologies promoted free-enterprise medicine at the expense of professional privilege. (➤ Ch. 28 Unorthodox medical theories)

Within little more than a generation, all this had diametrically changed. In 1888, the Supreme Court of the United States defended the right of states to require a professional licence to practise medicine, and several years later the court explicitly rejected the argument, dear to sectarian medical beliefs, that religious freedom could be invoked to legitimate irregular healers.[68] By then, medical sects were in decline or being incorporated into the regular profession. Those that would arise in the twentieth century, like osteopathy, were exceptions to medical monopoly, rather than serious threats to it as their nineteenth-century predecessors had been.[69]

The formation of a corporate monopoly in American medicine resulted from a multiplicity of contributing factors coming together in the last decades of the nineteenth century. Once again, specific professional change depended upon a larger political and cultural context. A general movement toward regulation, including effective federal government controls as seen in the passage of the Pure Food and Drug Act (1906), limited unrestrained competition at the same time as reliance on experts and bureaucratic efficiency superseded the ideal of democratic individualism. Cultivation, if not a cult of professionalism, rested upon revitalized and new institutions of higher learning, which, in turn, emerged out of the economic prosperity of industrialists-turned-philanthropists.[70] (➤ Ch. 63 Medical philanthropy after 1850)

More specifically, the American medical profession realigned and consolidated itself around a new scientific ideal. Beginning in the 1870s and extending until the outbreak of the First World War, perhaps as many as 15,000 American physicians pursued postgraduate studies in the German-speaking world – then the foremost centre for science and medicine. Not only did their numbers dwarf those of earlier generations of medical migrants to Paris (well under 1,000 during the first half of the century), but the type of medicine they brought back was anchored in experimental science.[71] This was the case whether they had worked on medical science at a university laboratory such as the renowned physiological institute at Leipzig or, as with the majority, acquired experience in a clinical speciality at a hospital centre, of which the leading exemplar was Vienna.

Furthermore – and this was a crucial difference from the pre-Civil War period – the German-trained American physician returned to a society and culture prepared to welcome scientific medicine. Neither the hospital infrastructure nor indigenous American medical culture had permitted the earlier Parisian-trained élite to introduce significant reform of medical education or professional organization. Despite their enthusiasm for Paris-style empiricist epistemology, their own professional identity conformed with that of their less-privileged colleagues in being shaped by expectations of patients and stiff competition from sectarians. The identity of the regular profession remained defined essentially in terms of therapeutic behaviour. In contrast with the homoeopaths and most other sects, regular professional therapy tended to be aggressive and productive of obvious visible effects, even though 'heroic' practices, such as copious bloodletting and purging, gradually yielded to milder 'conservative' interventions during the middle decades of the century.[72] Only after professional and public consensus around science-based medicine did therapeutic behaviour decline as the hallmark of professional identity. Professional medicine now became a matter of knowledge of the putative causes of disease, knowledge in principle obtainable in the laboratory by sophisticated theories and techniques, of which germ theory and the microscope were prototypes. On the basis of aetiological knowledge rather than therapeutic practice, professional physicians claimed to distinguish themselves from lay people and unqualified healers who lacked access to such matters. Although the claim implicitly promised future therapeutic rewards for public confidence in medical science, the American profession ironically found itself in the comfortable position of no longer being judged on its practical performance. Indeed, for the first time, therapeutic scepticism, long fashionable in European medical scientific circles, became acceptable doctrine in America.

The process by which scientific medicine took hold in the United States involved élite-driven reforms on several fronts. On the educational front, a few eastern university medical schools moved to upgrade entrance requirements and make the curriculum longer, more demanding, and scientific. Inspired by the German model of graduate education, the Johns Hopkins University, founded in Baltimore in 1876 with the legacy of a railroad magnate, pioneered the close integration of hospital training (Johns Hopkins University Hospital opened in 1888) and medical school (1893) with university graduate departments. The transformation of American medical schools according to a scientific model, presided over by university presidents and medical school deans, and generously funded by private foundations like the Rockefeller, was firmly in place by the turn of the century. By 1910, when the provocative survey of medical schools appeared, funded by the Carnegie Foundation and known after its author, Abraham Flexner (1866–1959), as the Flexner Report, the tremendous growth in non-university proprietary schools (a peak of 154 medical schools was attained in 1904), so decried in the report, had been stemmed and reversed.[73]

Meanwhile, on the licensing front, the precedent of the Illinois Board of Health (1877) reasserted state jurisdiction over medical practice. By the turn of the century, more than twenty states required an independent examination as well as a medical degree, and had laws on their books to prosecute unlicensed healers. The AMA, itself reorganized to expand its membership nearly ninefold and promote professional reform, led the campaign to establish high standards of state licensing. Through its Council on Medical Education, working closely with the academic medical élite, the AMA in effect drove the remaining proprietary schools out of business. Between 1910 and 1930, the doctor-to-population ratio fell by more than 20 per cent, although at 12 per 10,000, it remained substantially higher than European counterparts.[74]

By the 1920s, the American medical profession had emerged as a powerful corporate monopoly, probably the most influential profession in the country and a leader internationally. Its cultural authority rested on the prestige of experimental science. Appropriated by the academic élite, implanted in the modern medical school and in the university research and teaching hospital, scientism transformed medicine into the most sought-after career and respected profession in the United States. Even those who did not partake directly in the material success of urban specialists – by the early 1940s, specialists constituted a majority of American practitioners – shared the aura of professional prestige. Technological innovations like the telephone and automobile enabled general practitioners to double and triple their clientele, while licensing laws reduced the ranks of outside competitors, and reformed educational standards 'purified' the profession from within. The shift in location of middle-class practice from patients' private homes to doctors' offices and hospitals made possible a much-greater volume of clients even as it symbolized a shift in power relationships toward physicians.[75]

But the darker side to this 'golden age' of the American medical profession ushered in by realization of the ambitious goals called for in the Flexner Report became visible to critics of medical power in the 1960s.[76] The drive toward universalization of élite standards – national board examinations and completion of a post-doctoral hospital internship for licensing were in place by 1930 – made access to the profession much more difficult for disadvantaged minorities. Discrimination against blacks, Jews, and other ethnic or religious minorities took the form of quotas restricting their entry into medical schools, exclusion from medical societies, and denial of hospital privileges to the few who managed to qualify.[77]

The case of women physicians is instructive in this respect. (➤ Ch. 38 Women and medicine) In 1910, the proportion of women in the American medical profession peaked at six per cent of the total, more than double what it had been in 1880, and thereafter declined.[78] Overcoming considerable prejudice, American women had achieved significant gains during the second half of the nineteenth century. In 1849, Elizabeth Blackwell (1821–1910) pioneered by earning a medical degree from a proprietary school in upper New York state, thus breaking the age-old barrier against licensed women physicians in the West. (European centres, like Zurich and Paris, did not follow this precedent until the 1860s.) The following year, the first women's medical school came into being in Philadelphia; women physicians were welcomed by homoeopathic institutions, admitted to local and state medical societies, and continued to establish their own professional structures. They cultivated a presumed 'natural' capacity for healing, believed to be particularly pertinent when it came to ministering to their own sex and to children. (➤ Ch. 45 Childhood) Society, including the male medical profession, legitimated the female physician as an extensions of woman's nurturing role.[79]

The transformation of American medicine undermined this status. Not until 1950 did women recoup the numerical proportion they had attained in the profession at the beginning of the century; dramatic increases in their admission to medical schools only took place in the 1970s after the resurgence of the feminist movement. With Johns Hopkins a somewhat reluctant exception, many élite medical schools refused to admit women until well after the First World War, while separate women's institutions languished or collapsed. That the ethos of nurturing care, which had motivated and benefited women doctors, passed over to nurses is suggested by the spectacular numerical growth of that profession, by nearly tenfold, during the last two decades of the nineteenth century.[80] Female nurses, clearly subordinate to male physicians in the hospital and professional hierarchy, helped define and facilitate the authority of the physician as clinical scientist while they provided inexpensive labour to carry out the day-to-day functioning of hospital patient care.[81] (➤ Ch. 54 A general history of nursing 1800–1900; Ch. 55 The emergence of para-medical professions)

By the 1960s and 1970s, sweeping advances in technologies for diagnosing and treating disease had obviously altered the conditions of medical practice. But the structure of the American profession remained remarkably congruent with what Flexner had prescribed, this despite important changes like the advent of private and limited federal health-insurance schemes and large-scale admission of women medical students. By the early 1990s, medical education and thus the portal of entry to and primary means of socialization of medical professionals continues to espouse a paradigm that began to transform it at the end of the last century, although signs of transition have appeared. Other developed countries, most of which had adopted comprehensive public-health insurance by the post-war years, nevertheless followed a similar pattern of granting considerable autonomy and effective monopoly to a medical profession that rooted its claim to these privileges in the ideology of scientific research and technological progress.[82] Even the entry of large entrepreneurial private corporations into American health care over the last decade has not fundamentally altered this situation. (➤ Ch. 68 Medical technologies: social contexts and consequences)

CONCLUSION

As a result of the perceived and real power of the medical profession, it, along with other 'establishment' institutions, came in for criticism from diverse and often overlapping constituencies. Movements advocating the cause of women, consumers, blacks, psychiatric patients, and counter-cultural critics, epitomized by Ivan Illich's *Medical Nemesis* (1975), attacked organized medicine as insensitive to needs of patients and the collective welfare of society. Mounting health-care costs amid economic hard times have added to the malaise of the medical profession as it strives at the end of the twentieth century to adjust to changing cultural values and expectations. (➤ Ch. 57 Health economics)

This historical survey has illustrated the complexity of such cultural factors in shaping the profession at any given time and place. Generalizations by way of conclusion are elusive. But it has been suggested that in the tension between corporate monopoly at one extreme and 'free field' at the other, political radicalism, economic liberalism, and religious dissent have tended to favour the medical 'free field'.[83] The prestige accorded science and the success of organized medicine in aligning itself around this cognitive base furthered claims to professional monopoly. One may thus interpret the crucial transition whereby mediation of medical knowledge and power shifted from the control of patients to that of professionals in terms of the interaction of science with culture.

NOTES

1 Louis Cohn-Haft, *The Public Physicians of Ancient Greece*, Northhampton, MA, Smith College, 1956.

2 O. Temkin, *Galenism: Rise and Decline of a Medical Philosophy*, Ithaca, NY, Cornell University Press, 1973.

3 Vivian Nutton, 'Murder and miracles: lay attitudes towards medicine in classical antiquity', in Roy Porter (ed.), *Patients and Practitioners*, Cambridge, Cambridge University Press, 1985, pp. 23–53; Vern L. Bullough, *The Development of Medicine as a Profession. The Contribution of the Medieval University to Modern Medicine*, Basle, Karger, 1966, pp. 28–31.

4 Paul O. Kristeller, 'The School of Salerno: its development and its contribution to the history of learning', *Bulletin of the History of Medicine*, 1945, 17: 138–94.

5　Bullough, op. cit. (n. 3).

6　Nancy Siraisi, *Taddeo Alderotti and His Pupils*, Princeton, NJ, Princeton University Press, 1981.

7　Katherine Park, *Doctors and Medicine in Early Renaissance Florence*, Princeton, NJ, Princeton University Press, 1985.

8　Pearl Kibre, 'The faculty of medicine at Paris. Charlatanism, and unlicensed medical practices in the later Middle Ages', *Bulletin of the History of Medicine*, 1953, 27: 1–20.

9　Paul Delaunay, *La Médecine et l'Église*, Paris, Hippocrate, 1948, pp. 64, 76–82.

10　Margaret Pelling, 'Occupational diversity: barber-surgeons and the trades of Norwich, 1550–1640', *Bulletin of the History of Medicine*, 1982, 56: 484–511.

11　Allen G. Debus, *The English Paracelsians*, London, Oldbourne, 1965; P. M. Rattansi, 'The Helmontian-Galenist controversy in Restoration England', *Ambix*, 1964, 12: 1–23.

12　Richard Palmer, 'Physicians and the state in post-medieval Italy', in Andrew W. Russell (ed.), *The Town and State Physician in Europe from the Middle Ages to the Enlightenment*, Wolfenbüttel, Herzog August Bibliothek, 1981, pp. 47–61; José Maria Lopez-Piñero, 'The medical profession in sixteenth-century Spain', ibid., pp. 85–98.

13　Palmer, op. cit. (n. 12).

14　Carlo M. Cipolla, *Public Health and the Medical Profession in the Renaissance*, Cambridge, Cambridge University Press, 1976, pp. 71–2.

15　Ibid., pp. 79–85, 92, 94–6.

16　George N. Clark, *A History of the Royal College of Physicians of London*, Oxford, Clarendon Press, 1964, pp. 54–66.

17　Harold J. Cook, *The Decline of the Old Medical Regime in Stuart London*, Ithaca, NY, Cornell University Press, 1986.

18　Ibid., pp. 20, 276–80.

19　Rattansi, op. cit. (n. 11).

20　H. Cook, 'The Rose Case considered: physicians, apothecaries, and the law in Augustan England', *Journal of the History of Medicine*, 1990, 45: 527–55.

21　Jacques Gélis, *La Sage-femme ou le médecin: une nouvelle conception de la vie*, Paris, Fayard, 1988; Adrian Wilson, 'William Hunter and the varieties of man-midwifery', in W. F. Bynum and Roy Porter (eds.), *William Hunter and the Eighteenth-Century Medical World*, Cambridge, Cambridge University Press, 1985, pp. 343–69.

22　Theodore M. Brown, 'The College of Physicians and the acceptance of iatromechanism in mid-seventeenth century England', *Bulletin of the History of Medicine*, 1970, 44: 12–30.

23　Cook, op. cit. (n. 17), pp. 257–9.

24　Howard M. Solomon, *Public Welfare, Science, and Propaganda in Seventeenth-Century France: the Innovation of Théophraste Renaudot*, Princeton, NJ, Princeton University Press, pp. 162–200.

25　Toby Gelfand, *Professionalizing Modern Medicine: Paris Surgeons and Medical Science and Institutions in the 18th Century*, Westport, CT, Greenwood Press, 1980.

26　Colin Jones, 'The *Médecins de Roi* at the end of the *Ancien Régime* and in the

French Revolution', in Vivian Nutton (ed.), *Medicine at the Courts of Europe,*
1500–1837, London, Routledge, 1990, pp. 209–61, esp. 228–30.

27 Gelfand, op. cit. (n. 25), Chs 4, 5.

28 Toby Gelfand, 'Empiricism and eighteenth-century French surgery', *Bulletin of*
the History of Medicine, 1970, 44: 40–53.

29 Bynum and Porter, op. cit. (n. 21); William S. Heckscher, *Rembrandt's Anatomy*
of Dr. Nicolaas Tulp: an Iconological Study, New York, New York University Press,
1958.

30 Toby Gelfand, 'The origins of a modern concept of medical specialization: John
Morgan's *Discourse* or 1765', *Bulletin of the History of Medicine,* 1976, 50: 511–35;
Eric H. Christianson, 'Medicine in New England', in Ronald L. Numbers (ed.),
Medicine in the New World, Knoxville, University of Tennessee Press, 1987,
pp. 101–53.

31 Guenter B. Risse, *Hospital Life in Enlightenment Scotland: Care and Teaching at*
the Royal Infirmary of Edinburgh, Cambridge, Cambridge University Press, 1986;
Othmar Keel, 'The politics of health and the institutionalization of clinical
practices in Europe in the second half of the eighteenth century', in Bynum and
Porter, op. cit. (n. 21), pp. 207–56.

32 Toby Gelfand, 'Gestation of the clinic', *Medical History,* 1981, 25: 169–80.

33 Louis S. Greenbaum, 'Science, medicine, religion: three views of health care in
France on the eve of the French Revolution', *Studies in Eighteenth-Century Culture,*
1981, 10: 373–91.

34 Toby Gelfand, 'A "monarchical profession" in the Old Regime: surgeons,
ordinary practitioners, and medical professionalization in eighteenth century
France', in Gerald L. Geison (ed.), *Professions and the French State,* Philadelphia,
University of Pennsylvania Press, 1984, pp. 149–80.

35 David L. Cowen, '*Laissez-faire* and licensure in nineteenth-century Britain', *Bull-*
etin of the History of Medicine, 1969, 43: 30–40.

36 Susan C. Lawrence, 'Entrepreneurs and private enterprise: the development of
medical lecturing in London, 1775–1820', *Bulletin of the History of Medicine,*
1988, 62: 171–92; Toby Gelfand, ' "Invite the philosopher as well as the charitable": hospital teaching as private enterprise in Hunterian London', in Bynum
and Porter, op. cit. (n. 21), pp. 129–51.

37 Matthew Ramsey, *Professional and Popular Medicine in France, 1770–1830,* Cambridge, Cambridge University Press, 1988.

38 Ivan Waddington, *The Medical Profession in the Industrial Revolution,* Dublin, Gill
& Macmillan, 1984, Ch. 8; Gelfand, op. cit. (n. 25), p. 151.

39 Christianson, op. cit. (n. 30); Susan C. Lawrence, ' "Desirous of improvements
in medicine": pupils and practitioners in the medical societies at Guy's and St
Bartholomew's hospitals, 1795–1815', *Bulletin of the History of Medicine,* 1985,
59: 89–104; Caroline C. Hannaway, 'The Société Royale de Médecine and
epidemics in the Ancien Régime', *Bulletin of the History of Medicine,* 1972, 46:
257–73; Cook, op. cit. (n. 17).

40 Nicholas Jewson, 'Medical knowledge and the patronage system in eighteenth-
century England', *Sociology,* 1974, 8: 369–85; T. J. Johnson, *Professions and Power,*
London, Macmillan, 1972; Roy Porter, 'Laymen, doctors, and medical knowledge
in the eighteenth century: the evidence of the *Gentleman's Magazine*', in Porter,

op. cit. (n. 3), pp. 283–314; Jonathan Barry, 'Piety and the patient: medicine and religion in eighteenth-century Bristol', ibid., pp. 145–75.

41 Ramsey, op. cit. (n. 37), p. 74; Michel Foucault, *The Birth of the Clinic: an Archaeology of Medical Perception*, trans by A. M. Sheridan Smith, New York, Pantheon Books, 1973, Ch. 3.

42 Gelfand, op. cit. (n. 25), Chs. 8–10.

43 Russell C. Maulitz, *Morbid Appearances: the Anatomy of Pathology in the Early Nineteenth Century*, Cambridge, Cambridge University Press, 1987; Erwin H. Ackerknecht, *Medicine at the Paris Hospital, 1794–1848*, Baltimore, MD, Johns Hopkins Press, 1967.

44 Charles E. Rosenberg, 'The therapeutic revolution: medicine, meaning, and social change in nineteenth-century America', in Morris J. Vogel and Rosenberg (eds), *The Therapeutic Revolution*, Philadelphia, University of Pennsylvania Press, 1979, pp. 3–25.

45 Matthew Ramsey, 'The politics of professional monopoly in nineteenth-century medicine: the French model and its rivals', in Geison, op. cit. (n. 34), pp. 225–305, esp. p. 237.

46 Jan Goldstein, *Console and Classify: the French Psychiatric Profession in the Nineteenth Century*, Cambridge, Cambridge University Press, 1987; George Weisz, 'The politics of medical professionalization in France, 1845–1848', *Journal of Social History*, 1978–9, 12: 3–30.

47 Russell C. Maulitz, 'Channel-crossing: the lure of French pathology for English medical students, 1816–36', *Bulletin of the History of Medicine*, 1981, 55: 475–96; Susan C. Lawrence, 'Science and medicine at the London Hospitals: the development of teaching and research, 1750–1815', unpublished Ph.D. thesis, University of Toronto, 1985.

48 Irvine Loudon, *Medical Care and the General Practitioner, 1750–1850*, Oxford, Clarendon Press, 1987, p. 172; Lawrence, op. cit. (n. 47), Ch. 7; S. W. F. Holloway, 'The Apothecaries Act, 1815: a reinterpretation', *Medical History*, 1966, 10: 107–29, 221–35.

49 Loudon, op. cit. (n. 48), pp. 7, 301.

50 Ramsey, op. cit. (n. 45), p. 248; Loudon, op. cit. (n. 48), pp. 298–300.

51 M. Jeanne Peterson, *The Medical Profession in Mid-Victorian London*, Berkeley, University of California Press, 1978.

52 M. Jeanne Peterson, 'Gentlemen and medical men: the problem of professional recruitment', *Bulletin of the History of Medicine*, 1984, 58: 457–73.

53 Rosemary Stevens as quoted in Loudon, op. cit. (n. 48), p. 301.

54 Ramsey, op. cit. (n. 45), pp. 249–50.

55 Ramsay, op. cit. (n. 45), pp. 255–9, 269–74; Paul Weindling, *Health, Race and German Politics between National Unification and Nazism, 1870–1945*, Cambridge, Cambridge University Press, 1989, pp. 20–5.

56 Ramsey, op. cit., (n 45), pp. 251, 265–6.

57 Nancy M. Frieden, *Russian Physicians in an Era of Reform and Revolution, 1856–1905*, Princeton, NJ, Princeton University Press, 1981, pp. 5–11, 313.

58 Bernard Shaw, *Doctors' Delusions, Crude Criminology and Sham Education*, London, Constable, 1931, p. 1.

59 Gelfand, 'Medical nemesis, Paris, 1894: Léon Daudet's *Les Morticoles*', *Bulletin of the History of Medicine*, 1986, 60: 155–76.

60 Judith R. Walkowitz, *Prostitution and Victorian Society: Women, Class, and the State*, Cambridge, Cambridge University Press, 1980, Ch. 4; Alan M. Brandt, *No Magic Bullet: a Social History of Venereal Disease in the United States since 1880*, New York, Oxford University Press, 1985, Ch. 1.

61 Jules Worms, 'Le médecin dans la société moderne', *Le Scalpel*, 1887, 39: 229–30.

62 Judith W. Leavitt, *Brought to Bed. Childbearing in America 1750–1950*, New York, Oxford University Press, 1986; Evelyn B. Ackerman, *Health Care in the Parisian Countryside, 1800–1914*, New Brunswick, NJ, Rutgers University Press, 1990.

63 Ignaz Semmelweis, *The Etiology, Concept, and Prophylaxis of Childhood Fever*, ed. and intro. by K. Codell Carter, Madison, University of Wisconsin Press, 1983, intro.

64 Goldstein, op. cit. (n. 46).

65 Ramsey, op. cit. (n. 45), pp. 250–54; Richard H. Shryock, *Medical Licensing in America, 1650–1965*, Baltimore, MD, Johns Hopkins Press, 1967, Ch. 1.

66 Shyrock, ibid., pp. 31–2.

67 Alex Berman, 'The Thomsonian movement and its relations to American pharmacy and medicine', *Bulletin of the History of Medicine*, 1951, 25: 405–28, 519–38; Martin Kaufman, *Homeopathy in America*, Baltimore, MD, Johns Hopkins Press, 1971; William G. Rothstein, *American Physicians in the Nineteenth Century*, Baltimore, MD, Johns Hopkins Press, 1972.

68 Ramsey, op. cit. (n. 45), p. 276.

69 Norman Gevitz, 'Sectarian medicine', *Journal of the American Medicial Association*, 1987, 257: 1636–40.

70 Burton J. Bledstein, *The Culture of Professionalism. The Middle Class and the Development of Higher Education in America*, New York, Norton, 1976; E. Richard Brown, *Rockefeller Medicine Men*, Berkeley, University of California Press, 1979.

71 Thomas N. Bonner, *American Doctors and German Universities*, Lincoln, University of Nebraska Press, 1963; Russell M. Jones (ed.), *The Parisian Education of an American Surgeon: Letters of Jonathan Mason Warren, 1832–1835*, Philadelphia, PA, American Philosophical Society, 1978, intro.

72 Rosenberg, op. cit. (n. 44); John Harley Warner, *The Therapeutic Perspective: Medical Practice, Knowledge and Identity in America, 1820–1885*, Cambridge, MA, Harvard University Press, 1986; Martin S. Pernick, *A Calculus of Suffering: Pain, Professionalism, and Anesthesia in Nineteenth-Century America*, New York, Columbia University Press, 1985.

73 Kenneth L. Ludmerer, *Learning to Heal. The Development of American Medical Education*, New York, Basic Books, 1985, esp. Chs 5, 9, 10.

74 Ibid., Ch. 13.

75 Paul Starr, *The Social Transformation of American Medicine*, New York, Basic Books, 1982; Rosemary Stevens, *American Medicine and the Public Interest*, New Haven, Yale University Press, 1971.

76 John C. Burnham, 'American medicine's golden age: what happened to it?', *Science*, 1982, 215: 1474–9.

77 Edward H. Beardsley, *A History of Neglect. Health Care for Blacks and Mill Workers*

in the Twentieth-Century South, Knoxville, University of Tennessee Press, 1987, Ch. 4; George Rosen, *The Structure of American Medical Practice, 1875–1941*, Philadelphia, University of Pennsylvania Press, 1983, pp. 66–78.

78 Mary Roth Walsh, *'Doctors Wanted: No Women Need Apply'*, New Haven, CT, Yale University Press, 1977, Ch. 6, esp. p. 186.

79 Gina Morantz-Sanchez, *Sympathy and Science. Women Physicians in American Medicine*, New York, Oxford University Press, 1985, esp Chs 5–7.

80 Ibid., pp. 240–9, 262.

81 Susan M. Reverby, *Ordered to Care. The Dilemma of American Nursing, 1850–1945*, Cambridge, Cambridge University Press, 1987, Ch. 4; Charles E. Rosenberg, *The Care of Strangers*, New York, Basic Books, 1987, pp. 212–28.

82 Eliot Freidson, *Profession of Medicine*, New York, Dodd, Mead, 1970, pp. 5, 39, 42–3.

83 Ramsey, op. cit. (n. 45), p. 280.

FURTHER READING

Cook, Harold J., *The Decline of the Old Medical Regime in Stuart London*, Ithaca, NY, Cornell University Press, 1986.

Edelstein, Ludwig, *Ancient Medicine*, ed. by O. Temkin and C. Lilian Temkin, Baltimore, MD, Johns Hopkins Press, 1967.

Gelfand, Toby, *Professionalizing Modern Medicine. Paris Surgeons and Medical Science and Institutions in the 18th Century*, Westport, CT, Greenwood Press, 1980.

Loudon, Irvine, *Medical Care and the General Practitioner 1750–1850*, Oxford, Clarendon Press, 1986.

Ludmerer, Kenneth M., *Learning to Heal: the Development of American Medical Education*, New York, Basic Books, 1985.

Peterson, M. Jeanne, *The Medical Profession in Mid-Victorian London*, Berkeley and Los Angeles, University of California Press, 1978.

Porter, Roy (ed.), *Patients and Practitioners*, Cambridge, Cambridge University Press, 1985.

Ramsey, Matthew, *Professional and Popular Medicine in France, 1770–1830: the Social World of Medical Practice*, Cambridge, Cambridge University Press, 1988.

——, 'The politics of professional monopoly in nineteenth-century medicine: the French Model and its rivals', in G. L. Geison (ed.), *Professions and the French State, 1700–1900*, Philadelphia, University of Pennsylvania Press, 1984.

Russell, Andrew W. (ed.), *The Town and State Physician in Europe from the Middle Ages to the Enlightenment*, Wolfenbütteler Forschungen, vol. 17, Wolfenbüttel, Herzog August Bibliothek, 1981.

Shryock, Richard H., *Medical Licensing in America, 1650–1695*, Baltimore, MD, Johns Hopkins Press, 1967.

Siraisi, Nancy G., *Taddeo Alderotti and His Pupils*, Princeton, NJ, Princeton University Press, 1981.

Starr, Paul, *The Social Transformation of American Medicine*, New York, Basic Books, 1983.

Stevens, Rosemary, *American Medicine and the Public Interest*, New Haven, CT, Yale University Press, 1971.

Warner, John Harley, *The Therapeutic Perspective: Medical Practice, Knowledge, and Identity in America 1820–1885*, Cambridge, MA, and London, Harvard University Press, 1986.

48

MEDICAL EDUCATION

Susan Lawrence

Medical education, taken in its broadest sense, includes any means by which a person absorbs the knowledge and skills that a community recognizes to produce a healer, one entrusted to treat the sick. Such education refers not only to the process that makes a practitioner, but also to the continuing acquisition of information and technical expertise throughout a lifetime of experience with other practitioners, with the ill and the injured, and with the medical media of lectures, texts, reports, updates, and advertisements. Much medical training concentrates on conveying well-established (or 'safe') material to the novice, including appropriate professional behaviour. Yet debates have also raged on how to organize a curriculum that concurrently transfers skills needed to evaluate new theories or therapies, to adopt new techniques, even to produce new knowledge, given contemporary standards for valuing and assessing novel medical ideas.

This sweeping definition encompasses the wide variety of ways that people have, historically, become medical personnel. A handful of examples evokes this diversity: the midwife of classical Athens, trained by attending childbirth with experienced midwives; the late fourteenth-century university doctor of medicine, learned in ancient texts; the eighteenth-century surgeon-apothecary, indentured to a master for seven years; the itinerant herbalist of Jacksonian America, self-taught from cheap books; the late twentieth-century American urologist, graduated BS and MD, who served a four-year hospital residency, became board-certified through standardized examinations, and filled a required quota of credits in continuing medical education by attending special courses, reading journals, and participating in medical conferences. These examples evoke the close connections between medical training and medical knowledge, occupations, institutions, and mobility; and between changing medical education and shifting social, economic, political, religious, and cultural organizations, beliefs, and norms.

Training medical practitioners has always required conveying two kinds of knowledge from one generation to another: a body of theory, by which practitioners and patients conceptualize disease; and a set of skills, with which the healer can name the patient's illness, decide on an appropriate treatment and carry it out, whether by regimen, drugs, or surgical manipulation. From antiquity, debates on how best to educate medical practitioners, and the actual methods and curricula established to do so, have centred on the relative importance placed on theory versus techniques, on the philosophical versus the empirical, on science versus clinical experience. Yet, despite this heuristic dichotomy, theory and practice have also always been intertwined. Teaching a particular theoretical position on physiological or pathological processes shapes how practitioners think they might alter those bodily mechanisms. Applying a specific remedy or surgical procedure similarly embodies a host of theoretical assumptions about the body and illness, even if not coherently articulated.

In Western society, the social and cultural value placed on theoretical knowledge, be it philosophy or science, has frequently transformed this dichotomy into a hierarchy. Self-proclaimed élite practitioners have separated themselves from others, particularly those labelled empirics, quacks, or irregular healers, through claims about the importance of theoretical knowledge for understanding and treating disease. As such knowledge is obtained through access to technical material, such as classical texts or anatomical demonstrations, and to institutions, such as universities, hospitals, and laboratories, the structures of medical education both reflect and reinforce practitioners' social status, economic position, and potential political influence. Restricting entry into universities, connecting specific degrees or curricula to expensive medical licensing and, finally, accrediting medical schools by professional organizations under government supervision, are all means through which medical occupations have used education both to define themselves as professions and to establish their social authority via specialized knowledge. Historically, such social, economic, and professional boundaries on medical education have excluded various groups from practising élite medicine, whether a particular medical institution deliberately formulated restrictions or unwittingly conformed to contemporary assumptions about appropriate social roles and abilities. Thus women, members of racial and ethnic minorities, religious non-conformists, and the physically handicapped, all of whom practised medicine in the past millennia, could be informally trained in healing, but often not formally educated.

Indeed, for most of those who have cared for the sick in the past, training was an informal process, in the sense of being unregulated and unstandardized by medical or educational institutions. Learning through private study of texts (if literate), experience with the ill and injured, and, above all, by watching an established practitioner, encapsulates the medical education of most healers, from infirmary monks to frontier surgeons. Particulars about *how* they learned are thus frequently bound up with *what* they learned, via theoretical treatises, customs, and familiar techniques. (➤ Ch. 41 Surgery (traditional); Ch. 44 Childbirth; Ch. 30 Folk medicine; Ch. 61 Religion and medicine; Ch. 28 Unorthodox medical theories; Ch. 53 History of personal hygiene; Ch. 54 A general history of nursing 1800–1900) In contrast, focusing on medical education from the perspective of formal procedures designed to create both a socially and professionally recognized practitioner highlights intellectual and cultural assumptions about what kind of knowledge and skills a healer should have, his or her expected social niche, and the authority of her or his expertise. The history of modern Western medical education, characterized by a specific curriculum, a monetary relationship between student and teacher or school, and directed towards professional licensing, is thus intimately correlated with the history of the medical professions, (➤ Ch. 47 History of the medical profession), related medical institutions, and the state (➤ Ch. 49 The hospital; Ch. 50 Medical institutions and the state) This chapter concentrates on such formal medical education, but with the caveat that informally trained practitioners had, until the twentieth century, a significant proportion of patient care. (➤ Ch. 4 Medical care)

MEDICAL EDUCATION BEFORE 1500

Six developments central to Western medical education occurred well before 1500. By early antiquity, literate practitioners and scholars created a corpus of authoritative medical texts. At the same time, a hierarchy of medical practitioners, from an archetypal philosopher-physician to a host of more-mundane healers associated with craft training, emerged. By late antiquity in the Eastern Roman Empire, and later in the West, Christian religious orders established infirmaries and hospitals as institutions to care for the sick, although in the West such foundations frequently gave other disabled and indigent folk charitable comfort. Organized schools and, later, universities, which established formal foundations for advanced learning, appeared by the twelfth century. Similarly, urban guilds, which set entrance requirements and regulated local practice, emerged by the thirteenth century in Italy, and had considerable influence in northern Europe by the fourteenth century. Finally, from the thirteenth century, both secular and ecclesiastical authorities began to license medical practitioners, often demanding evidence of qualifications, examinations, or testimonies that distinguished the 'legitimate' practitioner from self-proclaimed healers.

Throughout the Graeco-Roman period, medical education centred on three shifting poles: the ubiquitous training-by-doing, instruction at a 'school' surrounding a well-known physician, and dipping into the texts and discussions demarcating the physician-philosopher from the unlearned empiric. By the fifth century BC in the Greek city-states, tensions between learning by following a master, in a craft tradition, and acquiring knowledge from texts seemingly available to anyone who could read, reflected both the hierarchial social divisions amongst practitioners and the emergence of competing medical sects, each with its own body of doctrine about disease and therapeutics. Texts particularly intruded, at least in the retrospective view of Galen (AD 129–200/210), on the ancient tradition of training within families of physicians, which the Hippocratic Oath evokes: the new practitioner swore 'to give a share of precepts and oral instruction and all the other learning to my sons and to the sons of him who had instructed me'.[1] As the Oath and other evidence from the Hippocratic Corpus demonstrates, however, 'physicians' already instructed pupils for fees, although there is little known about how much such teaching cost or precisely how paying disciples were accepted. Hints from various non-medical sources, including comments from Herodotus (c.484–c.430/420 BC), Plato (427–347 BC) and Aristotle (384–322 BC), point to the contemporary fame of several medical 'schools'. These centred around groups of practising physicians, such as those at Cos, Cnidos, and, later, at Hellenistic Alexandria, and presumably involved payment of some kind from those not considered family. Depending upon the physicians at hand, the disciples who came for instruction learned by watching practice, discussing medical principles, studying texts, and writing their own notes and commentaries. The extensive collection of Hippocratic writings itself emerged in part from student copies of cases, lectures, and readings, which suggest the diversity of pedagogical methods. Yet these classical 'schools' by no means had a fixed curriculum or, as far as is known, procedures by which disciples marked the end of their training.[2]

When Aristotle remarked that 'Even medical men do not seem to be made by a study of text-books',[3] he suggested the vital role that observation and personal experience served to produce a practitioner, not just a philosopher. Yet Aristotle's own life work underscores the increasing significance of philosophical knowledge for the healer who aspired to be more than adept at diagnosis, prognosis, and treatment, and, at the same time, the importance of knowledge about the body for the philosopher seeking to understand nature. The debate over how *much* philosophy a practitioner needed to become a 'physician', particularly in fields such as cosmology, logic, mathematics, and ethics, continued throughout the Graeco-Roman era. From the third century BC, for example, healers later labelled 'empirics' deliberately distanced themselves from over-philosophizing sects and emphasized founding all training and practice on direct experience. The dominant textual voice of this period, nevertheless, was Galen's. Surveying the proliferation of sects, of theoretical positions and methods, Galen insisted that the true physician be a philosopher. Training in the abstract disciplines, including anatomy and physiology, in addition to the traditional areas of therapeutics, dietetics, and surgical procedures, created a practitioner who could explain disease as well as treat it. Galen thus linked literate philosophical study with informed experience as the best method to produce a physician, despite his lip-service to depreciating texts that had corrupted ancient medicine. Like that of so many critics, Galen's legacy was to insist upon the limitations of book knowledge by authors with whom he disagreed, while simultaneously promoting textual authority in medicine through his own works.

The literate tradition established in Greek, Hellenistic and Graeco-Roman antiquity erected a corpus of medical knowledge that shaped medical education in the Eastern Roman (Byzantine) Empire, Islamic territories, and western Europe throughout the medieval period. Byzantine compilers, such as Oribasius (AD 325–403), provided abridgements of authoritative texts in Greek; Arabic scholars, from the seventh century, incorporated Hippocratic, Aristotelian, and Galenic works into their medical corpus; and, in the west, translators and Latin encyclopedists, such as Isidore of Seville (d. 636), conveyed the basic outline of Graeco-Roman theory and practice to literate practitioners and scholars. Preserving texts, through copying, translating, and commenting upon them, using various scholarly conventions, also served a pedagogic purpose, especially when these tasks became institutionalized in schools and universities.

Between the fourth and tenth centuries, however, the most significant innovations in medical education centred on the emergence of hospitals and relatively stable medical schools. The former originated in the late fourth or early fifth century in the Eastern Roman Empire. Such *nosokomeia* (places to care for the sick) or *xenon* (hospice/'hospital') differed from potential hospital prototypes, such as Roman *valetudinaria* (military infirmaries) in that physicians staffed them and they were open to all the sick. While primarily supported by church alms or state donations, these Byzantine hospitals served local lay communities as well as travellers and clergy. From indirect evidence, primarily references to libraries within the hospitals and a hierarchy of medical assistants and students, aspiring healers could attend them for clinical experience under officially appointed physicians. Certainly by the early twelfth century, some hospitals in Constantinople had elaborate facilities for instruction, including a specially selected physician-teacher.[4] Similarly, hospitals-cum-medical schools appeared in major Islamic cities by the late eighth century. (➤ Ch. 31 Arab-Islamic medicine) References to 'meeting rooms', libraries, and medical discussions at the hospitals in Baghdad and Damascus point to a fairly elaborate training for élite practitioners. In addition to studying the

'Sixteen Books of Galen', an Arabic compilation dating from the ninth century, physicians advised students to learn mathematics and logic, and to read widely in all fields of Arabic literature. Yet again, however, both the hospital 'schools' and the literate advice appealed to creating a practitioner culturally distinguished from empirics and charlatans.[5]

In contrast, 'hospitals' in the cities of Western Christendom well into the thirteenth, and sometimes into the seventeenth century, cared largely for the indigent poor or those without servants or kin, not only for the ill.[6] Arising from monastic infirmaries first built to shelter monks too sick to participate fully in religious life, European hospitals retained an intensely religious character, following Christ's injunction to assist the sick as a charitable act. (➤ Ch. 62 Charity before c.1850) Before the thirteenth century, these institutions, such as the Hôtel Dieu in Paris or St Thomas's Hospital in London, rarely called upon lay physicians and surgeons to treat their charges, concentrating instead upon basic nursing support. While an enterprising surgeon or physician might have taken his apprentices into the hospital wards for clinical experience, in western Europe this practice remained sporadic at best throughout the medieval period. No hospital in this area acquired a contemporary reputation as a 'school' as those in Constantinople or Baghdad did, even in the centuries after the Crusaders reported on eastern hospitals to western religious orders, which inspired a renewed interest in this charitable work.

In Western Christendom, formal medical education developed instead around two other urban medieval institutions: the university and the guild. These organizations overshadow less structured schools, primarily because the former have left records of curricula, matriculations, disputations, and degrees, while the latter appear at least in civil documents, with urban responsibilities and rituals. Hints about non-university schools appear most clearly for the presumed precursors of later universities, such as those at Salerno, Parma, and Bologna. The school of Salerno, the earliest known centre for medical education in western Europe, emerged in southern Italy by the late tenth century. Like the schools of Cos or Cnidos, Salerno's reputation first centred on a group of practitioners, not upon textual study. By the twelfth century, however, Salernitan authors had begun to compile collections of Hippocratic, Galenic, and translated Arabic texts that served as a core curriculum. Gathered together under the title *Ars medicinae* or *Articella*, these anthologies summarized the major theses of Graeco-Arabic medical philosophy and practice. Equally significantly, these later Salernitan instructors promoted teaching by commentary on these texts, by organizing series of 'questions' upon theoretical points derived from them and by once again stressing the connections between medical theory and general topics in natural philosophy. By the time that Salerno became an officially recognized university in the late thirteenth century, however, its reputation for medical teaching had precipitously declined. Yet the 'Salerno' model of academic study and disputations appears to have influenced the medical curricula that emerged at northern universities, although direct importation of Salernitan methods has been difficult to trace.

During the first wave of university formation, from the late eleventh through the twelfth century, medical 'masters' congregated with other teachers and students and established official relationships with secular and church authorities. Major medical faculties were founded at Bologna, Montpellier, and Paris by the early thirteenth century. Although university organizations varied widely throughout Europe, those faculties that received the power to award medical degrees had a fairly standard curriculum, order of advancement through the academic levels, and only matriculated men. The aspiring candidate ideally first obtained a bachelor's degree through an arts faculty, where he learned logic, Aristotelian natural philosophy, mathematics, and music theory, all in previously acquired Latin.[7] Then he began the bachelor's degree in medicine. This was obtained in conjunction with the arts degree at Bologna, but was a distinct degree in Paris; thus these universities became the paradigms for two rather different models for physicians' studies. During the bachelor's work and, later, for the licentiate and then doctoral degrees in a medical faculty, he studied texts ascribed (accurately or not) to Hippocrates and Galen. In addition, depending upon the university, he heard lectures derived from commentaries on these ancient authors, especially the work of Avicenna (980–1037), whose *Canon of Medicine*, an extensive Arabic analysis of classical theory, was first translated into Latin in the late twelfth century. Masters lectured, too, on their own interpretations of the texts at hand, and organized disputations on particular points of doctrine and procedure.

Doctoral graduation ultimately rested, after four to seven years of study beyond the arts degree, on having attended the requisite lectures, disputations, and oral examinations, and, at some universities including both Bologna and Paris, on having fulfilled a period of supervised practice under a physician for six months to two years. The student had to obtain this experience 'extramurally', making his own arrangements with a suitable practitioner, as no medieval university retained a 'clinical' staff. About 1300 at Bologna, 1340 at Montpellier, and at least from 1465 at Padua, moreover, university requirements demanded that students attend a dissection of a human cadaver, a procedure that only gradually supplemented anatomical lessons on animals. (➤ Ch. 5 The anatomical tradition) This fairly rigid outline, nevertheless, constrained only those who were determined to achieve degrees; since matriculants regularly outnumbered degree candidates, quite a few reasonably well-to-do practitioners attended universities for grounding in their field, but found the ultimate teaching degree unnecessary for their careers.

At many medieval universities, medicine shared the honours of being a higher faculty, one beyond the arts curriculum, with law (civil and/or canon) and theology. All three trained men to practise their chosen discipline, primarily through scholarly work, consultations, and teaching. Even though most faculty physicians had a private practice, civic post, or medical appointment to a local secular or ecclesiastical ruler, and spent some time directing students in bedside care on their own patients, university instruction centred on textual study. Degrees marked expertise in understanding ancient authorities, in commenting upon theoretical positions on disease causation, physiology, and rationales for practice, not directly upon clinical acumen. As this doctrinal approach became institutionalized and accepted as the appropriate way to produce a learned and élite physician, one who could teach as he had been taught, it established a tradition then adopted by universities founded in the thirteenth through early seventeenth centuries across western Europe.

Most European universities, especially in the north, focused their curricula on medicine, not surgery. The division between 'internal' medicine, the physician's province, and 'external' manual manipulation, the surgeon's territory, was frequently upheld as both an intellectual and practical demarcation, although frequently blurred in patient care. Despite having a surgical faculty at Bologna, surgeons as attendants to the politically powerful, and an increasingly Latinate surgical élite in various European cities, all from the twelfth century on, surgery had a very precarious position as an academic discipline in the medieval period. Some have argued that consiliar prohibitions against clergy shedding blood, promulgated in the twelfth century and again specifically in the Lateran decrees of 1215, forced clergy-physicians to forego practising surgery. It seems more likely, however, that university physicians, especially those at clerically dominated Paris, used these decrees to enforce a division between medicine and surgery that kept surgeons off the faculty. Elsewhere, as at Montpellier, the faculty failed to adhere to similar regulations. At secular universities like Bologna (and, later, Padua), such religious restrictions had little influence, and learned men lectured on surgery.[8]

Surgery's absence from many universities rested, instead, upon the differing status that it had both socially, as a manual, craft-oriented occupation, and intellectually, as it did not have the same weight of textual and philosophical authority from classical authors to be absorbed by its practitioners. Furthermore, surgeons, especially in northern Europe, formed urban guilds at the same time that medical masters joined to create university faculties. These separate institutions, patterned after other craft and trade organizations, both legitimized surgical training and provided some control over competing practitioners in various cities, including Paris, Montpellier, and London. Although rarely granted monopolies over surgical practice, membership in a barber-surgeons' guild signified that the candidate had passed an oral examination set by the guild's master-surgeons and, usually in university towns, by a university-trained physician. By the fourteenth century, many such guilds required documentation of apprenticeship to a practitioner, further demarcating those 'bred' to the occupation from non-guild surgeons. Paralleling secular and ecclesiastical permission to dissect human bodies at certain universities, moreover, surgeons' guilds or corporations obtained the right to perform anatomies to instruct their members. During the late Middle Ages as well, a growing vernacular literature on surgical topics supplemented the young surgeon's potential education, although there are no references to guilds demanding an examination on textual knowledge.

Secular and ecclesiastical authorities gave weight to the universities' and guilds' claims to produce qualified medical practitioners by recognizing the privileges to teach and practise that membership in each granted. Infrequently between the twelfth and early sixteenth century, however, monarchs and bishops also licensed practitioners directly, primarily basing their approbation on the testimony of other practitioners, but also seeking ways to recognize healers whom universities and guilds excluded. King Peter of Aragon briefly licensed Jewish practitioners in the 1340s, for example, as they could not obtain medical degrees from Christian universities.[9] Such decisions confirm that lay culture acknowledged diverse routes in medical training, which neither universities nor guilds could control.

ANCIENTS AND MODERNS: 1500–1730

During the next few centuries, the institutions and traditions established during the medieval period dominated European medical education. While relatively little changed in university, guild, or hospital structures *per se*, or in the routines of training by apprenticeship, medical education shifted along with transformations in European culture, political alignments, and intellectual innovations. The invention of printing with movable type, which began to make an impact on the production and distribution of texts in the early sixteenth century, spawned a new reverence for ancient knowledge at the same time that it stimulated the creation of more vernacular literature on health, disease, and treatment. Early modern monarchs and princes founded more universities, urban colleges – with non-academic 'faculties' empowered to license local practitioners – of physicians and/or surgeons (such as London's Royal College of Physicians in 1518), and encouraged academies and societies devoted to investigating natural philosophy. The religious controversies of the Protestant Reformation and its fallout, in turn, contributed to battles within medical circles on the implications of the new iatrochemical and iatromechanical philosophies. These challenges to Graeco-Arabic medical theory and practice emerged during the sixteenth and seventeenth centuries from complex roots in the rejuvenation of alchemy, rediscovery of other classical texts, and in the cosmological reorientation commonly labelled the Scientific Revolution.

The content of what was taught thus changed within institutions that remained superficially stable. Universities, especially those at Paris and Oxford, appeared conservative, if not reactionary, when their medical faculties reluctantly modified their medieval curricula to accept new theories and practices. At others, however, new professors found it relatively easy to introduce innovations, as long as they stayed within the confines of university statutes. At Padua, one of the leading centres of medical education in Europe by the early sixteenth century, medical humanists championing a return to Greek ideas and methods unsullied by centuries of interpolation turned not only to newly edited Galenic texts, but also to what they believed were Galenic teaching precepts, including student experience with medicines, anatomy, and diseases. None of these was strikingly new, in principle. But the *emphasis* put upon this experience through demonstrations of materials, the range of required exposure, and the results of shifting the balance of the students' time profoundly altered this institution.

The Paduan medical faculty lobbied their Venetian patrons to establish a botanical garden specifically for teaching purposes in 1545. Several years before Andreas Vesalius (1514–64) arrived there in 1537, both the surgical masters, such as Nicolò de Musicis, and medical professors had begun to transform the traditional annual 'anatomies'. Again following Galen's insistence on the importance of anatomy, the medical teachers started a series of textually oriented anatomical lectures distinct from dissection, while the surgeons responsible for the demonstration of the human cadaver extended their exercises beyond the usual three days. With the help of a cohort of humanistic physicians, Vesalius managed both to give the physicians' lectures on anatomy and to perform the dissections.[10] This solidly Galenic procedure inspired both Vesalius's *De Corporis Humani Fabricae* and a method for teaching anatomy that was much praised and, at least in most northern universities, regularly ignored.

Admiration for classical physicians also shifted Paduan attention to the bedside. As noted above, most medieval universities required some period of practice for granting the licentiate or doctoral degrees, but neither regulated the content of such clinical experience nor provided a structure for it in university facilities. The aspiring physician, instead, served a mini-apprenticeship to a practitioner that he himself arranged, which may or may not have included access to hospital patients, depending upon the practitioner's own affiliations and routines. Beginning in 1539 at Padua, however, with the appointment of Giambatista da Monte (d. 1551) to the Chair of the Practice of Medicine, this extramural model began to change. Da Monte, already a prestigious Galenic scholar and physician, regularly gave bedside discourses on his patients to his students. More important, he served as physician to the nearby Hospital of St Francis and 'deliberately [used] the hospital to teach practice not just in the sense of therapy, but in its more formal academic sense of a survey of particular diseases'.[11] Da Monte's clinical discourses became so admired that they were posthumously published from student notes. After da Monte, it became customary for members of the Paduan medical faculty to serve simultaneously as hospital physicians, thus regularly linking university lectures at least in principle with explanations of particular diseases seen in the local charity.

Padua justly deserved its contemporary reputation in the sixteenth and seventeenth centuries as major centre for 'advanced' medical education. It attracted students from all over Europe. Those who could afford it took degrees there; others attended the lectures, anatomical demonstrations, and clinical discourses before going elsewhere for their MD or simply returning home to practice. As significant as Padua was for inculcating both a revived academic rigour, especially in anatomy and physiology, and a scholarly approach to case histories, following da Monte, adoption of its classical reforms occurred slowly in other universities. Advocates for reformed anatomical teaching or regular access to hospital patients (or both) had often trained at Padua and came home applauding humanist medicine, but their ideas for reviving medical curricula then depended entirely on their own resources and vociferousness. At Cambridge, for example, John Caius (1510–73; MD Padua 1541), inspired by studying anatomy with Vesalius, co-founded a college (1558), endowed medical fellowships, and managed to obtain a royal grant for the annual dissection of two felons' bodies there in 1565. At Leiden, Paduan alumni proposed hospital instruction in the late sixteenth century. Yet the university only founded the *collegium medico-practicum* in the 1630s, finally responding to worries that Dutch students travelled to foreign countries (like Italy) and to rival universities (the new university at Utrecht) for such teaching.

Leiden, although unusual in its impressive reputation for bedside medicine, represents a common pattern in seventeenth- and early eighteenth-century Europe. The university arranged for clinical instruction to take place first at the city hospital, whose medical attendants were not university faculty members. These men were present during the professors' visits and may have offered some separate instruction. Shortly thereafter, the medical faculty organized two small wards in a local charity, where six men and six women, chosen from the general hospital population, were moved as demonstration material for formal clinical lectures. As the university did not require this experience for the medical degree, interest in it depended directly upon the enthusiasm of the university professors. In Franciscus de le Boë Sylvius (1616–72) c.1658, and then Hermann Boerhaave (1668–1738) from 1714 to his death, Leiden had two faculty physicians who actively – and successfully – promoted the *collegium medico-practicum* as central to academic medicine.[12]

Historians have described the Leiden model, with small wards holding sample cases about whom practitioners didactically lectured to illustrate diseases, as the 'proto-clinic'. Like anatomical dissections in the medieval period, these cases primarily served to display the application of textual knowledge, rather than to offer students raw material for independent observations. Whatever the limitations of such formal academic exercises, they nevertheless underscored the importance of seeing real patients during university studies, and, in the hands of a master like Boerhaave, in turn inspired Leiden's matriculants to seek more-official connections between hospitals and universities in the eighteenth century. At the same time, moreover, hospitals continued to provide experience for some surgeons' apprentices, physicians' pupils, and other practitioners' students informally, as they had done for centuries.

Hospitals barely encroached upon the traditional means for medical education via the university, apprenticeship, or *ad hoc* practice in this period. More potent rivals to the literate monopoly over élite, scholarly medical knowledge which the universities claimed appeared instead in published texts, around royal courts, at evolving learned societies, and with non-university lectures. Critics of Galenic medicine, whether religiously inspired to reject pagan or Catholic theories, aroused by discoveries of ancient mystics and magicians, or stimulated by the mechanical currents of the Scientific Revolution, found print an alternate avenue for enlightenment. The radical religious and alchemical medicine of Paracelus (c.1493–1541) is only one example of a new physiological and therapeutic system spread for decades by books, studiously ignored in official university curricula and read and debated assiduously in medical circles. Later in the seventeenth century, the experimental physiology of William Harvey (1578–1657), the mechanical philosophy of Pierre Gassendi (1592–1655), Robert Boyle (1627–91), and Isaac Newton (1642–1727), and the revamped Hippocratic clinical method of Thomas Sydenham (1624–89), similarly influenced medical theory and medical practitioners as much outside as within university settings. The foundation of royal botanical gardens and learned societies, in addition to informal teaching at universities and urban salons, expanded the sites for extracurricular, yet 'academic', medical education. Lectures on chemistry and botany at the Jardin du Roi (founded 1640) in Paris, for example, threatened the Paris medical faculty; private elaboratories and lectures at Oxford subverted Galenic interpretations of the body and treatment expected of orthodox students.[13]

By the early eighteenth century, the public procedures for medical training at universities and through apprenticeship remained superficially the same as they were in 1500. Yet revived admiration for the ancients and then their challenge by the moderns both modified the content of medical education and gradually shifted some teaching methods, notably in a greater role for clinical observations in hospitals. At the very least, academic medicine had become, both in training and in practice, more eclectic. While still revering classical authorities, few literate (and likely few illiterate) practitioners could ignore the competing theories and practices that would, over the next centuries, drive a self-conscious élite to establish firm boundaries on medical orthodoxy and banish uneducated irregulars from the professional marketplace.

THE CLINIC, THE LABORATORY, AND THE UNIVERSITY: 1714–1914

In the two hundred years between Boerhaave's appointment as Professor of the Leiden *collegium medico-practicum* and the outbreak of the First World War, Western medical education underwent its most revolutionary changes. In broad terms, four major, interdependent transitions occurred.

First, surgeons and other traditionally craft-oriented practitioners joined the academy. Replacing apprenticeship and guild certification with collegiate or university courses, medical degrees, and hospital internships, gradually made surgery, obstetrics, and ophthalmology medical specialities rather than distinct (and lower-status) occupations. Second, university and collegiate educators increasingly melded instruction in theory, via lectures in classrooms, with practical training, via supervised experience on hospital wards or in outpatient clinics. Third, the ideology of 'new' science repeatedly reconstructed what a proper practitioner should know and how he or she should be taught. In the eighteenth century, science meant eradicating medical superstitions, folklore, and religious healing, denouncing their practitioners as charlatans. In the early to mid-nineteenth century, science meant the rigours of objective observation, following disease from the bedside to the autopsy to tissues and cells. In the later nineteenth century, science meant the laboratory, with objective observation enhanced by the experimental method. (➤ Ch. 8 The biochemical tradition) Finally, state interest in a population's health, often prodded by medical élites, led governments to require ever more stringent criteria for licensing practitioners and restricting unlicensed competitors, a process that regularly directed changes in medical curricula.

During the eighteenth century, élite surgeons adopted the physicians' form of education through lectures and texts, while retaining their traditional emphasis on supervised practical training. Neatly dubbed the 'rise' of the surgeon, this process occurred in various forms throughout Europe. In several cases, surgeons expanded existing organizations, adding or revamping teaching privileges (usually anatomical dissections) to introduce longer, more formal courses. Thus, in 1724, Louis XV granted the College of Saint-Côme in Paris (a small organization of academic surgeons dating from the sixteenth century) support for five public courses in surgical subjects. Senior Parisian surgeons used this royal favour to establish a school, lecturing on anatomy, surgery, and the surgical materia medica.[14] Elsewhere, as in London, surgeons and their non-university colleagues offered private lecture courses throughout the eighteenth century, where students paid the instructor directly and obtained certificates of attendance, but no official recognition for such extra-apprenticeship education.[15] This trend further undermined guild-induced attitudes towards training: instead of ostensibly 'secret' surgical knowledge passed from master to apprentice, lectures outside university walls opened surgical theories and techniques to public and professional scrutiny.

Lectures extended an academic polish that aspiring practitioners sought, yet it was their conjunction with the hospital that transformed both surgical apprenticeship and medical teaching clinics between the mid-eighteenth and mid-nineteenth centuries. In England, Scotland, Russia, Spain, Portugal, Denmark, Sweden, Prussia, and other European nations and colonial possessions, the state – often through the military – and/or private interests established (or transformed) hospitals into specifically medical institutions, whether for childbirth or chronic or acute illnesses and injuries. Their founders frequently claimed that these state or private charities served to care for the sick poor or ill soldiers *and* to educate medical practitioners – primarily surgeons. Hospital training centred (at least in the ideal) on regularly walking the wards with hospital staff, performing minor tasks, listening to and preparing case histories, and observing autopsies. This procedure combined the surgical apprentice's *ad hoc* hospital experience with the medical pupil's structured introduction to patients and the theoretical analysis of their cases. With formal in-house lecture courses (as in the Russian hospital schools), nearby private or corporate lectures (London, Paris, Edinburgh, Berlin), or with access to university courses taught by hospital clinicians (Edinburgh, Vienna), clinical instruction and didactic teaching further intertwined. By 1800, those discussing medical education considered that having a university hospital or other student access to patients was absolutely vital.

Mingling surgery's and physic's pedagogical approaches was both a methodological and a cognitive shift. Variously described as medicine adopting 'the surgical point of view', the 'birth of the clinic', or the emergence of the 'hospital *problèmatique*', this shift focused the physician's attention to the anatomical localization of disease, away from individualized holistic causation, be it humoral, iatrochemical, or disseminated imbalances in the nervous powers.[16] (➤ Ch. 14 Humoralism) The physician began to see internal disease as the surgeon did: situated in organs and correlated with specific signs and symptoms. Gradually, in hospitals and clinics throughout Europe, physicians started to visualize *pathological* anatomy, discovered through extended experience with dissection and post-mortems. In turn, practical anatomy became a much more important medical subject, as did experience with patients from the bedside to the autopsy-table. Several mid-century hospital physicians (for example, William Cullen (1710–90) in Edinburgh) championed this approach, while a few, notably Giovanni Battista Morgagni (1682–1771) of Padua in his *On the Seats and Causes of Disease* (1761), incorporated it into the way they dealt with disease. Similarly, surgeons continued to absorb the 'physicians' point of view', both by seeking to make surgery more academic and systematized and to emphasize the importance of knowing physiology, physic, and the whole materia medica in order to be rational and gentlemanly practitioners. (➤ Ch. 7 The physiological tradition; Ch. 9 The pathological tradition)

Found sporadically and only partially articulated throughout the mid- to late eighteenth century, the unification of medicine and surgery has its emblematic marker in Revolutionary Paris. There, in the years between 1789 and 1815, reformers openly dismantled the old system of physicians in the universities and surgeons in the hospitals. Instead, aspiring physicians and surgeons attended a single medical school, sharing the same early curriculum and then developing a medical or surgical speciality in the later academic years and through the now-mandatory clinical experience in Parisian hospitals. The 'revolution' lay in officially making the surgeons and physicians have the same pattern of training, even if the content differed: at once didactic, textual, observational, and practical. From 1803, legal French practitioners had to hold a degree: either that of *Officier de Santé* (designed for rural practice), or a doctorate in medicine or surgery (in 1892, these three degrees merged into a single MD). Formal unification of the two professional branches of physic and surgery (and other medical proto-specialities) under a single preliminary curriculum occurred gradually at other Western universities and associated hospitals well into the nineteenth century. As nearly all degree-granting bodies and hospital wards admitted only men, and had other religious, economic, or racial expectations, the decades after 1800 also saw a severe narrowing of the diversity of socially tolerable practitioners.

In the 'new' hospital experience available to medical pupils, attention increasingly focused on learning clinical skills, including techniques for physical diagnosis as well as oral history-taking. The fairly rapid acceptance of the 1816 invention by R. T. H. Laënnec (1781–1826) of the stethoscope, and the number of students who flocked to learn this new technology from him in Paris, traditionally marks a crucial shift in medical perceptions. Thereafter, as physician-researchers invented new diagnostic devices for internal pathologies, instructors had to incorporate them into clinical training. Starting as advanced techniques for graduate specialists, use of innovative devices moved to junior levels as they became part of standard practice. The method – repeated hands-on, supervised experience – is as ancient as medicine, but the growing technological array, from the ophthalmoscope (invented in 1850–1 by H. von Helmholtz (1821–94)) to X-ray photography (invented in 1895 by W. C. Roentgen (1845–1923)), fought for space and time in clinical courses while frequently creating their own disciplinary experts. (➤ Ch. 35 The art of diagnosis: medicine and the five senses; Ch. 36 The science of diagnosis: diagnostic technology)

From the stethoscope on, training students in new diagnostic and therapeutic skills meshed with contemporary claims that medicine was finally creating clinical *science*. According to its promoters, all medical disciplines became more rigorous as practitioners adhered to collecting objective observations of disease in and among patients, organs, tissues, and fluids. Pierre C.-A. Louis (1787–1872), working at La Charité hospital in Paris, championed the 'numerical method'. He made both clinical acumen and the range of individual variations more precise by correlating thousands of clinical symptoms, signs, treatments, and post-mortem reports. Like Laënnec and many other nineteenth-century medical researchers, Louis urged the accountability that made other sciences – especially physics, chemistry, and biology – proffer certain knowledge: replication, measurement, and systematic and standardized methods to gather 'facts'.

The on-going debate over how best to educate medical practitioners to be 'scientific' centred on the bedside, the clinic, and the autopsy-table (with the appropriate lecture-learned knowledge of anatomy, chemistry, and physiology) during the first decades of the nineteenth century. Yet already the basic sciences began to challenge the sufficiency of watching science demonstrated during lectures to create a physician with enough observational and experimental discipline. Instead, medical chemists, physiologists, and cellular pathologists advocated hands-on training in their own realm: not at the bedside, or at autopsy, but in the laboratory. From at least the 1840s in German countries, the 1860s in France, and the 1870s and 1880s in the United Kingdom and the United States, intense controversies raged around reforming the medical curriculum to include the 'right kind' of science in the 'right way'. These conflicts bred multiple factions, but in broad terms they fell along now-familiar lines: bedside clinical science versus laboratory science; skills for practice versus knowledge for research; humanistic versus technical pre-qualifications; generalists versus specialists; practitioners versus academics; universities versus hospitals versus institute laboratories.[17] (➤ Ch. 11 Clinical research)

With the growth of several biomedical sciences into laboratories funded by universities and academic institutes, particularly when these expanded as distinct disciplines pursued by non-practitioners, rifts between academic clinicians and laboratory scientists intensified, as did those between the academics, clinical specialists, and general practitioners. On the one hand, laboratory scientists and specialists promised rapid medical advancement, emphasizing both the potential utility of theoretical research by specialists and the 'objective' mind that scientific training should foster among rank-and-file physicians, which would allow them to appreciate and apply new medical advances. On the other hand, non-academic practitioners argued that science courses were a waste of time: theories, experiments, and arcane data had little to do with most care for the sick, far from laboratories and libraries. The scientists' claims, they argued, represented a new élitism in medicine, one that led academics to dominate the profession and universities to dictate all forms of medical education.

The specific issues, actors, political implications, and economic complications varied considerably between institutions in the Western world from the 1860s well into the twentieth century. Yet many eyes turned towards German universities and institutes as key models for scientific medical education and research. Universities in Heidelberg, Leipzig, Munich, Göttingen, and Berlin, among others, competed for government support, affiliation with advanced institutes, scientific talent, and laboratory facilities for medical students. They largely succeeded in implementing laboratory science as the *sin qua non* of pre-clinical medical education and elevating the physician-researcher to the peak of medical prestige. At Heidelberg, for example, government reforms in 1858 simultaneously required those seeking medical licensure to have taken laboratory courses in physiology and chemistry, and established a chair in physiology to offer to Hermann Helmholtz.[18] The biomedical science produced in German institutions – and their later imitators in Britain, France, and the United States – certainly dazzled the world, particularly in physiology and bacteriology after the 1870s. Bacteriology, with its potential applications in clinical medicine and public health, spurred even reluctant physicians to recognize a new role for laboratory science in medical curricula, even without immediate therapeutic benefits. (➤ Ch. 16 Contagion/ germ theory/specificity)

Until the 1890s to 1910s, nevertheless, arguments over why and how to introduce laboratory science into general medical education remained largely a university issue, hence largely one on the European continent. In Germany, mandatory state licensing examinations were closely tied to medical study at universities, the institutions that also educated the social élite and professional bureaucrats. Even when German states did not require a doctorate to sit their licensing examinations, students still prepared for their examinations through university courses. The majority went on to write the necessary thesis, for the MD conferred significant professional and social status. In France, Spain, and other nations with relatively strong central governments and state-supported medical schools, medical faculties similarly controlled medical practitioners by their degree-granting monopolies, although influenced by the scope of state examinations. In France, however, the powerful hospital hierarchy – and much clinical teaching and prestige – remained outside direct faculty control and lent its weight to teaching clinical, rather than laboratory, science and practice.

In the Anglo-American world, governments were far more interested in citizens' freedom to choose nearly any sort of medical care than in centrally regulating medical education. Throughout the later 1800s and early 1900s, orthodox practitioners continued to argue that ill-trained healers brought illness and death, rather than cured diseases. Only near the turn of the century, however, did public acclaim for biomedical science begin to convince Anglo-Americans that the state should restrict medicine to the regularly educated and licensed practitioner for the health of all. In both the United Kingdom and the United States, restriction first meant privileging certain practitioners who had evidence of a regular medical education. Thus, in Great Britain and Ireland after 1858, practitioners who signed death certificates or worked for the state (including quite nominal appointments) had to be listed on the Medical Register. Other healers could still treat patients without state sanction, as long as they did not proclaim themselves 'physicians', 'surgeons', or members of other 'registered' medical occupations. Over the next decades, registration (ideally) allowed the public knowingly to choose an 'irregular' practitioner (however qualified) or a 'real' professional. The latter registered after passing one of the nineteen possible licensing examinations given by the traditional corporate bodies throughout the United Kingdom. In keeping with past conventions, neither the Royal College of Surgeons of England (for the MRCS) nor the Society of Apothecaries (for the Licentiate of the Society of Apothecaries (LSA)), for example, required the MD. Instead, the General Medical Council, which oversaw the licensing examinations, regulated the number of years and subjects of study for examination candidates. In the process, it imposed a 'voluntary' standardization on medical curricula across Britain and Ireland. In the United States, medical licensing and medical education varied considerably from state to state into the twentieth century, with very little state control until the 1880s. By the 1890s, aspiring practitioners could take a college BA, graduate MD, do postgraduate years in Germany, and return hoping for an élite, perhaps even academic, practice; all they usually *needed*, however, was two years' study at a school that granted medical degrees, be it orthodox or sectarian, connected to a hospital or not, equipped with laboratory space or simply a few lecture rooms and a collection of anatomical specimens.

At the turn of the twentieth century, bacteriology had made enough of a public and professional impact for science to be more closely identified with the laboratory than the bedside. In France, Great Britain, and the United States, pro-laboratory reformers rallied. In France (1890, 1892, 1912) and Great Britain (1900, 1912–13), for example, ministerial inquiries and medical committees reported on the inadequacies of medical education compared with that of Germany, linking perceived research productivity and utility with scientific training for undergraduate medical students. A series of reforms followed, most of which focused on forcing more basic and biomedical science on to all medical students. In the United States, the American Medical Association (AMA) had been advocating higher standards in medical education – and effective state licensing – since its formation in 1846. The Association of American Medical Colleges (1876), and then the AMA's Council on Medical Education (1904), regularly announced ideal standards; in 1905, these included one year of basic sciences, two years of laboratory biomedical science, two years of clinical training, plus a sixth year of hospital internship.[19] The council's survey committee, which began collecting data in 1906, found that a minority of schools were ready or willing to implement this European-style programme. Although several medical schools had introduced laboratory courses in the 1880s and 1890s, when states began to require an examination in addition to a medical degree, poor pay for European-trained graduates and even less funding for laboratories made advanced departments difficult to develop. One major exception to this was Johns Hopkins University, deliberately designed to have the most up-to-date (and Germanic) medical school across the Atlantic. Opened in 1893, Johns Hopkins Medical School required a preliminary bachelor's degree for entering medical students. Heavily endowed, the university could build and equip laboratories, establish a teaching hospital, and fund full-time academic positions for researching biomedical scientists and a few clinical faculty, freeing both from the private practice such men previously needed in order to survive. (➤ Ch. 53 Medical philanthropy after 1850)

Others soon found medical research and teaching causes worthy of private endowment, much as generous patrons had done in Germany, France, and Britain. The Rockefellers and Andrew Carnegie (1835–1919), in particular, began foundations to champion modern medicine, education, and philanthropy. Among their fruits was the famous investigation by Abraham Flexner (1866–1959) into medical education. Flexner, educated at Johns Hopkins in liberal arts, Harvard in psychology, and Berlin in comparative education, came to his project already prepared to favour the German model of university-centred medicine. His reports, *Medical Education in the United States and Canada* (1910) and *Medical Education: a Comparative Study* (1925) received enormous attention throughout the Western world. Flexner, quite aware of the complexities involved in creating schools that could foster science, clinical teaching, *and* patient care, nevertheless championed science as the key to success in all three arenas. Critical of the French system (too clinical), the British system (far too unscientific and decentralized), and certainly of most existing American schools (non-clinical, unscientific, and decentralized), Flexner articulated a new German–American ideal. For him, a medical school must be part of a university, with basic sciences taught in liberal-arts departments; it must have its own departments for the biomedical sciences to encourage research and advance instruction; it must have a teaching hospital, with full-time faculty staffing clinical departments in both the medical school and the hospital; it must have high entrance requirements, a graded curriculum, and end with the doctoral degree. The 1910 report, in short, unquestionably embodied a vision of élite medicine, a profession much less accessible than the one available through most contemporary schools and hospitals. While not entirely responsible for reforming American medical education – a process already underway in the 1890s – Flexner gave a strong voice to the vision of scientific medical training and a profession with fewer but 'better' doctors.[20]

To succeed in the twentieth century, the signposts were clear. A medical school – and the educational experience – required a university affiliation, lecture-theatres, dissection-tables, laboratories, researching faculty, full-time clinical instructors, up-to-date technology, a teaching hospital, and lots of interesting diseases; in short, a synthesis of the innovations of the previous four centuries. Henceforth, five distinct institutions warily worked together to provide modern medical education: the state, the hospital, the university, the medical school, and the private funding agency.

SCIENCE AND STANDARDIZATION: FROM 1914

The First World War interrupted the reforming movements begun before 1914. Yet the war offered further support for those seeking to modernize medical education. Medical and surgical successes, such as better control of the typhus-carrying body-louse, blood transfusions, and refined operations, all demonstrated scientific knowledge and training in action. Medical failures, during and after the war, as with the influenza pandemic, spurred optimists to call for more research in response to those critical of bacteriologists' grandiose claims. The Second World War marked a similar juncture. The post-1945 world enthused over medical progress, symbolized most obviously by the commercial availability of penicillin. (➤ Ch. 39 Drug therapies) The processes set in motion before both wars to rationalize and renovate medical education thus continued, fuelled by a new public eagerness to have science solve humanity's ills. Five broad trends characterize the period since 1914, all of which have brought new concerns and new urgencies to how to produce the practitioners that a nation wants or – often a different matter – those it might need.

First, the near-omnipresent crisis of the 'expansion of knowledge' has repeatedly challenged the medical curriculum. Second, increasing specialization and sub-specialization, another consequence of expanding sets of information, therapies, and techniques, has multiplied the years and the programmes available for postgraduate training. Specialization, for many, has compromised the education and role of the general practitioner; it has also spawned an empire of related health occupations, from dieticians and technicians to counsellors and salaried patient advocates. (➤ Ch. 55 The emergence of para-medical professions) Third, Western medicine has expanded geographically, clearly becoming a world-wide system and demanding radical changes in non-Western medical education, certification, and practice. Fourth, social and political movements have insisted that medical schools respond to cultural concerns: access to women and minorities, ethical dilemmas posed by medical technologies, and public accountability for the quality of care provided. Finally, medical education, like so many parts of the twentieth-century bureaucratic state, has become enmeshed in public and private funding networks that inevitably influence national and institutional priorities. (➤ Ch. 68 Medical technologies: social contexts and consequences; Ch. 38 Women and medicine; Ch. 57 Health economics)

A 'crisis' of knowledge has arisen whenever critics claim that the educational process, be it apprenticeship or a university curriculum, is not producing well-qualified practitioners, or, in more polemical terms, is producing too many ill-qualified ones. Although a long-term complaint, the problem of too much information and too little time to acquire it became acute in the twentieth century. By the 1920s, most Western medical degrees required four to five years of specifically medical study in biomedical science and clinical experience. Dealing with the demand for more in the medical curriculum generally pushed the basic sciences into required pre-medical training enforced by entry qualifications. By the 1940s in the United Kingdom and Canada, for example, where students begin medical school without completing a bachelor's degree, those intending a medical career needed to decide early in secondary school to finish the necessary science courses, or, in Britain, to complete a full year of pre-medical work. In nations where medical schools demanded a bachelor's degree before entry, undergraduate course work and/or separate exit or entrance examinations served to demonstrate adequate preparation. As a consequence, medical schools then focused on teaching the biomedical sciences most relevant to medical research and practice. Raising pre-medical standards served both to increase professional expectations and status, while reducing the number of legally recognized practitioners. At the other end, pushing training for any speciality into the postgraduate years ideally meant that the single, unified medical degree produced a practitioner nearly ready to be licensed, after having been responsible for clinical work during a year of hospital internship. As speciality certification developed, however, the disjunction between the medical degree and actual peer and/or state recognition for licensing has again widened.

Squeezing basic science and clinical work into undergraduate and postgraduate years offered a temporary respite for medical schools before the Second World War. Yet already the number of medical fields, and hence the number of subjects the student should at least be introduced to, multiplied. Medical curricula from the 1920s on reveal the addition of courses, from hygiene, public health, biochemistry, and statistical methods, to paediatrics, cardiology, haematology, and emergency medicine. Where courses were not added, administrators often increased the hours allotted to existing fields to cover new sub-fields, a less overt addition to burdened schedules. Recognizing the growing demand for postgraduate training, in 1920 the AMA Council on Medical Education created fifteen committees to study graduate work in medical specialities. Most of the fields, such as urology, neuropsychiatry, and dermatology and syphilology, either had, or rapidly established, formal requirements for peer certification. The AMA's Committee on Graduate Education then evaluated hospitals and university programmes, regularly issuing reports such as the 1928 'Essentials of Approved Residencies'.[21] Approximately every decade since the Second World War, either government-sponsored commissions in centralized nations, or national advisory and accreditation boards in less centralized ones, have re-evaluated the medical curriculum and other educational experiences, such as clinical work and standardized examinations, to reach a new consensus on how to create a suitable practitioner. The issue has been, and continues to be, what the 'basic' practitioner, the one acknowledged by the first medical degree, should know before becoming a specialist destined to interact with other highly specialized medical personnel. This goal, in turn, increasingly depended upon each nation's health-care system, particularly in the relationship between the general practitioner and the specialist.

From the early twentieth century, reforming medical education in the West has been caught up in the political and economic transformation of the delivery of health care. In Europe, where a variety of government-sponsored national health systems developed by the 1940s, the general practitioner became the primary care-giver, determining when patients should be referred to specialists. (➤ Ch. 50 Medical institutions and the state)In contrast, in the private system in the United States, patients sought specialists directly, as they competed for clientele, leading to the demise of the general practitioner and the creation of a new speciality in 'family practice'. In both systems, specialists received more income and prestige, hence higher places in the professional medical hierarchy and often more influence with political leaders. In both systems, too, access to postgraduate training – whether determined by professional speciality groups or government committees – limits the number and type of specialists. As postgraduate education for practitioners centres on hospitals, the relation of the hospital (state, private, religious) to the medical system (state versus private) and the internal distribution of power and resources within any particular hospital shapes what is essentially a final apprenticeship phase of medical training. As specialities split and subdivide (for example cardiology within internal medicine, plastic surgery within general surgery, proctology from gastro-enterology), so too do training programmes and certifying qualifications.

The ideal of the first medical degree as both common ground for all medical practitioners and sufficient – with a year or so of postgraduate hospital training – for practice remains in the Western world, although this ideal has been increasingly illusory since the 1960s. Cost and competing knowledge claims have restimulated other health professionals, such as nurse-midwives and physicians' assistants, to offer primary care and referral services, a trend that is likely to characterize late twentieth-century rural and inner-city care. Similarly, the ideal of the first medical degree as a staging-point for a research career – the general practitioner as scientist – has been tempered considerably since the Second World War and the growing specialization within biomedical sciences. Throughout the world, the Ph.D. demarcates the researcher in all but the clearly defined clinical fields. Generous government and private support for biomedical research in the 1950s to 1970s, particularly in the United States, further enmeshed the university, hospital, and medical school by supporting non-practising or part-time faculty through research grants that simultaneously enhanced the researchers' prestige and local power.[22]

The Western model of medical education, indeed of higher education, has become the world model. From the beginning of Western trade with, and colonization of, India, South-East Asia, Africa, China, and the Americas, Europeans exported their medical personnel, theories, and methods to serve their own communities. (➤ Ch. 58 Medicine and colonialism) Missionaries brought Western medicine along with Western religion. Indigenous systems, however, continued to thrive as long as local populations trained and supported their practitioners. Thus in India, for example, although the British East India Company allowed Indians to train as assistants and 'native doctors' by informal apprenticeship in the eighteenth century, and established a training school for 'native' practitioners in the early nineteenth century, the British made little attempt to import Western medicine into the subcontinent for the general population. The scholarly Ayurvedic and Unani systems, along with popular domestic medicine, flourished throughout the nineteenth centuries (and continue into the present). (➤ Ch. 33 Indian medicine) In 1835, however, the Governor-General of Bengal, William Bentinck (1774–1839) established the Calcutta Medical College specifically to bring European-style medical education to Bengal for Indians. With British faculty, instruction in English, a laboratory course in chemistry from 1837, and 'a virtually unlimited supply of cadavers', the school was an Anglo-Indian success once the middle-class Hindu students showed the tense founders that they would dissect human bodies, despite their cultural and religious abhorrence for the practice.[23] The Calcutta Medical College, and its twentieth-century imitators, typify the gradual importation of Western methods and ideology into colonial non-Western countries, as the educated Indian élite increasingly supported Western science as evidence of modernization and self-determination. In the Americas, in contrast, as indigenous populations were conquered or died out, native medicine had a precarious base, surviving only by an oral tradition and apprenticeship. The colonists, in turn, imported their own European educational system of the eighteenth and nineteenth centuries. (➤ Ch. 29 Non-Western concepts of disease; Ch. 2 What is specific to Western medicine?)

The creation of a world medicine along Western lines, tentatively begun by colonists, expanded enormously in the twentieth century. The export of Western industrialization, technology, and trade meant for many the export of Western science and medicine. In China, for example, the Rockefeller Foundation included the establishment of a Western-style medical school in Peking as vital for its programme of medical assistance and modernization. The organizers explicitly aimed their 'secular philanthropy' to expose China to the influence of Western science. The Peking Union Medical College opened in 1921 and, by 1937, had graduated 166 élite practitioners. They were well-versed in Western theories and therapies, but found it next to impossible to deal with China's health problems.[24] (➤ Ch. 32 Chinese medicine)

After the Second World War, independence and revolutionary movements throughout the non-Western world spurred newly autonomous governments to establish health-care systems, including programmes for medical education. Depending upon the nation's political and economic orientation, these systems have included hopes to continue to imitate Western educational models or to adopt some forms of indigenous care into a partly westernized programme. The United Nations World Health Organization (WHO), by spearheading worldwide disease-control projects, furthered the absorption of Western medicine. Several impoverished nations and areas have sought to keep abreast of Western medicine by sending students to train in the West, while simultaneously creating second-tier practitioners to serve rural and poor populations. As a result, many non-Western nations face a severe form of the polarization between the rural versus urban, and poor versus wealthy, practice seen in the West. As the full extent of Western medical education requires an infrastructure of hospitals, universities, and research funding, in addition to medical schools, it has been easier for the West to export specific medications, procedures, and visiting physicians than viable ways to produce resident medical practitioners that Western organizations can accept as health professionals. (➤ Ch. 59 Internationalism in medicine and public health)

The brief post-Second World War golden age of science-oriented Western medical education found its international critics in countries trying to create cadres of 'barefoot doctors'. It also found vocal critics closer to home after mid-century. Various social and political movements in Europe and North America challenged the perceived *status quo* on a number of fronts, and scientific medicine symbolized for many a new form of élitism, exclusivity, and paternalism that was not responsive to social needs. Such critics saw the very selectivity and monopoly for which physicians had lobbied so long, in the interests of producing well-qualified, orthodox practitioners, as barriers to reform in affluent cultures. In these decades, both practitioners and lay people confronted the overt and hidden restrictions on entry to medical school and advancement in the medical hierarchy based particularly on gender, race, and religious affiliation. Women, people of colour, and Jews (among others) had not been uniformly excluded from university-based medical education in all of Europe or the Americas. Certainly, from the 1860s, women could matriculate at – and graduate from – the predominantly male universities of Zurich and Paris. Elsewhere, as in Great Britain and the United States, women established separate medical colleges and hospitals for training, occasionally gaining entry into male medical schools. Similarly, in the United States, Afro-Americans established Howard University (1868) and Meharry College (1876) to produce more black physicians than those who could afford a European education or a rare chance to study at a white college. Jews, and members of other ethnic and religious groups, lived with unspoken quotas for access to various European and North American institutions.

The outspoken and sometimes violent student movement throughout the West, in conjunction with the Civil Rights movement and the mid-twentieth century women's movement, directly affected medical education in two ways. First, diversity among medical students increased as medical schools acknowledged some of their restrictions and sought to admit women and minorities; second, students voiced considerable concern for social issues, such as poverty, access to medical care, and the fear that technology overly distanced the practitioner from his or her patient. (➤ Ch. 34 History of the doctor–patient relationship) Curriculum response to the latter apprehensions, at least when the faculty shared them, included more attention to preventive medicine and more emphasis on human skills in patient interactions. Both of these changes, nevertheless, are still active late twentieth-century processes.[25] Indeed, the bioethics movement, which is more visible in the United States than in other Western nations because its health-care system idealizes patient autonomy, continues to fuel the public desire for socially aware, 'humanized' physicians: the new practitioner should eschew paternalistic authority while compassionately applying all the scientific knowledge at her or his disposal. (➤ Ch. 37 History of medical ethics)

Interwoven among all the twentieth-century changes in medical education are the central themes of funding and cost. Public support for medical training before the mid-nineteenth century consisted entirely of limited state patronage for universities and hospitals (as in Italy, Spain, and German nations) and religious or private donations for medical charities where some pupils learned from the sick. Since 1914, but especially since the Second World War, Western governments began to fund medical education on a massive scale, directly and indirectly. In nations with a national health system that runs hospital services and a public-grants programme that supports qualified students through post-secondary education, as in the United Kingdom or the former Soviet Union, financing medical training depends upon co-ordinating several government departments. In nations with more privatized systems, most obviously the United States, federal, state, and private funding has had an equally significant role, although often a less overt one. Private philanthropists like the Rockefellers and Carnegie invested considerable amounts in universities seeking to upgrade their medical schools to meet Flexnerian standards in the 1920s and 1930s. The federally funded National Institutes of Health, created after the Second World War, directed medical-school expansion through the generous grants provided for research, which indirectly supported faculty positions, laboratories, and equipment used in teaching medical and postgraduate students. This support, moreover, encouraged specialization in both clinical fields and the biomedical sciences, which, in turn, continued to crowd the medical curriculum.[26]

By whatever means the public finances medical instruction, in all Western (and westernized) nations the power imparted by fiscal jurisdiction shapes the values and priorities expressed in medical schools and their relationship to universities, hospitals, and lay communities. State-administered grants for student support, for example, ideally signify the equalization of opportunity for any qualified person, no matter what class, gender, race, or ethnic origin, to enter medicine. Funding for technology-dependent research instead of community-care residency programmes, or vice versa, similarly reflects a decision to opt – in any particular case – for future cures or present care. The question of cost dominates late twentieth-century medicine worldwide. Lay perspectives (via government, the press, or the courts) on the importance of laboratory and clinical science, access to technology and specialists, preventive medicine and patients' rights, increasingly challenge the medical profession's recently acquired status, autonomy, and unquestioned allegiance to science. The process of medical training will thus inevitably change as new social and professional consensus emerges on what, among so many competing needs, just might produce the 'best' practitioner for a price that the body politic can afford. In the end, no system of medical education can automatically create a healer, who has always been a mythological figure envisioned in the past for polemical use in the present. A formal mechanism for medical training can only supervise the mastery and application of specific knowledge and manipulative skills, in hopes to invite trust among patients and peers.

NOTES

1 Ludwig Edelstein, 'The Hippocratic Oath', in Edelstein, *Ancient Medicine: Selected Papers*, ed. by O. Temkin and C. L. Temkin, Baltimore, Johns Hopkins University Press, 1967, p. 6.

2 A. Thivel, *Chide et Cos? Essai sur les doctrines médicales dans la collection hippocratique*, Paris, Les Belles Lettres, 1981.

3 Aristotle, *Nicomachean Ethics* 1181b 2ff, in J. Barnes, *The Complete Works of Aristotle*, 2 vols, Princeton, NJ Princeton University Press, 1984.

4 Timothy S. Millar, *The Birth of the Hospital in the Byzantine Empire*, Baltimore, MD, John Hopkins University Press, 1985.

5 Gary Leiser, 'Medical education in Islamic lands from the seventh to the fourteenth century', *Journal of the History of Medicine and Allied Sciences*, 1983, 38: 48–75.

6 The following section on medieval hospitals, universities, and guilds relies heavily on Nancy Siraisi's excellent survey, *Medieval and Renaissance Medicine: an Introduction to Knowledge and Practice*, Chicago, IL, University of Chicago Press, 1990.

7 For the later arts curriculum, see P. Kibre, 'Arts and medicine in the universities of the later Middle Ages', in J. Ijsewijn and J. Paques (eds), *The Universities in the Late Middle Ages*, Louvain, Leuven University Press, 1978, pp. 213–27.

8 A. Goddu, 'The effect of canonical prohibitions on the Faculty of Medicine at the University of Paris in the Middle Ages', *Medizinhistorisches Journal*, 1985, 204: 342–62.

9 Siraisi, op. cit. (n. 6), p. 18.

10 Jerome J. Bylebyl, 'The School of Padua: humanistic medicine in the sixteenth century', in C. Webster (ed.), *Health, Medicine and Mortality in the Sixteenth Century*, Cambridge, Cambridge University Press, 1983, pp. 335–70.

11 Ibid., p. 348.

12 G. A. Lindeboom, 'Medical education in the Netherlands, 1575–1750', in Charles D. O'Malley (ed.), *The History of Medical Education*, UCLA Forum in Medical Science (no. 12), Los Angeles, University of California Press, 1970, pp. 201–16.

13 Allen G. Debus, 'Chemistry and the universities in the seventeenth century', *Mededelingen van de Koninklijke Academie voor Wetenschappen Letterenen Schone Kunster van Belgie*, 1986, 48: 15–33; Laurence Brockliss, 'Medical teaching at the University of Paris, 1600–1720', *Annals of Science*, 1978, 35: 221–51.

14   Toby Gelfand, *Professionalizing Modern Medicine: Paris Surgeons and Medical Science and Institutions in the 18th Century*, Westport, CT, Greenwood Press, 1980, pp. 21–2, 62–3.

15   S. C. Lawrence, 'Entrepreneurs and private enterprise: the development of medical lecturing in London, 1775–1820', *Bulletin of the History of Medicine*, 1988, 62: 171–92.

16   Oswei Temkin, 'The role of surgery in the rise of modern medical thought', *Bulletin of the History of Medicine*, 1951, 25: 248–59; Michel Foucault, *La Naissance de la clinique*, Paris, Presses Universitaires de France, 1963; Othmar Keel, 'The politics of health and the institutionalization of clinical practices in Europe in the second half of the eighteenth century', in W. F. Bynum and Roy Porter (eds), *William Hunter and the Eighteenth-Century Medical World*, Cambridge, Cambridge University Press, 1985, pp. 207–56.

17   The following discussion of nineteenth- and twentieth-century medical education relies on: Robert E. Kohler, *From Medical Chemistry to Biochemistry: the Making of a Biomedical Discipline*, Cambridge, Cambridge University Press, 1982; Timothy Lenoir, 'Science for the clinic: science policy and the formation of Carl Ludwig's institute in Leipzig', in W. Coleman and F. Holmes (eds), *The Investigative Enterprise: Experimental Physiology in Nineteenth Century Medicine*, Berkeley, University of California Press, 1988, pp. 139–78; Arlene Tuchman, 'From the lecture to the laboratory: the institutionalization of scientific medicine at the University of Heidelberg', in ibid., pp. 65–99; Kenneth M. Ludmerer, *Learning to Heal: the Development of American Medical Education*, New York, Basic Books 1985; Russell Maulitz, 'Physician versus bacteriologist': the ideology of science in clinical medicine', in M. J. Vogel and C. E. Rosenberg (eds), *The Therapeutic Revolution*, Philadelphia, University of Pennsylvania Press, 1979, pp. 91–108; Paul Starr, *The Social Transformation of American Medicine*, New York, Basic Books, 1982; George Weisz, 'Reform and conflict and French medical education, 1870–1914', in Robert Fox and Weisz (eds), *The Organization of Science and Technology in France 1808–1914*, Cambridge, Cambridge University Press, and Paris, Éditions de la Maison des Sciences de l'Homme, 1980, pp. 61–94.

18   Arlene Tuchman, 'Experimental physiology, medical reform and the politics of education at the University of Heidelberg', *Bulletin of the History of Medicine*, 1987, 61: 203–15.

19   'History of accreditation of medical education programs', *Journal of the American Medical Association*, 1983, 250 (12): 1502–8.

20   Daniel Fox, 'Abraham Flexner's unpublished report: foundations and medical education, 1909–1928', *Bulletin of the History of Medicine*, 1980, 54: 475–96.

21   'History of accreditation', op. Cit. (n. 19), p. 1505.

22   Robert H. Ebert, 'Medical education at the peak of the era of experimental medicine', *Daedalus*, 1986, 115: 55–81.

23   P. K. Chatterjee, 'Medical education in India since independence', *Journal of Indian Medicine*, 1981, 77: 91–5; Mel Gorman, 'Introduction of Western science into colonial India: role of the Calcutta Medical College', *Proceedings of the American Philosophical Society*, 1988, 132: 276–98.

24   E. Richard Brown, 'Exporting medical education: professionalism, modernization and imperialism', *Social Science and Medicine*, 1979, 13A: 585–95.

25 See, for example, S. Shea and M. T. Fullilove, 'Entry of black and other minority students into US medical schools: historical perspectives and recent trends', *New England Journal of Medicine*, 1985, 313: 933–40.
26 Ebert, op. cit. (n. 22).

FURTHER READING

Ackerknecht, Erwin, *Medicine at the Paris Hospitals, 1794–1848*, Baltimore, MD, Johns Hopkins University Press, 1967.

Bynum, W. F. and Porter, Roy (eds), *William Hunter and the Eighteenth-Century Medical World*, Cambridge, Cambridge University Press, 1985.

Dow, D. and Moss, M., 'The medical curriculum at Glasgow in the early nineteenth century', *History of Universities*, 1983, 3: 227–57.

Edelstein, Ludwig, *Ancient Medicine: Selected Papers*, ed. by O. Temkin and C. L. Temkin, Baltimore, MD, Johns Hopkins University Press, 1967.

Foucault, Michel, *La Naissance de la clinique*, Paris, Presses Universitaires de France, 1963.

Gelfand, Toby, *Professionalizing Modern Medicine: Paris Surgeons and Medical Science and Institutions in the Eighteenth Century*, Westport, CT, Greenwood Press, 1980.

Harvey, A. M., *Science at the Bedside: Clinical Research in American Medicine, 1905–1945*, Baltimore, MD, Johns Hopkins University Press, 1981.

Jackson, Ralph, *Doctors and Diseases in the Roman Empire*, Norman, University of Oklahoma Press, 1988.

Ludmerer, Kenneth M., *Learning to Heal: the Development of American Medical Education*, New York, Basic Books, 1985.

Morantz-Sanchez, Regina, *Sympathy and Science: Women Physicians in American Medicine*, New York and Oxford, Oxford University Press, 1985.

O'Malley, Charles D. (ed.), *The History of Medical Education*, Berkeley, Los Angeles and London, University of California Press, 1970.

Poynter F. N. L. (ed.), *The Evolution of Medical Education in Britain*, London, Pitman, and Baltimore, MD, Williams & Wilkins, 1966.

Purcell, Elizabeth (ed.), *World Trends in Medical Education: Faculty, Students, and Curriculum. Report of a Macy Conference*, Baltimore, MD, Johns Hopkins University Press, 1971.

Rothstein, William G., *American Medical Schools and the Practice of Medicine: a History*, New York and Oxford, Oxford University Press, 1987.

Shapiro, Karen, 'Doctors or medical aids – the debate over the training of black medical personnel for the rural black population in South Africa in the 1920s and 1930s', *Journal of Southern African Studies*, 1987, 13: 234–55.

Starr, Paul, *The Social Transformation of American Medicine*, New York, Basic Books, 1982.

49

THE HOSPITAL

Lindsay Granshaw

INTRODUCTION

The hospital in the late twentieth century epitomizes modern medicine. It is crucial to patients, where the most invasive life-saving procedures are seen to be carried out. It is also crucial to the medical profession, where élite doctors practise, training is carried out, and most status accrues. The perceived heroism of modern medicine is inextricably linked to hospitals. Hospitals, too, account for large proportions of health-care budgets in the West. Their staff, equipment, drugs, and administrative and building requirements seem to drive costs ever upwards. Not surprisingly, those who are critical of modern medicine have often had hospitals, in particular, in their sights.

But hospitals were not always central in this way: their centrality has been very much a nineteenth- and twentieth-century development. Hospitals in earlier times did not play the same part as their descendants today. They tended to be few in number, treating a restricted social group for a limited range of complaints. They employed few, if any, medical staff, and used few resources. They were one small part in a patchwork of health care, formal or informal. Thus, the hospital has meant different things at different points in history. (➤ Ch. 4 Medical care)

The study of hospitals used to be the preserve of practitioners from the institutions themselves, who tended to emphasize the role of doctors and the uniqueness of the institution. Each hospital seemed to exist alone, even though its development might, in fact, closely parallel that of others. The society within which the hospital was set often seemed not to impinge on or give any context to the hospital's activities or explain changes within it. Such histories tended to be positivist in approach: medicine seemed so effectively to fit the model. Despite drawbacks, such histories nevertheless serve as useful source material for comparative studies of hospitals.[1]

Social historians of medicine have recently directed their attention to the history of hospitals. It is not assumed that hospitals played a central role in health care in the past, nor that they are the obvious and necessary loci of modern medicine. The place as well as the structure of the hospital has been examined. Historians have looked beyond the doctors to the governors, administrators, nurses, technicians, and the patients, who so seldom featured in the older histories. These tended to assume that hospitals were established in answer to need among the poor as perceived by the better-off. More recently, the function of the hospital for the philanthropists themselves has been examined. In addition, there has been a debate over epistemological changes that may have stimulated the hospital's growth.[2]

ANCIENT AND MEDIEVAL HOSPITALS

Tracing hospitals in ancient times depends a great deal on the definition of 'hospital'. Very occasionally in ancient Greece, a patient might be treated away from home: for example, overnight in a doctor's surgery, or at a healing shrine (*Asklepieia*). There were also facilities (*valetudinaria*) for the treatment of slaves and soldiers in Roman times. There was often provision for the welfare of strangers attending festivals, just as there were hostels for Jewish pilgrims visiting Jerusalem, where welfare might also be provided. However, there is no evidence of buildings devoted to the reception, care, and treatment of the sick among the population at large until well into the Christian era, around AD 350.

Charity was part of Christian theology: taking care of the sick was one of the seven corporate works of mercy. By about AD 250, there is evidence of Christian leaders taking in the sick and giving them refuge, if not treatment. From about a century later, this was institutionalized, although the most important feature of such 'institutions' was their smallness and variety. The continuity between hospices caring for the elderly, travellers, or the sick persisted well into the Middle Ages, with 'institutions' serving all or none of these purposes. They were often transitory, existing for a few years and then dying away with their founder or sponsor. Nor were they of significant size, except in major cities. By AD 500, hostels capable of accommodating 500 people could be found in major pilgrim towns such as Rome, Antioch, Alexandria, or Jerusalem, but any medical care was likely to be tangential to their main aim of housing pilgrims. However, by the seventh century in Constantinople, there were some hospitals sufficiently well established that, in addition to dividing men and women into different wards, there were special wards for surgical patients and for eye cases. The foundation charter

(1136) of the Pantokrator hospital in Constantinople expected that there would be formal teaching within the hospital, and this was certainly known to be taking place in the fifteenth century. In all these (limited) respects, Byzantium was more developed than Latin Europe.[3] (➤ Ch. 62 Charity before c. 1850; Ch. 61 Religion and medicine)

In the Arabic world, by the tenth century, there were complex hospitals (*bīmāristāns*) in large cities such as Cairo, Baghdad, and Damascus. Conrad has argued that Islamic hospitals first emerged in Baghdad in the ninth century.[4] (➤ Ch. 31 Arab-Islamic medicine) Certainly by the twelfth century, hospitals were frequently to be found in large cities, but evidence before this time cannot be relied upon. Some Arabic hospitals were divided into male and female sections, and in some, medical teaching took place. They mostly looked after the poor or others lacking support, such as the elderly. Despite claims to the contrary, given the size of the cities they served, hospitals can have played only a small part in health care. The questions of whether their origins were in Christian or Islamic culture, and whether medieval hospitals in Christian Europe took from the Arabic world or vice versa, remain unresolved among historians.[5] The formal provision of teaching in Western hospitals has been generally considered to have been an Arabic influence. In commenting on whether teaching in hospitals in the Arab and Byzantine worlds developed in parallel, or whether the Arabic example predated the Byzantine equivalent, Nutton notes that Arabic authors regularly associated hospitals with medical teaching, whereas Byzantine writers did not.[6]

In medieval Europe, the number of 'hospitals' expanded in parallel with the growth of population, trade, and towns. It was the areas in which economic expansion was most marked (for example, the Italian cities) where institutions of any scale were chiefly to be found. They reflected, above all, their endowers' wishes, not necessarily any particular needs of the population. Throughout the history of hospitals in Europe runs the theme of action taken by the better-off in offering appropriate charity to the poor. Overt Christian charity was a necessary virtue to be manifested by all, especially those who had the means to do so, buying grace in heaven through earthly good works. Since it therefore became a mark of wealth itself, more secular social pressures might also manifest themselves: philanthropy was a means of demonstrating wealth and social position.

Institutions were usually associated with a church or monastery, with religion underpinning life within them. Hospices, from the Latin for 'a guest', provided care and hospitality for the poor, aged, infirm, and travellers, and were not necessarily devoted only to the sick. Even if they were, they might later metamorphose into something else: thus St John's, Cambridge, gradually became a college for poor students.[7] Institutions were often very small and short-lived, almost never (except in some Italian hospitals) offering care from a doctor, and with little distinction, say, between care for the elderly and care for the sick. A main aim for the many leprosaria was simply to segregate lepers from society. After the death of an endower, hospitals often foundered. These fluid institutions might look after a few members of the poor when sick: clearly, they were but one small part of the patchwork of help offered by family or community.

Although the pattern of tiny institutions, coming and going, changing into other forms within a religious and philanthropic context, probably held good for most western-European towns and communities, in the larger towns of Italy, and in Paris, more sizeable hospitals could be found, where a group of benefactors rather than a single person might be supporting each institution. Some of these hospitals may have served the growing number of tradespeople and merchants by caring for employees when sick. Continuity in the work-force was perhaps a new necessity, and increased geographical mobility meant that an employee no longer had other members of his or her family around for support. Whereas hospitals in other parts of Europe cannot be regarded as other than a small element in support for the poor, or even in philanthropic activity, in late-medieval and Renaissance Italy hospitals served a much more important function. As elsewhere, they were closely linked to other charitable initiatives, but they differed in that they were larger, and offered significant support to those whom they tended, including groups outside the sick poor. The confraternity and guild system was more highly developed in sizeable towns such as Florence. Confraternities had as a duty the practice of charity, though how far this extended beyond their own members depended on will and wealth. Consisting of lay people, but with strong links to churches and religious houses, they existed at many social levels, and a few managed hospitals.[8] In providing a kind of social insurance for their members and dependants when sick, they were performing a function beyond that of the smaller almshouses and hospitals elsewhere, something on which members of a group could rely.

Henderson has estimated that by the fifteenth century there were over thirty hospitals in Florence, giving a ratio of about one hospital for 1,000 inhabitants.[9] The size of these hospitals varied enormously, however, from under ten beds to 230 at the largest and most important, S. Maria Nuova (founded 1288). Moreover, hospitals served a wide variety of purposes, with care for the sick being only part of this. Thus the poor, orphans, pilgrims, or widows had institutions dedicated to them, with only seven of the thirty-three early fifteenth-century 'hospitals' being devoted to the sick. However, doctors were associated with these institutions, no doubt because they played a more central part in the community than elsewhere. Thus at S. Maria Nuova there were six visiting physicians, a surgeon, and three junior staff members. Patients tended to suffer from acute diseases, and most were returned home 'cured' after a hospital stay averaging eleven to fifteen days.

Perhaps not surprisingly, countries elsewhere in Europe looked to the Florentine hospitals as models. General provision for the poor in late medieval and Tudor England was, however, mainly provided by fraternities or guilds, and parishes. Hospitals and almshouses supplemented this. Knowles and Hadcock indicated that there were about 470 such institutions in the 1390s, and a further 325 earlier institutions had become moribund.[10] Numbers of inmates varied from around two or three to about thirty, with an average of ten. There were few hospitals of any size: those that existed were adversely affected by the Reformation, at least in the short term.

EARLY MODERN AND MODERN HOSPITALS

In Britain, a few institutions were, often with a break, re-established shortly after the Reformation. For example, St Bartholomew's (founded 1123), St Thomas's (founded between 1106 and 1212), Christ's and Bethlem (both founded 1247) were sold to the City of London after the dissolution of the monasteries. The city corporation claimed that the sick poor would suffer unless the hospitals continued to exist, but also had an eye to the lands with which they were endowed. In keeping with its medieval origins as an orphanage, Christ's evolved into an institution caring for poor scholars. St Thomas's and St Bartholomew's, once reopened, expanded as hospitals for the sick poor, with Bethlem continuing to cater for the mad. Although religious links had in theory been thrown off, much of the same ethos surrounded the hospitals, but this time it was Protestant in nature. Philanthropy was no longer intended explicitly to buy grace in heaven, but still was an appropriate act of Christian charity (and, as ever, demonstrated social position). In other respects the hospitals were laicized: those taking daily care of patients were likely not to belong to a religious order, but to be recruited from among the patients themselves, or were poor men and women from outside the hospital who sought an institutional home. Importantly, too, the hospitals were refounded with medical staffs: in the case of St Bartholomew's, three surgeons (1549) and a physician (1568). A few years later, these were increased to four surgeons and four physicians, and stood at this level until 1895. Even so, as London's population grew, it had only two hospitals of significant size. (In 1569 St Thomas's housed 203 patients.) Outside the capital, there was little or no institutional support.[11]

In Catholic countries, undisturbed by the Reformation, it might be expected that there would be greater continuity between medieval and early-modern establishments. Pullan certainly found that there was no radical break after 1500 in the way that charity was provided.[12] The poor continued to be served in Florence, Genoa, Rome, and Venice by private lay institutions of religious confraternities and hospitals. However, this did not mean that religious authorities dominated in controlling hospitals, nor that that had been the case earlier. The endowers of such institutions had long had the greatest influence over them. Thus Cavallo, looking at the late seventeenth- and eighteenth-century Turin hospitals, emphasized that charity was very closely tied to local protection, patronage, and social conflict. While the Reformation was severing religious ties with hospitals elsewhere in Europe, in Catholic Turin the city government was becoming involved in hospital administration, and other hospitals in the city were closely associated with the court and military authority. Merchants, bankers, and masters used their power through the city-influenced hospital to provide relief for those of the urban poor whom they favoured. In addition to the main hospitals, there were a number of smaller institutions that received large amounts of charitable support and, in turn, provided relief for particular groups of the poor. In Turin, beds were set aside for incurables, in a pattern not generally found elsewhere.[13]

Just as the trading centres had hosted larger hospitals in the Middle Ages, as other countries expanded economically so their hospitals grew. Thus, in Britain, the wave of establishments of general hospitals came in the eighteenth century, with the expansion of the middle classes. As in earlier centuries, the founders were usually lay people, often linked by particular social ties. The Westminster (the model for eighteenth-century London hospitals) was established in 1719, Guy's soon followed in 1721, St George's in 1733, the London in 1740, and the Middlesex in 1745. Similar institutions were established in the provinces: the Edinburgh Royal Infirmary in 1729, Winchester (the model for many of the others) in 1736, and about twenty more in major towns thereafter. Hospitals tended to be established in the older towns first, with new manufacturing cities such as Manchester and Birmingham following later. From the beginning, medical staff were appointed to these hospitals. The Edinburgh Royal Infirmary indeed planned from the outset to accommodate not just doctors but students as well. At mid-century, a handful of other hospitals were established for cases excluded from the general hospitals. Thus in London, the Lock Hospital (for venereal disease) was set up in 1746; and four lying-in hospitals, the British (1749), the City (1750), the General (1752), and the Westminster (1765), founded within a few years of each other.

Hospitals published lists of donors, in the hope of attracting further support. The inclusion of a few aristocratic names in the list would be used to lure in those of middle-class standing. These hospitals, like their medieval predecessors, were set in the context of charity: they were for the poor, or more particularly the 'deserving' poor. Social, not medical, criteria were to determine admission, and donors were given rights proportionate to donation to admit patients. Donors, as hospital governors, had far greater power over affairs in the hospital than the doctors whom they appointed. Patients received treatment free of charge, but first had to secure an admission ticket from a benefactor. The benefactors sought to exclude the socially 'undeserving' such as prostitutes or drunks, but also a range of other 'inappropriate' cases. The hospital, if it was to use its charity well, was intended to help as many of the poor as possible. From this, it was concluded that incurables should not be admitted, nor should fever cases, lest fever spread to other patients. Once in hospital, patients had to obey a strict set of rules; and if disobedient, they would be ejected from the institution. Convalescent patients had to help their sicker neighbours, mend sheets, clean the ward, or tend the fire.

For some historians, the end of the eighteenth century marks a watershed in the way in which the hospital was used and viewed. According to this perspective, changes in the concepts of disease were vital in altering the hospital's role. As Ackerknecht put it, the French Revolution saw the rise of hospital medicine, typified by observation, physical examination, pathological anatomy, statistics, and the concept of the lesion. Hospital medicine then dominated until the mid-nineteenth century, when it came to be replaced by laboratory medicine.[14] Foucault put the change in even stronger terms. Medicine changed radically, entering, taking over, and drastically altering the hospital. Previous medical thinking had relied on book-learning: as the past was rejected in Revolutionary France, so it was in medicine too. Blinkers fell from medical eyes and doctors suddenly saw clearly.[15] For Foucault, the new anatomico-clinical medicine that replaced the old classificatory medicine was based not in the lecture-theatre but in the hospital, where real experience could be gained. The clinic had become central to medicine in a way that it had never been before. The new medicine was reductionist and analytical: post-mortem findings were correlated with pathology in the living. Diseases were identified as afflictions which beset a range of individuals in the same kind of way, rather than unique to each, and statistics were used to establish the patterns of each disease entity. (➤ Ch. 9 The pathological tradition; Ch. 5 The anatomical tradition)

However, others do not see such disjunction at the French Revolution, or that ideology explained all. Doctors were already increasingly active within many hospitals, and the development of the medical profession itself is seen as crucial to some historians.[16] As doctors grouped together and sought to improve individual and collective status, they used hospitals as institutional bases on which they could consolidate. (➤ Ch. 47 History of the medical profession) Since it was the better-off in society who supported the hospitals, gaining a hospital appointment brought a doctor to the attention of potential patients who could help him establish a lucrative practice. However, patterns varied from country to country, and even where doctors were associated with hospitals they did not necessarily seek, nor achieve, greater influence there. Colin Jones, for example, looking at French provincial hospitals, finds far greater continuity between *ancien régime* and Revolutionary France than Foucault would have admitted.[17] Nor does he see increased attendance by medical practitioners at hospitals as necessarily implying that they had greater control over their institutions, with consequent effects. He argues that the nursing staff, in particular, had a firm grip well into the nineteenth century. (➤ Ch. 54 A general history of nursing: 1800–1900)

Social historians are sceptical of Foucault's notions of humoral ideas of disease simply being swept away by clear-thinking nineteenth-century doctors. (➤ Ch. 14 Humoralism) Patients and doctors shifted their views only very slowly over the nineteenth century.[18] However, it is undeniable that certain changes were introduced into some of the Paris hospitals, which had a major influence on medical ideas elsewhere in Europe and the United States over the nineteenth century, an influence overtaken later by German patterns and ideas. The practices and ideas explored in Paris did not necessarily originate there. In the seventeenth and eighteenth centuries, a strand of thinking emphasized that diseases were distinct natural historical entities that could be classified like plants. (➤ Ch. 17 Nosology) Physicians such as Thomas Sydenham (1624–89) began to describe particular diseases in this way. These nosologies were based on symptoms, but from the late eighteenth century, particularly in Paris, symptoms and signs in the living patient were increasingly correlated with pathological changes observed at post-mortem. Such an approach was pioneered by Philippe Pinel (1745–1826) at the Salpêtrière in Paris; R. T. H. Laënnec (1781–1826) (who also devised the stethoscope and promoted auscultation) at the Hôpital Beaujour and then the Hôpital Necker; and Pierre Louis (1787–1872) (who was considered the founder of medical statistics and who worked particularly on tuberculosis and typhoid) of the Hôtel Dieu. (➤ Ch. 19 Fevers) Their emphasis was on lesions rather than symptoms, with the focus gradually shifting from organ to tissue and to cell. By mid-century, new work was being undertaken in physiology by Claude Bernard (1813–78), from 1852 first Professor of Physiology at the Sorbonne; and in cellular pathology by Rudolf Virchow (1821–1902) at the Charité Hospital in Berlin, subsequently Professor at the university and Director of its pathological institute. (➤ Ch. 7 The physiological tradition)

Since leading medical thinkers in Paris in the early nineteenth century emphasized the relationship between physical diagnosis in the living and post-mortem appearances, hospital appointments became crucial, as it was here that large groups of patients whose symptoms and signs could be studied were gathered together. Moreover, the poor were less likely to make effective protest at post-mortems being carried out on their relatives. Thus for doctors who were keen to be at the forefront of medical thinking, hospitals were of increasing importance.

This did not necessarily dictate a marked change within institutions; as has been seen (see p. 1179), medical practitioners were already closely associated with hospitals, and had been in Italy, for example, since medieval times. Despite Foucault's claims, teaching had been carried on within hospitals from at least early modern times. In Britain, students were walking the wards in the eighteenth century. By the end of that century, large groups of students were following in the wake of leading surgeons and physicians, paying handsomely for the privilege. The Apothecaries' Act of 1815 in effect formalized the requirement that hospital experience should be part of a general practitioner's training, and by the mid-nineteenth century, hospital medical schools dominated medical education. (➤ Ch. 48 Medical education)

As cities grew, so the number and size of hospitals increased. As London's population expanded from half-a-million in the early eighteenth century to 5 million by 1900, its hospitals multiplied. In 1800, America's population was just over 5 million, with only a tiny proportion of that number living in sizeable communities. There were a couple of hospitals, the Pennsylvania Hospital (founded 1752) and the New York Hospital (founded 1771). By 1920, America's social organization and economy had radically changed, and there were now almost 5,000 hospitals, with few towns without one.[19] The increasing importance of hospitals for doctors is apparent. In Britain, doctors played a key role in the newly established eighteenth-century hospitals. From the late eighteenth century, medical practitioners began to found their own institutions. A model for such institutions was the Aldersgate Street Dispensary, established in London by John Coakley Lettsom (1744–1815) in 1770. (Lettsom also established the Medical Society of London in 1773, and the Royal Sea Bathing Hospital at Margate in 1779.) Lettsom was a Quaker who had practised abroad and, struggling against the closed world of the London medical profession, on his return established his own institutions. Dispensaries, which treated patients in their own homes rather than institutionalizing them, and which were cheaper to run, were subsequently set up, mostly by less-established medical practitioners in towns and cities all over Britain. The first Scottish dispensary was opened in 1776 in Edinburgh by Andrew Duncan (1744–1828), Professor of the Institutes of Medicine, to be used for teaching purposes.[20]

Not all dispensaries were as long-lasting as Aldersgate Street, but that did not prevent other doctors attempting a similar formula. A short-lived institution might indeed serve the founder's purpose if the aim was simply to gain recognition in a field. The out-patient dispensary for sick children established in 1769 by George Armstrong (1720–89) in London lasted only until 1782. Nevertheless, it spawned children's institutions elsewhere in Britain and on the European continent. The Kinderkrankeninstitut, established by Joseph Johann Mastalier (1757–93) in 1788 in Vienna, looked to the earlier British version.[21] (➤ Ch. 45 Childhood)

The nineteenth century saw a further expansion in the number of hospitals set up in Britain, again largely by medical entrepreneurs who were challenging traditional patterns and drawing their financial support from the trading classes. Setting up specialized institutions seemed one way to justify disrupting the *status quo*: patients could be offered special expertise, which the new localized explanations of disease helped to underpin. The model for this new wave of establishments was Moorfields or the Royal Ophthalmic Hospital, set up in 1804 by John Cunningham Saunders (1773–1810). Blocked from promotion at St Thomas's Hospital, he set up a dispensary, which shortly afterwards established a few beds, calling it an 'infirmary' for the treatment of ear and eye diseases, later for eye diseases alone.[22] So successful was the new infirmary, attracting subscribers as well as patients, that replicas of it were established over the next decades in all the major towns and cities in Britain, as well as on the European continent and in the United States.[23]

From the 1830s there was a great expansion in the number and type of special institutions in Britain. By 1860, there were at least sixty-six special hospitals and dispensaries in London alone. Some of the best-known British specialist hospitals had been established during the first two-thirds of the nineteenth century: for example, the Royal Hospital for Diseases of the Chest (1814); St Mark's Hospital for Diseases of the Colon and Rectum (1835); the Royal National Orthopaedic Hospital (merged from two institutions founded respectively in 1840 and 1864); the Brompton (1841); the Royal Marsden (1851); the Hospital for Sick Children, Great Ormond Street (1852); the National Hospital, Queen Square (1860), for nervous diseases; St John's Hospital for Diseases of the Skin (1863); and St Peter's Hospital, for urological disorders (1864). Although these hospitals were opposed by the general hospitals for taking cases from them, by the end of the nineteenth century the élite were seeking appointments within them, either as part of their training or indeed to complement a general-hospital appointment. In addition, the general hospitals began to set up special departments.[24]

The special hospitals were 'medicalized' earlier than the general hospitals, serving as a model for the latter. Doctors controlled patient admission, staff appointments, and policy. Donors' letters were simply granted to patients after, not before, they were admitted. Staff at the special hospitals also seem to have spent more time within their institutions: a patient undergoing surgery there was more likely to receive the attention of a full member of staff rather than a junior.

Although special hospitals were particularly numerous in Britain, hospitals also served the cause of specialization on the European continent and in the

United States. Thus children's hospitals were set up in Paris in 1802, in Berlin in 1830, St Petersburg in 1834, and Vienna in 1837; and other special hospitals also appeared. In the United States, the Massachusetts Eye and Ear Infirmary was established in 1824, on the model of Moorfields; the Boston Lying-In Hospital in 1832; the New York Hospital for Diseases of the Skin in 1836; a children's hospital in 1855 in Philadelphia; an orthopaedic hospital in 1867.[25] The Infirmary for Haemorrhoids, Fistula and Other Diseases of the Rectum (subsequently St Paul's Infirmary), established in New York in 1879 (and closed in the mid-1880s), was modelled on St Mark's Hospital in London. However, it is striking that whereas the institutions in Britain found fertile soil, in the United States, with its different social make-up and differently organized medical profession, special hospitals often did not last long.[26] In keeping with American society, the more successful specialist hospitals were those established for particular groups of people – Germans, Italians, Jews – reflecting and solidifying social ties among them. In Germany and Austria, as hospitals became closely associated with universities and the teaching of medical science, special departments tended to develop in preference to special institutions.

The establishment of institutions specifically for teaching purposes can be seen on the European continent more clearly than in Britain. However, University College London, set up in 1828 in opposition to the Anglican discrimination practised by Oxford and Cambridge, established its own hospital in 1834, the (now) necessary adjunct to its medical school. King's College was the Anglican response to this development, and King's College Hospital was set up in 1839.

While teaching had a major effect in bringing hospitals to the forefront of medical practice, so too did changes in surgery. In the early nineteenth century, a mere handful of operations were carried out in hospital. (➤ Ch. 41 Surgery (traditional)) By the end of the century, that was changing rapidly, although it was after the First World War that the change was most noticeable. In the Paris hospitals, there had been a greater emphasis on surgery, but further expansion came after the introduction in the late 1840s of general anaesthesia into medicine. (➤ Ch. 42 Surgery (modern)) Expansion did not simply follow this development. In fact, in both Europe and America at mid-century there was a crisis of confidence in hospitals: infection seemed to be endemic, and deaths from hospital diseases (so-called because they seemed to arise from the institutions themselves), particularly in the surgical wards, seemed by the 1850s unacceptably high. The phenomenon was dubbed 'hospitalism'. Various schemes were undertaken to reduce the incidence of hospital disease, many along lines that had been followed for generations – whitewashing the walls, disinfecting the wards, and encouraging good ventilation to blow away the miasma which was believed to spread infection. (➤ Ch. 15 Environment and miasmata) Ignaz Semmelweis (1818–65), a Hungarian obstetrician working in Vienna at the Allgemeines Krankenhaus, insisted that students entering his ward thoroughly washed their hands with disinfectant. He had concluded that puerperal fever was spread by staff and students who attended the mothers immediately after working in the dissecting room. Although rejected by colleagues at the time, his attempt was in keeping with those of others trying to combat hospital infections. Florence Nightingale (1820–1910), speaking from her post-Crimean platform, strongly advocated good ventilation. Drawing from leading opinion among sanitary reformers, she advocated the construction of pavilion-plan hospitals, with blocks of wards well separated to allow good ventilation, and built on sandy soil on an elevated site, so that dank airs did not collect. Her influence was strong, and many subsequent hospitals in Britain and America were built on that plan.[27] (➤ Ch. 64 Medicine and architecture)

To some, the only way to relieve hospital mortality was to disband the hospitals. Not surprisingly, the medical profession made great efforts to combat this perception. Many different plans for the reduction of surgical mortality were proposed before Joseph Lister (1827–1912) put forward his antiseptic scheme, based on the germ theory of Louis Pasteur (1822–95), arguing that it was the presence of specific germs that caused putrefaction in wounds. Lister is given much of the credit for transforming hospitals and surgery, although it was 'asepsis', an amalgam of earlier practices of great cleanliness, together with an amended version of the theory behind antisepsis, that came to be widely practised in hospitals. (➤ Ch. 16 Contagion/germ theory/specificity)

Undoubtedly anaesthesia, antisepsis, and asepsis allowed surgeons to undertake more-complex and more-frequent operations. Although such procedures were carried out in places other than hospitals, there was a marked increase in the number of hospital operations. Leading the way in the development of surgery were the German-trained surgeons, who initiated radical operations such as opening the abdomen under aseptic conditions. Theodor Billroth (1829–94), a German surgeon who later became Professor of Surgery in Vienna, pioneered abdominal surgery using antiseptic and, later, aseptic methods. Richard von Volkmann (1830–89), Professor of Surgery in Halle, Theodor Kocher (1841–1917), Professor of Clinical Surgery in Berne, Johann von Mickulicz-Radecki (1850–1905), Professor of Surgery at Breslau, and Johann von Nussbaum (1829–90), Surgeon at the Allgemeines Krankenhaus in Munich, contributed to the expansion of surgery. All worked in association with major hospitals, and many also held professorships of surgery within important medical schools. The German medical-science model, closely linking universities and hospitals, was imported to Johns Hopkins University in the United States. William Halsted (1852–1922), who had trained in Germany, began to undertake radical surgery there, strongly influencing his American colleagues.

Operating theatres in the leading surgical centres were quite distinct from the primitive facilities found in patients' homes. With all features designed to be sterilized – from glass operating tables to metal instruments – and special gear for the surgeons and, later, other staff members, hospital theatres clearly offered something new and different.[28]

Just as the extension of aseptic surgery encouraged surgeons to see the hospital as a fitting place in which to work, so expansion in the range of investigations also fostered the growth of the hospital. From the 1860s, chemical laboratories came to be associated with larger institutions, and from the 1880s and 1890s bacteriological investigations were also carried out in hospital laboratories. (➤ Ch. 8 The biochemical tradition; Ch. 11 Clinical research) The germ theory was further elaborated beyond Pasteur's notions by Robert Koch (1843–1910), who isolated the bacterial causes of tuberculosis in 1882, identified the cause of cholera in 1883, and put forward four postulates to be satisfied before accepting that an organism was the cause of a specific disease. His work, in particular, ensured that bacteriological laboratories became an integral part of the large hospitals, used especially for diagnosing tuberculosis. Pathology laboratories were added later. Increasingly, doctors did not only diagnose by examining the patient, but by sending samples to the laboratory to identify the disease, the state of a bodily fluid, or extent of a tumour. Private laboratories certainly backed up practice in consulting rooms, but the presence of such facilities in hospitals increasingly meant that they could offer something extra, something different from general practice. The discovery of X-rays in 1895 by Wilhelm Roentgen (1845–1923) was quickly harnessed for medical purposes. X-ray departments were established in many hospitals by the time of the First World War, and certainly by the 1920s. (➤ Ch. 36 The science of diagnosis: diagnostic technology) With all of these new investigative techniques available, not only were patients attracted to hospital, but hospital staffs were growing: technicians and other workers were added to the occupational groups that a hospital now needed to employ. (➤ Ch. 55 The emergence of para-medical professions)

The changing position of the hospital is not explicable without substantial reference to patient demand. A number of reasons can be given for this change. In a process that lasted well into the twentieth century, hospitals were gradually losing their charity stigma. Several factors certainly made hospitals more desirable – or at least less undesirable – in the eyes of patients. Increasingly, the hospital was seen as offering something different from what might be gained by visiting a doctor or pharmacist. But in other ways, too, hospitals became more attractive to patients. This can be linked to a number of developments, from the reform of nursing to the introduction of aseptic surroundings.

In Britain, there was the additional factor of the growth of poor-law infirmaries,[29] which was stimulated by the 1834 Poor Law Act, according to which relief outside an institution was deemed inefficient, and removed. The semi-destitute now had to choose between no additional support within the community or entering the workhouse: many families chose for them. Predominantly, it was the sick and elderly who were institutionalized, and the workhouse infirmaries rapidly expanded. By the 1860s, hospitals were being built alongside workhouses. They housed the poorest patients, taking them, in theory, away from the voluntary hospitals, and reducing the stigma attached to the latter.[30]

The position of nursing has been much debated. Although it has been argued that nursing was not as bad before the reforms as was often made out, nor as spotless afterwards, it was undoubtedly true that the image of the nurse underwent radical transformation. Nightingale herself had stressed the darker side of nursing – drunkenness, dishonesty, immorality – no doubt to contrast with what she intended for the future. Reform movements, for example at Kaiserswerth in Germany, preceded the Nightingale Training School (1860), and things did not change quite as much as she later implied. However, hospital nurses had tended earlier to be recruited from among patients, and although the new nurses might continue to be little more than cheap labour, at least cleanliness and basic literacy were now stressed in their training. Nursing was similar to domestic service. It recruited from much the same social strata, despite a few well-known 'lady' nurses. A great deal of housework was entailed in the work, and the emphasis was on discipline. Even after nurse training was introduced, most hospitals would have had untrained staff, although many claimed that they offered their own 'training'. As medical intervention became more intensive, so the nursing ratio went up. At various stages over the next hundred years, it was predicted that all female school-leavers would have to become nurses, such was the increasing demand. However, the reforms in nursing and the image of the young, uniformed nurse changed patients' views of the hospital, making it much more acceptable to the middle classes. Hospital managers were not averse to using pictures of nurses when they wished to attract either subscriptions or, indeed, patients.[31] (➤ Ch. 38 Women and medicine)

An apparent change in the class of patients – from the labouring poor to the better-off – was noted by those concerned with hospitals from the mid-nineteenth century. For some, this represented charity abuse which should be thwarted. Doctors outside hospitals complained that they were losing patients – and income – to hospitals. In many cases, it was denied that any such change was occurring, but in Britain some enterprising general practitioners sought to harness increased demand for hospital care by establishing their own institutions. The model for these 'cottage' hospitals was established in Cranleigh in Surrey, in 1859. Employers or local gentry might help to subsidize such hospitals, but patients were expected to contribute as well, and since the general practitioner received fees, he no longer lost out. It was also argued that the cottage hospitals gave country patients and their doctors access to hospital beds. In 1896, it was estimated that several hundred cottage hospitals were in operation, and that they had spawned many replicas in the United States.[32] (➤ Ch. 63 Medical philanthropy after 1850)

Other changes were affecting hospitals by this stage. The late nineteenth century saw the introduction into numerous areas – from the civil service to large institutions – of ideas and practices designed to increase institutional efficiency. In the United States in particular, the idea of 'scientific management', applying the lauded logicality of science to running businesses or institutions, was also applied within hospitals. In Britain, the expansion in the number of clerks, administrators within the colonial service, and the stress on efficiency through meritocracy all had their impact on the hospital. The change was slow, with lay governors often reluctant to give up their control, even to their own appointees. Long debates occurred over whether hospitals, as they became more complicated, larger, and employed more staff, should continue to be run by gentlemen recruited from among the governors, or by a professional manager with army or civil-service experience, for example. In the United States, hospital administrators were beginning to professionalize by the beginning of the twentieth century, with an association, a journal, and their own agenda.[33]

As the lower middle classes increasingly came to the hospitals, institutions began to set beds aside for paying patients. A small charge might be made of those in general wards, with a larger fee extracted from those in private rooms. Although the change was slow, it was significant: hospitals began to advertise their facilities, ensuring that private rooms were enticing, and widening the social pool from which they drew their patients. Such a development ran alongside the establishment in Britain of numerous nursing-homes: effectively small private hospitals for the middle classes. By paying for admission, patients were claiming a right that had always been conveyed on the poor as a favour. But the labouring poor themselves were increasingly securing a 'right' to hospital admission. The Hospital Saturday Fund, set up in the 1870s, collected small subscriptions from workers and, in return, secured admission tickets from the hospitals.[34] Employees would group together as well, buying tickets and distributing them amongst themselves to those in need. Such insurance schemes served to place hospitals in a more central position in health care.

The First World War reinforced this development across Europe. There were casualties among troops on a massive scale, and all, whatever their rank, expected to be treated in hospital if necessary. Surgery was greatly extended, and specialization advanced. Some of the effects can be seen in post-war planning for health care in Britain. When Lord Dawson of Penn (1864–1945) produced a report on the future provision of medical services in 1920, he envisaged that patients would be treated in the first instance at primary health centres, largely staffed by general practitioners. If their problems were more severe, they would pass down the line, after the wartime model, to a secondary health centre based on a hospital. Only by such an arrangement, he thought, could the benefits of modern medical science be brought to all.[35]

It is impossible to give anything like precise figures for the number of hospitals in the nineteenth century (or before), let alone beds and numbers of patients using them. Hospitals often wildly exaggerated the numbers of patients they were treating as they competed for philanthropy and sought to demonstrate their usefulness. However, some indication of the scale of growth can be given: St Thomas's estimated that its out-patient department saw 10,000 patients in 1800 and 100,000 by 1890. From the patchy evidence available, it may well be that patient demand in Britain grew at least tenfold, though from what to what is less clear. For Britain, Pinker, relying particularly on Burdett's *Year Books*, estimated that there were 254 hospitals in 1861 containing something like 14,772 beds. Perhaps a further 50,000 beds were available in the poor-law hospitals. There are significant problems with the nature of the data, and substantial variations between different sources. However, the scale of the increase is clear. By 1891, Pinker found almost 30,000 beds in the voluntary sector and over 83,000 in the public; by 1921, this had reached over 56,000 in voluntary hospitals and 172,000 in public hospitals, with over 87,000 beds in voluntary hospitals by 1938, and almost 116,000 in local authority hospitals. In addition, there were about 22,000 beds in private nursing-homes, and perhaps 26,000 in voluntary convalescent homes. This meant that the number of beds per thousand of the population rose from around 4 in 1861 to 7.64 by 1938, about half of current numbers. Looking only at voluntary hospitals, in London the number of beds available per thousand of the population stood at 1.63 in 1861 and had risen to 2.38 by 1938, while in the provinces it increased from 0.56 to 2.04.[36]

By the 1920s, the pattern had been set in which hospitals played a central role in health care. Between the wars, surgery became much more invasive, investigations extended, medical technology became increasingly important, and staff costs rose. (➤ Ch. 68 Medical technologies: social contexts and consequences) The development of ambulance services to transport the sick and injured to the hospital helped to make it the focus of emergency care. The medical staff by now had firm control of the hospital, although in many instances at teaching hospitals there were battles between clinicians and those primarily concerned with teaching over the nature of that control. As costs escalated, hospitals that had been funded on a voluntary basis ran into problems. In the United States, hospitals were already developing business strategies and, in conjunction with burgeoning insurance schemes, were attracting well-off patients. A two-tier system was rapidly developing in which the hospitals in the suburbs, with wealthy patients, were prospering and developing rapidly at the expense of poorer inner-city institutions. Local doctors would buy rights to hospital beds, which the hospitals were only too willing to sell. In turn, hospital beds were seen as a necessary arm of a leading doctor's practice.[37]

The financial underpinning of the American hospitals by insurance hardly existed in Britain, and this feature probably helps to explain why a national health service was introduced in Britain. And if so, this reveals a great deal about the importance of hospitals by the Second World War. In Britain, the voluntary hospitals seemed to stagger from one financial crisis to another, looking, in some ways, in envy at the former workhouse infirmaries, which by 1929 were cared for by local government. The voluntary hospitals' annual budget in 1938 ran at £16 million.[38] Although the voluntary hospitals did not relish the idea of low-status local-authority control, it was increasingly felt that, in return for the numbers of patients treated, the state should make some contribution. (➤ Ch. 57 Health economics)

The Second World War dictated a change in how things were arranged. The government prepared for a massive blitz with vast civilian casualties, assigning almost all hospitals particular tasks, and remunerating them for the beds they set aside. There were two main effects of such an arrangement: hospitals began to rely on the government payments, and they became more adjusted to forced co-operation within a government-planned scheme. When a national health service was seriously mooted in 1942 by William Beveridge (1879–1963) as the necessary complement to his social security plans, the reaction of those within the voluntary hospitals was mixed. In general, they opposed the idea of being taken into state service, but it was agreed that some sort of financial help was crucial. After the Labour victory in the 1945 General Election, with Aneurin Bevin (1897–1960) as Minister of Health, it was evident that a national health service would be introduced, despite opposition from the medical profession. Bevan exploited the division between hospital doctors and general practitioners, seeking to divide the profession and win over the former, in particular, by the favourable status given to hospitals. Teaching hospitals kept their endowments, and were answerable directly to the Ministry of Health. Private practice was retained. When the President of the Royal College of Physicians, Lord Moran (1882–1977), came out in favour of the service, it marked the beginning of the end for the doctors who opposed it. (➤ Ch. 50 Medical institutions and the state)

In the British National Health Service (NHS), hospitals formed the most important arm, followed by general practice, and a long way behind, community medicine. The service absorbed the provision that already existed. There were at the time over 900 voluntary hospitals, but many of them were small: over 250 had fewer than thirty beds. Most were taken into the NHS, with the ownership of buildings and land passing to the state. The teaching hospitals retained control of their endowment funds: all other funds went to the Ministry of Health. England and Wales were divided into regions, and hospitals were grouped under regional hospital boards. Teaching hospitals were managed by their own board of governors. In the 1950s and 1960s, new District General Hospitals were built to give more systematic hospital coverage around the country. In 1974, the service was reorganized to try to integrate all three arms in each local area. More recent changes (1991) seeking to establish an internal market, with hospitals being granted the right to opt for self-governing status and relatively free to decide what services to sell other parts of the sector, once again put great emphasis on hospitals.

Hospitals have come to be seen as the essential loci for medical advances. The increased interest of the medical profession in hospitals in the nineteenth century had indeed related in some way to 'research', at least in terms of gaining greater operative skills. In the twentieth century, medical research sat uneasily beside clinical practice in British hospitals, was more closely integrated in German university hospitals, and again fitted with some difficulty into American institutions with their public stress on individual patient care. Within the medical schools in Britain, so-called 'basic' medical science was undertaken by departments involved in pre-clinical teaching, but there was a significant division (despite attempts by the (American) Rockefeller and other foundations to fund bridges) between their work and that of the clinicians. However, trials were particularly a feature of clinical work in teaching hospitals in Britain after the Second World War, using the hospital base for their material. Like the governors of the pre-NHS hospitals, the NHS did not support research: that was left to the Medical Research Council or to pharmaceutical companies, whose own research and drug development should not be underestimated. (➤ Ch. 39 Drug therapies)

By the post-war period, hospitals, whether in the United States or Europe, were seen as quintessentially part of modern medical care: high-tech, invasive, the subject of high drama, or at least soap operas. Yet from the 1960s, critiques of hospitals and their doctors emerged. Particularly in the United States, medico-legal cases and third-party payment fuelled costs, as numerous investigations were undertaken and more and more capital was spent on medical equipment. (➤ Ch. 69 Medicine and the law) Remuneration was closely linked to the number of investigations undertaken. Some critics argued that modern hospital medicine had contributed little except cost: it was public-health measures in the nineteenth century that had actually brought down mortality and, at most, modern medical claims were simply based on the use of penicillin. (➤ Ch. 51 Public health) Historically, hospitals might even have increased mortality.[39] After the introduction of Medicaid and Medicare by Lyndon B. Johnson (1908–73) in the mid-1960s to aid the very poor, American politicians increasingly addressed the question of medical costs. Between 1960 and 1980, the daily cost of a hospital bed rose almost ninefold, in comparison to the consumer price index rise of threefold. Hospitals had become businesses, fuelled by third-party insurance payments. Establishing cost controls in the 1980s for government-paid treatments, based on an average cost of particular procedures, under the Diagnosis Related Groups (DRGs) system, had its effect on the insurance companies too, as they endeavoured to control costs. Few doubted that holding costs in hospitals was the key to controlling costs in health-care provision as a whole.

CONCLUSION

By the post-war years, hospitals were clearly central to modern medicine, and those seeking to extend the benefits or otherwise of modern practice to developing countries have seen the hospital as a key part of their armamentaria. Hospitals have played a variety of roles over the centuries, depending on their social setting. First introduced in the Christian era, much of their early history was dictated not necessarily by those cared for within them, or the population as a whole, so much as by the needs and desires of the philanthropists who founded them. Often short-lived, varied in their forms, it was only as towns grew that hospitals of any size can be seen. By the seventeenth century, they were taking on a more secular role, but still one dictated by the donors who supported them. Doctors were playing a larger part within them, offering philanthropy of their own. As economies grew, so the hospital, like other institutions, grew with them. During the nineteenth century, hospitals began to take a greater part in health care, first for the poor, and later for other classes as well. By 1920, many of the patterns of the modern, high-tech hospital were in place: professionally managed, depending on third-party payment, with trained nurses, interventionist doctors, medical students, investigations, and a very recognizable antiseptic aura, hospitals were seen as offering something distinct and additional to other sources of health care. Although the post-war period has seen a rapid expansion in costs, together with mounting criticism both of modern medicine and its hospitals, in public esteem there is little evidence that their reputations are under any real challenge.

NOTES

1   See, for example, Roy Porter, 'The gift relation: philanthropy and provincial hospitals in eighteenth-century England', in Lindsay Granshaw and Roy Porter (eds), *The Hospital in History*, London, Routledge, 1989, pp. 149–78.

2   See, in addition to the works cited in the Further Reading section, Robert Pinker, *English Hospital Statistics, 1861–1938*, London, Heinemann, 1966; F. N. L. Poynter (ed.), *The Evolution of Hospitals in Britain*, London, Pitman, 1968; John Woodward, *To Do the Sick No Harm. A Study of the British Voluntary Hospital System to 1875*, London, Routledge & Kegan Paul, 1974; Harry F. Dowling, *City Hospitals: the Undercare of the Underprivileged*, Cambridge, MA, Harvard University Press, 1982; Dieter Jetter, *Wien von dem Anfängen bis um 1900*, Wiesbaden, Steiner, 1982; V. G. Drachman, *Hospital with a Heart. Women Doctors and the Paradox of Separatism at the New England Hospital, 1862–1969*, Ithaca, NY, Cornell University Press, 1984; Geoffrey Rivett, *The Development of the London Hospital System*, London, King's Fund, 1986; Hilary Marland, *Medicine and Society in Wakefield and Huddersfield, 1780–1870*, Cambridge, Cambridge University Press, 1987.

3   T. S. Miller, *The Birth of the Hospital in the Byzantine Empire*, Baltimore, MD, and London, Johns Hopkins University Press, 1985; Vivian Nutton 'Essay review', *Medical History*, 1986, 30: 218–21. I am very grateful to Vivian Nutton for his help with this section.

4   Lawrence I. Conrad, 'The institution of the hospital in medieval Islam: ideals and realities', paper given to the Wellcome Institute for the History of Medicine, 13 November 1985. See also Michael W. Dols, 'The origins of the Islamic hospital: myth and reality', in *Bulletin of the History of Medicine*, 1987, 61: 367–90.

5   Lawrence I. Conrad and Vivian Nutton, *Jundishapur. From Myth to History*, Princeton, NJ, Darwin Press.

6   Nutton, op. cit. (n. 3).

7   See Miri Rubin, *Charity and Change in Medieval Cambridge*, Cambridge, Cambridge University Press, 1987; Martha Carlin, 'Medieval English hospitals', and Rubin, 'Development and change in English hospitals: 1100–1500', in Granshaw and Porter, op. cit. (n. 1), pp. 21–39, 41–59, respectively; K. Park, *Doctors and Medicine in Early Renaissance Florence*, Princeton, NJ, Princeton University Press, 1985. See also R. M. Clay, *The Medieval Hospitals of England*, London, Methuen, 1909; C. Dainton, *The Story of England's Hospitals*, London, Museum Press, 1961; D. Knowles and R. Neville Hadcock, *Mediaeval Religious Houses, England and Wales*, London, Methuen, 1909; Walter H. Godfrey, *The English Almshouse*, London, Faber & Faber, 1955; Carol Rawcliffe, 'The hospitals of later medieval London', *Medical History*, 1984, 28: 1–21; Peregrine Horden, 'A discipline of relevance: the historiography of the later medieval hospital', *Social History of Medicine*, 1988, 1: 359–74.

8   B. Pullan, 'Support and redeem: charity and poor relief in Italian cities from the fourteenth to the seventeenth century', *Continuity and Change*, 1988, 3: 177–208.

9   John Henderson, 'The hospitals of late-medieval and Renaissance Florence: a preliminary survey', in Granshaw and Porter, op. cit. (n. 1), pp. 63–92. See also B. Pullan, *Rich and Poor in Renaissance Venice. The Social Institutions of a Catholic State to 1620*, Oxford, Blackwell, 1971; John Henderson, 'The parish and the

poor in Florence at the time of the Black Death: the case of S. Frediano', *Continuity and Change*, 1988, 3: 247–72.

10 Marjorie K. McIntosh, 'Local responses to the poor in late medieval and Tudor England', *Continuity and Change*, 1988, 3: 209–45; Knowles and Hadcock, op. cit. (n. 7).

11 Dainton, op. cit. (n. 7); for lack of institutional provision in the provinces see, for example, Margaret Pelling, 'Illness among the poor in an early modern English town: the Norwich census of 1570', *Continuity and Change*, 1988, 3: 273–90.

12 Pullan, op. cit. (n. 8).

13 Sandra Cavallo, 'Hospitals in Turin in the eighteenth century', in Granshaw and Porter, op. cit. (n. 1), p. 95.

14 Erwin H. Ackerknecht, *Medicine at the Paris Hospital, 1794–1848*, Baltimore, MD, Johns Hopkins University Press, 1967.

15 Michel Foucault, *The Birth of the Clinic. An Archaelogy of Medical Perception*, trans. by A. M. Sheridan, London, Tavistock, 1976.

16 Park, op. cit. (n. 7); Cavallo, op. cit. (n. 13); Toby Gelfand, *Professionalizing Modern Medicine, Paris Surgeons and Medical Science and Institutions in the Eighteenth Century*, Westport, CT, and London, Greenwood Press, 1980.

17 Colin Jones, *The Charitable Imperative: Hospitals and Nursing in Ancien Régime and Revolutionary France*, London, Routledge, 1989.

18 See, for example, Charles Rosenberg, 'The therapeutic revolution. Medicine, meaning and social change in nineteenth-century America', *Perspectives in Biology and Medicine*, 1977, 20: 485–506.

19 Charles Rosenberg, *The Care of Strangers: the Rise of America's Hospital System*, New York, Basic Books, 1987, pp. 18, 341.

20 See Z. Cope, 'The history of the dispensary movement', in Poynter, op. cit. (n. 2), pp. 73–6; and T. Hunt (ed.), *The Medical Society of London, 1773–1973*, London, Heinemann, 1973; I. S. L. Loudon, 'The origins and growth of the dispensary movement in England', *Bulletin of the History of Medicine*, 1981, 55: 322–42.

21 Eduard Seidler, 'An historical survey of children's hospitals', in Granshaw and Porter, op. cit. (n. 1), pp. 184–5.

22 J. R. Farre, *A Treatise on Some Practical Points Relating to the Diseases of the Eye by the late John Cunningham Saunders . . . [and] A Short Account of the Author's Life*, London, 1811, pp. ix-xlii; B. Abel-Smith, *The Hospitals, 1880–1948. A Study in Social Administration in England and Wales*, London, Heinemann, 1964, p. 26; E. Treacher Collins, *The History and Tradition of Moorfields Eye Hospital: One Hundred Years of Ophthalmic Discovery and Development*, London, H. K. Lewis, 1929.

23 For Britain, see Richard Kershaw, *Special Hospitals*, London, George Putnam, 1909, pp. 62–4.

24 Lindsay Granshaw, ' "Fame and fortune by means of bricks and mortar". The medical profession and specialist hospitals in Britain, 1800–1948', in Granshaw and Porter, op. cit. (n. 1), pp. 199–220.

25 Joseph B. Kirsner, *The Development of American Gastroenterology*, New York, Raven Press, 1990, p. 141; George Rosen, *The Specialization of Medicine*, New York,

Froben Press, 1944; C. E. Rosenberg, 'The practice of medicine in New York a century ago', *Bulletin of the History of Medicine*, 1967, 41: 233–53; Rosenberg, 'Social class and medical care in nineteenth century America. The rise and fall of the dispensary', *Journal of the History of Medicine and Allied Science*, 1974, 29: 32–54.

26 Lindsay Granshaw, *St Mark's Hospital, London: a Social History of Specialist Hospital*, London, King's Fund, 1985, p. 72: Lone Banov, 'St Paul's Infirmary for Haemorrhoids, Fistula, and Other Diseases of the Rectum', *Southern Medical Journal*, 1978, 71: 1559–61.

27 J. D. Thompson and G. Goldin, *The Hospital: a Social and Architectural History*, New Haven, CT, Yale University Press, 1975; Jeremy Taylor, *Hospital and Asylum Architecture in England, 1840–1914: Building for Health Care*, London, Mansell, 1991; Lindsay Granshaw, 'St Thomas's Hospital, London, 1850–1900', unpublished Ph.D. thesis, Bryn Mawr College, PA, 1981, pp. 110–90; Florence Nightingale, *Notes on Hospitals*, 3rd edn, London, Longman, Green, 1863.

28 For Vienna, see Erna Lesky, *The Vienna Medical School of the Nineteenth Century*, trans. by L. Williams and I. S. Levij, Baltimore, MD, Johns Hopkins University Press, 1976. For antisepsis, see Lindsay Granshaw ' "Upon this principle I have based a practice": the development and reception of antisepsis in Britain, 1867–1890', in John Pickstone (ed.), *Medical Innovation in Historical Perspective*, London, Macmillan, 1992; Joseph Lister, 'On the antiseptic principle in the practice of surgery', *Lancet*, 1867, 2: 353–6.

29 See Rosenberg, op. cit. (n. 19), for the American case.

30 Gwendoline M. Ayers, *England's First State Hospitals and the Metropolitan Asylums Board, 1867–1930*, London, Wellcome Institute for the History of Medicine, 1971; Ruth Hodgkinson, *The Origins of the National Health Service: the Medical Services of the New Poor Law, 1834–1871*, London, Wellcome Historical Medical Library, 1967.

31 Monica E. Baly, *Nursing and Social Change*, London, Heinemann, 1982, pp. 64–75; Baly, *Florence Nightingale and the Nursing Legacy*, London, Croom Helm, 1986; B. Abel-Smith, *A History of the Nursing Profession*, London, Heinemann, 1982, pp. 1–35; Robert Dingwall, Anne Marie Rafferty and Charles Webster, *An Introduction to the Social History of Nursing*, London, Routledge, 1988; Perry Williams, 'Religion, respectability and the origins of the modern nurse', in Roger French and Andrew Wear (eds), *British Medicine in an Age of Reform*, London, Routledge, 1991, pp. 231–55.

32 Henry Burdett, *Cottage Hospitals, General, Fever, and Convalescent. Their Progress, Management, and Work in Great Britain and Ireland, and the United States of America*, 3rd edn, London, Scientific Press, 1896; Meyrick Emrys-Roberts, *The Cottage Hospitals, 1859–1990*, Motcombe, Wilts., Tern, 1991; see also Henry C. Burdett, *Hospitals and Asylums of the World: Their Origin, History, Construction, Administration, Management, and Legislation*, 4 vols, London, J. & A. Churchill, 1891–3.

33 David Rosner, *A Once Charitable Enterprise: Hospitals and Health Care in Brooklyn and New York, 1885–1915*, Cambridge, Cambridge University Press, 1982; Morris Vogel, *The Invention of the Modern Hospital. Boston, 1870–1930*, Chicago, IL, University of Chicago Press, 1980; Vogel, 'Managing medicine: creating a

profession of hospital administration in the United States, 1895–1915', in Granshaw and Porter, op. cit. (n. 1), pp. 243–60; Granshaw, op. cit. (n. 27); Rosenberg, op. cit. (n. 9). For Taylor's scientific management, see F. W. Taylor, 'A piece-work system', *Transactions of the American Society of Mechanical Engineers*, 1895, 16: 856–903. For commentary, see D. F. Noble, *America by Design: Science, Technology and the Rise of Corporate Capitalism*, New York, Knopf, 1979.

34 Rivett, op. cit. (n. 2).
35 Charles Webster, *The Health Services since the War*, Vol. I: *The Problems of Health Care: the National Health Service before 1957*, London, HMSO, 1988.
36 Pinker, op. cit. (n. 2).
37 Rosemary Stevens, *In Sickness and in Wealth: American Hospital in the Twentieth Century*, New York, Basic Books, 1989; Rosenberg, op. cit. (n. 19); Daniel M. Fox, *Health Policies, Health Politics: the British and American Experience, 1911–1965*, Princeton, NJ, Princeton University Press, 1986.
38 Webster, op. cit. (n. 35), p. 3.
39 I. Illich, *Limits to Medicine*, London, Pelican, 1977; B. Inglis, *The Diseases of Civilization*, London, Hodder & Stoughton, 1981; I. Kennedy, *The Unmasking of Medicine*, London, Allen & Unwin, 1981; T. McKeown, *The Modern Rise of Population*, London, Edward Arnold, 1976.

FURTHER READING

Abel-Smith, Brian, *The Hospitals 1880–1948. A Study in Social Adminstration in England and Wales*, London, Heinemann, 1964.
Ackerknecht, Erwin H., *Medicine at the Paris Hospital, 1794–1848*, Baltimore, MD, Johns Hopkins University Press, 1967.
Conrad, L. I. and Nutton, V., *Jundishapur: from Myth to History*, Princeton, NJ, Darwin Press.
Foucault, Michel, *The Birth of the Clinic. An Archaeology of Medical Perception*, trans. by A. M. Sheridan, London, Tavistock, 1976.
Granshaw, Lindsay, *St Mark's Hospital, London: a Social History of a Specialist Hospital*, London, King's Fund, 1985.
—— and Porter, Roy (eds), *The Hospital in History*, London, Routledge, 1989.
Jetter, Dieter, *Geschichte des Hospitals*, Wiesbaden, F. Steiner, 1966.
——, *Das Europäische Hospital: von der Spätantike bis 1800*, Cologne, DuMont, 1986.
Jones, Colin, *The Charitable Imperative: Hospitals and Nursing in Ancien Régime and Revolutionary France*, London, Routledge, 1989.
Mollat, Michel et al., *Histoire des Hôpitaux en France*, Toulouse, Privat, 1982.
Murken, Axel Hinrich, *Vom Armenhospital zum Grossklinikum: die Geschichte des Krankenhauses vom 18 Jahrhundert bis zur Gegenwart*, Cologne, DuMont, 1988.
Park, Katharine, *Doctors and Medicine in Early Renaissance Florence*, Princeton, NJ, Princeton University Press, 1985.
Pickstone, John V., *Medicine and Industrial Society: a History of Hospital Development in Manchester and its Region, 1752–1946*, Manchester, Manchester University Press, 1985.
Risse, G. B., *Hospital Life in Enlightenment Scotland. Care and Teaching at the Royal Infirmary of Edinburgh*, Cambridge, Cambridge University Press, 1986.

Rosenberg, Charles E., *The Care of Strangers: the Rise of America's Hospital System*, New York, Basic Books, 1987.

Rosner, David, *A Once Charitable Enterprise: Hospitals and Health Care in Brooklyn and New York, 1885–1915*, Cambridge, Cambridge University Press, 1982.

Stevens, Rosemary, *In Sickness and in Wealth: American Hospitals in the Twentieth Century*, New York, Basic Books, 1989.

Thompson, J. D. and Goldin, G., *The Hospital: a Social and Architectural History*, New Haven, CT, Yale University Press, 1975.

Vogel, Morris, *The Invention of the Modern Hospital. Boston, 1870–1930*, Chicago, IL, University of Chicago Press, 1980.

50

MEDICAL INSTITUTIONS AND THE STATE

Daniel M. Fox

This chapter interprets the history of interrelationships between the institutions of medicine and the state. It addresses events between the sixteenth century, when the modern concept of the state was first enunciated and used in political practice, to the present. Space and the author's knowledge limits its geographic range to western Europe and North America, although relationships between medicine and the state have also been important elsewhere in Europe and on other continents.

The argument of this chapter is that continuing negotiations occur between medicine and the state. The purpose of these negotiations is to establish consensus, or, failing that, a workable compromise about what the institutions of medicine and those of the state owe to each other. These negotiations take place not only over time but also in particular countries or their component sub-parts. The negotiations are influenced by numerous factors, which include:

1 the political culture of the country in which they occur;
2 the overt and covert goals of the state in negotiating with the institutions of medicine;
3 the overt and covert goals of the institutions of medicine; and
4 perceptions on the part of the persons negotiating on behalf of medicine and of the state of their relative power and authority.

The last point, that history is made by people, requires emphasis because most of this chapter will necessarily address abstractions. These abstractions are, however, grounded in primary-source data about what people thought, said, and did that have been gathered by historians, doctors, and political scientists over many years. The author's debt to this substantial body of historical research is summarized at the end of this chapter.

This chapter proceeds as follows. An initial section on definitions clarifies the terms used in this chapter. Then, chronological sections generalize about continuity and change in negotiations involving the institutions of medicine and states. These sections are divided as follows: sixteenth through eighteenth centuries; nineteenth century; the twentieth century to 198;, and contemporary history, defined as the last decade (1980s) and the immediate present.

DEFINITIONS

THE STATE

The definition of the state, either in general or in the case of particular states, has three elements: what it does, what justifies its existence, and its history. These elements overlap, but using any one of them alone as a definition is simplistic, for three reasons. The first reason is that states have had common attributes since the sixteenth century, when the theory of the modern state and its normative role was first enunciated by the Florentine Nicolò Machiavelli (1469–1527) and elaborated in France by Jean Bodin (c.1530–96). Second, the purpose and work of the state cannot be separated from the reasons its inhabitants do or do not accord it legitimacy. Third, the state is the result of its history, which is constantly being made and remade.

WHAT STATES DO

Here are two similar definitions of the state from the recent literature of political science that build on scholarship in political theory since the sixteenth century. The first, published in 1968, defines the state as a 'geographically delimited segment of human society united by common obedience to a single sovereign'.[1] The second, from a 1991 monograph, expands the definition to include a network of institutions through which authority is negotiated and exercised: 'The state is the corporate structure, coextensive with a political society, which is the locus of supreme political authority and can command an effective force monopoly to assure compliance with its decisions.'[2]

WHAT JUSTIFIES THE EXISTENCE OF STATES

Theorists and public officials have used a variety of justifications for the existence of states. The oldest of these are the divine and the patriarchal justifications. These hold that the state, and especially its rulers, are legitimized by a deity or by descent from a founding family that maintains sovereignty. Three more-modern justifications are organicism (the state is rooted in the intrinsic nature of human beings), force (the state is created by the deliberate action of human groups), and consent (the state is the result of voluntary agreement among its members). Some theorists hold that the normative concept of the state has been eroded since the late eighteenth century. The justification by consent led to concepts of popular sovereignty which, in turn, reduced the prestige of rulers. In this formulation, the state has become a less useful framework than the concept of government.

THE HISTORY OF STATES

A leading twentieth-century political scientist asserted that 'no theory of the state is ever intelligible save in the context of its time. What men think about the state is the outcome always of the experience in which they are immersed.'[3] Definitions and theories are approximations that are either normative or descriptive. Whatever their purpose, they are abstracted from the data of human experience. Thus generalizations about medical institutions and the state will at best capture only some of the ideas, words, and actions in any place at any moment in time.

POLITICAL CULTURE

Every state has a unique way of conducting its public affairs. In recent years, many scholars have characterized this uniqueness using the concept of political culture. This concept includes the structure of government and politics, styles of acceptable political behaviour, and what some scholars call the 'psychological orientations' of the actors in political situations.[4] The concept of political culture is particularly important when studying medical institutions, since a great deal of the substantive content of medical practice is regarded as transnational. This transnationality has been particularly pronounced since the mid-nineteenth century, as a result of advances in biological, chemical, statistical, and social-scientific knowledge as they apply to medical education, research, and practice. Thus the relationships between particular medical institutions and individual states has often been the result of the refraction, to use a somewhat loaded metaphor, of scientific and technological ideas and findings by political culture.

MEDICAL INSTITUTIONS

With this background in historically informed political theory, it is possible to define more precisely medical institutions as they relate to states. Medical institutions have two different meanings. The first is the conventional use of the word 'institution' to mean a place or an organization. For medicine, such institutions might be hospitals, medical schools, research establishments, and professional societies. The second and more elusive meaning of institution is a generally accepted mode of behaviour. For medicine, such institutions, as they relate to states, might include fee-setting and billing practices, services to the state in times of emergency, and obtaining informed consent from patients before performing procedures that carry risks. As is the case with most definitions that help to clarify historical events, these two overlap. Thus most institutions as modes of behaviour take place in institutions defined as places or organizations.

FROM THE SIXTEENTH TO THE EIGHTEENTH CENTURY

The history of medical institutions and states is inseparable from general social and economic, as well as political, history. The years from roughly 1500 to 1800 were characterized by the growth and consolidation of city, regional and local economies in Europe, the centralization of government, whether of nation- or city-states, and the elaboration of the structures of bureaucracy, the establishment of European settlements in the Western hemisphere, and the growth in size and power of urban middle classes whose incomes derived from commerce, manufacture, and the practice of the professions.

Three major themes characterize the relationships between medical institutions and states in these years. The first is regulation of the medical profession. The second is the role of medical institutions in making states wealthier and more powerful. The third is the mobilization of medical institutions in times of perceived state emergencies, particularly the threat of epidemics.

REGULATING THE MEDICAL PROFESSION

The major issues involving the regulation of doctors were admission to practice, the limitation of competition, normalizing a range of fees and charges, and policing professional misconduct. The dominant regulatory policy was to permit the continuation of forms of professional self-regulation that had been devised, especially in the cities of Italy, in the later Middle Ages. In states in which these mechanisms – generally guilds, but occasionally universities – did not have medieval origins, they were established, generally in the sixteenth century. For instance, in Venice, a guild for physicians and surgeons existed by 1258; and in Florence, a guild of physicians and apothecaries had been established by 1296. In England, however, a college of physicians on the Italian guild model was not established by royal charter until 1518, and then only accorded regulatory authority in the City of London and within seven miles of it.

Variations on this general pattern occurred in each state. Surgeons and apothecaries generally organized separately from physicians and were accorded regulatory authority over their members by the state. In most states, conflicts or at least tensions occurred between guilds or colleges and universities, especially around issues of certification for admission to practice.

Most of the medicine practised on most members of the population probably went unregulated in this period. There is a rich secondary literature about the prominence of unlicensed healers of various sorts, especially among the poorer classes in both cities and rural areas. Medical institutions and states concerned themselves mainly with the regulation of practice among the middle and upper classes, for which the stakes of income and prestige were the highest.

The case of France in the eighteenth century is instructive, in large measure because it has been the subject of vigorous research by historians in recent decades. As one of them wrote in 1988, 'France in the 18th century was legally a society of orders, of which the three medical *corps* formed an integral part, together with the corporations of the various urban crafts and trades.'[5] Physicians were the most prestigious and, in broad theory, surgeons and apothecaries were subordinate to them. But in practice, the system was considerably more complex. The medical profession was divided into several groups, one of which, the *licenciés*, were confined to practising in the countryside and in towns where no local monopoly had been established by a medical corporation. There were several other types of lesser doctors. Surgeons, who outnumbered physicians, practised a great deal of internal medicine. Apothecaries had considerable competition.

This system was breaking down in the decades before the French Revolution. Thus, under the various governments that held power after 1789, the regulation of medical practice was subject to vigorous negotiations with the state. Although some characteristics of the regulation of medicine under the Old Regime survived into the early nineteenth century, the new system that emerged under Napoleon became a model for other countries in Europe: 'a uniform (if two-tiered) national profession, with a coordinated national licensing system'.[6] (➤ Ch. 47 History of the medical profession)

THE ROLE OF MEDICAL INSTITUTIONS IN THE GROWTH OF STATES

There is a rich secondary literature on theories of mercantilism in the seventeenth and eighteenth centuries and on the contribution of members of the medical profession to the development of 'political arithmetic', the use of numbers to assist the state in enlarging its population and its wealth. In George Rosen's classic formulation of this theory, 'The welfare of society was regarded as identical with the welfare of the state.'[7] A more recent commentator has said that 'From the 17th century onwards it became customary to see the number of sovereign's subjects as a measure of his strength.'[8] The great medical names associated with mercantilist theory and practice include Sir William Petty (1623–87) and John Graunt (1620–74) in England, and Johann Peter Frank (1745–1821) in various cities of Italy and Austria. All three had a wide influence on the theory and practice of public health through their writings as well as their public work. (➤ Ch. 51 Public health)

It is difficult to describe the relationship between medical institutions and the state in this elaboration of mercantilist public-health theory and practice. On the one hand, the subject appears to belong entirely within the chapters in this encyclopedia on public health, demography, epidemiology, and the medical profession. (➤ Ch. 71 Demography and medicine; Ch. 52 Epidemiology)

On the other hand, aspects of the history of negotiations between medical institutions and states are inseparable from the story of what is generally called 'medical police'. In an important account of the subject of 'policing public health' in France, L. J. Jordanova disentangles the many concepts that are too easily simplified as public health. She describes medical police as including instances of committees of medical practitioners who 'worked closely with the municipal authorities on whom their licence to practise and form professional associations depended'. Moreover, legal medicine 'associated medicine with the execution of existing laws principally through the use of practitioners as expert witnesses at trials'. (➤ Ch. 69 Medicine and the law) Finally, 'medical police in the sense of controlling practice entailed not just the hounding of so-called charlatans and empirics but the elaboration of precise rules of conduct between various groups of licensed practitioners and between those of different ranks.'[9] (➤ Ch. 37 History of medical ethics)

MOBILIZING MEDICAL INSTITUTIONS IN CRISES

The third area of major importance in negotiations between medical institutions and states in these years was mobilization in times of crises. These crises included wars and, more frequently, outbreaks of epidemic disease, notably bubonic plague, smallpox, and yellow fever.

The story that follows examines the history of epidemics from the point of view of relationships between medical institutions and the state, deliberately ignoring the larger question of the development of public-health policy in Europe and North America. Two themes stand out in accounts of the mobilization of the medical profession during epidemics between the fourteenth and nineteenth centuries. First, civic leaders and doctors negotiated about who would treat those who were stricken, especially patients in the lowest social classes. Second, since these negotiations offered doctors opportunities as well as risks, the medical institutions were actively involved in the distribution of both the patronage and the burdens that accompanied epidemics.[10]

These themes are closely linked. In instance upon instance, the lay and medical leadership of a state jointly chose particular doctors to carry out the most onerous duties during an epidemic. The doctors who were chosen through these negotiations knew from the beginning of their service that they were balancing personal risks against potential benefits in status and income. They worked under contract to the city-state. In return for a salary, they carried out the plague-control regulations adopted by the civic authorities. These regulations included quarantine of outsiders and goods seeking admission to the city, and isolation of the sick within its boundaries. The 'plague doctors' were also obligated to care for the sick in their homes and in temporary hospitals.

The most important benefit a plague doctor could receive was permission to practise in a particular city after the epidemic: that is, the right to participate in the professional monopoly. This was the benefit most closely guarded by the guilds or corporations that regulated medical practice, by permission of the state.

THE NINETEENTH CENTURY

Both states and medical institutions experienced unprecedented changes in the years between the French Revolution and the First World War. Much of the enormous literature on the impact of these changes on the history of medicine is synthesized in other chapters in this encyclopedia.

This section focuses on seven issues that dominated the negotiations between the leaders of medicine and their counterparts in government throughout the nineteenth century and remained important in the twentieth century. Three of them bear on the demand for medical care; three on the supply of services; one was a tension between the dominant institutions of medicine and the state. The three issues on the demand side were matters of great concern to leaders of medicine and the state, and of direct interest to the general – increasingly a voting – public:

1 providing medical services for the poor;
2 spreading more predictably and equitably the cost of illness for the working and middle classes, both in lost income and medical services; and
3 addressing the impact of the work environment on morbidity and mortality.
   (➤ Ch. 72 Medicine, mortality, and morbidity)

The three supply-side issues were discussed mainly between leaders of medicine and the state. These issues were:

1 how to govern and subsidize hospitals;
2 how to organize and subsidize medical education and research; and
3 how to regulate entry into medical practice and restrain dangerous practitioners, both within medicine and in other occupations that claimed to heal.

The seventh issue, the tension between medicine and the state, involved core values. The scientific advances of the century made medicine a more international profession than ever before. The first international medical institutions were created. At the same time, states became increasingly nationalistic, competing aggressively for economic opportunity, colonial territory, military superiority, and symbols of national prestige in science and the arts.

Each of these issues will be examined in the following paragraphs. Readers are cautioned once again that the purpose of this chapter is to describe negotiations between leaders of medical institutions and those of the state. For details of, for example, the history of hospitals, or public-health practice or medical economics, other chapters, indicated by the cross-references, should be consulted.

PROVIDING MEDICAL SERVICES FOR THE POOR

The leaders of medical institutions and of most states agreed that serving the poor was a residual function for the medical profession. Consequently, out-patient care for the poor was provided in each country, either by volunteer doctors, usually newcomers to the profession or the city, or by low-paid full- or part-time practitioners who worked for municipal or regional government or for philanthropic agencies. In-patient care for most acute illnesses and injuries was provided in hospitals maintained by some combination of charity and public subsidy, depending on the country or, within countries, the region. Medical services in these hospitals were provided by low-paid, or unpaid, trainee doctors or newcomers, supervised by leading practitioners who thereby had opportunities to increase their prestige as teachers or researchers. An exception to these generalizations were the salaried doctors who served the mentally ill, mainly the mentally ill poor, in public asylums located, by therapeutic design, in rural areas. (➤ Ch.62 Charity before c. 1850; Ch. 63 Medical philanthropy after 1850)

State officials and doctors regarded medical services for the poor as residual in large measure because of the influence of the sanitary movement on social policy for the alleviation of poverty. Such leading sanitarians as Edwin Chadwick (1800–90) in England, Max von Pettenkofer (1818–1901) in Germany, L. R. Villermé (1782–1863) in France, and Lemuel Shattuck (1793–1859) in the United States, accorded relatively low priority to most of the institutions of medicine in improving the condition of the poor. Chadwick, for example, had considerable disdain toward curative medicine. All of them believed that 'science must precede action',[11] in particular, science that examined the effects of clean water, better sewage, and improved housing.

The sanitary reformers created a new medical institution: the full-time or substantial part-time public-health doctor (or health officer, or medical officer of health). These doctors were appointed by political jurisdictions to oversee measures to prevent disease and to collect official statistics. They were civic agents whose job was to protect the health of the whole population, but who, in fact, worked mainly among the poor, who lived in poorly ventilated, crowded housing, and who were most at risk from contaminated water and poor waste disposal. Unlike earlier civic doctors, the role of the new health officers was mainly in prevention. In a short time, however, diagnosis and the administration of out-patient and in-patient treatment for the poor became important roles for public-health doctors.

In every country, therefore, a substantial number of doctors earned much or even all of their living by taking care of the poor in systems that were established or regulated by the state. These doctors negotiated their wages and working conditions in contexts that involved larger stakes for other members of the profession. Particularly in times and places where there were few restrictions on the numbers of doctors who could enter practice, public and philanthropic policy for the poor had a significant influence on medical incomes. In Britain, for example, the medical-care provisions of the New Poor Law of 1834, according to one historian, 'protect[ed] the whole profession against the rate-cutting of its weakest members'.[12] In the United States, where the amount of public and philanthropic subsidy for medical care to the poor varied among cities and states, who qualified as poor, which doctors took care of them, and how doctors were compensated for their services were matters of contention throughout the century. Moreover, in-patient medical care for the poor was an important item of élite medical patronage, as will be discussed below (see p. 1217).

MEETING THE COST OF ILLNESS

The second demand-side issue was paying the increasing costs of illness for the working-class and the poor. There were two categories of cost: lost wages; and the services of doctors, other practitioners, and hospitals. These costs rose throughout the century. Lost wages due to illness became an increasingly pressing problem, because in each country of Europe and North America the proportion of the population who worked for wages, and especially for low wages, increased during the century. The cost of services began to rise noticeably in the closing years of the century, as a result of the increasing incidence of surgical intervention and of hospitalization. (➤ Ch. 42 Surgery (modern); Ch. 49 The hospital)

The institutions of medicine had complex interests in issues involving the costs of medicine. Although these interests played out differently in each political culture, they were articulated in each of them. In theory, doctors would be delighted if their patients did not lose wages as a result of illness or injury and were, therefore, able to pay their bills. In theory, too, doctors should not mind if a third party paid the bills generated by their patients. Such third parties could be the state itself, or an insurance body sanctioned by the state, or an organization created by working people themselves (a trade union, a friendly society, an ethnic association).

But in practice, doctors, acting through medical institutions, had a great deal to worry about. First, they were concerned about threats to professional autonomy: their freedom to practise and to charge fees, subject only to sanctions by their peers. Second, they were worried that third-party payers would ultimately make doctors employees. If doctors became employees they would lose the monopoly status they had attained through hard political negotiations with each state. These monopolies not only gave doctors control over the internal affairs of their own profession: they also restrained, or in some cases eliminated, competition from other professions, either doctors with less training, as in France, or with different theories, as in the case of homoeopaths and other sectarians of the United States. (➤ Ch. 28 Unorthodox medical theories)

Negotiations between the medical profession and states about the costs of care for working people and their dependants took place in every country in western Europe and North America during the half-century preceding the First World War. The most complete system of social insurance for the costs of illness was adopted in Germany in the 1880s. In effect, the burden of the costs of illness of everyone in the state was spread over everyone who had earnings, with some attention to equity. In 1911, Britain, which had earlier devised a system of voluntary worker contributions to associations called friendly societies, adopted a National Health Insurance scheme, which replaced lost wages and paid the costs of general-practitioner care for the working population. Dependants, the middle class, and hospital care were outside the scheme. Other European countries negotiated analogous schemes. Canada and the United States did not move beyond agitation to rationalize payment for the cost of illness during these years. (➤ Ch. 57 Health economics)

THE WORK ENVIRONMENT

Another demand-side issue that arose in the nineteenth century was a result of the increasingly evident and well-documented connection between working environments and particular diseases. Much of the task of regulating work environments was assigned to public health, especially on the European continent. But in England and North America, the institutions of medicine became involved with the state around the certification of illness and the awarding of compensation to workers who claimed that they had disabilities related to work. This situation arose because, as a recent historian notes, '19th century public health experts like Chadwick and [John] Simon recognized that it was most appropriate for medicine to intervene where it interfered least with vested interests. Such considerations have resulted in compensation being preferred to preventive public health measures.'[13]

This default by public health required the institutions of medicine to become involved with the courts and bodies established to award compensation.In the English-speaking countries between the 1890s and the First World War, a case-by-case approach to claims for compensation was replaced by formal workers' compensation systems run by public agencies. As Edward Berkowitz has written, 'American legislators accepted the British practice of combining benefits for temporary and permanent disability and for uniting health service and income maintenance benefits within one social insurance program.'[14] These new workers' compensation systems involved the institutions of medicine both in setting standards for compensation awards and negotiating fees for the treatment of compensatable illness and injury. (➤ Ch. 69 Medicine and the law)

Negotiations between leaders of medicine and representatives of the state about these demand-side issues always took place with both sides quite conscious of the overwhelming importance of supply-side issues to the willingness of medicine to collaborate or even to co-operate with agencies of government. These issues were vital to medicine because they determined whether the profession would maintain monopolistic control over its work.

HOSPITAL GOVERNANCE

During the course of the nineteenth century, and especially in the years after 1880, hospitals became the central medical institutions in Europe and North America. They absorbed increasing amounts of the resources society allocated to medical care and public health. The increased importance of hospitals was a result of new opportunities for surgical intervention and new ways of treating infectious disease among the poor. Moreover, research conducted in the laboratories and medical schools adjacent to hospitals promised startling advances in diagnosis and treatment. (➤ Ch. 11 Clinical research; Ch. 36 The science of diagnosis: diagnostic technology)

At the beginning of the nineteenth century, the medical profession everywhere competed for control of hospitals. In some countries, hospitals were dominated by lay trustees; in others, by religious orders; in still others, by officials of government at various levels. By the end of the century, doctors everywhere had gained effective control of hospitals, although formal governance arrangements varied widely among states. In the English-speaking nations, the dominant model of hospital governance retained a lay board, whose members served as either philanthropic or public appointees. In theory, these lay people appointed doctors to a medical board, which made decisions affecting the profession, and an administration, which ran the financial and housekeeping services of the institutions. In the continential models, hospitals were owned by public bodies, which delegated crucial power and authority to a hierarchy of doctors, subject to procedures of accountability.

Whatever the model, and whatever the formal mechanisms of accountability, doctors ran hospitals. They ran them because they made the decisions that determined what resources would be used, on which patients, for what duration of time. Doctors, in other words, controlled the major uncertainties in a complicated new industrial environment that produced medical and nursing services. Their control of hospitals was reinforced by an ideology that was, increasingly, shared by doctors and lay people.

According to this shared ideology, the advances in biological and medical science that had occurred since the closing decades of the nineteenth century provided a model for medical progress in the future. New knowledge was created in the laboratories that were associated with hospitals. This knowledge was then transmitted to new practitioners through medical education, the clinical aspects of which, according to the ideology, should properly occur in hospitals. Then, the knowledge was passed down a hierarchy of practitioners and institutions and made available to the general public.[15]

Powered by both control over the work environment and by this new ideology, the leaders of medical institutions won almost every negotiation with the state about hospitals. Issues of hospital location, size, complexity, design, and staffing were usually decided according to doctors' preferences, contingent on the state having funds available. Because of the new ideology, moreover, states and philanthropists (who were usually chartered by the state) were eager to make increasing amounts of funds available for hospitals.[16]

MEDICAL EDUCATION AND RESEARCH

As a result of advances in science and technology and the new centrality of the hospital as a medical institution, the complexity and cost of medical education increased during the century. Negotiations between medicine and the state about the structure, content, and amount of subsidy for medical education resulted in a hybrid public policy that has persisted until the present. Unlike most institutions of higher education, medical schools were subsidized by the state to provide both education and services. Support for educational work came from whatever organizations in the state financed higher education (central, regional, or local government; religion; philanthropy). But indirect support for education also came from the public and voluntary organizations that financed the provision of medical care in hospitals, especially care for the poor. This support took the form of capital expenditures on buildings and equipment, operating grants to teaching hospitals, and payments on behalf of indigent patients. (➤ Ch. 48 Medical education)

The fees paid for instruction by medical students met a declining percentage of the costs of medical education in the course of the century. By the last third of the century, older apprenticeship models of medical education had disappeared almost everywhere in Europe and North America. Apprenticeship survived, greatly transformed, in clerkships and house-staff positions in hospitals. These new apprentices were part of the staff deployed by medicine, as a result of its negotiations with the state, to serve the severely ill poor.

By the closing decades of the century, research and education were inseparable, even though most countries in Europe maintained medical-research institutions that were separate from medical schools and their associated teaching hospitals. Research and education were inseparable because of the guiding assumption among the medical élite that scientific investigation had become the primary source of valid medical knowledge. (➤ Ch. 8 The biochemical tradition)

The power of this assumption was initially revealed in the teaching hospitals of Paris and several leading German states during the first half of the century. Such prominent investigator-clinicians as Pierre Louis (1787–1872) in France, and Rudolf Virchow (1821–1902) in Berlin and Würzburg became models for thousands of successors throughout Europe and North America. (Virchow was unique, however, in combining hospital-based investigation with a career in general politics and broad influence on public-health policy.) There is rich documentation of the dissemination of the concepts that linked research, education, and the belief in medical progress.

As these concepts were disseminated, medicine made new claims upon the state. The basis of these claims was the assertion that expenditures on research – on both infrastructure and personnel – would lead eventually to improvements in the health status of individuals. In the short run, such expenditures would contribute to the prestige of the state in international competition. The bill for these claims was relatively small in the nineteenth century, but the acceptance of its legitimacy by the state and philanthropic institutions made possible negotiations for much higher stakes a few decades later.

REGULATING MEDICAL PRACTICE

The guild became an obsolete form of medical organization by the nineteenth century, requiring medicine and the state to create new regulatory institutions. When the modern idea of the state emerged, in the sixteenth century, the medical profession, like other occupations, adapted the medieval institution of the guild to meet contemporary needs. The state, in fact or in effect, ceded to the medical guilds (or colleges or universities, depending on country and region) authority to control entry into the profession, or several branches of the profession, and to regulate the behaviour of practitioners. Over the next few centuries, the structure and work of the guild altered to meet changing requirements of the state and the economics of medicine.

By the nineteenth century, many leaders of medicine and the state perceived that new arrangements for the regulation of medical practice were required. Especially after mid-century, the institutions of medicine sought to assert and protect monopoly status for their services in increasingly competitive market economies.

During the nineteenth century, states and medical institutions explored a number of new ways to regulate medical practice. The most extreme adaptation to a market economy occurred in the United States during the 1830s and 1840s. Medical practice was, to use a twentieth-century word, deregulated in almost all the states of the Union. Licensure laws were repealed in order to open opportunities to ambitious men who lacked élite connections. Many medical sects, as they were called, flourished. This social experiment was gradually replaced by a system of licensing in which states issued, or revoked, licences on the basis of criteria set by medicine and by the hardiest survivors among its competitors (notably osteopathy, chiropody, and chiropractic).

European doctors achieved a similar accommodation between medicine and the state without an experiment in deregulation. The general agreement, with many national variations, was that the state, or bodies designated by the state, (for example, the General Medical Council established in 1858 in Britain) would take responsibility for licensing new entrants into medical practice and for revoking licences as a result of the most egregious breaches of correct professional behaviour. More specialized credentials would be awarded by organizations that resembled the former guilds (or colleges or universities). (➤ Ch. 37 History of medical ethics)

Medical associations also lost their guild status as a result of negotiations with the state about the wages and working conditions of doctors who treated the poor and, later in the century, members of the working – and in some states the middle – classes. F. B. Smith perhaps exaggerated slightly when, writing about England, he described 'medical trade unionism' as well established and 'peculiarly defensive' by the 1830s.[17] But his fundamental point is correct: especially in the later decades of the nineteenth and the beginning of the twentieth century, medical associations, in England and elsewhere, became dominant but not monopolistic. They were dominant because they generally spoke for most of the profession, or at least its most prominent members. They were not monopolistic because, increasingly, they were unable to set prices in negotiations with individual patients. The agents of the state, who bargained on behalf of the pooled payments of tax payers or insurance premiums, exerted countervailing power against medical associations.

INTERNATIONALISM VERSUS NATIONALISM

Medical institutions were both international and national. The new scientific and technological advances of the century flowed freely across national borders. This flow was speeded by advances in communications technology; for example, news about the successful treatment of rabies by Louis Pasteur (1822–95) or the development of the X-ray by Wilhelm Roentgen (1845–1923) spread to every country in a few days. Models of scientific organization and practice, and related changes in both basic science and clinical medical education, also moved freely across borders. International congresses met to discuss science, technology, and the control of particular diseases, especially tuberculosis. In some countries, notably the United States, by late in the century, success in academic medicine required advanced study in Europe, particularly in Germany. (➤ Ch. 59 Internationalism in medicine and public health)

This internationalism contrasted with growing nationalism, especially in Europe. Tensions and conflicts between states grew in intensity between the 1870s and the beginning of the First World War. Nevertheless, there is little evidence of medical nationalism before that war. Powered by a shared belief among their members that the methods of science would lead to vast improvements in human health, medical institutions transcended the increasing competitiveness among nation-states.

THE TWENTIETH CENTURY TO THE 1980s

By about 1920, the issues that had been the subject of negotiations between medical institutions and the state in the nineteenth century had been placed in a new context. For most of the twentieth century, the state has mediated the social contract between the institutions of medicine and of society.[18] (➤ Ch. 70 Medical Sociology)

This important change in the role of the state in its relationship with medical institutions is evident mainly in retrospect. Looking backward from 1993 to 1920, there is considerable evidence that every medical institution was inextricably tied to the state. Negotiations between medicine and the state determined who entered medical education, what that education consisted of, where and how further medical education occurred, how licences and advanced certification were awarded, how patients paid and doctors were reimbursed, the size, location, and equipment of the hospitals that had become central to medical practice, and how medicine interacted with the legal system around issues of malpractice, expert testimony, and forensic science.

Most doctors in 1920 would not, however, have agreed with the analysis in the preceding paragraph. They would have been highly aware of the autonomy they still possessed: to locate their practices where they saw good opportunities; to choose or reject patients who presented themselves; to diagnose and treat according to their own notions of best practice; and to charge higher prices to their more affluent patients. Moreover, many doctors and the leaders of medical societies jealously protected their work against what they considered to be further encroachments by the state on the autonomy of medicine.

But encroachment was an obsolete word to describe the relationship between medicine and the state by 1920. Medical institutions and states had become irrevocably intertwined. They needed each other. The state needed the institutions of medicine to care for the sick in order to make them productive and law-abiding, to educate new doctors, to conduct research that would lead to better health, and to deal with emergencies like wars and epidemics that produced an unprecedented incidence of injuries and illness. Medical institutions depended on the state for much of their authority and most of their financing.

The state needed medical institutions for another reason that was largely unrecognized in 1920, but would soon become increasingly evident. Unprecedented changes in demography and the epidemiological situation were placing new demands on the state. More people were living to older ages. Shifts in fertility meant that later in the century fewer people of working age must provide for the health and well-being of more elderly people. (➤ Ch. 46 Geriatrics) In part as a result of the social and economic changes that increased longevity, chronic degenerative disease was becoming the largest burden on the medical-care systems established in the past through the negotiations of medicine and the state. Indeed, it was in the early 1920s that, in most of the countries under review, the number of people who died of chronic diseases exceeded for the first time the number that died from infection and injury.[19] By the 1930s, wherever the health of populations was surveyed, the number of people reporting disabling conditions that interfered with work and household responsibilities was consistently around 20 per cent. (➤ Ch. 4 Medical care)

Throughout the twentieth century, then, medical institutions have been essential to the fundamental purposes of the state: defending its population from harm and producing wealth. Medicine absorbed an increasing share of each nation's total income throughout the century. In part, this increase was a result of the rising cost of producing medical care as its technology and organization became more complex. But the state, acting for society, demanded that more medical care be produced. The growth in the share of national wealth going to medical care has often been described as the 'industrialization' of medicine. Many social scientists and journalists have claimed that medicine became 'big business' in the twentieth century.

This formulation oversimplifies the complicated negotiations between medicine and the state. The institutions of medicine did not resemble all forms of business. They were most similar to public utilities: businesses (or public agencies) that control a natural monopoly (like water or electricity). Public utilities have always had a special relationship to the state. They are privileged to act on behalf of the state. But at the same time, they are constrained by the state from using their natural monopolies to exploit helpless citizens.

Medicine also has had a natural monopoly and hence has been required to relate to the state as if it were a public utility. Its natural monopoly has been different from that of utilities that control resources such as water. The natural monopoly of medicine has been a result of the imbalance of power in the encounters between individual doctors and their patients. This imbalance is caused by two factors, both of which have made patients extremely vulnerable during medical encounters. The first factor has been the fear and anxiety patients feel when presenting their symptoms. The second has been that doctors possess special knowledge that society has denied to patients, both because it is difficult to understand and because the institutions of medicine have, over the centuries, successfully negotiated to keep it to themselves. (➤ Ch. 34 History of the doctor–patient relationship)

Unlike other public utilities, however, the critical moment in medicine is not the provision of a specific commodity or service, but rather the encounter between particular doctors and individual patients. The centrality of the encounter to medical practice causes problems for the modern state. It is one thing to regulate the quality and price of drinking-water; quite another to regulate what hundreds of thousands of doctors say and do to millions of patients on any particular day.

This difference between medicine and other public utilities has been the principal reason that there is what eighteenth-century political philosophers usefully called (in a different context, of course) a 'social contract' between medical institutions and society. Under the terms of this contract, medical institutions provide services at a particular level of quality, to an agreed-upon number of people, at a generally acceptable price. In return, society guarantees to medical institutions degrees of autonomy in clinical decision-making, in selecting and certifying members of the medical profession, and in earning incomes that exceed those of most other highly trained experts.

This social contract, of course, existed before the twentieth century. Throughout most of the history described in this chapter, most doctors negotiated individual contracts with their patients. Guilds negotiated some aspects of social contracts with agents of the state: particularly around entry into the profession, medical education, the regulation of deviant practitioners, behaviour in times of epidemic, and residual responsibilities for treating the sick poor.

But the social contract assumed pre-eminent importance in the relationship between medical institutions and the state in the twentieth century. The negotiations between medicine and the state in the nineteenth and early twentieth centuries had formed stronger linkages between the two than ever before around issues involving the demand for and supply of medical services. These linkages became even stronger in the twentieth century for two reasons. The first was the pressure of the demographic and epidemiological situation, described on p. 1219 above. The second was the pervasiveness of the ideology of medical advance described in the previous section (pp. 1210–18) of this chapter.

Both doctors and government officials justified the centrality of the state in negotiating the social contract between medicine and society by the belief that medical advance would contribute enormously to progress and therefore to the general welfare. By the late 1920s, the recent promise of medical science seemed to be on the verge of realization. Bacteriology had identified the causes of many infectious diseases and had stimulated the invention of vaccines and antitoxins. Insulin treatment was proving to have a dramatic effect on diabetes. New surgical techniques saved lives, as had been dramatized by events during the First World War. It seemed logical to argue by analogy that the same scientific method that had produced such success against infections and wounds would, as with diabetes, soon alleviate the disabling consequences of chronic diseases. (➤ Ch. 10 The immunological tradition; Ch. 23 Endocrine diseases; Ch. 66 War and modern medicine)

The history of medical institutions and the state in the twentieth century has been primarily the story of how particular social contracts were negotiated in each country and with what results. A large literature in political science and a somewhat smaller one in history describes these negotiations in exhaustive detail. Most of this literature can be found in bibliographies under the general heading of the 'welfare state'. In it, readers will find descriptions of how and when each country has addressed the issues of the demand for and supply of medical services and what the results of these negotiations have been.

The issues under negotiation are again grouped, as they were for the nineteenth century, as issues of demand and of supply. However useful this formulation based on political economy, it emphasizes continuities rather than discontinuities between the past and the present. Readers should be aware that important debates occurred in each country about the relationship between medical institutions and the state that have been forgotten because they left a small legacy, mainly of sentiment rather than of policy. For example, in the 1920s and especially the 1930s, influential experts on health policy like Sidney Webb (1859–1947) and Beatrice Potter Webb (1858–1943) in Britain, and Henry Sigerist (1891–1957), a Swiss residing in the United States, praised the Soviet medical system and urged its adoption in western Europe and North America. Their ideas were debated seriously at the time because they were consonant with broader support in each country for state medical services, staffed by full-time salaried doctors. Both the Soviet model and full-time state-salaried medical services (except for the military) have been political failures everywhere (including, recent evidence suggests, in the former Soviet empire).

On the demand side, the issues under discussion in the twentieth century expanded on what had been important in the nineteenth century. The issue of how to provide medical care for the poor became, in different countries at different times, the problem of who should have access to care, by entitlement or other means, and what the quantity and quality of that care should be. The issue of how to pay the cost of illness for the working and middle classes became two larger questions. The first question was what proportion of medical care for everyone should be paid for by, respectively, tax receipts, insurance premiums, and individual payments? The second question was over what population base, and with what considerations of equity, should the cost of medical care for a state be spread? The issue of replacing income lost during illness, which had dominated negotiations in every state in the nineteenth and early twentieth centuries, by the 1920s became subordinate to the problems of organizing and paying for medical care.

The issue of the impact of the work environment on morbidity and mortality continued to be difficult to negotiate in every country, mainly because of the resistance of large employers, and of many trade unions, to state intervention. In most countries, this issue, though important in the lives of citizens, ceased to be a major subject of negotiations between the institutions of medicine and the agencies of the state.

Similarly, the supply-side issues of the nineteenth century were amplified and modified in the twentieth century. Negotiations in the nineteenth century had settled the major issue in the governance of hospitals. Henceforth, doctors would, everywhere and no matter what the hospital's charter said, exert the strongest influence on how these institutions allocated their resources. By 1920, moreover, public- and private-sector policy-makers in Europe and North America had decided that hospitals would be the dominant institutions of medical-care systems, and that they would be organized in hierarchies based on technical sophistication within geographic regions. By mid-century, hospitals and payments to doctors who practised in them absorbed about two-thirds of the resources each country allocated to medical care. As a result, the main work of medicine, according to the social contract of every state, was to intervene in the acute episodes of chronic diseases, according priority to postponing death and alleviating pain.

Medical education and research expanded as a result of the renegotiation of the social contract in each country. Depending on the country, researchers began to dominate medical education some time between the 1910s and the 1930s. As a result, the preparation of new doctors became subordinate to research and patient care in the work (and the budgets) of most medical schools and their associated teaching hospitals.

The states that invested most heavily in the institutions of medical research did so as a result of a deeply held conviction that this expenditure would lead, eventually, to successful intervention in disease processes, especially in chronic diseases. Although individual researchers often had different goals, related to answering scientific questions, policy-makers were consistent in expecting practical results from public and philanthropic investments in research. Perhaps the most extreme statement of this point of view was made in 1960 by a prominent American Congressman, who said that the budget of the National Institutes of Health was his country's national health insurance.

States also became deeply involved in the regulation of research involving human subjects. This involvement was the result of events during the Second World War (discussed on p. 1224), of growing public consciousness of the rights of patients and the responsibilities of scientific investigators, and of a number of well-publicized scandals about inappropriate testing of drugs and vaccines on human subjects. (➤ Ch. 39 Drug therapies)

The roles of the medical institutions and the state in the regulation of medical practice in the twentieth century expanded on the negotiated agreements of the mid- and late nineteenth century. In most countries, associations of doctors, with the active or passive concurrence of the state, set the rules for licensure, certified specialized expertise, and disciplined deviant members of the profession.

There were, however, two important differences in regulation. Both were the result of the more-active involvement of the state in paying the costs of medical care and in subsidizing the supply of human and physical capital to provide it. States became active in determining the size of the cohort that entered (or in some states, that completed) medical education, and thus the overall size of the profession relative to the population. Several states have tried, with varying degrees of success, to influence the geographic distribution of doctors and the number in each of the specialities. The second area of state intervention has been in disciplining deviance within medicine. Both the courts, through malpractice litigation, and state regulatory bodies, through inspection of facilities and programmes to treat or remove impaired doctors, have undertaken the policing of medical institutions to a greater extent than in the past.

The final nineteenth-century issue that reverberated in the twentieth century was the tension between internationalism and nationalism in medicine. The international institutions of medicine were strengthened during the century, especially exchanging information about research results and the technologies of diagnosis and treatment. On the other hand, the bitter events of the Second World War and the Cold War made plain that most doctors, and most medical institutions, gave their primary allegiance to the nation-state rather than to the international institutions of medicine. The participation of many German doctors in ethically questionable research during the Second World War, and the compliance of many others with Nazi terrorism, for example, made plain that nationalism, or simply survival, outweighed the expressed values of medicine. Similarly, in the most bitter years of the Cold War, some doctors, especially psychiatrists, in both the Soviet Union and the United States breached the confidentiality of the doctor–patient relationship to agents of the state.

CONTEMPORARY HISTORY: MEDICINE AND THE STATE SINCE 1980

This concluding section assesses the recent history of the ongoing negotiations between the medical institutions and the state. Its purpose is to comment on what appear to be both continuities and pressures for change in the social contract between medicine and society as mediated by the state.

CONTINUITIES

The relationship between medical institutions and the state continues to have most of the characteristics described in the previous section. On the demand side, the state is everywhere the payer and guarantor of access. In every country of western Europe and in Canada, the state has taken the lead in organizing systems of access and payment that guarantee a negotiated minimum standard of care to everyone in the population, and spread the cost of that care, with attention to equity, over every working person. The broad consensus on these principles is more important than technical details about the mix of taxes, premiums, and consumer payments that maintain different medical-care systems. For a variety of reasons, the United States remains the anomaly: spending the highest proportion of its national product on medical care, and the largest amount on a per capita basis, but leaving 10–15 per cent of its population with the insecurity of knowing that the state will pay for urgently needed care only if no other source of payment is available.

On the supply side, there is also considerable continuity. States continue to cede dominant control of hospitals, medical education and certification, and research to the medical profession and its associations. At the same time, most states set public budgetary ceilings for these activities.

PRESSURES FOR CHANGE

Four issues appear to be the most likely candidates for renegotiation between medical institutions and society in the coming years. This judgement is based on their growing salience during the decade of 1980s and the beginning of the 1990s. These issues are:

the probable, and until recently, unexpected emergence of new, virulent infectious diseases;
the shifting boundaries between hospitals and other institutions of medical care in response to changes in the goals of medical treatment;
uncertainties about the determinants of the health of populations and a growing body of evidence about the limits of medical intervention; and
uncertainties about the relationship between expenditures on the institutions of medicine and the economic well-being of states.

Viral Traffic

The first issue was brought to prominence by the AIDS epidemic, more recently identified as a chronic infectious syndrome called HIV infection and related diseases. When the first cases of what was later called AIDS were recognized in 1981, many prominent people, in medicine as well as among the public, believed that most of the problems of identifying, preventing, and treating infectious diseases had been solved. (➤ Ch. 26 Sexually transmitted diseases)

By the end of the 1980s, however, thoughtful medical scientists were talking about a new conception of the history of virulent infectious disease. This new conception required a deeper understanding of the events in human history that, by changing the environment of viruses and their mode of transmission, would continue to create unexpected disasters that would begin as epidemics and remain as expensive chronic problems. This new concept, summarized by one of its proponents in the phrase 'viral traffic', would likely require new negotiations between medicine and the state to create advance-warning programmes that went beyond the traditional sentinel systems of public health.[20]

Shifting Boundaries, Changing Goals

During the economic downturn of the 1970s, every country in western Europe and North America became deeply concerned about the rising costs of medical care. In the 1980s, this concern merged with deeper uneasiness about the increasing concentration of resources on high-technology medicine in particular as practised in hospitals. The concern with high-technology medicine was also fuelled by increasing frustration about the imbalance of expenditures between, on the one hand, prolonging life, particularly for an increasingly elderly population, and, on the other, assisting people to live more-productive lives by managing more effectively the disabling consequences of chronic diseases and injuries. (➤ Ch. 68 Medical technologies: social concepts and consequences)

These concerns became focused on the budgets and responsibilities of hospitals in every Western country in the 1980s. Although many leaders of medical institutions agitated strongly to preserve the rate of increase in hospital expenditures and the power of doctors within them, both expenditures and medical power have eroded in the past decade. The use of resources by hospitals in every country has remained stable or declined slightly relative to ambulatory and long-term care (nursing-homes, home- and community-based services). Similarly, states have become more active in negotiating a decline in the proportion of new doctors who choose to practise speciality or sub-speciality disciplines rather than primary care.

Population Health

The belief that medical research, properly applied through a hierarchy of providers and facilities, would lead to improving health status for populations was the underlying premise of the social contract between medical institutions and the state during most of the twentieth century. This premiss has come under accelerating attack since the 1950s. A considerable body of research claimed that most of the advances in longevity and decline in mortality from infectious disease since the nineteenth century were the result of changes in diet, in sanitary practices, in housing, in risk-taking behaviour, and in public capita income. Researchers disputed the proportion of each factor, and of medical intervention, in improved health status. But by the late 1970s, there was little disagreement that the institutions of medicine had oversold themselves to the state.

Since then, there have been continuing pressures on states to revise the social contract with medical institutions in order to redistribute resources away from clinical medicine and conventional biomedical research. An important purpose of this redistribution would be to learn more about the determinants of health and to devise policies and practices based on this knowledge. There has been considerable resistance to this redistribution from many of the institutions of medicine. The most recent research suggests the possibility that a new and more-sophisticated approach to understanding the determinants of population health is emerging, with vast potential impact on the social contract between medicine and the state.[21]

Health and Wealth

Medical care is a major sector of the economy in every country of western Europe and North America. In the United Kingdom, the National Health Service is the largest employer. Several countries, including the United States, Canada, and Sweden, may be approaching the limit to the amount that they can spend on medical care without sacrificing the productivity of their overall economies. A major, but not the only, reason for this limit is that increasing amounts of medical-care expenditures are made on persons outside the labour force, who can have gains in health status but not in industrial productivity.[22] If further research justifies this reasoning, it is likely that, for the first time in history, medical institutions and the state will negotiate a trade-off between expenditures on medical services and investments that offer outputs that will improve real wages and general living conditions. Although the newly independent countries of central Europe are outside the scope of this chapter, there is evidence that several of them, notably Czechoslovakia and Hungary, face such tradeoffs in the early 1990s.

CONCLUSION

This chapter has covered a wide sweep of the history of both medicine and the nation-state. The central point has been that people representing the institutions of medicine and those of the state have been negotiating with each other over a variety of important issues for many centuries. These negotiations necessarily produce results that are particular to time and place. But the negotiations are also cumulative. They build on previous negotiations, so that the historical record always presents evidence of both continuity and change. Moreover, the negotiations always take place in the context of larger issues than those pertaining to medicine. Such contextual issues include broad values: how one accords priority between individuals and collectives, or how a state values the poor in relation to other classes. The contextual issues also include matters of economic policy and war, and of religion and ideology. (➤ Ch. 61 Religion and medicine)

From time to time, especially in the twentieth century, various voices within medical institutions in western Europe and North America have lamented a lost golden age. In this wondrous time, medicine was comfortably auton-omous, and the state (and the people who comprised it) did not interfere with the relationship between doctors and their patients. This chapter demon-strates that such nostalgic statements are fanciful. The medical institutions and the modern state have never been able to avoid close, mutually dependent relationships. They have not been able to avoid them because both have been too important to human society and its history.

NOTES

1 Frederick M. Watkins, 'State: the concept', in David Sills (ed.), *International Encyclopedia of the Social Sciences*, New York, Macmillan, 1968, Vol. XV p. 150.
2 Martin Sicker, *The Genesis of the State*, New York, Praeger, 1991.
3 Harold J. Laski, *A Grammar of Politics*, London, George Allen & Unwin, 1925, p. 2.
4 For an account of the history and definitions of the concept of political culture, see Gabriel L. Almond and Sidney Verba (eds), *The Civic Culture Revisited*, Boston, MA, Little Brown, 1980, pp. 26 ff. The concept of political culture came under attack in the literature of political science in the 1980s. However, see R. Inglehart, 'The renaissance of political culture', *American Political Science Review*, 1988, 82: 1203–30.
5 Matthew Ramsey, *Professional and Popular Medicine in France, 1770–1830*, Cambridge, Cambridge university Press, 1988, p. 19.
6 Ibid., pp. 104–5.
7 George Rosen, 'Cameralism and the concept of medical police', in Rosen, *From Medical Police to Social Medicine: Essays on the History of Health Care*, New York, Science History Publications, 1974, p. 122.
8 Oliver Faure, 'The social history of health in France: a survey of recent develop-ments', *Social History of Medicine*, 1990, 3: 442.
9 L. J. Jordanova, 'Policing public health in France, 1780–1815', in Teizo Ogawa (ed.), *Public Health*, Proceedings of the Fifth International Symposium on the Comparative History of Medicine – East and West, Tokyo, Taniguchi Foun-dation, 1981.
10 This account draws heavily on Daniel M. Fox, 'The Politics of physicians responsibility in epidemics', in Elizabeth Fee and Fox (eds), *AIDS: the Burden of History*, Berkeley, University of California Press, 1988, pp. 86–96.

11 William Coleman, *Death is a Social Disease*, Madison, University of Wisconsin Press, 1982, p. 207.
12 F. B. Smith, *The People's Health, 1830–1910*, London, Croom Helm, 1979, pp. 348–9.
13 Paul Weindling, 'Linking self help and medical science: the social history of occupational health', in Weindling (ed.), *The Social History of Occupational Health*, London, Croom Helm, 1985, p. 10.
14 Edward Berkowitz, 'Domestic politics and international expertise in the history of American disability policy', *Milbank Quarterly*, 1989, 67 (suppl. 2, part 1): 1989, p. 200.
15 I have written about this model at length in Daniel M. Fox, *Health Policies, Health Politics: the Experience of Britain and America, 1911–1965*, Princeton, NJ, Princeton University Press, 1986.
16 The discussion of hospitals here and in the subsequent sections of this chapter are informed by two recent books: Charles E. Rosenberg, *The Care of Strangers: the Rise of America's Hospital System*, New York, Basic Books, 1987; and Rosemary A. Stevens, *In Sickness and in Wealth: American Hospitals in the Twentieth Century*, New York, Basic Books, 1989.
17 Smith, op. cit. (n. 12), p. 348.
18 Much of the discussion of the social contract between medicine and society that follows grows out of many conversations over several years between the author and Professor Rudolf Klein of the University of Bath. He would describe what he calls the 'policy system' of a country, rather than the state, as the mediating agency.
19 Daniel M. Fox, 'Policy and epidemiology: financing health services for the chronically ill and disabled', *Milbank Quarterly*, 1989, 67 (suppl. 2, part 2): 257–87; and *Power and Illness: The Failure and Future of American Health Policy*, Berkeley, CA, University of California Press, 1993.
20 For the concept of viral traffic and for the transformation of AIDS into a chronic disease, see the articles by Stephen Morse, Elizabeth Fee and Daniel M. Fox, and David J. Rothman and Harold Edgar, in Fee and Fox (eds), *AIDS: the Making of a Chronic Disease*, Berkeley, University of California Press, 1991.
21 Robert G. Evans, and Gregory L. Stoddart, 'Producing health, consuming health care', *Social Science and Medicine*, 1991, 31: 1347–63.
22 Ibid., p. 1359.

FURTHER READING

Cipolla, Carlo M., *Public Health and the Medical Profession in the Renaissance*, Cambridge, Cambridge University Press, 1976.

Coleman, William, *Death is a Social Disease*, Madison, University of Wisconsin Press, 1982.

Cook, Harold J., *The Decline of the Old Medical Regime in Stuart London*, Ithaca, NY, Cornell University Press, 1986.

Fee, Elizabeth and Fox, Daniel M. (eds), *AIDS: the Burdens of History*, Berkeley, University of California Press, 1988.

—————, *AIDS: the Making of a Chronic Disease*, Berkeley, University of California Press, 1991.

Fox, Daniel M., *Health Policies, Health Politics: the Experience of Britain and America, 1911–1965*, Princeton, NJ, Princeton University Press, 1986.

—————, *Power and Illness: The Failure and Future of American Health Policy*, Berkeley, CA, University of California Press, 1993.

Klein, Rudolf, *The Politics of the National Health Service*, 2nd edn, London, Longmans, 1989.

Leichter, Howard, *A Comparative Approach to Policy Analysis: Health Care Policy in Four Nations*, New York, Cambridge University Press, 1979.

Ogawa, Teizo (ed.), *Public Health*, Proceedings of the Fifth International Symposium on the Comparative History of Medicine – East and West, Tokyo, Taniguchi Foundation, 1981.

Ramsey, Mathew, *Professional and Popular Medicine in France, 1770–1830*, New York and Cambridge, Cambridge University Press, 1988.

Rosen, George, *From Medical Police to Social Medicine: Essays on the History of Health Care*, New York, Science History Publications, 1974.

Rosenberg, Charles, *The Care of Strangers: the Rise of America's Hospital System*, New York, Basic Books, 1987.

Smith, F. B., *The People's Health, 1830–1910*, London, Croom Helm, 1979.

Stevens, Rosemary A., *In Sickness and in Wealth: American Hospitals in the Twentieth Century*, New York, Basic Books, 1989.

Weindling, Paul (ed.), *The Social History of Occupational Health*, London, Croom Helm, 1985.

51

PUBLIC HEALTH

Dorothy Porter

INTRODUCTION

The health of its population is a prerequisite for the survival of every human society. Since ancient times, human groups have devised rules and protocols to enhance the chances of health. This essay focuses on strategies for collective rather than personal health, even though the two often overlap and are inherently related to each other. The ideas of personal health management are considered elsewhere in this volume. (➤ Ch. 53 History of personal hygiene)

Public health has often been portrayed as a heroic progress from ignorance to knowledge, darkness to light, squalor to cleanliness, barbarism to civilization. More recent historiography, however, has explored the complex web of forces underlying changing demographic distributions of disease; contradictory theories of causation and prevention and their relationship to conflicting interests in the enforcement of health; the relationship of epidemics to social disruption; and the politics of health and the state.

This chapter will draw a history with a broad sweep from ancient to modern times. There is a case to be made, however, for a high-period of public health – a time when the most intense activity took place with the widest scope and implications. I believe this period began around the end of the eighteenth century and lasted up to the First World War. At that time, public health expanded most rapidly in numerous national contexts and was linked to the changing role of the modern state in developing industrial societies. This was a time when public health was a major force in the historical processes of transition. It justifies, therefore, a greater amount of discussion.

HEALTH CODES AND PROTOCOLS OF THE WORLD WE HAVE LOST

Discourses on health have existed from ancient times such as the Hippocratic treatise on *Airs, Waters, Places* (*c.* fifth century BC). The treatise divided diseases into 'endemic', which were always present, and 'epidemic', which only occurred occasionally and excessively. It attempted to identify the environmental determinants of local endemicity and to provide practical advice for colonization, suggesting that climate, soil, and water were crucial. (➤ Ch. 15 Environment and medicine; Ch. 18 The ecology of disease) New settlements should avoid marshy lowlands, and houses should be built on elevated areas to be warmed by the sun and catch salubrious winds. The treatise also directed its readers towards healthy living habits and nutrition. Ancient medicine emphasized the importance of personal regimens and dietetics to ward off disease. This was affirmed by Galen (AD 129–*c.*200/210) in his discussion of the natural (innate constitutional), 'non-natural' (environmental), and preternatural (pathological) causes of health and disease, which produced variations in the pulse and affected the balance of humours within the body (➤ Ch. 14 Humoralism) According to Galen, both innate causes of variation in the pulse, such as sex, temperament, weight, age, pregnancy, sleep, awakening, ambient air, and 'non-natural', or optional, causes, such as hot and cold baths, large meals, wine and water, all had the potential to become pathological. Thus he advised that health regimens should be designed for the successful manipulation of determinants such as air, food and drink, motion and rest, sleep and wakening, inanition and repletion, and accidents of the soul.

The two themes of personal and public hygiene continued to influence collective action to regulate environmental conditions, and the regulation of individual behaviour for the benefit of the community. Health regulation has been greatly spurred by the impact of infectious diseases. Certain diseases were, from ancient times, perceived to be spread through contact. As a result, isolation of sufferers was frequently invoked to protect the healthy. For example, there are many Biblical allusions to the isolation and repulsion of lepers from the general community. The lazaretto – pest-house – was an institution set up initially as a leper colony, placed outside the city boundaries. Later, it came to be used for more-general quarantine purposes.

From the fourteenth century, isolation methods expanded in Europe when a number of Mediterranean city-states introduced quarantine to protect themselves against the major epidemic of bubonic plague that began in 1346 commonly known as the Black Death. The first systematic quarantine was established by the city of Venice when, on 20 March 1348, it closed its gates to all suspect vessels, travellers, and ships. Milan followed suit in 1350, and in 1374, Bernabò Visconti (1323–85), ruler of Milan, gave orders to the

Podestà of Reggio that all victims of the plague and anyone who had nursed them were to be housed in a pest-house established beyond the city walls. In 1377, Ragusa set up stations where travellers and merchandise from infected areas were isolated for thirty days. At Marseilles (1383), Venice (1403), and Majorca (1471) the period was extended to forty days.

Richard Palmer has suggested, however, that the most influential attempts to control plague were those of the Milan ruler, Gian Galeazzo Visconti (1351–1402), between 1398 and 1400.[1] When plague appeared in Soncino in 1398, he banned any person travelling from there from entering Milan. He used the river Adda as a natural *cordon sanitaire* by having all travellers stopped at bridges and ports, and in 1400 he created alternative routes for pilgrims journeying to Rome which kept them out of the city. In 1399, Gian Galeazzo decreed that all who fell sick were to be removed to two plague hospitals, their houses shut up, and contacts sent out of town. He rejected the idea of his city council that the sick should be kept in their houses, and insisted that in the hospitals patients be separated and provided with medical care. Families were quarantined in monasteries outside the town. Milan's regulations became the model of plague prevention in Italy for the succeeding centuries.

Quarantine protected cities from the importation of plague, but hindered the pace and free flow of trade. However, it was also used to enhance a disease-free reputation amongst trading states. For example, in nineteenth-century Egypt, an international Quarantine Board was set up by the viceroy, Muhammed Ali (1769–1849), in the belief that certification of healthiness would bolster confidence in its merchant traffic and eliminate Egypt's traditional reputation as the cradle of plague.

Methods of isolation and quarantine were further expanded in response to the plague epidemics of the early modern period. In seventeenth-century Europe, the *cordon sanitaire* became the standard method of preventing the rapid spread of the disease between settlements. In addition, the nature of the pest-house became transformed. In the Plague Act of 1604, the British Parliament made statutory a set of orders which had first been issued in 1578. Thus, in the 1665–6 epidemic, local authorities were empowered to enforce the house-arrest of entire families of plague-sufferers. Households suspected of containing sickness were marked with an insignia, and all were prevented from leaving or entering by militia posted outside, by force if necessary. In addition, all clothes and bedding of victims were burnt, and funerals took place after dusk to reduce the number of participants. The Act also allowed local authorities to raise a local rate to cover the costs of enforcing compulsory isolation. (➤ Ch. 53 Epidemiology)

ENLIGHTENMENT, LIBERALISM, AUTOCRACY, AND HEALTH

Plague gradually retreated from western Europe and was last seen in Marseilles at the beginning of the eighteenth century. Subsequently, there was a lull in the advent of shock invasions of epidemic disease. The eighteenth century witnessed rising levels of endemic infections and chronic sickness, which occasionally became epidemic, such as malaria, smallpox, and gout. The absence of disasters meant that no new emergency methods of prevention were developed. But the Age of Enlightenment, instead, was a period of reflection upon the health of populations, and of social scientific analyses of disease; it witnessed the evolution of new preventive methods of sanitation and immunization.

QUANTITATIVE METHODS OF SOCIAL ANALYSIS

The idea of assessing the strength of the state by counting the population was developed by the seventeenth-century physician, wealthy landowner, and early social scientist William Petty (1623–87). In the preface to his *Political Anatomy of Ireland*, he stated that he was inspired by an observation made by Francis Bacon (1561–1626) that the preservation of the body politic and the body natural were linked:

> and it is reasonable, that as anatomy is the best foundation of one, so also of the other; and that to practice upon the politick, without knowing the symmetry, fabric, and proportion of it, is as casual as the practice of . . . empyricks. Now, because anatomy is not only necessary in physicians, but laudable in every philosophical person whatsoever; I therefore have attempted the first essay of political anatomy.[2]

Petty produced a political arithmetic of social facts to enhance the state's chances of military defence, commercial and technological expansion, and social reform. He collected data on population, trade, manufacture, education, diseases, and revenue. He was the earliest market researcher: 'What are the books that do sell most?', he asked. But he studied the conditions under which prosperity flourished and was impeded. Thus he attempted to project the number of lives – and economic wealth – that might be preserved for the Crown if the supply of qualified medical practitioners were to increase. Petty's contemporaries, such as Nehemiah Grew (1641–1712), produced similar quantitative analyses.[3]

Petty's friend, a mercer, and a fellow of the Royal Society, John Graunt (1620–74), began to calculate health and disease. He scrutinized the London Bills of Mortality to discover the regularities of life-events such as births and deaths – noting the excess of male versus female births, and excess of male versus female deaths – and the proportion of individual disease mortality to the whole. He highlighted the higher urban versus rural death rates.

These were the early foundations of 'vital statistics' and epidemiology which, by the nineteenth-century, became prerequisite for systematic disease prevention. Quantitative methods continued to develop in the eighteenth century. One of the most important tools of vital statistics was the 'life table', which was first devised in 1693 by the English astronomer Edmond Halley (*c*.1656–1743). Equally important was demographic analysis, which was popularized by the Revd Thomas Malthus (1766–1834). The study of statistics advanced in Germany in the eighteenth century, where the term *Statistik* – derived from the term *Staat* – came to describe catalogues and surveys illustrating 'the condition and prospects of society'. Gottfried Achenwall (1719–72), Professor of Law and Politics at Göttingen, greatly contributed to this field. The subject was combined with the study of law, largely for students hoping to become civil servants, who would explore the comparison between states in terms of their populations, geography, climate, natural resources, trade, manufacturing, military strength, education, religion, and constitution. But statistics remained descriptive until transformed into a science of probability by the French and German mathematicians Pierre-Simon de Laplace (1749–1827) and Carl Friedrich Gauss (1777–1855) in 1810–12. Later (see pp. 1238–41), I shall discuss how probabilistic statistics was incorporated, in the early nineteenth century, into the study of social physics by Adolphe Quetelet (1796–1874). Social physics was used to analyze quantitatively the social and economic determinants of disease distribution.[4] (➤ Ch. 71 Demography and medicine)

A RENAISSANCE OF HEALTH

Enlightenment doctors revived the Hippocratic philosophy of prolonging life and preserving individual health through dietetics, regimen, and exercise. The massive increase in health-advice books throughout Europe in the eighteenth century testifies to the popularity of personal-health cults. The same classical revival encouraged concern with environmental-health regulation. John Bellers (1654–1725), a Quaker cloth-merchant who lived largely in London, wrote comprehensively on the health of towns in 1714, emphasizing the importance of population density to the propagation of disease. He recommended municipal street-cleaning, refuse collection, regulation of dairies, abattoirs, and noxious trades. He was especially concerned with the replacement of intermittent with constant water supply to towns. (➤ Ch. 27 Diseases of civilization)

Eighteenth-century health investigators began to identify dirt with disease. The philanthropist John Howard (*c*.1726–90) studied gaols, bridewells, lazarettos, and hospitals in Britain and on the European continent in the 1770s and 1780s. He concluded that their filthy conditions and closed contaminated atmospheres were lethal, responsible for such endemic conditions as 'gaol fever' (typhus). The naval and military physicians James Lind (1716–94) and John Pringle (1707–82) campaigned for ship and camp cleanliness to eliminate typhus – also referred to as spotted fever. The political radical, religious dissenter, and physician John Haygarth (1740–1827) argued that typhus fever's contagiousness was responsible for its prevalence amongst the urban poor living in congested slums. Eighteenth-century health campaigners equally believed that stench spread disease. When Pringle and the physiologist and inventor Revd Stephen Hales (1677–1761) were commissioned in 1750 to try and purify the noxious air of Newgate Prison, they recommended the introduction of ventilators. Hales had first devised new mechanisms for the ventilation of ships and gaols in the 1740s, consisting of hand-operated bellows. Later, he devised a type of windmill device to be placed on roofs.

In Enlightenment England, the campaign to avoid disease was based on social science. It was, however, only sporadically translated into public policy through the haphazard proliferation of urban Improvement Commissions. Philanthropic individuals set up commissions with responsibility for improving paving, lighting, street-cleaning, etc. But no central-government policy was developed. In this *laissez-faire* society, however, public health did become a commercial enterprise. Various trades began to clean the surface of towns. Scavenging, street-cleaning, night-soil collection, and the design of 'airy' dwellings grew as profitable enterprises. (➤ Ch. 64 Medicine and architecture)

But the most successful of all eighteenth-century disease-prevention campaigns was inoculation against smallpox. The wife of the British ambassador to Constantinople, Lady Mary Wortley Montagu (1689–1762), first introduced inoculation into Europe in 1718, when she reported on its common practice in the Ottoman Empire. First practised on condemned prisoners and orphaned children, it was popularized by the inoculation of the royal family. High-ranking intellectuals such as Sir Hans Sloane (1660–1753), President of the Royal Society, endorsed it, together with Charles Maitland (1668–1748), a leading surgeon. From the 1760s, it was commercialized with great success by operators such as Robert (1707–88) and Daniel Sutton (1735–1819), who inoculated whole towns and villages at once. Haygarth promoted a complete system of smallpox eradication for the poor.

In contrast to the *laissez-faire* and localist model in England, the people's health on the European continent was considered the responsibility of a paternalistic, absolute monarch. A comprehensive system of medical police was designed by Johann Peter Frank (1745–1821), Physician to the late eighteenth-century Habsburg Court, and Director of the general hospital in Vienna. In six huge volumes, Frank outlined methods for regulating intimate individual behaviour that might spread or engender disease, such as marriage, pregnancy, and personal hygiene. Equally, he proposed public-hygiene measures of drainage, pure water supply, street-cleaning, control of vice and overcrowding, and the sanitary order of hospitals. Frank's system reflected the paternalistic political philosophy of 'cameralism' of the Habsburg Empire, headed by enlightened despots since the reign of Maria Theresa (1717–80), who saw the role of the monarch as that of the parent of the people. Cameralism viewed a growing, healthy population as an inexhaustible source of power for the monarch seeking agricultural, industrial, and military expansion. Thus, the body and behaviour of the individual was the economic and political property of the state, to be utilized for its benefit through the science of police (*polizei*), a form of civil-service administration. This philosophy was equally expressed in Sweden's extensive state health interventions before 1800. Health reform in Sweden was made possible through the creation of a national census in 1749 which, together with that of Finland, was the first in Europe.

THE HEALTH OF DEMOCRATIC CITIZENS

Democratic revolution in America and France asserted new principles regarding the state and the health of its subjects. Thomas Jefferson (1743–1826) believed that a life of 'liberty and the pursuit of happiness' would automatically be a healthful one. Jefferson told his co-signer of the Declaration of Independence, the physician and patriot Benjamin Rush (1746–1813), that the iniquity of European absolutism was reflected in its peoples' wretchedly unhealthy and demoralized condition. Democracy was the source of the people's health. Democratic citizens, self-educated in exercising their political judgement, would secure a healthful existence. Jefferson claimed that the healthiness of the American people reflected the superiority of democratic citizenship.

But it was French revolutionaries who added health to the rights of human beings. In 1791, the Committee on Mendicancy, directed by the duc de la Rochelle, declared work to be a right of people and, if the state could not provide it, then it must ensure a means of subsistence to the unemployed. In 1793, the National Convention's Committee on Salubrity added health to the state's obligations to citizens. The committee believed this could be achieved by establishing a network of rural health officers who, while trained in clinical medicine, would also become responsible for reporting on the health of communities and monitoring epidemics among both humans and farm animals.

The citizen's charter of health, however, was double-sided. The idéologue Constantine Volney (1757–1820) raised the issue of the citizen's responsibility to maintain his or her own health for the benefit of the state. In the new social order, the individual was a political and economic unit of a collective whole. Thus, it was a citizen's duty to keep healthy through temperance, both in the consumption of pleasure and the exercise of passions, and through cleanliness.

INDUSTRIAL MASSACRE AND THE BIRTH OF THE EXPERT MANAGERIAL STATE

From the end of the eighteenth century, public health was inextricably linked to the changing role of the state in the transition to industrial society. Industrialization exponentially multiplied environmental threats to health, primarily through the massive growth of towns. In Britain for example, London had 800,000 people in 1801, and there were only thirteen towns with a population of over 25,000. By 1841, London's population rose by one million, and forty-two towns contained over 25,000 people. By 1861, six British cities contained more than a quarter of a million inhabitants. Some of the larger cities, such as Manchester and Glasgow, grew at the rate of nearly 50 per cent, but the growth rate of some small towns was even more staggering. Middlesborough grew from 154 to 40,000 people in less than forty years. No urban development could possibly accommodate such a demographic explosion, which resulted in mass overcrowding, inadequate housing, dramatic accumulation of human, animal, and industrial waste products, together with rising levels of industrial and domestic atmospheric pollution, and deadly pollution of insufficient potable water supply. The grotesquely squalid conditions imposed upon the slum-dwelling proletariat was revealed by a host of observers, from social reformers to investigative journalists, and soon produced dramatic rises in infant mortality; rising levels of epidemic diseases, such as 'fever' – both typhoid and typhus; and rising levels of dependency created through sickness.

SOCIAL PHYSICS

The connection between environment and disease required, however, new methods of analysis. Thus, as the historian G. M. Young suggested, 'It was the business of the thirties to transfer the treatment of affairs from a polemical to a statistical basis, from Humbug to Humdrum.'[5] As the new tool for measuring social inequality, statistics became inherently linked with social-reform movements, providing the foundation for what Quetelet defined as a science of 'social physics'.

Social physics produced the first systematic analysis of disease patterns. The 'Partie d'hygiène', in France, led by Louis René Villermé (1782–1863), and the British physician and civil servant William Farr (1807–83), mapped out the disease patterns of nineteenth-century society in transition and attempted to identify their determinants. Above all, what the quantitative methods and epidemiological analyses of Farr and Villermé achieved was to demonstrate that in urbanized, industrial society, death had become a definitively social disease.

After the Napoleonic wars, Villermé, an ex-Army surgeon, devoted himself to the social diagnosis of disease. He became a member of the Royal Academy of Medicine and President of the Academy of Moral and Political Sciences. At the former, Villermé was a member of the department of hygiene, which produced numerous seminal socio-medical studies and was chaired by the physiologist Jean Noel Hallé (1754–1822). Frédéric Villot, the Director of the Paris Census Bureau, and his old teacher from the École Polytechnique, J. B. J. Fourier (1768–1830), completed a massive demographic study of Paris, the *Recherches statistiques sur la ville de Paris* in 1821. The Royal Academy of Medicine subsequently appointed Villermé to a Commission to examine the health implications of Villot's tableaux.

In his 'Rapport' of 1826, Villermé analysed the differential mortality between Paris *arrondissements* (city districts).[6] First, he examined environmental factors such as elevation, the soil, movement of prevailing winds and other meteorological conditions, but none coincided with patterns of mortality. The commission then turned to the question of congestion, but found that densities were so mixed within *arrondissements* that, again, no clear pattern emerged. Similarly, distribution of open spaces did not fit the facts. Having exhausted the traditional environmental determinants, the commission analysed the financial status of inhabitants using rent levels, identifiable through tax liabilities, as an indicator of wealth. The result was that untaxed renters, who represented the poorest inhabitants, consistently showed the highest levels of mortality within *arrondissements*. Villermé proceeded to confirm the analysis through detailed studies of quarters and streets. He demonstrated that the rue de la Mortellerie, which heaved with some of the poorest Parisians, had a death rate of 30.6 per 1,000, while a short distance away across the river, the higher-taxed residents of more spacious and comfortable quays of Île-Saint-Louis had a death rate of only 19.1 per 1,000. These data, together with further correlations on births, marriages, and ratio of illegitimacy with poverty and wealth, demonstrated that the rich had reduced fertility, increasingly abandoned natural children, and lived longest; the poor had higher birth rates, more of their children died, recognized their natural children, and died younger – most frequently at the prime of life.

Following these conclusions, Villermé created life-tables for the working-class, studying the textile industry in particular, correlating mortality to income. He was joined in some of his socio-medical investigations by François

Joseph Victor Benoiston de Châteauneuf (1776–1856). But his 1826 report showed, above all, that the prime agent of premature death was economic. Villermé and his associates in the 'Parti d'hygiène' believed, however, that the health of populations could be solved not through the actions of the state, but through the moral regeneration of the poor, which would put an end to destitution and its cohorts, disease and death. The hygienists believed that the masters of industry bore the responsibility of seeing that workers lived in a respectable way and were educated in moral habits, through Christian example and instruction. There was no role for the state or legislative reform in the view of the economist hygienists, for this would undermine individual freedom and initiative. They feared the rise of socialism and its aims to overthrow the rule of property. They sought instead a programme of amelioration through religious indoctrination of the poor into the ways of moral behaviour. Their answer to the claim that civilization produced the ills of society, such as poverty, was simply to say that the poor were as yet uncivilized. Their answer to the question, 'what was the cause of poverty?' was the poor themselves and who, once they were educated into the ways of civilized behaviour, would eliminate it.

Villermé asserted that the social origins of disease and death lay with the poor as a 'race apart', a barbarian, uncivilized multitude, which bred in abundance and died equally excessively. The answer was to civilize them into the ways of moral correctness and responsible citizenship. This belief was shared by the most significant advocate of statistical investigation of disease and mortality distribution in England, William Farr. He had a vision of the poor as wretched but redeemable creatures. He was against the expansion of financial assistance to the poor in England because it would be 'expended indiscriminately upon the idle, reckless, vicious as well as the good but unfortunate'.[7] But unlike his French counterparts, Farr attributed a much greater role to environmental determinants of health and pursued a different programme of disease prevention and social amelioration.

Farr used social statistics for social reform in his analysis of mortality and urban salubrity. The compulsory registration of births, marriages, and deaths and the Registrar General's Office were created in Britain under the 1836 Registration Act. T. H. Lister (1800–42) was appointed as the first Registrar and, on the recommendation of Edwin Chadwick (1800–90), Farr was appointed Compiler of Abstracts in charge of statistics.

Farr studied medical statistics under the French clinician Pierre Louis (1787–1872) in the early 1830s. In his annual reports at the Registrar General's Office, Farr demonstrated that mortality increased with density, and he stressed that overcrowding was the main determinant of high mortality from what he classified as zymotic diseases. Farr argued that crude mortality rates could direct public-health policy by using the 'life-table' as a 'biometer' of health and a measure of salubrity, comparable to the barometer for meteorological measurement or the thermometer for measuring heat.

In his first five Annual Reports, Farr highlighted the unhealthiness of urban over rural environments, and compared poor with wealthy registration districts. He identified lack of sanitation rather than poverty as the primary cause of higher urban mortality because he believed that the price of the necessities for subsistence had to outstrip completely the ability to purchase them before income had any influence on death rates. As a result, he advocated the keeping of statistics, education in basic hygiene for the general public, and the reform of medical education to make physicians more aware and responsible for preventing illness. He was a great enthusiast for vaccination and supported the campaign for the provision of uncontaminated water.

Farr showed that the life-table could demonstrate how life expectation at different ages varied according to occupation, wealth, and hygiene conditions. Subsequently, it became the basic tool of every English public-health officer analysing the health of a district, with infant mortality the most important vital measure. 'Vital statistics' became the primary subject of all public-health education.

POLITICAL ECONOMY AND THE SANITARY STATE

The social physics of disease, poverty, and urbanism was taken up throughout Europe in the first half of the nineteenth century. Its influence upon governments varied. In France, little systematic or comprehensive state action was enforced until later decades. In united Germany, after 1871, the state programme for health reform was extensive. But the translation of expertise into public policy-making in industrial society took root most profoundly in the expanding bureaucracy of the mid-Victorian British state.

Public-health reform in Britain resulted from a mixture of philanthropic relief, political expediency and, most of all, from utilitarian principles of political economy. It is also important to remember that health reform, like political reform, in early nineteenth-century Britain took place against a background of fear and suspicion. The creation of an urban proletariat by an industrial economy generated more than just increases in production. It bred more sharply defined economic class division and political suspicion, potentially threatening underlying social stability. As the landowning aristocracy struggled to maintain their rule of parliament through political reform, radical elements of the proletariat challenged the entire political structure, and, while revolution was never a threat, flashpoints of civil unrest heightened unease.

The arrival of cholera in Britain in 1831–2 provided such a flashpoint and stimulated the first government attempt to manage an epidemic through the creation of a temporary Board of Health. Asiatic cholera, possibly transmitted by British troop movements from India, rapidly spread across west Asia and eastern and western Europe throughout 1830–1. It followed trading routes, military movements, and refugee populations displaced through war. (➤ Ch. 66 War and modern medicine) Isolation cordons proved ineffective, and their enforcement caused rioting from Russia to Paris, in which nobility, government officials, and doctors were attacked by peasantry who believed there was a conspiracy to poison them. In Britain, removal of victims for isolation in workhouse infirmaries caused riots in Bristol. Rioters believed the medical profession were using the epidemic as a great body-snatching opportunity, for anatomical dissection. But, despite the clear differentiation of the class distribution of the epidemic, it demonstrated an enormous stability within British society. A largely philanthropic middle class did not flee, but volunteered relief to the stricken in diseased localities, and a co-operative working class obeyed civil orders.[8]

The murderous mortality of the 1832 cholera in Britain highlighted the problem of disease and its connection with the increasing costs of poverty levied upon taxpayers. This connection was chiefly perceived by the main author of the New Poor Law, the utilitarian lawyer/civil servant, one-time Secretary to Jeremy Bentham (1748–1832), Edwin Chadwick. By the early 1800s, political economists believed that the Old Poor Law system of subsidizing low agricultural wages was stagnating the labour market and constituting the greatest national expense. Chadwick, as Secretary to the Poor Law Commission from 1832, devised a New Poor Law, enacted in 1834, aimed at enhancing the circulation of labour by deterring dependency, making it a less-eligible life, than any form of employment, through incarceration in a workhouse. Separating the labouring from the dependent poor would prevent them from the contamination of pauperization. Chadwick explored many avenues, besides decreased eligibility, to prevent destitution, investigating causes of pauperism like alcoholism, crime, overcrowding, and violence, and concluded that a great proportion resulted from disease.[9]

In 1837, he appointed three doctors sympathetic to sanitary reform, Neil Arnott (1788–1874), James Phillip Kay-Shuttleworth (1804–71) and Thomas Southwood Smith (1788–1861), to investigate London districts with the highest typhus mortality. In their reports in 1838, they revealed the full squalor of the London rookeries, where medical officers as well as the local inhabitants lost their lives from rampant 'fever'.[10] Chadwick then decided to study insanitary areas throughout Britain.

Chadwick loathed poor-law medical officers because he thought they prescribed useless philanthropy, but he used hundreds of their reports to compile a massive survey published in his *Report on the Sanitary Conditions of the*

Labouring Population of Great Britain (1842). The conditions described in London in 1838 were matched in Glasgow, Birmingham, Leeds, Manchester, and other major urban centres. The *Report* recommended implementation of what Chadwick called 'the sanitary idea', beginning with the creation of a central public-health authority to direct local boards of health to provide drainage, cleansing, paving, and potable water, and the sanitary regulation of dwellings, nuisances, and offensive trades, etc. The local authorities were to appoint a medical officer of health to supervise and co-ordinate all local sanitary work, and an inspector of nuisances. Sanitary regulation would be assisted by strengthened nuisance laws and building laws, and local authorities would be allowed to raise a rate for large engineering projects to provide new sewage-drainage and water supply.[11]

Chadwick was convinced that the construction of massive new drainage and sewage-removal systems was of primary importance. He believed that the existing square, bricked sewers with large tunnel pipes that did not flush or empty should be replaced by small egg-shaped sewers lined with glazed brick and connected by small earthenware pipes, which would be constantly flushed by pressurized water. Liquid sewage could be recycled as fertilizer to outlying farming districts. Street-widening, the removal of cesspools and all other noxious nuisances, together with an end to intermittent drinking-water, were considered fundamental.

Chadwick built his sanitary idea upon a miasmatic theory of disease aetiology: that is, disease causation through non-specific contamination of the atmosphere by gaseous material given off by putrefying, decomposing organic matter. In other words, disease was smell. His colleague and closest ally, Southwood Smith, was an enthusiastic advocate of atmospheric aetiology and, though it was contested by other members of the medical profession, it allowed Chadwick to pursue urban sanitary reform and abolish quarantine – the all-time greatest impediment to free trade. (➤ Ch. 16 Contagion/germ theory/specificity)

Reformers rallied to the cause of urban sanitation in the Metropolitan Health of Towns Association, founded in 1844 by Southwood Smith, and in scholarly forums such as the National Association for the Promotion of Social Science, the Royal Statistical Society, and the London Epidemiological Society. These groups brought reformers together with influential policy-makers and cabinet ministers. For example, the Health of Towns Association was supported by aristocrats and politicians such as the Marquis of Normanby (1819–90), who was its first president, Viscount Morpeth (1802–64), Lord Ashley (later 7th Earl of Shaftsbury) (1801–85), Benjamin Disraeli (1804–81), and élite doctors such as Sir James Clark (1788–1870) and John Simon (1816–1904). Their supportive propaganda, such as a Health of Towns Association's report in 1847, became crucial in the fight for new legislation.

Following Chadwick's 1842 *Report*, a Royal Commission on the Health of Towns was set up in 1843–5, which reinforced its recommendations and added new clauses regarding interments. In 1846, Liverpool created the first sanitary authority under a local Act and appointed the first Medical Officer of Health, a local physician named William Duncan (1805–63). The Liverpool administration provided a model for national legislation. The first British Public Health Act was passed in 1848. While comprehensive, it remained permissive. The potential for a national sanitary bureaucracy was available but left largely to the direction of individual local governments. The Act created a central authority, the General Board of Health, consisting of three members: the evangelical, philanthropic 7th Earl of Shaftsbury (Lord Ashley), its first president; Viscount Morpeth (Earl of Carlisle), who had been responsible for introducing the Act into Parliament; and Chadwick, its only salaried member. Southwood Smith was appointed as Medical Adviser under the Nuisance Removal and Disease Prevention (Cholera) Act 1848.

Any one-tenth of the ratepayers within a locality could petition the General Board for the adoption of the Act, or it could be imposed by the Board upon a local authority with an annual death rate above 23 per 1,000. The local town council or corporation became the sanitary authority, as a local board of health. The local boards of health were responsible for sanitary supervision and inspection, drainage, water and gas supplies, and could increase the local rates or raise mortgages to cover costs. They were to appoint local medical officers of health. Local boards had the power to regulate offensive trades; remove nuisances, as defined under the 1846–8 Nuisance Acts; regulate cellar dwellings and houses unfit for human habitation; and provide burial grounds, public parks, and baths. The Act applied to all districts outside the metropolitan boroughs of London, which had their own Metropolitan Commission of Sewers, set up in 1848. The City of London obtained its own private Sewers Act 1848, to keep it outside the jurisdiction of the General Board, and appointed its own medical officer of health, John Simon.

Chadwick believed that metropolitan London was more important to sanitary reform than all other localities. The internal conflicts and incompetence of the Metropolitan Sewers Commission, however, led to Chadwick's removal from it in 1849. He still attempted to bring London's interments system and water supply under the control of the General Board. He wanted to 'nationalize' burial and set up state cemeteries, but was opposed by the Treasury and the metropolitan vestries. Ultimately, an Interments Act of 1852 allowed the Home Secretary to close any metropolitan burial ground, and empowered local parishes to purchase new graveyard sites, but the General Board had no power to intervene.

Chadwick aimed to municipalize the private water companies and link water supply to drainage under one public authority. He was effectively opposed by the Metropolitan Sewers Commission and the water companies, which constituted a powerful Parliamentary lobby. A Water Act of 1852 allowed the metropolitan water companies to retain their separate existence, but forced them to abandon all sources below Teddington and to provide constant supply and to cover their reservoirs and filter their water. In both the interment and water questions, private interests and municipal government resisted public ownership and central control.

Between 1848 and 1853, 284 districts applied to adopt the Public Health Act, and it was established in 103 towns. Vigour varied between sanitary authorities. Some failed to make any improvements to mains-drainage or implement the Board's engineering schemes. In other districts, the same insanitary conditions persisted whether they adopted the Act or not. Some authorities, however, took up their new responsibilities and powers with a vengeance and instituted model reforms under the direction of the Board's inspectors.

Opposition to the whole measure came not just from 'Metropolitan Radicals', but from outraged defenders of local government autonomy and those who opposed 'despotic interference' in the lives of individuals and the free relations of the economic market. The Tory press raged against 'paternalistic' government. The *Herald* believed that 'A little dirt and freedom may after all be more desirable than no dirt at all and slavery', and the *Standard* suggested that the country had 'heard enough of the effect of centralization in the New Poor Law'. Local ratepayers resented being dictated to by a 'clean party'. The Institute of Civil Engineers disclaimed the arterial system, and supported the alternative designs of Sir Joseph William Bazalgette (1819–91).

The General Board's immense unpopularity forced its members to resign in 1854. A first chapter in the English experiment in state health regulation closed.[12] A new professional health management, however, followed Chadwick's downfall, directed not by an engineering but a medical model, and run not by philosopher-lawyer reformers but by doctors.

MEDICAL STATEMANSHIP AND THE EXPERT STATE

In the year of the first British Public Health Act, revolutions on the European continent were trying to sweep away the remnants of absolutism. Medical reform was on the agenda of the revolutionaries' rhetoric in both France and Germany. In the February edition of the *Paris Medical Gazette*, Jules Guérin (1801–86) called for the creation of 'social medicine' to identify the social inequalities that produce disease. Later in the year, Rudolf Virchow (1821–1902) began a campaign of reform which required that medicine take up its new political role in the creation of a democratic state. Earlier in 1848,

Virchow had been requested by the Prussian authorities to investigate a devastating epidemic of typhus in the occupied territories of Upper Silesia. Virchow's investigation led him to conclude that only what he called a 'socio-logical epidemiology' could explain its cause. Economically exploited, politically subjugated, and culturally dispossessed, the Polish inhabitants of the occupied region apathetically suffered the cruelly inadequate conditions that allowed the disease to spread so rapidly and fatally. Only political freedom, 'full and unlimited democracy', the establishment of universal education, and economic revival, Virchow claimed, would prevent a similar epidemic from occurring. This was what he and his collaborators in the medical-reform movement identified as 'political medicine', in which the physician's responsibility was to take up his natural role as an 'attorney for the poor'.[13]

Virchow was not alone, however, in advocating a role for the physician as a new 'saviour of humanity'. Medical reformers in Britain echoed this plea. In the 1870s, Parliament's chief medical spokesman, the chemist Lyon Playfair (1818–98), Member of Parliament for Edinburgh University, suggested that:

> The public officer of health has to deal with the body politic just as the private physician has to deal with the body of an individual . . . communities are acting like individual patients. They try to resist the admission that they are in a state which requires an abnegation of their own will, and a submission to the orders of their medical advisers. They kick against the need but yield while they kick.[14]

He predicted, however, that society would eventually become a well-behaved patient, and public health become 'a great field open to growing medical men'. Playfair was describing the rise of medical 'statemanship' in Britain. Even as Chadwick was leading sanitary reform, medical critics, such as Henry Rumsey (1809–76), were outraged that the health of the nation was being governed by 'two barristers and a Lord'. Rumsey, a prominent spokesperson amongst the British medical profession, drew upon continental European concepts of medical police to construct a theory which he identified as 'state medicine'. He believed that scientific health government needed a comprehensively planned system of integrated investigative, preventive, and palliative medicine, thus fulfilling, he suggested, 'Plato's principle – that the physician must reform part of the polity of his commonwealth'. The realization of these ideals, however, began with the appointment of John Simon to the chief government post in health.

Chadwick was ousted from office because of his desire to replace democratic with bureaucratic government, which would do away with what he believed was government by 'sinister interests'. What Lord Russell (1792–1878) identified as Chadwick's 'Prussian' approach to centralized political control proved incompatible with the English tradition of letting local government be. John Simon was appointed in 1854 to become Britain's first chief medical administrator, initially at the General Board of Health and, after it was abolished under the 1858 Public Health Act, to the newly created Medical Department of the Privy Council.

Simon's powers were ostensibly minimal compared to the mandate which had been given to Chadwick. In 1858, he had only the power of 'inspection and report' and direct control of the vaccination service, previously administered solely by the Poor Law authorities. As medical officer, he was the only employee of the Medical Department at the Privy Council, which was comparable to the education department in the Home Office run by Kay-Shuttleworth. By 1872, however, Simon had used various clauses in the 1858 Act for the appointment of part-time and temporary inspectors to create a staff of about thirty. He also managed to recruit the most eminent members of the Victorian scientific élite to work for the department on various investigations and to establish the first government funding for independent scientific research.

Simon did not limit his focus to legislative reform but rather concentrated on the expansion of administrative management. He first expressed his philosophy of medical management in the one area where he had direct responsibility, the vaccination service. On the basis of improved information, he intended to provide a 'better system',

> not indeed removing from the Poor Law Board the formal control over vaccination contracts, but providing, as in aid of the Board, that for all the medical requirements of the case, the medically-advised Lords of the Council should regulate and supervise the service.[15]

Simon believed that the key to medical management was massive documentation of health conditions through social, epidemiological, and scientific research. His administration was a period of Blue Books reporting the results of scientific investigations into the *Necessaries of Health*, which included reports on *Dangerous Industries, Hospitals of the United Kingdom, Accidental and Criminal Poisoning, Dwellings of the Poorer Labouring Classes in Town and Country, Specialised Mortuary Statistics*, and the *Average Annual Proportions of Deaths*.

Simon used the new data to develop a wide range of new legislation. Three new Nuisances Acts between 1855 and 1863 gave local authorities wider powers to enter and inspect both business and domestic premises and to tackle excrement accumulation, street refuse, industrial waste and smoke, polluted rivers, slaughter-houses, and further threats to health. The Sewage Utilization Act 1867 allowed authorities to dispose of sewage outside their boundaries and purchase land for the purpose. The Local Government Act 1858 permitted compulsory purchase for sanitary purposes.

Simon's legislative reforms culminated in the Sanitary Act of 1866. This Act imposed a duty upon local authorities to inspect their districts and remove nuisances. It gave them new powers to provide clean water supplies, to regulate tenements, and to impose penalties for breaking sanitary by-laws. Most importantly, a new 'grammar of common sanitary legislation' extended the coercive power of the central government over local authorities to a hitherto unprecedented degree. Simon admitted using the symbolic value of the 1866 Sanitary Act to stimulate rather than impose action upon local governments. But, a year later, the 1867 Vaccination Act, which greatly enlarged the penalties for failure to vaccinate infants and children, was fully enforced and dramatically opposed. Compulsory infant vaccination aroused minimum opposition when it was first established in 1853. But anti-vaccinationism gathered momentum after 1867, ultimately reducing the strictness of the law by the end of the century. In the 1860s, the grammar of compulsion was also extended to the control of sexually transmitted diseases, and an equally vigorous campaign was launched to repeal The Contagious Diseases Acts. (➤ Ch. 26 Sexually transmitted diseases)

The serious defect of the 1866 Sanitary Act was that it failed to bring together the scattered sanitary legislation developed since 1848. This need became the subject of the Royal Commission on Sanitary Administration set up in 1868 at the request of the joint public-health committee of the British Medical Association and the National Association for the Promotion of Social Science. The Commission's final report led to the great codifying Public Health Act of 1875 and the compulsory appointment of a medical officer of health to every sanitary district in England and Wales. Poor Law and public-health central administration was amalgamated in the Local Government Board under the Local Government Act of 1872. But linking public health to the poor law in a central authority proved disastrous for the influence of medical expertise. Simon resigned his position as Medical Officer to the Local Government Board in 1876, frustrated by the parsimony of its Poor Law Director, John Lambert (1815–92). The mid-Victorian concept of state medicine was eclipsed with Simon's retirement, but the role of the medical expert in government service had been irrevocably established.[16]

George Kitson-Clark described the changing role of civil servants in Victorian government as 'statesmen in disguise'.[17] Simon's career exemplified undisguised use of medical expertise to guide the development of both the creation and implementation of public-health policy. Simon outlined his philosophy of medical statesmanship as an obligation to ensure that the 'physical conditions of existence' were protected by the law. (➤ Ch. 69 Medicine and the law) The latter included sufficient supply of sanitary housing, wholesome unadulterated food and drugs, the control of epidemic diseases, and state regulation of qualified medical practice. Throughout his career, Simon proposed a government ministry of health with its own cabinet minister. Medical statesmanship should guide ministerial decisions toward rational, scientific policy. The arena for medical expertise, however, moved from central to local government in Britain in the last quarter of the century. The compulsory appointment of medical officers of health, first to metropolitan sanitary districts in 1855 and later to provincial districts throughout England and Wales in 1872, created a national service of doctors responsible for the health of the community rather than the treatment of individuals. They were employed by local sanitary authorities to monitor health conditions through inspection and report, and were responsible for the removal of nuisances, the sanitary regulation of overcrowded lodging-houses, offensive trades, building standards, the conditions of bakeries, dairies, and slaughter houses, and prevention of infectious diseases through notification and isolation procedures. Their annual reports are a rich historical source on the 'people's health'. The function of public-health officers was structured by Parliament, but the interpretation of policy was governed by their professional ideology, which they identified as a preventive ideal.

The professional identity of medical officers of health became crucial to the execution of policy by the turn of the century. All were doctors from the time of their optional appointment under the 1848 Public Health Act. The Metropolitan Association of Medical Officer of Health was founded in 1856, followed by numerous provincial groups that were eventually amalgamated into the Society of Medical Officers of Health in 1889, which began a professional journal *Public Health* the same year. But the occupation was stratified between those in full- and part-time service, and provincial and metropolitan districts. This led to intra-professional conflict, and medical officers of health failed to consolidate their position with either their employers, the Local Sanitary Authorities, or their political masters, Parliament and the Local Government Board. Lacking any political force, a caucus of medical officers of health used standards of expertise to enhance occupational security by supporting the regulation of the postgraduate Diploma of Public Health. In the early nineteenth century, public health in Britain was led by social reformers, but from the 1870s it became diffused into the piecemeal development of a national civil service. Social reformers were replaced by professional administrators of the public-health system. The entrenchment of medical officers of health into a civil service gave them the power to demand change and expand their ideological horizons.[18] This became critical at the end of the century, when the value of the entire function of preventive medicine came into question. (➤ Ch. 47 History of the medical profession)

The transition of public health in Victorian Britain from social reform to medical statesmanship, to a professional civil service, was not unique. In Germany, Sweden, and Holland, there were similar patterns of professionalization. Virchow himself became a central political figure in the Reichstag.

The growth of bureaucratic, medical administration of health policy in Europe, however, is completely contrasted with the development of public health in the ruggedly individual, federal democracy of the United States.

VOLUNTARISM, MILITARISM, AND MISSIONARY PUBLIC HEALTH IN THE USA

The Jeffersonian assumption that a healthy democratic state would inevitably result in a healthy population was not borne out by the massive mortality resulting from persistent invasions of yellow fever from 1793. At the outset of the nineteenth century, the new Republic was still predominantly a rural society. There were only thirty-three cities in the United States with populations over 2,500. Conditions in these small towns reflected the agrarian life-style that surrounded them. Town-dwellers kept livestock in their homes; stray pigs, goats, and dogs roamed the streets; horse manure littered unpaved by-ways; garbage, human wastes, and discarded animal carcasses were dumped in the streets and thrown on to undrained vacant land; primitive cesspits served as the most efficient form of sanitation. Under these conditions, subsoils became saturated and polluted, and water supplies from local wells and cisterns became contaminated. Malaria raged almost everywhere except New England; enteric fevers were endemic; and imported yellow fever returned again and again in one epidemic wave after another, becoming almost endemic in southern ports. (➤ Ch. 19 Fevers)

Tiny towns began to grow rapidly in the first half of the century, their populations vastly outgrowing the capacity of their primitive amenities. Rural migration to industrial centres and European immigration swelled the urban settlements, doubling, then quadrupling numbers within decades. As industrialization developed, the prosperous and the poor moved both physically and ideologically further apart. Poverty was no longer viewed as a charitable estate by the wealthy, who blamed the poor for their condition. Paternalism gave way to a rising tide of rugged individualism in which community responsibility was dismissed in favour of individual self-sufficiency. In Jacksonian America, government was kept to a minimum, maintaining law and order so that each person could fend for her- or himself.

The yellow-fever epidemics of the early nineteenth century stimulated the creation of emergency, but temporary, health boards in cities such as Washington and New Orleans. Temporary city health boards did pass ordinances for street-cleaning and nuisance regulation, but had no means of enforcing them. They did not, however, outlast the epidemics and were not revived until cholera replaced yellow fever as the grim reaper of the early 1830s. While most towns were virtually without any health governance during this period, there were some notable exceptions. New York State, for example, set up a permanent quarantine authority, and in 1804 New York City created a permanent health inspector who gathered information and reported nuisances. But both enterprises declined during the first decades of their existence with reduced funding and lack of enthusiasm. The Boston Board of Health was the first elected body created by the General Court in 1798. As a representative body, it was more responsive to the general community and able to resist special business interests in the enforcement of quarantine restrictions.[19]

As towns grew, the water supply became more problematic, especially since without proper sewage and drainage local wells became increasingly polluted. Philadelphia, Madison, New Orleans, Pittsburgh, and St Louis all began to have water piped from distant, clean sources by the 1840s. Often, the early piping systems intermittently failed so that the supply was haphazard. But the need for continuous water supply grew urgent as the burgeoning populations increased the risks of fire and disease.[20]

Amidst this stagnation, the Civil War, paradoxically, galvanized new action. The Civil War cost the lives of 600,000 soldiers, most of whom died from typhoid and dysentery in grossly insanitary encampments. A Civilian Sanitary Commission, created in 1861, headed by New York physician Elisha Harris (1824–84) and the landscape architect Frederick Law Olmstead (1822–1905), reported an appalling lack of fresh food, pitiful levels of medical care for the sick and wounded, and precious few hospital facilities. The Commission distributed fresh fruit and vegetables to all regiments and ensured the regular supply of vital medicines, but more importantly it converted the Army Medical Corps to sanitary reform. Initially faced with total hostility from the medical officers, the Commission shamed the army into cleaning up through its damning reports of encampments turned into cesspits by lack of latrines, and other gross insanitary practices. The army medical corps adopted new hygiene regulations to prevent typhoid and other infectious diseases, and began providing a plentiful supply of fresh vegetables to prevent scurvy. (➤ Ch. 22 Nutritional diseases)

The sanitary reform of the Army had a direct impact on the civilian population when occupying Union troops began to impose new sanitary programmes in southern towns. General Benjamin Butler (1818–93), for example, occupied New Orleans from April 1862 and enforced sanitary regulations in the city with military police. But the chaos of reconstructing a society torn apart by civil war with a rapidly industrializing economy, attracting ever-larger numbers of immigrants from Europe, made it difficult to maintain such programmes. For example, freed slaves became virtually a refugee population and suffered all the massive deprivations that traditionally accompany such social and geographical dislocation. But the sanitary programmes established during the war at least began to institutionalize reforms.

Some individual localities had established sanitary reforms before the war and became prototypes for American public-health development. These civilian reforms were undertaken, not by wartime martial health-law or political parties or factions, but by pious, philanthropic individuals. The ideology of evangelical piety was able effectively to incorporate the principles of sanitary reform without adopting the political radicalism that had motivated European reformers. For example, John H. Griscom (1809–74), an attending physician at the New York Hospital and a founding member of the New York Academy and Medical Society, was the health inspector of New York City who conducted a large-scale survey in 1845 on *The Sanitary Condition of the Labouring Population of New York*. Always interested in the popularization of physiology and hygiene, Griscom, a pious Quaker, believed that it had a spiritual as much as a material message, because morality and the physical world were inherently linked in God's Design of Nature. High mortality resulted from man's neglect of the laws of nature, and following the rules of hygiene was a moral act and a religious duty. The sanitary regeneration of modern life was truly a religious crusade because sanitary degeneration produced moral depravity. Griscom believed that the solution to the problems of lack of sanitation and moral degeneration was to educate the poor into moral and hygienic salvation. He worked with philanthropic organizations such as the New York Tract Society to disseminate the gospel of hygiene to the poor.[21]
(➤ Ch. 63 Medical philanthropy after 1850; Ch. 61 Religion and medicine)

The pious logic of Griscom's philosophy of health reform was reproduced by many notable early health reformers such as Lemuel Shattuck (1793–1859), Griscom's contemporary, who was the pioneer of public health in Massachusetts.[22] The significance of religious moralism for US health reform was reinforced in the American response to cholera. Cholera crossed the Atlantic in 1832, but its effects were far more limited than those of the epidemic that followed in 1848–9 and killed 5,017 in New York City alone. Its greatest impact was in the cities, towns, and landing-spots along the Mississippi, the Arkansas, and the Tennessee after cholera spread like wildfire from New Orleans during the mild southern winter weather.

In the absence of government authorities, voluntary associations of citizens organized refuse removal, street-cleaning, and emergency hospital facilities. Moreover, evangelical volunteers preached hygiene reform to the diseased and their neighbours. In 1849, President Zachary Taylor (1784–1850) ordered a day of fasting as a prophylactic against the epidemic to atone for the vicious appetites that had brought the miserable retribution of cholera upon the land. Amongst moralistic sanitary reformers, sin was believed to be the primary predisposing cause of cholera – intemperance, non-churchgoing, and immorality amongst the reckless, feckless poor. Above all, it was punishment for the sin of materialistic avarice. God-fearing and enterprising industry had turned America into a land of plenty. But enterprise had turned into ambition and material greed. Moralists warned that the exploitation of the South by the northern states, the enslavement of Africans, and the frenzied lust for gold had forced the hand of providential punishment. But if reformers believed sin was the primary cause, they also believed that this gave rise to secondary exciting causes such as filth – next only to vice as the worst of mortal sins – poor drainage, and lack of ventilation. Evangelicals began preaching the gospel of hygiene. Prayer was a necessary but not sufficient remedy: practical measures were also needed.

Responses to cholera reveal contrasting cultures of health reform on either side of the Atlantic. In Britain, and in most of Europe, cholera heightened tensions between social and economic classes and mediated their political values. In the USA, it gave expression to dominant cultures of religious moralism and individualistic voluntarism. Individualistic voluntarism, missionary zeal, and militarism subsequently dominated the development of US health policy. A society that prized self-sufficiency recoiled from paternalistic government, which undermined the sovereignty of individual rights. But, challenged by escalating urban squalor and disease, this predominant ideology was supplemented by moralistic and militaristic sanitary reform.

From the 1870s, individual cities and states began to establish permanent health boards responsible for registration of births and deaths and for instituting emergency measures during epidemics. Before 1900, however, they were still largely powerless, and the chief function of most state boards became, in fact, the licensing of physicians. New reforms came, however, from outside municipal and state administrations, as public health became professionalized through the new standards of expertise and the institutionalization of health administration throughout the national community.

In the early 1900s, public-health reform proved its value for economic imperialistic expansion when the US military eliminated yellow fever amongst its troops occupying Cuba, and again when America beat the French at building the Panama Canal through the aid of mosquito eradication. The lessons learnt in Cuba and Panama stimulated efforts to improve conditions in the southern states. For example, a campaign to eliminate the 'disease of laziness' from the sharecrop community began when the bacteriologist Charles Wardell Stiles (1867–1941), persuaded the Rockefeller Foundation to set up a five-year Sanitary Commission for the eradication of hookworm in 1909.[23]

The actions of the military in Cuba and of the Rockefeller Commission in the southern states strengthened health reformers' demands for a national health agency. A National Board of Health had been set up in 1879, following a yellow-fever epidemic in 1878, but was abolished in 1883 over the issue of the sovereignty of individual states. By 1900, the only federal agency that co-ordinated health activities was the Marine Hospital Service. Originating with the 1789 law that provided hospital facilities for sick sailors, by the 1870s the Marine Hospital Service established a commissioned corps of medical officers, which could be called upon by any city or state health authority at times of health crisis. In 1887, the service set aside a single room in Washington DC to be a hygiene laboratory, which eventually developed into the National Institutes of Health.[24]

By 1902, the Marine Hospital Service was renamed the Public Health and Marine Hospital Service but was governed by the Treasury as much as by its Director, the Surgeon-General. Other government departments had specific health responsibilities. The Interior Department dealt with the hygiene and sanitary conditions of schools. The Census Bureau and the Department of Commerce and Trade dealt with health relating to factories and housing. The War Office dealt with military health and maintained a library, a laboratory, and epidemiological research. In 1906, the Yale economists Irving Fisher (1867–1947) and J. Pease Norton (1871–1952) led a Committee of One Hundred on National Health, which lobbied for the unification of these disparate responsibilities into one government department independent of Treasury control. But their aims were opposed by advocates of States Rights, who had also opposed the Food and Drug legislation in 1906. Ultimately, the administration of Theodore Roosevelt (1858–1919) rejected the proposed department of health in favour of expanding the existing Marine and Public Health Service into the US Public Health Service in 1912, which continued as a sort of federal health salvation army without cabinet representation.[25]

The development of federal agencies increased the pressure to create a professional service of public-health officers, who could work effectively in either a national or local context. Progressive health reformers believed that bacteriology could create a new discipline of scientific disease control. American physicians and scientists who had studied in Berlin popularized bacteriology in the 1880s. This ideal soon influenced leading public-health progressives such as Charles Chapin (1856–1941), who established public-health laboratories in Providence, Rhode Island; Victor C. Vaughan (1851–1929), who created a hygienic laboratory in Michigan; and William Sedgwick (1855–1921), who established bacteriological examination of Massachusetts water supplies at the St Lawrence Experimental Station. (➤ Ch. 8 The biochemical tradition; Ch. 9 The pathological tradition)

Chapin believed that bacteriology completely differentiated the new public health from the old. He suggested municipal engineering should manage sewage and drainage, while medical teams should concentrate on identifying and isolating cases of infection and implementing the latest technologies of immunology. Chapin launched a New Public Health Campaign in 1888 to eliminate diphtheria in Providence through the isolation of all bacteriologically tested victims and healthy carriers of the disease. This was combined with compulsory antitoxin treatment, plus a comprehensive programme of disinfection of victims' dwellings. His hopes for stamping out diphtheria, however, were dashed when he observed that during the period of strictest control the disease was at its height. This led him to drop his programme back to the previous level of voluntary hospitalization and temporary quarantine of siblings. Chapin found that these measures improved the reduction of diphtheria morbidity, and that he no longer had the problem of massive levels of quarantine.[26]

The new public health and the adoption of a bacteriological model of disease prevention, however, dominated the subsequent development of public-health training. The largest and most important school of public health was set up at Johns Hopkins to pursue prestigious research in the biomedical sciences, rather than to train students in practical health administration. The new public health was the model for the future.

BIOLOGY AND HEGEMONY

If bacteriology was the motor force of professionalization of public health in America, in Europe it served only to reinforce a process that had already been underway from the 1870s. In Britain, the major contribution of bacteriology, apart from its practical value in early diagnostic testing and immunological inoculations such as diphtheria antitoxin, was its role in an ideological war between social-Darwinist and environmentalist models of public health. (➤ Ch. 10 The immunological tradition)

In the two decades before the First World War, as imperialism experienced its most expansive historical hour, it was haunted by darkest paranoia. From the late nineteenth century, European intellectuals contemplated the worm in the evolutionary bud that could lead to biological degeneration. Theories of inevitable biological decline were transformed through the work of the English founder of biometrical statistics, Francis Galton (1822–1911), into a creed of eugenics that claimed the only salvation of the 'civilized races' was through selective breeding.

Degenerationism and hereditarian theories of disease gained momentum throughout Europe, the United States, and the colonial world. Eugenists challenged the entire legitimacy of public-health reform, claiming that preventive medicine was saving the weakly with the robust, and raining racial suicide upon imperial breeds. Social amelioration should be abandoned in favour of letting the weak go to the wall and breeding out the sickly, the deformed, the demented, and the undesirable, all of whom were deemed eugenically 'deficient'. Eugenists throughout Europe advocated marriage regulation, sequestration of the mentally deficient, and sterilization, voluntary or compulsory, of the unfit. Britain, France, Sweden, Germany, and their colonial territories, such as Australia and New Zealand, adopted various combinations of these policies. In Britain, some eugenists flirted with the idea of the 'lethal chamber' for ridding society of its unwanted. In Germany, this became a reality during the Second World War. In the United States, eugenic converts achieved the first compulsory-sterilization laws, which were passed in forty-four states and promoted strict immigration laws.[27] (➤ Ch. 20 Constitutional and hereditary disorders; Ch. 37 History of medical ethics)

Britain's humiliations in the Boer War stimulated a debate on 'national efficiency', which eugenists seized as an opportunity to spread the gospel of racial improvement through selective breeding. Environmentalists countered eugenic arguments, however, with wider programmes of preventive medicine. For example, medical officers of health, who considered themselves professionals in preventive medicine, began to include social behaviour as much as the physical environment amongst the determinants of health. In the pre-bacteriological era, the 'sanitary idea' depended upon epidemiological methods to identify the environmental determinants of disease. Edwardian medical officers of health now asserted that bacteriology demonstrated that individual behaviour and habits were crucial to spreading infection. The Chief Medical Officer of the Local Government Board, Arthur Newsholme (1857–1943), stated in 1910 that from the 'social standpoint', public health depended upon changing habits of domestic hygiene, reinforcing public-hygiene education, and identifying groups at risk in terms of both their physiology and sociological characteristics. The solution to 'social efficiency', Newsholme claimed, was the public-health management of all community life. The Edwardian public-health agenda included welfare programmes for pregnant and postnatal mothers, tiny infants, school children, men and women at work, the acutely sick, the chronically infirm, the tubercular, and the aged. (➤ Ch. 44 Childbirth; Ch. 45 Childhood; Ch. 46 Geriatrics) This agenda culminated in public-health officers demanding a comprehensive health system, integrating preventive and therapeutic services, administered by local health authorities and funded by taxation. The British debate about an integrated service continued throughout the years leading up to the Second World War and, eventually, was partially realized in the creation of the National Health Service in 1946–8.[28]

PROVISION OF HEALTH SERVICES AND THE NEW MANAGERIAL ROLE OF PUBLIC HEALTH IN THE TWENTIETH CENTURY

In the twentieth century, questions of health and social-welfare provision changed throughout the world, varying dramatically between industrially developed and underdeveloped countries. Major historical upheavals, such as communist revolutions in eastern Europe, inaugurated entirely new perspectives. The most important response to changing health needs and expectations was the development of an international concern realized in the creation of the World Health Organization. (➤ Ch. 59 Internationalism in medicine and public health) In Western societies, the most important challenge came from an epidemiological transition from infectious to chronic diseases, rising standards of living, and major advances in medical science and technologies. (➤ Ch. 68 Medical technologies: social contexts and consequences) The way in which these factors affected the intricate development of public-health practice can be illustrated by the British experience.

The unification of health services in Britain before the First World War was thwarted by the adoption, in 1911, of the German system of social insurance to fund medical services. Social insurance had been developed by the Bismark administration in the 1880s, but discussion of its adoption throughout Europe is beyond the scope of this chapter. (➤ Ch. 50 Medical institutions and the state) In Britain, health insurance helped to change the role of public health. From the end of the First World War, public-health officers increasingly took on a managerial role, co-ordinating a multiple, and often overlapping, collection of local services, including local-authority hospitals. When medical services were nationalized and funded by taxation under the National Health Service Act, which came into force in 1948, the role of local health authorities was undermined by the introduction of regional organization. (➤ Ch. 57 Health economics)

The epidemiological transition to chronic diseases after the Second World War created interest in new methods of clinical prevention and overshadowed environmental public health. In the post-war years, local health officers found themselves trying to co-ordinate an ever-widening range of community services, from local-authority clinics to social work. By the end of the 1960s, the concept of public health was replaced by the idea of community-service planning. Medical officers of health were replaced in 1974 by 'community physicians'. Community-health planning, however, incurred major conflicts with various factions, especially when the élite clinicians felt their autonomy compromised. Community medicine as a discipline experienced increasing difficulties in defining its constituency, and faced mounting problems of implementation in practice.

In the 1980s the new, lethal pandemic of AIDS revived interest in environmental public health throughout the world. The AIDS epidemic and the mounting health crises of famine, war, and economic underdevelopment stimulated the World Health Organization to make its strongest demand yet for the international community to work for universal 'health for all'.

The most ironic development in public hygiene in Western societies in the late twentieth century, however, is that it has come full circle. The central focus of preventive medicine is now the mass communication of personal health-care advice, urging individuals to take responsibility not only for their vulnerability to chronic disease, such as coronary disease or lung cancer, but also to raise their level of athletic fitness. Equally, the individual is urged to be responsible for the health of others: for example, through the anti-passive-smoking campaign. But the new era of missionary health evangelism, especially successful in the United States where, for example, anti-smoking campaigns have had their greatest impact, owes more to long traditions of personal-health cultures and a new emphasis on clinical prevention than to state medicine.

CONCLUSION

The complex implications of the AIDS epidemic have been discussed elsewhere in this volume (➤ Ch. 26 Sexually Transmitted Diseases), but for all Western and Third World societies it highlights some of the most critical controversies of public-health regulation. The distribution of equal health opportunities required regulation of the behaviour of individuals, governments, and the market-place. Public-health regulation has consistently conflicted with individual interests, from the isolation of lepers in ancient times, through the clash between trade and maritime quarantine in the late Middle Ages, to disputes over compulsory immunization and detention for infectious diseases in the modern period. The enforcement of health by the state has cost the civil liberty of individuals to trade without regard to healthy passage; to indiscriminately contaminate the environment with toxic, industrial effluence; or indeed contract, die of, and indiscriminately spread a number of socially and sexually transmitted diseases. The price paid for what John Simon called the legal protection of the 'physical conditions of existence' has been the curtailment of civil rights. There have been occasions in the history of public health when this price was deemed too high, such as when the Contagious Disease Acts were repealed in Victorian Britain or when compulsory screening and notification of HIV infection has been opposed in many Western societies.

The philosopher Michel Foucault (1926–84) believed that the rise of certain forms of knowledge were inherently disciplinary, geared to new regulatory mechanisms in modern societies. The theories and practices of health regulation pre-date any such modern pretensions and reflect changes in beliefs about religious destiny, the natural world, and scientific determination over a long period of time. The resolution of conflict between regulation and health provision, however, has always been the negotiation of a complex dialectic of knowledge and human interests. (➤ Ch. 70 Medical sociology; Ch. 72 Medicine, mortality, and morbidity)

NOTES

1 Richard John Palmer, 'The control of plague in Venice and Northern Italy 1348–1600', unpublished Ph.D. thesis, University of Kent, 1978.

2 Quoted in George Rosen, *From Medical Police to Social Medicine*, New York, Science History Publications, 1974, p. 163.

3 Nehemiah Grew, *The Meanes of a Most Ample Encrease of the Wealth and Strength of England in a Few Years Humbly Represented to Her Majesties in the Fifth Year of Her Reign*, 1699.

4 Theodore M. Porter, *The Rise of Statistical Thinking 1820–1900*, Princeton, NJ, Princeton University Press, 1986; Lorraine Daston, *The Reasonable Calculus: Classical Probability Theory, 1650–1840*, Princeton, NJ, Princeton University Press, 1988; Stephen M. Stigler, *The History of Statistics: the Measurement of Uncertainty before 1900*, Cambridge, MA, Harvard University Press, 1986.

5 G. M. Young, *Victorian England: Portrait of an Age*, 2nd edn, London, Oxford University Press, 1963, p. 32.

6 L. R. Villermé, 'Rapport fait par M. Villermé, et lu à l'Académie de Médecine, au nom de la Commission de Statistique, sur une série de tableaux relatifs au mouvement de la population dans les douze arrondissements municipaux de la ville de Paris pendant les cinq années 1817, 1818, 1819, 1820, et 1821', Paris, 1826.

7 Quoted by John M. Eyler, *Victorian Social Medicine. The Ideas and Methods of William Farr*, Baltimore, MD, Johns Hopkins University Press, 1979, p. 24.

8 R. J. Morris, *Cholera, 1832: the Social Response to an Epidemic*, London, Croom Helm, 1976.

9 Derek Fraser, *The Evolution of the British Welfare State: the History of Social Policy since the Industrial Revolution*, London, Macmillan, 1973.

10 See T. Southwood Smith, 'Appendix to the Fifth Annual Report of the Poor Law Commissioners', London, HMSO, 1839.

11 Edwin Chadwick, *Report on the Sanitary Conditions of the Labouring Population of Great Britain*, ed. by M. Flinn Edinburgh, Edinburgh University Press, 1965.

12 S. E. Finer, *The Life and Times of Sir Edwin Chadwick*, London, Methuen, 1952.

13 Rudolf Virchow, *Public Health Reports*, ed. by L. J. Rather, 2 vols Maryland, Science History Publications, 1986; K. Figlio and Paul Weindling, 'Was social medicine revolutionary? Rudolf Virchow and the revolutions of 1848', *Society for the Social History of Medicine Bulletin*, 1984, 34: 10–18; E. H. Ackerknecht, *Rudolf Virchow, Doctor, Statesman, Anthropologist*, Madison, University of Wisconsin, 1953.

14 Quoted in Dorothy Porter, 'How soon is now? Public health and the BMJ', *British Medical Journal*, 1990, 301: 738–41.

15 Quoted in Dorothy Porter and Roy Porter, 'The politics of prevention: anti-vaccinationism and public health in nineteenth-century England', *Medical History*, 1988, 32: 231–52.

16 R. Lambert, *John Simon and English Social Administration*, London, MacGibbon & Kee, 1963.

17 G. Kitson Clark, 'Statesmen in disguise: reflections on the history of the neutrality of the Civil Service', *Historical Journal*, 1959, 2: 19–39.

18 Dorothy Porter, 'Stratification and its discontents: professionalization and conflict

in the British public health service, 1848–1914', in E. Fee and Roy M. Acheson (eds), *A History of Education in Public Health*, Oxford, Oxford University Press, 1991, pp. 83–113.

19 John Duffy, *The Sword of Pestilence. The New Orleans Yellow Fever Epidemic of 1853*, Baton Rouge, Louisiana State University Press, 1966; Duffy, *A History of Public Health in New York City 1625–1866*, 2 vols, New York, Russell Sage Foundation, 1968.

20 Letty Anderson, 'Hard choices: supplying water to New England', *Journal of Interdisciplinary History*, 1984, 15: 211–34.

21 Charles Rosenberg and Carol Smith-Rosenberg, 'Pietism and the origins of the American public health movement', *Journal of the History of Medicine and Allied Sciences*, 1968, 23: 6–34.

22 B. G. Rosenkrantz, *Public Health and the State. Changing Views in Massachusetts, 1842–1936*, Cambridge, MA, Harvard University Press, 1972.

23 John Ettling, *The Germ of Laziness: Rockefeller Philanthropy and Public Health in the New South*, Cambridge, MA, Harvard University Press, 1981.

24 Fitzhugh Mullan, *Plagues and Politics. The Story of the United States Public Health Service*, New York, Basic Books, 1989.

25 Alan I. Marcus, 'Disease prevention in America: from a local to a national outlook, 1880–1910', *Bulletin of the History of Medicine*, 1979, 53: 184–203; Manfred Wasserman, 'The quest for a national health department in the Progressive era', *Bulletin of the History of Medicine*, 9: 353–80.

26 James Cassedy, *Charles V. Chapin and the Public Health Movement*, Cambridge, MA, Harvard University Press, 1962.

27 Daniel Kevles, *In the Name of Eugenics. Genetics and the Uses of Human Heredity*, New York, Knopf, 1985.

28 Dorothy Porter, 'Biologism, environmentalism and public health in Edwardian England', *Victorian Studies*, 1991, 34: 159–78.

FURTHER READING

Coleman, William, *Death is a Social Disease. Public Health and Political Economy in Early Industrial France*, Madison, University of Wisconsin Press, 1982.

Duffy, John, *The Sanitarians. A History of American Public Health*, Urbana, University of Illinois Press, 1990.

Evans, R. J., *Death In Hamburg. Society and Politics in the Cholera Years 1830–1910*, Oxford, Clarendon Press, 1987.

Lewis, Jane, *What Price Community Medicine? The Philosophy, Practice and Politics of Public Health since 1919*, Brighton, Sussex, Harvester, 1986.

Porter, Dorothy and Porter, Roy, 'The enforcement of health', in E. Fee and D. Fox (eds), *AIDS: the Burdens of History*, Berkeley, University of California Press, 1988, pp. 96–120.

Riley, James C., *The Eighteenth-Century Campaign to Avoid Disease*, Basingstoke, Macmillan, 1987.

Rosen, George, *A History of Public Health*, New York, MD Publications, 1956.

Rosenberg, C., *The Cholera Years 1832, 1849 and 1866*, Chicago, IL, University of Chicago Press, 1962.

Slack, Paul, *The Impact of Plague in Tudor and Stuart England*, London, Routledge & Kegan Paul, 1985.

Smith, F. B., *The People's Health 1830–1910*, London, Croom Helm, 1979.

Webster, Charles, *Problems of Health Care, The National Health Service before 1957*, London, HMSO, 1988.

Wohl, Anthony S., *Endangered Lives: Public Health in Victorian Britain*, London, Dent, and Cambridge, MA, Harvard University Press, 1983.

52

EPIDEMIOLOGY

Lise Wilkinson

INTRODUCTION

Epidemiology suggests etymologically a science of something falling upon the people, and statistics suggests the study of states; as originally used the word statistics had no necessary connection with arithmetic. Epidemiology came to mean the study of disease, any disease, as a mass phenomenon.[1]

Thus wrote Major Greenwood (1880–1949), first Professor of Epidemiology and Vital Statistics at the London School of Hygiene and Tropical Medicine (LSHTM), and one of the founders of the modern approach to epidemiology. Although the word 'epidemic' can be traced back to the texts of classical Greece, 'epidemiology' as a term, as a concept, and as a recognized discipline of medical science has existed for little more than 150 years. It was only in the second quarter of the nineteenth century that the work of the 'sanitary physicians', searching for aetiologies in prevailing outbreaks of cholera, typhoid, typhus, and smallpox, and the ever-present threat of tuberculosis, began to be seen in its social context. The foundation of the London Epidemiological Society in 1850 set the seal on the arrival of the concept of epidemiology as an integral part of burgeoning medical science and public-health movements.

Greenwood's historical perspective tended to focus on the interrelationship between epidemiology and statistical science, and on the people who first introduced, and the ones who later perfected, statistical methods. Yet he yielded to none in his admiration for the observations and conclusions on epidemic situations contained in the Hippocratic writings, produced two millennia before a system of vital statistics and statistical methods became available.

EPIDEMICS IN ANTIQUITY

Three books in the Hippocratic Corpus are of particular relevance in attempts to look for sources for early epidemiology: the first and third books of *Epidemics*; and the treatise *On Airs, Waters, Places*. Here may be found attempts to determine the influence of external and environmental factors on the patterns of distribution of endemic and epidemic diseases which form the essence of epidemiology. In the absence of a statistical framework, the factors discussed in these writings as important variables in different communities are climate, prevailing winds, water supply and soil, geographic location, and the habits and life-styles of the populations in question. Having become familiar with all these circumstances, a physician arriving in a previously unknown place '. . . would not be at a loss to treat the diseases' of local inhabitants; and with time and change of seasons, '. . . would know what epidemics to expect, both in the summer and in the winter, and what particular disadvantages threatened an individual who changed his mode of life'.[2] Such was the writer's confidence in his text, and in his readers. (➤ Ch. 18 Ecology of disease)

More than five centuries after the death of Hippocrates in the fourth century BC, Galen (AD 129–*c*.200/210) also considered an epidemic constitution of the surrounding air the most important factor in the initiation of epidemics. The influence of the atmosphere would vary with climate and season, and would also depend on the presence or absence of miasmas, which, in turn, were due to filth, putrefaction, swampy conditions, and sometimes astronomical phenomena. In discussing the characteristics of different fevers, Galen also introduced the idea of 'seeds' of disease carried by the air.[3] (➤ Ch. 15 Environment and miasmata; Ch. 19 Fevers)

The Hippocratic approach to the problem of epidemics was essentially that of a theoretician looking for causes, whereas Galen, ever the clinician and observer, favoured a more practical approach. It is in the Old Testament that one finds more specific guidelines for control of outbreaks of communicable disease. The Book of Leviticus contains three chapters of directions aimed specifically at preventing the spread of 'leprosy' by isolating 'unclean' sufferers, requiring them to cleanse themselves and their clothes and belongings, and imposing a period of quarantine followed by inspection to determine their 'clean' or 'unclean' state. The biblical sense of 'leprosy' is not clear, but it was almost certainly not identical with today's definition of the disease, and probably covered more than one ailment: herpes, syphilis, and gonorrhoea have been suggested.

Nothing essential was added to the basic epidemiology of antiquity for more than a thousand years. The importance of empirically devised isolation procedures and quarantine arrangements was emphasized also in treatises on epizootics among domestic animals, although the veterinary practitioner had a last resort not available to his colleagues in human medicine: disposal of infected individuals, and hence of the source of infection, by slaughter, and burning or deep burial of carcasses.

THE MIDDLE AGES

In these classical writings are represented all the putative causes that were to dominate epidemiological thinking and perception until rational scientific experiments of a different order became possible in the nineteenth century. During subsequent centuries, throughout the Middle Ages, different authors placed different emphases on the relative parts played in the causation of epidemics by atmospheric factors, miasmas, and contagion, as well as individual susceptibility. In addition, especially during the Dark Ages, there were frequent returns to pre-classical mystical thinking and practices, increasingly clothed in Christian respectability.

Nowhere are these concepts set out with greater clarity than in the plague tractates, the numerous treatises written during and after the Great Plague of 1348–50. Variously described as 'the greatest single calamity ever visited upon the human race', a catastrophe 'marking the real close of the mediaeval period and the beginning of the modern age', and the 'Great Teacher', the Black Death was certainly all of those. Above all, it taught and impressed on the minds of lay and medical writers alike the lesson of contagion, and the value of isolation and quarantine. For more than three centuries after 1350, bubonic plague, singly or accompanied by pneumonic plague and other more immediately transmissible diseases, continued to create havoc in Europe. Smallpox, measles, influenza, diphtheria, dysentery, and cholera all took their toll. Through it all, the principle of contagiousness became firmly established in the lay and professional minds alike. Quarantine stations became a permanent feature of major Mediterranean ports, and the Venetian Republic, which had early assumed a leading role in public-health legislation and maritime sanitation, had the first such station in 1403; ninety years later, the Venetians went so far as to fumigate letters and to wash money received from infected areas.[4] (➤ Ch. 16 Contagion/germ theory/specificity)

FROM THE SIXTEENTH TO THE EIGHTEENTH CENTURY

In the mid-sixteenth century, Girolamo Fracastoro (1478–1553) firmly dismissed the ideas of humoral imbalance as the cause of pestilential fevers. (➤ Ch. 14 Humoralism) Healthy persons, he wrote, 'whose humours have suffered no depravity, nevertheless catch the contagion from merely associating with the plague-stricken or from his clothes', concluding that 'The principles of contagion *per se* are the germs themselves.'[5] Fracastoro's use of the term 'germs' (*seminaria*) has caused writers inclined to Whiggish interpretation to claim for him a brilliant preconception of later principles of bacteriology; but it is clear from careful reading of the text that Winslow accurately assessed his contribution when he wrote that Fracastoro 'worked out a clear and essentially accurate analysis of the way in which living "germs" operate, without ever suspecting that they were living'.[6] To the sixteenth-century mind of Fracastoro, epidemics spread by means of 'germs' transmitted from person to person either by direct contact, or by fomes, or through the air over a distance. Particularly severe and widespread epidemics could be explained only by invoking unusual astrological phenomena and unfavourable conditions on Earth and in its surrounding atmosphere.

During the seventeenth and eighteenth centuries, there were a number of very different developments that were to influence the study of epidemics. One with far-reaching consequences in the future was the introduction of a system of statistical treatment of such records of births and deaths, and specifically infant and disease mortality, as were then available, by John Graunt (1620–74). Graunt was a self-made statistician and early member (on the insistence of Charles II) of the Royal Society with no formal training in either medicine or science; there have been later disputes among historians as to the extent of the influence of Sir William Petty (1623–87) on his writings. Graunt's *Natural and Political Observations* were first published in 1662, a remarkable first analysis of the Bills of Mortality, which had been appearing as records of burials and christenings at regular weekly intervals since 1603. Graunt was concerned with ratios of the sexes at death and at birth; from numerical regularities of death and of births, he progressed to determining the proportion of deaths from certain causes to all deaths in successive years and in different areas. W. F. Wilcox has called his achievement the determination 'in general terms, [of] the uniformity and predictability of many important biological phenomena taken in the mass'.[7] Graunt's theory and methods were largely ignored by his medical contemporaries, although put to good use by exponents of exact science: Edmond Halley (1656–1742) at home; and abroad by Abraham de Moivre (1667–1754), author of *Doctrine of Chances* (1716) and *Annuities upon Lives* (1724), and by Jean (1710–90) and Daniel (1700–82) Bernoulli.

Graunt's work was certainly ignored by Thomas Sydenham (1624–89); it had no place in his doctrine of epidemic constitutions. Sydenham and his French predecessor, Guillaume de Baillou (1538–1616), built on Hippocratic foundations to justify their belief in cosmic influences as determinants in the causation and spread of epidemics. Explaining the effects of epidemic constitutions, Sydenham warned his readers 'that diseases ... more especially the continued fevers, differ from one another like north and south, and that the remedy which would cure a patient at the beginning of a year, will kill him perhaps at the close'; and 'There are different constitutions in different years. They originate neither in their heat nor their cold, their wet nor their drought; but they depend upon certain hidden and inexplicable changes within the bowels of the earth.'[8] John Freind (1675–1728) pointed out that Sydenham did not necessarily practise what he preached, but tended to treat continued fevers in identical ways, regardless of the prevailing 'epidemic constitution'.

Progress in epidemiology in a different context, in a different corner of Europe, was made in the closing years of the seventeenth century, and the early decades of the eighteenth century. Initially, it owed little to statistics; it owed everything to the social context of medicine, and was later to be known as occupational medicine. First published at Modena in 1700, the pioneering treatise of Bernardino Ramazzini (1633–1714) bore the title of *Diseases of Workers*. It chronicled a wide variety of cases of disease that could reasonably be assumed to have been caused by the patient's occupation. The forty-one initial categories – another twelve were added later in a supplement – ranged from miners of metals, chemists, potters, and oil-pressers (and 'other workers at dirty trades'), to athletes, farmers, sailors, and curiously, 'Jews'. A separate tract dealt with 'diseases of learned men'. It formed a comprehensive introduction to a subject previously available only as specific advice to selected groups, especially miners and workers exposed to metal fumes. Concerned with individual professions rather than incidence and patterns of particular diseases, Ramazzini's work was a timely warning. It established in the minds of patients and doctors the need for caution in handling materials and situations, and the possibility of prevention by elimination of avoidable causes.

Ramazzini had earlier been occupied with more conventional, indeed Hippocratic, epidemiology. In the 1690s, he had recorded current epidemics in the northern Italian provinces where he lived and taught, looking for causes in prevailing winds and climate, and in the plant diseases attacking cereals and other crops. Towards the end of his life, ten years after the appearance of *Diseases of Workers*, circumstances forced Ramazzini to become involved in a different kind of epidemiological battle. The protagonist this time, of notable influence in developing epidemiology in the early eighteenth century, was not an epidemic in humans at all, but an epizootic decimating cattle in Italy and eventually throughout Europe. Waves of the viral infection rinderpest, specific to horned animals and commonly known as cattle plague, had for centuries periodically invaded Europe from the east, often with cattle transports through Dalmatia. The outbreak that began in northern Italy in 1711 and which spread eventually to all Europe, provided salutary lessons in patterns of spread of contagion and in the value of case tracing; however, the initial working theory, that the entire epidemic derived from the introduction of one sick individual among a herd introduced from Dalmatia, seems in retrospect open to question.[9] In certain areas, notably the Netherlands, the disease became endemic; it was periodically reintroduced elsewhere from such areas until the end of the century. The alarm with which the initial Italian outbreak was perceived was reflected in the choice of two highly respected physicians of the period to attempt to control it: Ramazzini in the Venetian territories, and Giovanni Lancisi (1654–1720) in Clement XI's Papal States.

The resulting treatises emphasize the necessity for cool and ruthless measures in the face of natural disasters on such a scale. Quarantine, isolation of infected herds, slaughter and enforced restrictions on the movement of animals became the order of the day, and effectively ended the outbreak in the Italian states concerned. Given the positions of Ramazzini and of Lancisi as leading authors and thinkers on medical matters, and the obvious contagious nature of the disease, the outbreak also gave impetus to contemporary speculation concerning the nature of contagious agents. Ramazzini now had little difficulty in accepting ideas of multiplying 'seeds' of disease in the Fracastorian sense as explanation for the spread of epidemics and epizootics. When Lancisi wrote his own account in 1715, the year after Ramazzini's death, he could draw on his experiences in Rome, and could discuss other literature that had appeared in the meantime. By 1715, a framework was in place for discussion of the question which was to be a subject of lively debate for the next century and a half: were contagious and infectious diseases caused by invisible living organisms, or by inanimate entities of a 'poisonous' nature? Lancisi was to return to the problem in a tract on swamp fevers two years later.

The overwhelming problems of destructive outbreaks of cattle diseases in Europe, which continued throughout the eighteenth century, were matched in human medicine by the disasters caused by smallpox. In the second decade of the century, the method of inoculation, as practised in the Near and Middle East, was brought to the attention of the Royal Society of London and the medical profession by the works of Emmanuel Timoni (fl. 1714) and of Giacomo Pylarini (1659–1718), and by the personal efforts of Lady Mary Wortley Montagu (1689–1762) and the Princess of Wales. It was not long before attempts were made to evaluate the new method by mathematical means.

In 1722, Thomas Nettleton (1683–1742), Halifax physician and friend of Daniel Defoe, reported to the Royal Society his own calculations of ratios of mortality to morbidity in natural and in inoculated smallpox in a number of towns and communities in his district. The then Secretary of the Society,

James Jurin (1684–1750), extended Nettleton's studies, and the title of his first paper on the subject, read to the Society in January 1723, summed up his own and Nettleton's earlier results: 'To give a plain Proof from Experience and Matters of Fact that the Small Pox procured by Inoculation (even by the Accounts of those who oppose that Practice) is far less Dangerous than the same Distemper has been for many years in the Natural Way.'[10] On their own terms, however primitive by later standards, the studies of Nettleton and of Jurin were pointers to later methods of statistical evaluation of immunizing procedures.

In the second half of the eighteenth century, there was renewed interest in the London Bills of Mortality. In his *Observations* in 1662, Graunt had explained their origins as a result of the plague epidemics of the time: 'the rise of keeping these Accompts, was taken from the *Plague*: for the said *Bills* (for ought appears) first began in the said year 1592 being a time of great *Mortality*; And after some disuse, were resumed again in the year 1603, after the great *Plague* then happening likewise.' From 1603 onwards, the Bills were printed and published weekly, and gradually included more and more diseases. By 1632, the recorded 'Diseases and Casualties' numbered a total of sixty-three, and included in addition to plague, smallpox, and measles such varied causes of death as 'Aged', 'Stillborn', 'Consumption', 'French Pox', 'Scurvy', 'Teeth', 'Vomiting', and 'Worms'. Nearly a century after Graunt's pioneering work, Thomas Short (c.1690–1772) published *New Observations on the Bills of Mortality* in 1750. Others took up the call for more-complete mortality returns, both in London and elsewhere. With the work of John Haygarth (1740–1827) on the Bills of Mortality for Chester in 1773 began the practice of comparing different specific diseases on the basis of their respective mortality figures. His remarks on the awesome effects of consumption on members of a population 'in their most vigorous perfection'[11] were to echo ominously through tuberculosis statistics in the following century. (➤ Ch. 71 Demography and medicine)

At the same time, in France, observations were made which began gradually to open up a growing and increasingly important part of the diseases of workers defined by Ramazzini: industrial medicine, in the industrialized nations of Europe. In 1769 appeared a work on anthrax which described in detail an outbreak among textile workers in factories at Montpellier producing woollen blankets. The author, one Jean Fournier (*fl.* 1742–81), was a practising physician and medical officer in the Duchy of Burgundy. He wrote on a number of diseases occurring in epidemic form in animals and in humans at the time. In the case of anthrax, he warned against transmission both by ingestion of contaminated meat offered cheaply by unscrupulous shepherds and butchers and, in the blanket factories, by handling of wool from infected animals. A hundred years later, the latter form became known as 'woolsorters' disease' in the industrial north of England.

The literature of the latter half of the eighteenth century reflects the growth of European nations, especially France and Britain, as colonial powers. There is a notable preoccupation with patterns of 'fever' abroad, and their relative impact on Europeans, as compared with native inhabitants, in far-flung outposts of empires, and exotic climates. The adverse effects of living under stressful conditions in foreign latitudes and confined spaces forced those responsible for the health of both civilians and the armed forces to confront the problems with what Bynum has called an 'enlarged geographical sensitivity'. The epidemiology of 'fevers', vaguely defined though they might be, became an integral part of a larger canvas and took their place alongside epidemics of more definitive disease entities such as smallpox and cholera. (➤ Ch. 58 Medicine and colonialism)

THE NINETEENTH CENTURY

By the end of the eighteenth century, a number of strands, old and new, were beginning to emerge which were eventually to provide a radical influence on the shaping and understanding of the study of crowd diseases. Above all, mathematicians were becoming aware of the possibilities inherent in the calculus of probability. Ten years into the nineteenth century, Pierre-Simon Laplace (1749–1827), French astronomer and mathematician, published a treatise on the analytical theory of probabilities, and suggested that such analysis could be a valuable tool to solve medical problems. In the following decades, his ideas were discussed in the Paris academies of science and of medicine. The combination of progress in mathematical methodology with the developing public-health and sanitary legislation initiated during the years of the Revolution, gave France an advantage over its European neighbours during the first half of the nineteenth century. The French physician who first adopted the use of mathematical methods in quantitative analysis of patients and aspects of their diseases was Pierre Charles-Alexandre Louis (1787–1872). His seminal use of *la méthode numérique* in his classic study of tuberculosis influenced a whole generation of students, and their students in turn, who became leaders in a new epidemiological science firmly rooted in statistical method. In Louis's recommendations for evaluation of different methods of treatment can be found the seeds of clinical (even randomized clinical) trials developed a century later. (➤ Ch. 11 Clinical research) In defending his numerical method against his critics in 1835, Louis stressed the import-ance of comparisons of sufficient numbers of patients: if, in an epidemic situation, one could subject 500 patients, picked at random, to one kind of treatment, and 500 others to a different one, then surely a significant result could be deduced from the relative mortality figures. He told his critics: 'It is precisely because of the impossibility of judging each individual case with any sort of mathematical accuracy that it is necessary to count.'[12]

Louis's contemporary, Louis René Villermé (1782–1863), gave up clinical practice after having followed Napoleon's armies in all the European campaigns, and turned to the application of statistics to problems in public health. In 1826, he used Parisian mortality statistics in a pioneering essay on the relation between poverty and disease. In 1840, he had turned his attention to the deplorable conditions endured by workers in the French silk industry, many of whom were children. His exposure of the iniquities of the system of labour in the factories, and its influence on patterns of disease, led to legislation restricting child labour in the following year. In his application of vital statistics to sociological problems, he was joined by his younger friend Adolphe Quetelet (1796–1874), who explored the relations between the theory of probabilities and the 'sciences morales et sociales'. (➤ Ch. 51 Public health)

From Fournier to Villermé, the concern with the effects of poverty and poor working conditions on the health of the people, in general and as reflected in vital statistics, had been given expression in France before, during, and after the Revolution for more than fifty years before comparable social documents began to appear elsewhere in Europe. When the young Rudolf Virchow (1821–1902) gave vent to his feelings in comments on his experiences during the devastating epidemic of typhus fever among poor weavers in Upper Silesia in 1848, his call for public-health measures and financial assistance for the stricken workers was accompanied by political sentiments unacceptable to the Prussian government. In that year of revolution, Virchow lost his job and left for Würzburg. Seven years later, he was back in triumph, with an institute of his own, and a lasting commitment to the politics of democracy as well as to the rapidly developing medical science in nineteenth-century Europe.

Thus during the 1840s, epidemiology in France and in Germany was becoming inextricably linked to public-health campaigns with a distinctly political flavour, at a time of political upheaval. Much further north, in a political backwater, epidemiology was fortuitously presented with an opportunity for unique observations of the pattern of spread of a contagious disease under naturally controlled conditions. At the beginning of April 1846, a cabinet-maker from Copenhagen arrived in the remote Faroe Islands, in apparently good health; a few days later, he went down with an attack of measles. Through his friends and other contacts, the disease spread; within weeks it involved all communities in the islands. Peter Ludwig Panum (1820–85) was sent by the Danish government to investigate. In a model study, relying on observation, case-tracing, and simple analysis of data, Panum's material consisted of a constant population, contained in a restricted area, of just over 6,600 inhabitants. Of these, 98 survivors from a previous epidemic in 1781 were immune; 1,500 individuals were protected by effective quarantine arrangements; of the remaining *c.*5,000 inhabitants, 99.5 per cent, according to Panum's calculations, caught measles. Significant relative mortality values were notoriously difficult to obtain, and Panum handled the available statistical material with appropriate caution. Summing up towards the end of the decade which had begun with F. G. J. Henle the essay by (1809–85) on miasmas and contagia, Panum came down heavily in favour of the concept of contagiousness as opposed to the theory of miasmas, and of the consequent importance of quarantine regulations. His study of an isolated island community, he concluded, could well serve as an example to provide some insight into the 'possible power of epidemics to decimate populations'.[13]

The growing perception of crowd diseases as directly related to social conditions, to poverty, and to squalor and long hours in the workplace, was also coming to the fore in Britain in mid-century. Following the first official census-taking in the United Kingdom in 1801, the office of Registrar-General of Births, Deaths and Marriages in England had been established in 1837; William Farr (1807–83) became its first Compiler of Abstracts two years later. Already in the second *Annual Report*, published in 1840, Farr declared his intention of defining laws governing the course of epidemics, and began his attempt by charting the rise and subsequent decline of mortality in the recent smallpox epidemic of 1838–9. He wrote:

> *Laws of Epidemics.* – Epidemics appear to be generated at intervals in unhealthy places, spread, go through a regular course, and decline; but of the cause of their evolutions no more is known than of the periodical paroxysms of ague. The body, in its diseases as well as its functions, observes a principle of periodicity; its elements pass through prescribed cycles of changes, and the diseases of nations are subject to similar variations.[14]

Farr's declaration of intent was accompanied by series of mortality numbers, and calculations of rates of acceleration and deceleration of deaths in the epidemic. His terse conclusion was that 'The small-pox would be disturbed, and sometimes arrested, by vaccination, which protected a part of the population, and by inoculation, which there is reason to believe led to the extension of the epidemic by diffusing the infection artificially.'[15] At this stage, in 1840, Farr was aware of Henle's arguments for contagion and its 'close analogy with fermentation'; in the absence of proof, he was not ready to accept the 'infusorial hypothesis' of the action of animalcules. Almost three decades, and twenty-eight *Annual Reports*, later, Farr by the end of the 1860s had accepted the evidence that had accumulated in the meantime. He now believed that the spread of epidemics required a dual explanation, and that to prevent spread, both factors must be controlled.

> The primary object to aim at, is placing a healthy stock of men in conditions of air, water, warmth, food, dwelling, and work most favourable to their development. The vigour of their own life is the best security men have against the invasion of their organisation by low corpuscular forms of life.[16]

During the severe outbreak of cattle plague imported with transports from Russian ports in 1865–6, Farr saw an opportunity to test the accuracy of his 'laws governing the course of an epidemic'. His prediction for the course and eventual decline of the epizootic proved, if not perfect, at least reasonably close to the observed facts.[17]

When at last he accepted the idea of contagion as a factor in the spread of epidemics, Farr referred to the work of his contemporary, William Budd (1811–80). Like Farr, Budd had studied in Paris and had been influenced by Louis, whose authority he acknowledged. A promising career in London, on the Seamen's Hospital Society's ship *Dreadnought*, was cut short by a near-fatal attack of typhoid fever, and Budd retired to hospital practice and teaching in Bristol. From there, he published a number of papers on epidemiology, especially of anthrax in humans, until then ignored in Britain, and of typhoid fever, which had so nearly killed him in London. He agreed with Louis that it was a contagious disease, and added the opinion that it could be transmitted by means of contaminated water. Earlier, he had made a study of cholera, published in the same year as the first paper by John Snow (1813–58) on the subject. There were never priority disputes between Farr, Budd, and Snow; there was a concerted effort to master the epidemiological problems of typhoid fever and cholera, and to devise effective means of preventing future outbreaks. Their individual approaches to epidemiology were all different: Farr was the medical statistician *par excellence*; Budd was among the few authors in Britain at that time whose interest was focused on the role of contagious agents; Snow, wholly committed to the study of transmission patterns of cholera by contaminated water in specific instances, used much material from Farr's reports to prove the danger of polluted Thames water supplied by private companies in the cholera outbreaks in London in 1848–9 and 1854. The implication of the Broad Street Pump in the London outbreak of 1854, and the control achieved by the simple expedient of removing the pump handle, has perhaps become better known than other equally important aspects of Snow's work on epidemiology and natural water filtration.[18] (➤ Ch. 27 Diseases of civilization; Ch. 53 History of personal hygiene)

The dilemmas of differing interpretations and their corollaries facing epidemiologists in the mid-nineteenth century are well illustrated by the controversy between Snow and his colleague, John Sutherland (1808–91), who analysed an outbreak of cholera in Manchester in 1849. Snow did not quarrel with Sutherland's statistical treatment; he did criticize the simplicity of his interpretation. For Sutherland was interested only in immediate practical results: if provision of clean water eliminated the risk of cholera, then there was no need for further discussion of the relative merits of miasmatic theories as opposed to theories of transmission by contaminated water.[19]

In 1850, epidemiology came of age in London with a society of its own. Its conceptual origins were obvious from the name first proposed: 'The Asiatic Cholera Society', reflecting the growing threat of the disease (main outbreaks 1832, 1848, 1854, and 1866). By the time of the first meeting, the name had become the more general 'Epidemiological Society'. The new society's manifesto made clear its aims to integrate all aspects of observation, investigation, and prevention of epidemic diseases. The five committees initially formed to pursue these intentions represent the topics then most in need of immediate study:

1 the Committee on Small Pox and Vaccination;
2 the Epizootic Committee;
3 the Cholera Committee;
4 the Hospitals Committee;
5 the Continued Fevers Committee.[20]

Snow was among the founder members of the Epidemiological Society. So were the two men in the forefront of the public-health movement in Britain in the nineteenth century: Edwin Chadwick (1800–90), whose works on Poor Law reform and on the health of the labouring poor were published in the 1830s and 1840s; and John Simon (1816–1904), the first Medical Officer of Health to the City of London and author of *English Sanitary Institutions* (1890). Also among the early membership was Snow's friend Benjamin Ward Richardson (1828–96), who founded the short-lived *Journal of Public Health and Sanitary Review* in 1855.

Farr, on the other hand, appears to have concentrated his efforts and channelled his influence through another London society founded sixteen years before the emergence of the Epidemiological Society: the Statistical Society, later the Royal Statistical Society. With a membership that included both Chadwick and Farr, and William Augustus Guy (1800–85), this society, over the years, placed an increasing emphasis on vital and medical statistics. Guy, who also acknowledged the influence of Louis, used statistics primarily as a tool in determining the influence of occupation and life-style on general health, and on susceptibility to specific diseases, especially tuberculosis. Between them, the two societies wielded considerable influence on epidemiological studies, with emphasis on statistical analysis, in the middle years of the nineteenth century.

During the Epidemiological Society's second decade, it became increasingly obvious that reliance on statistical analysis was not in itself a sufficient basis for epidemiological methodology. Other factors must be taken into consideration: above all, the possible existence of particulate, living, microscopic agents both causing initial cases and also acting as means of spread of transmissible disease. All but definitive proof of the causative role of 'bacteridia' in the aetiology of anthrax was delivered by Casimir Davaine (1812–82) in France in the 1860s; by the later 1870s, Robert Koch (1843–1910) had perfected the methodology and delivered unequivocal proof, and Louis Pasteur (1822–95) was developing a vaccine. Farr's reference to 'zymotic principles' and 'low corpuscular forms of life . . . propagating matters of zymotic diseases', and to their possible control by vaccination, in his thirtieth *Annual Report* in 1868, shows him on the way to acceptance of the germ theory.

In the last decades before the methods developed by Pasteur and by Koch, and the ensuing discoveries, forced general acceptance of the germ theory by all but a handful of die-hards, a few instances of imported yellow fever caused confusion among European epidemiologists. A mosquito-borne virus disease of complex aetiology, its behaviour in separate outbreaks in Gibraltar (1828), at Saint Nazaire (1861), and at Swansea (1865) proved hard to explain. The appearance of the disease in European ports was linked to the arrival and docking of ships from Cuba. At Gibraltar and Saint Nazaire, their cargoes were sugar; at Swansea, copper ore. All three outbreaks were studied at the time by competent investigators whose reports were models of case-tracing; but in the absence of knowledge of the true nature of the disease, they could contribute nothing to a deeper understanding. The investigations concluded that yellow fever was an imported disease, and that consequently it must be controlled at any port of entry, albeit without seriously interrupting international trade routes, so crucial to the socio-economic ethos of the times. It was the same regard for the vested interests of nineteenth-century commerce that worked against acceptance of the logic of quarantine in the politics of all the major powers. Emphasis remained, for the time being, on careful case-tracing and assessment of local environmental factors.[21]

The accelerating development of a final, scientifically based, germ theory was soon to change the overall approach to epidemiology. From 1880 onwards, the factual search for bacteria, and later for filterable viruses, replaced theoretical arguments for and against contagia and miasma. Epidemiology entered its second major phase, when morbidity and mortality statistics could be related not just to specific infectious diseases, but to specific diseases caused by specific identifiable agents. Another whole dimension was added by the possibility of developing vaccines that might prevent such diseases. Pasteur successfully demonstrated the protective action of a vaccine against anthrax in 1881; by 1886, he had also developed a post-exposure prophylactic treatment for rabies. The evaluation of vaccines against diseases already of great epidemiological complexity also called for the use of statistics. However, early euphoria and hopes for speedy control of any infectious disease once its agent was known were soon dashed – Koch's tuberculin was a case in point. The alternatives of vaccine development and distribution, and improved public-health measures, were to prove ultimately successful, but only on an extended time-scale.

If the emergence of bacteriology on a broad scientific basis changed the complexion of epidemiology from the late nineteenth century onwards, it did so in parallel with developments and increasing sophistication in medical statistics. Before the turn of the century, Karl Pearson (1857–1936), building on the work of Francis Galton (1822–1911), and on Quetelet's earlier theory of probabilities, consolidated the discipline of biometrics, the branch of statistics concerned with biological variation and inheritance. A barrister by profession, Pearson's grasp of higher mathematics as applied to statistics, their graphic interpretation, and the significance of correlations, opened the way to the use of vital and medical statistics in new interpretations of problems of wider social significance in the twentieth century.[22]

THE TWENTIETH CENTURY

The first attempts to marry the higher mathematics of statistical theory to emerging concepts of bacterial infectivity were made in the first decade of the twentieth century. Three very different quantitative problems were studied by three different authors: William Heaton Hamer (1862–1936) proposed a discrete time model in an attempt to explain the regular occurrence of measles epidemics; John Brownlee (1868–1927), first Director of the Medical Research Council, wrestled, not entirely successfully, for twenty years with problems of quantification of epidemiological 'infectivity'; and Ronald Ross (1857–1932) explored the mathematical application of the theory of probabilities, and his own 'theory of happenings', in attempts to determine the relationships between numbers of mosquitoes and incidence of malaria in endemic and epidemic situations.[23] (➤ Ch. 24 Tropical diseases)

Nevertheless, acceptance of the value of statistics in medical science was to prove a slow process. In the words of Lancelot Hogben (1895–1975), Pearson was 'a fine logician', but he was also blinkered by an obsession with logic and pure mathematics to an extent that made him a 'poor naturalist with little patience for good clinical judgement'.[24] The eventual successful application of Pearson's coldly efficient biometrics to clinical and to wider social problems came about through the humanizing influence of his pupil Major Greenwood.

It was, in the first instance, the work of Greenwood that to the medical world made statistics an acceptable and integral part of a new, broadly based, twentieth-century epidemiology. A reluctant physician with a penchant for history, Greenwood escaped from the family tradition of general practice in east London through association with the physiologist Sir Leonard Hill (1866–1952) and with Karl Pearson. The combination of training in experimental science in Hill's physiology department at the London Hospital, and the lessons learned in the hard school of Pearson's 'idolatry of measurement as an end in itself', made Greenwood the ideal choice for the new position of professional statistician at the Lister Institute in 1910. Here there was immediate scope for statistical treatment of the data from the Institute's plague investigations in India, and also of infant mortality rates and mortality rates in pulmonary tuberculosis. Among this early work in medical statistics was also a pointer to work later to be developed at the London School of Hygiene and Tropical Medicine (LSHTM): papers on statistical treatment and interpretation of mortality rates in possibly non-infectious, chronic diseases such as cancer. (➤ Ch. 72 Medicine, mortality, and morbidity; Ch. 25 Cancer)

During the First World War, concern for the health of workers in the munitions industry – inspired, it must be said, partly by the necessity to boost their efficiency – initiated the modern approach to the epidemiology of occupational health. As a first step, the Health of Munition Workers Committee (HMWC) was established by the government, its role to advise on questions of industrial fatigue, hours of work, suitable diets, etc. Leonard Hill, an early recruit to the Medical Research Committee, which in 1920 became the Medical Research Council (MRC), was also a member of the HMWC, and, through him, Greenwood joined its research team. From 1918, the committee's research work was taken over by the Industrial Fatigue Research Board (IFRB). By then, Greenwood was working for the Health and Welfare Section of the Ministry of Munitions. When a new Ministry of Health was created after the war, Greenwood became its first senior Statistical Officer. Vital statistics with medical, epidemiological statistics had arrived at government level. The Ministry of Health was created just before the Athlone Committee reported on postgraduate medical education in 1921. Both these events were factors in the wider influences, above all the intervention of the International Health Board of the Rockefeller Foundation, which led to the transformation, between 1923 and 1929, of the London School of Tropical Medicine into the LSHTM, and thus gave London a school of public health of international standing, to complement the Johns Hopkins School of Hygiene and Public Health in the United States.

After five years of planning and building, the LSHTM opened officially in 1929; and it was here that the ultimate stage of epidemiological science consolidated its twentieth-century concern with diseases beyond the obvious infectious ones, now rapidly coming under control. Above all, the concern was to be with finding means of preventing other such diseases, in the way that vaccines were beginning successfully to prevent common childhood diseases, and even tuberculosis. (➤ Ch. 10 The immunological tradition) This development had begun with Greenwood's wartime work. After the war, his position within the new Ministry of Health, as well as his connection with the MRC, gave impetus to the growing application of medical statistics to both occupational, industrial diseases and to less easily defined, stress-induced, cardiac and other illnesses. When Greenwood became the first incumbent of the Chair of Epidemiology and Vital Statistics at the LSHTM, the department worked in close co-operation with the MRC, often sharing personnel and facilities.

Following the First World War, Greenwood added another subject to his interests: experimental epidemiology, which had been initiated in the work of W. W. C. Topley (1886–1944). Topley's early work had been in pathology; wartime experiences, in particular an epidemic of typhus in Serbia, turned his attention to the study of epidemiology. (➤ Ch. 66 War and modern medicine) The result was pioneering studies and analyses of the spread of bacterial infection under controlled conditions in herds of laboratory mice, soon afterwards taken up by Simon Flexner (1863–1946) at the Rockefeller Institute. Topley's need for help with the finer points of statistical technique was met by his co-operation with Major Greenwood. From 1927, they were colleagues at the LSHTM: Topley in the Chair of Bacteriology and Immunology, Greenwood in that of epidemiology and Vital Statistics. Between them they perfected the methodology of experimental epidemiology, and established the relevance of its results from herds of laboratory mice for natural outbreaks in human communities.

The last, and most radical, change in direction for epidemiology in the twentieth century was initiated by a younger associate and protégé of Greenwood, Austin Bradford Hill (1897–1991). Son of Greenwood's erstwhile mentor, the young Bradford Hill was prevented by illness from taking up the study of medicine; overcoming this handicap with determination, he turned instead to mathematics and economics. Armed with a degree in economics, he was employed at first by the IFRB of the MRC. From then on, he built a career which was to change the face of the twin sciences of epidemiology and medical statistics, and also eventually to affect the life-style of considerable numbers of twentieth-century men and women.

For more than a decade, until the outbreak of war in 1939, Bradford Hill conducted a number of studies in occupational health, ranging over a wide area of industrial fatigue and ill health in workers in various industries, from cotton-weaving, pottery, and aluminium manufacture to London Transport. These studies relied on existing mortality and morbidity data, and carried a number of potential sources of error. The perfectionist in Bradford Hill was to find greater satisfaction in the more accurate observations of his seminal post-war work: clinical, and randomized clinical, trials of drugs and of vaccines, and, in collaboration with Richard Doll (b. 1912), the epic work on smoking and lung cancer. (➤ Ch. 39 Drug therapies) It was the latter which, together with work beginning almost simultaneously in America, brought about remarkable changes in public-health policies and private habits in a number of countries from the 1950s onwards. The change to a move socially conscious orientation, with closer links to the public-health movement, of later twentieth-century epidemiology, was reflected in Britain in the work of the Socialist Medical Association, which was founded in 1930, and of which Greenwood was a founding member.[25]

In the United States, similar changes in direction and emphasis in epidemiology had been taking place since the beginning of the twentieth century, coinciding with another recent development in medical science. Until the end of the nineteenth century, aspiring medical researchers in a number of fields, but especially in the new bacteriology, had visited European laboratories during their formative years. With the opening of the Johns Hopkins Medical School in 1893 and the Rockefeller Institute for Medical Research in 1904 – and later the Johns Hopkins School of Hygiene and Public Health during the First World War – American scientific medicine acquired a home-base. Within these centres, as well as in their European counterparts in Britain, France, Germany, and elsewhere, the early decades of the twentieth century brought disappointments as well as achievements in the wake of the hopes and enthusiasm of the bacteriological era.

Although some vaccination programmes were successful, and pasteurization of milk dramatically reduced infant morbidity and mortality in outbreaks of 'cholera infantum', or summer diarrhoea, (➤ Ch. 45 Childhood) the tuberculin fiasco and the uncertainties surrounding the efficacy of diphtheria antitoxin treatment were among the factors highlighting the limitations of bacteriological results in their practical applications. Those working in the forefront of epidemiological research were forced to realize that knowing the specific agents of individual infectious diseases did not necessarily solve problems of control. In the United States, as in Europe, less than perfect results of the efforts to control major outbreaks of a number of diseases, culminating in the 1918–19 pandemic of influenza, brought realization that identification of infectious agents as cause of disease was not the whole answer. There was a need to return to first principles, and to recognize

> that there is no single cause of mass disease, that causation involves more than the agent directly giving rise to the process, that cause lies also in the characteristics of the population attacked and in the features of the environment in which both host population and agent find themselves.[26]

In other words, the 1920s and 1930s saw a general merging of the views of the bacteriological era with ideas expressed in the nineteenth century.

Epidemiologists came to see their subject as a kind of medical ecology, and community disease as the result of ecological processes. Simon Flexner at the Rockefeller Institute for Medical Research, and Wade Hampton Frost (1880–1938) at the Johns Hopkins School of Hygiene and Public Health, were among those who moved from single-minded pursuit of infectious agents to a broader view of causes and effects.[27] As a young officer in the Public Health and Marine Hospital Service, Frost had earned his epidemiological spurs as one of a group assigned to control an outbreak of yellow fever in New Orleans in 1905 – the last serious epidemic of the disease in the United States, less than five years after Walter Reed (1851–1902) and his co-workers, in heroic experiments, had demonstrated the transmission of the filterable virus of yellow fever in humans through the vector *Aedes aegypti*. At least as important for the control of yellow fever, and for the successful completion of the Panama Canal, had been the public-health campaigns in Havana and on the Panamanian Isthmus, led by W. C. Gorgas (1854–1920) at the beginning of the century. The fact that the disease, and especially jungle yellow fever, continues to be a problem in other parts of the world, whereas smallpox has been eradicated, is a reminder of the difficulties presented by vector-borne diseases as opposed to those attacking only human hosts.

Like Greenwood and Bradford Hill at the LSHTM, Flexner and Frost in the United States presided over developing epidemiology during the crucial period, when preoccupation with diphtheria, influenza, poliomyelitis, tuberculosis, and other acute infections began to extend to non-infectious, chronic diseases. At the same time, a study of a well-known infectious agent in the 1920s and 1930s led to unexpected results of fundamental importance for biology as a whole. What began as a search for chemical differences between serologically different strains of pneumococci in the laboratories of O. T. Avery (1877–1955) at the Rockefeller Institute resulted in an improved classification of more than seventy known types with different epidemiological characteristics. Continued painstaking work during the Second World War on the chemical nature of induced transformation of pneumococcal types led Avery to the momentous discovery of DNA as the carrier of genetic information.

Since the foundation of the Johns Hopkins School in 1916, and the LSHTM in the 1920s, the two schools have been in the forefront of developments in epidemiology. At the same time, organizations such as the World Health Organization (WHO) have achieved practical results that once seemed beyond reasonable hope of success. The global eradication of smallpox in 1979, two hundred years after Jenner first drew attention to the protective powers of cowpox, was the happy outcome of a prolonged struggle.[28] (➤ Ch. 59 Internationalism in medicine and public health)

CONCLUSION

During the latter half of the twentieth century, the science of epidemiology has come full circle in its global concerns. The emphasis on infectious diseases and their causal agents which dominated epidemiological thinking in the Western world in the early decades of the century gradually lost its immediacy once means of control became increasingly available in the form of safe, efficient vaccines, sulphonamides, and antibiotics in the 1930s and 1940s. Epidemiologists and public-health authorities became increasingly preoccupied with hidden environmental causes in developed countries. In the developing world, on the other hand, common European diseases such as measles and tuberculosis began to overtake, in terms of morbidity and mortality, the traditional tropical parasitic illnesses as major health problems. Another couple of decades further on, tobacco-related lung cancer and cardiac disease are assuming in the Third World the importance registered in developed countries in mid-century. And only since 1980 has AIDS emerged as a simultaneous, global, epidemiological threat of formidable proportions. (➤ Ch. 26 Sexually transmitted diseases) The circle has closed; the problems of global epidemiology remain as acute as ever.

NOTES

1 Major Greenwood, *Epidemics and Crowd Diseases*, London, Williams & Norgate, 1935, p. 15.

2 'Airs, waters, places', in *Hippocratic Writings*, ed. by G. E. R. Lloyd, trans. by J. Chadwick and W. N. Mann, Harmondsworth, Penguin Classics, 1983, pp. 148–9.

3 Vivian Nutton, 'The seeds of disease: an explanation of contagion and infection from the Greeks to the Renaissance', *Medical History*, 1983, 27: 1–34; see esp. pp. 4–9.

4 C.-E. A. Winslow, *The Conquest of Epidemic Disease*, Madison, University of Wisconsin Press, 1980 pp. 88–116; orig. pub. 1943, Princeton, Princeton University Press.

5 Hieronymi Fracastorii, *De Contagione et Contagiosis Morbis et eorum Curatione*, trans. and notes by Wilmer Cave Wright, New York, G. P. Putnam's Sons, 1930, Book II, pp. 81, 85.

6 Winslow, op. cit. (n. 4), p. 133.

7 Peter Laslett, 'Introduction', *The Earliest Classics: John Graunt and Gregory King*, London, Gregg International, 1973, p. 2.

8 *The Works of Thomas Sydenham, M.D.*, 2 vols, London, Sydenham Society, 1848–50, Vol. I, p. 33.

9 L. Wilkinson, 'Rinderpest and mainstream infectious disease concepts in the eighteenth century', *Medical History*, 1984, 28: 129–50.

10 Genevieve Miller, *The Adoption of Inoculation for Smallpox in England and France*, Philadelphia, University of Pennsylvania Press, 1957, pp. 91–2, 111–14.

11 A. M. Lilienfeld and D. E. Lilienfeld, 'The epidemiologic fabric', *International Journal of Epidemiology*, 1980, 9: 199–206, 300–4; see p. 303.

12 P. Ch. A. Louis, *Recherches sur les effets de la saignée dans quelques maladies inflammatoires, et sur l'action de l'émétique et des vésicatoires dans le pneumonie*, Paris, J. B. Baillière, 1835, pp. 75–6.

13 P. L. Panum, 'Iagttagelser, anstillede under Maeslinge-Epidemien pa Faeröerne i Aaret 1846', *Bibliothek for Laeger*, 1847 (3rd series), 1: 270–344; see p. 324.

14 William Farr, *Vital Statistics: a Memorial Volume of Selections from the Reports and Writings of William Farr*, Metuchen, NJ, New York Academy of Medicine, Scarecrow Press, 1975, p. 317.

15 Ibid., p. 320.

16 Farr, op. cit. (n. 14).

17 John Brownlee, 'Historical note on Farr's theory of the epidemic', *British Medical Journal*, 1915, 2: 250–52.

18 D. E. Lilienfeld and A. M. Lilienfeld, 'Epidemiology: a retrospective study', *American Journal of Epidemiology*, 1977, 106: 445–59.

19 Lilienfeld and Lilienfeld, op. cit. (n. 11), pp. 299–300.

20 *The Commemoration Volume, Transactions of the Epidemiological Society*, London, Shaw, 1901, p. 10.

21 William Coleman, *Yellow Fever in the North*, Madison, University of Wisconsin Press, 1987.

22 George Rosen, 'Problems in the application of statistical analysis to questions of health: 1700–1880', *Bulletin of the History of Medicine*, 1955, 29: 27–45; see p. 45.

23 Paul E. M. Fine, 'John Brownlee and the measurement of infectiousness: an historical study in epidemic theory', *Journal of the Royal Statistical Society*, 1979 (Series A), 142 (3): 347–62; see pp. 348–349.

24 Lancelot Hogben, 'Major Greenwood 1880–1949', *Obituary Notices of Fellows of the Royal Society of London*, 1950–1, 7: 139–54; see p. 141.

25 Milton Terris, 'Epidemiology and the public health movement', *Journal of Chronic Diseases*, 1986, 39: 953–61; see p. 958.

26 John E. Gordon, 'The twentieth century – yesterday, today, and tomorrow (1920–)', in F. H. Top (ed.), *The History of American Epidemiology*, St Louis, MO, C. V. Mosby, 1952, pp. 115–16.

27 K. F. Maxcy, *Papers of Wade Hampton Frost. A Contribution to Epidemiological Method*, New York, Commonwealth Fund, 1941.

28 Frank Fenner, 'Smallpox, "the most dreadful scourge of the human species": its global spread and recent eradication', *Medical Journal of Australia*, 1984, 141: 728–35, 841–46; see p. 845.

FURTHER READING

Ackerknecht, E. H., 'Hygiene in France, 1815–1848', *Bulletin of the History of Medicine*, 1948, 22: 117–55.

Bynum, W. F. and Nutton, V. (eds), *Theories of Fever from Antiquity to the Enlightenment*, *Medical History* (supp. I, London, Wellcome Institute for the History of Medicine, 1981.

Cliff, A. and Haggett, P., 'Island epidemics', *Scientific American*, 1984, 250 (5): 110–17.

Coleman, William, *Death is a Social Disease: Public Health and Political Economy in Early Industrial France*, Madison, WI, University of Wisconsin Press, 1982.

Creighton, Charles, *A History of Epidemics in Britain*, 2 vols, Cambridge, Cambridge University Press, 1891–4.

Eyler, John M., 'William Farr on the cholera: the sanitarian's disease theory and the statistician's method', *Journal of the History of Medicine*, 1973, 28: 79–100.

——, *Victorian Social Medicine: the Ideas and Methods of William Farr*, Baltimore, MD, Johns Hopkins University Press, 1979.

Greenwood, Major, *Epidemiology, Historical and Experimental*, Baltimore, MD, Johns Hopkins University Press, 1932.

——, *The Medical Dictator*, London, Keynes Press, 1986.

Hamer, William, *Epidemiology Old and New*, London, Kegan Paul, 1928.

Lilienfeld, Abraham M. (ed.), *Times, Places and Persons: Aspects of the History of Epidemiology*, Baltimore, MD, Johns Hopkins University Press, 1980.

Lilienfeld, David E., ' "The greening of epidemiology": sanitary physicians and the London Epidemiological Society (1830–1870)', *Bulletin of the History of Medicine*, 1979, 52: 503–28.

McNeill, William H., *Plagues and People*, Oxford, Blackwell, 1976.

Pelling, Margaret, *Cholera, Fever and English Medicine 1825–1865*, Oxford, Oxford University Press, 1978.

Sand, René, *Vers la médecine sociale*, Paris, J.-B. Baillière, 1948.

Sticker, Georg, *Die Bedeutung der Geschichte der Epidemien für die heutige Epidemiologie: ein Beitrag zur Beurteilung des Reichsseuchegesetzes*, Giessen, Töpelmann, 1910.

Tröhler, Ulrich, 'Quantification in British medicine and surgery, 1750–1830, with special reference to its introduction into therapeutics', unpublished Ph.D. thesis, University of London, 1978.

53

THE HISTORY OF PERSONAL HYGIENE

Andrew Wear

The meaning of 'hygiene', literally 'health' in Greek, has undergone radical change over time. In the classical period, Galen (AD 129–*c*.200/210) wrote that medicine was divided into hygiene and therapeutics, into the art of staying healthy and preventing disease, and into the art of treating disease.[1] Today, hygiene means cleanliness, and has a narrower scope. It is still associated with health for, since the nineteenth-century germ theory of disease, to be unclean is to be full of germs, hence unhealthy. However, there are many illnesses such as cancers, heart disease, and chronic neuromuscular conditions which are not normally explained using modern ideas of hygiene, cleanliness, and germs. The classical view of hygiene, however, was that it was concerned with the prevention of all types of disease.

The art of hygiene from the Greek period to the eighteenth century was primarily concerned with a person's life-style and relationship to the environment. Geographical location, climate, food, water, the emanations of the body, sexual activity, exercise and rest, sleeping and waking were taken into account when preserving health or when explaining and curing illness. This holistic approach to the health of the body (typical of Hippocratic and Galenic medical theory) was transformed in the nineteenth century. As the medical view of disease changed, so did hygiene. In the first half of the nineteenth century in the Paris hospitals, disease came to be perceived as localized in specific organs and parts of the body, and in the second half of the century, specific agents such as bacteria were seen as causing disease. In this way, medicine lost its holistic aetiology of disease as a malfunction of the whole body (expressed in humoral theory as a general imbalance or excess of the humours produced by the environment and/or life-style). (Ch. 14 Humoralism) Hygiene similarly lost its holistic viewpoint and came to reflect the new specificity of medicine. Dirt became the visible manifestation

1283

of the invisible, of the hidden bacterial agents of disease, and cleanliness was a first approximation towards preventing disease. (➤ Ch. 9 The pathological tradition)

However, not all the components of what previously constituted hygiene have been lost. Aspects of life-style still form part of medicine: for instance, exercise in heart disease, types of food or environmental pollutants in cancer; but they are parts of the older hygiene, which has now lost its name.

Changes in medicine were not the only reason for the transformation of hygiene; social movements were also responsible. Developments in manners amongst the nobility in the eighteenth century altered standards of cleanliness. In the nineteenth century, these trickled down to the middle classes. Cleanliness, or the lack of it, came to be associated with moral worth or with immorality. To be clean had a double sense: the physical and the moral. The campaigns to inculcate cleanliness amongst the working classes came to combine religious and social motives with the imperatives of post-Pasteurian medicine. Indeed, those who sought to impose or provide from above the means to cleanliness sometimes associated medical reasoning with theories of racial hygiene and progress. The history of hygiene, therefore, touches upon types of history (such as social and cultural history) which are usually thought to lie outwith the traditional remit of the history of medicine.

THE CLASSICAL VIEW OF HYGIENE AND ITS CONTINUATION

Hygiene in the Hippocratic and Galenic writings shaped the Western medical tradition on hygiene into the nineteenth century. They provided a template for later writers, which from the start was flexible, and which over time became even more so. But until the birth of modern scientific medicine, the main features of classical medical hygiene remained recognizable across the centuries.

Hygiene, the preservation of health and prevention of illness, in the Hippocratic and Galenic writings was concerned with the individual. Engineering works such as Rome's *cloaca maxima* attest to an interest in the mechanics of public health such as sewage disposal (as do the aqueducts and pipes that supplied water). But in classical hygiene the emphasis was on the individual and not on the community, the *polis* or *urbs*.

Various Hippocratic treatises (*c.* fifth century BC) gave instructions and hints on how to stay healthy. Some of the advice was of a general nature, applicable to all. *Regimen in Health* stated:

> The layman ought to order his regimen in the following way. In winter eat as much as possible and drink as little as possible: drink should be wine as

undiluted as possible, and food should be bread, with all meats roasted; during this season take as few vegetables as possible, for so will the body be most dry and hot.[2]

Behind Hippocratic hygienic advice there often lay the goal of achieving a qualitative and humoral balance within the body. (➤ Ch. 14 Humoralism) So in the passage above, winter with its cold and moist qualities had to be countered by food and drink of opposing qualities. Individual characteristics were taken into account, for each person had an innate constitution that tended towards particular qualities and humours that had to be brought back into balance:

> Those with physiques that are fleshy, soft and red, find it beneficial to adopt a rather dry regimen for the greater part of the year. For the nature of these physiques is moist. Those that are lean and sinewy, whether ruddy or dark, should adopt a moister regime for the greater part of the time, for the bodies of such are constitutionally dry.... Older people should have a drier kind of diet for the greater part of the time for bodies at this age are moist and soft and cold. So in fixing regimen pay attention to age, season, habit, land, and physique, and counteract the prevailing heat or cold. For in this way will the best health be preserved.
> Walking should be rapid in winter, slow in summer.[3]

The treatise also set out how procedures such as the use of emetics and clysters should be used in a regular prophylactic way by the healthy, according to the season and the types of bodily constitution. Hygiene and therapeutics shared not only theories as to the causes of health and illness, but also had medical procedures in common. The annual springtime bleeding undertaken in the Middle Ages and Renaissance to lessen the increase in blood at this time is another example. (➤ Ch. 40 Physical methods)

More detailed and extensive hygienic advice was given in the Hippocratic treatise *Regimen*. Its discussion of the effects upon the health of specific environments and regimens were to be repeated, echoed, and amplified into the eighteenth century. Places such as marshy grounds and mountains; the different winds; the various kinds of food such as grains, pulses, meats, fishes, birds, milk products, vegetables, herbs, and fruits, are all considered in terms of their qualities and the effects of those qualities upon the body and its evacuations. (➤ Ch. 15 Environment and miasmata; Ch. 18 Ecology of disease)

As the examples below show, advice seems to have been based on a mixture of commonsense experience and on maxims less obviously founded, wrapped around by the humoral-qualitative theory:

> The winds which strike regions from off the sea, or from snow, frost, lakes or rivers all moisten and cool both plants and animals, and are healthy unless they be cold to an excess when they are hurtful by reason of the great changes of cold and heat which they make in bodies.
> As to animals which are eatable you must know that beef is strong and

binding, and hard of digestion because this animal abounds with a gross thick blood. . . . Dog's flesh dries, heats and affords strength, but does not pass by stool. The flesh of puppies moistens and passes by stool, still more by urine. Wild boar's flesh is drying and strengthening, and passes by stool.

Thyme is hot, passes easily by stool and evacuates phlegmatic humours. Hyssop is warming and expels phlegmatic humours.[4]

Regimen did not only consider food and drink in their simple states. The different qualities and powers of meats preserved in wine, vinegar, and salt were described, as were those of different cooking methods, such as boiling, grilling, and roasting, that would weaken, moisten, dry, and bind. Food and medicine were closely associated. The Hippocratic treatise *On Ancient Medicine* asserted that medicine was a specialized form of dietetics, that trial and error found out which foods were good for health, and that the same process of discovery could turn some foods into therapeutic medicines. Hygiene, in a sense, took a medical view of food as it did of topology, climate, and much else.

Advice was given in *Regimen* on sleep and sexual activity, on the types of baths that should be taken, and on exercise. In winter, for instance:

It is beneficial to sleep on a hard bed and to take night walks and night runs, for all these things reduce and warm; unctions should be copious. When a bath is desired, let it be cold after exercise in the palaestra; after any other exercise, a hot bath is more beneficial. Sexual intercourse should be more frequent at this season, and for older men more than for the younger.[5]

There was a great deal of advice on exercise, an important part of the culture of free-born Greeks. It was one of the most visible and deliberate aspects of hygiene and, as Galen was to write, the hygienist could be called a gymnast, though, he added, it would be a mistake to do so, as a hygienist was more than a gymnast.[6]

The Hippocratic treatises were largely silent about the type of people they were writing for. *Regimen in Health* addressed itself to the 'ordinary' lay person (ἰδιώτης), and *Regimen* 'to the great mass of mankind, who of necessity live a haphazard life without the chance of neglecting everything to concentrate on taking care of their health'.[7] Galen, the great synthesizer of Greek medicine, who, in terms of authority, was for the Middle Ages and Renaissance 'Prince of Physicians second to Hippocrates', wrote a treatise on hygiene which followed the Hippocratic writings in many but not all respects (see p. 1287 on the theory of ageing). In the *De Sanitate Tuenda* (Greek: *Hygieina*) Galen was more specific about his readership. Only those with leisure, who could set everything aside to look after their health, and who also possessed from the start a perfect constitution, could achieve perfect health (at the end of the treatise there were some chapters for those with less than perfect constitutions). Galen was not interested in reforming social conditions in the name of hygiene. The connection between work and health was, however, clear in his mind: 'the life of many men is involved in the business of their occupation, and it is inevitable that they should be harmed by what they do and that it should be impossible to change it.'[8] Galen was aware that as well as slavery and poverty, the single-minded pursuit of a job by the reasonably well-off could be harmful: 'those who through ambition or zeal have chosen some form of life so involved in affairs of business that they can have little leisure for the care of their bodies are also willing slaves to hard masters.'[9] Unlike nineteenth-century writers, Galen did not belong to a culture that could use medical reasoning to urge a change or amelioration in working conditions. Galen's client, like Aristotle's philosopher, was leisured, rich, and in the top ranks of society.

The *De Sanitate Tuenda* discussed at length the different types of exercise and bathing regimes, as well as dealing with environmental factors such as airs and waters. It was loosely organized on a birth-to-old-age basis. In the case of infants, Galen advised that their natural moisture should be preserved with moistening measures such as warm baths and foods such as milks, and that the principle that 'opposites are remedies of opposites' was not appropriate to infants (that is the use of drying remedies).[10] (➤ Ch. 45 Childhood) In the case of old age, he did apply the principle. Unlike the Hippocratic *Regimen*, which stated that old age was characterized by cold and wet qualities, Galen argued that ageing was the process of becoming progressively colder and drier. The regimen of the old had to consist of moistening and warming agents, especial care being taken that the flickering intrinsic warmth of the aged was not extinguished.[11] (The Greek image of life as a flame, a natural heat nurtured by a radical moisture or humour as oil feeds the flame of a lamp, was to be repeated down the centuries.[12])

The contents and structure of classical hygiene never became totally fixed even in the Middle Ages and Renaissance, when the aggregators and then the compendium-makers of classical knowledge flourished. Writers on hygiene tended to emphasize a particular aspect of the environment or of a person's life-style. However, some time after Galen, the 'six non-naturals' came to provide the canonical categories that made up hygiene.[13] These were air, food and drink, sleep and waking, movement and rest, retention and evacuation including sexual activity, and the emotions or the passions of the soul. These categories were not fixed in the Hippocratic writings, and a slightly different list was given in Galen's *De Sanitate Tuenda*. But Galen did set them out in his *Ars Medica*, and he explained why they were necessary for the health of the individual (though he did not coin the mysterious term 'non-naturals'):

Of necessity we are immersed in the surrounding air, and we eat, drink, wake and sleep. We are not necessarily thrust against swords or beasts. Hence in the first category of causes but not in the second there is an art devoted to the protection of the body. Now that these matters have been set forth, we shall find in each of these items which necessarily alter the body, its own kind of healthful causes. One comes from contact with the surrounding air, another from movement and rest of the whole body or its parts, a third from sleep and waking, a fourth from things taken into the body, a fifth from those that are excreted and returned, a sixth from the affections of the mind.[14]

Fourteen centuries later, Robert Burton (1577–1640) echoed Galen when he wrote that physicians would tell us that the 'six non-natural things . . . are the causes of our infirmities', and that they are necessary 'because we cannot avoid them, but they will alter us, as they are used or abused'[15] (a point of view that could easily lead to advocating modern, alcohol-centred temperance, as John Wesley (1703–91) began to do in the next century).

Much of the content of classical hygiene remained the same through the Middle Ages and Renaissance. A key text was the *Regimen Sanitatis Salernitanum*, composed around the thirteenth century and attributed to the medical school of Salerno, one of the first in Europe after the fall of Rome. The verses of the *Regimen* were added to or amended over time in numerous manuscripts, and then in printed editions that attest to its popularity. Hygiene was usually placed first, and there followed verses on materia medica; then anatomy, physiology, and the therapeutics of particular types of fevers and diseases. The *Regimen* was not clearly structured. Though it referred to the six non-naturals, it was an *omnium gatherum* of medical knowledge, uncomplicated, often witty, and translated from Latin into many European languages, which ensured that it had a wide readership.

The illustrated health handbooks of the Middle Ages known as the *Tacuina Sanitatis* also referred to the six non-naturals but, as in the *Regimen Sanitatis Salernitanum*, the distinction between hygiene and therapeutics was not clearly made. This illustrates the point that there was a continuum between diet for health, and diet as part of therapeutics to cure illness. Some herbs and foods were treated as remedies. Wheat opened abscesses, lettuce relieved insomnia and spermatorrhoea; other foods combined both hygienic (health-giving) and therapeutic properties. Rue sharpened the eyesight and dissipated flatulence; pasta was good for the chest and for the throat; whilst grapes nourished, purified, and fattened.[16] By the Middle Ages, the qualitative-humoral theory of using opposites to achieve balance was being expressed in degrees of qualities (from one to four, with four being the most intense). The pulp of oranges was cold and humid in the third degree, whilst the skin was dry and warm in the second. The winds and seasons also had particular degrees of qualities. (The south wind was warm in the second degree, dry in the first, and spring had moderate humidity in the first degree – and they were good for the chest and for all animals, respectively).[17] The quantification of qualities gave an impression of exactness, and it probably added to the sense of expert esoteric knowledge surrounding medicine.

The difference between modern hygiene and that of the pre-Pasteurian era is indicated by the way in which the *Tacuina* dealt with clothing. Rather than emphasizing that clothes should be clean, the treatises focused upon their qualitative properties, the aim being to achieve a qualitative-humoral balance rather than to avoid the as-yet undiscovered agents of disease. Woollen clothing was warm and dry. The best was the thin cloth from Flanders, which protected the body from cold and held warmth, although it could cause skin irritation. Linen clothing was cold and dry in the second degree; the best was 'the light, splendid, beautiful kind', which moderates the heat of the body, but can be dangerous as 'it presses down on the skin and blocks transpiration'.[18]

The richly illustrated *Tacuina* could have been afforded only by the wealthy. Despite the popular appeal of the *Regimen Sanitatis Salernitanum*, most books on regimen were aimed at the well-off or at the middling members of society. For instance, Odericus of Genoa (d. 1505) at the end of the fifteenth century wrote his *De Regenda Sanitate Consilium* for the Genoese patrician Pietro Sali; in 1493 Bartholomäus Scherrenmuller (*fl.* 1476) composed the *Regimen und Uffenthalt der Gesunthait von demm Tag der Entpfengnuß in Mutter leyb bis an End des Alters* for Graf Eberhard (1445–96) (who two years later, became Duke of Württemberg).[19] More generally, Marsilio Ficino (1433–99) published in 1489 his often-printed *Liber de Vita* (of *De Vita Triplica*) 'for the health of students or those who work in letters'; and Gugliermo Gratarolo (1516–68) wrote in 1555 a treatise on the health of students and magistrates.[20] As in Galen's time, leisure helped to determine who could benefit from treatises on hygiene. The sedentary and the studious comprised a new focus for writers on hygiene. Robert Burton's *Anatomy of Melancholy* (1621) reflected this trend, being aimed at the mental health (and ills) of students and the studious (the melancholy humour being thought to predominate in the constitution of scholars). (➤ Ch. 21 Mental diseases)

Despite the limitations of readership (the greatest of which was literacy) health-advice books were very popular in the sixteenth century. Paul Slack has calculated that in England, between 1486–1604, 115 editions of explanatory textbooks on medicine and books of regimen were issued in the vernacular out of a total of 392 editions of books in English dealing with medicine.[21] For example, between 1536 and 1595, sixteen editions were published of the *Castel of Health* by Thomas Elyot (*c.*1490–1546); other publications included a translation by Thomas Paynel (*fl.* 1528–68) of the *Regimen Sanitatis Salerno* (1528), a *Breviary of Health* (1547) by Andrew Boorde (b. 1490), *Government* *of Health* (1558) by William Bullein (d. 1576), and *The Haven of Health* (1584) by Thomas Cogan (*c.*1545–1607). These works found eager buyers, and their popularity is a clear sign of interest in self-help and hygiene amongst a considerable section of the population.

Old topics were given a fresh airing in the Renaissance. Exercise, which figured largely in Galen's *De Sanitate Tuenda*, had not been emphasized in the Middle Ages, but the humanist endeavour of Thomas Linacre (*c.*1460–1524) in producing a scholarly Latin version of the Greek text of the treatise in 1517 gave it a new prominence. Hieronymus Mercurialis (1530–1606) in *De Arte Gymnastica* (1569) related classical gymnastics and exercises to health, as did Massilio Cagnati (1543–1612) in the second part of his *De Sanitate Tuenda* (1605).

There was also an emphasis on the relationship between hygiene and ageing, reflecting Galen's view that different hygienic measures have to be taken according to the age of the individual. As Richard Palmer has pointed out, from the time of Roger Bacon (*c.*1214–94), a new strand enters into this relationship – the aim of prolonging life.[22] (➤ Ch. 46 Geriatrics) The Galenic view was that one's life-span was fixed by nature (the aim of hygiene being to attain the allotted number of years), and Christian teaching stressed the next world and the transience of this (to which can be added the Thomistic emphasis on God's foreknowledge through his providence of the future). (➤ Ch. 61 Religion and medicine) But in the Middle Ages and the Renaissance, there developed slowly a more active and manipulative view of nature and of the body, in which nature itself could be mastered. Roger Bacon, in his *De Retardatione Accidentium Senectutis* and *De Conservatione Juventutis*, looked back to human beings' extended life-span (a thousand years) that was attained in the early years after the Fall. Regimen and secret remedies could ensure a long life (which God had originally authorized). Similarly, Arnold of Villanova (d. 1311) in his *De Conservanda Inventute et Retardanda Senectute* advocated diet, baths, exercises, and alchemical remedies to conserve youth.[23]

Despite such changes in emphasis, the content of the books on hygiene or regimen remained largely unaltered from Greek times. Why was this so? At a banal yet true level, one can reply that nearly all classical knowledge lasted well into the sixteenth century, and that this was ensured by the authority of the written word, by the assimilations in the Middle Ages of classical learning into Christianity and into its institutions, the church-run schools and universities, and by the Renaissance veneration of classical knowledge. Also, the medical hygienic teachings of the Greeks made sense to the Renaissance and to the eighteenth century in material terms, for the world of the Greeks had much in common with later, pre-industrial societies. The metaphor of old age as a lamp whose oil was giving out was as recognizable to eighteenth-century society as to the Greeks, as both used oil lamps.

Moreover, both in classical Greece and enlightenment Europe, the health dangers of the environment had to be judged by an individual's senses. Before the age of detailed chemical analysis of air, water, or food, and science-based inspectorates, which would validate their quality, people had to use their own senses. The advice on what constituted good water (clear, crystalline, from swift-flowing sources and uncontaminated by stagnant or marshy water), or good air or food was therefore useful advice, addressed to practical needs. It was related to personal hygiene and not to public health. For it was the individual who assessed the healthiness of the environment, and in the case of food, the advice was directly related to the individual's constitution. The Italian Health Boards set up by the city-states of Venice, Florence, Milan, and Genoa to deal with plague went on to take, in the sixteenth century, some powers for inspecting food markets, as did city authorities in England. However, this was a fragmentary and embryonic form of public health.

Classical ideas of hygiene also helped Europeans from the early sixteenth to the late nineteenth century to cope with foreign lands and climates, especially those of the tropics. (➤ Ch. 24 Tropical diseases) A person's constitution was partly determined by the constitution of the place in which he or she was born and had resided. A move to a different climate meant that one's body no longer fitted its environment and so was more liable to ill health. A process of 'seasoning', of gradual acclimatization, not only to climate but also to new foods and drinks, could re-establish the fit. Europeans struggling to adapt to new environments such as those in America,[24] and then in India and Africa, found these ideas very congenial. For example, James Johnson (1777–1845), in *The Influence of Tropical Climates, More Especially the Climate of India on European Constitutions* (1812), was not sanguine about the ability of Europeans to survive in India, but he wrote that seasoning would be helped by the long sea-voyage to India, by imitating the example of native Indians and eating vegetarian Hindu dishes in the first year and Moslem meat dishes in the second; and again, like the Indians, clothing lightly and keeping houses cool. The use of classical ideas of hygiene which directly related environment and life-style to health gave a sense to new settlers that they had a degree of direct, personal control over their health, despite new and hostile climates. This helps to explain why such ideas lasted so long. (➤ Ch. 58 Medicine and colonialism)

Much of the advice for both Europe and the Tropics was repeated in book after book. Some of it undoubtedly mirrored experience and folk knowledge. For instance, the prohibition on living in low-lying marshy areas, drinking stagnant waters, and breathing thick vaporous air (after plague hit Europe, this was sometimes termed pestilential air) reflected the high mortality of such malarial regions, which modern historical demographers have high-

lighted.[25] Again, the assumption in the health-advice books that the country-side was healthier than the city and that its life-style should be emulated is backed up by the findings of demographers. Other long-lasting traditions of a cultural sort probably helped to reinforce such views. The pastoral tradition emphasized the country over the town, and the Garden of Eden, man's and woman's natural place, gave Biblical authority to a classical idea. There were other underlying assumptions that helped to structure some of the advice. A recurrent theme was that swift motion was healthy, whether of water, of air, of animals (and of humans) and of fish, and this also emphasized the point that the wild parts of nature were best. City life was seen as unhealthy (its air was dark with smoke and polluted, people and houses were crowded too close together, and its inhabitants under-exercised). Similarly, the food produced from animals that were penned up, crowded, in dark conditions, and fed kitchen scraps, was unhealthy for humans. The spectrum of unhealthiness continued into certain places, climates, and animals in nature. For instance, as well as stagnant air and low-lying marshy ground, fish that swam in slow-moving, muddy dark waters produced ill flesh. Not all of nature was healthy. It seems that motion, light, uncrowded and airy sweet-smelling environments were considered healthy, whilst the stagnant and the slow-moving, the dark and the murky, and the crowded and evil-smelling were seen as unhealthy qualities (a view that continues to the present).[26] These characteristics and qualities, together with the traditional four qualities (hot, cold, dry, and wet) of Hippocrates and Galen, were used when the health of air, water, or food was being judged. What is not very prominent until the sixteenth century in the health-advice books is a strong link between morality and hygiene, especially dirt (though there was condemnation of the too-indulgent patient).
(➤ Ch. 27 Diseases of civilization; Ch. 71 Demography and medicine)

Christianity had helped to give a specific moral and even ascetic tone to hygiene. From the days of the early church, the sins of gluttony and drunkenness had been condemned; the health of the body (the house of the soul) had been linked to the health of the soul, and the Christian was enjoined to care for the body as well as for the soul. (The injunctions of Leviticus have a specifically hygienic flavour, but they were religious and not medical in intent – though their existence could have made the medical injunctions of classical hygiene easier to assimilate for a Christian world.)

In the sixteenth century, Luigi Cornaro (c.1463–c.1566) made the link between hygiene, Christianity, and temperance very explicit. His *Trattato de la Vita Sobria* of 1558 was popular, and was translated into French, English, and German. It looks forward to late seventeenth- and eighteenth-century developments in hygiene discussed below (see pp. 1286 ff.), for, as well as taking a religious approach, Cornaro produced a very personal, even idiosyncratic, treatise, rather than a traditional or canonical account of regimen.

Cornaro ascribed his longevity (he stated he was over 80 years old at the time of writing) to moderation, plenty of exercise, keeping his mind occupied with pleasurable activities, and particularly to discovering what foods and drinks suited his health and then sticking faithfully only to them. This eclectic and traditional approach was modified by a religious note and by a great emphasis on the exact measurement of the quantity of food and drink to be taken at each meal or during each day (twelve ounces of solid food, fourteen ounces of wine). The stress on precision was the equivalent to the specific remedy of the empiric: Cornaro emphasized that the secret of his longevity lay in the measured sparseness of his diet. He used the language of vice and virtue to unite religion with diet and health:

> coming then to that evil concerning which I propose to speak – the vice of intemperance – I declare that it is a wicked thing that it should prevail to such an extent as to greatly lower, nay, almost abolish, the temperate life. For though it is well known by all that intemperance proceeds from the vice of gluttony, and temperance from the virtue of restraint, nevertheless the former is exalted as a virtuous thing and even as a mark of distinction, while temperance is stigmatised and scorned as dishonourable, and as befitting the miserly alone.[27]

Cornaro went on to make the connection between sin and becoming ill. People crave, he wrote, 'to gratify the appetites', and 'abandoning the path of virtue, they have taken to following the one of vice – a road which leads them, though they see it not, to strange and fatal chronic infirmities through which they grow prematurely old.'[28] The appeal of his treatise undoubtedly lay in its autobiographical content. His story was analogous to a genre of writing, popular with both Catholics and Protestants – that of the religious conversion. Through intemperance, Cornaro wrote, he lay at the age of 40 at death's door; he took stock, reformed himself, and became a new, healthy man. Dissipation, ruin, seeing the light, and conversion to a new and good life were found, not only in lives of saints, but in many biographies and autobiographies of the time. It is a highly personal type of writing, in which the individual takes charge of his own destiny. This is reflected in Cornaro's views of what role the physician should play in giving advice on regimen. The physician, Cornaro stated, should act like a friend, encouraging and sympathizing with the patient, but only the patient can discover what is good for him- or herself: 'It is impossible for anyone to be a perfect physician of another. Since, then, a man can have no better doctor than himself, and no better medicine than the temperate life, he should by all means embrace that life.'[29] (➤ Ch. 34 History of the doctor–patient relationship)

Cornaro's religious note, his recipe of self-help, and his emphasis on the methodical and exclusive use of a meagre and precisely measured diet, establish a distance between himself and orthodox medicine. His treatise looks forward to the fragmentation of the consensus on hygiene and to a number of idiosyncratic treatises, which were *sui generis* to their authors and often united morality with hygiene.

Change in ideas of regimen occurred in the seventeenth century (and, as with Cornaro, even earlier). The non-naturals continued to be used to organize writings on hygiene, but some of the contents changed. (John Wesley, the founder of Methodism, preached the new theme of temperance whilst using the non-naturals to order his comments on regimen in the beginning of his *Primitive Physick* (1747).) What was orthodoxy in medicine remained unclear from the late seventeenth until the nineteenth century. Galenic medicine was replaced by iatrochemistry, iatromechanics, and the medical systems emanating from Leiden and then Edinburgh, which jostled and succeeded each other, none of them establishing any long-lasting dominance. At the same time, quack or empirical medicine, with its specific medicines tailored not to the individual patient but to the illness (or to all illnesses, in the case of panaceas), came into prominence, although it had always been on the medical scene. (➤ Ch. 28 Unorthodox medical theories)

Hygiene reflected these wider changes in medicine. There was no consensus as to what constituted a proper diet (other aspects of classical hygiene still continued: for instance, ideas on healthy places, airs, and waters). Moreover, diets were proposed that could be employed by everyone, instead of being individually tailored to the particular patient. Different diets were promoted, just as different panaceas were advertised by empirics. In the process, the range of what was allowable to eat narrowed; diet became more specific. Classical ideas on diet had been eclectic; they were inclusive rather than exclusive. This was ensured by the belief that different foods suited different constitutions and different ages, and by the Hippocratic injunction of moderation in everything.

As Virginia Smith has shown, one of the traditional four qualities came to be emphasized to the exclusion of the others. Cold regimens, in the form of cold baths, cold foods (often vegetarian-only diets), and cold drinks were prescribed.[30] Asceticism and temperance were associated with such regimes, whilst hot baths, hot foods such as meats and rich spices, and hot drinks such as wines and spirits had connotations of luxury and intemperance.

Sir John Floyer (1649–1734), student of baths and spas and proponent of cold-bathing, wrote in 1697 of the corrupting and enervating effects of a hot regimen:

> Brandy, spirits, strong wines, smoking tobacco, strong ale, hot baths, wearing flannel and many clothes, keeping in the house, warming of beds, sitting by great fires, drinking continually of tea and coffee, want of due exercise of body, by too much study or passion of the mind, by marrying too young, or by too much venery (which injures eyes, digestion, perspiration and breeds wind and

crudities); and for all the effeminacy and niceness and weakness of spirits that is produced in the hysterical and hypochondrical.[31]

Here, morality was associated with hygiene (Floyer was probably reflecting popular ideas). His strictures were taken up by eighteenth- and nineteenth-century proponents of cooling regimens, who argued that they helped to harden and to make manly the constitution and to protect it from illness. Children, especially, were seen as being in need of such hardening. John Locke (1632–1704), in *Some Thoughts Concerning Education* (1693), stressed that the earlier this happened the better, so babies should be kept from warm rooms and swaddling-clothes. Instead, they were to be toughened by cold air, cold baths, and few clothes. The analogues of such ideas can be found in the earlier health-advice books, where a tough country labouring life was seen as healthy, and in the eighteenth-century idealization of the primitive or noble savage, as well as in eighteenth- and nineteenth-century ideas of manliness.[32]

Changing ideas of human relationships with the natural world, as well as beliefs in cooling regimens, helped to shape views on diet. As Keith Thomas has pointed out, vegetarianism was taken up by people who felt that the suffering of animals (which they saw as akin to humans) precluded their slaughter as food. The view that the world and its creatures had been created for humans' use came into question, especially by radicals and nonconformists. Thomas Tryon (1634–1703), a follower of the teachings of Jakob Boehme (1575–1624), was a noted proponent of vegetarianism in the second half of the seventeenth century. A strict vegetarian himself (he refused to wear shoes made from leather), he advised his readers to limit their consumption of meat rather than giving it up altogether. He combined the ethical view of not harming God's creatures with the old hygienic belief that the food that we eat affects our own body and mind (red meat, Tryon thought, made its eater aggressive and unpleasant – an antidote to the praise heaped upon the red beef of old England).[33] George Cheyne (1671–1743), the author of the popular *Essay of Health and Long Life* (1724) and who at one time weighed over 32 stones, recommended moderation in meats and alcoholic drinks, but not total abstention. His motto was moderation in everything, but he could also advise his patients to go on specialized excluding diets. Lord Hervey (1696–1743) was told by Cheyne to eat no meat for six weeks, and then to go on a total milk diet for two months. In fact, Hervey was put on a three-year diet in which 'I ate neither flesh, fish nor eggs, but lived entirely upon herbs, roots, pulses, grains, fruits, legumes and all those sorts of foods, which before I left off meat and wine, I would never eat of, though in the smallest degree, without feeling a pain in my stomach in half an hour after they were lodged there.'[34]

Although Cheyne's work was aimed at the well-to-do, hygiene came to be targeted at a wider section of society. Tryon's writings, as befitted his radical religious beliefs, were aimed at the poor as well as the better-off. Growing consumerism in the medical market-place at this time also helped in the wider dissemination of new hygienic ideas. James Graham (1745–94), the purveyor of the magneto-electrical 'Celestial Bed' for the cure of impotency and sterility, was an evangelical Christian and entrepreneur who popularized vegetarianism. However, there were more far-reaching attempts to bring hygienic knowledge and practices to the poorer parts of society.

In the sixteenth and seventeenth centuries, a sense of charity had led to the publication of treatises on medicine for the poor. These were usually collections of inexpensive recipes for medicines, as the immensely popular *Le Médecin des pauvres* (1669) by Paul Dubé, or ΠΤΩΧΟΦΑΡΜΑΚΟΝ ... *Help for the Poor* (1653) by Robert Pemel. Sometimes, as in the *Traité de la conservation de santé* by Philibert Guybert (*c.*1579–1633), part of his *Oeuvres du médecin charitable* (1653, 6th edn), advice on regimen, in this case structured on the non-naturals, was given to the poor.

In the eighteenth century, there was added to simple charity, a sense that the poor needed to be educated, to be enlightened out of their 'ignorance' and 'superstitions' in matters of health. For John Wesley, this was a religious as well as a medical ignorance. In his *Primitive Physick*, as well as providing medical prescriptions and hygienic advice (the latter drawn from Cheyne), Wesley put health and illness into a religious context. The Fall of man produced 'the Seeds of Weakness and Pain, of Sickness and Death ... now lodged in our inmost Substance: Whence a thousand Disorders continually spring'.[35] Some of the non-naturals were placed in a biblical context:

> The Heavens, the Earth and all things contain'd therein, conspire to punish the Rebel against their Creator. The Sun and Moon shed unwholesome Influences.... The Air itself that surrounds us on each side is replete with the Shafts of Death. Yea, the food we eat, daily saps the Foundations of Life, which cannot be sustain'd without it. So has the Lord of All secured the Execution of his Decree 'Dust thou art, and into Dust thou shalt return'.[36]

Preventive measures were also seen as having religious origins and legitimations. For instance, exercise:

> One Grand Preventive of Pain and Sickness of various kinds seems intimated by the Great Author of Nature in the very Sentence that intails Death upon us. 'In the Sweat of thy face shalt thou eat bread, till thou return unto the ground.' The Power of Exercise both to preserve and restore Health, is greater than can well be conceiv'd; Especially in those who add Temperance thereto.[37]

Wesley's religious and hygienic message was still personal hygiene rather than public health. But groups and populations started to come under medical scrutiny. In 1700, Bernadino Ramazzini (1633–1714), Professor of the Practice of Medicine at Padua, published his *De Morbis Artificium*, translated into English five years later as *A Treatise of the Diseases of Tradesmen*. He studied a variety of trades and occupations and showed how the specific working conditions of chemists, gilders, glassmakers, painters, blacksmiths, copper and tin workers, surgeons treating venereal cases with mercury, bakers, and many others were conducive to diseases. The poor, as a group, were also seen as more susceptible to disease. Simon-André Tissot (1728–97), Professor of Medicine in Lausanne, stated that the poor in the countryside of Switzerland suffered the highest mortality and morbidity rates of all – thus reversing the traditional view of the healthiness of the countryside and of those who laboured in it. In his *Avis au peuple sur la santé* (1761), Tissot (founder of the famous cuckoo-clock firm) used a traditional environmental and life-style approach when discussing hygiene or the prevention of disease. The ills of country people were caused by excessive work, by great poverty and not enough food, by drinking cold water when hot, or lying in a cold place, by having dunghills under their windows and not airing their rooms, and by building houses on low-lying marshy land. Some of these causes could be avoided, but excessive work and famine could not, though they might be ameliorated. Some of the habits of country people, Tissot believed, were still examples for the healthy life. Exercise, if moderate, staying in the open air, going to bed early and rising very early, could be models for people in the cities. Tissot's hygiene was still concerned with life-style and environment as determinants of health, but it does mark a shift in which traditional hygienic theory is put to the use of public health. Tissot's work reflects one component of public health, the emphasis on the group or population rather than on the individual. But another component is not present. It is not until the state enforces the norms of hygiene upon a group of people or a country that we can properly talk of public health (it had happened earlier during the outbreaks of plague and was to happen again in the nineteenth century). (➤ Ch. 50 Medical institutions and the state)

The popular work by William Buchan (1729–1805) entitled *Domestic Medicine* (1769) occupies a similar half-way stage between private and public hygiene. The work allows us an insight into the reasons for the shift and a look forward to nineteenth-century developments. Buchan's was a work of the Enlightenment. The need to educate, to enlighten, the poor into health was present in Tissot's work, but Buchan made it very explicit. The social framework into which he placed the poor was a traditional one: they could not afford doctors and had to rely on themselves, on others equally ignorant, or on the charity of 'the better sort of people in the county in assisting their poor neighbours in distress', for, 'it never was, and, in all probability, never will be in the power of one half of mankind to obtain the assistance of physicians, what must they do?'[38] In a typical Enlightenment vein, redolent with the sense of knowledge fighting ignorance through education, Buchan wrote that:

> The ignorant rustic puts little confidence in any endeavours of his own. All his hopes of a cure are placed in something which he does not understand, something mysterious and quite above his capacity, as herbs gathered under the influence of some planet, charms, the nostrums of quacks and conjurers. Such are the ridiculous and destructive prejudices, which prevail among the inhabitants of this country, even in this enlightened age, and such is their entire ignorance of medicine, that they become the easy dupes of every pretender to it.[39]

The solution was that the 'better sort of people' would bring light where there was ignorance:

> the ladies, gentlemen, and clergy who reside in the country . . . will teach the poor the importance of a proper regimen both in health and in sickness; the danger of trusting their lives in the hands of quacks and conjurers, and the folly of their own superstitious notions.[40]

It was no longer the rich or the studious who needed hygienic advice and education.

Diatribes against quacks and refutations of popular errors and ignorance had been written in previous centuries, but there is a new note here. The identification of the poor with ignorance and superstition is very strong, as is the wish to educate them in an almost coercive sense, something that is found even more strongly in the nineteenth-century campaigns that were concerned with the physical and moral hygienic cleanliness of the poor. Buchan connected dirt with the poor, as did writers in the next century, for instance, during the cholera outbreaks of the nineteenth century. (➤ Ch. 19 Fevers; Ch. 16 Contagion/germ theory/specificity; Ch. 52 Epidemiology) Buchan used a mixture of the theory of contagion and environmental (miasmatic) and dietary reasoning drawn from traditional hygiene to associate the poor with dirt, disease, and danger to others:

> One common cause of putrid and malignant fevers is the want of cleanliness. These fevers commonly begin among the inhabitants of close, dirty houses, who breathe bad air, take little exercise, use unwholsome food and wear dirty cloaths. There the infection is generally hatched, which often spreads far and wide to the destruction of many. Hence cleanliness may be considered as an object of public attention. It is not sufficient that I be clean myself, while the want of it in my neighbour affects my health as well as his own. If dirty people cannot be removed as a common nuisance, they ought at least to be avoided as infectious.[41]

The wish for state involvement and for coercion, its frequent accompaniment, is clearly present. Buchan's move towards public health is also evident in his concern with groups of people. As well as the poor, he wrote of the Navy, Army, and especially of 'mechanics', 'that useful set of people, upon whom the riches and prosperity of Britain depend, can never be too much regarded. Their valuable lives are frequently lost for want of due attention to circumstances which both to themselves and others may appear trifling.'[42]

This is not quite the same as Edwin Chadwick (1800–90) in the nineteenth century justifying the cost of public health with the argument that it pays a country to have a healthy workforce. The help to be given to Buchan's mechanics was either self-help or small-scale charitable help, reflecting a society in which ties of mutual obligation and reciprocity had not yet been replaced by the large-scale anonymous, uniform, and standardizing public-health measures of the state. (➤ Ch. 62 Charity before 1850)

Buchan's hygiene and therapeutics was traditional; he wrote that

> in the treatment of diseases we have been chiefly attentive to diet, drink, air and the other parts of regimen. Regimen seems to have been the chief, if not the only medicine of the more early ages, and to say the truth it is the most valuable part of medicine still.[43]

The transformation in hygiene that occurred between the later eighteenth century and the nineteenth century was not essentially in its theories (though the theory of contagion was apparent in Buchan's work and, before him, in the plague policies of governments). The change was that a theory that had applied to individuals was applied to groups and to populations. As Philip Curtin has shown, the mortality rate in the British Army abroad improved during the eighteenth and nineteenth century. In its stations in the British West Indies, India, and the West African coast, the Army focused on the environment of its troops. It improved ventilation in its buildings, built hill stations in airy situations and tried to ensure purer water supplies.[44] The hygiene theory that acted as the motor for these measures was the environmental and climatological one drawn from classical hygiene.

Elsewhere in this *Encyclopedia* the reader can find further aspects of the transition from private to public hygiene. (➤ Ch. 51 Public health) For instance, the increased use of statistics as seen in the works of Thomas Short (d. 1772); or in the massive inquiry organized by Vicq d'Azyr (1748–94) and the Société Royale de Médecine, carried out in the last thirty years of the eighteenth century in France, which tried to relate health and disease to topology, climate, and people's life-styles. As James Riley has pointed out, the number of variables in such studies was unmanageably high, but this was part of the nature of traditional hygiene.[45] These statistical and epidemiological studies are further indications that medicine was adding a public dimension to hygiene. However, the theoretical basis of hygiene also underwent change, gradual and hardly visible at first, but very apparent in the nineteenth century. (➤ Ch. 59 Internationalism in medicine and public health)

HYGIENE AND CLEANLINESS

Cleanliness had never been absent from traditional classical hygiene. Dirt in air, perhaps coming from the exhalations and miasmas of dunghills, latrines, and sewers, was considered harmful to the constitution, as was dirty water or the food produced from animals living in dirty conditions. Moreover, bathing, both for pleasure and for medicinal purposes (here, I include both hygiene and therapeutics), had been common from classical times. However, social historians have pointed out that a strong argument can be made that the emphasis on personal cleanliness in the eighteenth and nineteenth centuries came about for social rather than medical reasons. Georges Vigarello, in *Concepts of Cleanliness*,[46] has traced the decline of public bathing from the Middle Ages and especially the Renaissance to the eighteenth century, as it came to be associated in the mind of authority with tumults, prostitution, and crime. Bathing did continue at some spas for medicinal purposes. But private bathing, which from classical times was undertaken infrequently and which had connotations of luxury and effeminacy (it was also felt to be medically dangerous, as it opened up the pores and so allowed miasmatic pestilential air to invade the body), was taken up by the eighteenth-century French nobility. At the same time, clothing and cleanliness changed their relationship. Vigarello shows how cleanliness in the Middle Ages and early Renaissance was concerned with the outermost clothes: if they were clean and bright that was enough. When linen begun to be used and to be changed more frequently in the sixteenth and seventeenth centuries, the whiteness and cleanliness of the linen, hidden by the outer clothes and lying next to the skin, became a necessary mark of good breeding (though the quotation from the *Tacuinum* cited on p. 1289 suggests that the association between linen and brightness – that is, cleanliness – was even earlier). This interiorization of cleanliness proceeded until it reached the skin, with the use of baths in the eighteenth and nineteenth centuries. A clean or dirty skin was normally hidden from sight: perfumes and powders had often been used to disguise bodily smells. Keeping one's skin clean was, therefore, policed not by others but by oneself, by an internal sense of what were good manners (or by an internal sense of guilt), to which the discoveries of Pasteurian medicine were to give added weight. Underlying this account is the work of Norbert Elias (*The Civilizing Process*, and *The Court Society*),[47] who shows how the French nobility developed more elaborate and more civilized manners from the later seventeenth century to distinguish themselves from the up-and-coming French bourgeoisie (and in the process were changed, so that they were no longer a powerful group able to threaten the French Crown). The irony is that the middle classes did continue to ape the manners of the nobility. In the nineteenth century, baths and washbasins (and, in France, bidets to some extent) were given their own room in middle-class homes, and the wider availability of water, and the encouragement to use it, made cleanliness a sign of civilized gentility and of good social order. Those who were not clean (the poor) lay outside the pale of society. Wesley had used the rabbinical phrase 'cleanliness is next to Godliness', and the moral and hygienic benefits of cleanliness came to be closely associated.

The sociologists' case for the cleanliness craze of the nineteenth century might be overstated. The cleanliness and dirt of air, water, and food was of concern to hygiene from Greek times on. The regulations for street-cleaning, for the disposal of nuisances such as dung-heaps, and for food markets in European cities from the Middle Ages onwards also attest to a civic concern with cleanliness (though in practice, it was not very effective). Nevertheless, it is true to say that until recently, Europe was a dirty place; certainly, other cultures thought so. The Dutch, at the beginning of the seventeenth century, described with some wonder the clean habits of the Africans of the Guinea coast:

> They are curious to keepe their bodies cleane, and often wash and scoure them ... they are very careful not to let a Fart, if any bodie be by them; they wonder at our Netherlanders, that use it so commonly, for they cannot abide that a man should Fart before them, esteeming it to be a great shame and contempt done unto them; when they ease themselves they commonly goe in the morning to the Townes end (where there is a place purposely made for them) that they should not be seene, as also because men passing by should not be molested by the smell thereof, they also esteeme it a bad thing that men should ease themselves upon the ground, and therefore they make houses which are borne up above the ground, wherein they ease themselves, and every time they done it they wipe; or else they goe to the water side, to ease themselves in the sand, and when these Privie-houses are full, they set fire in them, and let them burne to ashes.[48]

This contrasts with the Roman habit that lasted into the Middle Ages of communal latrines and the communal use of a sponge placed on a stick. Or, with Samuel Pepys (1633–1703), who noted 'I was forced ... to rise and shit in the chimny twice' when he visited a strange house and was not provided with a chamber-pot for the night. (Or, again the contrast can be made with the court of Charles II, which had fled the plague in 1665 for the colleges of Oxford, 'leaving at their departure their excrements in every corner, in chimneys, studies, coal houses, cellars'.)[49] The distaste of other cultures for European ideas of cleanliness is also reflected in the curse of the nomadic Tartars who, as Richard Johnson recounted in the sixteenth century, when they cursed their children wished them to 'tary so long in a place that thou mightest smell thine owne dung, as the Christians doe'.[50]

By the nineteenth century, the situation had reversed itself. Westerners perceived themselves as clean and the rest of the world as dirty. Edward S. Morse (1838–1925), in his article 'Latrines of the East', saw the filth of the Orient as a menace to Europe and proposed that oriental countries should be invaded with missionaries of hygiene:

> The nations of Europe stand in periodical dread of cholera from the regions lying east of them. The Orient stands as a continual menace to the nations of Europe, and the time may not be far distant when a propaganda in the interests of sanitary science shall invade these countries with their missionaries of hygiene to teach the people the gospel of cleanliness. That the masses might be ready to receive such teaching is shown by the success accompanying the efforts of medical missionaries beyond that of those who teach dogma alone.[51]

As with other aspects of colonialism, the non-white races were viewed as analogous to the poor whites: dirty, uneducated and of a low moral and hygienic standard (and so potentially dangerous). The association of dirt and faeces with foreign, non-European races is illustrated by the ethnographic work of the American John G. Bourke (1846–96), whose *Scatalogic Rites of All Nations* (1891) takes an interest in faeces to be a cultural characteristic of 'primitive' races. (➤ Ch. 60 Medicine and anthropology)

How did Europe's perception of dirt change so radically in the nineteenth century? As well as the social origins of a concern with cleanliness discussed on pp. 1300–1, and the discovery in the second half of the nineteenth century of pathogens such as bacteria which were associated with dirt, the development of public health is a major factor. For, as well as clean water supplies, food, cities, and houses, people also had to be clean in their habits. Up to the time of Pasteur (1822–95) (and beyond), traditional environmental and miasmatic theory was the vehicle for the new emphasis on cleanliness. Education, it was believed, would play a crucial role. For instance, in 1882, hygiene was included in the curriculum of French primary schools, and the proper use of the toilet and of washing was taught. At the same time, regular inspections of the cleanliness of children was instituted. Jean-Pierre Goubert has shown how, in the schools, morality was inseparable from hygiene. As the Director of Primary Education expressed it in a circular to the primary schools of Paris in 1872: 'Cleanliness is almost always an element in an indication of moral attitudes.'[52]

The association between cleanliness and morality became very general and pervasive as the nineteenth century progressed. In the process, the old meaning of hygiene as health in general changed and fragmented. Cleanliness became a constant theme, but it could be social, moral, and racial as well as physical cleanliness. For example, at the beginning of the nineteenth century, Thomas Beddoes (1760–1808) had written his *Hygëia or Essays Moral and Medical on the Causes Affecting the Personal State of our Middling and Affluent Classes* (1802–3). Beddoes condemned the affluent life-style of the commercial classes that flourished in newly industrialized imperial England. Too many comforts and too much wealth created anxiety and illness. In Beddoes's three volumes, hygiene still meant health, and though the amalgam of morality and medicine was already present, it was mainly directed at the rich.[53] When in 1876 Benjamin Ward Richardson (1828–96) produced his Utopian vision of *Hygëia. A City of Health*, there was also medical moralizing, but its context and target were very different. His was a city to be built mainly for the less well-off; in it, there would be no alcohol, tobacco, or gambling, it would be 'a total abstainers town'.[54] Richardson's ideal city, constructed in the aftermath of Chadwick (one of his heroes) on the principles of sanitarian science and technology, produced morally ideal citizens. (In the nineteenth century, it became a truism amongst reformers that if the physical conditions of the poor, both in terms of public and personal hygiene, were made clean, then their morals almost inevitably would also be sparkling white.) And elsewhere, Richardson wrote: 'Let us cleanse our outward garments, our bodies, our food, our drink, and keep them cleansed. Let us cleanse our minds, as well as our garments and keep them clean.'[55]

The 'Great Unwashed', the poor, were the objects of the new hygiene, and as the phrase indicates, of stigmatization. They were given the means to become clean. In the second half of the nineteenth century, municipalities built a large number of public baths, often ornate palaces of the sanitary ideal. By this means, public health facilitated private hygiene. In 1852, almost 2,778,400 baths were taken in the public baths of Paris; in London, by 1912, there were over 3,000,000 visits to the public baths. Housing, sewerage, and water regulations also had the indirect effects of providing the conditions that would enable a personal hygiene of cleanliness to be put into practice. At the same time, the use of soap spread from the middle classes to the working classes. Men such as William Lever (1851–1925), who began by selling Sunlight soap in 1886, made fortunes from soap manufacture, which became an industrial commodity in its own right. More slowly, other practices, such as the use of toothpaste and toothbrushes, spread through Western society. Underpinning the emphasis on personal cleanliness was the fear of infection. Miasmatic and environmentalist theories had stressed that dirt at both the public level (dunghills, poor sewers, etc.) and the personal level (not washing hands) led to infection. Then, the work of Lister (1827–1912) and Pasteur in the second half of the nineteenth century and the emphasis on aseptic operating-theatres and hospitals also acted as a powerful example for domestic and personal cleanliness. (➤ Ch. 42 Surgery (modern); Ch. 49 The hospital)

Today, there may be less awareness of the need for cleanliness, for the discovery of antibiotics means that we no longer have to fear that the slightest infected cut might be fatal.

Not only did cleanliness reach the skin, it also went deep into the body. The creed of inner cleanliness was a popular one. The London surgeon William Arbuthnot Lane (1856–1943) believed that the body's wastes could poison it. In the 1900s and 1910s, he advised ileosigmoidostomy and colectomy, or the use of paraffin oil, to avoid the ills which he believed were caused by the autointoxication from the faeces that civilized men and women retained too long in their gut (was there an analogy here with the dangers that cesspits and sewers were thought to pose in the larger public world?). At a more popular and enduring level, John Harvey Kellogg (1852–1943) made his fortune by selling cereals such as All-Bran, so that Americans could avoid the same dangers.[56] Beauty as well as health was associated with inner cleanliness. An advertisement for Andrews' Liver Salts claimed in 1939: 'and finally – to complete your Inner Cleanliness – Andrews gently cleans the bowels, sweeping away impurities that thicken your figure and coarsen your skin'.[57]

However, the strong social and religious components of the new hygiene indicate that we are faced with a large-scale cultural transformation (something hinted at by the advertisement quoted above) and not just a change in medical knowledge and technology (such as the invention and provision of flush-toilets). A sign of this is the way hygiene entered into debates on the 'fitness of the race', that so concerned commentators in the nineteenth and early twentieth centuries (and later the 'racial hygiene' or 'purity' of the Nazi period). Dirt, poor hygiene, and slum conditions could produce a population of poor stature permeated by ill health. In the first half of the nineteenth century, it was argued that changing sanitary conditions and hygienic habits could improve the situation. On the other hand, some eugenicists, in the aftermath of concern with the possible physical deterioration of recruits to the British Army (sparked by the Army's performance in the Boer War), argued the opposite. As Dr J. B. Haycraft put it, 'I do not see how we can shirk the fact that preventative medicine and civilization between them have already deteriorated in a marked degree the healthy vigour of our race.'[58] Behind such sentiments lay the belief that Darwinian natural selection should be allowed to operate within human society. (➤ Ch. 37 History of medical ethics)

One irony is that the European peasant, terrified of baths and their debilitating effects, would, from his or her cultural viewpoint, have heartily agreed with the eugenists' conclusion. Another irony is that it does appear as if a combination of public and personal hygienic measures, together with better diet, transformed the European regime of mortality and morbidity (the precise contribution to this represented by diet and public and personal hygiene is a matter of debate). But as Thomas McKeown pointed out, infectious diseases, the killers of the young, began to disappear before the advent of effective medical drugs like sulphonamides and antibiotics.[59] (➤ Ch. 39 Drug therapies) Europe made the transition to a demographic regime in which people lived longer and died from chronic rather than acute diseases. It partly did so because people washed their hands, their bodies, and their houses; learned not to spit in public, killed flies, kept food from going bad, and learned through education to do those things which today help to keep us well and alive and which we almost do automatically and without thinking. If the new hygiene represents a cultural change, it was also a change with profound medical consequences. (➤ Ch. 72 Medicine, mortality, and morbidity)

NOTES

1 Galen, *A Translation of Galen's Hygiene (De Sanitate Tuenda) by Robert Green*, Springfield, IL, C. C. Thomas, 1951, pp. 5, 17.

2 Hippocrates, *Regimen in Health* (I), in *Works*, Vol. IV, trans. by W. H. S. Jones, London, William Heinemann, and Cambridge, MA, Harvard University Press, 1931, p. 45.

3 Ibid. (II), pp. 47–9.

4 Hippocrates, op. cit. (n. 2) (II: XXXVIII, XLVI, LIV), pp. 305, 317–19, 333.

5 Hippocrates, op. cit. (n. 2) (III: LXVIII), p. 371.

6 Galen, op. cit. (n. 1), p. 80.

7 Hippocrates, op. cit. (n. 2) (I), pp. 44–5; op. cit. (n. 4), (III: LXIX), p. 381.

8 Galen, op. cit. (n. 1), p. 51.

9 Ibid., p. 51.

10 Galen, op. cit. (n. 1), p. 23.

11 Galen, op. cit. (n. 1), p. 195.

12 On this see T. S. Hall, 'Life, death and the radical moisture', *Clio Medica*, 1971, 6: 3–23; Peter H. Niebyl, 'Old age, fever and the lamp metaphor', *Journal of the History of Medicine*, 1971, 26: 351–68; Michael McVaugh, 'The "humidum radicale" in 13th century medicine', *Traditio*, 1974: 259–83.

13 See L. J. Rather, 'The "six things non-natural": a note on the origins and fate of a doctrine and a phrase', *Clio Medica*, 1968, 3: 337–47; Saul Jarcho, 'Galen's six non-naturals: a bibliographic note and translation', *Bulletin of the History of Medicine*, 1970, 44: 372–7.

14 Jarcho, ibid., p. 376 (Kühn 1, 367).

15 Robert Burton, *The Anatomy of Melancholy*, London, 1621, part 1, sec. 1, memb. 1, subs. 1, and part 1, sec. 2, memb. 2, subs. 1, cited in Rather, op. cit. (n. 13), p. 337. The first passage goes on to state that the six non-natural things 'are the causes of our infirmities, our surfeiting and drunkenness, our immoderate insatiable lust and prodigious riot'. The potential of the six non-naturals for moralizing and for discourses on temperance is clear.

16 Luisa Cogliati Arano, *The Medieval Health Handbook. Tacuinum Sanitatis*, New

York, George Braziller, 1976, Pl. XIV, XVIII, XXXV, XLII, XLIII, (refers to a number of different manuscripts).

17 Ibid., Pl. VIII, XLIV, XLV.

18 Ibid., Pl. XLVI, XLVII.

19 Oderico da Genova, *De Regenda Sanitate Consilium*, ed. by Fortunato Cirenei, Vol. XXV: *Scientia veterum*, Genoa, University of Genoa, 1961; Wolfram Schmitt, 'Bartholomaüs Scherrenmüllers Gesundsheit Regimen (1493) für Graf Eberhard im Bart', unpublished MD thesis, Ruprecht-Karl-Universität-Heidelberg, 1970.

20 Gugliermo Gratarolo, *De Literatorum et eorum qui Magistratibus funguntur Conservanda Praeservandaque Valetudine*, Basle, H. Petri, 1555.

21 Paul Slack, 'Mirrors of health and treasures of poor men: the uses of the vernacular medical literature of Tudor England', in Charles Webster (ed.), *Health, Medicine and Mortality in the Sixteenth Century*, Cambridge, Cambridge University Press, 1979, pp. 237–73.

22 Richard Palmer, 'Health, hygiene and longevity in medieval and renaissance Europe', in Íosio Kawakita, Shizu Sakai and Íasuo Otsuka (eds), *History of Hygiene*, Proceedings of the 12th International Symposium on the Comparative History of Medicine – East and West, Tokyo, Ishiyaku EuroAmerica, 1991, pp. 75–98.

23 Ibid., pp. 87–9.

24 On southern parts of North America, see Karen Kupperman, 'Fear of hot climates in the Anglo-American colonial experience', *William and Mary Quarterly*, 1984, 41: 213–40.

25 See Mary Dobson, 'Mortality gradients and disease exchanges: comparisons from old England and colonial America', *Social History of Medicine*, 1989, 2: 259–97; and Dobson, ' "Marsh fever": a geography of malaria in England', *Journal of Historical Geography*, 1980, 6: 359–89.

26 See Andrew Wear, 'Making sense of health and the environment in early modern England', in Wear (ed.), *Medicine in Society, Historical Essays*, Cambridge, Cambridge University Press, 1992, pp. 119–47.

27 Louis Cornaro, *The Art of Living Long*, trans. by W. F. Butler, Milwaukee, WI, William Butler, 1903, p. 40.

28 Ibid., p. 41.

29 Cornaro, op. cit. (n. 27), p. 58.

30 Virginia Smith, 'Prescribing the rules of health: self-help and advice in the late eighteenth century', in Roy Porter (ed.), *Patients and Practitioners. Lay Perceptions of Medicine in Pre-industrial Society*, Cambridge, Cambridge University Press, 1985, pp. 249–82; Smith, 'Physical puritanism and sanitary science: material and immaterial beliefs in popular physiology, 1650–1840', in W. F. Bynum and Roy Porter (eds), *Medical Fringe and Medical Orthodoxy 1750–1850*, London, Croom Helm, 1987, pp. 174–97.

31 John Floyer, *An Enquiry into the Right Use and Abuses of the Hot, Cold and Temperate Baths in England*, London, R. Clavel, 1697, preface; cited by Smith, 'Physical puritanism', op. cit. (n. 30), pp. 179–80.

32 See Roy Porter and Dorothy Porter, *In Sickness and in Health*, London, Fourth Estate, 1988, pp. 27–9.

33 Keith Thomas, *Man and the Natural World. Changing Attitudes in England*

1500–1800, Harmondsworth, Penguin, 1984, pp. 287–302; also Smith, op. cit. (n. 30).

34 Dorothy Porter and Roy Porter, *Patient's Progress. Doctors and Doctoring in Eighteenth-Century England*, Oxford, Polity Press, 1989, pp. 93–4 (from D. A. Ponsonby, *Call a Dog Hervey*, London, Hutchinson, 1949, p. 48).

35 John Wesley, *Primitive Physick*, London, T. Trye, 1747, p. iii.

36 Ibid., pp. iv-v.

37 Westley, op. cit. (n. 35), p. v.

38 William Buchan, *Domestic Medicine*, Edinburgh, Balfour, Auld & Smellie, 1769, pp. xii-xiii.

39 Ibid., p. xiii.

40 Buchan, op. cit. (n. 38), p. xiii.

41 Buchan, op. cit. (n. 38), p. 89.

42 Buchan, op. cit. (n. 38), p. xi.

43 Buchan, op. cit. (n. 38), p. xii.

44 Philip D. Curtin, *Death by Migration*, Cambridge, Cambridge University Press, 1989.

45 James C. Riley, *The Eighteenth-Century Campaign to Avoid Disease*, London, Macmillan, 1987, pp. 47–8, 146–50.

46 Georges Vigarello, *Concepts of Cleanliness. Changing Attitudes in France from the Middle Ages*, Cambridge, Cambridge University Press, 1988.

47 Norbert Elias, *The Civilizing Process*, 2 vols, Oxford, Blackwell, 1978–82; Elias, *The Court Society*, Oxford, Blackwell, 1983.

48 Samuel Purchas, 'A description and historical declaration of the golden kingdome of Guinea. . . . Translated out of Dutch', in *Hakluytus Posthumus or Purchas his Pilgrimes*, 20 vols, Glasgow, James MacLehose, 1905, Vol. VI, p. 265.

49 Robert Latham and William Matthews (eds), *The Diary of Samuel Pepys*, London, Bell & Hyman, 1972, Vol. VI p. 244 (28 September 1665); Terence McLoughlin, *Coprophilia or a Peck of Dirt*, London, Cassell, 1971, p. 89, citing Anthony à Wood.

50 'Certain notes unperfectly written by Richard Johnson . . . 1556', in Richard Hakluyt, *The Principal Navigations, Voyages, Traffiques and Discoveries of the English Nation*, London, George Bishop, Ralph Newberie & Robert Baker, 1599, Vol. I, p. 284.

51 Edward S. Morse, 'Latrines of the east', *American Architect*, 18 March 1893: 1–18.

52 Jean-Pierre Goubert, *The Conquest of Water. The Advent of Health in the Industrial Age*, Oxford, Polity Press, 1989, p. 153.

53 On Beddoes, see Roy Porter, *Doctor of Society. Thomas Beddoes and the Sick Trade in Late-Enlightenment England*, London, Routledge, 1992.

54 Benjamin Ward Richardson, *Hygeia. A City of Health*, London, Macmillan, 1876, p. 29.

55 Lloyd G. Stevenson, 'Science down the drain', *Bulletin of the History of Medicine*, 1955, 29: 1–27; citing Benjamin Ward Richardson, *Biological Experimentation: its Function and Limits*, 1896, p. 101.

56 See James C. Whorton, 'Inner hygiene: the philosophy and practice of intestinal

purity in Western civilization', in Kawakita, Sakai and Otsuka, op. cit. (n. 22), pp. 1–31.

57 *Picture Post*, 1939, 3, (5): 67.

58 Anthony S. Wohl, *Endangered Lives. Public Health in Victorian Britain*, London, Methuen, 1984, p. 334.

59 Thomas McKeown, *The Modern Rise of Population*, London, Edward Arnold, 1976; for modifications and disagreements see Simon Szreter, 'The importance of social intervention in Britain's mortality decline *c.* 1850–1914: a re-interpretation of the role of public health', *Social History of Medicine*, 1988, 1: 1–37; Alex Mercer, *Disease, Mortality and Population in Transition*, Leicester, Leicester University Press, 1990.

FURTHER READING

Corbin, Alain, *The Foul and the Fragrant. Odour and the French Social Imagination*, Leamington Spa, Berg, 1986.

Goubert, Jean-Pierre, *The Conquest of Water. The Advent of Health in the Industrial Age*, Oxford, Polity Press, 1989.

Kawakita, Yosio, Sakai, Shizu, and Otsuka, Yasuo (eds), *History of Hygiene. Proceedings of the 12th International Symposium on the Comparative History of Medicine – East and West*, Tokyo, Ishiyaku EuroAmerica, 1991.

McLoughlin, Terence, *Coprophilia or a Peck of Dirt*, London, Cassell, 1971.

Reyburn, Wallace, *Flushed with Pride. The Story of Thomas Crapper*, London, Macdonald, 1969.

Sigerist, Henry, *Landmarks in the History of Hygiene*, Oxford, Oxford University Press, 1956.

Temkin, Owsei, 'An historical analysis of the concept of infection', in Temkin, *The Double Face of Janus and Other Essays in the History of Medicine*, Baltimore, MD, Johns Hopkins University Press, 1977, pp. 456–71.

Tomes, Nancy, 'The private side of public health: sanitary science, domestic hygiene, and the germ theory, 1870–1900', *Bulletin of the History of Medicine*, 1990, 64: 509–39.

Vigarello, Georges, *Concepts of Cleanliness. Changing Attitudes in France in the Middle Ages*, Cambridge, Cambridge University Press, 1988.

54

A GENERAL HISTORY OF NURSING: 1800–1900

Christopher Maggs

INTRODUCTION

We can, with relative precision, date the emergence of modern nursing as a paid and trained occupation in the United Kingdom, from 1880. The significance of this date, which does not deny the prior existence of nurses nor ignore the fact that in other countries it happened later, lies in the rapid expansion of hospital-based training programmes and of the rise in the number of women recorded as nurses within the census. These changes coincided with and were predicated on the re-emergence of the hospital as the ideological and epistemological centre of medical activity.[1]

In 1801, there were approximately 4,000 general hospital beds in the whole of the United Kingdom, most of then in England and Wales, serving a population of some 10 million. By the end of the century, there were 28,000 general beds in England and Wales, for a population of about 32 million. So far as we can estimate, before 1861 there were less than 1,000 'nurses'; by 1901, the estimated number of nurses was approaching 70,000. Of these, only 10 per cent were working in the hospital sector – in general, fever, special, Poor Law, or voluntary hospitals.[2] However, the majority of these 'new' nurses had either experience of working in a hospital or were 'trained' nurses, with a certificate from the training institution. By 1901, nurses could receive formal training not just in the voluntary and teaching hospitals, but throughout the Poor Law service itself. Indeed, the state had quietly begun the regulation of its nursing work-force long before the emerging profession began its demands for registration. (➤ Ch. 49 The hospital; Ch. 50 Medical institutions and the state)

Whilst similar chages can be seen in other countries, including the United States of America, they differ in the degree to which the state itself became involved in the production of the new nursing workforce. Reverby has chronicled the development of nursing in the USA, using the Boston area as a case study.[3] Other scholars, including Melosh, have added to our understanding of the separate and distinct pattern of development of nursing in the USA. These authors draw attention to the virtual absence of state intervention, reflecting the federal structure of government in the North American continent. Another important difference between the UK and USA experience has been the involvement of universities in the development of nursing through education.[4] According to Davies, this led to an emphasis on 'education for excellence' in the USA, compared with an emphasis on achieving the minimum standards in the UK. As a consequence, the growth of a body of nursing knowledge has tended towards being USA-centred and -led, whilst in the UK, the emphasis has been largely on the daily practice of nursing.

This is clearly shown in early nursing textbooks. In England, they resembled manuals for improving the skills of the middle-class housewife with whom the nurse was compared, and consequently authors stressed the importance of diet, quiet, decorum, and cleanliness. By the end of the century, and under the influence of the contacts with North American nursing leaders and programmes, nursing textbooks included chapters on anatomy and physiology, drugs and measurement, physics and chemistry, bandaging, care of tracheostomies, the use of inhalations and steam therapies, and the origins of nursing and nursing ethics.

Popular fiction of the early nineteenth century provides an additional source for the study of nursing. Popular novels from Dickens to Trollope portrayed the nurse either as a selfless wife or relative, a drunkard, or a potential mistress. In turn-of-the-century novels, the nurse was often depicted as a woman choosing to follow a career, perhaps after rejecting a marriage proposal, but a career for which she needed to be educated and trained. No longer was nursing something that any woman could do; it was an occupation that only the trained could do well.

The introduction of the notion of nursing as an occupation and as a career was aided by public debate about the pay and conditions of employment for women in general, and nurses in particular. Women working as nurses before the reforms – before nursing laid claims to professional status – were employed and paid as casual labour, by the case. There was little opportunity to develop any allegiance other than to the individual patient and family or, for a few, to a particular doctor or 'consultant'. (➤ Ch. 38 Women and medicine) With training and career came a structured wage system and relatively standard conditions of employment. New entrants often rceived no pay for the first one or two years of their training; thereafter, they received a small allowance of an average £18 per annum. As trainees, they were required to be in residence, and most (but not all) received free board and lodgings and uniform. Once qualified, the pay rose by annual increments from an average of £20 per annum to £35 per annum as a senior nurse. Qualified nurses had to pay for their board and lodgings, although most continued to receive free uniforms.

Those nurses who left the hospital sector for the community returned to the tradition of piece-work, generally being paid by the case. Growing numbers turned to working for agencies in an attempt to maintain a steady income rather than having to rely on the vagaries of the market. Others sought further qualifications – such as midwifery or massage – to extend the range of skills they could offer and thus increase their periods of employment. (➤ Ch. 40 Physical methods)

Between 1860 and 1900, nursing was transformed from being small-scale, mainly untrained and freelance work for a few women into an organized and controlled occupation, employing a growing number of lower-middle- and upper-working-class women.[5] How did such a shift take place? What factors contributed to this change, which many contemporaries and some historians labelled a 'revolution'? Was it simply the fortuitous coincidence of reformers and the need for reform, or were there more significant processes at work?

BACKGROUND

There can be no single 'History of Nursing, only histories'.[6] This aphorism is worth remembering as we embark on this particular study of the development of modern nursing. It may well prove impossible to disengage the historical development of nursing from other, perhaps more important, social, political, and economic changes. The impact of industrialization has had a more significant role in nursing than advances in medical science. Indeed, there may be less direct relationship between medical science and nursing, and rather more between the changing position of men and women in society.[7] Nevertheless, there is a need to try and uncover key events and processes that have brought about contemporary nursing.

It is also the case that most histories of nursing so far published are, in fact and in the main, histories of nurses. Whether the concern has been with reformers and leaders, such as Elizabeth Fry (1780–1845) or Florence Nightingale (1820–1910), or with the institutionalization of nursing care, we know more about nurses than about the practice of nursing. We know, that is, who the nurses were, where they came from, and their intraprofessional rivalries with each other, with doctors, and with lay administrators. However, we still know very little about what they did for patients. Where our knowledge of practice is better, it is often only because it has emerged as evidence for professional demarcation disputes. Indeed, as current concerns with measuring the outcomes of nursing interventions show, we know very little about what effect nursing has had on 'health gains'.

This is not to say that contemporaries themselves ignored practice. Indeed, the opposite is the case. Even for those individuals for whom state regulation of nurses became a passion, the starting-point had been difficulties in ensuring safe practice. Ethel Manson (Mrs Fenwick, 1857–1947), a leading state regulationist, began her campaign in the late 1880s with a belief that regulation would ensure safe practitioners for the middle classes in their own homes, a process which would eventually lead to ensuring safe practitioners for the working classes in the hospitals.[8]

The gap in our understanding of the development of nursing is primarily the fault of historians who have ignored what nurses do. For example, Holcombe's study of *Victorian Ladies at Work*,[9] includes a section subtitled 'The working life of hospital nurses', which concerns not 'work' but conditions of service: pay, hours of duty, pensions, and holidays. The case is not as bad as it might be. There are numerous accounts of nursing work in the literature, which provide some evidence for a historical critique of the labour process in nursing. For example, Castle, in a study of the development of nursing at one Australian hospital between 1926 and 1982, draws attention to the use of oral testimony to recreate nursing work.[10] Her respondents recalled using techniques such as linseed poultices, applying dressings, and massage. Vera Brittain (1893–1970) and Enid Bagnold (1889–1981), both Voluntary Aid Detachment (VAD) nurses during the First World War, gave a non-professional insight into nursing duties, which provides a lay perspective on what it was that nurses did.[11]

With perhaps the exception of F. B. Smith, in his study of *The People's Health*,[12] few authors have attempted to chronicle patients' experiences of nursing care. There are a few accounts left by patients themselves which give some insight into nursing practice, although most concern bad rather than good practice.[13] In almost all such accounts, there are many references to the way in which nurses were expected to clean and tidy wards and equipment, and about the imposition of order – real and ideological. Throughout the late nineteenth and early twentieth centuries, the nursing press carried articles and correspondence about the proper duties of the nurse – a less than veiled attack on scrubbing and cleaning. Occasionally, such attacks found their way into a wider press, particularly the growing market of women's journals, where they questioned nursing as a 'respectable career'. In part, this was as a result of the belief, propounded most vociferously by Florence Nightingale, that nursing consisted of two functions. First, nursing the environment in which the patient lay and, second, nursing the patient or assisting the doctor. In organizational terms, nurses could be expected to clean and dust as well as carry out instructions given by doctors.

More recently, feminist historiography has provided a more theoretical evaluation of nursing work. Gamarnikow has deconstructed the cleaning and tidying tasks so frequently discussed and commented upon by nurses, to show how gender relations are manifest in nursing.[14] In some early nursing textbooks, the first role of the nurse became elevated to a science, the science of hygiene, whilst the second became translated as learning about scientific medicine in order to carry out orders better. Linking the two was an ideo-logical bridge of obedience and discipline based on male power and female support. There are also studies in the history of nursing that do not have an explicit conceptual framework but, nevertheless, are part of a theoretical tradition. The prime example is Abel-Smith's seminal study of the growth of professional nursing, now thirty years old.[15] Writing in the tradition of social policy analysis, Abel-Smith provides a detailed account of professional-ization, which includes discussion of key factors such as exclusion of particular groups from full membership of the profession and the challenge of trade unionism versus professional value systems. Others have linked the develop-ment of modern nursing with changes in religion and religious value systems or the impact of war on the broad social fabric. Such theoretical contributions are essential if our understanding of the development of nursing is to pro-gress. (➤ Ch. 61 Religion and medicine; 66 Medicine and modern war)

This essay attempts an overview of the development of modern nursing in the United Kingdom, taking into account the reservations outlined above. It focuses, for example, on examining the relationships between industrialism and nursing work rather than on biographical detail of the leading reformers. It is only through such synthesis that a fuller picture may emerge. In so doing, the essay outlines a historiography for nursing history that provides one model for understanding developments in other countries and societies.

NURSING BEFORE INDUSTRIALIZATION

In its broadest sense, nursing is providing care to those who are ill or suffering. It is, in that sense, a universal human activity, which finds an echo in most human moral codes, whether religious or humanist. However, if we are concerned with nursing as an economic activity, as work, rather than as part of humanity, we need to look for its separation from the universal to the particular. That task is not as straightforward as it might appear. In part, it is difficult because we do not know enough about large tracts of history; in part, it is because to undertake such a quest assumes that nursing is no longer a universal but has indeed become a particular economic activity. In other words, the experience of the development of nursing in our society and those closest to it in structure and beliefs may not be the same as in societies which have evolved in different ways. And, in some senses, to take this approach may mean that we distort what has happened in our own social framework as well. For example, to see nursing as work, as an economic activity, may mean concentrating on waged work to the exclusion of other forms of work. The wise-women who provided nursing care in small communities and within networks (including pregnant women and the dying) in return for payments in cash or in kind may be omitted if we over-emphasize nursing as waged work. Where such people do inhabit historical accounts of the development of nursing, they may be consigned to the backwoods of 'unreformed' nursing to join real and fictional characters like Sairey Gamp and Betsy Prig.[16] (➤ Ch. 65 Medicine and literature)

There is also a danger that, in revising the history of nursing, we may ignore the real contribution made by religion to nursing and to caring. Late nineteenth-century debates about pay and conditions – and indeed, training itself – owe something to this legacy. Baly has chronicled the influence of religious thought and communities, as well as individuals, on the development of nursing in Great Britain.[17] Rose points out that Elizabeth Fry's contribution to nursing was predicated on her Quaker beliefs.[18] The wish to preserve at least some vestige of the religious commitment to care was expressed in statements such as 'nursing is a vocation'. This belief could be pervasive, even in the face of other obvious 'facts'. The introduction of what was becoming the standard three-year nurse training course was held up at the London Hospital until the death of its most influential matron, Eva Luckes, in 1919: McGann notes that 'Miss Luckes believed that nursing was a vocation' and that to become a nurse required a particular 'character' or 'spirit'. In this, she was opposed by members of the London Hospital Board of Governors. Less than one year after her death, they introduced the three-year programme.[19]

Until recent times, it may also be difficult to separate the caring from the curing – the conventional split between nursing and medicine. There are eighteenth-century medical biographies and textbooks which appear to maintain caring as part of curing, at least for patients treated in the community rather than in hospital. This may have something to do with contemporary medical science as well as practice. (➤ Ch. 4 Medical care) Whilst care and cure might be philosophically and conceptually inseparable, the tasks associated with aspects of treating patients could be separated. Novice doctors and surgeons, slaves, the family, friends, and neighbours of the sick or injured person took on the role of caring, leaving the role of curing to the doctor or surgeon. Occasionally, someone might be paid to watch the sick.

This division of labour was not simply based on gender, as it clearly became in the eighteenth and nineteenth centuries. Rather, it was a division based on skill, knowledge, expertise, rank, and time-as-money. With more patients to be seen, the ability of the physician to provide the whole caring/

curing process (if it ever existed) became severely curtailed. Others were needed to take over some of the physician's functions, and these were the tasks and duties which did not require the physician actually to carry them out. They were the tasks that could be dropped from the medical curriculum, as it became crowded with medical science.

INDUSTRIAL CHANGE: THE CONTEXT FOR THE DEVELOPMENT OF NURSING

It is with the impact of industrialization and the growth of industrial society that we can more clearly see and describe the division of labour in health care which explains the development of modern nursing. Despite debate about the nature and timing of industrialization, most historians are agreed that Britain (and perhaps some continental European and North American societies) underwent a fundamental change in the period between 1750 and 1850. That change was not just an economic change but involved the entire social system, from art and culture through education, to politics and beliefs. Once altered, the social structure never returned to its pre-industrial character, and social organizations such as health care were permanently transformed.

A number of reasons may be cited for the emphasis on industrialism. First, the general growth of population not only created more sick people but also provided a greater source of labour to care for them. Second, industrialization brought with it an emphasis on waged work within a new form of work organization. Even where work continued in traditional settings, the impact of the factory system on production transformed the whole world of work. Third, industrialization forced a growing separation of work and home, which contributed to the growth of institutional care for the sick. Fourth, industrialism brought into being a new class structure, a society divided between the working and middle classes, whose experiences and values were radically different. Despite some overlap, the interests of the two classes were irreconcilable, and relationships flared into protest on more than one occasion. One consequence of this new class structure was a resurgence of conscience in those who gained most from the effects of industrial society – the emerging middle class. Finally, although wars are part and parcel of history, the wars and campaigns in the period of industrialization and after resulted in major health-care crises for which the traditional health-care system was unable to provide. Flowing through many of these strands of social change was the changing role of the state and local and central government. Far from being a period of non-interventionist, *laissez faire* government, much of the nineteenth century saw a growing expansion of the role of central government in social affairs, from citizenship through education to health.

The nineteenth century saw the first modern explosion in populations. The population of England and Wales virtually trebled in total between 1801 and 1901. More importantly, the population growth was generally amongst those living in the towns and cities, many of which came into existence as a result of industrialization. Similar events took place in continental Europe and North America.[20] Not only did more people lead to overcrowding and slums, with disease following in its wake, but there was a growing imbalance in the ratio between men and women in the total population. The middle decades became the first of several periods of the 'woman question', as contemporaries struggled to come to terms with the 'surplus of women' in their midst.

Associated with this rapid growth was the mobility of the population which caused social stress and added to the burden of ill health. In particular, migration towards towns and cities and away from rural communities which continued throughout the nineteenth century led to stress on the conventional systems of care. In the towns and cities, in particular in the new industrial areas of the north and the midlands, the industrial climate quickly subverted any attempts to maintain traditional social relationships. Work and family life became increasingly separated for all members of the working-class family unit. Even had it been possible before, industrialization reduced the ability of the working-class family to care for itself. (➤ Ch. 27 Diseases of civilization)

At the same time, within the middle class the separation of home and work expressed itself most starkly in the 'separate spheres' of culture between men and women. Men left the world of work at the door, whilst within, women were expected to create and sustain an ideal of family gentility. Servants were employed to carry out the tasks needed to sustain the tranquility of family life, freeing the women of the middle-class households to develop their skills in household management, and to acquire 'accomplishments' such as music and the arts. For some, there was time to become educated, within the family or, as the century unfolded, in the growing number of schools for middle-class girls which mirrored the characteristics and some of the aspirations of the boys' schools. For most, some form of charitable social-welfare work was obligatory.

The new cities, such as Manchester, Leeds, London, New York, and Chicago, acted as magnets for single men and women in search of new work opportunities. Nursing was one area that offered more than the opportunity to work. Nurse training in the expanding and new hospitals provided accommodation and safety in what were potentially threatening communities.

Industrial society brought with it new ways of working and new areas of employment, in the industrial sector and in the expanding commercial and service sectors. The expansion in the non-industrial sectors was most dramatic after the 1860s and towards the end of the nineteenth century, when inventions such as the sewing-machine and the typewriter coincided with the availability of a new labour force, predominantly female, which was not necessarily preconditioned by what were viewed as outmoded values of the pre-industrial age. These new workers were usually born in the industrial towns and cities and had few, if any, links with traditional, pre-industrial culture. Whilst contemporary explanations for introducing more women to such occupations as clerical work appealed to their dexterity and their predisposition to repetitious and routine work, their true value lay in their lack of attachment to any pre-industrial social values.

The nineteenth century also saw major changes in the way in which Western societies were governed. In Britain, the growing importance of local government was aided by the introduction of the New Poor Law in 1834, and by a series of public-health, housing, and education measures that followed. (➤ Ch. 51 Public health) The very gradual extension of the franchise enhanced the power of local government by broadening its base in society, as well as increasing its ability to control, or attempt to control, local expenditure. At the same time, new central-government departments were created to co-ordinate and act as channels for financial and political accountability for these local-government activities. An expanding and increasingly professional civil service collected information and statistics as part of the accountability process. In turn, central government was more ready, for whatever reasons, to use Commissions of Inquiry and Select Committees of both Houses of Parliament to provide information for the conduct of government. The eventual conflict of interest between local and central government contributed to the relatively slow development of social medicine and health care in Britain.

Just as efficiency became the guiding principle of legislation like the Poor Law and the work of the civil service, so it became the guiding principle in social conscience. Early nineteenth-century philanthropy had been highly individual, a matter between the individual's private conscience and God, although never divorced completely from public approbation. Philanthropy and charity formed an essential aspect of the Christian doctrine and many felt an obligation to do good works. (➤ Ch. 62 Charity before c.1850) By mid-century, reaction was beginning to set in against uncoordinated charity-giving. The scale of need, changes in the needs themselves, an apparent lack of gratitude by some recipients, concern on the part of the middle class to prevent the respectable poor from becoming tainted by welfare, and changed economic circumstances of many donors forced a reappraisal of charity. Under the auspices of the Charity Organization Society, many middle-class benefactors moved from individual acts of philanthropy to organized charity, directed not at highly individualized causes, but at the roots of poverty. Charitable bodies themselves were regulated by the introduction of the Charity Commissioners in 1853, although this was aimed more at reducing fraud than co-ordinating philanthropy. Regulation of philanthropy, whether formal or informal, contributed to making donors more aware of the need to be involved in the disposal of charitable funds. The growth of committees to organize and regulate charity provided the middle class with further opportunities to utilize their industrial and commercial (and in the case of women, their domestic) management skills. (➤ Ch. 63 Medical philanthropy after 1850)

The impact of war on health care and, specifically, nursing and nurses throughout the nineteenth century is problematic. Recent research has demonstrated that the army and navy had well-developed medical and nursing systems for dealing with wounded personnel, although the experience of the Crimean War called even those facilities into question.[21] Tierney, in looking at the impact of the Civil War on nursing developments, suggests that the same was not true for the USA.[22] There, the largest army hospital had forty beds, nursing was given by recuperating soldiers or soldiers' wives, and 'hospitals were understaffed, insanitary, near polluted areas, on damp ground, and sometimes near unburied bodies'.

It was not always the sheer numbers of the wounded that stretched military medical services almost to breaking-point, but the camp fevers, such as dysentery and typhoid. (➤ Ch. 19 Fevers) This was almost certainly the case during the Civil War in the USA, when the prisoner-of-war camps witnessed catastrophic levels of deaths through starvation and fevers, rather than battle injuries. Tierney argues that whilst public attention had been drawn to the women's rights movement and to the work of Florence Nightingale, 'it took the crisis created by the Civil War to unsettle traditional attitudes and propel women into the role of hospital nurses'. Until the full horrors of the wartime conditions became known and fully appreciated, training for military nursing was rudimentary and brief. The Civil War, Tierney concludes, 'created the stage and the essential need for employing women in heretofore untried ways'. It 'necessitated the construction and development of more and better hospitals', which in turn necessitated a new approach to the profession of nursing and the employment of nurses.

The expansion of the British empire was achieved not only by war, but by diplomacy and through the export of institutions and practices. The most obvious were the military and the civil service. By the turn of the century, aspects of the health-care system were part of the process of expansion of empire, particularly in the Commonwealth and the Middle East. (➤ Ch. 58 Medicine and colonialism)

Perhaps the more relevant impact of war on nursing lies in the way in which the public was able to receive reports from the front about the progress of the campaigns and the plight of the armed forces. Public awareness was aided by the development of faster communication using the telegraph and, in the case of the Crimean and South African campaigns, the presence of war correspondents and other observers whose writings and illustrations stirred public opinion and forced the Government to react. The publication of letters between 'observers' at the battle front and influential people at home added to the general knowledge of the medical problems of the armed forces, and added weight to calls for reform from individuals such as Florence Nightingale.

It is within these general and specific contexts that we need to situate the development of modern nursing in the nineteenth century. Whilst in different societies nursing took different routes to modernity, we can see that in the Western cultural tradition it has many common themes.

THE DEVELOPMENT OF MODERN NURSING

Three key themes emerge from a review of the development of modern nursing in the nineteenth century, themes which have a resonance in other countries and societies. First, the impact of reformers and pressure groups; second, the role of the state; and third, the changing experience of women in society.

In keeping with the late eighteenth- and early nineteenth-century tradition, we can find a number of individuals who involved themselves in the care of the sick and in the provision of nursing services. Many were motivated by religious conviction, whether High Anglican or Dissenting tradition, and their concern for the sick was but one aspect of an overall Christian commitment to humankind. Thus, Elizabeth Fry, a Quaker, sought to alleviate the conditions in a number of hospitals, in the same way as she attempted to alleviate the plight of convicts and deportees, in the main, through personal example and by appeal to Christian virtues.[23] Such motivation lay behind the work of later 'nurses', including Agnes Jones (1832–68) and other 'nightingales'.[24] Nightingale herself began her work for the sick as part of her Christian duty, and even contemplated encouraging one or more religious order of women to take a more active role in developing a nursing service.[25] Indeed, several mid-century women's orders did take on the responsibility of providing a nursing service, including the group organized by Mary Jones (1812–87), Nightingale's 'Dearest Friend', at King's College Hospital, London.[26]

Towards the latter part of the century, reformers were less likely to stress the Christian mission, in which the sick were usually regarded as passive. In keeping with the changing approach to charity and philanthropy, and to social welfare, latter-day reformers (who still included Nightingale) looked to transforming the health-care system, and therefore the nursing system itself, rather than individual hospitals or local domiciliary nursing services.

It is in that light that we can view the work of reformers and pressure groups, who included Sir Henry Burdett (1847–1920), Ethel Manson (Mrs

Fenwick), Rosalind Paget (1855–1948), the Society for the Registration of Nurses, and the Midwives Institute. Burdett was instrumental in developing hospital administration along sound business principles, which included the regulation of the nursing work-force. Ethel Manson sought to protect the middle-class public from dangerous nurses through state registration, and helped start the Society for the Registration of Nurses. Her cause was duplicated in the USA, but was based on experiences in other countries including New Zealand, Belgium, Germany, and Finland.[27] Rosalind Paget founded the Midwives' Institute and was instrumental in obtaining state registration for midwives in England by 1902, setting a model that nurses could attempt to follow. (➤ Ch. 44 Childbirth)

In the main, these reformers and pressure groups took part in campaigns across a broad front, rather than a single issue. Burdett, for example, linked his commitment to liberal economics to a desire for efficiency in the public services, which included health, old-age pensions, and hospitals. There was also considerable cross-fertilization of ideas and exchange of information between reformers and pressure groups. Occasions such as the World Fair (Chicago, 1891) provided important opportunities for influential people to meet and develop plans for reform. So far as nursing (or midwifery) was concerned, reformers argued for two main platforms. First, education, which included developing personal and moral responsibility; and, second, organizational change which, for some, meant the need for the state to intervene in social affairs.

The recognition that not all women were naturally nurses, but that nursing required education and training, coincided in the later decades of the nineteenth century with a major demographic shift: the problem of 'surplus women' of the middle classes. Contemporaries sought ways of opening up the world of work to such women, whilst retaining some of the trappings of middle-class women's non-work experiences. Nursing, as well as teaching and some areas of commerce, were areas of employment which were potentially able to absorb women from the middle classes looking for entry into the labour force. (➤ Ch. 71 Demography and medicine)

Initially, reformers were concerned to introduce into the hospitals women of strong personal and moral character from their own ranks who would, by dint of those characteristics, reform the nursing services and attract the new type of recruits. These, once trained, could go on and spread the message of reform and efficiency throughout the world of the sick. That approach failed for two reasons. First, sufficient numbers of such strong characters were not forthcoming and, of those who did come forward, not all were as strong as had been supposed.[28] Second, the demand for change outstripped the supply of such women and, more importantly, the supply of women to train under them. Allied to this was a reluctance on the part of middle-class women to enter nursing, coupled with a reluctance by some middle-class matrons to recruit from their ranks because of the bad experiences with such women.[29] Many matrons preferred women from the respectable working class, preferably those with some experience of paid employment before nursing.

Linked to the failure to recruit their original nursing staff, matrons and reformers quickly recognized that training could not be accomplished merely by example, but that it needed a structure. Early experimentation with a combined role of matron and teacher led quickly to new appointments as assistant matron/tutor, and eventually to separation of the teacher role from the service (matron) role, although matrons retained administrative and professional control over the nurse-teachers, if not the curriculum. The separation was completed when schools of nursing were built as institutions apart from the host hospital rather than as part of the nurses' home.

Within the curriculum, the nursing emphasis was complemented by a medical orientation, with lectures on anatomy, physiology, and pharmacology. Some medical practitioners objected that in some schools, such as the Manchester Royal Infirmary, there was not sufficient medical input, and the matron and teachers were forced to revise the training programme accordingly. Many recruits welcomed this development, not just because it was linked to the increasing interventionist role for the practising nurse, but because it clearly linked nursing knowledge to medical knowledge. Nursing gained in status from this association, at least within the medical world, although some die-hard medical and nursing professionals objected that nurses were not there to be surrogate doctors, but to carry out medical orders. It also clearly signalled to others that nursing was becoming a trained profession. (➤ Ch. 48 Medical education)

In the transition from one system to another, to one that emphasized training, reformers needed to look at the knowledge and practice base of nursing, in order to define the content of the training programme. As has been noted, there was some anxiety about the balance of 'medical knowledge' within the nurse-training syllabus, although few objected to its inclusion in some degree. It was, however, in the arena of practice that most debates and arguments took place. The professional and public debates about nurses' cleaning duties were one aspect of this transitional stage in the development of nursing. Another aspect was the professional relationship between doctor and nurse. This debate centred around the need to maintain gender relationships whilst acknowledging that the nurse worked as an informed doer with the doctor. The nurse-teachers and the matrons instituted regimes that created and sustained ideas of subordination, obedience, and respect for medicine, if not always medical practitioners. Davies has referred to the roles of the home sister/assistant matron or sister tutor as that of a 'moral police' force.[30] Nurses were expected to inculcate habits of order and discipline in all aspects of their lives. The living-in requirement for trainees and for qualified nurses added to the pressure for conformity to the culture of obedience. That there was the need for a moral police force demonstrates, in part, the tensions created by what were essentially middle class led ideologies of male–female relationships.

The regime percolated the clinical as well as the training and off-duty worlds. Textbooks devoted considerable space to 'professional ethics', including the need for order and discipline. The rituals of practice, including the performance of the 'doctor's rounds' – later mimicked by nurses themselves as 'matron's rounds' – aided the process of indoctrination. A clear hierarchy of duties and responsibilities, beginning with the lowly duties of cleaning sluices and sinks, and ranks within nursing supported the distinction between the medical and nursing staffs, since they taught the importance of obedience.

The tasks performed by the nurses, sharply divided according to time served, changed as the needs of doctors changed. The introduction of anaesthesia, for example, required more and more nurses to develop general skills in dealing with postoperative patients. (➤ Ch. 42 Surgery (modern)) New techniques and medical regimes necessitated that the nurse learn how to manage patients in traction or in steam-tents. In all of this, developments in nursing practice came about in response to changing medical expectations of the nurses' role. Any reference to an original and separate nursing role was largely forgotten or subsumed under the vague notion of 'nursing art'.

A number of nursing leaders and reformers of nursing, or the health-care system itself, developed nursing knowledge and practice by publishing articles and textbooks for trainee nurses. The early tracts on nursing by Nightingale provide a base-line for this development because they generally offered a polemic in justification of transformed nursing. Later writers concentrated less on the philosophy and more on the practicability of nursing as science and art. Henry Burdett, in particular, as owner of the Scientific Press and editor of *The Hospital*, wrote manuals and guides and helped a number of the new nursing leaders like Eva Luckes at the London Hospital publish influential nursing texts. Ethel Manson (Mrs Fenwick) owned and published the *Nursing Record* which, in addition to being the main vehicle for pro-state registrationist views, also carried a growing number of clinical and education features.

Unlike the early nineteenth-century 'reformers', those working to reform nursing in the UK at the end of the century, including Burdett and Manson, looked to organizations and groups rather than example to carry through their plans. The period from about 1880 saw the emergence (and frequently the demise) of many organizations aimed at reforming nursing. In midwifery, for example, the Midwives' Institute (later the Royal College of Midwifery) was formed in 1881 to seek legislation to regulate the training and employment of midwives. The Matrons' Association and the Hospital Association, both influential bodies in the drive for the regulation of nursing and health care, were formed in the mid-1880s. This development was particularly significant where reforms required state regulation, as in the case of the registration of nurses. Individuals were no longer able, by whatever means, to bring about legislative change; the role of the pressure group in the political process was coming to the fore. (➤ Ch. 47 History of the medical profession)

This is not to suggest that the change to organization rather than example was always, or frequently, successful. The campaigns for state regulation of midwifery and of nursing lasted over twenty years and almost thirty-five years, respectively, despite having very powerful backing from key politicians and public figures. In the main, the state was reluctant to intervene in a process which it regarded as best regulated by professionals. It was only likely to intervene when, as in the case of nursing, no internal agreement could be reached between competing professional groups or, as in the case of midwifery, where the public-health consequences of non-intervention (high infant mortality, poor health in children leading to inefficiency in adulthood) were likely to cause a major public outcry as well as potential economic failure.

The state was also reluctant to intervene in nursing because of the structure of government and of the separation of political responsibilities between local and central government. Central government was regarded as concerned with raising national revenues for defence, for example, and for macro-legislation. Local government had fought throughout the nineteenth century for the right to raise local revenues to meet local needs, including health care and social welfare. Any attempt at altering the balance of powers and responsibilities was not likely to succeed. The Poor Law authorities, for example, began to regulate and expand the provision of nursing services once central government had clarified the national legislation about the use of local rates in mid-century.[31] The local regulations covered terms and conditions of employment, pensions and, eventually, training to an agreed standard throughout the Poor Law service. Outside the Poor Law service, voluntary hospitals lacked an umbrella body to facilitate such changes. Individual hospitals set their own terms and conditions, and their own training programmes. But even here, the forces of the market made their influence felt. Competition for recruits, denied by contemporaries but nevertheless part and parcel of the nursing world,[32] forced hospitals and matrons to move towards standard contracts and training programmes.

These processes, although not without their problems, meant that the need for state intervention was not as acute as the protagonists claimed. Indeed, in retrospect, it is unclear what state regulation would have achieved other than creating, as some reformers demanded, a licensing body for nurses along the lines of the General Medical Register. Whilst the regulatory bodies did specify minimum criteria for registration and thus have some influence on training, it was some time before either the General Nursing Council (GNC), set up in 1919, or the Central Midwives' Board, set up following the Midwives' Act of 1902, actually extended their work into the standard and content of training programmes.[33] As late as 1930, one matron of a large voluntary hospital in London was sceptical of the value of 'state registration' and state examinations, and advised her nurses not to bother to register with the GNC but to rely on their certificates from their training hospitals as proof of their ability and professional expertise.[34]

The influence of individual matrons, as this last example shows, was considerable. They determined not only the 'moral climate' in nursing, but also shaped the work lives of the nurses themselves. The training school and the matron became important indicators of professional worth. Some nurses were able to point to leaders who were nationally well known, like Eva Luckes at the London Hospital. Where the matron was not known outside of the immediate area, her role and the way she performed it took on the trappings of these relatively few national figures. Eventually, the matron became The Matron, as though all were equal in status and power.

Unlike the early reformers, most matrons and their nurses did not have private means and needed paid employment. This meant that they tended to adopt the line of their employing institution. Few were able to challenge publicly the views of the hospital administrators and senior doctors, had they so wished. Instead, many looked to collaboration with other nurses and the establishment of pressure groups or representative organizations such as the College (later Royal College) of Nursing. In such forums, they formulated their professional codes and common pathways, contributing to the development of a cohesive professional group. Nursing journals became important transmitters of this developing consensus, just as they were contributing to the growth of a common nursing-knowledge base through the clinical and educational articles.

PSYCHIATRIC AND DOMICILIARY NURSING

The foregoing has dwelt on the changes that took place in the acute general areas of care. In part, this reflects the way in which general nursing took the professional high ground and contemporaries regarded nursing in other spheres, such as mental health and community care, as 'second class'. Evidence for the 'professional imperialism' of general nursing over other branches comes from the increasing expectation that nurses working in psychiatry or domiciliary nursing would have dual qualifications: general nursing and the 'specialist' training. Dual qualifications were not mandatory and there were cases of the general (single-qualification) nurse being appointed over the head of the 'specialist' (single-qualification) nurse.[35] No matter, it was the possession of the general qualification that was paramount. The trend was towards using the specialist qualification as a means of more-assured or more-rapid career development, rather than a means of providing particular skills or knowledge in the specialism. Church has noted that Nightingale's influence on the development of nursing in the psychiatric field in the USA was perhaps more important than the development of psychiatry as a medical discipline, although there would continue to be enormous and professionally draining tensions between the nursing model and that of medicine.[36]

We know little about psychiatric nursing and psychiatric nurses.[37] This explains, in part, why we know so little about male nurses, since it was in psychiatry that men found employment as carers and nurses. (➤ Ch. 56 Psychiatry) Nolan has begun to explore the role of men in psychiatric nursing, their origins (often as ex-servicemen), and the strong ties between the work and the families of male nurses.[38] Carpenter has provided some insights into male nurses and the tensions between them as men, and nursing as women's work.[39] Men were employed as 'servants' to the insane, and for cases involving violent behaviour, much of which was due to alcohol abuse or syphilis. More work needs to be carried out before we have a more representative picture of the male nurse; that work will be essential if we are to undertake a critique of the nursing ideology of caring.

In contrast, domiciliary nursing and midwifery have attracted more attention. There are a number of studies that deal with the development of community based nursing services and, especially, services for the poor.[40, 41] In Britain, domiciliary nursing services were the first to be 'organized' and 'professionalized' because of the links to poverty and the need to rescue the poor from the potential trap of pauperism. Visiting the sick in their own dwellings was part of the 'duty' of the middle classes, as Nightingale herself experienced.[42] Domiciliary nursing or sick-poor visiting was important because, despite significant growth in the provision of in-patient care, hospitals were never able to satisfy the need for nursing (or medical) care. Provident, charitable, and philanthropic societies existed alongside local government and state provision for health care, and all recruited from the new nurses produced by the reforms. It was also important as the arena in which the full force of the predominantly middle-class values of nineteenth- and twentieth-century society could be brought to bear on the most important social unit and its key 'worker', the family and the wife/mother. It is no coincidence that the title of Loane's study of domiciliary nursing care was *An Englishman's Castle*, and that in its case studies of sick-poor nursing the author (herself a health visitor and eugenist) sought to portray moral rectitude among the deserving poor.[43] (➤ Ch. 70 Medical sociology)

CONCLUSION

There is no doubt that nursing altered radically after 1880. In Britain, that process took place and was largely completed, except for state regulation, by the outbreak of the First World War. The same is generally true of North America. In other Western societies, the process probably began a little later, at least in those countries with a stronger tradition of the involvement of the religious orders in nursing the sick. Beyond the Western societies, change tended to follow imperialism, whether economic or military.

In the majority of cases, common themes can be identified, themes with which this overview has been concerned. The change from individualism towards collective activity by reform-minded people and the development of pressure groups and professional organizations is one theme. That, in turn, required the development of a common culture and shared tradition, to which we can add the development of a nursing literature. At the same time, the demand for change in terms of health care required a major push, and in many cases this was provided by industrialization and urbanization. In turn, the changing position of women, both working class and middle class, provided the focus for new work opportunities and opened up health and welfare as possible new economic sectors. The third theme is the political structure that encouraged the growth of health care, but did not necessarily involve regulation, either of health services or of health professionals.

In looking at the ways in which nursing has changed in almost all societies, historians will need to move away from concentrating on individuals, no matter how important they were, and towards the contexts within which change took place. Taken together, a clearer picture of the development of modern nursing can emerge. A historiography of nursing must begin with recognizing these themes and testing them in specific cases. That approach begins to question what sources will provide the information needed to develop that critique. Secondary accounts come under the microscope, and can be seen to be as much about constructing a particular (or The ...) history as about understanding how change occurred. Primary materials need to be expanded to take in literature, personal experiences and, for the recent past, oral testimony. More importantly, the development of a historiography forces the historian to consider the issue of periodization and the possibility of discontinuity. New approaches to nursing history will show that there is little to be gained from seeing nursing as a universal phenomenon with origins far back in antiquity. Nursing means different things in different periods. Nursing, as it has been described in this essay, has just passed its centenary and is unlikely to celebrate another.

NOTES

1   B. Melosh, *The Physician's Hand: Work Culture and Conflict in American Nursing*, Philadelphia, PA, Temple, 1982.

2   C. Maggs, *The Origins of General Nursing*, London, Croom Helm, 1985.

3   S. Reverby, *Ordered to Care: the Dilemma of American Nursing 1850–1945*, Cambridge, Cambridge University Press, 1987.

4   O. M. Church, 'The development of nursing at the Bellevue and Yale hospitals', in C. Maggs (ed.), *Nursing History: the State of the Art?*, London, Croom Helm, 1987; C. Davies, (ed.), *Rewriting Nursing History*, London, Croom Helm, 1980.

5   Maggs, op. cit. (n. 2).

6   Davies, op. cit. (n. 4).

7   E. Gamarnikow, 'The sexual division of labour: the case of nursing', in A. Kuhn and A. M. Wolpe (eds), *Feminism and Materialism*, London, Routledge, 1978; Melosh, op. cit. (n. 1).

8   W. Hector, *Mrs Bedford Fenwick*, London, Royal College of Nursing, 1973.

9   L. Holcombe, *Victorian Ladies at Work*, Newton Abbot, David & Charles, 1973.

10   J. Castle, *Nursing at the Wollongong Hospital 1926–1982*, Australia, Univeristy of Wollongong, 1984.

11   V. Brittain, *Testament of Youth*, London, Gollancz, 1933; E. Bagnold, *Diary without Dates*, London, Heinemann, 1918.

12   F. B. Smith, *The People's Health*, London, Croom Helm, 1979.

13   B. Aronovitch, *Give it Time: an Experience of Hospital 1928–1932*, London, Gollancz, 1974; R. Hawker, 'A day in the life of a patient', *Nursing Times*, 12 June 1985, 43–4; Hawker, 'For the good of the patient', in C. Maggs: op. cit. (n. 4).

14   Gamarnikow, op. cit. (n. 7).

15   B. Abel-Smith, *A History of the Nursing Profession*, London, Croom Helm, 1960.

16   C. Dickens, *Martin Chuzzlewit*, London, Hazell, Watson & Viney, 1844.

17   M. Baly, *Florence Nightingale and the Nursing Legacy*, London, Heinemann, 1986.

18   J. Rose, *Elizabeth Fry*, London, Macmillan, 1980.

19   S. McGann, 'Eva Charlotte Luckes: pioneer or reactionary?', *History of Nursing Society Journal*, 1991, 3, 5: 30–2.

20   M. Ryan, *Womanhood in America from Colonial Times to the Present*, New York, Watts, 1975.

21   A. Summers, *Angels and Citizens: British Women as Military Nurses 1854–1914*, London, Routledge & Kegan Paul, 1988.

22   R. Tierney, 'The beneficent revolution: hospital nursing during the Civil War', in V. Bullough, B. Bullough and M. Stanton (eds), *Florence Nightingale and her Era: a Collection of New Scholarship*, New York, Garland, 1990.

23   Rose, op. cit. (n. 18).

24   F. B. Smith, *Florence Nightingale: Reputation and Power*, London, Croom Helm, 1982; O. Banks, *Faces of Feminism*, Oxford, Martin Robertson, 1981.

25   Baly, op. cit. (n. 17); Bullough, Bullough and Stanton, op. cit. (n. 22).

26   Smith, op. cit. (n. 24).

27   L. Boyd, *State Registration for Nurses*, London, Saunders, 1911.

28   Baly, op. cit. (n. 25).

29   Ibid.; Baly, *Nursing and Social Change*, London, Heinemann, 1973.

30   C. Davies, 'Experience of dependency and control in work', *Journal of Advanced*

Nursing, 1976, 1; Davies, 'The regulation of nursing work: an historical comparison of Britain and the USA', *Research in the Sociology of Health Care*, 1982, 2.

31 R. White, *Social Change and the Development of the Nursing Profession: a Study of the Poor Law Nursing Service 1848–1948*, London, Kimpton, 1978.

32 Maggs, op. cit. (n. 2).

33 N. Radford and A. Thompson, *Direct Entry: a Preparation of Midwifery Practice*, Guildford, University of Surrey, 1988.

34 Maggs, op. cit. (n. 2).

35 Maggs, op. cit. (n. 2).

36 Church, op. cit. (n. 4).

37 Church, op. cit. (n. 4); R. Dingwall, 'The place of men in nursing', in M. College and D. Jones (eds), *Readings in Nursing*, Edinburgh, Churchill Livingstone, 1979; P. Nolan, 'Psychiatric nursing in the nineteenth and twentieth centuries', unpublished Ph.D. thesis, University of Bath, 1990.

38 Nolan, ibid.

39 M. Carpenter, 'Managerialism and the division of labour in nursing', in R. Dingwall and J. McIntosh (eds), *Readings in the Sociology of Nursing*, Edinburgh, Churchill Livingstone, 1977; Carpenter, 'Asylum nursing before 1914: a chapter on the history of labour', in C. Davies (ed.), *Rewriting Nursing History*, London, Croom Helm, 1980; Carpenter, 'The labour movement in the National Health Service', in A. Sethi and S. Dimmock (eds), *Industrial Relations and Health Services*, London, Croom Helm, 1982.

40 P. Allan and M. Jolley, *Nursing, Midwifery and Health Visiting since 1900*, London, Faber, 1982; J. Brickman, 'Public health, midwives and nurses 1880–1930', in H. Lagemann (ed.), *Nursing History: New Perspectives, New Possibilities*, New York, Teachers' College Press, 1983; D. Dwork, *War is Good for Babies and Other Young Children: a History of the Infant and Child Welfare Movement in England 1898–1918*, London, Tavistock, 1986.

41 J. McIntosh, 'District nursing: a case of political marginality', in R. White (ed.), *Political Issues in Nursing: Past, Present and Future*, Chichester, Wiley, 1985; L. Peretz, 'Infant welfare in Oxford City 1919–1939', in R. Whiting (ed.), *Cities and their People*, Manchester, Manchester University Press, 1991; P. Robson, 'Health visiting: a brief history', *Radical Health Visitors' Newsletter*, 1983, 4.

42 Baly, op. cit. (n. 17).

43 M. Loane, *An Englishman's Castle*, London, Scientific Press, 1909.

55

THE EMERGENCE OF PARA-MEDICAL PROFESSIONS

Gerald Larkin

A growth in the numbers of health professions in this century, and linked changes in their relationship with the medical profession, have attracted relatively limited attention from historians and related scholars. Some particular occupations in addition to the medical profession, such as nursing and midwifery, have drawn very considerable interest (➤ Ch. 44 Childbirth; Ch. 54 General history of nursing), but in other cases there is little to match the extensive range of literature concerned with the history of doctors and their forebears. The delivery of modern medicine, however, has become increasingly dependent upon a complex web of allied occupations, each with its own history of evolving skills and professional ambitions. In particular, over the past century medical practitioners have come to form a minority, albeit premier, group, amongst the normal range of state-registered or -licensed health-care professionals. In addition to the nursing profession, many other numerically smaller occupations have provided essential technical, therapeutic, and diagnostic services across a variety of health-care contexts. (➤ Ch. 4 Medical care)

The full diversity of processes of historical development amongst these 'para-medical' professions cannot be addressed in this chapter, which instead will examine some examples of major themes common to all of them. Before this discussion, however, a few particular issues of terminology require some initial clarification. The term 'para-medical' is not meant to imply, in this usage, any judgements on hierarchies of status found amongst health-care occupations, or, for example, that those included within it are ancillary rather than integral to the modern history of medicine. Also, whilst it is virtually impossible to avoid using the term 'profession' in the ensuing text, no attempt will be made to enter into the extensive sociological and historical debates as to whether this specific term has any precise and enduring general meaning, which any particular occupation might reflect. Rather, as the medical division of labour has expanded in line with the evolution of modern health care, in practice a significant variety of descriptive usages for its occupations has developed. The para-medical group in a generic sense has graduated over the past century from a nominal status of being 'unskilled assistants' or in some instances 'untrained rivals' to doctors, to 'medical auxiliaries', and on to 'professions supplementary to medicine' or 'allied health professions'. In perhaps a few cases, an almost 'coequal' or complementary stage is detectable, certainly amongst those occupations such as pharmacy or dentistry which accompanied, rather than post-dated, the occupational ascendancy of doctors. In this chapter, without judgement on these historical and cultural relativities of esteem, the term 'para-medical' will be used as a shorthand description of

1 any occupation that has organized itself in connection with medical work, and thus shares its conventional concepts of disease; and
2 has successfully sought or clearly aspired to state registration, licensing, or some form of recognized certification, principally in this century.

By contrast to this definition of the term 'para-medical', chiropractors, osteopaths, and others have sought, and in some countries achieved, state licensing, but they have also held heterodox concepts of disease causation and treatment. Their histories, albeit intimately interwoven with para-medical occupations such as physical therapy and aspects of medical specialization, cannot be considered here. (➤ Ch. 28 Unorthodox medical theories; Ch. 40 Physical methods) Within the broad scope of full-time health labour, only the 'planets' surrounding the 'sun' of medicine will be considered. These have achieved formal recognition through a variety of legal processes, which may vary: for example, the British system of nationally determined statutory provision for occupational self-regulation, compared to the more common European practice of direct supervision by an appropriate ministry or state authority. These processes may also be locally based, as is customary in the myriad complexities of American and Australian state-based, or Canadian provincial government based, systems for registering or licensing occupations. To this extent, there are numerous local para-medical histories. Any particular occupation may be unique to one setting, or at least not recognized elsewhere, as in the latter-day emergence of a speciality of 'respiratory technologists' in North America. Indeed, nomenclature for the same occupation may vary, as in the Anglo-American usages of chiropodist/podiatrist or ophthalmic optician/optometrist. According to American state legislation, for example, physical therapists may work directly with clients or only through medical referral, and are subjected to other arrangements in Canada. Whatever these variations, however, they usually represent different legal and administrative responses to the evolution of a fundamentally similar occupational structure.

Different national and local traditions rest upon recognizably similar social, technical, and cultural forces that create an internationally recognizable cluster of occupations. This is at its clearest in the internationally varying nursing and medical professions, and a group of widely recognized para-medical professions such as physical and occupational therapy, radiography, medical laboratory technology, chiropody, and varying types of optician. These latter examples broadly represent those para-medical occupations with a longer history, although processes of occupational specialization over the second half of this century have created groups as diverse in character as clinical psychologists and hospital physicists. Amongst the older groups, however, there is an internationally evident shared period of initial formation and organization: for example, the foundation of the first Society of Optometrists in New York state in 1892, and the British Optical Association in 1895; the inception of the American Physical Therapy Association in 1921, and the chartering of the British Society of Physiotherapists in 1920; the start of both the American Society of Radiologic Technologists and the British Society of Radiographers in 1920; and the foundation of both the first podiatry college in America and the British Society of Chiropodists in 1912.

Reliable historical information on these and similar events is variable in quality, but the above list indicates a complex and diverse range of development which in turn is linked to many aspects of the evolution of different medical and surgical specialities. There are variations between these occupations, in their origins, in their location and types of practice, in their patterns of training, and in the social and gender characteristics of their members both within groups and between them over time. It is, however, possible to detect some fundamental similarities within these many differences, and thus to impose an elementary range of classifications. First, some of the more established para-medical occupations are linked in origin directly to the scientific development of modern medicine. Their beginnings date from the processes of applying those enhanced diagnostic technologies, which were either newly invented or refined and improved through the latter years of the nineteenth century. This connecting feature is evident in occupations such as radiography and laboratory science, or, a little earlier, in ophthalmic science as the invention of the ophthalmoscope began to open new market prospects for opticians. (➤ Ch. 36 Science of diagnosis: diagnostic technology)

This latter occupation within the scientific group, however, did not entirely develop as did the other two at the end of the nineteenth century, which requires some comment. Its forebears in the English-speaking world were members of the Worshipful Company of Spectacle Makers, founded by royal charter in England in 1629. The company drew upon still earlier and broader origins in the spectacle-makers' guilds of the late medieval period also found in Paris, Nuremberg, and other European cities. The company's charter essentially continued the guild activities of cultivating the market, through regulating the length of training, the numbers of apprentices, and the quality of products. Masters who took on 'too many' apprentices, or sold spectacles with improperly ground lenses, were fined, and cheap or substandard foreign imports were banned. In 1671, for example, ten dozen pairs of spectacles made in France were confiscated from a vendor and publicly smashed with a hammer. The earlier charter petition, asserting that makers with seven years' apprenticeships were 'almost utterlie undone' by unqualified competition, prefigured many licensing debates of later centuries, particularly in its claim that 'All such trades, misteries and manufacturers as are incorporated into a bodie politique doe still subsist in a comlie and commendable manner and those subject to noe certaine ordinances, rules or government are proved by experience to be in shorte time utterlie subverted'.[1]

As an early trade-protection agency, the company's writ extended only to the boundaries of the City of London. By the nineteenth century, unlike the barber-surgeons' and apothecaries' companies in the meantime, its influence had declined substantially. Typically in Europe and North America through the eighteenth and nineteenth centuries, jewellers, watch- and instrument-makers, chemists, itinerant peddlers, variously qualified doctors, oculists, and wonder-working quacks of all kinds provided a range of optical services and products.[2] Despite this trading diversity, optical sciences and linked aspects of medical knowledge were developing. In particular, the invention by H. L. F. von Helmholtz (1821–94) of the ophthalmoscope in 1851 followed shortly by the ophthalmometer, and then the pioneering study of F. C. Donders (1819–89), which was published in 1864 and established comparative standards of visual acuity, together began to change matters. These diagnostic and technical improvements brought the more reputable end of optical practice within the boundaries of scientific medicine, although not, as will be seen, under medical professional control.

A second major para-medical occupational group may be seen initially to have a principally therapeutic rather than scientific origin, although again it is internally varied. It is composed of occupations that developed in response to treatment needs, rather than through the application of particular technological innovations. For example, physiotheraphy began its modern growth from the 1890s. It drew upon ancient techniques of massage and manipulation, as well as a renewed European interest in physical culture and exercise through the late nineteenth century. In Sweden, this was regulated through the Central Institute of Stockholm, which, under state supervision, certificated men and women trained in massage and remedial gymnastics. Their migration elsewhere, together with nurses beginning to specialize in techniques of 'rubbing' with support from progressive doctors, began to stimulate the new occupation. Traditional practices tempered by insights from medical science also provided, as in the reforming nursing profession, a respectable career for 'educated girls from the Victorian home'.[3] These could safely enter a medico-moral complex quite separate from some of the contemporary salacious features of massage.

At the same time, within the broader medical profession, expanding areas such as orthopaedics created new requirements. Safer surgery led both to an increase in operations and ever more surviving patients whose recuperative treatment required supervision. (➤ Ch. 42 Surgery (modern)) Similarly, other newly emergent specialities, such as electrology and therapeutic radiology, although now partly superseded, also required aides for the fashionable administration of 'medical' electricity and (usually ill-judged, by today's standards) exposures of radium. The range of conditions thought to benefit from extensive irradiation of their unfortunate victims was somewhat more extensive than that considered appropriate in later decades. In response to medical and popular demand, new assistants were recruited for these tasks and shared the work with radiographers, physicists, engineers, electricians, and others adept at setting up and employing the appropriate machinery.

On both sides of the Atlantic, the advent of the First World War drew many of these disparate developments together, and, as with many medical areas, gave them a particular impetus. As American involvement in the conflict grew, approximately 800 women were trained through military-sponsored short courses, as 'physical therapy aides'. They, in turn, were dispersed through military hospitals by the end of the war, and received the unofficial title of 'rubbing angels' from appreciative recipients of their services amongst the wounded.[4] This was matched by similar developments within the nascent physical-therapy movement in Britain. In 1914, Miss (later Lady) Essex French, who was a trained masseuse and a daughter of the Commander-in-Chief of the British Expeditionary Force, with others founded a Massage Corps responsible to the War Office for work amongst the wounded. 'Society' connections were strong amongst the first British pioneers, but, as in the American case, patriotic services valuably demonstrated their organizing abilities and, coincidentally, the respectability of the new occupation. (➤ Ch. 66 War and modern medicine)

In addition to a growth in physical therapy, the enormous casualty rates of the 1914–18 war further widened the development of a range of therapeutically oriented para-medical occupations. In 1912, the first conference on speech therapy was held in London and was concerned mainly with stammering. However, early members of the proto-profession, particularly in the ensuing years, were progressively involved in the management of recovery processes following head injuries and other forms of psychological trauma. By 1918, the American military had also established a training programme for occupational therapists, following a request from General J. J. Pershing

(1860–1948) commanding its Expeditionary Force in Europe. Programmes for the 'reconstruction aides' proliferated over the next three years to assist veterans with adjustment to their injuries. This again provided a nucleus of similarly trained early practitioners for the emerging profession, and a basis for diversifying their work between the two world wars.[5] Alongside the circumstances of war, patient survival rates improved through the first decades of the century, further contributing to rising requirements for restorative types of occupation. As medical and surgical skills progressed, a further realization gathered force, namely that enhancing the fullest degree of recovery and functional capacity after both short- and long-term illness needed skills beyond the particular roles of the doctor and nurse.[6] Thus in the inter-war years, a growing understanding of rehabilitation as part of the treatment became linked to the more widespread and civilian development of the specialities of physical and occupational therapy. Indeed, a widening of the concepts of health, healing, and treatment beyond a concern with immediate medical activities can be seen as a major force operating over many decades. Occupations of all kinds, both orthodox and fringe, exploiting the 'narrowness' of medical practice, have secured a niche in the division of labour. Variants of 'holism' and 'health promotion' or 'healthy living' creeds are now linked to diffuse sects, occupations, and movements.

Whether their origins were principally associated with diagnostic improvements or developments in therapeutic practices, all the above-mentioned para-medical occupations have shared a similar historical ambition for professional recognition. Much as the pre-modern medical profession through the nineteenth century campaigned for reformed legal privileges, so these later groups sought to unify their early divisions, to standardize and upgrade their training patterns, and thus to define their occupational terrain. The prior experience of the medical profession was a notable exemplar in these matters, and the later and contemporary efforts of nurses and dentists to secure state registration (in the UK successfully in 1919 and 1921, respectively) provided further important stimuli to their quest. In this process, both medical and para-medical groups ubiquitously have argued across history that the 'properly trained' practitioner, as opposed to less-qualified rivals, has to be evident to colleagues, employers, and clients. A licensing authority to regulate standards of entry, training, and practice was thus required, preferably staffed by their own practitioners. Such measures, apart from the general public benefit ensuing, also benefited those within the new order by giving them a market edge over the unlicensed competitor. Thus the attraction of state registration, whether in the rare strong form of a total monopoly over an area of medical labour or more usually in the recognized custody of the title of 'qualified', is regarded as evidence of a full professional status. Its advantages have been such as to ensure its centrality to most occupational histories in health care.

In fundamentally similar ways, all professions seek special forms of recognition. However, this pursuit by one group usually brings conflict, not only with those 'cast out' as unqualified, but also with existing and otherwise-qualified groups. These are usually very anxious to conserve, protect, and even to extend their historically secured advantages. Thus the formalized stages of occupational evolution in the medical division of labour and the sharper articulation of issues of inter-professional rivalry are ultimately linked. Through its historical precedence in most countries, the medical profession has played a major role in the emergence of allied occupations, by positively and negatively trying to shape their development to correspond with its own central, but also evolving, position in health care. (➤ Ch. 47 History of the medical profession) In this sense, there are no separate medical and para-medical histories, but rather a linked process of contructing, formalizing, and dividing skills and responsibilities between them. Tasks and skills regarded as the preserve of medical practitioners in any one era or context may be para-medical in another, depending upon the specialities and circumstances involved. In particular, the premier profession has fought hardest to retain control over the diagnosis and prescription of treatment. In particular areas, this generalization does not hold, particularly where medical specialities for whatever reason fail to flourish: for example, the sharing of manipulative treatments by osteopaths, physical therapists, and others.

Despite many revisions of occupational 'frontiers' through time, however, there are again some detectable patterns or stages evident in the closely connected histories of medical and para-medical specialization. These take the forms of an initial mixture of patronage and suspicion. Most generally, this is evident as para-medical practitioners begin to come together for mutual advancement, protection, or to pool and up-grade knowledge. Medical interest, or indeed aversion at this stage, begins to coalesce in forms of conditional sponsorship and help, or sometimes excoriation and bitter rivalry. An ensuing stage of elaboration or codifying of inter-occupational relationships usually follows, to fix controls and various task boundaries. This may take the usual form of overt medical professional authority being buttressed, or occasionally a separate and often uneasy course of divergent development. Finally, there is an emergence of more autonomous and looser relations within the by now more codified medical hierarchy of occupations. This creates further tensions, typically requiring in most countries some form of state intervention and regulation. (➤ Ch. 50 Medical institutions and the state) Some examples taken from these overlapping phases of evolution, reflecting its varied and slightly different progress according to national conditions, will guide the following discussion.

EARLY YEARS

Many of today's health-related professions began as small and elementary organizations established around the turn of the century. In their early years, they were typically composed of very small numbers of activists, initially concerned to provide mutual contact, support, and pressure for improvements in training and practice. At this stage, relationships with the medical profession were often harmoniously based upon a mixture of deference on the one side and patronage from the other. For example, the Society of Trained Masseuses, founded in the UK in 1895, emphasized from the outset that its members would not initiate their own treatments, and could only work under medical direction in conditions of 'strictest loyalty'. Its royal charter, granted in 1920, reinforced this provision, as did the founding terms of the American Women's Physical Therapy Association, formed in 1921. Members were to carry out only prescriptions given by doctors, who were prominent in the early years of both organizations.[7] In particular, diagnosis and prescription were the responsibilities of medical practitioners, and respectability for massage and other treatments or practices, together with access to clients, depended on compliance with these constraints. Prominent doctors played active and leading honorary roles only in those associations which, in their view, acknowledged a pre-existing hierarchy of knowledge and skills, such as, in Britain, the Pathological and Bacteriological Laboratory Assistants' Association founded in 1912, and the Incorporated Society of Chiropodists founded in 1916, (now the Institute of Medical Laboratory Science and the Society of Chiropodists); and in the United States, the American Associations of Occupational Therapists and Medical Technologists, which developed in the ensuing years. Medical involvement on these initially restrictive terms added credibility and employment advantages to members of these nascent associations struggling to establish their early position.

There were, however, tensions from the start, most notably in cases where a medical speciality was itself in its infancy and thus also marginal in status. For example, two years after W. C. Röntgen (1845–1923) discovered the potential diagnostic uses of X-rays in 1895, a Röntgen Society was formed in England. The production and administration of X-rays was still very much in the hands of lay scientists, and thus physicists and engineers were invited to join the new society. The American Röntgen Society, founded in 1900, at first also actively encouraged all kinds of lay scientists and technicians to join. Although radiology as a medical speciality was only in its infancy, by 1903 the *British Medical Journal*, following complaints in the medical press, began to enunciate a standard policy to govern co-operation between these different groups. This was echoed in 1905 by the Académie de Médecine in France, and was to become familiar in many countries. As the *British*

Medical Journal put it, there was 'no reason for professional prejudices against the practice of radiology by laymen, so long as they confine themselves to the more mechanical act of producing a picture and abstain from assuming a scientific knowledge of the bearings of their radiographs on diagnosis or prognosis'.[8] (➤ Ch. 68 Medical technologies: social contexts and consequences)

Early inter-occupational relationships were uneasy where the division of responsibilities was at first unclear, and where none the less both medical and para-medical groups were mutually dependent upon one another in their work. In particular, where both lay and medical practitioners claimed the same skills and were both male groups, as in the case of ophthalmic opticians and medically qualified ophthalmologists, they were less than cordial. The General Medical Council, for example, in a detailed memorandum to the Privy Council, opposed a British Optical Association attempt at state registration in 1906. This, it argued, was sponsored by an inferior, dishonest, and venal class of tradesmen seeking to trespass upon medical innovations and responsbilities.[9] The possible licensing of direct competition in the marketplace posed particular problems for both sides which could not be contained within patron-client relationships. Dentists, by contrast, partly through carefully defining their role so as not to compete with the medical profession, established more amicable relationships and secured state registration in Britain in 1921, following an earlier registration of élite dentists through the Royal College of Surgeons.

Whilst ophthalmic opticians in Britain were at first unsuccessful in pursuing recognition as an autonomous profession, the history of optometry in North America up to the 1920s contains similar conflicts with the medical profession, but a rather different outcome. Optometry's expansion, and the American Medical Association's (AMA) growing interest in controlling eye care, led in 1892 to New York ophthalmologists accusing a Mr Charles Prentice, an optometrist, of breaching the state's medical acts. This challenge stimulated the growth of the American Optometric Association (AOA), which began affiliating smaller state-based groups into its midst. Its case, in defiance of the ophthalmologists' charges, was that 'a lens is not a pill', and thus its members' activities in examining and prescribing were outside contemporary legal definitions of reserved medical responsibilities. An ensuing and widening series of legal battles on these points resulted in all states passing licensing laws recognizing optometry by the 1920s. Despite, or perhaps because of, this setback, the AMA, like its British counterpart in attitude, continued a policy of non-cooperation with the AOA up to the 1950s.[10] (➤ Ch. 69 Medicine and the law)

INTER-WAR YEARS

Despite the relatively rapid rise of optometry in North America, in most cases the 1920s and 1930s saw a more limited codifying and stabilizing of occupations, usually under medical control. This occurred at first in pathology and radiology, given their increasingly central role in sustaining the diagnostic credibility of doctors. In the former case, conventional practice now rested on complex laboratories, located in hospitals, clinics, and commercial agencies. Their control and the nature of professional authority within them, by contrast with the days of the single doctor with microscope and slides, rapidly came to the fore. The American College of Surgeons insisted through the 1920s that its 'certified' hospitals had to have a laboratory headed by a physician. This measure alone prevented laboratory technologists from assuming a competitive entrepreneurial role in this rapidly expanding area of practice.[11] In 1929, the American Society of Clinical Pathologists, representing the ascendant medical speciality, capitalized on this position by launching its own system for directly certifying laboratory personnel. Through this mechanism, the association was able to determine the extent of technologists' practice. Any advisory, diagnostic, or interpretive work could be prohibited, in effect creating quite separate superior and inferior occupational castes. It also enabled the association to determine, via the content of training courses, the future role and knowledge levels of technologists. The Pathological Society of Great Britain, through its analogous links with technicians, also closely monitored their training. This, again, was aimed at ensuring a proficiency in routine procedures, rather than a more threatening acquisition of medical knowledge or interpretative competence. In the longer term, highly trained lay scientists became essential to the development of pathology's contributory disciplines, but their forebears, perhaps inevitably in the circumstances of the 1920s, were notably constrained. (➤ Ch. 9 The pathological tradition; Ch. 11 Clinical research)

In the case of radiographers and radiologists, relationships in the post-1918 years also came under increasing strain. In Great Britain by 1917, a purely medical society, the Association for the Advancement of Radiology and Physiotherapy, had been founded with plans for a postgraduate diploma in radiology. Its first secretary, Dr Hernaman-Johnson, sought from the outset to redefine the roles of both doctor and technician and their relationship:

> what can be done ... is to control the timing, and insofar as may be, the practice of such people – to secure, in a word, that they shall be competent and shall not accept patients except in conjunction with a medical man.... It will be said with truth that in some cases the radiographer will dominate the doctor who seeks his aid. We should welcome lay assistance and seek to

organize and guide it. It is too late in the day to make a mystery of taking plates but the interpretation of them is ours for ever.[12]

Thus the Society of Radiographers, founded in 1920, with matching numbers of medical practitioners, electrical engineers, and radiographers on its council, soon became subject to forces of division. Its founding terms emphasized that radiographer members were to work under medical direction and supervision. However, in practice through the early 1920s, they continued to report on X-ray examinations, which was not specifically forbidden by the original terms of incorporation. This practice of 'lay reporting', to other doctors rather than directly to patients, was resented by radiologists anxious to promote both their speciality and livelihood. Thus, in 1925, the General Medical Council was pressed to find a formula that strengthened the position of medical radiologists over technicians, whilst also allowing other doctors with a 'pre-Röntgen' training to rely on radiographers without a formal breach of medical prerogative. Consequently, radiographers were forbidden to interpret plates, but on request were to 'describe their appearances' to any medical practitioner incapable of perceiving their shadowy portents.[13]

Beneath such legalistic formulae lay a basic and wider unease about the ownership of new technologies and the professional sovereignty of both the medical specialist and general practitioner in many settings. Thus in both Britain and North America, any further licensing of para-medical groups was strongly opposed, and strained patronage and informal means of influence were replaced by a policy of direct supervision by doctors' professional associations. The AMA, for example, through its Council on Medical Education, was able to extend its existing role in accrediting medical schools and teaching hospitals to the inspection of an increasing range of para-medical facilities and training standards. In 1931 and 1933, respectively, both the American Occupational and Physical Therapy Associations, in the context of the times, voluntarily entered into these arrangements. In effect, unlike less orthodox practitioners such as osteopaths and chiropractors, at that point they valued medical recognition above any possible but perhaps unattainable autonomy.[14] Similarly, the British Medical Association (BMA) in 1932 started a Board of Registration for Medical Auxiliaries, strongly supported by the medical patrons of para-medical organizations. Given that both chiropodists and opticians had failed in the 1920s to secure the progress of state registration bills through Parliament, leading radiographers and physiotherapists hoped that affiliation to the Board would enhance their legitimacy. This, in turn, could eventually bring state registration in some form.

Whatever the plausibility of these calculations, both the nature of medical control and the seeds of its demise some years later were to be seen in its founding terms. The Board's Council, vetting applicants and training programmes, had a permanent medical majority membership. This agency insisted on all para-medical groups being registered as working only under doctors' orders. Amongst others, psychiatric social workers were rejected in 1938, given their preference in some instances for seeing clients directly without medical referral. (➤ Ch. 43 Psychotherapy) Tensions were also particularly evident with chiropodists, who wanted some autonomy in both diagnosis and treatment, which historically they had enjoyed. Whilst some doctors recognized those chiropodists closest to medical influence, few accepted the chiropodists' analogy of their mutual relationship as being similar to that between medicine and dentistry. The issue of recognising an area of diagnostic autonomy for chiropodists, which did not encroach on medicine and surgery, divided the BMA's membership for over ten years up to 1939. A system of 'prescribed limitations' was finally agreed, governing depths of surgical incisions, anaesthetic procedures, treatable conditions, and practice ethics. This, however, only attracted one section of practitioners. It also alienated other practising chiropodists from the new register, which was already faltering in other occupational areas. By only admitting those who would agree to such subordinate terms, the Board limited the growth of formal medical control in the years building up to the National Health Service.

Whilst some limited and transitory settlements occurred, this did not extend to ophthalmic opticians, who were only too aware of the earlier successes of their American and Australian counterparts in securing the separate licensing of optometry. In Britain, as elsewhere, they had their own commercial premises outside of hospitals and clinics, and thus direct access to clients. Although a Health Ministry enquiry in 1927 had declared that whatever the skills of trained refractionists, no training could be 'sufficiently thorough to avoid the danger which is involved in the possession of a little medical learning',[15] within a few years official, rather than medical, attitudes changed. As at an earlier stage in America, medical ophthalmologists, as opposed to general practitioners pursuing eye-testing fees, were too few in number. Also, their preferred para-medical grade of 'dispensing optician' was too limited in role to meet the rising demand for eye-tests and reliably prescribed spectacles. Through the 1936 Insurance Act, ophthalmic opticians secured some recognition, thereby signalling a diminution in state support for overt medical dominance.

THE POST-WAR YEARS

Like the 1914–18 war, the Second World War had a major and widespread impact on para-medical professions, through expanding and more centrally organizing their services. However, again, this contributed in the post-war period to a further heightened sense of professional identity in a context of changing economic circumstances and social assumptions. 'Traditional' but, in fact, very recent links with the medical profession were questioned in a process that continues to the present day. For example, in the United States the AMA was able at first through its Council on Medical Education, to carry forward its system of directly accrediting and thus substantially controlling a range of subordinate health professions. None the less, tensions gathered force in subsequent decades as AMA influence was perceived to be an excessive constraint upon para-medical groups trying to pursue their professional advantage in the expanding health-care market.[16] By 1970, the American Society of Medical Technologists was attempting to reverse its previous practice constraints. The society successfully petitioned the Justice Department to free its members from at all times having to work under the control of qualified doctors or pathologists. This was judged to be a restraint on trade, and was matched by numerous tensions within other occupations previously more acquiescent to the medical profession authority.[17] Under these pressures in the early 1970s, the AMA, the American Hospital Association, and the Federal Government began to call for a moratorium on the pursuit of licensing issues. Their immediate concerns, focusing upon excessive specialization and fragmentation, overlay the growing difficulty of one premier profession controlling a complex occupational evolution.

This loosening of links had gathered force earlier in Britain, particularly as direct state management of health care developed at a faster pace than elsewhere. The 1940s processes of intensified planning for a new national health service forced para-medical professions to examine the future, not least as the BMA lobbied the government for statutory powers over allied professionals in the new era. Ministry policy by this time was to reject granting state support for any form of strengthened BMA control over other para-medical occupations. It should be noted, however, that this was not in itself a rejection of medical dominance.[18] Its reform and realignment, rather than end, was required, particularly as the state's own role in managing health care was strengthened. A more effective type of medical control was to be linked to overall state supervision, a policy that found expression in the establishment in 1949 of the Cope Enquiry into Medical Auxiliaries.[19] This was formally concerned with mechanisms for managing the future supply and training of radiographers, chiropodists, laboratory technicians, almoners, and speech and occupational therapists. It was, however, the first of a number of similar attempts by various governments in the post-war era to address a growing concern about the 'fragmentation of medicine'.

The report recommended the establishment of one statutory body to oversee the training and practice of all medical auxiliaries. A two-tiered system was proposed, consisting of a policy-making council and a range of occupationally specific administrative subcommittees. The unitary approach of Sir Zachary Cope (1881–1974) to the issues at least accelerated the growth of a sense of strategic co-operation across auxiliary professions. However, medical auxiliaries were to be in a permanently fixed minority to doctor membership of 'their' council. This proved, in changing times, to be an affront to a number of para-medical organizations, which attacked the assumption that doctors could, by virtue of their training and experience, satisfactorily plan and control the curricula of training and methods of work of the professions under review. In their very different view, the everyday relationship was that of specialists in a team, with the doctor as a leader but not as a supervisor of other professions. The structural relationship more generally was to be one of historically linked and co-operating but separate 'sovereignties' within health care. In Britain, this emphasis marked the emergence of seeds of an occupational 'commonwealth' rather than imperial mode of hierarchical relationships. Cope's proposals were not carried forward by the government of the day, given what it termed 'an insufficient agreement on fundamental matters'.

A new debate, however, had been opened within and between professional communities, particularly as the abandoning of Cope's proposals intensified medical concerns. The *British Medical Journal*, for example, defensively reasserted a traditional position, that 'as more and more skills develop, and as the division of labour grows ever more refined in the field of health, the more necessary it becomes to co-ordinate all this work under medical guidance'.[20] However, some medical professional opinions were also changing, and the *Lancet*, whilst reasserting the doctor's predominance over technicians, recognized the validity in part of auxiliaries' aspirations, and the 'developing stresses in the structure of medicine associated with them'. Also, less confrontational attitudes were evident in the words of Sir Russell Brain (1895–1966), then President of the Royal College of Physicians:

> these disciplines are the children of medicine in the sense that if it were not for medicine these disciplines would not exist. On the other hand if it were not for them medicine would be in many respects where it was fifty years ago. It rests on this generation to work out a pattern of relationship which would be satisfying for all concerned.[21]

Para-medical resolve in Britain to press for less medical domination and some form of state registration was enhanced in the interim by the publication in 1952 of the separate Crook Report on Opticians.[22] This recommended a General Optical Council, with registers variously for ophthalmic and dispensing opticians, and for those qualified in both branches of work. The council, made up of a majority of opticians, was to oversee training and ethical standards, and progress was also made on the issue of eye examinations. It was recognized that a proper training for ophthalmic opticians, in fact, enabled them to 'suspect the presence of disease' rather than conclusively confirm its presence, a clearly medical responsibility. This distinction between suspecting and diagnosing satisfied all parties, and after a half-century of dispute, led on relatively non-controversially to the 1958 Opticians' Act. This resembled the earlier optometry licensing in North America and Australia, although optometrists in some American states have themselves successfully resisted any formal recognition of 'dispensing opticians'.

However, despite these developments, any willingness of representatives of the medical profession in Britain to come to some wider terms of settlement with other occupations was not immediately evident. In response, and by contrast with their previous policy of working with the profession, government officials began negotiations over state registration directly with the remaining major para-medical associations in 1954. The Royal Colleges objected to any scheme that might create what were by now termed 'Professions Associated with Medicine'. After some terminological negotiations, the final settlement of 'Professions Supplementary to Medicine' emerged. This new generic title, through implying both traditional hierarchy and change, appeared to address the concerns of both parties, rooted in wider feelings that social hierarchies, which medical structures reflected, were under question. A prevalent and continuing strong sense that other health workers were both technically subordinate and socially inferior to doctors was, however, also criticized from within the medical profession. Notably Theodore Fox (1899–1989), then editor of the *Lancet*, argued for a fundamental re-evaluation of the links between medicine and related professions.

Fox's concept of the 'Greater Medical Profession' offered a positive picture, one of capitalizing upon rather than trying to refute the inevitable social, technical, and educational changes affecting medicine and all social spheres at the time. He argued that 'medicine' and 'doctors' were unfortunately conflated in the minds of too many medical practitioners, which was associated, in turn, with a mentality demanding unique and in this way unmerited forms of respect. Contrary to these views, the interdependency of medicine, in Fox's argument, had to be acknowledged as a product of an ever more complex division of labour. The co-ordination of health care as a consequence was only possible by training doctors in the skills of leading rather than subordinating related skilled workers, even if this might lead in the longer term to a reduction of status and income differentials. Instead of a rigid solid hierarchy of the medical profession and the 'others', a 'commonwealth' of senior and emergent professions was required, not only for the future but equally for a resolution of immediate conflicts. As Fox put it:

On the analogy of political empires, we should be well advised to avoid making our concessions too small or leaving them too late. We should show ourselves as reasonable elder brothers, not as rulers who are being pushed. For my part, I believe that, if we want our medical commonwealth to hold together, it is safer to err on the side of too much self-government than of too little. I believe that our greater medical profession will run better if we go as far as is reasonably possible towards granting full professional status to every kind of person in it.[23]

These sentiments, and the associated warnings of offering 'too little too late', proved relevant in the case of one group with ambitions beyond any accolade of acknowledgement as a 'profession supplementary to medicine'. By this stage, speech therapists wished to be totally free of any lingering attenuated medical tutelage and thus pressed for their exclusion from the impending Act, on the grounds that their links were at least as much with disciplines such as phonetics and psychology as with medicine. They had previously joined the BMA's auxiliary board as recently as 1942, but by the 1950s were very reluctant to stay within even a weakened and reformed medical embrace. The College of Speech Therapists argued instead for complete professional autonomy, and hoped, incidentally, for pay parity with teachers, thought at the time to be an advantageous tactic. Ministry of Health officials opposed their policy, on the grounds that the ultimate diagnosis of the causes of speech disorders must rest with the medical profession, but they were overruled by their then Minister. State registration was to be presented as a prize, an accolade for development, and not as a constraint upon an occupation seeking finally to distance itself from the premier profession and a fixed para-medical identity.

Despite the *Lancet*'s support for changes in attitudes, opposition to legislation continued up to 1960 amongst leading doctors. The BMA's official position was that any registering body for para-medical professions should be 'predominantly medical in composition'. This, as ministry records indicate, was not to be conceded, and a final supervisory council balanced doctors and 'auxiliaries' in equal numbers. The associated professional boards were dominated by the newly recognized professions, and disputes within the council or between the council and boards were to be subject to government adjudication. Thus the eventual Act, in operation and principle, was a compromise, insofar as it reduced both 'excesses' of medical power and para-medical ambition. The state, in an increasingly common international pattern, became an umpire, or to further Fox's analogy, an appeal court functioning jointly across a range of professional jurisdictions. In this new role, British government calculations were that the medical profession would display its feelings rather than co-ordinate any outright challenge. This calculation proved to be correct, and the Professions Supplementary to Medicine Act came into effect in 1960. The *British Medical Journal*, noting a concern that the case for medical control had failed, proffered a warning about 'specialization outside the control of the doctor going too far'. The *Lancet* was more welcoming to the new professions, albeit claiming that 'the application rather than the development of science' distinguished their training from that of doctors and dentists. Naturally, it was hailed as the start of a new era by the professions themselves, and little concern was expressed about continuing medical participation on a reduced basis in their affairs or the now more formal and direct involvement of the state in professional jurisdictions.[24]

CONCLUSION

Various social, political, economic, and technological changes, as they impact upon complex health-care systems, stimulate the growth of a proliferating range of para-medical occupations. By the mid-1970s, for example, the eight core supplementary professions recognized by the 1960 Act in Britain – that is, radiography, chiropody, dietetics, medical laboratory technology, occupational therapy, orthoptics, physiotherapy, and remedial gymnastics – formed only a proportion of the approximately forty occupations classified as paramedical in government statistics.[25] In the same period in the USA, new roles also appeared, such as 'physician assistants', although this particular development has perhaps been overtaken by a growing concern about an 'oversupply' of doctors in the 1980s. Other relatively new occupations in the USA include inhalation therapists, electroencephalograph technicians, cytotechnologists, and orthotists.[26] The involvement of the modern state in health care, whether directly as in Britain or through controlling the limits of a 'free market', inevitably extends in these circumstances to attempts to regulate its labour supply and character. The issue extends beyond health professions into the regulation of all professional or 'expertise-based' services. The attempt, for example, of the Quebec government to establish an overall framework for 'professional corporations' in 1973 resulted in the formal recognition of twenty-five health occupations.[27] A similar review in Ontario, limited to health occupations, in 1989 led to seventy-five submissions from aspiring groups and twenty-four recognized professions. Medicine in Canada, as elsewhere, has faced a whole series of occupations in recent decades 'either defending or seeking to establish their autonomy and/or actively chipping away at medical territory'.[28] The eventual state licensing of radiographers in the Australian state of Victoria, finally overcoming protracted medical opposition in 1983, further exemplifies the process of inevitable state regulation to some degree moderating earlier types of medical dominance.[29]

As occupational relationships with the state and the character of interprofessional controls changed in the post-war period, at the same time particular para-medical occupations have gone through a number of internal changes. As technologies and the social context of practice evolve, some have followed the nursing profession and undergone internal restructurings creating new lesser-trained permanent 'assistant' grades. This may be favoured by employers as creating cheaper labour and as an antidote to professionally dominated 'over-long' training periods. It may also add to the scarcity value of the 'real', fully trained professional, particularly if unskilled competition can be eliminated by para-medical control of the new subordinate group. American laboratory technologists have developed, for example, a certified assistant programme based on a shorter training period under their supervision. In this respect, previous historical patterns evident between medicine and its 'satellite' occupations appear again within the latter as the century closes. Technological change, as well as labour-cost pressures, also creates both 'de-' and 're-professionalizing' changes. For example, in the case of radiographers, continuing technical changes arguably may have de-skilled their work. Equipment has continued to improve, so that X-ray production, dosimetry, and exposures are in part automatically governed. In some instances, compared to fifty years ago, arguably little skill beyond 'button-pushing' may be left. On the other hand, rising public concerns over safety, new types of ultrasonic, nuclear magnetic, and computer-enhanced imaging, in conjunction with ever-sophisticated medical and surgical procedures, all call for notably enhanced knowledge and training. The full impact of an on-going revolution in diagnostic imaging, with its clearer location and representation of ever-smaller *in vivo* tissue damage and change, largely remains to be seen. This could embrace a host of occupations and specialities in health care seeking access to, control of, and benefits for their own evolving identities.

These developments, in turn, continue to strain the social, legal, and professional codes associated with earlier social and technical phases in the medical division of labour. The pattern of past social divisions, as exemplified, for instance, in the distinct phases of producing and assessing an X-ray film or plate, can no longer encompass and divide the emergent technologies. Patients, however, have also changed in their types of morbidity and, in particular, their expectations concerning health and the boundaries of lay and professional knowledge. These latter aspects of change call for enhanced psychological and social skills of interaction and communication from all in the wider medical profession. (➤ Ch. 34 History of the doctor–patient relationship) Thus, whilst some technical changes, as in the broader context of industry, may render occupational practices obsolete, in health care the balance is towards an extension and deepening of the range of skills and competences required of its occupations.

As para-medical occupations widen their particular roles as well as their numbers under forces of social and technical change, the 'turf-disputes' of the past, however archaic to the modern eye, seem set to continue. The surfacing of associated controversies has been muted of late by another internationally evident tendency. Various national governments, most particularly through the 1980s, have sought to reduce or at least to hold costs and the ever-growing rate of state involvement in the overall management and financing of health and welfare.[30] In a climate of cost-containment, renewed claims to professional identities in particular may be viewed as attempts to escape paymaster scrutiny. Ironically, health-service managers, charged with profit/cost responsibilities in these circumstances, have an interest in incorporating an anti-professional rhetoric in their own recent occupational ascendancy. Accountants and professional managers perhaps inevitably prosper, even in a period with echoes of some of the more jaundiced eighteenth- and nineteenth-century perceptions of the pretences and conceits of occupational monopolies. (➤ Ch. 57 Health economics)

It is perhaps one other major change, more lasting than the mutations of government policies, which in recent decades has gathered force, and will impact upon all para-medical professions and the pattern of interprofessional relationships. It mirrors what occurred in the case of the medical profession itself, which in preceding centuries was able progressively to eliminate an apprenticeship type of training for its practitioners. By the early 1900s, doctors qualified through a university-based education and qualification system, whatever their clinical training in hospitals during it. In previous centuries, access to the universities varied across the separate interrelated castes of the pre-modern profession, evident in Britain in the convergent but once separate apprenticeship training of apothecaries and barber-surgeons in contrast to élite physicians. (➤ Ch. 48 Medical education) This process was virtually complete by the time of the emergence of the para-professions, and indeed was intimately linked to it by providing a new apprentice group or occupational class guaranteed to retain rather than eventually to transcend responsibilities for routine and less-attractive work.

Thus through the period mostly discussed in this chapter, the emergent hierarcy of medical labour was at first firmly based upon differences in educational, social, and very often gender status across a graduate/non-graduate divide. Typically, doctors were university trained and male, whilst para-medical workers, like nurses, were very often female and trained in hospital schools or working units as part of the labour force in a shorter apprentice mode. (➤ Ch. 38 Women and medicine) Access to longer university-based qualifications, rather than relatively short on-the-job training, was also associated with professions such as optometry and dentistry, which were able to establish more autonomous spheres of practice. In periods and countries where graduates in general, and in particular female graduates in medicine, were few, para-medical training provided a respectable alternative for women and lower-class men competing to secure their livelihoods. As general educational opportunities have widened, in turn, para-medical preparation has extensively moved to a university or equivalent base. Whilst very far from being complete, this tendency, more advanced in North America and Australia than in Europe, is unlikely to be reversed. It is fuelled by forces outside of and reflected within the world of medicine, emanating from the functional and administrative requirements of complex modern societies. Whether a medical 'commonwealth' of notionally equal but really status-divided professions can everywhere flexibly accommodate these gathering changes remains to be seen. Interprofessional co-ordination, as required to offset the fragmenting effects of increasing occupational specialization may, as the century closes, prove to be more elusive than in the more-clearly status-ranked era of its dawn. (➤ Ch. 70 Medical sociology)

NOTES

1 E. W. Law, *The Worshipful Company of Spectacle Makers. A History*, London, Worshipful Company of Spectacle Makers, 1978, p. 81.

2 J. W. Begun and R. C. Lippincott, 'The politics of professional control, the case of optometry', in J. A. Roth (ed.), *Research in the Sociology of Health Care*, Greenwich, CT, JAI Press, 1980.

3 J. H. Wickstead, *The Growth of a Profession*, London, Edward Arnold, 1948.

4 G. Gritzer and A. Arluke, *The Making of Rehabilitation. A Political Economy of Medical Specialization 1890–1980*, Berkeley, University of California Press, 1985, p. 53.

5 H. L. Hopkins, 'A historical perspective on occupational therapy', in Hopkins and M. D. Smith (eds), *Occupational Therapy*, 7th edn, Philadelphia, Lippincott, 1988.

6 L. Cooper *Occupational Therapy, an Emerging Profession in Health Care*, College of Occupational Therapists, London, Duckworth, 1990.

7 G. Gritzer, 'Occupational specialization in medicine, knowledge and market explantions', in Roth, op. cit. (n. 2).

8 *British Medical Journal*, 1903, 1: 831.

9 General Medical Council Minutes, London, 1906, p. 198.

10 R. C. Number, 'The fall and rise of the American medical profession', in N. O. Hatch (ed.) *The Professions in American History*, Notre Dame, Indiana, University of Notre Dame Press, 1988.

11 P. Starr, *The Social Transformation of American Medicine*, New York, Basic Books, 1982, p. 222.

12 Hernaman-Johnson, 'The place of the radiologist and his kindred in the world of medicine', *Archives of Radiology and Electrotherapy*, 1919, 24: 181.

13 G. V. Larkin, 'Medical dominance and control, radiographers in the division of labour, *Sociological Review*, 1978 26: 843–58.

14 Gritzer, op. cit. (n. 7).

15 *Report of the Committee on the Optical Practitioners Registration Bill*, Cmnd 2999, London, HMSO, 1927, p. 13.

16   C. A. Brown, 'The division of laborers, allied health professions', *International Journal of Health Services*, 1973, 3: 435–44.

17   M. R. Williams, *An Introduction to the Profession of Medical Technology*, Philadelphia, Lea & Febiger, 1971.

18   Public Record Office, London, MH 58: 234.

19   Report of the Committees on Medical Auxiliaries (chaired Z. Cope), Cmnd 8188, London, HMSO, 1952.

20   'Medical Auxiliaries', *British Medical Journal*, 1953, 1: 1267–8.

21   *Journal of the Chartered Society of Physiotherapy*, 1953, 52.

22   *Inter-departmental Committee on the Statutory Registration of Opticians*, Cmnd 8531, London, HMSO, 1952.

23   T. Fox, 'The greater medical profession', *Lancet*, 1956, 779.

24   G. V. Larkin, *Occupational Monopoly and Modern Medicine*, London, Tavistock, 1983.

25   B. Donald, 'Professions auxiliary, supplementary or complementary to medicine', *Health Trends*, 1978 10: 5–9.

26   Brown, op cit. (n. 16).

27   L. Soderstrom, *The Canadian Health System*, London, Croom Helm, 1978, p. 82.

28   D. Coburn *et al.*, 'Medical dominance in Canada in historical perspective: the rise and fall of medicine', *International Journal of Health Services*, 1983, 13 (3): 407–33.

29   J. Daly and E. Willis, 'Technological innovation and the labour process in health care', *Social Science and Medicine*, 1989, 28 (11): 1149–57.

30   Cf. the range of international papers in the *Milbank Quarterly*, 'The changing character of the medical profession', 1988, 66 (2).

FURTHER READING

Gritzer, G. and Arluke, A., *The Making of Rehabilitation. A Political Economy of Medical Specialization 1890–1980*, Berkeley, University of California Press, 1985.

Larkin G. V., *Occupational Monopoly and Modern Medicine*, London, Tavistock, 1983.

Willis, E., *Medical Dominance, the Division of Labour in Australian Health Care*, Sydney, Allen & Unwin, 1983.

56

PSYCHIATRY

Jan Goldstein

Although the attempt to heal madness goes back in the Western medical tradition at least to Hippocrates (*c*.450–370 BC), psychiatry as a medical speciality – that is, a gainful form of medical practice that occupied its practitioners full-time and to the exclusion of other branches of healing – was the invention of the late eighteenth century. It had, at the level of ideas, two major prerequisites: a new technique for treating madness, called the moral treatment, which was believed to bring about cure on a more regular and reliable basis than anything that had preceded it; and a new institution, the asylum, conceptualized both as the appropriate setting for the cure of madness and as itself an active instrument of cure. A third factor, the increase of population density, was a prerequisite not only for psychiatry, but for the phenomenon of medical specialization more generally. (➤ Ch. 47 History of the medical profession)

Modern medical specialization differed fundamentally from the traditional tripartite division of the healing art into medicine, surgery, and pharmacy that could be found everywhere in Europe under the guild system of the Old Regime. The traditional division assumed a hierarchical superiority of medicine, as a liberal art marshalling knowledge and requiring intellectual capability, over the other two, as merely mechanical arts. By contrast, medical specialization, which parcelled out different diseases to different types of doctors, assumed intellectual parity among the specialities. The idea for such specialization appears to have come from the model of craft manufacture,[1] where the strategy of assigning to different workers the different operations entailed in producing a commodity evolved naturally as changing market conditions dictated the production of goods on an increasingly large scale. This spontaneous economic development was then theorized – for example, by Denis Diderot (1713–84) in the *Encyclopédie* in the early 1750s[2] – and held up as a desideratum on the grounds of the greater efficiency and degree of expertise that it brought about. Eventually, Adam Smith (1723–90) in his *Wealth of Nations* (1776), with its celebrated example of the pin-factory, labelled the principle the 'division of labour' and gave it canonical status.

The division of medical labour, however, lagged behind its craft precursor by many decades. For one thing, the theory of humours, still prevalent during the eighteenth century, construed every disease as an event of the entire body, and its holistic perspective discouraged focus on any single disease. (➤ Ch. 14 Humoralism) By contrast, early nineteenth-century pathological anatomy, or the theory of disease as a localized organ lesion, offered a congenial intellectual underpinning for a restriction of medical focus. (➤ Ch. 9 The pathological tradition) 'Each organ has its priest', as one German physician colourfully described the situation of medical specialization in Paris in the 1840s.[3] For another thing, the Old Regime healing art had developed a rudimentary form of specialization with highly pejorative connotations. The riskiest operations – those most likely to fail and hence to bring obloquy upon the practitioners who performed them – were abandoned by legitimate surgeons and fell instead to a floating body of unlicensed practitioners, who were called (among other things) specialists. (➤ Ch. 41 Surgery (traditional)) Hawking their services in the early-modern town and countryside, these specialists included itinerant oculists and 'cataract couchers', lithotomists, and hernia-operators.[4] Owing to their familiar presence, the notion of medical specialization became confused with and tainted by that of quackery, and this taint impeded the acceptance of specialization by accredited medical men. (➤ Ch. 28 Unorthodox medical theories)

Eventually, however, the victory of medical specialization was assured not only by the victory of pathological anatomy, but also by a series of demographic factors: the increasing size of urban populations, the glut of professionals during the first half of the nineteenth century,[5] and the increasing competition for patients among the disproportionate number of physicians who chose to practise in cities. (➤ Ch. 71 Demography and medicine) The division of medical labour was, as the sociologist Emile Durkheim (1858–1917) would describe it in 1893:

> a result of the [occupational] struggle for existence, but it is a mellowed denouement. Thanks to it, opponents are not obliged to fight to a finish, but can exist one beside the other.... The oculist does not struggle with the psychiatrist, nor the shoemaker with the hatter.[6]

Durkheim's 'mellowed denouement' was, of course, the final result; specialization-in-process, by contrast, almost always generated intensely bitter feelings within the ranks of the medical profession as the claims of the new specialists increasingly forced generalists out of previously shared turf. Thus, for example, when the Paris city hospital system in 1840 created a new position devoted solely to the treatment of the urinary tract and appointed a specialist to fill it, the general surgeons of the Paris hospitals wrote a long and irate letter of protest against this 'introduction of specialities'; the editors of the prestigious medical journal which published the letter applauded the efforts of the generalists and urged them to take even stronger measures in defence of their cause.[7] A popular French career guide of the same period warned the young doctor that electing to follow one of the specialities would require living with the unceasing 'opprobrium or at least low esteem of his colleagues'.[8]

If psychiatry participated in the delicate and conflict-laden process that attended the formation of all modern medical specialities, its formation also had features peculiar to it alone. An examination of its founding therapeutic strategy – the moral treatment – and its correlative institution – the asylum – will make these peculiarities clear. (➤ Ch. 21 Mental diseases)

MORAL TREATMENT

Cursorily defined (and we shall need to elaborate that definition in the course of this chapter), the moral treatment for the cure of insanity meant the use of methods that engaged or operated upon the intellect and emotions, as opposed to the traditional methods of bleedings, purges, and vomits applied directly to the lunatic's body. While it did not entail a complete abandonment of the old stock of physical remedies, it did entail an acknowledgement of their grave insufficiency. (➤ Ch. 40 Physical methods)

The moral treatment was of combined Anglo-French provenance and quickly became the subject of a muted priority dispute between those two nations. When French practitioners began to cultivate it, they routinely cited previous English successes with the method and credited their counterparts across the Channel (for example, Francis Willis (1718–1807), who had assumed the weighty responsibility of treating the madness of King George III during the period 1788–9) with having provided them with inspiration. The French physician Philippe Pinel (1745–1826), who codified the moral treatment in his *Traité médico-philosophique sur l'aliénation mentale* (1801), fitted this pattern, but Pinel added to his grateful acknowledgement of the English precursors a rather damning critique of them. Nowhere, he said, had they provided a written description of the moral treatment detailed enough to guide the novice; instead, they perversely kept 'impenetrably veiled' the new therapeutic technique that they so enthusiastically recommended.[9] Pinel proposed to fill this gap by clearly specifying the components of the method. For their part, the English regarded Pinel with disdain; noting the 'decided superiority [of] the practice towards maniacs in Great Britain', the *Edinburgh*

Review opined in 1803 that 'readers in this country' would find the discussion of the moral treatment in Pinel's book 'neither new nor profound'.[10] By the 1830s, when French alienists had acquired a firmer sense of professional identity, their rehearsals of their collective history omitted all mention of the British origins of the moral treatment. They represented their history as a wholly French one, and they even transformed Pinel's alleged invention of the moral treatment into a dramatic founding moment of mythic proportions. Pinel was said to have literally unchained the furious lunatics of the Bicêtre during the radical republican phase of the French Revolution, and by this emancipatory act to have rendered them instantly calm and tractable. Memorialized in paintings, this founding myth of the psychiatric profession has only recently been exposed by scholars as largely fictive.[11]

But what, precisely, was the moral treatment? Pinel never gave a formulaic or even an explicit answer to that question; however, from the account embedded in the case histories in his *Traité*, several points emerge as salient.[12] First, in therapeutic interventions, the alienist was to prefer use of the 'ways of gentleness'. This strategy of gentleness, rooted in the optimism associated with the Enlightenment, assumed that insanity did not entail a full-scale obliteration of the patient's rational faculties and a descent into bestial status, but that a vestige of 'humanity' always remained and could be appealed to and reinforced. Second, in those cases where gentleness had little impact on the lunatic, the alienist was obliged to undertake – regretfully and without anger – the task of 'repression' or 'subjugation'. For this purpose, the alienist's very physical presence was supposed to exude authority. Sometimes, the authority might inhere a particular aspect of that presence. For example, Francis Willis, whose talents Pinel described in this context, was renowned for a piercing gaze that infallibly conveyed to lunatics the message that he was their master; as Willis himself put it, he commanded 'by the EYE!'.[13] The third principle of the moral treatment was to combat and destroy the erroneous idea that had lodged in the patient's mind and was, according to the theories of sensationalist psychology prevalent in western Europe in this period, responsible for the condition of insanity. To this end, the alienist needed either to have gained the confidence of the patient by employing gentle means or to have coerced the patient's respect by employing repressive and fearsome ones. Once this groundwork was laid, the idea-combat took two basic forms. The alienist could attempt to distract the patient from the pathological idea, usually by engaging him or her in useful labour or having him or her listen to music. Or the alienist could subject the patient to a startling or jolting experience – to 'strike the imagination strongly', in Pinel's parlance – in a manner calculated to discredit a particular idea. This second technique frequently lent the moral treatment an element of theatricality, as when Pinel staged a mock-trial to acquit a patient suffering from delusional guilt, or enlisted a convalescent patient to tell a joke that made a patient in the throes of delirium suddenly aware of the ludicrous illogic of his or her assertions. A final aspect of the moral treatment concerned the management of disordered and disabling passions. (In contrast to the sensationalist psychologists, who represented insanity in purely intellectual terms as a type of error, Pinel insisted that the viscerally based passions also played a part in the aetiology of that disease.) Like other aspects of the moral treatment, passional management relied upon the extraordinary authority presumed to emanate from the figure of the alienist, who as a pedagogue of the passions was cast in the almost omnipotent, world-restructuring role of the tutor in the *Emile* (1762) of Jean Jacques Rousseau (1712–78).

A technique composed of such diverse elements was obviously open to diverse interpretations. While early nineteenth-century proponents of the moral treatment stressed that its leitmotiv was gentle humanitarianism coupled with enlightened rational optimism, late twentieth-century historians have tended to offer very different characterizations. One, focusing upon the British origins of psychiatry and especially the care for insane Quakers instituted at the York Retreat, saw the moral treatment as an effort to develop the lunatic's powers of self-control and thus to 'remodel him into something approximating the bourgeois ideal of the rational individual'; as such, the moral treatment was part of a larger cultural movement toward the internalization of disciplinary norms, a movement necessitated by industrial capitalism.[14] Another scholar, studying the French data, reached the similar conclusion that the moral treatment fused a moralizing discourse with a medical one; it was a forced inhalation of 'the pure oxygen of bourgeois morality, alone capable of resuscitating for the social order those subjects who have failed in it'.[15] While there are undeniable areas of congruence between the moral treatment, on the one hand, and such global historical phenomena as the bourgeois ethos and the need to discipline the new factory labour force, on the other, this chapter will focus on a more limited problem: the significance of the moral treatment for the professionalization of psychiatry.

In this regard, one attribute of the moral treatment stands out as having profound implications for the formulation of a medical speciality of psychiatry: in terms of both its origin and content, the moral treatment was decidedly non-medical. Before its adoption by medical practitioners, it had been informally developed by lay people; and insofar as medicine meant in the eighteenth century 'Physick', or the application of physical remedies, the moral treatment stood outside its purview. These facts were hardly a secret. William Tuke (1732–1822), who ran the York Retreat and instituted the moral treatment there, was a layman – a wholesale tea and coffee merchant highly vocal about his distrust of medical practitioners who pretended to treat insanity.[16] Although Pinel was himself an accredited physician, he trumpeted the degree to which he had relied upon lay caretakers of the insane – *concierges*, he called them – in formulating his ideas about the moral treatment. For Pinel, this point was a political one. Associating himself with the French Revolutionary attack upon the exclusivity of the privileged corporations, he wanted to show that members of the élite faculties of medicine could not be counted upon to foster medical progress, that the contributions of humble outsiders like the *concierges* of the insane were equally, if not more, necessary.[17] But whatever the reasons for adopting it, the moral treatment saddled the emergent psychiatric speciality with a practical problem: how to turn a non-medical technique into the basis of a medical claim for monopolistic control over the care of the insane.

This problem was handled differently in Britain and in France, as a reflection of the different political cultures of those two nations. In Britain, with its precocious constitutional government, Parliament had become involved in lunacy policy at an early date, primarily to curb civil-rights abuses in connection with the wrongful incarceration of individuals on grounds of insanity, or the inhumane treatment of those rightfully incarcerated. Thus already in 1774, a parliamentary act set down conditions for the regulation of the private, profit-making madhouses flourishing in the British *laissez-faire* economy.[18] The moral treatment had achieved a certain renown when Samuel Tuke (1784–1857) published his *Description of the Retreat* (1813), but it was brought to national attention by a parliamentary Select Committee in 1815–16, charged with investigating allegations of maltreatment in public institutions for the insane, including the famous Bethlem in London. Dr Thomas Monro (1759–1833) of the latter institution testified under pressure that, while respect for tradition had led him to rely heavily on the putative medical remedies for madness (bleedings, purges, vomits), such remedies had little effect, and any cures he obtained were rather the result of techniques of moral management. This and similar, highly publicized testimony by other eminent physicians – as well as William Tuke's own testimony against the medical treatment of mental derangement – necessitated that those members of the British medical profession intent on exercising control over insanity find some way to accommodate the moral treatment within their therapeutic arsenal. After a long period of uneasy debate between the alternatives of medical and moral therapy, the official line of British psychiatry became by the 1840s that a judicious *combination* of the two was more valuable than the exclusive use of either.[19] Thus, in Britain, parliamentary muckraking was instrumental in bringing about the medical adoption and legitimation of the moral treatment.

In France, by contrast, a medical profession centralized in Paris adopted the moral treatment on its own initiative, beginning in the 1790s, and used it to ground claims for the establishment of a new psychiatric speciality. To be sure, the founding-father, Pinel, did not accept the moral treatment in its pristine, lay form but attempted to raise it to fully scientific status by translating it into the language of sensationalist psychology and demonstrating its efficacy statistically.[20] None the less, reliance upon the moral treatment proved a mixed blessing for Pinel's successors, who were left extremely vulnerable to competition from traditional Catholic healers of the insane. The latter shrewdly turned the alienists' own arguments against them, pointing out the decided superiority of priests, monks, and nuns in offering emotional support and consoling words to the mentally disturbed; such clerics could invoke the promises of the Gospel, a resource abandoned by thoroughly secular French alienists.[21] (➤ Ch. 61 Religion and medicine) Thus the pivotal place of the moral treatment in French psychiatric discourse encouraged a protracted boundary dispute between the nascent psychiatric profession and the Catholic clergy over which group would be entrusted by society with the care of the insane. The dispute was not resolved until the closing decades of the nineteenth century when, as part of its general anti-clerical crusade, the Third Republic lent strong support to the professional claims of a scientific *médecine mentale*.[22] The contest between psychiatry and religion was less marked in Britain. In refusing completely to relinquish physical remedies for insanity in either theory or practice, nineteenth-century British alienists exhibited a certain tactical shrewdness, for they explicitly recognized that an exclusive embrace of moral remedies would suggest 'the clergyman rather than the physician as the logical person to treat insanity'.[23]

In the German lands, where physicians first coined the term 'psychiatry' (*Psychiatrie*) from the ancient Greek roots meaning a medicine of the mind, and where the publication of psychiatric periodicals (albeit short-lived ones) began in 1805 – earlier than anywhere else – the actual practice of the new medical speciality lagged notably behind the theory.[24] German medicine of the first half of the nineteenth century developed under the aegis of Romantic *Naturphilosophie*, an application of philosophical idealism to the realm of nature which assumed a fundamental identity between mind and nature and sought to bring the latter to consciousness of itself. As a result, German physicians frequently rejected as methodologically impoverished the empirical, observational bent of their French and British counterparts, and the self-styled psychiatrists of the pioneering German generation found the espousal of some version of the moral treatment – that is, of a treatment for madness that ministered to the mind rather than the body – entirely congenial and unproblematic. The *Rhapsodien über die Anwendung der psychischen Curmethode auf Geisteszerrütingen* (1803) of Johann Christian Reil (1759–1813) proposed to adapt the Anglo-French moral treatment to German conditions. The book, generally regarded as the beginning of German psychiatry, included many of the 'gentle' strategies we have already seen (the tall, majestic alienist with stentorian voice impressing on the patient's imagination; the staff trained in play-acting in order to second the alienist's efforts to unseat the patient's fixed ideas). But it also recommended a dose of brutality (application of sealing-wax to the palms, whipping with nettles, submersion in a tub full of eels) to render the patient entirely receptive to the good offices of the healers.[25] J. C. A. Heinroth (1773–1843), who unlike Reil had some first-hand experience with the insane and who taught psychiatric medicine at Leipzig from 1811, presented his variant on the moral treatment in his *Lehrbuch der Störungen des Seelenlebens* (1818). Unlike French alienists of the period, who typically shunned the language of religion, Heinroth drew an analogy between insanity and sin. Both were voluntary and hence transgressive renunciations of the rational capacity for free choice, God's original gift to humans. According to Heinroth, the moral treatment forced the mad person back into the norm of reason by subjecting him to the healthy, religious, and hence stronger personality of the alienist.[26] But because the Germans of this period were more energetic about developing psychiatric theory than about applying it, they were largely spared the professional problems associated with the implementation of the moral treatment in Britain and France.

The American proponent of the moral treatment was Benjamin Rush (1746–1813), an ardent Pennsylvania democrat who was among the signatories of the Declaration of Independence, served as a military surgeon during the American Revolution, and described fellow citizens who refrained from active revolutionary participation as afflicted with 'Tory rot'. Never a full-time psychiatrist, from 1787 Rush had exclusive care of the maniacs in the wards of the Pennsylvania Hospital. At the end of his life, he published his *Medical Inquiries and Observations upon the Diseases of the Mind*, the first and for many years the only American textbook on the nature and treatment of insanity. Like Pinel, Rush believed in psychosomatic reciprocity; but more physiological in orientation than the French, he emphasized the influence of body over mind more than that of mind over body. Accordingly, Rush's rendition of the moral treatment included the requisite gentle and theatrical psychological interventions, but he put more stock in physical treatments designed to cure madness by altering the flow and pressure of the blood. Hence his famous 'tranquilizer', a restraining armchair with a box for the patient's head intended to reduce both external sensations and the activity of the cerebral arteries; and its complementary contraption, the 'gyrator', whose centrifugal action was supposed to carry blood away from the brain.[27] As in the case of Germany, there was a temporal disjunction in the United States between the theoretical articulation of the moral treatment and the wide-scale development of psychiatric practice in the asylum.

THE ASYLUM

The insane asylum is one of a group of institutions which, in the 1960s, the American sociologist Erving Goffman labelled 'total institutions'. While found in many historical eras, they proliferated noticeably in the West during the late eighteenth and early nineteenth centuries. Other total institutions invented during this peculiarly fertile period include the prison and the poorhouse. Total institutions, according to Goffman, defy the ordinary, compartmentalizing arrangement of modern society whereby individuals 'sleep, play and work in different places, with different co-participants [and] under different authorities' and instead locate all three spheres of life in a single place and under a single authority. They prescribe and rigorously enforce from above a tight schedule of activities; and their population is divided between the inmates, who reside in the institution, and a small supervisory staff, who spend the workday there but reside outside. The total, all-encompassing nature of the institution is symbolized by 'a barrier to social intercourse with the outside and to departure that is often built right into the physical plant, such as locked doors, high walls . . .'.[28]

Twentieth-century commentators have viewed the remarkable efflorescence of the total institution during the late eighteenth and early nineteenth centuries as a response to the social disorder attendant upon industrialization and the breakdown of a traditional, fixed social hierarchy. The anxiety produced by the appearance of large and conspicuous numbers of wandering lunatics, criminals, and paupers could be allayed by building incarcerative institutions which, it was firmly believed, would not only keep such deviants out of sight and prevent them from inflicting harm, but would also, by dint of a rehabilitative regimen, prepare them for eventual re-entry into society in a normal, productive capacity.[29] It must be stressed that the incarceration of deviants was not in itself the novelty of this period. At least since the 'Great Confinement' of the mid-seventeenth century, western European nations had made a concerted effort to remove deviants from the streets. The novelty lay rather in an unprecedented confidence in the therapeutic efficacy of certain forms of incarceration and in a fresh taxonomic sensibility that led to the division and strict segregation of deviants according to type. By contrast, the French *hôpital général* of the age of Louis XIV, and its counterparts, the German *Zuchthaus* and British workhouse, had entertained no therapeutic ambitions and had indiscriminately lumped together madness, idleness, debauchery, venereal disease, and old age as fully comparable species of unreason.[30] Like the embrace of the moral treatment, so, too, the wedding of psychiatry to the institutional form of the asylum imposed special professionalization problems on the emergent psychiatric speciality. In order to survive collectively, psychiatrists needed a governmental or private agency that was willing to make a large capital investment in the construction of asylums and was persuaded also that the key personage on the asylum staff was the physician.

If the Germans coined the term 'psychiatry', the self-conscious appropriation for psychiatry of the old term 'asylum' (*asile*), meaning a place of refuge, was a French contribution – the linguistic work of Pinel's student, Jean-Etienne-Dominique Esquirol (1772–1840). During the second decade of the nineteenth century, Esquirol embarked on a series of systematic, self-financed tours of the facilities for lunatics throughout France. Describing these fact-finding missions in a memoir presented to the Minister of the Interior in 1818, and urging the amelioration of the 'revolting barbarism' he had observed (lunatics detained in jails, chained in dark cellars, or mixed pell-mell with people suffering from other afflictions), Esquirol remarked, 'I would like these [new] establishments [housing only the insanc] to be given a specific name which conjures up no painful idea; I would like them to be called asylums.'[31]

Esquirol's 1818 memoir was his first overture to the state bureaucracy on behalf of the nascent medical speciality of psychiatry. In it, he argued that the care of lunatics in France should be everywhere entrusted to a 'special physician with special expertise' who, having renounced all other clientele, would have complete personal dominion over a newly created asylum. By dint of such architectural features as a courtyard for promenades and a minimum of bars and padlocks, the asylum would function not merely as a segregated depot for lunatics, but also as 'an instrument of cure'.[32] (➤ Ch. 64 Medicine and architecture)

The brunt of Esquirol's professional project was realized only later in the Law of 30 June 1838 on the asylums. As part of the lobbying for that Law, Esquirol fine-tuned his assertions about the therapeutic efficacy of the asylum. He put forth the theory of isolation, which quickly came to overshadow the moral treatment as the chief basis of the alienists' bid for public authority. Isolation consisted, said Esquirol, in 'removing the lunatic from all his habitual pastimes, distancing him from his place of residence, separating him from his family, his friends, his servants, surrounding him with strangers, altering his whole way of life.' The technique was grounded, like the moral treatment, in eighteenth-century sensationalist psychology. The sudden, radical change in environment was supposed to alter the stimuli impinging on the lunatic's mind and thus to shake up and dislodge the pathological ideas entrenched there, leaving the psychiatrist in a position to provide the lunatic with new stimuli productive of new and sane ideas. Some of the therapeutic benefits of isolation might be accomplished through travel to distant lands, especially in the company of a stranger. But clearly, the standard form of isolation was a stay of some duration in an asylum.[33]

In the legislative debate leading to the passage of the Law of 1838, the theory of isolation was frequently mentioned on the floor of the Chambers as a medical-scientific justification for the political measure at hand. Indeed, the Law resulted from a close collaboration between politicians and psychiatrists – the former expressly committed to a humanitarian mode of handling the insane that would also be protective of public order ('philanthropy and police', the slogan ran), the latter offering their medical-scientific expertise in return for a massive enhancement of their public role and status. In other words, the Law provided a context in which politicians of a liberal stamp and psychiatrists legitimated one another. In the form in which it was finally approved, it mandated the creation of a nationwide network of asylums staffed by full-time medical doctors. It thus brought into existence a race of psychiatric functionaries: appointed by the Minister of the Interior, removable by him, and paid salaries in accordance with a fixed bureaucratic scale. In addition, the Law made provision for students attached to the asylums, thus formalizing the latter's status not merely as a hospital for patients, but also as a training institute to ensure the transmission of psychiatric knowledge. It placed privately run madhouses under state supervision and mandated their medicalization. That the Law also played a critical, if indirect, role in solidifying a sense of collective professional identity among French alienists is shown by the fact that it supplied the impetus for the founding of the first psychiatric journal in France, the *Annales médico-psychologiques* (founded 1843).[34]

The Law of 1838 proved truly comprehensive, and is still in force in the late twentieth century.[35] During the first fifteen years after its passage, compliance generally took the form of makeshift measures; the rash of construction of new public asylums began only in the 1850s, leading one historian to observe: 'It was the same for the asylums as for the railroads: the regime of Louis-Philippe [the constitutional monarchy of 1830–48] devised the plans, but the Second Empire [1852–70] and early Third Republic actually laid the rails and erected the psychiatric institutions.'[36]

Although the British began legislating on institutions for the insane considerably earlier than the French, they carried out the task in piecemeal fashion. Most important for our purposes, British reformers – the usual early nineteenth-century mix of Benthamites and Evangelicals – achieved their goals without either enlisting the psychiatrists as collaborators or naming them as beneficiaries. Thus an Act of 1808 providing for the construction of county asylums financed by the county rate did not specify that these new institutions be run by physicians, or even that they include a physician on their staffs. After its passage, disgruntled British medical practitioners were forced to mount independent and frequently unsuccessful campaigns to convince local magistrates of their indispensability to the functioning of asylums. From the French medical standpoint, this absence of physicians was so odd, professionally maladroit, and incongruous with a public institution that in 1827 the alienist in charge of the Paris men's asylum of Bicêtre left a note in the visitors' book of the Bedfordshire county asylum advising the director that the place was sorely in need of a resident medical attendant.[37]

Only with the passage of the Lunatics Act of 1845, which set all institutions for the insane under a full-time national inspectorate, did the British introduce even an implicit force for the medicalization of the asylum. The new Act installed an inspectorate composed of five lay, three legal, and three medical commissioners; and in practice, the medical contingent proved sufficiently influential that the inspectorate manifested a steadily growing hostility to non-medically run asylums and helped to establish medical hegemony over them.[38] An important factor in this shift to the medicalized asylum was the celebrity acquired by John Conolly (1794–1866) when he was appointed in 1839 as Superintendent and Resident Physician of the county asylum of Hanwell and introduced the non-restraint system there. This successful renunciation of bodily coercion in the treatment of lunatics, hailed as a continuation of the tradition of the Tukes and as another British contribution to the triumph of humanity, was effectively invoked during the agitation for the 1845 Act by Anthony Ashley Cooper, later 7th Earl of Shaftesbury (1801–85), the leader of the parliamentary movement for lunacy reform.[39]

That the asylum movement in the disunited Germany of the first half of the nineteenth century has thus far attracted less attention than the comparable movements in France and Britain may be a historiographical quirk or an accurate reflection of the importance that the Germans themselves attached to that movement. It is perhaps noteworthy in this regard that, unlike the French and British, the Germans never, during the entire course of the nineteenth century, produced a uniform legislative code about the procedures for asylum admission; indeed they did not do so until after the Second World War.[40]

At the beginning of the nineteenth century, Germany found itself in a situation of theoretical precocity and practical backwardness: professors of philosophy and medicine were lecturing and writing on mental therapeutics 'before the subjects themselves – the insane poor – [had] gained social visibility'.[41] As Cabinet Minister to the Prussian king, the enlightened reformer Karl August von Hardenberg (1750–1822) established in Bayreuth in 1805 the Psychic Cure-Institution for the Mentally Ill (*Psychische Heilanstalt für Geisteskranke*), generally regarded as the beginning of the modern treatment of the insane in German-speaking countries.[42] (After Napoleon defeated Prussia in 1806, the same von Hardenberg and his fellow-aristocrat, Karl vom Stein (1757–1851) overhauled and modernized the structure of the Prussian state – an indication of the synchrony between the rhythms of political and psychiatric development.) The German asylums founded in the next several decades generally bore the imprint of Romanticism. They catered to a small number of patients and were situated in the countryside, where the natural, harmonious, and idyllic environment could exercise its presumably salutary effect on minds gone awry.[43] The increase in the number of asylums enabled the creation of a psychiatric journal with staying power: the *Allgemeine Zeitschrift für Psychiatrie*, which still survives, was founded in 1844 by three asylum administrators: H. P. A. Damerow (1798–1866), C. F. Flemming (1799–1880), and C. F. W. Roller (1802–78).[44] But the real flowering of German psychiatry occurred not during the heyday of the asylum, but only in the latter part of the century, when that discipline switched its primary institutional locus in Germany to the university.[45]

The birth of the asylum in early nineteenth-century America has been traced to the influence of European models and to the contemporary critique of Jacksonian society.[46] These two factors operated sequentially. During the opening decades of the century, direct transatlantic links, especially with the Tukes in England, as well as the availability in English translation of key texts by Tuke and Pinel, inspired the foundation of a number of privately funded eastern-seaboard institutions devoted to implementing the moral treatment: the Friends' Asylum near Philadelphia (1817), the McClean Hospital in Boston (1818), the Bloomingdale Asylum in New York (1821), the Hartford Retreat in Connecticut (1824). Since the rationale for these institutions was well publicized by their founders' fund-raising efforts, and their subsequent success made known in their officers' annual reports, they set the ground rules for later American asylums.[47] But not until the Jacksonian period did a veritable 'cult of asylum [sweep] the country', and then it was supported not by private benefactors but by the taxpayer and the state legislature. By 1850, almost every state in the north-east and Midwest had erected a public asylum, and by 1860 this was true of twenty-eight of the thirty-three states. According to the historian David J. Rothman, the asylum cult derived from the prevalent belief that the social conditions of American democracy – especially the frenetic competition for wealth and power and the ambition unleashed by omnipresent opportunity – actively bred insanity and that the new American republic had to vindicate itself by restoring to its damaged citizens the mental equilibrium of which it had inadvertently robbed them. The environmentalist assumption that the aetiology of insanity was largely social led in turn to the faith that removal *from* society and into the carefully structured world of the asylum would bring cure. Faith in the technique of 'isolation' (Americans used the same term as the French psychiatrist, Esquirol) was further bolstered by statistics, by the 'incredible number of cures' to which pre-Civil War asylum doctors routinely testified. By 1844, American psychiatrists had achieved the rudiments of professional organization. The Association of Medical Superintendents, composed exclusively of heads of asylums, dated from that year; its focus on administrative and architectural issues rather than medical-scientific ones evinces the aptness of 'medical superintendent' as the early term for psychiatrist in the United States.[48]

RECONFIGURATIONS OF THE LATE NINETEENTH CENTURY

The second half of the nineteenth century saw important changes in the institutional and intellectual models that had launched professional psychiatry. Most dramatically, the regnant optimism about the therapeutic efficacy of the asylum gave way to a deep-seated pessimism as asylum populations swelled with chronic patients demonstrably impervious to moral management. The asylum found itself transformed from a therapeutic to a fundamentally custodial institution.[49] Coincident with this institutional shift was an intellectual one. Psychiatrists came to theorize insanity not as a psychological or psychosomatic disorder (a conceptualization appropriate to the therapeutic asylum), but rather as an irreversible brain condition and as a product of degeneration – that is, a 'taint' or sickly deviation from the norm initially caused by a pathogenic environment, poor nutrition, or alcoholic abuse, and subsequently transmitted in the Lamarckian manner through heredity, becoming progressively more severe with each generation until the family line became sterile and, finally, extinct. (➤ Ch. 20 Constitutional and hereditary disorders; Ch. 15 Environment and Miasmata; Ch. 22 Nutritional diseases) Each European nation had its psychiatric theorists of degeneration. France led the way with Bénédict-Augustin Morel (1809–73), author of the seminal *Traité des dégénérescences* (1857), and Valentin Magnan (1835–1916); their ideas were diffused in Britain by Henry Maudsley (1835–1918), who gave them a Darwinian twist, and in Austria and Germany by Richard von Krafft-Ebing (1840–1902), who applied them to the sexual perversions.[50] A scene in *L'Assommoir* (1877), a novel of the Paris working class by Emile Zola (1840–1902), epitomized the psychiatric trend of the day. Shortly before the roofer, Coupeau, dies gruesomely in the Sainte-Anne asylum of a chronic alcoholic delirium, the unnamed 'specialist', probably Dr Magnan, seeks confirmation of psychiatry's basic theoretical tenets by asking the patient's wife 'in the hectoring manner of a police inspector, "Did this man's father drink? . . . Did the mother drink?"'[51]

The shift to an organicist conception of insanity was coupled with a shift in psychiatry's international centre of gravity from France to Germany. By mid-century, German scientists and physicians had repudiated with a vengeance their earlier affinity for Romantic *Naturphilosophie*. A strict and sober positivism came into vogue, evidenced in the area of psychiatry by the success of *Pathologie und Therapie der psychischen Krankheiten* (1845), the textbook by Wilhelm Griesinger (1817–68), which equated psychiatry with the study of cerebral disease and definitively severed that discipline's previous ties with speculative philosophy. Griesinger's status as the consummate German psychiatrist of his era was a function not only of the scientific cachet of his theory, but also of the new psychiatric career pattern he forged. He was not an asylum doctor, but rather a university psychiatrist bearing the title of professor – an inordinately prestigious title in nineteenth-century Germany, conferring admission into the cultivated bourgeois élite, or *Bildungsbürgertum*. Initially, Griesinger held a professorship in internal medicine, treating mental patients in his medical clinics; his authority increased still further when, in 1865, he was appointed to the newly created, specialized Chair of Psychiatry and Neurology at the University of Berlin.[52] University psychiatry enhanced the potential attractiveness of the pscyhiatric career. It offered the practitioner the possibility of a less reclusive, more sociable life-style than was afforded by full-time residence in an (often rural) asylum. It also changed the intellectual content of the career: psychiatric knowledge was now assumed to be generated less from cumulative daily contact with the insane than from neuroanatomical research in a university laboratory.

Karl Jaspers (1883–1969), the German psychiatrist and philosopher who first conceptualized the historical movement from asylum to university psychiatry, believed that it entailed roughly equal measures of gain and loss. In return for becoming a 'pure science', he said, psychiatry also became 'more cold-blooded [and] impersonal, less humane'.[53] To varying degrees, other nations followed the Germans' lead in situating psychiatry within the university matrix. In France, where co-ordinated, research-oriented universities of the modern type were not even created until 1896, anxiety over German competition (especially in the wake of the French defeat in the Franco-Prussian war) prompted the creation of the first academic Chair of Psychiatry, not at a university but at the Paris Faculty of Medicine, in 1878.[54] In Britain, Maudsley gave an endowment to the City of London in 1907 to establish a university psychiatric clinic on the German model; opened in 1915, it is now the teaching hospital in psychiatry for London University.[55]

A second reconfiguration of psychiatry in the latter nineteenth century likewise occurred in both the domains of theory building and career structure. Asylum psychiatry had worked with a simple binary conception of insanity: either one was insane, or one was not. After mid-century, however, psychiatrists began to blur the edges of this binary opposition and to speak of an intermediate zone, a large grey area, occupied by a population of potential new patients: the *demi-fous*, or half-mad. This conceptual move eventually led to the articulation of two categories fundamental to the enterprise of twentieth-century psychiatry: the 'psychotic', whose contact with reality is severely ruptured, and the 'neurotic', whose minimal maladaptations do not preclude getting on in ordinary society. The former required institutionalization and hence fit the older model of asylum psychiatry; the latter, who could safely remain in the outside world but would benefit from scheduled visits to the doctor's office, made possible the practice of out-patient psychiatry, thus freeing the speciality for the first time from its dependence upon the institutional form of the asylum.

This link between theory and career structure was especially clear in the case of Jean-Martin Charcot (1825–93), nicknamed the 'Napoleon of the neuroses'. His internationally celebrated work on hysteria enabled him to open the first out-patient clinic at the old Paris asylum of the Salpêtrière in 1879.[56] In the United States, out-patient care of the neurotic initially fell to the neurologists who, shortly after the formation of the American Neurological Association in 1875, began to vie openly with asylum superintendents for recognition as experts on insanity. By contrast to the asylum superintendents, who were often identified with pietistic Protestantism and moral issues, the neurologists defined themselves in terms of their allegiance to science and European scientific medicine. Lacking an institutional base, they typically set up in private practice and, as a consequence, acquired a clientele that included a large number of (usually affluent) patients suffering from neurotic ailments – residual patients who perplexed other doctors.[57] Hence, it is hardly accidental that two American neurologists of this period, George M. Beard (1839–83) and S. Weir Mitchell (1829–1914), pioneered the out-patient treatment of a catch-all neurosis known as neurasthenia or (following the title of one of Beard's books) American nervousness. The work of Beard and Mitchell enabled the private practitioner of neurology in the United States to redefine and to wrest from the hands of the clergy what the sociologist Andrew Abbott has called the 'personal problems jurisdiction'. And by 1920, when psychiatry and neurology had been loosely knit together in a joint speciality, such private practice entered the purview of the old-style psychiatrist as well.[58]

An informal international division of labour seems to have governed research on the neuroses and the psychoses. If *fin-de-siècle* French psychiatry under the aegis of Charcot took the lead with the neuroses, *fin-de-siècle* German psychiatry retained its newly acquired predominance by means of the psychoses. In this regard, the central figure was Emil Kraepelin (1856–1926), who secured his first university professorship in psychiatry (in Dorpat in Estonia) at the age of 30 and later moved on to more prestigious posts in Heidelberg and Munich.[59] Kraepelin delineated and made a psychiatric staple of the diagnostic category, dementia praecox, a disease that characteristically appeared during adolescence and left the intellect fundamentally intact while producing detachment, a lack of strong feelings, and a propensity to vacant laughter and silly, meaningless word-play. A diagnosis of dementia praecox automatically constituted a prognosis: incurable mental infirmity. Kraepelin credited the new institutional conditions of German psychiatry with providing the necessary preconditions for his discovery. The small size of the asylums of the Romantic era had, he said, simply not furnished sufficient material for clinical observation, but in the years between 1859 and 1917 the patient population of the Munich asylum and its annexes had increased sixteenfold, and the connection between asylum and university psychiatric clinic had encouraged and facilitated research.[60]

Dementia praecox was not an entirely novel discovery. As *démence précoce*, it had been identified by Morel as early as 1852,[61] but had failed to entrench itself in the diagnostic arsenal of French psychiatry. By contrast, the description of dementia praecox that initially appeared in the fifth edition (1896) of Kraepelin's *Lehrbuch* was a psychiatric landmark in Germany and elsewhere.[62] According to Smith Ely Jelliffe (1866–1945), who had studied with Kraepelin in Munich, American psychiatry during the first quarter of the twentieth century was 'preeminently Kraepelinian psychiatry'.[63] The command of German-language psychiatry over the psychoses was subsequently continued and strengthened by the Swiss-born, German-trained Eugen Bleuler (1857–1939). From his position as Professor of Psychiatry and Director of the picturesquely situated Burghölzli asylum in Zurich, Bleuler first articulated in 1911 the concept of schizophrenia which, both an elaboration and a critique of Kraepelinian dementia praecox, emphasized that the disease did not necessarily progress to dementia but could have a favourable outcome.[64]

TWENTIETH-CENTURY TRENDS

In broad outline, psychiatry in the twentieth century has been marked by three main trends:

1 the emergence of Freudian psychoanalysis;
2 the discovery and use of pscyhotropic drugs; and
3 the antipsychiatry movement.

The creation of the Viennese neurologist Sigmund Freud (1856–1939), psychoanalysis was at its inception marginal to institutionalized psychiatry; indeed, Freud's explanation of his own 'dream of the uncle with the yellow beard' in his *Interpretation of Dreams* (1900) frankly revealed his frustrated preoccupation with obtaining the coveted status of university professor.[65] Freud's professional overtures to Bleuler and to Carl Gustav Jung (1865–1961), Bleuler's assistant at the Burghölzli, can be read as an effort to acquire a psychiatric imprimatur for the new discipline of psychoanalysis.[66] Freud never fulfilled this ambition in Europe; but it was otherwise in the United States where, he noted with some distaste, the 'absence of any deep-rooted scientific tradition' and the 'much less stringent rule of official authority' prompted an easy receptivity to psychoanalytic theory on the part of professors and asylum superintendents.[67] Eventually, American psychiatry fully embraced psychoanalysis. As superintendent of St Elizabeth's Hospital, William Alanson White (1870–1937) had in 1914 introduced psychoanalytic psychotherapy for schizophrenic patients. When White became President of the American Psychiatric Association in 1924, that organization and the American Psychoanalytic Association began holding their annual meetings at the same time and place. This arrangement lasted until 1974, by which time the Freudian ardour of American psychiatrists had cooled.[68] (➤ Ch. 43 Psychotherapy)

Waning interests in psychoanalysis on the part of American psychiatrists was accompanied by rising expectations for psychopharmacology on the part of the international psychiatric community. The first psychotropic drug, lithium, was successfully used to manage manic-depression in Australia in 1949. A variety of antipsychotic and antidepressant compounds, most notably the phenothiazines and imipramine, were developed in France and Switzerland in the early 1950s. Psychopharmacology brought a new wave of self-confidence and therapeutic optimism to the psychiatric profession. It promised a relatively safe, cost-effective method of alleviating mental suffering without recourse to lengthy hospital stays or time-consuming pschoanalytic reconstructions of the repressed traumas of early childhood. It also revived psychiatry's identity as a 'hard' and exact science, the identity cultivated in the second half of the nineteenth century.[69] (➤ Ch. 39 Drug therapies)

Somewhat ironically, then, the reliance on psychotropic drugs was one of the causes of the antipsychiatry movement of the 1960s. The movement, which began in Britain, had three main tenets: that madness was not an objective behavioural or biochemical phenomenon, but rather a completely context-dependent label; that modern Western culture was peculiar in its total devaluation of madness, its rationalist refusal to recognize that madness, as an experience of another order of reality, has something important to teach us; and that under the right circumstances, psychotic experience can be a form of self-healing and, hence, should not be pharmacologically altered or suppressed. The most charismatic proponent of antipsychiatry was R. D. Laing (1927–89), a British psychiatrist influenced by such continental European philosophers as Martin Heidegger (1889–1976) and Jean-Paul Sartre (1905–80). In 1965, Laing established an antipsychiatric community (the word 'hospital' was deliberately avoided) at Kingsley Hall in a working-class neighbourhood in London. Patients and psychiatrists lived under the same roof, and nothing in their dress or demeanour distinguished one group from the other – a lack of markers that created visible anxiety in medical personnel visiting from conventional mental hospitals. Psychiatrists at Kingsley Hall were said to 'assist' patients in living through the full-scale regression entailed by schizophrenia; they most emphatically did not 'treat' them. Kingsley Hall's star patient was Mary Barnes, who emerged from full-scale regression to become an abstract painter whose paintings were exhibited in a London gallery. But for the most part, the techniques of anti-psychiatry were not so successful. The movement spread beyond Britain. Its chief American spokesperson was Thomas Szasz (b. 1920); and in France, Michel Foucault (1926–84), recognizing the similarity between certain of his own ideas and the principles of anti-psychiatry, lent his support to it. Anti-psychiatry gave impetus to the deinstitutionalization of the insane, which occurred in the late 1970s and the 1980s. A less controversial outcome of the movement was recognition of the patient's right to refuse antipsychotic drugs or electro-shock therapy.[70]

The anti-psychiatry movement has now largely spent its force. But as the end of the twentieth century approaches, psychiatry, while the oldest of the medical specialities, lacks the stability that age would seem to confer. It remains, in a sense, hostage to the mind–body problem, buffeted back and forth between psychological and physical definitions of its object and its techniques.

NOTES

1 This suggestion is made by Toby Gelfand, 'The origins of a modern concept of medical specialization: John Morgan's *Discourse* of 1765', *Bulletin of the History of Medicine*, 1976: 50.

2 See the article, 'Art', in Denis Diderot and Jean le Rond d'Alembert, *Encyclopédie, ou dictionnaire raisonné des sciences, des arts et des métiers*, 36 vols, Lausanne and Berne, Société Typographique, 1778–81, Vol. III, p. 342.

3 K. R. A. Wunderlich, quoted in Erwin H. Ackerknecht, *Medicine in the Paris Hospital, 1794–1848*, Baltimore, MD, Johns Hopkins University Press, 1967, p. 163.

4 George Rosen, *The Specialization of Medicine*, New York, Froben, 1944.

5 See Lenore O'Boyle, 'The problem of an excess of educated men in western Europe, 1800–1850', *Journal of Modern History*, 1970, 42: 471–95.

6 Emile Durkheim, *The Division of Labor in Society*, trans. by George Simpson, New York, Free Press, 1933, pp. 267, 270.

7 'De l'admission des spécialités dans les hôpitaux de Paris. Réclamation des chirurgiens', *Archives générales de médecine*, 1840 (3rd series), 7: 373–4.

8 Edouard Charton, *Guide pour le choix d'un état*, Paris, Lenormant, 1842, p. 398.

9 Philippe Pinel, *Traité médico-philosophique sur l'aliénation mentale, ou la manie*, Paris, Richard, Caille & Ravier, An. 9 [1801], p. 47.

10 Anon., review of Pinel, *Traité*, in *Edinburgh Review*, 1803, 2: 161.

11 On this process of myth-making, see Gladys Swain, *Le Sujet de la folie: naissance de la psychiatrie*, Toulouse, Privat, 1977, pp. 41–7. On paintings depicting the

mythic event, see Dora B. Weiner, 'The apprenticeship of Philippe Pinel: a new document', *American Journal of Psychiatry*, 1979, 136: esp. 1128.

12 This analysis of the moral treatment derives from Jan Goldstein, *Console and Classify: the French Psychiatric Profession in the Nineteenth Century*, New York and Cambridge, Cambridge University Press, 1987, ch. 3. Most of the same features can be found in British variants of the moral treatment; for example, see Roy Porter, *Mind-Forg'd Manacles: a History of Madness in England from the Restoration to the Regency*, Cambridge, MA, Harvard University Press, 1987, pp. 206–28.

13 Willis is quoted in Ida Macalpine and Richard Hunter, *George III and the Mad-Business*, New York, Pantheon, 1969, p. 272.

14 Andrew Scull, 'Moral treatment reconsidered: some sociological comments on an episode in the history of British psychiatry', in Scull (ed.), *Madhouses, Mad-Doctors, and Madmen: the Social History of Psychiatry in the Victorian Era*, Philadelphia, University of Pennsylvania Press, 1981, pp. 105–18, esp. 111, 113.

15 Robert Castel, 'Moral treatment: mental therapy and social control in the nineteenth century', in Stanley Cohen and Andrew Scull (eds), *Social Control and the State*, New York, St Martin's Press, 1983, pp. 248–66, esp, 254, 258.

16 Andrew T. Scull, 'From madness to mental illness: medical men as moral entrepreneurs', *Archives européennes de sociologie*, 1975, 16: 218–51, esp. 225–6.

17 Goldstein, op. cit. (n. 12) ch. 3, esp. pp. 72–8.

18 On parliamentary regulation, see Kathleen Jones, *Lunacy, Law and Conscience, 1744–1845*, London, Routledge & Kegan Paul, 1955; on private madhouses, see William L. Parry-Jones, *The Trade in Lunacy: a Study of Private Madhouses in England in the Eighteenth and Nineteenth Centuries*, London, Routledge & Kegan Paul, and Toronto, University of Toronto Press, 1972.

19 Scull, op. cit. (n. 16), esp. pp. 229–34, 255–6.

20 Goldstein, op. cit. (n. 12), ch. 3, esp. pp. 89–105.

21 Goldstein, op. cit. (n. 12), ch. 5.

22 Goldstein, op. cit (n. 12), ch. 9.

23 Forbes Winslow, *On Insanity* (1854), cited in Andrew T. Scull, *Museums of Madness: the Social Organization of Insanity in Nineteenth-Century England*, New York, St Martin's Press, 1979, p. 167.

24 See 'The word "Psychiatry"', *American Journal of Psychiatry*, 1951, 107: 628–9, 868–9; the word was coined in 1808 by Johann Christian Reil in one of the periodicals he edited, *Beiträge zur Beförderung einer Curmethode auf psychischem Wege*. On the disjunction between psychiatric theory and practice in Germany in this period, see Klans Doerner, *Madmen and the Bourgeoisie: a Social History of Insanity and Psychiatry*, trans. by Joachim Neugroschel and Jean Steinberg, Oxford, Basil Blackwell, 1981, pp. 197–200.

25 Doerner, ibid., pp. 199–206; Hannah S. Decker, *Freud in Germany: Revolution and Reaction in Science, 1893–1907*, New York, International Universities Press, 1977, pp. 27–36.

26 Doerner, op. cit. (n 24), pp. 238–45.

27 Carl Binger, *Revolutionary Doctor: Benjamin Rush, 1746–1813*, New York, Norton, 1966, pp. 177–8, 248–60, 270–4.

28 Erving Goffman, 'On the characteristics of total institutions', in *Asylums: Essays*

on the Social Situation of Mental Patients and Other Inmates, New York, Anchor Books, 1961, esp. pp. 3–8.

29 Somewhat differently inflected versions of this story are told about France by Michel Foucault, *Discipline and Punish: the Birth of the Prison*, trans. by Alan Sheridan, New York, Pantheon, 1977; and about the United States by David J. Rothman, *The Discovery of the Asylum: Social Order and Disorder in the New Republic*, rev. edn, Boston, Little, Brown, 1990; orig. pub. 1971.

30 The *locus classicus* of this thesis about the 'Great Confinement' and the subsequent change in the mode of classifying deviants is Michel Foucault, *Madness and Civilization*, trans. by Richard Howard, New York, Random House, 1956, chs 2, 8. The thesis is a controversial one and has recently been criticized as inaccurate with respect to the British experience by Roy Porter, 'Foucault's great confinement', *History of the Human Sciences*, 1990, 3: 47–54. On the German *Zuchthaus*, see Theodore Ziolkowski, *German Romanticism and its Institutions*, Princeton, NJ, Princeton University Press, 1990, pp. 141–2.

31 J.-E.-D. Esquirol, *Des Établissements des aliénés en France et des moyens d'améliorer le sort de ces infortunés*, Paris, Huzard, 1819, p. 26.

32 See ibid., pp. 23, 27, 30, 38–41; and Goldstein, op. cit. (n. 12), pp. 129–38.

33 J.-E.-D. Esquirol, *Question médico-légale sur l'isolation des aliénés*, Paris, Crochard, 1832, pp. 31, 54, 74–5; see also Goldstein, op. cit. (n. 12), pp. 276–7, 285–92.

34 Goldstein, op. cit. (n. 12), ch. 8, esp. pp. 276–85, 292–4, 297–307.

35 On some efforts to reform the Law of 1838, see Robert A. Nye, *Crime, Madness and Politics in Modern France: the Medical Concept of National Decline*, Princeton, NJ, Princeton University Press, 1984, ch. 7.

36 G. Lantéri-Laura, 'La chronicité dans la psychiatrie française moderne', *Annales E.S.C.*, 1972, 27: 548–68; see p. 562.

37 Jones, op. cit. (n. 18), pp. 74–7; and Scull, op. cit. (n. 16), pp. 246–8, 250.

38 Jones, op. cit. (n. 18), ch. 10; Scull, op. cit. (n. 16), p. 257. For a more detailed and nuanced account, see N. Hervey, 'A slavish bowing down: the Lunacy Commission and the psychiatric profession 1845–60', in W. F. Bynum, Roy Porter and Michael Shepherd (eds), *The Anatomy of Madness: Essays in the History of Psychiatry*, 3 vols, London and New York, Tavistock, 1985–8, Vol. II, pp. 98–131.

39 See Andrew Scull, 'John Conolly: a Victorian psychiatric career', in Scull (ed.), *Social Order/Mental Disorder: Anglo-American Psychiatry in Historical Perspective*, Berkeley and Los Angeles, University of California Press, 1989, pp. 162–214, esp. 187–92.

40 Peter Berner, 'L'Allemagne', in Jacques Postel and Claude Quétel (eds), *Nouvelle histoire de la psychiatrie*, Toulouse, Privat, 1983, pp. 194–201, esp. 196.

41 Doerner, op. cit. Pn. 24), p. 207.

42 Ziolkowski, op. cit. (n. 30), pp. 138–9, 144.

43 Berner, op. cit. (n. 40), p. 195.

44 Decker, op. cit. (n. 25), pp. 33, 35.

45 Berner, op. cit. (n. 40), p. 197.

46 The second factor is emphasized by David J. Rothman in his influential *The Discovery of the Asylum*, op. cit. (n. 29). Rothman's American exceptionalism is criticized, and the importance of European antecedents stressed, by Andrew

Scull, 'The discovery of the asylum revisited: lunacy reform in the New American Republic', in Scull, op. cit. (n. 39), pp. 95–117.

47 Scull, ibid., *passim*.

48 Rothman, op. cit. (n. 29), chs 5–6, esp. pp. 128–34.

49 For this development in France, see Lantéri-Laura, op. cit. (n. 36), pp. 554–5; for England, see Scull, op. cit. (n. 23), for the United States, see Rothman, op. cit. (n. 29), pp. 237–40.

50 See Robert Castel, *The Regulation of Madness: the Origins of Incarceration in France*, trans. by W. D. Halls, Berkeley and Los Angeles, University of California Press, 1988, ch. 7; Daniel Pick, *Faces of Degeneration: a European Disorder, c.1848–c.1918*, Cambridge and New York, Cambridge university Press, 1989; and Ian R. Dowbiggin, *Inheriting Madness: Professionalization and Psychiatric Knowledge in Nineteenth-Century France*, Berkeley and Los Angeles, University of California Press, 1991.

51 Emile Zola, *L'Assommoir* trans. by Leonard Tancock, Harmondsworth, Penguin, 1970, ch. 13, esp. p. 413; orig. pub. 1877.

52 Decker, op. cit. (n. 25), pp. 36–43.

53 Karl Jaspers, *General Psychopathology* trans. by J. Hoenig and Marian W. Hamilton, Chicago, IL, University of Chicago Press, 1963, pp. 846–7; orig. pub. 1913.

54 Goldstein, op. cit. (n. 12), pp. 345–50, 367.

55 Pick, op. cit. (n. 50) p. 206.

56 Goldstein, op. cit. (n. 12), pp. 332–4, 337–8. For Charcot's nickname, see Henri F. Ellenberger, *The Discovery of the Unconscious: the History and Evolution of Dynamic Psychiatry*, New York, Basic Books, 1970, p. 95.

57 Gerald N. Grob, *Mental Illness and American Society, 1875–1940*, Princeton, NJ, Princeton University Press, 1983, pp. 51–5.

58 Andrew Abbott, *The System of Professions: an Essay on the Division of Expert Labor*, Chicago, IL, University of Chicago Press, 1988, ch. 10, esp. pp. 285–9, 294. On Beard and Mitchell, see for example, George Frederick Drinka, *The Birth of Neurosis: Myth, Malady, and the Victorians*, New York, Simon & Schuster, 1984, ch. 8.

59 On Kraepelin's biography, see Erwin H. Ackerknecht, *A Short History of Psychiatry*, trans. by Sulammith Wolff, New York and London, Hafner, 1959, pp. 67–70.

60 Emil Kraepelin, *One Hundred Years of Psychiatry*, trans. by Wade Baskin, New York, Citadel, 1962, pp. 33, 148.

61 See the description in B.-A. Morel, *Études cliniques: Traité théorique et pratique des Maladies mentales*, 2 vols, Paris, Baillière, 1852–3, Vol. I, pp. 36–8.

62 The description can be found in English translation in Kraepelin, *Lectures on Clinical Psychiatry*, rev. and ed. by T. Johnstone, New York, Wood, 1904, Lecture 3.

63 Louise Brink and Smith Ely Jelliffe, 'Emil Kraepelin, psychiatrist and poet', *Journal of Nervous and Mental Disease*, 1933, 77: 134–52; see p. 135.

64 Ackerknecht, op. cit. (n. 59), pp. 70–1; Manfred Bleuler, 'Schizophrenia: review of the work of Prof. Eugen Bleuler', *Archives of Neurology and Psychiatry*, 1932, 11: 610–27.

65 See Carl E. Schorske, 'Politics and patricide in Freud's *Interpretation of Dreams*', *American Historical Review*, 1973, 78: 328–47. Freud's discussion of the dream is found in ch. 4 of *The Interpretation of Dreams*.

66 See Sigmund Freud, *On the History of the Psycho-Analytic Movement*, trans. by Joan Riviere, New York, Norton, 1966, pp. 26–7; orig. pub. 1914.
67 Ibid., p. 32.
68 Walter E. Barton, *The History and Influence of the American Psychiatric Association*, Washington, DC, American Psychiatric Press, 1987, p. 111.
69 Ross J. Baldessarini, *Chemotherapy in Psychiatry*, Cambridge, MA, Harvard University Press, 1977.
70 See Mary Barnes and Joseph Berke, *Mary Barnes: Two Accounts of a Journey through Madness*, New York, Harcourt Brace Jovanovich, 1972; and Peter Sedgwick, *Psycho-Politics: Laing, Foucault, Goffman, Szasz and the Future of Mass Psychiatry*, New York, Harper & Row, 1982.

FURTHER READING

Ackerknecht, Erwin, *A Short History of Psychiatry*, trans. by Sulammith Wolff, New York and London, Hafner, 1959.

Barnes, Mary and Berke, Joseph, *Mary Barnes: Two Accounts of a Journey Through Madness*, New York, Harcourt Brace Jovanovich, 1972.

Bynum, W. F., Porter, Roy and Shepherd, Michael (eds), *The Anatomy of Madness: Essays in the History of Psychiatry*, 3 vols, London and New York, Tavistock, 1985–8.

Castel, Robert, *The Regulation of Madness: the Origins of Incarceration in France*, trans. by W. D. Halls, Berkeley and Los Angeles, University of California Press, 1988; orig. pub. as *L'Ordre psychiatrique*, 1976.

Doerner, Klaus, *Madmen and the Bourgeoisie: a Social History of Insanity and Psychiatry*, trans. by Joachim Neugroschel and Jean Steinberg, Oxford, Basil Blackwell, 1981; orig. pub. as *Bürger und Irre*, 1969.

Foucault, Michel, *Madness and Civilization*, trans. and abr. by Richard Howard, New York, Random House, 1965; orig. pub. as *Histoire de la folie* (1961).

Goffman, Erving, *Asylums: Essays on the Social Situation of Mental Patients and Other Inmates*, New York, Anchor, 1961.

Goldstein, Jan, *Console and Classify: the French Psychiatric Profession in the Nineteenth Century*, New York and Cambridge, Cambridge University Press, 1987.

Grob, Gerald, N., *Mental Illness and American Society, 1875–1940*, Princeton, NJ, Princeton University Press, 1983.

Pick, Daniel, *Faces of Degeneration: a European Disorder, c.1848–c.1918*, Cambridge and New York, Cambridge University Press, 1989.

Porter, Roy, *Mind Forg'd Manacles: a History of Madness from the Restoration to the Regency*, Cambridge, MA, Harvard University Press, 1987.

Rothman, David, *The Discovery of the Asylum: Social Order and Disorder in the New Republic*, rev. edn, Boston, MA, Little, Brown, 1990;: orig. pub. 1971.

——, *Conscience and Convenience: the Asylum and its Alternatives in Progressive America*, Boston, MA, Little, Brown, 1980.

Scull, Andrew, *Museums of Madness: the Social Organization of Insanity in Nineteenth-Century England*, New York, St Martin's Press, 1979.

Still, Arthur and Velody, Irving (eds), *Rewriting the History of Madness: Studies in Foucault's* Histoire de la folie, London, Routledge, 1992.

57

HEALTH ECONOMICS: FINANCE, BUDGETING, AND INSURANCE

Nick Bosanquet

The public-health movement of nineteenth-century Britain stimulated interest in social accounting. The first complete system of physician payment based on insurance principles was of German origin in the 1880s: and the United States has been the twentieth-century leader in financial management and accounting systems for hospitals. Since the early 1980s, the influence of ideas originating in America has grown. Old distinctions between centrally funded, insurance-based and market-orientated systems have become blurred as policy-makers have sought to introduce similar techniques of financial control and economic analysis.

Social accounting for public health showed up the cost of premature mortality in loss of earnings and poverty for dependants. The main case for insurance systems from 1900 onwards was put in terms of improving access to services for working-class patients. Insurance systems, private or public, increased the demand for access to hospital services. From 1918 onwards, financial priorities in Britain and the US began to show marked differences. The UK system concentrated on the finance of low-tech general-practitioner care, while the US concentrated on access to hospital care. The problem of access to hospital services was resolved in very different ways. For the US, there was the development of the Blue Cross system with its local hospital base, beginning in the 1930s. This linked access to local premiums rather than to national taxation. Within Britain, dependence on national tax-funding became complete after the nationalization of the hospitals in 1948. (➤ Ch. 49 The hospital) This created new and unexpected problems of access, which led in turn to further centralization through such techniques as programme budgets, cash limits, and performance indicators.

Current measures of activity and commitment show very different results between health systems. Thus in 1987, total health expenditure as a proportion of gross domestic product (GDP) was 11.2 per cent in the US, 8.6 per cent in France, 8.2 per cent in Germany, and 6.1 per cent in Great Britain. The role of primary care and the numbers of specialist contacts also varies widely between systems. Such differences are not of recent origin, but have deep roots in the working of different financial incentives and systems over long periods of time. As between Britain and the US, finance established and then reinforced very different strategies for care, with the accent in Britain on primary care and in the US on advance of hospital care through intensive methods of treatment. (➤ Ch. 4 Medical care)

Innovation in financial techniques used to be by the few. Even countries such as Japan, Sweden, and France were followers, not leaders. Over the last two decades, the culture has become more international. The influence of international organizations such as the Organization for Economic Co-operation and Development (OECD) and the World Health Organization (WHO) has grown. The WHO has promoted budgeting and planning systems for developing countries. The OECD has provided a firmer base for international comparison. Health economics was initially concentrated in the US and in the UK, but has now been diffused. By 1990, a common economic language and culture across the globe was coming into use in all types of health system.

MEDICINE 1760–1860

Before 1860, most medical treatment to the social élite in the US and in the UK was given by physicians working from consulting rooms in a few larger cities. The development of a medical career structure had begun in the eighteenth century long before legislation to set standards for medical qualification. (➤ Ch. 47 History of the medical profession) The individual physician took decisions about his or her own career, and charged fees to patients who could afford to pay. The pursuit of income by individual physicians – and later, surgeons – supplied a strong economic motive force in medical care, although most doctors remained poorly paid. The main expenditure was in fees by the more affluent. In Britain, economic progress after the Industrial Revolution created new markets for higher quality medical services in provincial cities, as well as expanding the centuries-old market in London. It also created more opportunities for practice in country areas with the patronage of the old squirearchy, the new landowners, and richer yeoman-farmers. The poor sought treatment from apothecaries, unqualified practitioners, or quacks. (➤ Ch. 30 Folk medicine; Ch. 28 Unorthodox medical theories) There was fairly general cynicism about the benefits of medical treatment. The career path to high fees lay through the voluntary hospital. In both Britain and the US, the voluntary hospital before 1860 benefited from important subsidies in kind from the free services of honorary consultants. In the UK, career development was linked to scientific interest. Medicine was affected by the Scientific Revolution of the eighteenth century. There was increased activity in teaching and research, which led, in the first half of the nineteenth century, to greater problems in finance and fund-raising. 'In the first half of the nineteenth century, the average number of patients in hospitals in England and Wales increased from about 3,000 to nearly 8,000.'[1] For the US, there was less local development of teaching and research, and for some there was reliance on study in Paris and later Germany in career development. As in the UK, the work of honorary consultants supplied an important subsidy, but the incomes of hospitals remained low and conditions poor. 'Limited income and continued marginality to medical care meant that voluntary hospital policies and priorities could change little in the antebellum years.'[2] Hospitals provided minimal diet, dressing, and medical attention, and the main economic incentive was to prevent any expenditure above a very low minimum. The main sources of income in the US were to be found in charitable donations, the fees of paying patients, and payments on behalf of seamen. (➤ Ch. 62 Charity before 1850)

PUBLIC HEALTH: THE RISE OF THE HOSPITAL AND GROWING COMPETITION IN THE MEDICAL MARKET 1860–1914

The public-health movement began to gain momentum in the UK from the Liverpool Sanitary Act of 1846, the Public Health Act of 1848, and the researches of John Snow (1813–58) linking cholera to defective water supplies in 1854. From then to 1914, there was a growing programme of investment in sanitation, water supplies, and latterly in improved housing for the poor. (➤ Ch. 64 Medicine and architecture) The public-health movement worked through inspection and regulation. It stimulated expenditure on social infrastructure rather than directly on health services. The vaccination programme had also worked mainly through regulation, although there was some direct national expenditure on the production of vaccines and local expenditure under the Poor Law on vaccination of the children of the poor.[3] (➤ Ch. 51 Public health)

The vaccination and public-health programmes led to early work on measuring benefits. New official statistics collected by William Farr (1807–83) in the UK made it possible to assess benefits of public health in terms of reduced mortality on a small area basis. Such local calculations often suggested that the returns to investment could be huge. (➤ Ch. 71 Demography and medicine) US thinking followed this work. The Yale economist Irving Fisher (1867–1947) was commissioned by the progressive administration of President Theodore Roosevelt (1858–1919) to examine National Vitality. His report argued in 1910 that 'The economic loss to Philadelphia caused by the smallpox epidemic of 1871–2 has been estimated by Doctor Lee at $22m. . . . A vaccine bureau with physicians, a disinfecting station and the inauguration of a campaign of education capable of forestalling the whole epidemic would have cost $700,000.'[4] Fisher's report concluded that public-health measures produce 'tangible returns on the investment of several thousand per cent as a rule'.[5]

In 1860, Florence Nightingale (1820–1910) started the training school at St Thomas's Hospital, which was to carry her model of nursing around the world. (➤ Ch. 54 A general history of nursing: 1800–1900) The model involved not just staff-training, but better sanitation, an improved environment on the wards, and accommodation of the new nurses in nurses' homes. The pressure towards better funding of hospitals was felt both in America and in Britain. In the US, it was intensified by the Civil War experience, which showed that better ventilation and sanitation could lead to much better results from hospital treatment. Between the end of the Civil War and 1914, the American hospital system was transformed. Investment to meet the requirements of greater hygiene and of the Nightingale nursing system was only the first step. After 1880, there was pressure to invest in new technology and in improved surgery, pathology laboratories, and, after 1895, in X-ray departments. (➤ Ch. 42 Surgery (modern); Ch. 9 The pathological tradition; Ch. 36 Science of diagnosis: diagnostic technology)

This transformation brought changes in funding and budgeting. Most of the new beds were in community hospitals, so that there was much more intensive local fund-raising, especially for the endowment of beds. Fees from private patients supplied the most important source of additional income: 'America may be regarded as the home of the pay system'.[6] However, in spite of subsidy through staff vocation, hospitals before 1914 had great difficulty in keeping pace with rising expenditure. Patients were asked to pay itemized bills with separate charges for anaesthesia and X-rays. By the 1920s, the American hospital had become a market-orientated institution serving a large middle-class public, well beyond the span of the voluntary hospitals in a few large cities.

The Nightingale revolution had a different impact in Britain. Its main financial effect was to stimulate improved conditions in the Poor Law hospitals and the building of new hospitals for infectious diseases by the Metropolitan Asylums Board.[7] The main new finance was from rates and taxes, and the new financial systems were concerned with auditing rather than with the active pursuit of higher income. Improvements were sought in nurse staffing. A report in the British Medical Journal of 1880 wrote of how there had been 'a vast amelioration of the condition of the sick poor in workhouses' over the previous decade but that 'there was still much room for improvement especially it was believed in the nursing department.'[8] (➤ Ch. 63 Medical philanthropy after 1850) There was much less development of new technology or improvement in medical education than in the US. (➤ Ch. 48 Medical education)

The main financial innovation affecting the voluntary hospitals in Britain was in co-ordinated fund-raising by the Prince of Wales (later King Edward's Hospital Fund). This was a new foundation formed in the 1890s which tried to promote rationalization of hospitals in London, but with little success. The concern about maldistribution of hospitals in London led to the collection of comparative data in which the hospital administrator Henry Burdett (1847–1920) was a pioneer. The main focus for finance was on groups of hospitals – Poor Law or voluntary – rather than on more-intensive management of single hospitals. The large role of public authorities and the small role of direct payment by patients provided distinctive differences from the US. According to Burdett, 'Free relief has now become so general that the majority of the population in England consider it not only not a disgrace, but the most natural thing in the world when they fall ill, to demand and receive free medical treatment without question or delay.'[9] Infectious-disease hospitals continued to be more important in the UK than in the American system. The predominant financial basis of hospital care had, up to 1880, been based in Britain and in the US on the old model of the voluntary hospital, with hospitals for the poor run by local government (US) or the Poor Law (UK) in large cities. For the voluntary hospital, funding and budgeting were rather similar, with dependence on charitable funds and budgets covering relatively simple care. Between 1880 and 1914, the basis of funding of the two systems diverged. The American hospital system came to be funded largely through private-patient contributions. The British system came to be more dependent on voluntary donations. There was a contrast in the level of finance between the two systems. Funding in the US could finance technical innovation and increasing scientific research. Hospitals in Britain came to be affected by the same problems of inadequate response to new technology as affected British industry in the late-Victorian and Edwardian periods. The financial problems of the voluntary hospitals in Britain also stimulated the growth of Poor Law hospitals financed by local tax funding.

The period from 1860 to 1914 also saw distinctive changes in the 'market' for medical services. Numbers of doctors increased, and in Britain intense competition restricted medical incomes. The process of competition was described in the autobiography of Alfred Cox (1866–1954), later Secretary of the British Medical Association (BMA), in describing his early apprenticeship in Carlisle to Dr Abbott in the late 1880s:

> Dr Abbott had ... spent a couple of years as assistant to a man in London who farmed out a number of cheap cash-on-attendance branch practices. The

principal work of the owner of these businesses was to go round each branch every day to inspect the books, collect the money and keep an eye on his assistants. Abbott who was essentially a money-maker, was greatly attracted by this system and made up his mind to try it out on his own account. . . . He selected Carlisle for the experiment, partly because his father had gone there, but mainly because it had a large industrial population who had never been catered for on a cash basis. The other doctors in the place strongly resented his intrusion and his methods; they were strictly orthodox and apparently preferred to do a lot of work for nothing rather than to resort to cheap fees or contract work. Carlisle was therefore virgin soil for Abbott's methods and the result fully justified his choice. He took a shop in a main street, painted the front window with the word Dispensary, and a list of his consulting hours and circulated handbills announcing his terms.[10]

Competition was the reality behind the fee levels offered by club practice, where friendly societies and groups representing miners and other employees were able to drive a hard bargain in fees for medical services for groups of employees.

The American medical profession was also affected by increased competition, although in rather different ways from the UK experience. By 1910, there was one physician for every 568 patients.[11] Abraham Flexner (1866–1959), comparing these figures with the German ratio of one physician for every 2,000 inhabitants, concluded in 1910 that there was a national surplus. However, later studies by the American Medical Association (AMA) showed that the surplus was much greater in the West and in medium-sized communities. In large cities, the problem seemed to be the inability of poorer people to afford fees. One survey showed that 21.7 per cent of the sick were treating themselves exclusively with patent medicines and home remedies. In the US, moves to improve standards in medical schools after 1910 suggested that the size of the profession might well grow more slowly than in the past.[12] Even before the Flexner reforms of medical education, the ratio of physicians to patients had shown little change. The population rose 138 per cent from 1850 to 1910, while the medical profession grew by 153 per cent. Rising population and the growing middle-class market helped to give American doctors a very different perspective. The profession in Britain sought to escape from market pressures through state subsidy. US doctors looked to solutions in terms of practice development and geographic mobility expressed in a large increase in numbers of doctors taking State Board examinations. The American profession had greater confidence in security through fee income, helped even as early as 1910 by the beginnings of private insurance.

THE RISE OF NATIONAL HEALTH INSURANCE: 1910–48

In Britain, politics rescued the profession from its persecution or even imminent prostration by the market. Before 1886 there were few qualified medical practitioners in the House of Commons. Over the next two decades, increasing numbers were elected during a period of growing concern about national efficiency.[13] The profession itself provided prime evidence, which fed the growth of this concern through the results of medical inspections of school-children. (➤ Ch. 45 Childhood) In the UK, increased public intervention in education prepared the way for public intervention and tax-funding in health. Concern for national efficiency supplied the context for new insurance-based plans for improving access to personal health services. The problem of medical incomes became a focus for national concern in a way that would not otherwise have been so.

The main prototype for the insurance model was from imperial Germany, where the first national compulsory sickness insurance law was passed in 1883 and covered most employees. The range of benefits provided was wide, including the services of general practitioners, specialists, and hospital care. The administrative responsibility for the system rested with the sickness insurance societies (*Krankenkassen*), which could be based on localities such as Leipzig, or industries, or large firms. Control was in the hands of a body of representatives, of whom two-thirds were elected by the insured persons and one-third by the employers.[14] Employers and employees contributed to the cost, and there was no direct contribution from the state. The scheme provided for a free choice of doctor, and payment was by a mixture of fee for service and capitation elements. The UK scheme came some three decades later in 1911, and was universally regarded as much inferior. It covered only 40 per cent of employees, as compared to 77 per cent who were covered in the German scheme by 1911. The UK scheme covered wage-earners, while the German scheme allowed the funding agencies to extend coverage to dependants. By 1914, 37 per cent of the *Krankenkassen* had done so, covering 4 million dependants. The UK scheme provided exclusively (except for patients with tuberculosis) for access to medical treatment by doctors drawn from a local panel, or list of doctors willing to take insurance patients. Local administration was in the hands of insurance committees, a system partly established in order to prevent direct management of medical services by approved societies. These committees, in fact, limited their scope to clerical work. They did not develop the managerial functions which in Germany fell to the *Krankenkassen*. Any central managerial role in the system came to be exercised after 1918 by the Ministry of Health, which also watched over the finances of the system. It employed some eighty

Regional Medical Officers, whose main concern was with excessive prescribing. The role of the Ministry provided a further pressure towards central funding and ultimately towards a tax-funded National Health Service. Already in the 1930s, the Ministry was actually paying grants to local government to develop community midwifery services first, and then planning grants for specialized services for patients with cancer, although the 1939 Cancer Act was never implemented because of the outbreak of the Second World War.

The BMA had sought to have Six Cardinal Points included in the 1910 insurance scheme. These were:

1 an income limit of two pounds per week for the insured;
2 free choice of physician by the patient;
3 administration of the medical benefit by local health committees composed of doctors;
4 method of payment to be decided by a vote of district physicians;
5 adequate remuneration with the aim of 8s. 6d. per patient;
6 adequate medical representation on all administrative bodies.

The Government agreed to most of these demands, although the income limit was set at £3 rather than £2 and the capitation fee at 6s. 6d. There was a small additional fee of 1s. 6d. to cover drug treatments. The insurance scheme thus reflected the consensus views of the profession at the time, although this may have been somewhat obscured by a political battle, which was partly the product of personality factors, with the political titan Lloyd George (1863–1945) pitted against the mass-membership of the BMA.

The British scheme was comparable to the German one only in its provision for payments when the insured were absent from work, although even these were on a less generous scale. Rising expenditures on this account provided the main source of controversy about the scheme in the inter-war period. The link between budget and individual practice was through the capitation payment. This was raised to 9s. in 1923 after a national arbitration, and covered medical attendance. The system set up considerable incentives to minimize costs, and shrewdly organized practices were able to raise their net returns.[15] Local competition continued, although reduced in its effects because the panel payments set a floor to the incomes of doctors in industrial areas. From 1910 onwards, the development of national insurance schemes came to be crucial in health-service funding across Europe. From 1918 onwards, France adopted an insurance scheme, initially on similar lines to the German one so as to ensure that the *status quo* was preserved in the newly recovered provinces of Alsace and Lorraine.[16] However, the French system came to include some special features of its own, such as cost-sharing by which the patient paid 15–20 per cent and the insurance fund or *caisse* 80–85 per cent. Insurance schemes in this period had distinctive features that were important in setting long-term future directions for health services. The UK system covered a limited range of services and stressed direct consultation between the patient and the panel doctor. The capitation system of payment, which was chosen by the profession in preference to fee-for-service in all areas except Manchester, carried on over to the National Health system of financing general practice. The UK insurance system encouraged the separation of specialist services from general practice and a low rate of referral to specialists. The German and French systems, on the other hand, covered access to specialist services and led to a high rate of referral to specialists. The UK insurance system had the long-term effect of increasing the role of primary care. It encouraged practices to compete for patients, and it also encouraged patients to conceive medical service in terms of visits to general practitioners. Already under the inter-war panel system, variations in practice income widened as the more successful practices developed as small firms, and consultation rates rose from two to four per year for each patient on the panel. There was considerable concern, however, about the quality of service, with the view being taken by independent observers that the panel system had encouraged superficial treatment through the quick consultation and the bottle of medicine.[17] (➤ Ch. 34 History of the doctor–patient relationship)

The development of the US system diverged further from that of the UK and of Europe after 1910. There was an active campaign for health insurance in the US from 1910 to 1920, which seemed at one time to be assured of success. It drew on a background of concern about low incomes, especially as this affected general practitioners who felt that their incomes were not even keeping pace with rising costs. 'One reason for this was that they were losing their patients; the rich to specialists, the contagious to public health doctors and the poor to dispensaries and hospital out-patient departments.'[18] There was also concern about access to care. 'For the first time in history, the value of medicine was indisputable; yet rising costs were tending to limit adequate care to the well-to-do who are able to pay, and to the very poor who accept medical care as charity.'[19] Yet the case for health insurance was lost by 1920, and its supporters had failed to win enactment even in states such as Wisconsin, New York, and Massachusetts with strong records of social legislation. The opposition was partly an instinctive reaction of the medical profession to increased government activity, but it also reflected the recovery of medical incomes that followed the peace and continued into the boom of the 1920s. The complex and more developed relationships between American doctors and hospitals may have also played a role in pointing to a professional future of closer involvement with a hospital system that was much larger and better financed than those in Europe.

THE US 1910–65: THE RISE OF THE VOLUNTARY HOSPITAL

From 1910 onwards, a series of changes began to strengthen the position of the larger voluntary hospital in professional terms. The Flexner Report on medical education in 1910 and the accreditation activities of the AMA set higher standards for staffing and medical education. The organization of the American medical effort in the First World War was through base hospitals attached to particular university medical schools: Harvard, Yale, Pennsylvania, and others. Even before American entry into the war in 1917, there had been a considerable contribution from volunteers, including some of the future leaders of the profession such as the neurosurgeon Harvey Cushing (1869–1939).[20] American medicine had gained a reputation for advanced technology in treatment of the severely wounded. The effect of American involvement in the First World War was to strengthen the prestige of the leading hospitals and to encourage the development of hospital medicine.[21] This was a great contrast to its impact in Britain, where the main conclusions drawn from the war were of the primacy of public health and primary care and the need for controlling referral through hospital specialization, lessons spelled out in the post-war Dawson Report on the future of health services.[22] These conclusions reflected the different British experience of protecting health in a long siege rather than the main US experience of a short period of active hostilities. (➤ Ch. 66 War and modern medicine)

By 1920, larger American hospitals had secured professional legitimacy. They were well placed to expand funding and to set up an investment in hospital medicine, which was to set the pattern for the future.

> Hospital construction boomed in the 1920s, buoyed up by successful hospital fund-raising efforts and by an increasing number of bequests. . . . When prices are held constant, the real value of hospital construction in the late 1920s was not to be reached again until the 1950s. . . . This investment made hospitals one of the largest enterprises in the United States, outstripped only by the iron and steel industry, the textile industry, the chemical industry and the food industry.[23]

This was a radical change from the 1860s, when American cities had much lower ratios of hospital beds to population than found in Europe.

The investment of the 1920s led to serious problems after the Great Depression of 1931, when many hospitals had great difficulty in covering the costs of this expansion. The 1920s set patterns for intensive capital investment and hospital activity. The 1930s established a recession-proof method of funding these services through group hospitalization plans or the Blue Cross. These were prepayment plans 'which offered subscribers the opportunity to receive specified hospital services, without cost at the time of need, for a small on-going monthly payment'.[24] The sales of the plans were targeted at middle-income groups in sales and clerical work. A related smaller scheme, Blue Shield, provided for prepayment of physicians' bills. The Blue Cross system of reimbursement related health care to occupation rather than to the local community, and established a fee-for-service system which stimulated the growth of surgery and of in-patient care. It also established the principle of third-party payment in American hospital care. After the Second World War, insurance companies also entered the market in a big way. The effects were long-lasting, and carried over to shape the Medicare programme introduced in 1965 which introduced federal funding for the health care of elderly Americans. This continued with the same principles of fee-for-service and third-party payment.

From 1935 onwards, American voluntary hospitals developed financial systems that were well in advance of those found elsewhere, although they were often idiosyncratic to an individual institution. They had procedures for planning new developments and for raising finance through bond issues. The most popular textbook from 1935 to 1950 was MacEachern's *Hospital Organization and Management*. This set out the functions of the business department in some detail, covering control of income, expenses, assets, liabilities, equities and information on hospital activities. It also had guidance on how 'To arrive at a budget for future operation based on experience of the past which shows results produced, income incidental to their production and expense involved. The budget thus arrived at will form the basis for future expenditures and possibly determine the extent of the activities of the hospital.' The hospital's accountants were expected to produce detailed analyses of costs, not just for budgetary control but for setting rates to patients. 'Hospital rates should be arrived at by the logical process of first making detailed studies of all costs involved. The increasing emphasis upon cost as the basic element in rates has led to the current importance attached to cost accounting.'[25]

With financial stability came confidence in expansion and political power. After 1946, the voluntary hospitals were able to win a programme of federal subsidy to new hospital construction through the Hill–Burton Act. They also opposed effectively any new government initiative in health insurance. The system ran smoothly until the early 1960s, when concern began to grow about access of elderly Americans to health care. From then on, government funding and new systems run by government agencies were to become much more important.

THE UK AND EUROPE 1945–90

The reconstruction of Europe changed many aspects of European society, but not its health services. The model of national health insurance introduced by Otto von Bismarck (1815–98) was exceedingly durable and provided the basis for major expansion in services and funding. It was only in the early 1980s that there were major changes in the system in France; and only at the end of the decade that there were some signs of change in Germany.

Only Britain opted for fundamental changes in the financing and budgetary organization of health services after 1945. The National Health Service (NHS) implemented in 1948 involved principally the nationalization of the hospital system, which was henceforth to be funded through national taxation. Other areas of health services were much less changed. Financial incentives in general practice only showed major differences from the panel system after the Family Doctor Charter in 1965, and some services, especially community nursing and public health, continued to be funded through local taxation until 1974. From 1948 to 1974, the main focus was on funding and activity in the hospitals. The main financial problem was that of staying within annual budgets, and financial planning was aimed at improving budgetary information for revenue spending.[26] There were also some pioneering attempts to improve value for money by putting inter-hospital comparisons on a standardized basis.[27] Accounting for capital assets was not carried out, and when a Hospital Building Plan was begun in 1961, it had little or no basis in financial information. (➤ Ch. 50 Medical institutions and the state)

The Family Doctor Charter of 1965 represented a significant innovation and an early experiment in a new private/public mix.[28] The old system had made global payments to family doctors to cover costs and income. Under the new system, they were given specific subsidies to employ receptionists, nurses, and other staff such as practice managers. Family doctors were also given access to capital on preferential terms through the so-called cost rent scheme to encourage investment in premises. The system was further developed by extending fee-for-service payments for family planning and immunization. From 1974, the pace of financial innovation increased throughout the NHS. The nationalization of the former community health services in 1974 stimulated interest in health planning. Between 1974 and 1976, there was a development of programme budgeting, by which expenditure was related to activity. One effect of this was to give a clearer picture of how expenditure was divided between different demographic groups, especially elderly people. (➤ Ch. 46 Geriatrics) It also made it possible to choose priorities between services, so that from 1976 onwards the NHS was committed to spending more on the so-called priority services for people who are elderly, mentally ill, or mentally handicapped.[29]

The 1980s brought more use of local comparisons through performance indicators for costs and activity. The decade also saw progress in improving choice among capital projects through use of option appraisal, which set up standard procedures for comparing alternative projects.[30] There were proposals for introducing valuation of capital assets and depreciation, but little progress had been made by 1990. Above all, the 1980s saw more use of annual budgetary estimates or cash limits to compare financial performance. Managers had to work to the immediate incentive of staying within the annual budget and, if an over-run seemed likely, to reduce activity. At the national level, new guidelines were debated for relating the appropriate rate of increase of public spending to need as measured by demographic change, change in treatment methods, and in technology. Before the 1990 NHS Act, the main direction of change was to strengthen financial controls from the centre and to raise the importance of the annual cash limit.

CONVERGENCE IN FINANCIAL SYSTEMS?

Analysis of post-war health services has usually stressed a tripartite division between national insurance-based systems, national health services with tax funding from the centre, and the US system with its stress on individual entrepreneurship. During the 1980s, all three systems faced different crises, which led to consideration of types of reform. For the first time, there were signs of the development of a common language and common culture in health financing. By 1990, the Health Care Financing Administration was spending a considerable amount of the American taxpayers' money on a special OECD study of health systems across the developed world.[31] The growth of health economics itself as a discipline, and its spread from a US and UK base to France, Sweden, and Spain (although not to Japan), was also important, as was the OECD, in promoting international comparisons. (➤ Ch. 59 Internationalism in medicine and public health) The first phase of interest by economists in health problems was from 1890–1914 in the US, where Irving Fisher wrote about the costs of illness, and other economists were involved in advocacy of health insurance as part of the wider concern with protective labour legislation. For decades, there was little further interest shown by economists in health care, apart from a large study published in 1945 by Milton Friedman (b. 1912) and Simon Kuznets (1901–85) of monopoly effects in raising medical incomes.[32] Since 1960, health economics has become a major field, first in the US and later in the UK. Early US work was on the special nature of the choice and information problems presented by the demand for health care.[33] The state of the subject in the early 1960s is well summarized in a survey by Klarman commissioned by the Ford Foundation.[34] Much later work arose from the successive crises of cost-containment in the US system. Economists detected a bias towards high-tech and to excessive production of expensive care, as opposed to mundane medium-tech services. Some also saw a contribution from supplier-induced demand in raising health-care costs. Economists contributed assessments of the costs and benefits of particular programmes, beginning with early studies of renal dialysis and renal transplantation. They carried out many studies of reasons for variability in hospital costs and of differences in local rates for surgical operations.[35,36] From the 1970s, there was much work on the demand for health, stressing the role both of individual choice and of social factors for influencing health outcomes. Economists performed a service function in providing data for decision-makers aiming to make choices and to reduce costs in health systems. They carried out some large-scale empirical studies, especially the controlled study of the effects of different insurance systems on consumer choice, financed by the Rand Corporation in the 1970s.[37] This study confirmed that financial incentives had a strong influence on patient behaviour, with almost any direct payment reducing demand by 20 per cent or more. Economists also acted as outside critics of the low productivity of health care as compared to the importance of individual decisions about smoking and life-style.

The UK contribution in health economics was a distinctive one from the early 1970s onwards. To begin with, it tended to be far less concerned with the supply and cost problems of health services and more with the special problems of collective choice and welfare economics that justified public intervention.[38] Later, it stressed the need to assess benefit and to make more effective choices of how to use scarce resources, with economists from the University of York advocating the use of the Quality Adjusted Life Year (QALY), as a measure of benefit.[39]

There was also substantial work on the problems of choice in health programmes in developing countries. For poorer countries, much early work going back to the 1950s stressed the evaluation of preventive programmes such as malaria eradication in terms of gains in reduced mortality and economic productivity. There was also work on the economics of primary care, using nursing aides and medical assistants in the context of the WHO Programme for Health for All in the Year 2000. Planners in middle-income countries came to be concerned with the introduction of health-insurance schemes, which had spread by the early 1990s throughout most of Latin America and Asia. By the early 1990s, there was a swing in most countries towards greater direct payment by consumers, a move strongly advocated by the World Bank for services other than those with large social benefits or externalities.[40]

The US system moved from decades of consensus to a serious crisis of cost containment in the 1970s.[41] Employers began to complain bitterly about the rising cost of health insurance. Hospitals and professionals showed little restraint, as federal funding of Medicare for the elderly and Medicaid for the poor after 1966 added to the demand for services. Medicare, in particular, stimulated higher hospital expenditures for all social groups, and had a continuing influence on the hospital system. The Government sought to control costs by encouraging the development of competition among health-care providers and by giving tax incentives to the growth of the Health Maintenance Organizations, which undertook to provide full health services in return for annual subscription. It also tried to stimulate efficiency by reimbursing hospitals for treating patients on a fixed-price basis, with the prices set for 467 diagnosis-related groups (DRGs). The shift to provider-competition certainly changed the character and strategy of the voluntary hospital, which became much more capital-intensive and concerned with community needs only if they were also backed by ability to pay. All US hospitals approximated to the for-profit hospitals that had flourished in the 1970s. This diverted development into the area of ambulatory care, where reimbursement continued to be on a cost-plus basis rather than on rates set by DRGs. But it was not successful in containing costs or in reducing total activity. By the early 1990s, major new problems of access and ability to pay had emerged, with one-third of Americans not fully covered by health insurance. The wheel had come full circle to proposals for national health insurance.

Insurance-based systems also faced problems of rising activity and cost. These were dealt with in the early 1980s by concerted action or improved collusion between professions and insurance funds in Germany. France adopted more far-reaching changes towards the use of cash-limited budgets and DRG systems within the hospital service. By the end of the 1980s, these changes seemed to have stabilized expenditure, but they had not led to a more efficient or effective pattern of services.

By the end of the 1980s, the most extensive reforms were to be found in the UK health system, which opted for provider-competition while retaining tax-funding. The 1990 NHS Act provided for the development of an internal market, where purchasers would receive funds on a capitation basis for their resident population.[42] They would then contract with providers on activity and quality of care. These providers might be independent agencies (NHS Trusts), directly managed services, or the private sector. For family doctors, there was a new performance-related contract, stressing more payment by fee for service. They were also given the option of becoming miniature health-maintenance organizations or fund-holding practices. The main inspiration for the plan was to be found in the work of Professor Alain Enthoven of Stanford University.[43]

Similar ideas were under discussion in Denmark and the Netherlands.

The convergence of health systems, which had seemed likely from their common base in technology and professions, seemed at last to be coming about, although driven by the mechanics of funding rather than by the needs of patients. The main national differences were coming to be in the degree of urgency with which the problems were addressed, reflecting the very different shares of GDP committed to health services.

ACKNOWLEDGEMENTS

I would like to thank Rosemary Stevens and Charles Webster for helpful comments on an earlier draft, Anna Zajdler for research assistance, and Frances Daniels for her unfailing patience and cheerfulness.

NOTES

1   B. Abel-Smith, *The Hospitals 1800–1948*, London, Heinemann, 1964, p. 18.
2   C. Rosenberg, *The Care of Strangers*, New York, Basic Books, 1988, p. 33.
3   W. M. Frazer, *A History of English Public Health 1834–1939* London, Ballière, Tindall & Cox, 1950, pp. 70–2.
4   N. I. Fisher, *A Report on National Vitality: Its Wastes and Conservation*, Washington, DC, Government Printing Office, 1909, p. 744.
5   Ibid., p. 745.
6   H. C. Burdett, *Hospitals and Asylums of the World*, London, Churchill, 1893, Vol. III, p. 55.
7   Abel-Smith, op. cit. (n. 1), pp. 119–32.
8   'Trained nurses in workhouse infirmaries', *British Medical Journal*, 1880: 99.
9   Burdett, op. cit. (n. 6), p. 56.
10   A. Cox, *Among the Doctors*, London, Christopher Johnson, 1951, pp. 21–2.
11   Ronald Numbers, *Almost Persuaded. American Physicians and Compulsory Health Insurance, 1912–1920*, Baltimore, MD, Johns Hopkins University Press, 1978, p. 4.
12   Abraham Flexner, *Medical Education in the United States and Canada: a Report to the Carnegie Foundation for the Advancement of Teaching*, New York, Carnegie Foundation for the Advancement of Teaching, 1910.
13   Bentley B. Gilbert, *The Evolution of National Insurance in Great Britain*, London, Michael Joseph, 1966, pp. 72–81.
14   I. S. Falk, *Security Against Sickness. A Study of Health Insurance*, New York, Da Capo Press, 1972, pp. 71–92; orig. pub. Garden City, Doubleday Doran, 1936, pp. 71–92.
15   A. Digby and N. Bosanquet, 'Doctors and patients in an era of national health insurance and private practice 1913–38', *Economic History Review*, 1988, 2 XLI 1: 74–94.
16   Falk, op. cit. (n. 14), pp. 205–39.
17   J. Collings, 'General practice in England today: a reconnaissance', *Lancet*, 1950, 1: 555–85.

18 Numbers, op. cit. (n. 11), p. 9.

19 Numbers, op. cit. (n. 11), p. 10.

20 Harvey Cushing, *From a Surgeon's Journal 1915–18*, London, Constable, 1936, pp. 1–511.

21 Rosemary Stevens, *In Sickness and in Wealth. American Hospitals in the Twentieth Century*, New York, Basic Books, 1989, pp. 90–5.

22 Ministry of Health, *Consultative Council on Medical and Allied Services*, Interim Report on the Future Provision of Medical and Allied Services, London, HMSO, Cmd 693, 1920, p. 5.

23 Stevens, op. cit. (n. 21), p. 111.

24 Stevens, op. cit. (n. 21), pp. 182–9.

25 M. MacEachern, *Hospital Organization and Management*, 2nd edn, Chicago, IL, Physicians' Record Co., 1947, p. 728.

26 C. Webster, *Health Services since the War*, London, HMSO, 1988, pp. 1–479.

27 C. Montacute, *Costing and Efficiency in Hospitals*, London, Nuffield Provincial Hospital Trust, 1962, pp. 35–41.

28 N. Bosanquet and B. Leese, *Family Doctors and Economic Incentives*, Aldershot, Dartmouth/Gower, 1989.

29 Department of Health and Social Security, *Priorities for Health Services in England*, London, HMSO, 1976, pp. 1–83.

30 Department of Health and Social Security, *Option Appraisal*, London, HMSO, 1982, pp. 1–42.

31 OECD, *Health Care Systems in Transition. The Search for Efficiency*, Paris, OECD, 1990.

32 M. Friedman and S. Kuznets, *Income from Independent Professional Practice*, New York, National Bureau of Economic Research, 1945.

33 K. J. Arrow, 'Uncertainty and the welfare economics of medical care', *American Economic Review*, 1963, 53: 941–73.

34 H. Klarman, *The Economics of Health*, New York, Columbia University Press, 1965.

35 M. Feldstein, *Economic Analysis for Health Service Efficiency*, Amsterdam, North Holland Publishing 1967.

36 V. Fuchs, *The Health Economy*, Cambridge, MA, Harvard University Press, 1986.

37 J. Newhouse *et al.*, 'Some interim results from a controlled trial of cost sharing in health insurance', *New England Journal of Medicine*, 1981, 30: 1501–7.

38 A. Culyer, *Need and the National Health Service*, Oxford, Martin Robertson, 1976.

39 A. Williams, 'The economics of coronary artery by-pass grafting', *British Medical Journal*, 1985, 291: 326–9.

40 D. de Ferranti, *Paying for Health Services in Developing Countries*, Washington, DC, World Bank, 1988.

41 A. Califano, Jr, *America's Health Care Revolution*, New York, Random House, 1986, pp. 58–68.

42 Department of Health, *Working for Patients*, London, HMSO, 1989.

43 A. Enthoven, *Reflections on the Management of the National Health Service*, London, Nuffield Provincial Hospitals Trust, 1985, pp. 1–51.

FURTHER READING

Abel-Smith, B. *The Hospitals 1800–1948*, London, Heinemann, 1964.

Berman, Howard and Weeks, Lewis, *The Financial Management of Hospitals*, 4th edn, Ann Arbor, MI, Health Administration Press, 1979.

Bosanquet, N. and Leese, B., *Family Doctors and Economic Incentives*, Aldershot, Dartmouth/Gower, 1989.

Brend, W. A., *Health and the State*, London, Constable, 1917.

Califano, J. A. Jr, *America's Health Care Revolution: Who Lives? Who Dies, Who Pays?*, New York, Random House, 1986.

Cox, Alfred, *Among the Doctors*, London, Christopher Johnson, 1951.

Falk, I. S., *Security Against Sickness. A Study of Health Insurance*, New York, Da Capo Press, 1972; orig. pub. Garden City, Doubleday Doran, 1936.

Fox, D., 'From reform to relativism: an intellectual history of economics and health care', *Milbank Memorial Fund Quarterly*, 1979, 57: 279–336.

Frazer, W. M., *A History of English Public Health 1834–1939*, London, Baillière, Tindall & Cox, 1950.

Gilbert, Bentley, *The Evolution of National Insurance in Great Britain*, London, Michael Joseph, 1966.

Lee, K. and Mills, A., *The Economics of Health in Developing Countries*, Oxford, Oxford University Press, 1983.

MacEachern, M., *Hospital Organization and Management*, 2nd edn, Chicago, IL, Physicians Record Co., 1947.

McGuire, A., Henderson, J. and Mooney, G., *The Economics of Health Care. An Introductory Text*, London, Routledge & Kegan Paul, 1988.

Nightingale, F., *Notes on Hospitals*, London, 1863.

Numbers, R., *Almost Persuaded. American Physicians and Compulsory Health Insurance, 1912–1920*, Baltimore, MD, Johns Hopkins University Press, 1978.

OECD, *Health Care Systems in Transition. The Search for Efficiency*, Paris, OECD, 1990.

Rosenberg, C., *The Care of Strangers*, New York, Basic Books, 1988.

Stevens, Rosemary, *In Sickness and in Wealth. American Hospitals in the Twentieth Century*, New York, Basic Books, 1989.

PART VII

MEDICINE, IDEAS, AND CULTURE

58

MEDICINE AND COLONIALISM

David Arnold

The tradition of representing the history of medicine as a heroic struggle against disease has enjoyed a long and powerful reign in the history of European colonialism, as it has in the history of Europe itself. But it has been accentuated in the colonial context by the tendency to see history only in terms of the colonizers and to ignore the experience of the colonized; it has been heightened, too, by the frequency with which medical practitioners and imperial proconsuls cited medicine as evidence of the humanitarian zeal and high-minded benevolence of colonial rule, and even to justify the very fact of colonialism itself. The history of tropical medicine, in particular, has been presented as the story of white races' achievements against a background not only of fell disease and hostile environments but also of the ignorance, superstition and inertia of the 'natives'. (➤ Ch. 24 Tropical diseases) In treating medicine as scientific objectivity rather than as a political construct and cultural artefact, it has conventionally been seen as a panacea, a means of liberation, not a regulatory or repressive device. Even at a time when European colonialism was itself in rapid decline, many scholars still held to the idea that medicine was one of colonialism's nobler and more redeeming features, evidence that, whatever the 'political disadvantages' of colonialism, it had brought real benefits to the people of Africa and Asia.[1]

Recent scholarship has been more sceptical and more probing. Discussion of colonialism and medicine has veered away from the triumphalist visions and hagiographic histories of the past, and sought the closer integration of medicine with the economic, political, and cultural history of colonialism. Scholars have become wary of the professed objectivity of colonial medicine and have linked it instead with the material objectives and ideological imperatives of colonial rule. Medicine has come to be identified as a colonizing force in its own right, a potent source of political authority and social control.

While this reinterpretation has credited medical practitioners with considerable influence over the ideology and practice of colonial rule, there has, on the other hand, been a tendency to question many of the medical achievements once confidently attributed to them. Nowadays, disease (and naturally acquired, rather than medically conferred, immunities) often figures as a more potent dynamic in the history of European conquest and colonization overseas than the apparently puny exertions and ill-informed speculations of medical practitioners. Social history and anthropology have also made their mark. Historians today are more willing than their predecessors to view colonial medicine through the experiences and perceptions of those who actually came under its sway; more willing, too, to see European medicine as but one (and not necessarily the most acceptable or efficacious) among several competing systems of health and healing. Conclusions differ, but there appears to be a growing gulf between the sweeping claims once made for Western medicine and its actual historical record.

It is important to note at the outset, however, the enormous variety of political, social, and geographical situations that the term 'colonialism' has encompassed over the last four or five hundred years. For all its apparent familiarity, colonialism remains an elusive phenomenon. Given the diversity of political doctrines, economic activities, and cultural practices that have sheltered under its broad umbrella at different times, it would be hard to find a single typology of colonialism – or of colonial medicine – that would convincingly fit them all. A possible solution is to argue that there was not one colonialism but two. There were white-settler colonies like Canada and Australia, located mainly in the temperate zones, where colonialism marked an almost complete break with the pre-European past. The introduction of European peoples, languages, institutions, and diseases, and the accompanying devastation or marginalization of indigenous societies, brought a drastic and lasting transformation that was reflected in a history of medical ideas, agencies, and practices modelled on those of Europe itself. By contrast, there were many (mainly tropical) territories, particularly in Africa and Asia, where colonialism was a more transient, if traumatic, episode: a brief encounter, lasting in some instances no longer than a generation or two and arguably having only a limited or localized impact upon indigenous society. Despite the presence of a formal colonial administration, indigenes (or, as in the Caribbean, immigrant non-whites) formed the great majority of the population, while the European élite remained socially aloof and confined to positions of economic, military, and bureaucratic control.

For all its general utility, however, this simple division of the world into temperate and tropical colonies can be misleading. Many colonies did not fit neatly into either category, but occupied a position somewhere between the two extremes, as in French Algeria, where European settlers ultimately failed to oust native Algerians, or in New Zealand, where the Maori survived white immigration and retained a separate ethnic and cultural identity. Potentially, there could be several different typologies and chronologies of colonial medicine reflecting different geographical locations, different social and cultural mixes, and varying time-scales. A typology of colonial medicine based on the experience of the Thirteen Colonies of British North America, beginning in the early seventeenth century but concluding in the late eighteenth century and dealing almost entirely with the history of a white immigrant population, would necessarily be very different from that of French West Africa or Indochina, beginning in the early or middle decades of the nineteenth century and covering the medical ideas and activities of both a white ruling class and a far larger indigenous population. On the other hand, although there may appear to have been enormous differences between the medical history of, say, Senegal and Canada or New Zealand and Jamaica, any simple dichotomy between temperate and tropical colonies is likely to obscure the extent to which all colonies, by virtue of their physical distance from the centres of imperial power and their political, economic, and cultural dependency, might share similar characteristics that set them apart from Europe and alike placed them in a 'frontier' situation. The extent to which colonial medicine is thus merely a variant of a metropolitan archetype (itself subject to historical change and competing pressures) or represents something distinctive has thus been an important underlying issue in recent debates about colonialism and medicine. The argument here, which will draw particularly on British India, will be that tropical or semi-tropical colonies with a largely non-European population were most likely to represent colonial medicine in its most distinctive form. In part, this reflected the degree to which tropical or subtropical territories presented disease problems unfamiliar in Europe and other temperate areas. But it was also that in a situation where Europeans constituted a small ruling élite, Western medicine was closely tied to the colonial state itself and this manifested itself in close co-operation across a wide range of military, economic, and administrative activities. Not only was medicine more state-oriented or -dependent than in white-settler colonies, it also served an important role in enunciating imperial ideology and in negotiating or imposing the terms on which colonialism related to indigenous peoples and cultures.[2]

THE ROLE OF MEDICAL WORKERS IN COLONIAL EXPANSION

There can be no denying the European origins of colonial medicine. It sailed in the ships of the explorers; it marched with the armies of the colonizers. This automatically set it apart from the medical beliefs and healing practices of the indigenous population, helped sustain cultural and professional ties with Europe, and, depending upon the context, cast medicine in a defensive, antagonistic, or evangelical role. Although there were individuals in the vanguard of European expansion – like Hernando Cortés (1485–1547) in Mexico or Jacques Cartier (1491–1557) in Canada – who valued local remedies and held native healers in high esteem, historically such moments were rare and short-lived or dictated only by the absence of European surgeons and physicians. More commonly, especially in the nineteenth century, Western medicine was present from the outset and implicated in all the subsequent phases of colonialism: from exploration and conquest, to state formation and the exploitation of human and natural resources. (➤ Ch. 2 What is specific to Western medicine?; Ch. 29 Non-Western concepts of disease)

This involvement partly reflected the multiple roles assumed by individual medical practitioners. In advance of formal colonization, doctors might figure as explorers, their medical training an aid to their own survival and to their skills as scientific reporters. Mungo Park (1771–1806), the Edinburgh-trained surgeon whose travels in the 1790s 'opened the classic age of European exploration in West Africa', like David Livingstone (1813–73) in southern and Central Africa half a century later, was a pioneer in the discovery and scientific reconnaissance of lands hitherto beyond Europe's reach.[3] Doctors doubled as diplomats, their medical skills and reputation winning them privileged access as physicians and confidants to Mogul emperors or North African beys, enabling them to secure economic and political concessions for European merchants and would-be colonizers.[4]

With few other scientific experts and trained naturalists at its command, an incoming colonial power might turn to medical practitioners to conduct surveys of its new territories and to report on the natural resources and assets of the country and on diseases that might threaten European health or hinder agricultural productivity. As in Europe and North America in the late eighteenth and early nineteenth centuries, but with a belief in the greater potency of disease-causing miasmas in tropical climates, medical practitioners in the West Indies, West Africa, and India carried out topographical surveys and experimented with the use of vital data in an attempt to quantify the relationship between environment, disease, and demography. They described climate, soils and vegetation, but also speculated on the incidence and causes of prevalent diseases. Although a large part of this literature addressed questions of European health and the ability of Caucasians to survive as 'exotics' in an alien land, this was seldom completely separated from consideration of the health of the local inhabitants, which even allowing for 'constitutional' differences between races might be a useful guide to the nature and causes of specific diseases. These pioneers included Thomas Trapham (1673–1702), whose *Discourse on the State of Health on the Island of Jamaica* of 1679 has been identified as the first English-language account of tropical disease and medicine; Thomas Winterbottom (1765–1859), whose two-volume *Account of the Native Africans in the Neighbourhood of Sierra Leone*, published in 1803, drew upon seven years' experience and observation in West Africa; and James Johnson (1777–1845), a naval surgeon and the author of *The Influence of Tropical Climates, More Especially the Climate of India, on European Constitutions* (1813), which went through several editions and revisions by the 1860s. Through their medical interests, doctors became authorities on ethnography, recording the habits and customs of indigenous or slave populations, the diseases that afflicted them, and the medicines they employed. While some doctors wrote purely for the guidance of local planters or newly arrived surgeons, others saw themselves as privileged observers at the out-stations of an expanding scientific empire, serving the wider community through their books and scholarly papers, many of which were published in the scientific capitals of Europe.[5] (➤ Ch. 15 Environment and miasmata; Ch. 18 The ecology of disease; Ch. 71 Demography and medicine)

The responsibility of medicine for the practical needs of the colonizing power meant that the doctor or surgeon's first priority was to preserve or restore the health of European soldiers and sailors, merchants, planters, and officials. Some new colonies, like Australia and New Zealand in the nineteenth century, appeared to be blessed with a favourable climate (in an age when climate seemed a major determinant of health and disease), and to offer an environment that compared favourably with Victorian England. But many tropical regions rapidly (and, the statistics suggest, deservedly) acquired an awesome reputation for sickness and mortality: as far as European health was concerned, the Caribbean and East Indies came close to rivalling West Africa's claim to be 'the white man's grave'. Since Europe's commercial and political presence in these areas was dependent upon maritime power, the health of Europeans at sea or visiting tropical coasts and islands was a primary cause for concern in the eighteenth and early nineteenth centuries: the *Treatise of the Scurvy*, published by James Lind (1716–94) in 1753, was but one example of the extensive naval medical literature that arose from Europe's Atlantic slave trade, its commerce with the East Indies, and the maritime rivalry between the British, French, and Dutch. In view of their enormous commercial and strategic significance, the sugar-producing islands of the West Indies featured prominently in the early English and French literature on 'the diseases of warm climates'. However, with the abolition of slavery in the British Empire in 1834 and the slump in the islands' prosperity, the focus shifted by the 1850s to Algeria and Senegal for the French and to India for the British: these became the new colonial observation posts and laboratories. A further expansion and partial reorientation of the literature on colonial (or 'tropical') medicine came in the late nineteenth century with the growing political and economic involvement of the imperial powers in

South-East Asia (Malaya, Java, and French Indochina), and in northern and sub-Saharan Africa.[6]

STATE MEDICAL SERVICES IN THE WHITE-SETTLER COLONIES

In white-settler colonies, where Europeans rapidly came to form the bulk of the population, Western medicine could find a ready and expanding constituency, though it might face some unwelcome competition from 'bush medicine' and homoeopathy. (➤ Ch. 28 Unorthodox medical theories) Private practice could survive and even flourish without being dependent upon state patronage. But elsewhere, as in nineteenth-century Algeria, India, or Java, the state long remained the principal provider of employment for Western medical practitioners. Where the power of the state rested heavily upon the army, and where the absence or paucity of white planters, traders, and settlers created few opportunities for the growth of an independent medical profession, colonial medicine was largely a military affair. The army served several medical roles. It provided a trained medical cadre for the military's own high-priority health needs and a route for professional advancement; it was a primary site of medical observation and experimentation at a time when most of civilian society lay beyond medical scrutiny and surveillance; and, as in French West Africa, it was often also the only agency capable of mounting extensive public-health campaigns against malaria, yellow fever, and sleeping sickness. (➤ Ch. 19 Fevers) In British India, mainly for want of any alternative agency, colonial doctors were pressed into service as prison superintendents and forestry officers. There, the relationship between the army and the medical profession was typically close. Members of the Indian Medical Service (IMS), the premier medical agency, combined military and medical rank and, in times of war, were likely to be switched from civilian posts back to military duties. As late as 1924, the IMS was referred to as 'primarily a military service', and much the same description could be applied to other colonial medical services in Africa and Asia at that date.[7]

Many recent writers have stressed the limited impact of colonial medicine on indigenous societies and the extent to which it was confined to serving the needs of the colonialists themselves. Ramasubban has argued that in British India in the nineteenth century, the protection of the army and the European civilian population was 'at all times the highest priority' of colonial health policy. In her view, colonial medicine was 'enclavist' in character, directed almost exclusively to the medical needs of white civilians and military garrisons and ignoring the bulk of the Indian population.[8] There is much evidence to support this line of argument, not only for India but for many other colonial territories in Africa, Asia, and the Pacific in the nineteenth and early twentieth centuries. Indeed, many measures that were introduced during this period in the name of public health (such as the contagious diseases acts, which attempted to control venereal disease and prostitution) barely concealed a central preoccupation with the health of white soldiers and civilians. (➤ Ch. 26 Sexually transmitted diseases; Ch. 51 Public health) Even though epidemics of cholera, smallpox and malaria were hugely destructive of human life in India before the First World War, it was the perceived threat to the health of British troops (particularly from cholera) that first provided the impetus for sanitary reform and the beginnings of a public-health administration. (➤ Ch. 52 Epidemiology; Ch. 53 History of personal hygiene) One of the ways in which improvements to army health in India were achieved was by turning cantonments into sanitary 'oases', cut off as much as possible from the surrounding disease environment. Not all soldiers benefited equally from such measures. Non-white troops – Indian, African, and West Indian – seldom received such privileged attention, though they might be better protected than white soldiers by inherited or acquired disease immunities, and were sometimes deliberately deployed for this reason in localities where experience had shown Europeans to be particularly at risk. This was one of the ways in which colonialism shifted the disease burden from whites to blacks. Only gradually did measures introduced to provide better medical care and improved sanitary conditions for white soldiers extend to those of other races.

Another way in which the health of European soldiers and civilians was privileged was through strategies of avoidance and segregation. The miasmatic theories that dominated nineteenth-century thinking about disease causation and transmission encouraged recourse to evasive measures. When epidemics of smallpox, cholera, or malaria threatened, troops were moved from their barracks into temporary camps in more salubrious locations. Hill resorts were established in many parts of the tropics to preserve the health or speed the recovery of European soldiers and civilians. By the mid-1890s, nearly a quarter of British troops in India were stationed in the hills.[9] Avoidance strategies took on additional significance towards the close of the nineteenth century under the influence of the germ theory of disease. (➤ Ch. 16 Contagion/ germ theory/specificity) As bacteriological research began to reveal how malaria and other diseases were transmitted from one human host to another, disease came to be identified not, as in the past, with pathogenic landscapes, but with living 'native reservoirs' of diseases. One way of protecting European health was accordingly to locate white residential areas as far as possible from 'native' quarters or to throw a sanitary cordon around the urban areas inhabited by non-white populations seen as harbouring plague, smallpox, and other diseases.[10]

HEALTH CARE FOR INDIGENOUS POPULATIONS

However, privileged though the health of European soldiers and civilians undoubtedly was, it would be erroneous to see colonial medicine as intended for their consumption alone. Even the logic of protecting white health might require medicine to leave its sanitary enclaves and infiltrate surrounding populations. Some degree of intervention might be necessary if only to vaccinate and inoculate those servants, camp-followers, and employees with whom white soldiers and civilians came into frequent contact. One of the main incentives for the expansion of European medicine beyond a white/military enclave was in order to make colonial labour more productive and profitable, though in practice the capitalist profit motive often needed the additional impetus of outside political pressure. Like the army, colonial plantations and mines were often sites of exceptionally high sickness and mortality: the harsh treatment of labourers, deficient diets, and crowded, insanitary living conditions, unhealthy locations, and the mixing of people from different disease environments all contributed to a state of endemic ill health. High rates of mortality and absenteeism due to sickness might persuade employers of the desirability of providing elementary health care for their workers or slaves. Doctors might be an adjunct to more-effective labour management, for example by distinguishing those who were genuinely ill from 'shirkers' who could be punished or sent back to work. Soaring sickness and death rates might also arouse humanitarian indignation in Europe and so force medical and sanitary reforms on reluctant slave-owners and planters. The colonial state might itself be driven to intervene to prevent further scandals or to ensure that the supply of labour did not dry up and paralyse enterprises that were vital to its own revenues. The imposition of certain minimal health standards was one of the ways in which colonial regimes in effect sanctioned coercive and exploitative modes of labour control.

Medicine's role in the management and legitimation of labour was established as early as the 1780s and 1790s in the Atlantic slave trade. With humanitarian objections to the slave trade mounting, the British Parliament laid down its own conditions for allowing the trade to continue. 'Guinea surgeons' were required by law to inspect slaves before their embarkation in Africa and on arrival in the Americas, and were also expected to help slaves survive the ordeal of the 'middle crossing'. A similar combination of commercial and political pressures operated in the West Indies themselves, where planters were obliged to establish 'sick houses' or hospitals for slaves.[11] Following the abolition of slavery in the British Empire in 1834, the recruitment of Indian indentured labourers for plantations in South Asia and elsewhere also attracted concern and led to the imposition of similar legal and medical controls. In the plantation and mine economies of the Dutch East Indies, British Malaya, and western and southern Africa, local or migrant workers also received a degree of medical attention generally unavailable to the surrounding population, though seldom sufficient to protect them from the hazards of their working environment.[12]

Involvement in the management of colonial labour was thus one of the ways in which Western medicine reached out to include sections of the non-white population. This involvement was, in turn, duly reflected in the way in which diseases such as yaws, beriberi, and ankylostomiasis, the characteristic diseases of plantation labour, came to occupy a prominent place in the annals of tropical medicine. (➤ Ch. 22 Nutritional diseases) But in focusing upon the needs of plantation and mine labour, colonial medicine merely created a new set of 'enclaves' to set alongside those of the white civilians and the army. And, as with the army, the concentration of scant medical resources on estate and mine workers emphasized the male bias of colonial health provision and the general neglect of women's and children's health and of rural society as a whole.

THE EFFECTS OF EPIDEMICS ON PUBLIC-HEALTH SERVICES

Gradually, colonial medicine cast its net more widely. As in Europe, epidemic diseases were a powerful stimulus to the development of public health and improved medical services. Colonies in temperate as well as tropical zones shared in a series of epidemic episodes during the course of the nineteenth and early twentieth centuries: cholera and smallpox between the 1830s and 1880s; plague in the 1890s and 1900s; influenza in 1918–19. The medical histories of many colonies, and no less significantly the popular experience and perception of medicine, has to a large extent been written in terms of these epidemiological crises and the attempts of colonial health authorities to contain them. In East and Central Africa, sleeping sickness in the early years of the twentieth century was quickly followed by epidemics of influenza, plague, and malaria. In India, cholera prompted the appointment of a Royal Commission on the sanitary state of the army which, in turn, gave rise to the first serious attempts to draw up a public-health system for India. The plague epidemic that erupted in Bombay in 1896 was met with state-backed medical intervention on an unprecedented scale, and forced a major review of the country's sanitary and medical services.[13] (➤ Ch. 50 Medical institutions and the state)

Coming at a time of new-found confidence in the capacity of medical science to conquer disease, the epidemics of the late nineteenth and early twentieth centuries hastened the growth of the colonial state and exemplified its expansion into previously untouched areas of society. This was particularly the case in tropical colonies where private practice and public philanthropy contributed relatively little, and the role of the state was correspondingly greater. But the pace of change varied markedly from one part of the colonial world to another. In white-settler colonies, developments in private medical practice and public health might be rapid and in line with (or even in advance of) contemporary developments in Europe. Like other areas of white settlement, the influx of poor migrants into New Zealand during the Otago gold rush of 1861 provided the stimulus for early public-health legislation. Similarly, the threatening plague pandemic of the 1890s and 1900s caused alarm in New Zealand and led to the assumption of drastic public-health powers by the Government: it also forced the colonial authorities into a belated concern for Maori health. Constitutionally a dominion from 1907 and so moving away from conventional colonial status, New Zealand had a Ministry of Health nearly twenty years before Britain, and in such fields as child welfare proved itself in many respects more innovative and far-sighted than Britain.[14] (➤ Ch. 45 Childhood) Such developments are a reminder that colonial medicine was not always derivative of, and dependent upon, metropolitan forms and practices.

But elsewhere, especially in the tropics, colonial governments might baulk at the expenditure and administrative effort needed to take Western medicine to an indigenous and possibly resistant population. In India, part of the responsibility for public health was transferred in the 1880s to local government boards, partly in emulation of the municipalization of public health in Victorian Britain, but without either the funds or the civil zeal necessary to make it very effective. In East Africa, significant expansion of state medical services came only after the First World War when colonial governments began to accept responsibility for African as well as European health. Hospitals were a feature of colonial medicine from the outset, but in their urban location and sometimes, too, in their racial exclusivity, they tended to reflect its more enclavist characteristics. It was only from the 1850s in India and later in many other colonies that dispensaries and clinics began to be established in the countryside, and from the 1920s to be supplemented by mobile dispensaries and itinerant medical squads. It was late in the colonial day before Western medicine began to turn its attention to problems of poverty and malnutrition, rural hygiene and sanitation, and women's and children's health – in short, to see medicine in terms of public health rather than the narrow priorities of the colonial state. Even then, Western medicine might be very thinly spread. On the eve of Britain's departure from India in 1947, there was only one registered doctor (of Western medicine) for 6,300 people and only one nurse for every 43,000, as compared with one doctor per 1,000 people and one nurse for every 300 in Britain. In the rural areas of the

United Provinces in northern India there was only one hospital or dispensary for every 106,000 people. It was not surprising that an official investigation into the state of health in India in the mid-1940s concluded that the existing health services were 'altogether inadequate to meet the needs of the people'.[15] Many African and South-East Asian colonies were as badly or even worse off when independence came.

The limited out-reach of Western medicine was exacerbated in many colonies by the extent to which Europeans monopolized professional appointments and denied all but the most junior positions to members of indigenous communities. The close relationship between the medical profession and the colonial state, the pressure exerted by empire-wide organizations like the British Medical Association, and racist arguments against the employment of Africans and Asians, largely restricted non-whites to the lowly ranks of vaccinators, nurses, dressers, and assistant surgeons. Even in India, where medical education for Indians dated back to the opening of Calcutta's Medical College in 1835, it took a century to overturn the racial exclusiveness of the Indian Medical Service.[16]

THE DISEASE FACTOR IN EUROPEAN EXPANSIONISM

From a position of relative obscurity, disease and medicine have come to occupy a central place in the history of European expansionism. Scholars have argued forcefully in favour of disease and (to a lesser degree) medicine as formative factors in the establishment and evolution of European empires overseas. To a degree that appears startling when compared with the historiography of even a few decades ago, disease and medicine have come to be recognized as arbiters in the fate of Europe's expansionist drives overseas, in dividing up the globe between areas of white and non-white settlement. Epidemic diseases like smallpox and measles are now widely credited with having devastated and demoralized indigenous populations in such previously isolated regions of the globe as the Cape of Good Hope, Australia, New Zealand, and the Pacific Islands, thereby clearing the way for European conquest and colonization. Where once the courage and daring of the Spanish *conquistadores* were thought to have toppled the Aztec and Inca empires of Mexico and Peru, the historian now looks to a more insidious and deadly invader: the smallpox virus. Without the disease factor working in their favour, it is doubted that the Spanish and subsequent European intruders in the Americas would have met with such success or found Indian resistance so ineffectual. Conversely, endemic diseases are seen to have been largely responsible for holding back Europe's expansion into Africa for several centuries until, in the second half of the nineteenth century, quinine opened the floodgates to European power. Yellow fever and malaria, unwittingly imported from Africa, combined with racial patterns of immunity and susceptibility, are now seen as dictating the ethnic composition and distinctive history of colonization and labour in the Caribbean.[17]

It may be argued that the trend towards biological determinism has been carried too far and is in danger of overlooking the complex interplay of means and motive that shaped European expansionism over several centuries. But one of the apparent consequences of the current stress upon disease invasions and immunities rather than conscious human agency has been to detract from the role of medicine. With disease so strongly in the ascendant, Western medicine appears by contrast a rather feeble adversary. Indeed, European colonialism, once praised for having freed much of Africa, Asia, and the Pacific from the scourge of disease, is now widely regarded as having been (as Donald Denoon puts it) a 'health hazard', unleashing a crisis of mortality that it was medically powerless, until relatively recently, to efface. The forging of new epidemiological links between previously isolated regions of the globe, the movement of fleets and armies and of many millions of slaves and indentured labourers, the spread of disease through ecological change and social dislocation, the misery bred by shanty-towns and cities, all these have been implicated in the apparent explosion of mortality that followed hard on the heels of European rule.[18] (➤ Ch. 27 Diseases of civilization; Ch. 72 Medicine, mortality, and morbidity) Medicine, by contrast, was less profligate with its favours – at least as far as non-settler colonies were concerned. In tropical territories, where unfamiliar climates and diseases were thought to call for drastic remedies, Western medicine probably had little beneficial effect on the health of its hapless patients, white or black. With its grim enthusiasm for violent purges and copious bleedings, before the 1850s it probably wrecked many more lives than it saved. Although some scholars like Philip Curtin write with confidence of the effectiveness of certain hygienic and sanitary measures in curbing European mortality from the middle of the nineteenth century, or stress the life-saving contribution made by quinine as a prophylactic against malaria from roughly the same date, others remain understandably sceptical about the practical achievement of Western medicine in the tropics before the Second World War.[19]

Some medical measures were surely more effective than others. Two of the most widely discussed have been smallpox vaccination and quinine prophylaxis. Vaccination against smallpox is particularly interesting: this was one of the first Western medical measures to be extensively employed outside Europe (it was introduced to colonies as far distant as Mexico and Ceylon within a decade of Edward Jenner (1749–1823) discovering it); it was also an attempt to curb the ravages of a disease that Europeans had themselves been instrumental in spreading to many parts of the globe. Some writers see vaccination as having had an almost immediate impact on smallpox mortality, and for the first time affording the medical profession a reliable means of protection against one of the commonest and most deadly diseases. However, doubts remain both about its actual effectiveness in the face of technical problems (such as the preservation of the lymph in hot and humid climates), and the capacity of colonial governments to deliver vaccination on an adequate scale, given popular opposition and the difficulty of creating reliable vaccination agencies. Studies of vaccination in the West Indies, Asia, and Africa suggest that, in the long term, it was effective in reducing indigenous as well as European mortality, but that it took rather longer and encountered more obstacles than was previously recognized.[20]

Controversy continues, too, to surround quinine prophylaxis. More than any other single medical discovery, the use of quinine in the prevention and treatment of malaria has been cited as the vital breakthrough that allowed Europeans to penetrate Africa and to extend their mastery over tropical Asia. Following severe mortality in earlier West African expeditions, the successful use of quinine by William Baikie (1825–64) on the Niger expedition of 1854 has been taken as proof that disease was no longer a barrier to European exploration and control. Quinine, writers like Oliver Ransford have averred, was the 'prime factor in allowing the whiteman's conquest of Black Africa'.[21] And yet the evidence seems equivocal. Forty years after the Niger expedition, Europeans were still dying from malaria, or becoming seriously incapacitated by it. Although white mortality in tropical Africa began to decline significantly from the 1890s, this was partly due to the adoption of insect-control measures introduced following the discovery by Ronald Ross (1857–1932) of the role mosquitoes played in malaria transmission. The use of quinine was by no means universal among Europeans in the tropics in the second half of the nineteenth century, and for a long time there was no agreement about the appropriate dosage required. Moreover, while quinine, taken regularly and in sufficient doses, might give valuable protection to Europeans, it was not necessarily available to, or popular with, other denizens of the tropics. Despite government attempts to popularize the use of quinine, malaria continued throughout the colonial period to be a major (if not *the* major) cause of mortality in British India.[22]

But while much recent attention has been directed towards attempts to quantify the demographic impact of medicine and disease, medicine's contribution to empire should surely not be understood solely in terms of its demonstrable effects on health and mortality. Medicine was also an integral, if unquantifiable, part of the ideological apparatus of empire. In an age when colonialism was confidently equated with civilization, medicine was given a prominent place among the benefits that European civilization could bestow upon the benighted rest of the world. Speaking in 1899, when imperial power in India was at its zenith, the Viceroy, Lord Curzon (1859–1925), claimed that the British had come to India not simply as conquerors but also as benefactors, bringing their religion, law, literature, and science with them. Critics might cavil about the value of Britain's laws and religion, but about science, especially medical science, he believed there could be 'no two opinions'. Medicine was 'the most cosmopolitan of all sciences'; it embraced 'in its merciful appeal every suffering human being in the world': it transcended boundaries of caste, creed, and gender. Medicine was itself sufficient justification for British rule in India.[23] Curzon was not alone in choosing to single out the benefits of medicine and its identification with Europe's 'civilizing mission'. For Rudyard Kipling (1865–1936), it was part of the 'white man's burden' and the philanthropic ends of empire to 'bid the sickness cease', much as Hubert Lyautey (1854–1934), one of the principal architects of the French colonial medical service, declared in a phrase reminiscent of Curzon that 'La seule excuse de la colonisation c'est le médecin'.[24]

RELATIONSHIPS BETWEEN WESTERN AND INDIGENOUS MEDICAL SYSTEMS

For regimes that rested heavily upon the army, the police, the tax-collector, and the judiciary, it was encouraging to believe that effective control could be won and maintained more cheaply through doctors and surgeons, and that medicine, along with education, could do more than anything else to break down cultural resistance to colonial rule. It was sometimes reckoned that as a 'civilizing and pacifying force' one skilful doctor was worth more than a company of infantry, and that a well-run hospital had 'greater power in the long run than a battery of maxim guns'.[25] The importance attached to its 'civilizing and pacifying' role is a further reason for not seeing colonial medicine in purely enclavist terms. Medicine also acted as a powerful force in the ideological subordination and cultural representation of indigenous peoples. By the mid-nineteenth century, medicine had acquired the authority of an impartial and objective science, a stature that gave considerable weight to its often highly partisan pronouncements. Western medicine was cited as indisputable evidence that colonial rule stood for rationality and progress, while indigenous society foolishly cherished superstition and witchcraft, was ruled by ignorance and cruelty, and held beliefs and practices Europe had left behind with the Dark Ages. Sometimes openly, sometimes subliminally, medical science conducted a protracted struggle with social and religious practices that Europeans did not understand or found deeply repugnant. (➤ Ch. 60 Medicine and anthropology) In an age of social Darwinism and high empire, medical discourse and practice were impregnated with the language of race, preoccupied with the need to preserve and protect the health of the white population, while attributing to other races all kinds of vices and abominations. Medicine stamped its authority upon the physical and cultural stereotypes of non-white races – their weakness, lethargy, promiscuity, and so forth – and endorsed Europe's claims to cultural and racial supremacy. Medical practitioners could be critics of empire, but more commonly, their influence was to be found as part of the intellectual driving-force behind policies of ideological incorporation and political subordination.[26]

In its more hegemonic ambitions, Western medicine was allied with religious agency and 'spiritual conquest'. This was particularly evident in regions where the state's own medical agencies were absent or weak. In the colonies of Spanish America, where Franciscans, Dominicans, and other religious orders founded hospitals and cared for sick and needy Indians, one of the motives was to win converts to Christianity. This was a strategy of acculturation previously employed among the Moors of southern Spain.[27] Evangelization through medicine was important, too, in nineteenth-century colonialism in Africa, Asia, and the Pacific Islands, though its role varied greatly from one situation to another. Missionaries were excluded from India until 1813, and even after that date the colonial administration considered it politic to distance British rule as much as possible from the evangelists: failure to do so was seen as a contributory cause to the Mutiny and Rebellion of 1857. There, missionary medicine played second fiddle to state medicine, or found itself restricted to areas that were low on the state's list of priorities, such as the care and treatment of lepers. By the 1880s 'zenana missions', established to provide medical help for Indian women in their own homes, were beginning to break down the hitherto heavily male bias of colonial medicine in India.[28] (➤ Ch. 33 Indian medicine; Ch. 61 Religion and medicine)

In many parts of Africa, state medical provision was almost entirely confined to European civilians and soldiers before the 1920s, thus leaving missionary medicine to fill the void in African health care. At first, medicine was seen principally as a means of preserving the missionaries' own health, but when their evangelical efforts were rebuffed, missionaries turned to medicine to open doors otherwise closed to them. Christianity's 'healing' doctrine and humanitarian practice was a deliberate challenge, too, to the power of local 'witch-doctors'. Dispensaries and hospitals helped attract converts, to establish and maintain viable Christian communities, even to stave off competition from rival missionary societies. Although after the First World War colonial administrations took over part of the missionaries' medical work, there remained a broad compatibility between the 'civilizing' ambitions of the state and the evangelizing activities of the mission doctor.[29]

The cultural and political assertiveness of Western medicine was evident, too, in attitudes towards indigenous medicine. In the Americas, Africa, and Asia, it functioned in contradistinction to indigenous medical practices and healing beliefs. It was characteristic of medicine's colonizing nature that it sought to establish its superior or monopolistic rights over the body of the colonized. The vigorous denunciation of indigenous healers, from the 'witchdoctors' and spirit mediums in Africa to the *vaidya*s and *hakim*s of Hindu and Islamic medicine, was supported by claims that their practices were grounded in superstition, or at best mere empiricism, and were often dangerous. (➤ Ch. 31 Arab-Islamic medicine) Although initial encounters between Western and indigenous medicine might be fairly open and egalitarian,[30] it was more common for practitioners of Western medicine to assume a hostile attitude, especially in the second half of the nineteenth century as Western medicine became more than ever convinced of its uniquely scientific basis and superior therapeutic powers. In further evidence of the close ideological and functional relationship between medicine and the state, colonial authorities intervened to prohibit practices and cults that they saw as medically or politically objectionable – hence the outlawing of 'black magic' in Jamaica following its implication in the slave rebellion of 1760, the prohibition of variolation in parts of India in the second half of the nineteenth century, the suppression of the Sopona smallpox cult in Nigeria in 1917, and the witchcraft ordinances in Britain's African colonies in the 1920s and 1930s.[31] The colonial state thus made itself the arbiter of what was 'good' or 'bad' medicine.

But the relationship of Western with indigenous medicine could be one of appropriation and not merely of intolerance. In many parts of the expanding colonial world, the arrival of Western medicine was accompanied by a search for new drugs that might be added to Europe's pharmacopoeia or serve as cheap and convenient substitutes for imported medicines. This quest was further encouraged by a belief that in every region God (or Nature) would provide the cures for local fevers and fluxes. This pharmacological investigation was more important in some areas and times than in others. One aspect of the 'Columbian exchange' between Europe and the Americas was the former's acquisition of many valuable New World medicinal drugs. Although some drugs were taken up in North America from Indian usage or through experimentation, central and northern South America proved a far richer source, including balsam, cinchona, and ipecacuanha.[32] There was a prolonged investigation in nineteenth-century India of the plant and mineral extracts used by Ayurvedic practitioners, but fewer of these were new to Europe or found lasting favour with European practitioners.[33] (➤ Ch. 39 Drug therapies) But while Europe freely pillaged native pharmacies in search of suitable drugs (along with other 'useful' plants and minerals), there was no corresponding incorporation of the cultural ideas and religious practices which had surrounded the use of them in their places of origin. When Aztec drugs were taken over by the Spanish, their properties were understood solely in terms of the humoral pathology then prevalent in Europe (➤ Ch. 14 Humoralism):

there was little interest in how the Aztecs had used them or why they believed them efficacious.[34] It was rarer for therapeutic practices other than drugs to be taken up in this colonizing process. Variolation (inoculation against small-pox) was a rare example of how a practice widespread in many parts of Africa and Asia might be incorporated into European medicine, and even that was to be quickly superseded by Jennerian vaccination.[35]

Because colonial medicine was so closely aligned with state power and appeared generally so antagonistic towards indigenous healing practices, the two might become in the popular view virtually indistinguishable – alike alien, coercive, malevolent. Even vaccination, so confidently hailed by nineteenth-century colonialists as one of Europe's greatest boons, might be interpreted as a painful and sinister process by which the state puts its 'mark' on those it intended to conscript for indentured labour, convert to Christianity, or offer up as sacrifices to its own merciless gods. For many indigenes in the first generation or two of their encounter with colonialism, medicine was a potent source of rumour and distrust, evasion and, occasionally, resistance.[36] The conflict between colonial medicine and indigenous societies was accentu-ated by the growing tendency for the state to take charge of many areas of social and cultural life that had formerly been part of local traditions of disease control and community medicine, but which had probably never been part of any ruler's responsibility. While white-settler colonies were able to evolve fairly decentralized and voluntaristic medical systems, in the colonies of Africa, Asia and the Pacific, medicine was one of the most intrusive expressions of state power. Partly for this reason, Western medicine often became a critical issue in the growth of anti-colonial movements. Some nationalists and traditionalists sought the restoration of old medical beliefs and practices as part of their assault on Western colonialism and cultural hegemony, but there were also Western-educated politicians and indigenous practitioners of Western medicine who resented the racial exclusiveness and narrow priorities of colonial medicine and argued instead for a freer distri-bution of its benefits, and who assigned medicine and public health a more-central place in nation-building and economic development than colonialism allowed.

In practice, though, the monopolistic ambitions of Western medicine often went unrealized, defeated by indigenous evasion and resistance, or thwarted by bureaucratic lethargy and financial stringency. This often left a cultural and social space within which pre-existing idioms of disease and medicine could quietly continue or peacefully coexist with colonial practice. One example of this was among the black populations of the New World. Despite the abrupt and brutal manner in which they were torn from their home societies in Africa and shipped off to the Americas, the slaves and their descendants retained some of their medical links with Africa or worked them into a new and syncretic medical culture. Although plantation hospitals were established in the West Indies and in the southern United States, black medical beliefs and practices were tolerated or survived in quiet defiance of the medicine of their masters.[37] In India, where indigenous culture was too tenacious for more than a century of colonialism to erase, the Hindu Ayurvedic and Islamic Yunani systems of medicine, after a period of decline and official hostility, found fresh patronage from the middle classes in the late nineteenth and early twentieth centuries and became part of the country's revivalist movements. Even while taking on some features of Western medicine, Ayurvedic and Yunani medicine presented themselves as culturally more-acceptable alternatives to Western medicine.[38] Moreover, in the Indian countryside, the slow advance of Western medical practice had done little even by 1947 to dent popular belief in disease-deities and folk medicine. (➤ Ch. 30 Folk medicine) Monopolistic by inclination, in much of the tropical world, colonial medicine was obliged to accept pluralism in practice.

CONCLUSION

The old assumption that Europe's medicine was transferred wholesale and unmodified to the colonies is now viewed more critically. Of late, there has been much stress upon the innovations dictated by 'frontier' conditions, by remoteness from the centres of metropolitan medicine, and by the absence in backwoods or veldt of qualified physicians. Conversely, it has been argued that when colonial practice is actually examined alongside that of contemporary Europe, the differences are in fact not very great: the medical institutions and the forms of medicine practised in colonial America before 1800, for instance, were probably much like those in Europe at the time.[39] For centuries, European universities and medical schools supplied doctors and surgeons to medical establishments abroad, and this presumably served to give a high degree of standardization to Western medicine abroad as well as in Europe. The traffic in trained medical personnel was mostly one-way – from Europe to the rest of the world – for the colonies were important outlets for doctors unable or disinclined to seek employment at home. But there are at least some notable instances of physicians – like James Ranald Martin (1793–1874), who, after forty-four years in India, served on two royal commissions in England and helped establish the Royal Victoria Hospital at Netley, and Edmund Parkes (1819–76), whose brief service as an army surgeon in India helped launch him as 'the founder of the science of modern hygiene' – who successfully moved back from the 'periphery' to influential careers in Britain.[40]

The expansion of European empires in the late nineteenth century, the rise of new economic and political imperatives, and the growth of new networks of transport and communications made medicine more than ever an empire-wide project. Individuals like Patrick Manson (1844–1922) and Ronald Ross, and research institutes in Algeria, India, Malaya, and Indochina, could contribute the results of their field research to metropolitan science, while roving experts and commissions from specialist institutions in Europe were able to relay news of the latest medical discoveries to even the remotest colonies. This rapid movement of people and ideas was indicative of the importance of professional and scientific linkages within imperial systems and the role of the colonies as research stations and laboratories; but it was also expressive of the way in which on the eve of the First World War colonial medicine, like the colonies themselves, had become a source of intense rivalry, as well as occasional co-operation, between imperial powers.[41] At this moment of high imperialism, perhaps more than at any other time, medicine occupied a central place in the ideological as well as the technological processes of colonial rule. (➤ Ch. 59 Internationalism in medicine and public health)

NOTES

1 L. H. Gann and Peter Duignan, *Burden of Empire: an Appraisal of Western Colonialism in Africa South of the Sahara*, Stanford, CA, Hoover Institution Press, 1967, pp. 282–92; Edmond Sergent, 'La médecine française en Algérie', *Archives de l'Institut Pasteur d'Algérie*, 1954, 32: 281–5. For a sharply anti-colonial critique, see Frantz Fanon, *A Dying Colonialism*, Harmondsworth, Penguin, 1970, ch. 4.

2 The absence of a more distinctive form of medicine in North America before 1820 is discussed by Richard Harrison Shyrock, *Medicine and Society in America, 1600–1860*, New York, New York University Press, 1960, pp. 84–5.

3 Philip D. Curtin, *The Image of Africa: British Ideas and Action, 1780–1850*, Madison, University of Wisconsin Press, 1964, pp. 144–6; Michael Gelfand, *Livingstone, the Doctor: his Life and Travels*, Oxford, Blackwell, 1957.

4 D. G. Crawford, *A History of the Indian Medical Service, 1600–1913*, London, W. Thacker, 1914, Vol. I, pp. 113–28; Nancy Elizabeth Gallagher, *Medicine and Power in Tunisia, 1780–1900*, Cambridge, Cambridge University Press, 1983, pp. 88–9; Jim Paul, 'Medicine and imperialism in Morocco', *MERIP Reports*, 1977, 60: 4–5.

5 M. T. Ashcroft, 'Tercentenary of the first English book on tropical medicine, by Thomas Trapham of Jamaica', *British Medical Journal*, 1979, 2: 475–7; Curtin, op. cit. (n. 3), pp. 182–3, 185–6, 190–1, 209–10; Richard B. Sheridan, *Doctors and Slaves: a Medical and Demographic History of Slavery in the British West Indies, 1680–1834*, Cambridge, Cambridge University Press, 1985, ch. 1.

6 Andrew Balfour, 'Some British and American pioneers in tropical medicine and hygiene', *Transactions of the Royal Society for Tropical Medicine and Hygiene*, 1925, 19: 189–229; P. Nosny, 'Propos sur l'histoire de la médecine coloniale française', *Médecine tropicale*, 1964, 24: 375–82; Sheridan, op. cit. (n. 5). See also the sources cited in August Hirsch, *Handbook of Geographical and Historical Pathology*, London, New Sydenham Society, 1883; and Philip D. Curtin, *Death by Migration:*

Europe's Encounter with the Tropical World in the Nineteenth Century, Cambridge, Cambridge University Press, 1989.

7 *The Army in India and its Evolution*, Calcutta, Superintendent of Government Printing, 1924, p. 117. Until 1911, '[Western] medicine in the Dutch Indies was virtually synonymous with military medicine': A. H. M. Kerkhoff, 'The organization of the military and civil medical service in the nineteenth century', in G. M. van Heteren, A. de Knecht-van Eekelen and M. J. D. Poulissen (eds), *Dutch Medicine in the Malaya Archipelago, 1816–1942*, Amsterdam, Rodopi, 1989, p. 12. For French military medicine, see J. H. Ricosseé, 'French West and Equatorial Africa', in E. E. Sabben-Clare, D. J. Bradley and K. Kirkwood (eds), *Health in Tropical Africa during the Colonial Period*, Oxford, Clarendon Press, 1980, pp. 228–38.

8 Radhika Ramasubban, *Public Health and Medical Research in India: their Origins under the Impact of British Colonial Policy*, Stockholm, SAREC, 1982, p. 9; Ramasubban, 'Imperial health in British India, 1857–1900', in Roy MacLeod and Milton Lewis (eds), *Disease, Medicine, and Empire: Perspectives on Western Medicine and the Experience of European Expansion*, London, Routledge, 1988, pp. 38–60. For a critique, see Roger Jeffery, *The Politics of Health in India*, Berkeley, University of California Press, 1988, ch. 3.

9 *Annual Report of the Sanitary Commission with the Government of India, 1894*, Calcutta, Superintendent of Government Printing, 1896, p. 47.

10 Raymond E. Dummett, 'The campaign against malaria and the expansion of scientific, medical, and sanitary services in British West Africa, 1898–1910', *African Historical Studies*, 1968, 1: 171–2; Leo Spitzer, 'The mosquito and segregation in Sierra Leone', *Canadian Journal of African Studies*, 1968, 2: 49–61; Maynard W. Swanson, 'The sanitation syndrome: bubonic plague and urban native policy in the Cape Colony, 1900–1909', *Journal of African History*, 1977, 18: 387–410.

11 Sheridan, op. cit. (n. 5), chs. 4, 10; cf. Todd L. Savitt, *Medicine and Slavery: the Diseases and Health of Blacks in Antebellum Virginia*, Urbana, University of Illinois Press, 1978.

12 Chee Heng Leng, 'Health status and development of health services in a colonial state: the case of British Malaya', *International Journal of Health Services*, 1982, 12: 397–417; G. T. Haneveld, 'From slave hospital to reliable health care: medical work on the plantations of Sumatra's east coast', in van Heteren, de Knecht-van Eekelen and Poulissen, Gerald op. cit. (n. 7), pp. 105–18; Mark W. De Lancey, 'Health and disease on the plantations of Cameroon, 1884–1939', in W. Hartwig and K. David Patterson (eds), *Disease in African History*, Durham, NC, Duke University Press, 1978, pp. 153–79; Randall M. Packard, *White Plague, Black Labor: Tuberculosis and the Political Economy of Health and Disease in South Africa*, Pietermaritzburg, University of Natal Press, 1990.

13 Geoffrey Rice, 'Christchurch in the 1918 influenza epidemic: a preliminary study', *New Zealand Journal of History*, 1979, 13: 109–37; Howard Phillips, 'The local state and public health reform in South Africa: Bloemfontein and the consequences of the Spanish 'flu of 1918', *Journal of Southern African Studies*, 1987, 13: 210–33; James W. Brown, 'Increased intercommunication and epidemic disease in early colonial Ashanti', in Hartwig and Patterson, op. cit. (n.

12), pp. 191–8; Harvey G. Soff, 'Sleeping sickness in the Lake Victoria region of British East Africa, 1900–1915', *African Historical Studies*, 1969, 2: 255–68; Ann Beck, *A History of the British Medical Administration of East Africa, 1900–1950*, Cambridge, MA, Harvard University Press, 1970, pp. 35–47, 105–11; I. J. Catanach, 'Plague and the tensions of empire: India 1896–1918', in David Arnold (ed.), *Imperial Medicine and Indigenous Societies*, Manchester, Manchester University Press, 1988, pp. 149–71; Terence Ranger, 'The influenza pandemic in Southern Rhodesia: a crisis of comprehension', in Arnold, ibid., pp. 172–88.

14   F. S. Maclean, *Challenge for Health: a History of Public Health in New Zealand*, Wellington, R. E. Owen, 1964, pp. 12–16, ch. 8; Arthur Porritt, 'The history of medicine in New Zealand', *Medical History*, 1967, 11: 334–44. For Canada, see Geoffrey Bilson, *A Darkened House: Cholera in Nineteenth-Century Canada*, Toronto, University of Toronto Press, 1980; and Bilson, 'Public health and the medical profession in nineteenth-century Canada', in MacLeod and Lewis, op. cit. (n. 8), pp. 156–75. For Australia, see Diana Dyason, 'The medical profession in colonial Victoria, 1834–1901', in MacLeod and Lewis, op. cit. (n. 8), pp. 194–216; Milton Lewis, 'The "health of the race" and infant health in New South Wales: perspectives on medicine and empire', in MacLeod and Lewis, op. cit. (n. 8), pp. 301–15.

15   *Report of the Health Survey and Development Committee*, Delhi, Manager of Publications, 1946, Vol. I, pp. 11, 13, 37.

16   Terence J. Johnson and Marjorie Caygill, 'The British Medical Association and its overseas branches: a short history', *Journal of Imperial and Commonwealth History*, 1973, 1: 303–29; Roger Jeffery, 'Recognising India's doctors: the establishment of medical dependency, 1918–39', *Modern Asian Studies*, 1979, 13: 301–26; Charlotte Searle, *The History of the Development of Nursing in South Africa, 1652–1960*, Cape Town, Struik, 1965; K. David Patterson, *Health in Colonial Ghana: Disease, Medicine and Socio-economic Change, 1900–1955*, Waltham, MA, Crossroads Press, 1981, pp. 12–14.

17   P. M. Ashburn, *The Ranks of Death: a Medical History of the Conquest of America*, New York, Coward-McCann, 1947; Alfred W. Crosby, *The Columbian Exchange: the Biological and Cultural Consequences of 1492*, Westport, CT, Greenwood Press, 1974; and Crosby, *Ecological Imperialism: the Biological Expansion of Europe, 900–1900*, Cambridge, Cambridge University Press, 1986, ch. 9; Kenneth F. Kiple, *The Caribbean Slave: a Biological History*, Cambridge, Cambridge University Press, 1984.

18   Donald Denoon, *Public Health in Papua New Guinea: Medical Possibility and Social Constraint, 1884–1984*, Cambridge, Cambridge University Press, 1989, p. 32; Ira Klein, 'Death in India, 1871–1921', *Journal of Asian Studies*, 1973, 32: 639–59; Hartwig and Patterson, op. cit. (n. 12).

19   Dennis G. Carlson, *African Fever: a Study of British Science, Technology, and Politics in West Africa, 1787–1864*, Canton, MA, Science History Publications, 1984, ch. 4; Kiple, op. cit. (n. 17), pp. 151–4; Sheridan, op. cit. (n. 5), p. 329 f.; Curtin, op. cit. (n. 6), L. J. and J. M. Bruce-Chwatt, 'Malaria and yellow fever', in Sabben-Clare, Bradley and Kirkwood, op. cit. (n. 7), pp. 43–62.

20   David Arnold, 'Smallpox and colonial medicine in nineteenth-century India', in Arnold, op. cit. (n. 13), pp. 52–61; Donald B. Cooper, *Epidemic Disease in Mexico*

City, 1761–1813: an Administrative, Social and Medical Study, Austin, University of Texas Press, 1965, ch. 4; Brown, op. cit. (n. 13), pp. 189–90; Gerald W. Hartwig, 'Smallpox in the Sudan', *International Journal of African History*, 1981, 14: 5–33; Bram Peper, 'Population growth in Java in the nineteenth century: a new interpretation', *Population Studies*, 1970, 24: 71–84; P. Boomgaard, 'Smallpox and vaccination on Java, 1780–1860: medical data as a source for demographic history', in van Heteren, de Knecht-van Eekelen and Poulissen, op. cit. (n. 7), p. 127.

21   Oliver Ransford, *'Bid the Sickness Cease': Disease in the History of Black Africa*, London, John Murray, 1983, p. 71; Gann and Duignan, op cit. (n. 1), p. 173; Daniel R. Headrick, *The Tools of Empire: Technology and European Imperialism in the Nineteenth Century*, New York, Oxford University Press, 1981, ch. 3.

22   Curtin, op. cit. (n. 6), pp. 136–40; J. A. Sinton, *What Malaria Costs India*, Delhi, Government of India [n.d.]; Michael Gelfand, *Lakeside Pioneers: Socio-medical Study of Nyasaland (1875–1920)*, Oxford, Blackwell, 1964, pp. 11–14; William B. Cohen, 'Malaria and French imperialism', *Journal of African History*, 1983, 24: 23–36.

23   *Indian Medical Gazette*, 1891, 34: 134.

24   D. Schoute, *Occidental therapeutics in the Netherlands East Indies during Three Centuries of Netherlands Settlement (1600–1900)*, Batavia, Netherlands Indian Public Health Service, 1937, p. iii.

25   Andrew Scott and Henry Harold Scott, *Health Problems of the Empire: Past, Present and Future*, London, Collins, 1924, p. 100.

26   David Arnold, 'Cholera and colonialism in British India', *Past and Present*, 1986, 113: 118–51; Malcolm Nicolson, 'Medicine and racial politics: changing images of the New Zealand Maori in the nineteenth century', in Arnold, op. cit. (n. 13), pp. 66–104.

27   Guenter B. Risse, 'Medicine in New Spain', in Ronald L. Numbers (ed.), *Medicine in the New World: New Spain, New France and New England*, Knoxville, University of Tennesse Press, 1987, pp. 37–42; for Spanish America, see also Suzanne Austin Alchon, *Native Society and Disease in Colonial Ecuador*, Cambridge, Cambridge University Press, 1991.

28   Margaret I. Balfour and Ruth Young, *The Work of Medical Women in India*, London, Oxford University Press, 1929, ch. 5.

29   J. F. Ade Ajayi, *Christian Missions in Nigeria, 1841–1891: the Making of a New Elite*, London, Longman, 1965, pp. 159–61; Beck, op. cit. (n. 13), pp. 14–20; Gelfand, op. cit. (n. 22).

30   Gallagher, op. cit. (n. 3), p. 39; Norman Etherington, 'Missionary doctors and African healers in mid-Victorian South Africa', *South African Historical Journal*, 1987, 19: 77–91.

31   Sheridan, op. cit. (n. 5), p. 78; David Arnold, 'Smallpox and colonial medicine in nineteenth-century India', in Arnold, op. cit. (n. 13), pp. 59–60; Tola Olu Pearce, 'Political and economic changes in Nigeria and the organisation of medical care', *Social Science and Medicine*, 1980, 14: 92; Beck, op. cit. (n. 13), pp. 136–9.

32   Gordon Schendel, *Medicine in Mexico: from Aztec Herbs to Betatrons*, Austin, University of Texas Press, 1968, pp. 74–80; Shyrock, op. cit. (n. 2), pp. 48, 84.

33 For example, Whitelaw Ainslie, *Materia Indica: or Some Account of those Articles which are employed by the Hindoos, and Other Eastern Nations, in their Medicine, Arts, and Agriculture*, 2 vols, London, Longman, Rees, Orme, Brown & Green, 1826; Udoy Chand Dutt, *The Materia Medica of the Hindus, Compiled from Sanskrit Medical Works*, Calcutta, Thacker, Spink, 1877.

34 Risse, op. cit. (n. 27), pp. 43–4.

35 Eugenia W. Herbert, 'Smallpox inoculation in Africa', *Journal of African History*, 1975, 16: 539–59; John Duffy, *Epidemics in Colonial America*, Baton Rouge, Louisiana State University Press, 1953, ch. 2.

36 Arnold, op. cit. (n. 31), pp. 55–7; P. Boomgaard, 'Smallpox and vaccination on Java, 1780–1860: medical data as a source for demographic history', in van Heteren, de Knecht-van Eekelen and Poulissen, op. cit. (n. 7), p. 127.

37 Sheridan, op. cit. (n. 5), ch. 3; cf. Savitt, op. cit. (n. 11), ch. 5.

38 Charles Leslie, 'The modernization of Asian medical systems', in John J. Poggie and Robert N. Lynch (eds), *Rethinking Modernization: Anthropological Perspectives*, Westport, CT, Greenwood Press, 1974, pp. 69–108.

39 John Duffy, *The Healers: a History of American Medicine*, Urbana, University of Illinois Press, 1979, chs 2–5; Edmund H. Burrows, *A History of Medicine in South Africa up to the End of the Nineteenth Century*, Cape Town, A. A. Balkema, 1958, pp. 67–8; Numbers, op. cit. (n. 27), *passim*.

40 Francisco Guerra, 'Medical colonization of the New World', *Medical History*, 1963, 7: 147–54; Neil Cantlie, *A History of the Army Medical Department*, Edinburgh, Churchill & Livingstone, 1974, Vol. II, pp. 220–4 for Martin and Parkes.

41 Michael Worboys, 'Manson, Ross and colonial medical policy: tropical medicine in London and Liverpool, 1899–1914', in MacLeod and Lewis, op. cit. (n. 8), pp. 21–37; Wolfgang U. Eckart, 'Medicine and German colonial expansion in the Pacific: the Caroline, Mariana, and Marshall Islands', in MacLeod and Lewis, op. cit. (n. 8), pp. 80–102; Anne Marcovich, 'French colonial medicine and colonial rule: Algeria and Indochina', in MacLeod and Lewis, op. cit. (n. 8), pp. 103–17.

FURTHER READING

Arnold, David (ed.), *Imperial Medicine and Indigenous Societies*, Manchester, Manchester University Press, 1988.

Curtin, Philip D., *Death by Migration: Europe's Encounter with the Tropical World in the Nineteenth Century*, Cambridge, Cambridge University Press, 1989.

Denoon, Donald, *Public Health in Papua New Guinea: Medical Possibility and Social Constraint, 1884–1984*, Cambridge, Cambridge University Press, 1989.

Gallagher, Nancy Elizabeth, *Medicine and Power in Tunisia, 1780–1900*, Cambridge, Cambridge University Press, 1983.

Hartwig, Gerald W. and Patterson, K. David (eds), *Disease in African History: an Introductory Survey and Case Studies*, Durham, NC, Duke University Press, 1978.

MacLeod, Roy and Lewis, Milton (eds), *Disease, Medicine, and Empire: Medicine and the Experience of European Expansion*, London, Routledge, 1988.

Numbers, Ronald L. (ed.), *Medicine in the New World: New Spain, New France, and New England*, Knoxville, University of Tennessee Press, 1987.

Owen, Norman G., *Death and Disease in Southeast Asia: Explorations in Social, Medical and Demographic History*, Singapore, Oxford University Press, 1987.

Sabben-Clare, E. E., Bradley, D. J. and Kirkwood, K. (eds), *Health in Tropical Africa during the Colonial Period*, Oxford, Clarendon Press, 1980.

INTERNATIONALISM IN MEDICINE AND PUBLIC HEALTH

Milton I. Roemer

As communications and trade have increased among nations in all parts of the world, people have come to recognize the interdependence of each country's health on the disease problems of all other countries. In its broadest sense, international health work concerns the many resultant health activities carried out across national boundaries.

COLONIALISM, RELIGIOUS MISSIONS, AND PHILANTHROPY

The beginnings of internationalism in medicine or cross-national health work must be traced to colonial expansion in Asia and Africa. In the sixteenth century, the Portuguese established settlements in China, India, and the Malay Peninsula in South-East Asia. Later, the Dutch and then the British became the principal European colonists in both Asia and Africa. Great Britain was the dominant imperial power in the eighteenth and nineteenth centuries. As colonial governments grew stronger and their military and civilian personnel increased, small garrison hospitals or medical stations were established for their care. Sometimes, special wards would be set up for the indigenous population. (➤ Ch. 58 Medicine and colonialism)

A customary course of events was illustrated by the British colonization of East Africa around 1890. The initial settlement was by the Imperial British East Africa Company, which soon engaged British doctors to take care of its employees. In 1894, the British Foreign Office took control of this work, including the medical services. A few years later, these services became a medical department in the British protectorate of Kenya and Uganda, but its resources were very small. In an account of policies in East Africa in 1895–1912, the medical services were considered necessary only to protect Europeans against tropical health hazards. Some attention was also given to workers imported from British India, but the health of native Africans was not considered a British responsibility. Colonial government medical services for the control of tropical diseases and for general medical care were generally not extended to the African population until after the First World War. (➤ Ch. 24 Tropical diseases)

The strategy of colonial health services was to provide support for the general objectives of colonial agriculture. The greatest emphasis was placed on growth and export of cash crops, through transfer of male workers to areas of commercialized agriculture, with consequent reduction of traditional food crops at home. The policy led to extensive malnutrition, even while the income from foreign trade increased. This was evident under the German, and later the British, colonial policies in what is now Tanzania.

Recent historical research on European imperialism, however, has recognized a complex mixture of motives and strategies in the role of Western medicine in Asian and African colonies. In the early nineteenth century, the health protection of European military personnel and civilian settlers was the main objective. Colonial medical services were largely confined to the main cities, where Europeans were concentrated. When quinine was used by Europeans in an African expedition of 1854, it was described as 'the prime factor in allowing the white man's conquest of Black Africa'. After the 1880s and the great breakthroughs in bacteriology, the discipline of 'tropical medicine' took shape, but its principal objective was to make tropical environments more congenial to European colonists. (➤ Ch. 15 Environment and miasmata; Ch. 18 The ecology of disease)

In the late nineteenth and early twentieth centuries, the rationale of colonial medical services gradually changed. It was increasingly appreciated that the health of soldiers and other Europeans depended largely on the health of native populations around them. As early as 1865, a British official in the Bengal region of India wrote:

> Even if we look no further than the protection of the health of the European soldiers, it will be evidently insufficient if we endeavor to improve the condition of our cantonments alone, and ignore the existence of the masses of the native population by which our troops are surrounded.

The Indian Medical Service, nevertheless, though started by the British in 1714, did not really begin to serve the Indian people until the twentieth century. In Africa, a Colonial Medical Service for the British colonies was started only in 1927.

In mining and agriculture, disease among indigenous workers was increasingly seen as an impediment to production. It was an obstacle, in later terminology, to economic development. Reduced output of commodities likewise meant lesser tax-collections. Also, as the political consciousness of native populations rose, health services were recognized as useful in displaying benevolent and paternalistic intentions by the foreign masters. For all these reasons, by the First World War and even before the 'national liberations' after the Second World War, colonial health services had acquired a much broader meaning: that is, to apply scientific medicine as well as public-health strategies to the needs of general colonial populations.

Medical services by religious missions were entirely separate from the colonial government, and these might help the Africans. A seventy-bed hospital was built in 1897, for example, by the Church Missionary Society in Uganda, principally to serve native Africans. The colonial government administration looked upon these mission services as a useful supplementation to the official programme. (➤ Ch. 61 Religion and medicine)

In the nineteenth and early twentieth centuries, missions came from Europe and North America to spread the doctrines of Christianity. As vehicles for their evangelism associated with humanitarianism, they developed hospitals or clinics in many small towns and villages. These facilities often provided the first contact of rural people with Western medicine. In several Latin American countries, hospitals, founded by religious groups (mostly Catholic) from Spain and Portugal, became the most numerous facilities. In the later twentieth century, most of these 'beneficencia' hospitals were subsidized and then taken over by governments.

In 1799, John Vanderkemp (1748–1811) had been the first medical missionary in Africa. He was a Dutch physician, whose work was sponsored by the London Missionary Society. Later in the mid-nineteenth century, a Scottish physician, David Livingstone (1813–73), served as a medical missionary in the area of South Africa that is now Botswana, and after 1850, he became a general explorer in Central Africa. In the late nineteenth and early twentieth centuries, Albert Schweitzer (1875–1965) established the hospital at Lambaréné in French Equatorial Africa, eventually attracting worldwide attention.

Missionary work by physicians started in China at Canton around 1840. These evangelical physicians brought to imperial, and later republican China, its first acquaintance with Western medical education. They introduced concepts of bacteriology and organ pathology, and demonstrated the role of nurses in caring for patients in hospitals. Several Western-type medical schools were founded, leading to the Peking Union Medical College, started with support from the Rockefeller Foundation in 1914. After 1949 under the Communist government, Western religious missions were terminated in

China, but the Peking College was continued as a high-level medical school. (➤ Ch. 32 Chinese medicine)

International health work was carried out in many countries by the Rockefeller Foundation from the United States. The Rockefeller International Health Divison (started in 1913) promoted health activities in Latin America and Asia involving:

1 basic health research;
2 training of health personnel through supporting graduate education; and
3 setting up of demonstrations of model health programmes.

Among its more notable achievements, the Rockefeller Foundation developed an effective yellow fever vaccine, mounted a campaign against the mosquito, and trained health personnel to carry out this preventive work.

Specific enterprises for mining, agriculture, or other forms of production often established medical units for the care of their employees and their families. In the nineteenth and early twentieth centuries, some colonial governments required business enterprises with more than a certain number of workers to establish medical-care units. This was the policy in India, Egypt, and Nigeria, for example. After national independence was gained, such requirements usually became more rigorous.

Aside from direct colonial domination, overt military hostilities promoted by foreign governments have seriously impaired health services in certain newly independent countries. This has been evident recently in the support of counter-revolutionary *contras* by the United States to erode the health gains of the Sandinista government of Nicaragua in the 1980s. It is seen also in the insurrections supported by the Government of South Africa against the FRELIMO (Mozambique Liberation Front) independence movement that gained control over Mozambique in 1975.

On a non-religious and non-governmental basis, another sort of international health work was done by heroic figures such as Norman Bethune (1890–1939) of Canada. In support of the republican (loyalist) cause in Spain, he performed surgery behind the battle lines in 1936, and then went to China in 1938 to work with the Red Army before its final victory in 1949. There can be little doubt that inspiration from religion or political conviction or a spirit of international goodwill has figured prominently in the extension of international health work.

INTERNATIONAL SANITARY CONFERENCES

The first truly international collaborative work, involving twelve European countries (including Turkey), was a meeting in Paris in 1851. It was designated as an International Sanitary Conference. Although it lasted from July

1851 to January 1852, the discussion of different policies on quarantine regulations at national borders failed to lead to any agreement. There were unresolved disputes among the delegates about the contagiousness of plague, yellow fever, and cholera: whether these dreadful scourges were communicated from the sick to the well or whether they were due to certain atmospheric, climatic, and soil conditions creating an 'epidemic constitution'. A majority of the delegates voted that cholera should be subject to quarantine regulations, but none of the participating governments acted to ratify such regulations. The only accomplishment of this six-month meeting was the basic experience of several countries in meeting together to discuss an international health problem.

After eight years, a second International Sanitary Conference was held in Paris in 1859. In the interim, an Italian microscopist, Filippo Pacini (1812–83), described clearly the cholera vibrio as the pathogenic agent of the disease, a discovery overlooked for thirty years until it was reaffirmed by Robert Koch (1843–1910). Also in 1854, John Snow (1813–58) demonstrated the contagiousness of cholera through ingestion of faecally contaminated water in London from the River Thames. After five months, the second conference adjourned with no resolution of the dispute between the contagionists and the miasmatists, and no subsequent ratification of the draft convention on quarantine of cholera by any country. (➤ Ch. 16 Contagion/germ theory/specificity)

The third International Sanitary Conference was held in Constantinople in 1866, followed by a fourth conference in Vienna in 1874. Still no effective agreements could be reached, despite a fifth conference in Washington in 1881 and a sixth in Rome in 1885. It was only at the seventh International Sanitary Conference, held in Venice in 1892, that agreement was finally reached. It had taken forty-one years of discussion to reach consensus of very limited scope on quarantine of west-bound ships with cases of cholera on board. This historic convention also provided that the Pan-Arab Quarantine Board of Health in Egypt should prepare compatible provisions regarding plague and yellow fever, although their aetiology and epidemiology were still quite unknown. (➤ Ch. 52 Epidemiology)

An eighth conference was held at Dresden in 1893, followed by a ninth at Paris in 1894. At the tenth conference, held in Venice in 1897, agreement was reached on a second international convention on plague (whose spread by rat fleas was not to be discovered until some years later). This conference of twenty-one nations also decided that an international committee should be constituted to codify the sanitary conventions and conclusions of the conferences of 1892, 1893, 1894, and 1897.

International Sanitary Conferences continued to be held periodically until the fourteenth in 1938, which brought to an end the international work of the Health, Maritime, and Quarantine Board. This had been functioning in Alexandria (although largely under the control of the Egyptian Ministry of Health) since 1881. Later, the structure that housed it became the site of the Eastern Mediterranean Regional Office of the World Health Organization (WHO). Another border quarantine agency, founded in 1838 at Constantinople (now Istanbul), with field offices throughout the Ottoman Empire, was completely terminated by the League of Nations (see pp. 1424–25) in 1923.

In 1902, as a sequel to these international quarantine efforts, the republics of Latin America, along with the United States, established the Pan-American Sanitary Bureau (PASB), with offices in Washington, DC. The strong voice of the United States in this body was reflected in its first several directors, each of whom was a recently retired Surgeon-General of the US Public Health Service. Other leading US figures succeeded to this post until 1958, when the first Latin American health leader was chosen: Dr Abraham Horwitz (b. 1910) of Chile. Since then, several notable Latin American figures have served in this role, while a US physician has always occupied a second place as Deputy-Director. In 1949, the PASB became the Regional Office for the Americas of the WHO.

Aside from this long series of international conferences to halt the spread of infectious diseases, the nineteenth century spawned international congresses on other medical and related subjects. In 1867, the first general medical congress, with representatives from many nations, was held in Paris; it was followed every two years by similar meetings in Florence, Vienna, and other European cities (except for 1887, when it was held in Washington) until 1913 (in London). International congresses on specialized health-related subjects had, in fact, been held earlier in Brussels: on statistics in 1851, demography and hygiene in 1852, and ophthalmology in 1857. Other international meetings took place in various European cities: on veterinary medicine (1863), pharmacy (1865), tuberculosis (1888), dermatology (1889), psychology (1890), gynaecology and obstetrics (1892), alcoholism (1894), leprosy (1897), dentistry (1900), surgery (1902), school hygiene (1904), physiotherapy (1905), cancer (1906), sleeping sickness (1907), epilepsy (1909), comparative pathology (1912), and the history of medicine (1920). These are only a sampling of the subjects of such international meetings, most of which were based on topics of interest to the newly emerging medical specialists.

THE RED CROSS AND GENEVA CONVENTIONS

Almost parallel with the International Sanitary Conferences and their development was another international initiative launched by private individuals. This was the Red Cross, founded by five leading citizens of Geneva in 1863. A Swiss philanthropist, J. Henri Dunant (1828–1910), had witnessed the bloody battle of Solferino (northern Italy) in 1859, and he formed the International Committee of the Red Cross, devoted to helping the wounded soldiers of any country. The impartial humanitarian spirit of the Comité International de Croix Rouge (CICR) was closely linked to traditional Swiss neutrality in international affairs; all members and employees of the CICR, therefore, had to be Swiss citizens. (➤ Ch. 63 Medical philanthropy after 1850)

Very soon, several European nations formed their own national Red Cross societies, and they met in Geneva in 1864. This First Geneva Convention agreed that 'sick and wounded soldiers will be collected and cared for *irrespective of nationality*'. This remarkable impartiality was confirmed and extended at subsequent Geneva Conventions held in 1906 and 1929. The Third Convention (1929) extended the Red Cross purposes to include help for prisoners of war and also for civilian victims of hostilities. (➤ Ch. 66 War and modern medicine)

The several national Red Cross (and later, in Muslim countries, the Red Crescent) societies grew and developed during periods of peace after wars. In peacetime, they devoted their voluntary efforts to helping their own citizens in the event of various natural disasters, such as floods, hurricanes, earthquakes, and fires; they also helped to care for people injured in civil wars or other types of mass violence.

By the end of the First World War, the national Red Cross societies, while still non-governmental, had attained sufficient stability and recognition to be noted in the Covenant of the League of Nations (Article 25) in 1918. Then in 1919, under the leadership of the American Red Cross, there was formed, for the first time, an international League of Red Cross Societies. Initially, there were member-societies from twenty-six countries; this grew to 113 countries in 1970, and to 164 in 1987. The League of Red Cross Societies headquarters is located in Geneva, but it is separate from the CICR, though obviously in close working relationship. The CICR is financed mainly by voluntary donations from the national societies.

The national members of the League meet every two years in Geneva, as a Board of Governors, with one vote per member (regardless of national population). In the Geneva secretariat, there are several sections, the most important of which are the Relief Bureau and the Health and Social Service Bureau. The latter has activities relating to:

1 first-aid and accident prevention;
2 blood transfusion services;
3 standardization of medical equipment; and
4 medical information and documentation.

The League of Red Cross Societies as a whole is devoted to: 1 assisting national societies in their development of programmes; and 2 co-ordinating collaborative international efforts of national societies. The League also maintains relationships with the WHO and the United Nations International Children's Emergency Fund (UNICEF), described on p. 1426.

OIHP AND THE LEAGUE OF NATIONS

Another milestone in international health was reached in 1907, when an agreement was reached in Rome among twenty-three European countries on the establishment of a permanent public-health office in Europe. This was the Office International d'Hygiène Publique (OIHP), to be located in Paris. Its functions concerned the collection and dissemination of new knowledge on infectious diseases that should be embodied in international quarantine regulations. The principal focus initially was on cholera, plague, and yellow fever, three diseases that had occupied the attention of the International Sanitary Conferences. Eventually, OIHP membership extended to nearly sixty countries, including Persia, India, Pakistan, and the United States. French was the only official language.

Soon the concerns of OIHP were broadened to other communicable diseases, such as malaria, tuberculosis, typhoid fever, meningitis, sleeping sickness, and the overall suppression of insect vectors. Interest was shown also in other public-health subjects, such as food hygiene, the management of hospitals, and the hygiene of schools and factories. Although OIHP did not do any fieldwork on these matters, it provided an international forum for their discussion among public-health leaders of different nations. With the outbreak of the First World War in 1914, all OIHP operations were suspended, except the publication of its *Bulletin*. Recommendations had been made to governments on environmental sanitation, notification of cases of tuberculosis, inoculation against typhoid fever, and isolation of cases of leprosy. The dissemination and discussion of such ideas had some value, in spite of no national action being taken for their implementation. (➤ Ch. 51 Public health)

After the First World War, a worldwide desire for peace resulted in the organization of the League of Nations. To carry out its activities relating to the 'prevention and control of disease', a subdivision was established, known as the Health Organization of the League of Nations. The United States was not a member of the League, and vetoed a proposal to move the Paris-based OIHP, of which it was a member, into the League. Therefore in 1921, there were three international agencies with very similar functions: the OIHP, the Pan-American Sanitary Bureau, and the League's Health Organization. Co-operative agreements among these were obviously necessary.

In 1919, typhus fever epidemics spread through Russia and Poland. Some 1.6 million cases were reported in Russia; in addition, the unprecedented world pandemic of influenza arose, estimated to have caused as many as 15 million deaths by 1920. In this catastrophic situation, an International Health Conference met in London, but it was attended by only five countries: Great Britain, France, Italy, Japan, and the United States. Eventually, the Health Organization of the League of Nations became a Health Committee of the League, and of its eight members, four served also as members of the Permanent Committee of the OIHP.

In spite of the diplomatic complexities of these relationships between the League's Health Committee and OIHP, several new international health activities were initiated by the League. Broadly speaking, these fell into two general categories: international health studies, expert committees on selected subjects, and proposed international standards on certain issues; and field assistance to countries with special health problems.

With modest funding, most League health activities fell into the first category. Studies were made and expert committees appointed on major diseases (malaria, syphilis, tuberculosis, leprosy, etc.), on aspects of health care (school health service, health centres, medical-care administration, health insurance, medical education, etc.), and on other matters. International classification of the 'Causes of Death and Disease', the standardization of biological substances and potent drugs, and the methods of control of narcotics were solid achievements. Especially important studies were made and conferences were held on nutrition, the health aspects of housing, physical education, and the general provision of public-health services in rural areas. As part of its epidemiological intelligence work, in 1925 the League Health Organization set up a field office in Singapore, to collect and disseminate reports on infectious diseases in the Far East.

The second main type of League health activities, field assistance to countries, was limited by insufficient funding. In 1928, Greece was assisted in reorganizing its public-health services, followed by a similar service to Bolivia. In 1929, China was helped to develop its public-health service, particularly for epidemic control. Smaller missions were sent to a few other countries, and study-tours were made by health administrative officials from many countries to observe public-health practices in selected European nations.

THE SECOND WORLD WAR

With the invasion of Poland by Nazi Germany in 1939, the League of Nations soon collapsed and, with it, the League's Health Committee. This gave a clear lesson to the group of public-health leaders, who later set out to establish a 'World Health Organization' (WHO). The fate of WHO should not depend on the survival of its parent body, the United Nations (UN). An Interim Commission was organized at an International Health Conference, held in New York in 1946. The WHO Constitution drawn up by the Commission was ratified and took effect on 7 April 1948, with the signatures of twenty-six member-states of the UN (but independent of the UN). By 24 June 1948, when the first World Health Assembly, held in Geneva, adjourned, the WHO Constitution had fifty-five national signatories.

In December 1946, the UN General Assembly established UNICEF, to be supported by the voluntary contributions of governments. The Interim Commission to plan a 'World Health Organization' had just been formed, and the directors of UNICEF did not wish to encroach on its jurisdiction. From the outset, therefore, UNICEF worked in close co-operation with WHO, using its own money essentially for the provision of supplies (food and drugs) and equipment. UNICEF is governed by the Executive Board of members from twenty-five countries, and comes under the general supervision of the UN Economic and Social Council. Although 'emergency' was soon deleted from the title of UNICEF, it was retained in the acronym, and the agency's robust performance has kept it alive to the present time.

In the years of the Second World War, other international organizations, with substantial health functions, were launched. To provide general relief, including health services, to the war-torn countries of Europe as well as to China, forty-three nations formed the UN Relief and Rehabilitation Administration (UNRRA) in 1943. This was an intentionally temporary agency, in which representatives from the United States played a major role. The Health Division of UNRRA was transferred to WHO by a vote of its Council in 1946.

Another specialized agency of the United Nations, intended also to be temporary, was the International Refugee Organization (IRO), established in 1948. The former Director of the displaced persons programme in the Health Division of UNRRA was taken on the IRO executive staff, based in Geneva. In January 1949, the UN Assembly terminated the IRO, but continued its important work through the UN High Commissioner for Refugees (UNHCR). UNHCR had a relatively small staff, and did no international health work directly, but looked to WHO for technical advice. Health services to refugees were left in the hands of the host countries. UNHCR still operates, with headquarters in Geneva, and works closely with WHO.

After the Second World War, a new type of international work was developed through the initiative of the United States and several European countries: namely, foreign aid from industrialized countries to developing countries on a one-to-one basis. These 'bilateral assistance programmes' were designed to assist in many fields, including health services. By 1980, expenditures by most industrialized countries (principally the seventeen member-states of the Organization for Economic Co-operation and Development – OECD) were larger through bilateral than through multilateral programmes.

Out of a total of about US$30 billion for all types of foreign aid in general, about $3 billion or 10 per cent was earmarked for health projects. Of this amount, about one-third was spent through WHO and other UN-affiliated agencies and two-thirds through bilateral aid programmes. The United States, for example, provided development assistance to eighty-eight countries in 1980, of which health assistance applied to sixty countries. In the first post-war decades, most bilateral US expenditures were focused on population control through family planning, but in the latter 1970s and the 1980s, US policy shifted toward the support of the WHO strategy of emphasizing primary health care.

THE WORLD HEALTH ORGANIZATION AND ITS WORK

In 1948, after its first World Health Assembly, the WHO took action to form a Secretariat in Geneva. It was given space for its initial years in the Palais des Nations, which had been the last home of the League of Nations. As stated in Chapter I of its Constitution, WHO was 'to act as the directing and coordinating authority on international health work'. This was a much broader scope than any other international agency in the orbit of the UN.

WHO's structure and functions expanded rapidly. Its programme initially included activities acquired from the International Sanitary Conferences, the OIHP, the Health Committee of the League of Nations, and the Health Division of UNRRA, plus many new projects affecting the overall development of national health systems.

Soon after the establishment of WHO headquarters in Geneva, steps were taken to set up regional offices. The first was the South-East Asia Regional Office, located in New Delhi, India, in January 1949. In July 1949, a second office for the Eastern Mediterranean Region was set up in Alexandria, at the seat of the original Pan-Arab Health, Maritime, and Quarantine Board.

In the same month, July 1949, negotiations with the Pan-American Sanitary Bureau in Washington resulted in its integration with WHO as the Regional Office for the Americas. In 1951, two more Regional Offices were established: for the Western Pacific Region, based in Manila, Philippines; and the African Region, based in Brazzaville, French Equatorial Africa (later the Republic of Congo). The last Regional Office, to be formed by the vote of a majority by its member states, was for Europe; located temporarily in Geneva in 1952, it was moved to its final location in Copenhagen in 1957. The WHO Constitution provides for election of the Regional Office directors by a majority of the countries in each region.

Within WHO, the highest authority is the World Health Assembly, convened once each year for about three weeks in May. The Assembly includes representatives of all member-states – some 166 countries in 1990 – with one vote each, regardless of size or financial contribution. Large countries, nevertheless, naturally have substantial influence. The Regional Boards in each of the six regions have a great deal of autonomy, since they are chosen by the constituent countries and they elect the Regional Director. In reality, the regions tend to follow policy decisions of the global headquarters, but they are free to implement these in their own way.

Between assemblies, there are two meetings per year of an Executive Board, composed of twelve to eighteen persons 'technically qualified in the field of health', but not representing their own countries. The Executive Board prepares the agenda for the World Health Assembly, and makes recommendations to it on all matters of world health policy.

For advice on almost every technical question considered by WHO, the headquarters Secretariat appoints Expert Panels, and from these are selected Expert Committees that recommend policies. In 1990, there were expert panels on forty-seven subjects – for example, malaria, maternal and child health, pharmaceuticals, environmental health, medical-care organization, health-personnel development, etc. – containing 2,600 persons from virtually all countries. The experts chosen for committees are intended to represent all countries concerned with the special problem under discussion.

In its first decade, WHO focused major attention on specific infectious diseases afflicting millions of people in the developing countries. These included malaria, yaws, tuberculosis, and venereal diseases. There was also a high priority for maternal and child health services, for environmental sanitation (especially safe water), and for standardization of drugs and vaccines. In these years, WHO developed close working relationships with other UN agencies.

The second WHO decade (1958–68) was much influenced by the national liberation in Africa of several former colonies, which became voting members of the Organization. In 1960, the departure from the newly independent Democratic Republic of the Congo of nearly all foreign doctors created a massive emergency. Working with the international Red Cross, WHO recruited 200 physicians and other health workers, and established a new fellowship programme to enable scores of Congolese 'medical assistants' to become fully qualified doctors. In this period, fellowships for health-personnel development became a major WHO strategy in almost all countries.

WHO stimulated and even collaborated with the world chemical industry in the 1960s to develop new insecticides for fighting the vectors of onchocerciasis ('river blindness') and for treating schistosomiasis. Demonstration that tuberculosis could be effectively treated, without expensive sanatorium care, was a great breakthrough of the late 1950s. Even the mundane standardization of the nomenclature of diseases and causes of death was an important contribution to international health communications.

The third WHO decade (1968–78) included the great victory of eradicating smallpox from the earth. In 1967, smallpox was still endemic in thirty-one countries, afflicting between 10 and 15 million people. The work was done by teams of public-health workers in all the countries affected, with WHO serving as leader, co-ordinator, and inspiration. Millions of dollars were saved worldwide by this achievement, which overcame various national rivalries and suspicions.

The momentum of this great campaign added strength to another drive, for expanding the immunization of the world's children against six once-ravaging diseases: diphtheria, tetanus, whooping cough, measles, poliomyelitis, and tuberculosis (with BCG vaccine). After long hesitation for political reasons, in this period WHO finally entered the field of family planning by promoting worldwide research and development on human reproduction. New efforts were also put into the control of malaria and leprosy. WHO also promoted the training of auxiliary health personnel, such as China's 'barefoot doctors' and India's traditional birth-attendants. Such training was a sounder investment in most developing countries than preparing physicians for predominantly urban medical practice.

The fourth decade (1978–88) was ushered in by a great world conference of WHO and UNICEF in Alma Ata, a city of the Asiatic part of the Soviet Union. Thirty years after its birth, 134 WHO member-states reaffirmed their commitment to equality, as embodied in the slogan 'Health for All'. In reaction against excessive attention to high-technology, the Alma Ata conference emphasized the great importance of primary health care, preventive and curative, as the best approach to national health policy. This approach, stressing community participation, appropriate technology, and intersectoral collaboration, became the central pillar of world health policy (see pp. 1430–1).

In this period, every country was encouraged to develop a list of 'essential drugs' for use in all public facilities, instead of the thousands of brand-name products sold in world markets. WHO's condemnation of the promotion of artificial infant-formula products in developing countries also attracted widespread attention. The worldwide control of infantile diarrhoea with oral rehydration therapy was another great advance, based on very simple principles.

Most of the estimated 500,000 maternal deaths each year are preventable through family planning – to avoid illegal abortions – and hygienic education of traditional birth-attendants. WHO has also mounted increasing efforts against cancer, which now takes as many lives in the developing countries as in the affluent ones. The fight against tobacco, the largest single cause of preventable death in both men and women, is part of WHO effort in every country. Disseminating the simple rules of diet, exercise, non-smoking, prudent use of alcohol, and hygienic working conditions are major objectives of health education in WHO everywhere. The worldwide epidemic of AIDS (acquired immune deficiency syndrome) has presented another challenge to WHO in mounting global efforts to stem the spread of this lethal sexually transmitted virus disease. (➤ Ch. 26 Sexually transmitted diseases) Underlying all these efforts is WHO's constant advisory activity to strengthen the official public-health organizations for health protection in all countries.

Interpreting the strategies of WHO during its first four decades reveals a broad trend from the specific to the general. In its early years, the objectives were defined by specific diseases and conventional categories – such as maternal and child health services and environmental sanitation – within the established domain of public health. The crisis in the Congo led to a broader approach there, but the principal efforts went to the eradication of smallpox and the expanded programme of immunization. In the first two decades, WHO was young, perhaps fragile, and dominated by a few Western industrialized countries. It was only in the third decade that it felt stable enough to explore the sensitive field of family planning, and even this was only to promote research in human reproduction.

In the fourth decade, WHO embraced a far-reaching objective of promoting worldwide equity for health. 'Health for all by the year 2000' was a slogan with the broadest possible political implications. The pathway to this goal was through 'primary health care', which included all principal strategies of prevention, as well as appropriate treatment of common diseases and injuries. The implications of this approach were not concealed, but called frankly for community participation and political commitment. No longer did WHO confine its interest to purely technical matters, but addressed openly the countless issues surrounding the organization of national health systems in every country.

After 1978, the great majority of WHO member-states were young developing countries. No longer were policies dictated by a handful of Western powers. The UN was firmly established and, even in the Security Council, veto power rested with the Soviet Union and the People's Republic of China, as well as with the US and the UK. Among the several UN specialist agencies, WHO was probably the most universally respected. Its performance had won plaudits from countries of every political persuasion. Its Director-General was an unhesitant idealist, born in a small country (Denmark) from a missionary family. The Regional Committees had become additional sources of political expression, and five out of the six were dominated by developing countries. To these countries, dramatic national health problems were more important than the ideologies of European or American medical associations.

Co-operation of WHO with other specialized agencies of the UN has been effective in avoiding jurisdictional disputes. Collaboration with the International Labour Office (also located in Geneva) has concerned activities in occupational health and in the health aspects of social-security programmes. Regarding nutrition and the control of animal diseases (zoonoses), there is substantial co-operation with the Food and Agriculture Organization, based in Rome. School health programmes and the health education of teachers involve reciprocal relations with the UN Educational, Scientific, and Cultural Organization (UNESCO), based in Paris. Collaborative arrangements were even made with the International Civil Aviation Organization on the disinfection of aircraft landing across national borders.

Official relationships were also established between WHO and various international non-governmental organizations (NGOs). Important among these is the International Committee of the Red Cross and the League of Red Cross Societies, but there are hundreds of others in special fields. Under the sponsorship of WHO and UNESCO, an overall NGO was established for maintaining relationships with various scientific bodies. It is known as the Council for International Organizations of the Medical Sciences (CIOMS), and its headquarters are in the WHO building in Geneva. The sixty-two international members of the CIOMS are reviewed every two years by WHO officials. Members of CIOMS include such NGOs as the World Federation for Mental Health, the International Planned Parenthood Federation, the World Medical Association, and the International Council of Nurses.

ALMA ATA AND PRIMARY HEALTH CARE

The International Conference on Primary Health Care, held in Alma Ata, has been noted (see p. 1429). Out of this conference there was issued the Declaration of Alma Ata, which states, among other things, that:

> A main social target of governments, international organizations and the whole world community in the coming decades should be the attainment by all peoples of the world by the year 2000 of a level of health that will permit them to lead a socially and economically productive life.

This 'primary health care' approach called for attention to major health promotive, preventive, and elementary-treatment aspects of common disorders. Several overall strategies were emphasized, such as appropriate technology, community participation, and co-ordination of health work with other social sectors (education, agriculture, housing, etc.) or intersectoral collaboration. The governments of nearly all countries soon affirmed their support of this primary health care approach in their national health systems.

The Alma Ata Declaration reaffirmed the high priority that countries should give to at least eight well-established programmes of health promotion and protection. These were:

1 education on prevailing health problems and the methods of preventing and controlling them;
2 promotion of an adequate food supply and proper nutrition;
3 an adequate supply of safe water and basic sanitation (waste-disposal);
4 maternal and child health care, including family planning;
5 immunization against the major infectious diseases;
6 prevention and control of locally endemic diseases;
7 appropriate treatment of common diseases and injuries;
8 provision of essential drugs.

As these elements were discussed, an even broader range of health activities was encompassed. As back-up for primary health care, there had to be small general hospitals at the 'first referral level'. Community health workers, with training of only a few months, had to be prepared in large numbers for work in rural districts. In district hospitals or health centres for ambulatory care, appropriate simple laboratory and even X-ray equipment should be available. Mental health problems should be identified by community health workers, if only for appropriate referral to other resources.

GENERAL PRINCIPLES OF INTERNATIONAL HEALTH WORK

By the latter 1980s, several basic principles for international health work had become widely accepted by WHO and other agencies in the UN family. Abiding by these principles helps to explain the high respect accorded to WHO and UNICEF throughout the world, especially in the developing countries:

1 international health work in any country is done only at the invitation of the country. Multi-national agencies are established by member-states and have no supra-national authority;
2 all international civil servants must be devoted only to the agency in which they work, and not to their country of origin;
3 an international health agency must respond to requests for help, without regard to the political ideology of the government in power. It must not pass judgement on the ethical values of that government (an exception to this policy has been applied to South Africa, because of its extremely unjust racial policies embodied in apartheid);
4 the development of national health systems has become generally recognized as contributing to overall social and economic development. Healthy

people are able to contribute more effectively to national productivity than people handicapped by disease and disability;

5 the health of a population is influenced by all social sectors, not only by the health services. Health objectives, therefore, demand the greatest possible emphasis on intersectoral collaboration;

6 in determining priorities among the countless health problems observed in all countries, the highest priority should be assigned to problems affecting the largest number of people. This criterion calls for lesser emphasis on high-technology tertiary hospitals and greater emphasis on primary health care in all countries;

7 international health policies should promote national health systems that assure the most equitable distribution of health services – preventive and curative – to all people;

8 while motivated initially by the objective of stopping the spread of communicable diseases, international health work has become increasingly concerned with all aspects of health and health services worldwide. The promotion of world health is recognized as being dependent on the prudent use of all types of health resources, the control of all types of disease and disability, and the provision of adequate economic support.

The heightened appreciation of international health work is matched by a greater recognition of the value of health services in virtually all countries. In the early decades of the twentieth century, health and medical activities, as reflected in national expenditures, absorbed only 1 to 5 per cent of national wealth (measured by GNP). The fraction was greater in the more-industrialized countries and less in the less-developed countries, where so much had to be spent on food and shelter. As the potentialities of the health sciences expanded after the Second World War, the share of GNP devoted to health systems increased almost everywhere, to a level of 6 to 11 per cent in the affluent countries and a level of 2 to 5 per cent in the developing countries. (➤ Ch. 57 Health economics)

These higher expenditures were both a cause and a result of collectivized methods of financing, through general taxation and earmarked social-insurance funding. They also provoked greater political interest in cost-containment through increasing the efficiency of health systems, deliberate planning of the supply of various health resources (personnel and facilities), and controlling the demand for services through different types of cost-sharing by patients. In all but a few industrialized countries, most health expenditures came from government, and therefore served to make health services economically accessible to nearly everyone. In many, if not most, developing countries, governmental programmes were seriously inadequate, and most health expenditures came from the private sector, with great resultant inequities. (➤ Ch. 50 Medical institutions and the state)

Toward the end of the twentieth century, these inequities became a major concern of international health work – a far cry from the original narrow focus on border quarantine. The WHO, the World Bank, UNICEF, and other international agencies have become concerned about how each country organizes and operates its own national health system. The horizon of good health is continually expanding, so that national health systems must become broader and stronger to achieve their goal.

One may wonder how this mounting interest in the overall national health system of each country has affected the global role of WHO. Has this focus constituted a departure from the sense of national interdependence that generated, for example, the early conventions to halt the spread of infectious disease? Not at all. In the modern world, the claim that 'disease knows no borders' has become a cliché that no mature health leader repeats. The goal today is now to assure *within* all countries – rich or poor, large or small – the full health benefits of modern science and civilization. This is not to avert the transmission of cholera from Asia to Europe, but to enrich the lives of Asian people for their own sakes. 'One world' should mean not merely to eliminate the need for border quarantine, but to endow each country with the resources and strategies to achieve maximum health for all its people. At this stage in world history, national sovereignty is still respected. Within this reality, the goal of world health means that all the people of every country will have equal opportunity to attain 'the highest possible level of health'. (➤ Ch. 72 Medicine, mortality, and morbidity)

FURTHER READING

Aitken, J. T., Fuller, H. W. C. and Johnson, D. (eds), *The Influence of Christians in Medicine*, London, Christian Medical Fellowship, 1984.

Allan, Ted and Gordon, Sydney, *The Scalpel, the Sword: the Story of Norman Bethune*, Boston, MA, Little, Brown, 1952.

Arnold, David (ed.), *Imperial Medicine and Indigenous Societies*, Manchester, Manchester University Press, 1988.

Beck, Ann, *A History of the British Medical Administration of East Africa, 1900–1950*, Cambridge, MA, Harvard University Press, 1970.

Council for International Organization of the Medical Sciences, *Organization, Activities, Members*, Geneva, CIOMS, 1989.

Dayton, Edward R., *Medicine and Missions: a Survey of Medical Missions*, Wheaton, IL, Medical Assistance Program, 1969.

Garrison, Fielding H., *An Introduction to the History of Medicine*, 4th edn, Philadelphia, PA, W. B. Saunders, 1966, p. 789.

Goodman, Neville M., *International Health Organizations and their Work*, London, Churchill Livingstone, 1971.

Howard, Lee M., 'International sources of financial cooperation for health in developing countries', *Bulletin of the Pan-American Health Organization*, 1983, 17 (2): 142–56.

Howard-Jones, Norman, *The Scientific Background of the International Sanitary Conferences 1851–1938*, Geneva, WHO, 1975.

—— *International Public Health between the Two World Wars – the Organizational Problems*, Geneva, WHO, 1978.

——, *The Pan-American Health Organization: Origins and Evolution*, Geneva, WHO, 1981.

Hume, Edward H., *Doctors Courageous*, New York, Harper, 1950.

Kohn, R. and Radius, S., 'International comparison of health services systems: an annotated bibliography', *International Journal of Health Services*, 1973, 3 (2): 295–309.

Linsenmeyer, William S., 'Foreign nations, international organizations, and their impact on health conditions in Nicaragua since 1979', *International Journal of Health Services*, 1989, 19 (3): 509–29.

MacLeod, R. M. and Lewis, Milton, (eds), *Disease, Medicine and Empire: Perspectives on Western Medicine and the Experience of European Expansion*, London, Routledge, 1988.

Mungeam, G. H., *British Rule in Kenya 1895–1912*, Oxford, Clarendon Press, 1966.

Musgrove, Philip, 'The impact of the economic crisis on health and health care in Latin America and the Caribbean', *WHO Chronicle*, 1986, 40 (4): 152–57.

Roemer, Milton I., *The Organization of Medical Care under Social Security*, Geneva, International Labour Office, 1969.

Turshen, Meredeth, 'The impact of colonialism on health and health services in Tanzania', *International Journal of Health Services*, 1977, 7 (1): 7–35.

World Health Organization, *The First Ten Years of the World Health Organization*, Geneva, 1958.

——, *The Second Ten Years of the World Health Organization 1958–1967*, Geneva, 1968.

60

MEDICINE AND ANTHROPOLOGY

Carol MacCormack

THE NINETEENTH CENTURY

The relationship between medicine and anthropology was very close in the nineteenth century when anthropology emerged as a distinct discipline. In the nineteenth century, key literature that was self-consciously entitled 'anthropological' or 'ethnological' was published, scholarly societies were organized, and influential people took up teaching posts at Oxford, Cambridge, London, and Columbia. But the birth was not without trauma. Racialist and colonialist politics clashed, not only with humanitarian and evangelical sentiments, but with the emerging secular scientific sentiments of the time as well. Many of the most articulate actors in this drama had been trained in medicine, including comparative anatomy, moral philosophy, and even comparative linguistics, classical literature, and history. Following exploration and emerging international trade in the eighteenth century, comparative anatomy became a focus of enquiry in the natural sciences. Were savages separate species? This question was seldom a purely scientific question, as it was often linked with economic and political debates about slavery. Anthropology, or ethnology as it was more commonly designated in Europe, began to give a framework for the study of physical and cultural attributes of non-European people. Today, anthropology still encompasses comparative ethnography, archaeology and comparative history, anthropological linguistics and physical anthropological studies of human evolution and adaptation to environments.

In the nineteenth century, empirical methods began to displace 'armchair speculation' about the variability of humankind and the process by which Europeans had become 'civilized'. Other themes that emerged by the end of the century were the psychology of rational versus magical or religious thought, and comparative kinship and state organization. But the most vital question of all was fuelled by the influence of Charles Darwin (1809–82) and his followers: did humanity originate from a unitary past or from a diversity of origins? The concept of polygenesis or separate creation of races goes back at least as far as Paracelsus (1493–1541), but it was opposed initially in the nineteenth century by people with a rational and emotional commitment to Christian teaching, especially those in the evangelical revival in the Church of England, much of which revolved around William Wilberforce (1759–1833) and the anti-slavery Clapham sect, and by nonconforming Christians such as Quakers committed to the concept of 'that of God in everyone'. (➤ Ch. 61 Religion and medicine)

These concepts and emotions were illustrated in the work of James Cowles Prichard (1786–1848), a Bristol physician. His Edinburgh thesis in medicine, written in 1808, included comparative anatomy, comparative philology, and comparative history. He had been influenced by the lectures of Dugald Stewart (1753–1828) in moral philosophy, in which Stewart vigorously opposed polygenic speculations about the origin of native Americans. Prichard's parents were Quakers, committed to the doctrine of human unity, and later in life he joined the evangelical wing of the Church of England. In 1813 he wrote the first edition of *Researches into the Physical History of Mankind*,[1] in which he tried to demonstrate that all humankind shared a single physical origin and were governed by the same religious and ethical imperative. He used both biological and historical evidence to explain physical differences between populations and also worked on biological mechanisms that might explain differences. He charted the geographical distribution of racial groups, attempting to trace them all back to a single root, giving full importance to the process of migration and environmental adaptation in accounting for racial diversity. In 1819, Prichard's *An Analysis of Egyptian Mythology* was published,[2] in which he explored similarities between Christian scripture and ancient Egyptian texts. This work was then carried on by cultural 'diffusionists', notably Grafton Elliot Smith (1871–1937) and William Perry (c.1888–1949) at University College London early in the next century.[3] Prichard did not use an evolutionary framework for his historical interpretation, but focused on similarities between different races in terms of physical type, language, customs, political organization, and religion. He suggested that Adam was black, a view in direct opposition to the 'degenerationist' view of other races popular among factions of French and British natural scientists.[4]

Late in life, in 1848, Prichard finished the third and final edition of *Researches into the Physical History of Mankind*. He elaborated the concept of the 'psychic unity of man', a theme that was especially elaborated in twentieth-century American anthropology by Franz Boas (1858–1942) and his students as they explored the limits of cultural universals *vis-à-vis* cultural relativism.

It is also a theme taken up perennially in anthropology and philosophy debates about rationality, and in psychology most notably by C. G. Jung (1875–1961). Prichard summed up his writing with the visual metaphor of a tree. Tribal differences constituted the twigs, but all grew from the same root.[5]

Following Prichard's death, his point of view was further developed by Robert Gordon Latham (1812–88), who had been trained in both medicine and comparative philology. His *Natural History of the Varieties of Man* was published in 1850, and the two-volume *Descriptive Ethnology* in 1859.[6] The polygenist point of view, however, was skilfully put forward in the 1850 publication by Robert Knox (1791–1862), *The Races of Men*.[7] Knox read medicine in Edinburgh, then served as an army surgeon at Waterloo and the Cape. In South Africa, he dissected bodies of fallen Africans, then went to study comparative anatomy in Paris under Georges Cuvier (1769–1832) and Geoffroy Saint-Hilaire (1779–1853). Although originally a political radical, he became associated with a scandal about cadavers supplied by murderers, and as his career went into decline, he became a political reactionary.[8] Taking a polygenist position, he specifically attacked Prichard, setting out to demonstrate that no race could overcome the limits of its hereditary destiny. For him, race explained everything in human history, and in the 1862 edition of *The Races of Men* argued that only certain races were within the human species.[9] Knox was supported by Joseph Barnard Davis (1801–81), who worked as a surgeon on an Arctic whaler, then settled as a medical practitioner in Staffordshire about 1825. He and John Thurnam (1810–73), another physician, excavated ancient British skulls to 'prove' the diversity of human origins. John Beddoe (1826–1911) trained in medicine at University College London, then went to Edinburgh where he studied Highland Scots. His *Races of Britain* was published in 1868, an attempt to demonstrate the permanence of racial type. He wrote that black people were physically distinct and mentally inferior, and offspring of blacks and Europeans were partially infertile.[10]

The debate between mono- and polygenists reflected conflicting attitudes to the impact of nineteenth-century colonial expansion. By 1835, humanitarian sentiments were clearly affecting colonial policy, with Lord Glenelg (1778–1866) and James Stephens, both of the evangelical Clapham sect, controlling the Colonial Office. (➤ Ch. 58 Medicine and colonialism) In 1835, Thomas Fowell Buxton (1786–1845), the man who had taken over leadership of the parliamentary anti-slavery group from William Wilberforce, called for a parliamentary select committee on aborigines. When its rather damning findings were published, Thomas Hodgkin (1798–1866), a Quaker physician, organized the Aborigines Protection Society. Its first objective was to collect 'authentic information concerning the character, habits and wants of uncivilized tribes'.[11] Humanitarian and empirical motives were at one as the society sought to influence public opinion which, in turn, would ameliorate the more exploitative aspects of colonial practice. In 1839, Hodgkin travelled to Paris and, shortly afterwards, the Société Ethnologique de Paris was founded. Richard King (c.1811–76), who had been Hodgkin's pupil at Guy's Hospital, and who had been on a two-year expedition to the Arctic, organized the Ethnological Society of London, which by the end of 1843 met regularly in Hodgkin's home. Although Hodgkin continued to be active in both the Aborigines Protection Society and the Ethnological Society of London, the former became more of a focus for humanitarian concerns, while the latter began to take on an overtly scientific character.

However, the debate between mono- and polygenic origins of humankind came to be reflected in competing learned societies. In 1863, James Hunt (1833–69) founded a rival Anthropological Society of London which was more interested in the anatomical aspects of ethnology. Within two years, it had over 500 members, and ultimately grew to almost 800 members. However, the eminent anatomists, including Charles Darwin and Thomas Huxley (1825–95), remained with the Ethnological Society, with Huxley becoming its President in 1868. He referred to Hunt's Anthropological Society as a nest of imposters.[12]

Many members of the Anthropological Society were polygenists and dismissed Darwin's theory of evolution as a restatement of the Prichardian doctrine of human unity. Hunt said that the questions of origins and evolution was unknowable and he was only interested in classifying living populations, particularly by the shape of the cranium. Francis Galton (1822–1911) eventually became head of the Anthropological Institute, and some of his racialist views were as extreme as those of Hunt. The Anthropological Society had scientific meetings criticizing missionary work among 'savage' races, and taunted the Christian Union in premises across the street by hanging an articulated 'savage' skeleton in the front window. Clearly, the difference between the two societies was more political than scientific. Hunt's first presidential address was 'On the Negro's Place in Nature', concluding that Negroes were a different species, closer to apes than Europeans. Since they were incapable of civilization, they were better off as slaves. The Anthropological Society gave public support to the harsh suppression by Governor E. J. Eyre (1815–1901) of a black farmers' rising in Jamaica in 1866; and Thomas Huxley, in the Ethnological Society, led the liberal and humanitarian public attack on Eyre. However, it was Huxley who was the ultimate peacemaker, and in 1871 the two societies, under the umbrella of the British Association for the Advancement of Science, merged as the Anthropological (later Royal Anthropological) Institute of Great Britain and Ireland. Because Huxley was not acceptable to many in the old Anthropological Society, he stepped aside, and John Lubbock (1834–1913), who wrote on comparative kinship structure, was a Liberal member of Parliament, Vice-Chancellor of the University of London, and a life-long friend of Charles Darwin, became the first President.[13]

By 1884, with reforms that allowed religiously nonconforming individuals to have university posts, Edward Tylor (1832–1917) had become Reader, then Professor in 1896, at Oxford. He was not trained in medicine, but he travelled widely, wrote learnedly, and had a lively empirical curiosity. For example, when he was given a Tasmanian skin-scraper, he immediately had it tested by his butcher.[14] Tylor's definition of culture is still the benchmark definition informing anthropology today, a concept which separates culture from race, the former being learned behaviour socially transmitted and the latter being biologically (genetically) transmitted.

EARLY TWENTIETH CENTURY

The turn of the century is characterized by the first large-scale rigorously empirical anthropological field studies. In the United States, the question of human origins and racial diversity had a different emotional and political urgency from that in Britain. Were the degenerationist views of the French zoologist Comte de Buffon (1707–88) correct, and would Europeans become savages if they remained in the physical environment of the Americas? Who were the native Americans: one of the lost tribes of Israel, perhaps? To gain insight into such questions, Franz Boas played a key role in the Jesup North Pacific Expedition which, between 1897 and 1902, explored the Asian and North American hinterlands of the Bering Sea which joins the two continents. The papers from the expedition began to document the process by which the New World was populated. Other papers, for example, included a detailed description of a Siberian shaman attending a woman who had been in labour for days. He used an iron instrument to remove the foetus in parts, thus saving the woman's life. Boas had founded the American Folk-Lore Society in 1888 (linguistics, myth, and culture), turned the journal *American Anthropologist* towards empirical research in 1898, founded the American Anthropological Association in 1900, and revitalized the American Ethnological Society in the same year. As Professor of Anthropology at Columbia University, he was active until his death (literally in the arms of the French philosopher and anthropologist Claude Lévi-Strauss (b. 1908) in 1942). Boas's academic background was in physics and geography rather than medicine. He had done fieldwork with Arctic Eskimo and sub-Arctic native Americans since 1883, some of the work funded by the British Association for the Advancement of Science in collaboration with Edward Tylor at Oxford. Boas and his students were more historically oriented than their British colleagues, and initially used comparative linguistics, archaeology, myth, comparative technology, and other techniques to chart migration of Asians across the ice-age land-bridge of the Bering Straits. Then their attention turned to documentation of the diverse native American groups being displaced by European settlers and in many cases dying out before their eyes. With the rise of the Third Reich in Germany, Boas, a German immigrant, and his student, Ruth Benedict (1887–1948), sorted with scientific clarity the concepts of race, language, and culture as independent variables in human society.[15]

The first major British empirical fieldwork, the Torres Straits expedition, was organized by Alfred Haddon (1855–1940) at Cambridge in 1898. Haddon had been trained in the Cambridge school of physiology of Sir Michael Foster (1836–1907) and took up a Cambridge University lectureship in physical anthropology in 1895, later becoming Professor. The Torres Straits expedition included two scientists trained in medicine, neurophysiology, and experimental psychology: C. S. Myers (1873–1946) and W. H. R. Rivers (1864–1922). Rivers especially did much to orient British anthropology toward collection of primary data, setting the discipline firmly into the empirical tradition. Following the Torres Straits expedition, Rivers worked with the Toda people in India in 1901–2, and in various areas of Melanesia in 1907. Initially, he was influenced by Darwin and interpreted his data in an evolutionary framework, but abandoned that perspective in 1911 and became more interested in the process of migration, trade, and cultural diffusion. Smith and Perry at University College London carried the diffusionist perspective to extremes, and the counterbalance came from the Boasian school in the United States, which tended to emphasize independent invention and cultural relativism. But Rivers was also the precursor of functional theory, which dominated most of British anthropology and much of American anthropology through the 1950s. Rivers observed that among 'simple' people a useful art was at the same time an aspect of religious rites, aesthetics, and a part of social organization. He demonstrated that all the different domains of culture are interconnected, and a change in one will bring change in the rest. In 1924, Rivers wrote *Medicine, Magic and Religion*, pointing out that indigenous medical systems are social institutions to be studied in the same way as kinship, politics, or other institutions.[16] He also argued that if one accepts the underlying causal premises or beliefs in a non-European medical system, then indigenous medical practices follow rationally from those logical premises. Rivers also developed the basic methodological technique for collecting and recording genealogies, a technique still used today in comparative kinship studies and medical genetics. (➤ Ch. 30 Folk medicine) In his work with soldiers during the First World War, Rivers observed that their battle-induced hysteria and anxiety neuroses occurred independently from sexual frustration. (➤ Ch. 66 Medicine and modern war) In 1920, his book *Instinct and the Unconscious* challenged Freud's libido theory.[17]

When Rivers died in 1922, he and Haddon had trained students at Cambridge who, in turn, came to dominate British anthropology. In 1906, Haddon and Rivers sent A. R. Radcliffe-Brown (1881–1955) to study the Andaman Islanders. Radcliffe-Brown had won an exhibition at Trinity College, Cambridge, in 1902, read the mental and moral sciences tripos, and studied experimental psychology with Myers and Rivers and philosophy of science with A. N. Whitehead (1861–1947). In 1904, he took a first and became Rivers's first research student. Radcliffe-Brown had also read the work of the French sociologist, Emile Durkheim (1858–1917), and in *A Natural Science of Society* blended sociological and biological concepts into a functional framework.[18] (➤ Ch. 70 Medical sociology) The separate institutions of a society (kinship, religion, etc.) were like the circulatory, digestive, and other systems of the body. One could use an analytical approach to 'dissect' these sub-systems to know their 'anatomy' (form) and 'physiology' (function). Like organisms, cultures evolved in the direction of increasing diversity and complexity. Radcliffe-Brown established anthropology as an academic discipline in Cape Town and Sydney. He lectured at the University of Chicago in 1931, where his functional paradigm had more lasting impact on American sociology than anthropology. American anthropology at the time was dominated by Robert Lowie (1883–1957) and Alfred Kroeber (1876–1960), who, like their mentor Boas, carried on his largely historical, linguistic, and cultural relativist approach.[19] Other students of Boas, notably Ralph Linton (1893–1953), Ruth Benedict and Margaret Mead (1901–1978), attempted to synthesize psychoanalytic, *gestalt*, and learning theory with cultural theory, a development that was largely resisted in Britain by Radcliffe-Brown and his students.[20] (➤ Ch. 43 Psychotherapy) Radcliffe-Brown was appointed to the Chair in Social Anthropology at Oxford in 1937, and headed the Royal Anthropological Institute in the 1940s.

Two of Radcliffe-Brown's Oxford students and colleagues, Meyer Fortes (1906–83) and E. E. Evans-Pritchard (1902–73), are of interest. Meyer Fortes came to anthropology from a background in psychology at Cape Town. He produced brilliant functional studies based on prolonged and meticulous fieldwork primarily in Ghana, and only late in his career wrote on the Oedipal complex in cross-cultural contexts. Meyer Fortes took the Chair in Social Anthropology at Cambridge in 1950, and Evans-Pritchard succeeded Radcliffe-Brown to the Oxford Chair in 1946.

Evans-Pritchard's *Witchcraft, Oracles and Magic Among the Azande*, published in 1937, returned to the rationality question posed by Rivers, Lucien Lévy-Bruhl (1857–1939) in France, and others. Why did Africans explain disease, death, and other misfortune as caused by witchcraft, and what was the role of the witch-doctor and the oracle in diagnosis and treatment? What was the relationship between their materia medica and witchcraft or sorcery concepts?

Evans-Pritchard asked: 'is Zande thought so different from ours that we can only describe their speech and actions without comprehending them, or is it essentially like our own though expressed in an idiom to which we are unaccustomed?'[21] He concluded, as had Rivers, that given the initial premise that harm can be caused by thoughts of envy, greed, malice, etc., then the rest of the beliefs follow logically.[22] Although 'expressed in an idiom to which we are unaccustomed', the Zande idea that a social environment of hate and other stress can impair health is now appearing in the medical literature in psychoneuroimmunology.[23]

LATE TWENTIETH CENTURY

In the latter half of the twentieth century, the relationship between medicine and anthropology has been diverse. There have been very detailed field studies carried out by people trained in both medicine and anthropology. For example, Una Maclean, now Reader in Community Medicine at Edinburgh, worked as a physician-anthropologist in the Yoruba area of Nigeria for seven years, and her publications, which appeared in the 1960s, set the standard for other studies that have followed.[24] More radically, Africans are writing their own medical anthropology. Harriet Ngubani, for example, was encouraged to come to Cambridge by Meyer Fortes. Her *Mind and Body in Zulu Medicine* is an excellent translation into Western thought of Zulu concepts of the cause of illness, sorcery, the relationship between ancestors and illness, ideas of pollution, treatment of disease, colour symbolism in medicine, and notions of spirit possession.[25] In the 1980s, with radical racial integration in the University of Cape Town, Ngubani was named to the Chair in Social Anthropology. Similarly, Gordon Chavunduka, while occupying the Chair in Sociology at the University of Zimbabwe, had apprenticed himself for several years to traditional practitioners, and came to head the Zimbabwe National Traditional Healers' Association. He is the author of *Traditional Healers and the Shona Patient*.[26] (➤ Ch. 29 Non-Western concepts of disease) The dialogue between Europeans and Africans has come a long way since the days of James Hunt and the Anthropological Society of London!

This contemporary ethnological approach focuses on how a particular group of people perceive and deal with illness. It strives for an insider's view at the descriptive level, but at the interpretive stage may transcend what local people actually say and do, trying to fit their thoughts and actions into broader theoretical patterns. Thus Ngubani and others, after a careful study of healing and fertility rituals, concluded that colour symbolism of red, black, and white speaks universally to the basic physiological truths of blood, semen, and breast milk; to birth, nurturing, and death. Often such symbolism is a metaphor for cosmological truths as well. Victor Turner described the richly metaphorical meaning of symbols used by Ndembu people in Zambia during healing and fertility rituals. The symbols, taken from nature, represent hot and cold, left and right, red and white, below and above, male and female, doctor and patient. The traditional healer mediates such opposites in rituals that seek health and fertility, at the same time ordering the entire Ndembu social and physical universe. It is difficult to put a label on such healers who are also ritual specialists, and Turner's 'A Ndembu doctor in practice' has become a classic in both medical anthropology and the field of symbolic and ritual analysis.[27] It is the kind of holistic perspective now being rediscovered by the holistic health movement in Western countries.[28]

Anthropologists have collaborated with epidemiologists to solve problems and plan public-health initiatives. For example, Robert Glasse and Shirley Lindenbaum, who had done extensive anthropological research in Papua New Guinea, collaborated with D. C. Gajdusek to solve the riddle of a widespread degenerative neurological disease among women and children in the South Fore area of Papua New Guinea. Gajdusek, who was awarded the Nobel Prize for his work, originally suspected a genetic disease. However, Lindenbaum and Glasse knew of mortuary ceremonies in which women and children ate the under-cooked brains of the deceased. This, then, was the route of transmission for the slow virus causing kuru disease and death. Glasse and Lindenbaum, in talking with old people, found that both cannibalism and kuru were relatively new to the Fore area. The custom of cannibalism began about 1910, and the first case of kuru some time later. Now, with the abolition of such rituals, there are no signs of the disease among children.[29] (➤ Ch. 2 What is specific to Western medicine?)

After hope of eradication in the 1960s, malaria is becoming an increasing public-health concern in tropical countries. (➤ Ch. 24 Tropical diseases; Ch. 52 Epidemiology) From a purely epidemiological perspective one might choose to chemosuppress non-immunes, or have an anti-malarial drug available for quick treatment. However, even when supplies are adequate and no resistance to the drug of choice is present, for a variety of cultural, social, political, and psychological reasons, the drug may not reach the target group. In areas with widespread drug resistance, much more innovative, small-scale, community-involved approaches to malaria control are being explored, often with essential collaboration from anthropologists.[30] The Special Programme for Training and Research in Tropical Diseases of the World Health Organization has particularly encouraged anthropologists and other social scientists from tropical countries to work collaboratively with medical scientists on intervention strategies. This collaboration is particularly fruitful when the focus is on the primary health care approach in preventing and controlling disease. Some foundations and bilateral aid agencies, particularly agencies in the Scandinavian countries and the Netherlands, have been very sensitive to cultural and social dimensions of health programmes in developing countries, and have funded anthropologists from those countries for higher education in anthropology and epidemiology. (➤ Ch. 59 Internationalism in medicine and public health)

Since the nineteenth century, there has been interest in health and nutrition related to environmental adaptation. In the 1960s, Richard Lee and his Harvard colleagues made important observations among the pygmoid Dobe !Kung of the Kalahari Desert. He made his observations during years of drought, but still found a population that was well nourished even though they only spent 1.2 to 3.2 days per week working to gather and hunt food. Subsequent studies have shown that the Dobe !Kung lack evidence of coronary heart disease, have one of the lowest serum cholesterol levels in the world, and show no evidence of blood pressure rising with age. There is a similar lack of death from cancer, and even dental caries are rare. The !Kung have the longest birth intervals of populations not using contraceptives, and low parity. However, the picture changes dramatically for those who have been displaced from their gathering and hunting range to which they are so well adapted, and who have settled on cattle posts. Birth intervals, for example, become half what they had been.[31]

Medical anthropology tends to overlap with medical sociology and community medicine when looking at domestic and international health-care systems. Some of the analysis has been informed by Marxian theory and some has not. All stress that sickness behaviour is never a purely personal matter. John Janzen's work in Lower Zaire described a 'therapy management group' of kin and others who took over the care of a sick person, deciding whether they should seek traditional or Western care, whether they should go to hospital, how long they should stay, and other matters.[32] Closer to home, Irving Zola, looking at 'the case of non-compliance', described the following ethnographic observation. The doctor, looking down at the chart and not the patient, says jocularly, 'Well Anne, how are you today?' The patient says 'Lousy, Robert, how are you?' The doctor, taken aback, responds 'My name is Dr Johnson, I only called you Anne to make you feel comfortable.' The patient replies, 'Well, my name is Dr Greene, I only called you Robert to make *you* feel more comfortable.'[33] Perhaps the most important recent development has been informed by the feminist critique in many academic disciplines, including anthropology, medicine, and the nursing profession. The literature deals with doctor–patient interaction, symbolic meanings of the body and its functions, and the politics of fertility management.[34] (➤ Ch. 34 History of the doctor–patient relationship; Ch. 38 Women and medicine)

CONCLUSION

In the nineteenth century, anthropology as an academic discipline became established in close relationship with the more humanitarian concerns that arose within medicine. It particulary spoke, with medicine, about racialist and exploitive aspects of nineteenth-century domestic and colonial life. Today, developing countries which are bound into a single economic system with industrial countries have not enjoyed humanitarian benefits commensurate with the rich countries.[35] When an anthropological voice is particularly needed, academic anthropology in Britain has barely held its ground, and medical anthropology has never had a secure academic footing. In the United States, the picture is different. The Society for Medical Anthropology, a sub-group within the American Anthropological Association, has just over 2,000 members, and medical anthropology has moved into the mainstream of the discipline, and into many medical schools as well.

NOTES

1 James Cowles Prichard, *Researches into the Physical History of Mankind*, 5 vols, London, 1836–47.
2 James Cowles Prichard, *An Analysis of Egyptian Mythology*, London, 1819.
3 G. Elliot Smith, *The Ancient Egyptians and the Origin of Civilization*, rev. edn, London, Harper, 1923.
4 George Stocking, *Victorian Anthropology*, New York, Macmillan, 1987; John Barnes, 'Anthropology in Britain before and after Darwin', *Mankind*, 1960, 5: 369–85.
5 Barnes, op. cit. (n. 2); Marvin Harris, *The Rise of Anthropological Theory*, New York, Columbia University Press, 1968; Robert Lowie, *The History of Ethnological Theory*, New York, Holt, Rinehart & Winston, 1937.
6 R. G. Latham, *Natural History of the Varieties of Man*, 1850; Latham, *Descriptive Ethnology*, 2 vols, 1859.
7 Robert Knox, *The Races of Man*, 1850.
8 Adrian Desmond, *The Politics of Evolution*, Chicago, IL, University of Chicago Press, 1989.
9 Ibid.
10 Stocking, op. cit. (n. 2); John Beddoe, *The Races of Britain*, Bristol, Arrowsmith, 1885.
11 Stocking, op. cit. (n. 2), p. 242.
12 Stocking, op. cit. (n. 2).
13 George Stocking, 'What's in a name? The origins of the Royal Anthropological Institute (1837–71)', *Man*, 1971, 6: 369–90.
14 Lowie, op. cit. (n. 3), pp. 68–85.
15 Harris, op. cit. (n. 3); Franz Boas, *Race, Language and Culture*, New York, Macmillan, 1948 (collection of papers published between 1887 and 1936); Ruth Benedict, *Race, Science and Politics*, New York, Viking, 1945.

16 W. H. R. Rivers, *Medicine, Magic and Religion*, 1924.

17 Ian Langham, *The Building of British Social Anthropology: W. H. R. Rivers and his Cambridge Disciples in the Development of Kinship Studies, 1898–1931*, Dordrecht, Reidel, 1981; Harris, op. cit. (n. 3); Adam Kuper, *Anthropology and Anthropologists: the Modern British School*, 2nd edn, London, Routledge, 1983.

18 A. R. Radcliffe-Brown, *A Natural Science of Society*, New York, Free Press, 1948.

19 Alfred Kroeber, *Anthropology*, New York, Harcourt, Brace, 1948.

20 Ralph Linton, *The Cultural Background of Personality*, New York, Appleton, Century, Crofts, 1945.

21 E. E. Evans-Pritchard, *Witchcraft, Oracles and Magic Among the Azande*, Oxford, Clarendon Press, 1937, p. 4.

22 See also, Brian Wilson (ed.), *Rationality*, Oxford, Basil Blackwell, 1969; Robin Horton and Ruth Finnegan (eds), *Modes of Thought*, London, Faber & Faber, 1973; Martin Hollis and Steven Lukes (eds), *Rationality and Relativism*, Oxford, Basil Blackwell, 1982; Stanley Tambiah, *Magic, Science and Religion and the Scope of Rationality*, Cambridge, Cambridge University Press, 1990.

23 See, for example, G. F. Solomon, 'Psychoneuroimmunology: interactions between central nervous system and immune system', *Journal of Neuroscience Research*, 1987, 18: 1–9.

24 Una Maclean, 'Traditional medicine and its practitioners in Ibaden, Nigeria', *Journal of Tropical Medicine and Hygiene*, 1965, 68: 237–44; Maclean, 'Traditional healers and their female clients: an aspect of Nigerian sickness behaviour', *Journal of Health and Social Behaviour*, 1969, 10: 172–86.

25 Harriet Ngubani, *Mind and Body in Zulu Medicine*, London, Academic Press, 1977.

26 Gordon Chavunduka, *Traditional Healers and the Shona Patient*, Gweru, Mambo Press, 1978. See also Murray Last and Chavunduka (eds), *The Professionalisation of African Medicine*, Manchester, University of Manchester Press, 1986.

27 Victor Turner, *The Forest of Symbols*, Ithaca, NY, Cornell University Press, 1967.

28 Patrick Pietroni, *The Greening of Medicine*, London, Gollancz, 1990.

29 John Mathews, Robert Glasse and Shirley Lindenbaum, 'Kuru and cannibalism', *Lancet*, 1968, 2: 449–52; Lindenbaum, *Kuru Sorcery: Disease and Danger in the New Guinea Highlands*, Palo Alto, CA, Mayfield, 1979.

30 Carol MacCormack and George Lwihula, 'Failure to participate in a malaria chemosuppression programme', *Journal of Tropical Medicine and Hygiene*, 1983, 86: 99–107; Robert Snow et al., 'Permethrin-treated bed nets prevent malaria in Gambian children', *Transactions of the Royal Society of Tropical Medicine and Hygiene*, 1988, 82: 138–42; MacCormack, Snow and Brian Greenwood, 'Use of insecticide-impregnated bed nets in Gambian primary health care', *Bulletin of the World Health Organization*, 1989, 67: 209–14. See also Craig Janes et al. (eds), *Anthropology and Epidemiology: Interdisciplinary Approaches to the Study of Health and Disease*, Dordrecht, Reidel, 1986.

31 Richard Lee, *The !Kung San: Men, Women and Work in a Foraging Society*, Cambridge, Cambridge University Press, 1979; Nancy Howell, *Demography of the Dobe !Kung*, New York, Academic Press, 1979. See also Alexander Alland, *Adaptation in Cultural Evolution: an Approach to Medical Anthropology*, New York,

Columbia University Press, 1970; Ann McElroy and Patricia Townsend, *Medical Anthropology in Ecological Perspective*, North Scituate, MA, Duxbury, 1979.

32 John Janzen, *The Quest for Therapy in Lower Zaire*, Berkeley, University of California Press, 1978.

33 Irving Zola, 'The case of non-compliance', in Leon Eisenberg and Arthur Kleinman (eds), *The Relevance of Social Science for Medicine*, Dordrecht, Reidel, 1981, pp. 241–52.

34 See, for example, Carol MacCormack (ed.), *Ethnography of Fertility and Birth*, London, Academic Press, 1982; Brigitte Jordan, *Birth in Four Cultures*, Montreal, Eden Press, 1978; Carolyn Sargent, *The Cultural Context of Therapeutic Choice*, Dordrecht, Reidel, 1982; Sargent, *Maternity, Medicine and Power: Reproductive Decisions in Urban Benin*, Berkeley, University of California Press, 1989; W. Penn Handwerker (ed.), *Births and Powers: Social Change and the Politics of Reproduction*, Boulder, CO, 1990; Yoyceen Boyle and Margaret Andrews, *Transcultural Concepts in Nursing Care*, Glenview, IL, Scott Foresman, 1989.

35 'Western economics and Third World health', *Lancet*, 2 September 1989: 551.

FURTHER READING

Chavunduka, Gordon, *Traditional Healers and the Shona Patient*, Gweru, Mambo Press, 1978.

Desmond, Adrian, *The Politics of Evolution*, Chicago, IL, University of Chicago Press, 1989.

Douglas, Mary, *Edward Evans-Pritchard*, London, Fontana, 1980.

Helman, Cecil, *Culture, Health and Illness*, 2nd edn, London, Wright, 1990.

Kuper, Adam, *Anthropology and Anthropologists: the Modern British School*, 2nd edn, London, Routledge, 1983.

Last, Murray and Chavunduka, Gordon (eds), *The Professionalisation of African Medicine*, Manchester, University of Manchester Press, 1986.

MacCormack, Carol (ed.), *Ethnography of Fertility and Birth*, London, Academic Press, 1982.

Medical Anthropology Quarterly.

Ngubani, Harriet, *Body and Mind in Zulu Medicine*, London, Academic Press, 1977.

Social Science and Medicine [journal].

Stocking, George, *Victorian Anthropology*, New York, Macmillan, 1987.

Tambiah, Stanley, *Magic, Science and Religion and the Scope of Rationality*, Cambridge, Cambridge University Press, 1990.

61

RELIGION AND MEDICINE

Roy Porter

Religion and medicine share a single aim, that of making whole. It is no accident that 'holiness' and 'healing' have a common etymology, rooted in the idea of wholeness; as do salvation and the salutary, cure, care, and charity. Certain highly unified or deliberately syncretist belief systems make little differentiation between modes of wholeness, just as small societies commonly have one single job description, such as 'witch doctor', for all thaumaturgical activities. But the world's great cultures have tended to create some sort of conceptual distinction ('dualism') between body on the one hand and, on the other, soul, mind, or spirit; and consequently have fostered the differentiation of medicine from faith, and of doctor from priest, the one attending to the cure of bodies, the other to the 'cure' of souls. All such distinctions are necessarily messy and unstable, since experience also shows the connections, no less than the divisions, between the somatic and the psychic, the this-worldly and the transcendental. Not surprisingly, therefore, physic and faith criss-cross and overlap at many points; though often complementary, there nevertheless remains great potential for conflict; though separate, there remains scope for unification.

Alternatively, it might be suggested that medicine and faith are, in the end, perhaps offering mutually exclusive paradigms of the human condition. *Tres medici, duo athei* was often flung in doctors' faces. There are no grounds for taking this taunt literally; indeed, individual physicians have often been eloquently pious, witness *Religio Medici* by Sir Thomas Browne (1605–82). But, surveying the whole development of human consciousness, it is arguable that it was the experience of suffering, sickness, and death which gave birth to religious devotion in the first place; and equally, that modern medical advances (the conquest of disease, the prolongation of life) have played no small part in widespread secularization.

Other contributions to this encyclopedia consider the religious impulses behind healing in China, Islam, and the Hindu world, as well as in preliterate societies. This chapter focuses upon the West, examining the interplay of a medical tradition born out of Classical philosophy and science, with Judaeo-Christianity. (➤ Ch. 31 Arab-Islamic medicine; Ch. 32 Chinese medicine; Ch. 33 Indian medicine)

THE BODY, SICKNESS, AND THE SOUL

Like many other great faiths and philosophies, Judaeo-Christianity articulates a generally dualistic cosmology that ennobles the soul (spirit, mind) while disparaging the body (flesh), sometimes seen as the soul's prison. The soul is immortal, immutable, and eternal: the flesh, by contrast, is weak and corruptible, and, thanks to Original Sin, theologically tarred with the brush of brutishness and evil. At the Fall, man's yielding to carnal lust, or, in a slightly different version, his disobedience, brought disease, pain, and death into the world. (➤ Ch. 12 The concepts of health, illness, and disease)

Such anxieties about the frailty of the flesh are reflected in the exacting regulation of the body demanded by the Old Testament and maintained ever since within Judaism, with its elaborate prohibitions and disciplines concerning hygiene, diet, and sexual habits. Purity necessitated such defences against defiling bodily pollutions (for example, the menstruating woman). It was a Talmudic requirement that Jews should not live in a city without a physician.

For their part, the early Christians responded to distrust of the body with rather different defences. Drawing upon Eastern religio-philosophical asceticism, the Desert Fathers praised virginity and cultivated mortification. Hermits pioneered heroic self-denial to quell the lusts of the flesh and free the spirit for godly service; through the regulations of St Benedict (c.480–c.547), such individual asceticism was eventually Taylorized into the collective discipline of monastic rule, for expiatory, propitiatory, and purificatory purposes. Fasting and self-flagellation became popularly identified in the medieval mind as the hallmarks of holiness, and chastity was increasingly expected of the Catholic clergy, albeit more honoured in the breach.

Belittling of the flesh is common to many faiths. Christianity, however, encodes unusually complex attitudes towards the body. More than most theosophies, it personalizes the Supreme Principle (God the Father), and involves Him intimately with the sublunary world. God has an only Son, who is born in the flesh (a conception widely thought scandalous amongst Ancient thinkers), before being crucified, in agony, in the flesh. Incarnation and sacrifice are, in turn, commemorated in the sacrament of the Eucharist, whereby, at least in Roman Catholic theology, ritual bread and wine are literally transubstantiated into the body and blood of the Saviour. Through this divine propitiation, believers are offered the hope, not (as in many faiths) of some rather amorphous, wishy-washy life after death, but of a palpable bodily resurrection at the Last Judgment, to be followed by a heavenly resumption of physical being for the saved, and eternal hellfire torments for the damned. In the conversion of peasant Europe from paganism, Christianity drew much credit from the fate of the body. Sudden deaths, unexpected reprieves, or the appearance of physical stigmata, were attributed to Providence. Medieval saint cults commonly sprang up when the corpse of a holy individual supposedly failed to decompose, or assumed preternatural healing properties.

In other words, while reviling the flesh as tainted by sin, Christianity also emphasized the sacred immanent therein. This double vision is central to orthodox theology, whose job was to map out a difficult middle ground. Thus while asceticism was prized, mortification was never to be driven to the point of death (after all, being God's creature, man was not the proprietor of his own body, hence Judaeo-Christianity's strict suicide prohibition). On the one hand, Gnostics and such Manicheans as the Albigensians, who deemed the flesh as the devil's work, and hence wholly evil, were denounced as heretics. On the other, Ranters in mid-seventeenth-century England, and other Antinomians who claimed that Christ dwelt within them – hence that the flesh could not sin – were equally anathematized. Down the centuries, churchmen typically enjoined the faithful to treat sickness as due punishment for the collective sinfulness of humankind, and also, to some degree, for personal sins. The medieval Black Death and, no less, the cholera pandemics of the nineteenth century, were standardly interpreted from the pulpit as visitations of divine wrath and vengeance, designed to edify and teach humility, patience, and faith. But while 'resignation' was in order, Christians despised the 'fatalism' in the face of disease that they observed in Islam. After all, God had set humans on earth to do His work, ultimately the saving of souls; hence it was the duty of humans to preserve their bodies using all proper 'means'. Though black magic and sorcery were thereby excluded, for both medieval scholastics and, later, Calvinists, medicine was clearly a godly instrument.

Over the centuries, certain Christian sects have condemned some or all aspects of medical practice as impious. In Britain and North America, various Presbyterians and Dissenters repudiated smallpox inoculation and vaccination on the grounds that the deliberate implantation of a disease into a healthy person (in however mild a form, and with however laudable a motive) risked breaking the Sixth Commandment. Jehovah's Witnesses originally denied the germ theory. Nowadays they still refuse blood transfusions, even at the risk of death, in the belief that the practice contravenes Scripture (Genesis 9: 4, etc.), though they happily accept organ transplants. Nevertheless, the great Christian churches have routinely accepted that medicine has its rightful role, alongside other human arts. After all, was not the evangelist Luke 'the beloved physician'? And did not the incarnate Christ Himself, while instructing physicians to heal themselves, give proofs of His own divine powers by acts of healing? Some thirty-five such miracles are recorded. The apostles subsequently exercised healing as 'a gift of the spirit' (1 Corinthians 12: 9). From the start, Christianity made its way in the world as a healing faith.

The vision of the body advanced in mainstream Catholic and Protestant theology – fallen, yet still the instrument of God – has suggested a *modus vivendi* involving coexistence and co-operation between the churches and the medical profession. Priests were to tend the tribulations and salvation of the soul, the ailments of the body became the prerogative of the faculty; above all, after the Fourth Lateran Council (1215) forebade clerics to shed blood through the practice of surgery, and warned against immoderate involvement in treating physical complaints. This practical division of labour was obviously question-begging and fragile. Some of its tensions will be explored in later sections (see pp. 1456 ff.).

CHRISTIANITY AND MEDICAL INSTITUTIONS

Christianity brought into the world no novel, exclusive theory of disease. The general tendency of Christian theology to emphasize personal accountability and guilt was easily superimposed upon the 'physiological', humoral aetiologies promoted by Classical medicine, which viewed an individual's state of health as hingeing upon personal life-style, constitution, and character. (➤ Ch. 14 Humoralism)

The success of the church, however, reoriented medical practice quite decisively. In the ancient world, the Aesculapian art was generally practised as a private trade; it was the duty of families to make provision for the needs of their own sick. Medicine had little public face or institutional embodiment, beyond the handful of temples where incubation therapy was practised, and the field and barracks hospitals that military needs inevitably called into existence. (➤ Ch. 4 Medical care)

This changed within Christendom. Charity was the supreme religious virtue. In the name of love, and with the conviction that every human was a soul to be saved, believers were enjoined to care for those in need: the destitute, the handicapped, the poor, the hungry, those without shelter, and, perhaps above all, the sick. Once the conversion of Constantine (d. AD 337) rendered Christianity the official imperial religion, 'hospitals' sprang up as pious foundations, and with them religious fellowships dedicated to serving fellow humans. Some hospitals were outgrowths of religious houses: after all, monasteries needed medical facilities to care for their own sick brethren. In time, certain abbeys assumed a more conspicuous medical role. Across the medieval centuries, thousands of 'hospitals' were thus established by pious bequest, under the rule of regular religious orders. Some were designated for particular diseases, especially the leprosaria. How far the majority of such establishments ever did, or even were intended to, perform functions which may strictly be called 'medical' remains warmly disputed. Research has shown that hospitals in late medieval and renaissance Italy were typically well endowed and administered, and played key roles in coping with disease. Elsewhere, many foundations fell into corruption; others, including the leprosaria, outlived their need. Most at best provided shelter, a bed, food, and perhaps pious prayers towards pious deaths.[2] (➤ Ch. 49 The hospital: Ch. 62 Charity before c.1850)

Whatever its shortcomings by later standards, it would be wrong, however, to take too negative a view of the medieval hospital. What is crucial is that it was (to use Colin Jones's term) the Christian 'charitable imperative', which, for the first time, led to the foundation of institutionalized public care for the sick.[3] It is not a foregone conclusion that, without such pious donations and religious vocations, alternative provision would automatically have been made. After the closure of practically all such 'hospital' foundations at the Henrician Reformation, England almost entirely lacked institutions designated for the sick until the eighteenth century, when a new wave of largely religious philanthropy, spearheaded by clergy, led to the setting up of major new general hospitals in London (Guy's, the Westminster, the Middlesex, the London, and St George's), infirmaries in the provinces, and specialist institutions besides.

Such religiously motivated and funded initiatives continued in the nineteenth century in response to massive demographic rise, industrialization, and urbanization. (➤ Ch. 63 Medical philanthropy after 1850) Throughout Europe and North America, 'missions', commonly led by clergy and staffed by nuns and sisters, addressed the needs of the sick, the old, the orphaned, the pregnant, the blind, deaf, and disabled. In all such rescue work, the aura of religion lent respectability to helping such dubious cases as the venereally afflicted, or unmarried mothers in lying-in homes. (➤ Ch. 58 Medicine and colonialism) In many nations, lunatic asylums developed on an essentially denominational basis. In the United States, thousands of voluntary denominational hospitals were established, their nursing staffs comprising women with religious vocations (in the mid-twentieth century, almost a thousand Catholic hospitals were handling some 16 million patients a year).

More spectacularly, Counter-Reformation zeal led to the founding of enormously successful religious orders devoted to hospital service beyond the cloister. Set up by Vincent de St Paul (1580–1660), the Daughters of Charity dedicated themselves to nursing as a Christian vocation. By the time of the Revolution, they were running 426 houses in France alone. Such hospitals were first and foremost focused upon piety, and only secondarily constituted centres of medicine. Physicians remained subordinate. The Daughters saw their mission as impressing religious duties upon those who recovered, and ensuring a pious death for the rest. Till well within this century, hospitals in Catholic nations depended utterly upon their dedication.

In institutionalizing such a sense of mission, and mobilizing female energies, Protestants lagged. In the nineteenth century, German Lutheranism gave rise to the Kaiserswerth school, set up to train women as nursing deaconesses. It was after her visit to Kaiserswerth in 1851 that Florence Nightingale (1820–1910) developed her own secularized nursing orders. (➤ Ch. 54 A general history of nursing: 1800–1900) Quakers such as Elizabeth Fry (1780–1845) initiated hospital visiting to succour the sick.

How far and how quickly industrializing nations would have developed hospital systems in the absence of multiform religious impulses is a moot point. An institution which, almost certainly, would not have developed without such impetus from Christian zeal was the medical mission overseas. From the sixteenth century, the Jesuits recognized the power of medical cures for winning converts in the Americas and Asia. In the nineteenth century, fired by the Evangelical movement, and accompanying new waves of colonial expansion, Protestant medical missions expanded rapidly, funded from the USA, Britain, Germany, and Holland. In Britain, the huge publicity attending the mission of David Livingstone (1813–73) in central Africa transformed the movement. Financed, if sometimes hamstrung, by mission societies at home, doctors typically embraced the dual aims of overcoming sickness and Satan – tasks seen as inextricably linked, especially in all-out campaigns against native magic healing systems and the hated witch-doctor. (➤ Ch. 30 Folk medicine) Medical missionaries faced a dilemma. They commonly protested against the exploitative excesses of colonial rule, while, by their very presence, being the agents who rendered possible the success of the 'white man's burden'.

Before the twentieth-century advent of state health systems and compulsory medical insurance, the eleemosynary impulse provided the impetus and the channels for the institutional care of the sick poor; it was the sense of religious vocation that staffed hospitals and mission societies. It would be too much to claim that piety typically also explains the choice of career amongst practitioners. Yet it is certain that the direction taken by élite medicine from medieval times onwards owed much to the emergent religious structures of Latin Christendom.

Contemporaneously with the general revival of learning gaining momentum from the eleventh century, Graeco-Roman medicine was received in the West, transmitted largely via Arab sources. Monastic houses were initially the chief centres for the preservation, copying, and study of manuscripts.

From the twelfth century, universities became foci for the teaching and interpretation of Classical and Arab medicine. Though Italian colleges were linked to municipalities, and hence grew up as relatively secular institutions, beyond the Alps, universities developed under ecclesiastical auspices, their syllabuses shaped by the programme of Christianized Aristotelianism given expression by Albertus Magnus (c.1200–80), Thomas Aquinas (1225–74), and other great Dominican pedagogue-philosophers. Study of the trivium and quadrivium provided the religio-philosophical basis upon which some proceeded to the study of medical texts. This intensely academic approach to medicine encouraged the establishment of the learned physician at the top of the professional tree, above lesser practitioners who learned their craft by experience or, later, formal apprenticeship. Prizing the head above the hand, physic established itself as an academic and liberal profession of intellectual acumen, one whose members were expert in the theory of disease, clinically well informed, and superior in diagnostic and prognostic ability – and, not least, did not stoop to the use of the knife or the mortar. In most nations, if in different ways, university-educated physicians succeeded in securing royal or municipal charters, and in establishing corporate bodies endowed with privileges and the right to exclude and prosecute interlopers. (➤ Ch. 48 Medical education; Ch. 47 History of the medical profession)

The making of the profession of the physician was thus deeply indebted to the specifically ecclesiastical form and content of higher learning forged in the Middle Ages and maintained through the early modern centuries. It was not until the dismantling of the religiously exclusive university in the nineteenth century that the prestige of the scholastically, or humanistically trained physician was undermined, and new, secular, educational attainments for the physician – to be achieved in the teaching hospital – became defined. Moreover, not till then did universities open their doors to women, thus permitting for the first time their entry into the upper echelons of the faculty. (➤ Ch. 38 Women and medicine)

Over the centuries, religio-humanist medicine made a point of emphasizing the accord between the teachings of medicine and the doctrines of the church. Prominent from the seventeenth to the nineteenth century, natural theology drew heavily upon anatomy for proofs of the perfectly harmonious adaptation between structure and function wrought by the Great Physician. (➤ Ch. 5 The anatomical tradition; Ch. 7 The physiological tradition) Charles Bell (1774–1842) contributed a Bridgewater Treatise on the human hand. In Prussia, medicine was given a decisively Pietist slant by the prime role played by Georg Stahl (1660–1734) in promoting medical education at the University of Halle. Just as the medieval physician was meant to ensure that the patient had first confessed, such early formulations of medical ethics as *Medical Ethics*

(1803), by Thomas Percival (1740–1804), argued that it was the physician's duty to point the sick and dying to religion. (➤ Ch. 37 History of medical ethics)

Religious constraints shaped, and limited, medical training and research. The medieval Vatican issued injunctions restricting medical dissections, thereby reinforcing a powerful religious antipathy – felt by most people – to tampering with the corpse (how, for one thing, could the dead rise at the Last Judgment, once they had been dismembered by the anatomist's knife?). Well into the nineteenth century, practical anatomy teaching through post-mortem dissection was commonly inhibited in the university environment. Demonstrating anatomy by the direct method had largely to be practised, and then often with dubious legality, in the hospital autopsy room and at private anatomy schools. In the nineteenth century, religious convictions fuelled opposition to vivisection experiments on animals for medical-research purposes. (➤ Ch. 9 The pathological tradition; Ch. 11 Clinical research)

CONFLICT

Doctors and priests mapped out for themselves 'separate spheres', a mutually agreeable compartmentalization. Galenism espoused a medical 'materialism', which explained physical sickness organically and treated it by physical means. Matters pertaining to the 'rational', or immortal, soul were rendered unto the church. This division of labour was never wholly sustainable.

For one thing, medieval Catholicism, while warning priests not to become engrossed in medicine, nevertheless upheld certain healing functions. Because it viewed God as immanent in the world, and because, for practical parochial purposes, it tended to sanctify popular magical beliefs, Catholicism offered succour for the sick, not just through consolation of prayer, but through the veneration of relics, the purchase of ex voto offerings, through pilgrimages and holy waters, and, above all, saints' shrines and cults. Saints gained reputations by the score for special healing talents: to cure toothache, you prayed to St Apollonia (d. 249), who had been martyred by having her teeth yanked out; sufferers from rabies were urged to hasten to the shrine of St Hubert (d. 727) in the Ardennes.

Moreover, individual holy people have claimed, down the centuries, to possess divinely vouchsafed healing gifts. In Stuart England, Valentine Great-rakes (1629–83) relieved by prayer and laying-on of hands (see pp. 1463–4); a century later, Bridget Bostock (fl. 1740) cured with her holy spittle. In mid-nineteenth-century France, the visions of Bernadette Soubirous (1844–79) led to the development of Lourdes as the leading healing shrine (today, it is visited by 3 million pilgrims a year).

'Miracle cures' were energetically denounced by Reformation Protestants as superstitious and magical. For its part, the post-Tridentine Catholic hierarchy grew more critical of such claims (it has authenticated only sixty-four of the thousands of 'miracles' wrought at Lourdes); and the medical profession has generally adopted a disbelieving, or, at least, a deeply sceptical stance. (Perhaps because of professional jealousy, as anthropologists might note, the modern medical profession has surreptitiously appropriated for itself much of the charisma of religious healing in its own High Temple, the high-tech hospital.) Nevertheless, holy healing has always maintained a popular appeal; and the less official churches and the medical profession are willing to countenance cures beyond reason and nature, the more such practices fall into the hands of rank charlatans.

If religion has claimed a healing mission of its own, certain currents in medicine have, for their part, been eager to dissect faith, contending that religious experience is not authentic but symptomatic of some (psycho)pathological condition. Medical scoffers could always argue that autopsies never discovered an organ of religion, a seat or site of will, of consciousness, of mind, or soul. Surely there must be some organic crossing-point between mind and body, and one more convincing than the Cartesian pineal gland? If not, were not conscience and soul, then, mere verbal fictions, bugaboos invented by priests to control the people? Research fuelled the assumption – greeted by some with anxiety, by others with anticipation – that the progress of anatomy and physiology, of biochemistry and genetics, would in time prove humans wholly material beings: no more, no less. This was the ambition of the soul-destroying *L'Homme Machine* (1749) Julien de La Mettrie (1709–51) – the atheistic, or, more precisely, naturalistic, implications of which were spelled out by the *philosophe*, the Baron d'Holbach (1723–89). And Enlightenment medical materialism of this kind reached its apogee in the *Rêve d'Alembert*, in which Denis Diderot (1713–84) used the eminent Montpellier physician Théophile de Bordeu (1722–76) as the mouthpiece for the view that consciousness is entirely organic in origin, and religion a sick person's dream. Certain late Enlightenment ideologues such as Condorcet (1743–94) and the British physician Erasmus Darwin (1731–94) entertained the possibility that medical science would one day abolish death, thereby initiating a secular heaven on earth. (➤ Ch. 13 Ideas of life and death; Ch. 46 Geriatrics)

Strands of nineteenth-century medical materialism furthered these lines of attack upon the religious concept of human beings. Phrenology and certain schools of neurophysiology argued that thought was a function of the brain, at least implicitly challenging the credibility of the immaterial self or soul. Religious experiences were themselves subject to medical analysis; in the anti-clerical atmosphere of *belle-époque* Paris, J. M. Charcot (1825–93) and P. M. L. P. Richer (1849–1933) examined images of religious ecstasies and put them down to hysteria. (➤ Ch. 21 Mental diseases) And radicals dreamed of a post-revolutionary society in which priests would be supplanted by doctors.

Such broad territorial rivalries between medicine and religion remained, however, exceptional. More important, especially during the early modern centuries, were recurrent and more-localized boundary disputes fought between doctors, priests, and the public over particularly ambiguous or dangerous sorts of sickness. Often, what was in dispute was the public concept of disease and the implications for appropriate action. The understanding of disease was traditionally multi-dimensional. Primarily medical and somatic causes (poor constitution, bad environment, miasmas, contagious germ seeds, etc.) dovetailed with the primarily personal and moral-religious (vicious life-styles, intemperance, etc). The idea of individual responsibility for personal sickness (what we often call 'victim blaming') was quite compatible with the medical model; theologians, for their part, did not deny natural causes. On occasion, however, medical and religio-moral frameworks of reference could be seriously at odds.

Plague epidemics often provoked such problems. Not surprisingly: bubonic plague was highly lethal, rapidly fatal, and spread like wildfire, threatening whole communities. Like leprosy, plague was heavy with scriptural references and religious metaphors. It was typically interpreted as a visitation, requiring atonement. The fourteenth-century Black Death sparked widespread flagellant movements, as well as anti-Semitic pogroms. In Renaissance Italy, faced with plague epidemics, church authorities commonly called mass processionals, intercessions, and propitiatory prayers. Municipal authorities, by contrast, ordered quarantine and isolation, banning the religious gatherings. As Cipolla has shown, the outcome often proved a test of strength between the church and the bureaucrats, the people typically siding with the priests (for official public-health measures such as quarantine were commonly economically disastrous to the community). On one occasion, the entire Florentine health board was excommunicated.[4] (➤ Ch. 51 Public health; Ch. 52 Epidemiology)

Plague led contemporaneously to tussles in England between medically endorsed royal authority on the one hand, and Puritan protest on the other. Central government and city corporations responded to epidemics by initiating measures of containment, shutting city gates, banning markets, and quarantining sufferers and suspects in their own homes. Calvinist preachers condemned such measures as misguided, medically worthless, and (because they seemed to contradict Providence) impious. 'It is not the clean keeping and sweeping of our houses and streets that can drive away this fearful messenger of God's wrath', argued Laurence Chaderton (c.1536–1640), 'but the purging and sweeping of our consciences from ... sin.'[5] True Christian fellowship demanded not sequestration, but mutual aid and trust in God.

The prime field of contention between medical and religious attitudes towards the afflicted was, however, that involving alleged witchcraft and possession. The baselines were well established. It was universally agreed in early modern Europe that the Devil had the power to produce physical evil, either personally, or through his minions, such as witches. One manifestation of such diabolical power was sickness or death, in humans or beasts. When someone fell sick in suspicious circumstances, without obvious physical cause, accusations of *maleficium* commonly followed and were investigated: was the victim possessed? Faced with symptoms such as swooning, fits, vomiting, incoherent speech, and delirium, ministers and medics agreed that there were three possible explanations: authentic disease; malingering and fraud; or demonic possession. To make a determination, doctors had their examination procedures. (Were there unambiguous lesions? Could the *stigmata diaboli* be disconcerned?) Priests had separate tests. (How did the victim respond to prayer, to the display of the Cross?) In most instances, religious and medical experts seem to have concurred.

But not always. In London in 1602, Mary Glover fell sick with fits, and Elizabeth Jackson, a charwoman, was accused of betwitching her. In testimony before the court, the physician, Edward Jorden (1569–1632), contended that the disorder was organic. Puritan counter-witnesses protested this was a cause of demonism, a view upheld by the judge, Sir Edmund Anderson (1530–1605), a noted hammer of witches. In response, Jorden published his *The Suffocation of the Mother* (1603), arguing that the accepted signs of possession were generally produced by the somatic disease called 'the Mother', or hysteria.

Jorden did not deny the reality of demonism. Nor did this case prove a clear-cut contest between medical and religious opinion. Other medical witnesses contradicted Jorden; but he was supported, in turn, by eminent pillars of the Church of England. For it was the policy of the bishops to champion essentially naturalistic readings in such cases. Catholics contended for true possession, since that vindicated their favoured recourse to exorcism; Puritans too, for they aimed to promote fastings and prayer. Countering both of these, Anglican authorities argued for disease.

In the long run, governments, church establishments and ruling élites Europe-wide, terrified by the anarchistic tendencies of the witch-craze, 'medicalized' demonism and possession, often dismissing them as cases of fraud or hysteria. Indeed, in the rationalist atmosphere of the Enlightenment, belief in diabolic powers was itself increasingly stigmatized as ignorant, superstitious, or psychopathological. This raises the question of religious insanity.

RELIGIOUS MADNESS

The key to the explanatory programme of Greek medicine is sometimes said to lie in the Hippocratic contention that the 'sacred disease' was not – contrary to traditional belief – a form of divine seizure but, despite its extraordinary manifestations, as natural as any other affliction: epilepsy. Greek medicine thus created the paradigm for treating insanity as somatic in aetiology: mania was due to an excess of choler; melancholy, of black bile; such imbalances in turn creating disturbances of the passions. Medieval and Renaissance Galenism upheld such organic theories of insanity. yet, all the while, and with abundant Biblical authority, from the fate of Nebuchadnezzar II (c.630–562 BC) through to New Testament demoniacs, the Christian churches also reinstated supernatural theories of insanity. On the one hand, madness could, albeit rarely, be divine, in the person of the holy fool, seer, or prophet, who might in his ecstasies receive the word of God or be vouchsafed visions. But, and far more commonly, delirium could be the mark of demonic possession.

Early modern specialists in insanity, such as Robert Burton (1577–1640), author of *The Anatomy of Melancholy* (1621), or Richard Napier (1559–1634), the contemporary Anglican parson-practitioner famed for his psychotherapeutic skills, endorsed both the organic and the spiritual models: individual cases needed exact diagnosis and personal treatment. Napier routinely had recourse to a package of herbal drug remedies, prayers, counsel, and, more occasionally, sigils and other quasi-magical means.[6] (➤ Ch. 43 Psychotherapy)

In subsequent centuries, eminent individuals such as William Blake (1757–1827) and Vaslav Nijinski (1890–1950) claimed to have been blessed with holy *furor*. Medical and theological opinion, however, increasingly discounted this possibility. The reality of diabolically induced insanity remained central to many religious sects. John Wesley (1703–91), the founder of Methodism, typically viewed the mad folks he encountered as satanically possessed, and conducted exorcisms to save their souls. In the great Ulster religious revival of 1859, the profound disturbances undergone by many of the gospellers' converts were interpreted, by the evangelical leaders, as marks of authentic wrestlings with the Devil.

Over the centuries, however, the medical profession increasingly set its face against the view that such transports could be due to anything preternatural. Supposed visions and voices were, after all, just delusions, due either to errors in the reasoning processes (for example, false associations of ideas) or, as was more commonly claimed, to physical lesions – above all, nervous disorders creating ocular or auricular sensory abnormalities. Indeed, often with the approval of governments and élite opinion, the emergent psychiatric profession ventured further, claiming that extreme and violent religious manifestations routinely betrayed signs of psychopathology, and were the marks of a religious lunatic fringe. (➤ Ch. 56 Psychiatry) Methodism itself was widely diagnosed as a form of insanity; and the category of 'religious madness' or 'religious monomania' became standard in asylum admissions. Even religiously oriented psychiatric hospitals, such as the Quaker Retreat at York, did not seek to treat such patients through religious means.

Heavily somatically oriented, nineteenth-century psychiatry became a branch of medicine notably cool towards Christianity. It was, of course, Sigmund Freud (1856–1939) who deemed religion either an illusion, or repressed sexual drives in their sublimated form. Other currents of modern psychodynamics, especially Jungianism, have rather chosen to emphasize the common ground linking religious and psychological consciousnesses: an endeavour supported, for example, by the Menninger Foundation at Topeka, Kansas, founded by the Presbyterian Karl A. Menninger (1893–1990).

ALTERNATIVES

This chapter has argued that regular faith and regular medicine have generally peacefully coexisted. Hospitals had their chaplains; churches have collected for medical charities. Over recent centuries, the major Christian confessions have had less to say about bodily health in general, confining themselves increasingly to the regulation of sexuality, and to related issues such as contraception and abortion.

Both pillars of orthodoxy have been challenged, however, by a series of heretical leaders and movements, critical of their professional, institutional, and monopolistic pretensions, and insistent, albeit in very diverse ways, that true faith and true health derive not from priests or doctors, but lie within the power of the individual. Their patriarch was Paracelsus (1493–1541), the 'Luther of the physicians'. A fervent Protestant, Paracelsus believed the essence of religion lay in faith, personal experience, and spirituality. Scholastic medicine was found wanting for much the same reasons as popery. It too relied upon the dry bones of authority and privilege; it was a racket, defrauding the people. In particular, Paracelsus decried Galenic medicine for its materialist, and implicitly atheistic, tendencies. Creation was pervaded with spiritual powers; humans could grasp and commandeer these through contemplation, through natural magic, and through a revitalized chemistry. Medicine itself offered a key to the spiritual understanding of being, and healing, in turn, had to be spiritualized and holistic, recognizing the interpenetration of the somatic and the spiritual.

Through the sixteenth and seventeenth centuries, Paracelsian ideas won followers in radical circles, combining variously with hermetic, astrological, alchemical, Behmenist and other spiritual and eirenical currents, and seeking to reinstate truly Christian healing. In Civil War and Interregnum England, Paracelsian reformers such as John Webster (1610–82) battled against Laudian Anglicans, College of Physicians Galenists, and orthodox Presbyterian Puritans alike, to promote the Christian reform of medicine, without success.

The triumph of the mechanical philosophy through Descartes (1596–1650), Newton (1642–1727), and their followers, on the contrary buttressed iatromechanistic models in medicine, viewing the body as a machine, and thus putting a practical medicine/religion dualism upon a new footing.

After this defeat, movements promoting the Paracelsian programme repeatedly surfaced, though relegated to the medical fringe. In his popular medical handbook, *Primitive Physick* (1747), John Wesley sought to make medicine 'a plain, intelligible thing, as it was in the Beginning', by providing simple cures bypassing the monopolistic, mystifying ramp operated by the physicians.[7]

In particular in North America – and surely in reaction to the early nineteenth-century vogue for 'heroic physic' – such health-reform causes were championed not by physicians but by lay people, disaffected equally with official creeds and regular medicine, and seeking to replace both with a unified, holistic philosophy of spiritual and bodily health, carved out of their own personal experience. Amongst such sects as the Grahamites and the Thomsonians, certain convictions have been widely shared. They have promoted a medical recension of original sin, arguing that civilized humans have brought disease upon themselves by the Fall, manifest in modern lifestyles: urbanism, greed, speed, excessive meat eating, and abuse of fermented liquor. (➤ Ch. 27 Diseases of civilization) By way of remedy, they have advocated – on grounds indistinguishably medical, moral, and religious – a return to 'natural' ways of living: vegetarianism, sexual restraint, temperance (in both its general and its specific senses), and abandonment of stimulants such as tea, coffee, and tobacco. They have generally urged an end to artificial and synthetic drugs, trusting to God-given, natural herbal remedies. Homoeopaths insisted upon ultra-pure medicaments, taken in minute quantities; Thomsonians and Coffinites restricted themselves to a few herbal preparations. Influenced by Swedenborgianism, some groups went a stage further, discarding medicines altogether, and trusting to the healing powers of Nature, aided by those of water, prayer, self-control, and spiritual illumination. (➤ Ch. 28 Unorthodox medical theories)

With its 'a plague on both your houses' attitude, the Christian Science movement exemplifies many of these features. Rejecting the strict Congregationalism of her parents, Mary Baker Eddy (1821–1910) spent much of her youth sick with non-specific nervous disorders. Regular physicians did her no good. Relieved by homoeopathy and the mesmeric treatments of Phineas Quimby (1802–66), she then undertook, a self-healing regime. Its success led her in 1866 to adumbrate her own system, whose creed declared that 'there is but one creation, and it is wholly spiritual'. Matter therefore was an illusion; hence there could be no such reality as somatic disease. As explained in her bestselling textbook, *Science and Health* (1875), true 'mind healing' would dispel the illusions of sickness and pain. Proclaiming itself the new scientific medicine of the new age, Christian Science owed its high rate of conversions to the 'patient: heal thyself' confidence it inspired.

In societies such as nineteenth-century North America, with rapid social change and beliefs in turmoil, and where orthodoxies – religious and medical – seemed irrelevant and outdated, a multitude of spiritual faiths shot up, centring upon the individual, and prizing the self-help experience of the lay person. Spiritualism and theosophy won followers. From their early days, both the Mormons and the Seventh Day Adventists voiced their antipathy to regular medicine, Joseph Smith (1805–44) recognizing only roots and herbs, and the Mormons, once in Utah, passing laws restricting the dispensing of most orthodox remedies ('deadly poisons'). Mormons, in particular, championed the constitutional right to resist compulsory smallpox vaccination. Growing out of the Millerite religious- and health-reform movement, with its emphasis upon abstemiousness and vegetarianism, the Adventists, led by Ellen White (1826–1915), proclaimed a 'gospel of health', which particularly valued hydropathic cures. (➤ Ch. 40 Physical methods) Their Health Reform Institute at Battle Creek, Michigan, was headed by John Harvey Kellogg (1852–1943), brother of the cereal manufacturer.

SECULARIZATION

The modern rise of irreligion has many sources. It is often suggested that highly rationalized and bureaucratized churches have helped dig their own graves by abandoning the miraculous aspects of revealed and scriptural Christianity. The rationalizing tendency has certainly been present amongst mainstream Christians over the last few centuries.

The scriptures present a multitude of events that defy natural assumptions about the body and its workings: raisings from the dead, miracle cures, healing by touch, supernatural afflictions, voices and visions, the remarkable longevity of the patriarchs, to say nothing of a talking snake. The Fathers and subsequent theologians added more, not least the virgin birth. Medieval pastoral religion embraced multitudes of popular practices designed to protect health and banish disease.

Hostile to the Catholic theology of 'works' and to what it denounced as popular paganism, the Protestant Reformation energetically embarked upon purging 'magic' and 'superstition', not least the efficacious thaumaturgical properties of the sacraments. Embrasing this outlook, Protestantism teamed up with the rationalism of the new science and with medical materialism, to demystify the wonders of the body and associated magical healing claims. Thus when, at the Restoration, Valentine Greatrakes, the Irish stroker, performed his healing ministry, such pious Christians as Robert Boyle (1627–91) discounted the possibility that the cures were preternatural (faith in these would only reflect ill upon the faith), preferring to conceptualize Greatrakes's healing in terms of the forces of particles set in motion by the laying-on of hands. Within fifty years, the English monarchy had abandoned its own theocratic privilege of 'touching for the king's evil'.

Similar changes surrounded reassessments of suicide. Traditionally, the churches regarded self-inflicted death as a mortal sin. Certainly in England, and probably elsewhere, doctors, public opinion, and ecclesiastics during the 'long eighteenth century' increasingly came round to the view that self-slaughter was typically, almost *definitionally*, committed in a state of mental imbalance, and so escaped the condemnation of sin and vice. Suicide was thus removed from the religious sphere; such medicalization actually suited the mood of a more pelagian theology. Likewise, faced with convulsionaries, eighteenth-century clergy, no less than scoffers, sought medico-pathological reasons to explain away so-called miracles or demonic manifestations. Nowadays, when faced with supposed cases of demoniacal possession, most Protestant churches advocate psychiatric counselling. The dilemmas posed by supernaturalism surface in their most acute form against Christian congregations in Third World countries, where many believers expect to find providential causes and cures for sickness, whereas their Western-educated ministers look to germs and antibiotics. (➤ Ch. 29 Non-Western concepts of disease)

This retreat from holy healing may appear a classic case of the *trahaison des clercs*, desacralizing theologians who have seemingly sold their birthright for a mess of pottage. (There is a nice irony in the fact that whereas, at their foundation, the Seventh Day Adventists were antipathetic to regular medicine, by 1984 the first implantation of a baboon heart into a human (Baby Fae) was performed in an Adventist hospital.) Yet it cannot be denied that circumstances have worked against the churches. When disease was rampant, and medicine incompetent to stay the Grim Reaper, the bleak Augustinian vision of the world as a hospital, and sickness as largely self-inflicted made eminent sense. Christianity did not mask these realities. Rather, it provided rituals enabling them to be borne. Confronting death, the man familiar with the *ars moriendi*, the art of dying well, would squarely confront his Maker, denounce the Devil and all his works, fervently pray, knowing he was but in the antechamber of life proper.

Things changed. From the eighteenth century, the development of narcotics – above all, opiates – increasingly permitted deathbeds to be tranquillized, sedated, relatively pain-free. (➤ Ch. 67 Pain and suffering) The comatose patient no longer acted out the histrionics of the good death. Increasingly, the quiet death was preferred, a peaceful falling asleep. The nineteenth-century minister, falling in with the family, developed new ways of orchestrating this 'beautiful' departure. Since Vatican Two, no longer are Catholic funerals accompanied by the *Dies irae*, with its agonized plea for deliverance 'from everlasting death on that day of terror'.

More generally, as life expectations have risen, and medicine has reduced suffering and the risk of being suddenly, unexpectedly, snatched from the world, the old consolatory role of Christianity has correspondingly diminished. And with it the traditional conviction, often expressed by clergy, that disease and pain were positively beneficial. As late as the mid-nineteenth century, it was not unusual for preachers to follow Paul and commend the virtues of the 'thorn in the flesh'. The great Victorian Baptist evangelist, Charles Haddon Spurgeon (1834–92), was convinced that 'the greatest earthly blessing that God can give to any of us is health, with the exception of sickness.... A sick wife, a newly made grave, poverty, slander, sinking of spirit, might teach us lessons nowhere else to be learned so well.'[8] This 'sweet are the uses of adversity' view, however, appeared perverse and, we might say, sick to that noble Victorian invalid Harriet Martineau (1802–76). In her *Life in the Sickroom* (1844), she condemned such views as mawkish: true religion should be healthy-minded.[9] Later theologians have mainly cast their vote on Martineau's side.

In doing so, they have swum with the tide of the twentieth century. Lives have grown lengthier, safer, less racked with pain; worldly blessings have increased. Yet not without costs. As Ivan Illich, amongst others, has noted, the higher the expectations of health, fitness, beauty, longevity, and physical fulfilment, the greater the stigmas of being sick, ugly, old, and disabled, and the less easy it is to face death: death, indeed, has become the 'new pornography'.[10] And if medicalized death in the terminal ward is free of the terrors of hellfire, it is also devoid of consolation. It is significant that, given scientific medicine's inability to give any meaning, and maybe any dignity, to dying, the hospice movement has arisen, as an essentially Christian framework to cope with our going out.

And all the while, from the mid-twentieth century, the star of such charismatic American evangelical preachers as Oral Roberts (b. 1918), with their much-ballyhooed healing mission, was rising. In 1978, the Pentecostalists established their $150 million City of Faith Medical and Research Center in Tulsa. At a time when it appeared that the established churches had opted out of their healing role, and were perhaps committing euthanasia in the process, the instinct for grander meanings denied by the disenchanted world and its interpreters reasserted itself.

NOTES

1   Thomas Browne, *Religio Medici and Other Works*, ed. by L. C. Martin, Oxford, Oxford University Press, 1964; orig. pub. 1642.

2   See Martha Carlin, 'Medieval English hospitals', in L. Granshaw and Roy Porter
    (eds), *The Hospital in History*, London, Routledge, 1989, pp. 21–40; Miri Rubin,
    'Development and change in English hospitals', ibid., pp. 41–60; John Hender-
    son, 'The hospitals of late-medieval renaissance Florence: a preliminary survey',
    ibid., pp. 63–92.

3   Colin Jones, *The Charitable Imperative: Hospitals and Nursing in Ancien Régime and
    Revolutionary France*, London, Routledge, 1989.

4   See Carlo Cipolla, *Faith, Reason and the Plague*, Brighton, Harvester, 1979.

5   Quoted in Richard Palmer, 'The church, leprosy and the plague in medieval
    and early modern Europe', in W. J. Sheils (ed.), *The Church and Healing*, Oxford,
    Basil Blackwell, 1982, pp. 79–100; see. p. 97.

6   See M. MacDonald, *Mystical Bedlam: Madness, Anxiety and Healing in Seventeenth-
    Century England*, Cambridge, Cambridge University Press, 1981.

7   J. Wesley, *Primitive Physick*, London, T. Trye, 1747.

8   Quoted in Timothy P. Weber, 'The Baptist tradition', in Ronald L. Numbers
    and Darrel W. Amundsen (eds), *Caring and Curing. Health and Medicine in the
    Western Medical Traditions*, New York, Macmillan, 1986, pp. 288–316; see p. 291.

9   H. Martineau, *Life in the Sick Room: Essays by an Invalid*, 2nd edn, London,
    Moxan, 1854.

10 Ivan Illich, *Limits to Medicine: the Expropriation of Health*, Harmondsworth, Pen-
    guin, 1977.

FURTHER READING

Two valuable collections first:

Numbers, Ronald L. and Amundsen, Darrel W. (eds), *Caring and Curing. Health and
    Medicine in the Western Medical Traditions*, New York, Macmillan, 1986. (An invalu-
    able volume, containing essays on all major Christian traditions).

Sheils, W. J. (ed.), *The Church and Healing*, Oxford, Basil Blackwell (for the Ecclesiasti-
    cal History Society), 1982. A major collection of essays, which includes the follow-
    ing: Richard Palmer, 'The church, leprosy and the plague in medieval and early
    modern Europe', pp. 79–100; Henry D. Rack, 'Doctors, demons and early Method-
    ist healing', pp. 137–52; J. V. Pickstone, 'Establishment and Dissent in nineteenth-
    century medicine: an exploration of some correspondences and connexions between
    religious and medical belief-systems in early industrial England', pp. 165–90; Logie
    Barrow, 'Anti-establishment healing: spiritualism in Britain', pp. 225–48; Terence
    Ranger, 'Medical science and Pentecost: the dilemma of Anglicanism in Africa',
    pp. 333–66.

OTHER RELEVANT BOOKS

Ariès, Philippe, *Western Attitudes Towards Death: from the Middle Ages to the Present*,
    Baltimore, MD, Johns Hopkins University Press, 1974; London, Marion Boyars,
    1976.

Brody, Saul Nathaniel, *The Disease of the Soul: Leprosy in Medieval Literature*, Ithaca,
    NY, Cornell University Press, 1974.

Brown, Peter, *The Body and Society: Men, Women and Sexual Renunciation in Early Christianity*, New York, Columbia University Press, 1988.

Browne, Thomas, *Religio Medici and Other Works*, ed. by L. C. Martin, Oxford, Oxford University Press, 1964.

Bynum, W. F. and Porter, Roy (eds), *Medical Fringe and Medical Orthodoxy, 1750–1850*, London, Croom Helm, 1987.

Camporesi, P., *The Incorruptible Flesh: Bodily Mutation and Mortification in Religion and Folklore*, Cambridge, Cambridge University Press, 1988.

Cipolla, Carlo, *Faith, Reason and the Plague*, Brighton, Harvester, 1979.

Cooter, R. (ed.), *Studies in the History of Alternative Medicine*, London, Macmillan, 1988.

Curl, J. S., *The Victorian Celebration of Death*, Newton Abbot, David & Charles, 1972.

Donat, J., 'Medicine and religion: on the physical and mental disorders that accompanied the Ulster revival of 1859', in W. F. Bynum, Roy Porter and Michael Shepherd (eds), *Anatomy of Madness*, London, Routledge, 1988, Vol. III, pp. 125–50.

Doob, Penelope E. R., *Nebuchadnezzar's Children: Conventions of Madness in Middle English Literature*, New Haven, CT, and London, Yale University Press, 1974.

Elmer, Peter, 'Medicine, religion and the Puritan Revolution', in Roger French and Andrew Wear (eds), *The Medical Revolution of the Seventeenth Century*, Cambridge, Cambridge University Press, 1989, pp. 10–45.

Gevitz, N. (ed.), *Other Healers. Unorthodox Medicine in America*, Baltimore, MD, Johns Hopkins University Press, 1988.

Granshaw, L. and Porter, Roy (eds), *The Hospital in History*, London, Routledge, 1989 (contains four relevant essays: Martha Carlin, 'Medieval English hospitals', pp. 21–40; Miri Rubin, 'Development and change in English hospitals', pp. 41–60; John Henderson, 'The hospitals of late-medieval and renaissance Florence: a preliminary survey', pp. 63–92; Roy Porter, 'The gift relation: philanthropy and provincial hospitals in eighteenth-century England', pp. 149–78).

Hill, A. W., *John Wesley Among the Physicians*, London, Epworth Press, 1958.

Illich, Ivan, *Limits to Medicine: the Expropriation of Health*, Harmondsworth, Penguin, 1977.

Inglis, Brian, *Natural and Supernatural*, London, Hodder & Stoughton, 1977.

Jones, Colin, *The Charitable Imperative: Hospitals and Nursing in Ancien Régime and Revolutionary France*, London, Routledge, 1989.

MacDonald, M., *Mystical Bedlam: Madness, Anxiety and Healing in Seventeenth-Century England*, Cambridge, Cambridge University Press, 1981.

——, 'The secularization of sucide in England, 1660–1800', *Past and Present*, 1986, 111: 50–100.

Martineau, H., *Life in the Sick-Room: Essays by an Invalid*, 2nd edn, London, Moxon, 1854.

Porter, Roy, 'Medicine and religion in eighteenth-century England: a case of conflict', *Ideas and Production*, 1987, 7: 4–17.

——, *Mind forg'd Manacles: Madness and Psychiatry in England from Restoration to Regency*, London, Athlone Press, 1987.

—— and Porter, Dorothy, *In Sickness and in Health: the British Experience 1650–1850*, London, Fourth Estate, 1988.

——, 'Death and the doctors in Georgian England', in R. Houlbrooke (ed.), *Death, Ritual and Bereavement*, London, Routledge, 1989, pp. 77–94.

Randi, James, *The Faith Healers*, London, Prometheus Books, 1989.

Slack, Paul, *The Impact of Plague in Tudor and Stuart England*, London, Routledge & Kegan Paul, 1985.

Stannard, D. E., *The Puritan Way of Death: a Study in Religion, Culture and Social Change*, New York and Oxford, Oxford University Press, 1977.

Thomas, K. V., *Religion and the Decline of Magic: Studies in Popular Beliefs in Sixteenth- and Seventeenth-Century England*, London, Weidenfeld & Nicolson, 1971; reprinted Harmondsworth and New York, Penguin, 1978.

Walker, D. P., *Unclean Spirits*, London, Scolar Press, 1980.

Wear, A., 'Puritan perceptions of illness in seventeenth-century England', in Roy Porter (ed.), *Patients and Practitioners*, Cambridge, Cambridge University Press, 1985, pp. 55–99.

Webster, C., *The Great Instauration*, London, Duckworth, 1975.

62

CHARITY BEFORE *c.*1850

Colin Jones

INTRODUCTION

The history of charity is often written in terms of three allegedly dichotomous relationships. First, Christian charity is counter-poised against non-Christian indifference to charitable activity, with it being assumed that charity is a highly specific and exclusive social and affective practice marking Christianity out from other world religions and ideological formations. Second, Christian voluntarism is contrasted with secular compulsion: it is held that the habits of voluntary giving so strong within the Christian – and particularly Roman Catholic – traditions contrast with a degree of state-driven compulsion in modern welfare states. Third, a dichotomy is posited between charitable 'caring' and secular 'curing': the rise of Western scientific medicine and its associated therapies are held to replace a tradition of caritative concern which had little or no specifically medical content. A great deal of research from the 1960s onwards on the history of charity has, however, highlighted how misleading all those dichotomous relationships are and emphasized the need for subtler and more nuanced conceptual frameworks for charting the historical links between medicine and charity in the period down to 1850.

It is certainly true that Christianity has always tended to follow the doctrinal cues of its founder, and to be associated with a high prioritization of charitable rhetoric and values, and an impressive range of caring activities. However, the assumption that charitable activities are quintessentially and exclusively Christian, and that the story of charity is thus the chronicle of Christian piety, is erroneous. Medieval hospitals, for example, which are often seen as an archetypal expression of a Christian Age of Faith, were paralleled by similar institutions in Islamic society, and indeed the Islamic hospital tradition may have influenced Christian institutions. Moreover, charitable institutions have habitually had social as well as religious objectives. Hospitals, the most enduring institutional form of religiously motivated charity, have also been a means whereby the wealthy could give to – and thereby control and dominate – the poor. (➤ Ch. 31 Arab-Islamic medicine; Ch. 49 The hospital; Ch. 61 Religion and medicine)

The putative dichotomy as regards charitable motivation, between Christian voluntarism in the field of health care and the element of compulsion and obligation inherent in modern welfare-state systems, is also shown to be ill-founded by much recent research. In the confessional states prevalent in medieval and early modern Europe, for example, where the spiritual and temporal influence of the church was strong, there was often, as I have argued elsewhere, a kind of 'charitable imperative' in place, which imposed significant pressures of social and moral conformity as well as religious orthodoxy on the faithful and impelled them towards charitable activity. Similarly, though many historians assume a long-term linear passage 'from charity to state welfare', with the rise of state welfare systems from the late nineteenth century onwards predicated on the putative decline and inadequacy of traditional Christian charity, recent research has underlined the vitality of the charitable impulse in industrial and post-industrial societies.

Third, the tendency to dichotomize 'caring' from 'curing' – with the charitable allegedly specializing in the former, scientific physicians (portrayed as indifferent or even hostile towards organized religion) in the latter – is similarly lacking in historical foundation. The dichotomy rests on Whiggish assumptions about the course of scientific advance, with 'medicine' essentially comprising 'What (usually male) Doctors Do'. When set within the context of the broad range of health-care provision of very different sorts of societies in the past in Europe and beyond, such assumptions achieve the not-inconsiderable feat of being at once doctor centred, ethnocentric, classist and sexist! Historians are increasingly sensitive to 'unlicensed medicine', including the medical activities and interests of the religiously motivated in monasteries, hospitals, and among the rural poor. They also recognize that medical practitioners have not invariably been anti-clerical or religiously indifferent. (➤ Ch. 4 Medical care)

MEDIEVAL CHARITY (TO THE BLACK DEATH)

The esteem of early Christians for charity owed much to the value attached to the virtue by their founder. The Works of Mercy (food for the hungry, drink for the thirsty, shelter for the homeless, clothing for the needy, visiting the sick and prisoners, burying the dead), outlined in Christ's own words in the Gospel, provided a charitable template for successive generations. From earliest times, as a result of the quasi-identification with them that Christ assumed in the Incarnation, paupers were singled out for special concern. This, moreoever, included care for health: Christ had used his healing powers over the body as well as the spirit of the afflicted.

In the early church, appointed officials of both sexes within each Christian community – deacons and deaconesses, working under the bishop – distributed alms to the needy and visited the sick; and from the fourth century, hospitals were established in the Eastern Empire. Many of the forms of this programme had antecedents and parallels in non-Christian environments: the Jews had always set great store by bodily health and concern for community members; the Greeks' houses of healing (known as temples of Asclepius) in some ways resembled early Christian hospitals; and the Roman army could boast military infirmaries and a system of health provision. The high priority accorded charity was new, however, and even pagan writers remarked on the particular concern that early Christians attached to these endeavours, viewing Christianity as a 'religion of healing' *par excellence.*

These charitable forms were considerably strengthened by Christianity's passage in the fourth century from obscure Jewish sect to orthodox cult of the Roman Empire. They survived the fall of that empire too in ways reflected by the different trajectories followed by hospitals in Western and in Eastern Christendom. In the East, a very wide range of hospital types continued to exist – hospitals for the sick, but also orphanages, old peoples' homes, centres for the blind, and so on – and the continued importance of urban centres permitted a lay medical profession to be available to staff hospitals and visit the sick poor. In the West, in contrast, urban decay after the fall of the Roman Empire reduced the vitality of medical professions, and hospitals were less functionally differentiated and less medically oriented.

In the West, medical care for the sick under the auspices of charity came increasingly to be focused on ecclesiastics with an interest in health care, notably in monasteries and under the authority of the bishops. The most common institution, the *xenodochium* (the term *hospitale* came to be used from the eighth and ninth centuries) offered board, lodging, and care for travellers and most varieties of the sick and decrepit. Hospitals retained this character throughout the Middle Ages, and even related institutions devoted to the segregation of lepers offered little in the way of specifically medical care. Formal medical knowledge survived in monasteries, which were repositories of the medical manuscripts of Antiquity: monastic infirmaries might be staffed by monks who read classical medical texts, perhaps adulterating them with folkloric remedies and spiritual healing.

The Western church in the Middle Ages accommodated medicine and theology, and was less hostile to medical intervention than is often claimed. The theological positions that emphasized the equation between sickness and sin, that valued bodily asceticism and self-abnegation, and which held that cure could only come from God, sat comfortably alongside a belief in the efficacy of human agency in care of health under divine grace. Regulated and refined in conciliar rulings, a tradition of *medicina clericalis* emerged. Any practitioner of medicine was to ensure a sick person had received confession before undertaking treatment. No ecclesiastic in holy orders was to engage in surgery, which involved the spilling of blood and whose effects might cast responsibility for death on the church. Ecclesiastics were enjoined to practise only if they were medically competent, kept up with medical knowledge, and consulted colleagues. They were not to harm patients through negligence, nor by experiments. The administration of medicine was to be viewed essentially as a charitable act and should not occasion personal enrichment. (➤ Ch. 37 History of medical ethics; Ch. 47 History of the medical profession)

Personal sanctity offered no armour-plating against contracting disease, and it was inevitable that the sick should be keen to achieve bodily health by any means clergy or physicians could offer. The latter were, however, few on the ground, while the former enjoyed prestige for healing powers. To a considerable extent, the Christianization of Europe had been grounded in the healing powers of the church – most clearly through the cults of saints and relics. Moreover, the emergence of lay brotherhoods in the numerous hospitals created in the course of the thirteenth and fourteenth centuries considerably expanded the parameters of ecclesiastical medical care. A degree of functional differentiation began to emerge in the dense network of institutions that developed throughout Western Christendom. Alongside the *hospitale*, there emerged institutions for abandoned children, the aged, repentant prostitutes, the blind, the insane, and so on. Medieval hospitals were often staffed by nursing communities, the most celebrated of which were international organizations such as the Hospitallers of Saint John of Jerusalem (*c.*1108), the Order of the Holy Spirit (1145) and (notably for lepers) the Order of Saint Lazarus (*c.*1120). Their activities were complemented by voluntary associations of the pious under the influence of Franciscan spirituality, such as the Beghards and Béguines in the Low Countries, as well as religious confraternities in Italian cities, both groups providing a variety of caring services. Some hospitals, especially in more-urbanized areas such as north Italy, received care from lay physicians. Yet this was still only exceptional, and overall throughout the Middle Ages, medically minded ecclesiastics and groupings of the pious far outnumbered lay medical practitioners in the provision of health care.

The growing profusion of ecclesiastical regulation in the domain of medical practice highlights the fact that, in the expanding urban economy of the High Middle Ages, medicine had again become a lay profession in the West. The emergence of the medical professions – university-trained physicians, guilds of surgeons and apothecaries, all putatively monopolistic in their branch of the trade and all enjoying privileges grounded in public law – was a major limiting factor on ecclesiastical medicine. In order to prevent interprofessional boundary disputes, *medicina clericalis* increasingly confined itself to charitable treatment of the poor and those beyond physical reach of town-based physicians. A rough and ready *modus vivendi* emerged between the two professions. When the Black Death hit Avignon in 1348, for example, Clement VI (Pope, 1342–52), resident in the city, encouraged the clergy's ministrations to the sick and ordered processions of public penance; but he also hired physicians to cope with the sick. Medical charity was routed through the medical professions; it did not seek to bypass them.

REFORMATION, COUNTER-REFORMATION, AND CONFINEMENT OF THE POOR (SIXTEENTH AND SEVENTEENTH CENTURIES)

The bifurcation of Western Christendom in the Reformation caused perhaps less of an impact on the charitable performance of different societies than might appear likely. Reformation thinkers, following Martin Luther (1483–1546), tended to shun 'good works' in favour of 'justification by faith', while some Protestant reforms – such as the dissolution of the monasteries in Henrician England – had an important impact on the availability of charity. Yet in broad terms, the social policies of both Catholic and Protestant societies were surprisingly similar. Both Protestant and Catholic zealots sought to activate a 'reformation of manners' – to achieve through a mixture of social discipline and proselytizing uplift a more docile and religiously orthodox laity. Throughout Europe, especially after the 1510s and 1520s, poor laws were reframed: sturdy beggars were chastized, the 'deserving poor' (especially the aged, the infirm, and defenceless children) were aided, and rationalization of charitable institutions achieved. The pauper, whose image in the Middle Ages had attained the aura of holy poverty, was refurbished in altogether more sinister guise as the godless, shiftless, and work-shy beggar who had to be whipped into line. The charity of the faithful had now, it was stressed, to be canalized away from indiscriminate almsgiving to such characters and towards approved centres of public assistance and social discipline.

It is tempting to see this important change in patterns of charitable giving as a response to the social problems associated with urbanization, the development of commercial capitalism, and the decline of feudalism. Popular revolt sometimes pushed ruling élites into major poor-relief reorganization; while the appearance of syphilis from the 1490s stimulated a number of initiatives, such as the *incurabili* hospitals which grew up in most Italian cities. However, the reform of poor relief owed much, too, to changes within the social and political élite. The growth of city governments from the late Middle Ages had already, for example, led to a greater degree of secular control over charitable institutions. New forms of charitable provision were often sponsored by emerging fractions of the élite – notably the mercantile classes – who saw in poor relief a means of symbolically marking their own raised social status, establishing patronage networks, and shaping provision to benefit their own material and political interests. Charity has often been an arena for power-struggles between rival fractions of the élite, and new poor relief policies were, in this period as in others, often as much about dispute between charitable donors as about pressure from below.

Throughout the early modern period, the model of charitable rationalization outlined in the early sixteenth century was never wholly successfully implemented for lengthy periods. Some obstacles were religious and attitudinal. Resistance to the prohibition on manual almsgiving to the visibly needy in face-to-face encounters was always tenacious. The policing and bureaucratic powers of the early modern state were limited too. The political context also needed to be right for these measures to stand a chance of working. Political instability and civil turbulence were recipes for failure. The spate of poor-law reform in the early sixteenth century in France, for example, was disrupted by the political turmoil of the Wars of Religion (1561–98), and it was only in the early seventeenth century that the socio-political context was right for reform to be taken up again.

The strengthening of the state over the course of the seventeenth and eighteenth centuries also favoured the attempted implementation of new poor-law methods. England's Elizabethan poor laws, based on a system of parish relief, were essentially in place by 1601; a similar system was adapted in the Netherlands down to the early seventeenth century; some Italian states, and then, from the 1620s, France, began a new wave of charitable reform, one of whose most striking features was the institutionalization of needy and incorrigible beggars in what were called 'general hospitals'. This direction of social policy reached its most celebrated heights in France during the reign of Louis XIV (r. 1643–1715) where a royal edict of 1656 established the Paris *Hôpital général*, and where over one hundred such institutions were created in subsequent decades, containing an inmate population soon in excess of 100,000 individuals. This shift in charitable forms and priorities in the sixteenth and seventeenth centuries made confinement the preferred mode of poor relief for a century or more. Yet the new 'general hospital' was less of a medical institution than its name suggests. Most were a mixture of orphanage and old peoples' home rather than clinical institutions.

Furthermore, although the medical professions now had all the trappings of corporative entities, their interest in charitable provision for the poor was more limited in many respects than the clergy's. The Catholic clergy in particular, revitalized and professionalized through the reforms of the Council of Trent, placed a new emphasis on the education and moralization of the poor. Although they were in theory forbidden to engage in any secular occupation, including medicine, in practice the emphasis on nurturing the spiritual and physical welfare of the laity proved a backdoor entrance for the post-Tridentine clergy into medical practice. Parish clergy increasingly engaged in physical as well as spiritual first aid on their parishioners. Indeed, an Italian manual for parish priests in 1745 even contained suggestions on how best to perform a Caesarean operation!

Pastoral commitment of the post-Tridentine clergy was the spawning-ground of one of the most remarkable initiatives in the tradition of *medicina clericalis*, namely the creation of nursing communities. A few of these were masculine, notably the Brothers of Saint John of God, or Brothers of Charity, founded in Spain in 1537, who came to specialize in institutionalized care for the insane and in sophisticated surgical practice throughout Europe. Most nursing communities were, however, female. The Daughters of Charity, established by Saints Vincent de Paul (1581–1660) and Louise de Marillac (1591–1660) in Paris in 1633, were strong-backed country women who acted as charitable intermediaries for the wealthy, and provided professional levels of patient care within the growing numbers of Europe's hospitals. Freed (unlike their medieval nursing forebears) from the confines of the cloister, they also renewed the traditions of home visiting and care for prisoners. Organized centrally and bureaucratically efficient, the Daughters of Charity constituted the prototype of numerous similar female communities that proliferated, especially in France, in the late seventeenth and early eighteenth centuries. Trained by apprenticeship and armed with only the (usually outdated) rudiments of medical theory, such women nevertheless provided more sophisticated pharmaceutical care and the elements of medical and surgical care for the vast numbers of paupers who passed through the social institutions of Counter-Reformation Europe.

The tradition of *medicina clericalis* was, moreover, particularly strong in the extra-European world. Female nursing communities on the model of the Daughters of Charity were established in Canada from the mid-seventeenth century. Male missionary orders also played a role, partly perhaps because the efficacious practice of medicine was viewed as a means of converting unbelievers as well as of succouring one's neighbour. Thus the Jesuits received permission in 1641 to practise medicine, provided that they only practised where no physicians were available, performed no surgery, and worked out of charity rather than a spirit of enrichment. Other missionary orders, such as the Lazarists in Madagascar, and Franciscans, Dominicans, and Brothers of Charity in the Spanish American colonies, also assumed medical functions. (➤ Ch. 58 Medicine and colonialism)

ENLIGHTENMENT AND PHILANTHROPY (EIGHTEENTH AND EARLY NINETEENTH CENTURIES)

The framework of charitably orientated medicine established by Reformation and Counter-Reformation militants lasted well into the eighteenth century. Indeed, the number of hospitals and religiously inspired nurses operating in the arena of medical charity was probably higher towards the end of the eighteenth century than at any previous time. Voltaire (1694–1774), Diderot (1713–84), and other anti-clerical writers might mock the contemplative orders, but they had nothing but praise for the charitable activism of the Daughters of Charity. The parish clergy too, both Protestant and Catholic, were frequently eulogized for their commitment to the welfare of their parishioners, and a number of rulers toyed with schemes to make them frontline agents of primary health care. This role was based on their skills in lay medicine rather than in spiritual healing. The latter was increasingly depreciated, even within the churches, in this period of growing rationalism and materialism. Indeed, the professionalized clergy were often in the vanguard of attempts to expunge 'superstitious' popular healing beliefs. The medieval practice of the monarchs of France and England 'touching for the king's evil' (scrofula) fell into disrepute and disuse.

There continued to be a good deal of parallelism in the charitable responses of both Catholic and Protestant states and communities. Indeed, there was a greater degree of reciprocal borrowing across the confessional divide than at any time since the Reformation. The order of nursing deaconesses established by the German Lutheran community at Kaiserwerth in the 1820s, for example, owed a great deal to the institutional example of the Daughters of Charity, and Florence Nightingale (1820–1910) and other nursing reformers of the mid-nineteenth century looked to both sources of inspiration. (➤ Ch. 54 A general history of nursing: 1800–1900) The revival of hospital and prison visiting instigated in England by Elizabeth Fry (1780–1845) similarly could be viewed as a Protestant imitation of established Catholic practice. The institutional cross-over worked both ways, moreover: when pre-Revolutionary France set about reforming its hospitals, it specifically tried to learn from English experience; the pavilion-style architecture of the Plymouth naval hospital was widely imitated throughout continental Europe and the New World in the nineteenth century. (➤ Ch. 64 Medicine and architecture)

Religious élites continued to make a considerable input into charitable foundations, though as always it is difficult to disentangle religious commitment from civic pride, personal aggrandizement, social fear, and other more mundane motivations. The spate of new charitable establishments in eighteenth-century England, for example, owed much to the local role of the 'godly': over a score of provincial infirmaries were created between 1736 and 1779; new dispensaries complemented their activity in most major provincial centres; and more specialized institutions (fever hospitals, lying-in hospitals, orphanages, asylums, etc.) highlighted the vitality of the charitable instinct. Significant in this respect too was the foundation in Paris in 1833 by Frédéric Ozanam (1813–53) of the Society of Saint-Vincent-de-Paul. Dedicated to an ideal of mobilizing the Catholic laity in the service of the poor through direct and face-to-face contact and assistance, the society spread throughout the Catholic world and provided a revitalized form of Catholic charitable commitment.

If religious motivation remained strong, the charitably minded had increasingly to accommodate inroads into their institutions from two directions: the state and the medical profession. Most states in Enlightenment Europe sought to extend their regulation and control over poor-relief provision. In the eighteenth century, enlightened absolutists prided themselves on their efforts in this sphere. Joseph II (r. 1765–90) of Austria, for example, closed contemplative monasteries in a campaign to shift charity towards more socially useful objectives, and reformed the Vienna hospitals wholesale. The efforts of the French state were even more far-reaching. Even before 1789, the Government had reduced the autonomy of charitable foundations, including hospitals. After 1789, it went further, as Revolutionary assemblies strove to establish a kind of 'welfare state' based on state pensions financed partly from the closure of supernumerary and newly nationalized hospitals. These efforts were accompanied by an anti-clerical attack on nursing communities, which were formally abolished. These efforts fell foul of rampaging inflation and political instablility, and by the late 1790s, the French state was engaging in a spectacular U-turn in its social policy. (➤ Ch. 50 Medical insitutions and the state)

The Revolutionary decade caused immense harm to the fabric of charitable institutions not only in France, but also in those neighbouring regions which France had militarily occupied in these years (the Low Countries, western Germany, north-west Italy). As a result, greater state intervention seemed essential. It would be wrong to imagine, however, that this necessarily signified a reduction in the role of private voluntaristic efforts. States tended to extend their welfare commitments by legislating into existence welfare requirements, provision of which was often left to private bodies, and by propping up rather than by replacing existing charitable bodies. The post-Revolutionary state in France, for example, permitted poor-relief institutions to reacquire their patrimony, stimulated the charity of the faithful, and permitted the Daughters of Charity and their ilk to re-form and recruit. The early nineteenth century was to see a remarkable efflorescence of female charitable and teaching communities on this model, whose role in the provision of care was immense. In the 1850s, two-thirds of France's hospital pharmacies were staffed and run by such female communities. Though their salary levels and conditions of service were increasingly regulated by the state, they retained the aura and the legal status of charitable bodies. These nursing communities became truly worldwide in their coverage. Numerous European states besides France saw the establishment of such bodies; Protestant analogues evolved; missionary efforts took religious nurses throughout the colonized world; and the foundation of the Sisters of Charity by Elizabeth Bayley Seton (1774–1821) in Emmitsburg, Maryland, in 1809, was the beginning of important developments on the North American continent. (➤ Ch. 38 Women and medicine)

If state intervention increasingly affected and regulated the activities of charities, the growing prestige of the medical profession was another factor limiting the free expression of the charitable impulse. It was in the eighteenth century that, mainly due to the growth of interest in clinical medicine, bedside observation and 'hands-on' teaching methods, the medical professions began to take a greater interest in having access to the bodies of the poor, most noticeably in hospitals. (➤ Ch. 48 Medical education) Whereas the post of hospital doctor had often in the past been a sign of gentility and benevolence, it came increasingly to be seen as a career desideratum and as a prerequisite for research. Moreover, the proven, if limited, efficacy of medicine made the presence of medical practitioners even more desirable than in the past. Scientific studies of nutrition throughout Europe and the New World, for example – witnessed in experiments on infant feeding patterns designed to reduce perinatal mortality, and on 'economic' or 'Rumford soups' for adult paupers – increased the prestige of medical practitioners within hospitals and in other charitable organizations. (➤ Ch. 45 Childhood)

These developments upset established patterns of territoriality within the hospital: doctors and charitably inspired nurses had to work out – often painfully – a new *modus vivendi*. Hospital management and charitable managers also had to defer to medical opinion where once they had condescended. Medicine and poor relief had, as we have seen, been intimately connected from earliest times. By 1850, the construction of the 'patient' – a sick person, not just a pauper suffering from infirmity, in the hands of a clinician rather than a charitably minded gentleman-doctor or religious activist – was well on the road to being effected. (➤ Ch. 63 Medical philanthropy after 1850)

FURTHER READING

Amundsen, D. W. and Numbers, R. L., (eds), *Caring and Curing. Health and Medicine in the Western Medical Traditions*, New York, Macmillan, 1986.

Andrew, D., *Philanthropy and Police: London Charity in the Eighteenth Century*, Princeton, NJ, and London, Princeton University Press, 1989.

Barry, J. and Jones C. (eds), *Medicine and Charity before the Welfare State*, London, Routledge, 1991; esp. S. Cavallo, 'The motivations of benefactors: an overview of approaches to the study of charity', pp. 46–62.

Foucalt, M., *Folie et déraison. Histoire de la folie à l'âge classique*, Paris, Plon, 1961 (part translated as *Madness and Civilization: a History of Insanity in the Age of Reason*, London, Tavistock, 1965).

Granshaw, L. and Porter, Roy (eds), *The Hospital in History*, London, Routledge, 1989.

Gutton, J. P., *La Société et les Pauvres en Europe, XVIe–XVIIIe siècles*, Paris, Presses Universitaires de France, 1974.

Jones, C., *Charity and Bienfaisance: the Treatment of the Poor in the Montpellier Region, 1740–1815*, Cambridge, Cambridge University Press, 1983.

——, *The Charitable Imperative. Hospitals and Nursing in Ancien Régime and Revolutionary France*, London, Routledge, 1989.

Lallemand, L., *Histoire de la charité*, 4 vols, Paris, 1910.

Lis, C. and Soly, H., *Poverty and Capitalism in Pre-industrial Europe*, Brighton, Harvester Press, 1979.

Miller, T. S., *The Birth of the Hospital in the Byzantine Empire*, Baltimore, MD, Johns Hopkins University Press, 1985.

Mollat, M., (ed.) *Études sur l'histoire de la charité*, Paris, Publications de la Sorbonne, 1974.

——, *The Poor in the Middle Ages*, New Haven, CT, and London, Yale University Press, 1986; orig. pub. as *Les Pauvres au Moyen-Âge*, Paris, Hachette, 1978.

Pullan, B., *Rich and Poor in Renaissance Venice: the Social Institutions of a Catholic State*, Oxford, Basil Blackwell, 1971.

——, 'Catholics and the poor in early modern Europe', *Transactions of the Royal Historical Society*, 1976 (5th series), 26.

——, 'The Old Catholicism, the New Catholicism and the poor', *Timore a Carità. I Poveri nell'Italia Moderna*, Cremona, 1982.

Riis, T. (ed.), *Aspects of Poverty in Early Modern Europe*, Alphen aan den Rijn and Stuttgart, Sijthoff, 1981.

Sheils, W. J. (ed.), *The Church and Healing*, Oxford, Basil Blackwell for the Ecclesiastical History Society, 1982.

Slack, P. *The English Poor Law, 1531–1782*, London, Macmillan, 1990.

Tierney, B., *Medieval Poor-Law: a sketch of Canonical Theory and its Application in England*, Berkeley, University of California Press, 1959.

Woolf, S. J., *The Poor in Western Europe in the Eighteenth and Nineteenth Centuries*, London, Methuen, 1986.

63

MEDICAL PHILANTHROPY
AFTER 1850

W. F. Bynum

FORMS AND FUNCTIONS OF MODERN
MEDICAL PHILANTHROPY

Charity is a New Testament word, signifying 'universal love'; *philanthropy*, a compound word of Greek derivation, means literally 'love of mankind'. Their etymological roots thus give them a close relationship, and in popular contemporary usage, a medical charity and a medical philanthropy are much the same thing. As this chapter seeks to demonstrate, there are striking historical continuities in the relationships between charity and medicine.

The vocabulary used to name philanthropic organizations is exceptionally varied. In Britain, for instance, the Association of Medical Research Charities (AMRC) consists of a group of philanthropies that spend a reasonable proportion of their disposable income supporting medical research. None of the association's constituent members has the word 'charity' in its title. Rather, they are described by such words as foundation (British Heart Foundation, Nuffield Foundation, Ciba Foundation); society (Parkinson's Disease Society, Multiple Sclerosis Society); campaign (Cancer Research Campaign, National Asthma Campaign); trust (Wellcome Trust, Migraine Trust, Leverhulme Trust); association (Chest, Heart and Stroke Association; Motor Neuron Association); or fund (Imperial Cancer Research Fund, National Kidney Research Fund).[1]

In the United States, usage is equally flexible. Thus, the Rockefeller Foundation, the Carnegie Corporation, the Commonwealth Fund, the American Heart Association, the American Cancer Society, the Community Chest, and numerous trusts, institutions, commissions, orders, clubs, lodges, benefits, and memorials have been involved in the support of medical research or care. The names do not always give a clue to the distinction between collecting charities (those that derive most or all of their income from voluntary gifts from the public) and endowment philanthropies (those with principal or total income from endowments or from a single source). Many foundations are of the latter type: Rockefeller, Ford, Sloan, Mellon, Nuffield. Nevertheless, the Infantile Paralysis Foundation, established in the wake of the bout of polio suffered by Franklin Roosevelt (1882–1945), was primarily a collecting charity, as is the British Heart Foundation.[2] Most trusts (but not the Migraine Trust), are the products of endowments. Sometimes, charities with large endowments make public appeals, or collecting charities cease their fund-raising activities and distribute only the interest from their capital. The King Edward Hospital Fund for London, for example, was a collecting charity until the nationalization of most of the voluntary hospitals under the National Health Service (1948). Since then, it has operated on the interest from the capital it had accumulated.[3] At the same time, the wealthier voluntary hospitals were permitted through trustees to retain control and use of the endowments that they had amassed over the decades. (➤ Ch. 49 The hospital)

Even if the distinction between endowed and collecting charities is not always precise, it was the former that traditionally posed most problems of regulation. The voluntary, collecting charities had to establish a relationship with the giving public who, it was assumed, would not contribute to mismanaged or corrupt organizations. In Britain, the Charity Commission, established in 1853, had responsibility for the endowed charities alone until 1960, when the brief was extended. In the United States, it was the endowed trusts and foundations of the late nineteenth-century industrial magnates that Congress viewed with suspicion and sought to police. Legislation governing the legal and financial status of charities, the appointment of trustees, public accountability, and capital accumulation has been passed periodically in many countries. No system can completely prevent fraud, excessive administrative costs, or ill-judged appropriation of charitable funds. Nevertheless, many charities and foundations can point to reasonable, even distinguished, records of involvement in large areas of public life, not least in medical care and medical research. (➤ Ch. 4 Medical care)

There are no sharp breaks in the forms of medical charity, or the motivations of the charitable, before and after c.1850. Not all charity before 1850 was religious in its organization or intended consequences; not all philanthropy after it the result of secular forces. Many of the features that characterize modern medical philanthropies were in place by the mid-nineteenth century. Already, a number of the more influential charities had complicated organizational structures, were run by a mixture of paid and unpaid staff, and had developed sophisticated publicity mechanisms and creative ways of encouraging the public to support them. Endowed charities were also in existence, using investments and interest to support their aims.

Many had briefs that included medical care, alongside housing, relief of poverty, education, religious instruction, reformation of prostitutes, and a thousand other areas of perceived need. People of particular religious persuasions established hospitals or sent out medical missionaries in the eighteenth as well as the present century. (➤ Ch. 62 Charity before c.1850)

Despite continuities, there have also been significant changes in the past century and a half. Medical charity/philanthropy is, after all, always the product of the same values and forces which had created the contemporary systems of medical care. As medical care has become more complex, expensive, and regulated, so has medical philanthropy. Escalating medical costs have made hospitals and comparable institutions require ever-larger sources of funding, to purchase a new piece of sophisticated equipment, open a new facility, pay salaries, or simply keep wards open. In the United States and Great Britain, in particular, medical education and medical research from the mid-nineteenth century posed new financial problems not met by traditional patterns of charitable giving or by the state. Supporting research seemed to several wealthy philanthropists a novel way of demonstrating a love of one's fellow human, for the laboratory might yield new drugs, vaccines, or a breakthrough in knowledge with widespread public benefit. In recent years, new ways for individuals to act philanthropically have emerged through schemes for blood donation or carrying organ transplant cards.[4]

Since the mid-nineteenth century, medical philanthropies and voluntaristic social agencies have developed and operated alongside a growing state involvement in medical research, health care and social services, philosophies of health rights and the welfare state, and formal publicly funded programmes of 'foreign aid'. Nineteenth-century savings banks and pension funds have largely passed from the charitable to the commercial sphere. Hospitals and schools are now more likely to be public institutions, or at least critically dependent on public moneys. Female penitentiaries and male reformatories are more commonly linked to the state's systems of law and order. Nevertheless, voluntarism remains an important aspect of modern life, and philanthropy remains big business. Like so much else, charities and philanthropies have increased dramatically in number and income in the past century, particularly in the English-speaking parts of the world.

In practice, even an ideal welfare state could not provide for every perceived health-related need: research into that particular disease; that piece of equipment for a local hospital; help for people (or their families) suffering from this disease or disability. Within the past decade or so, the philosophy of welfarism has been under assault, and in the name of 'Victorian values', citizens have been encouraged to fend for themselves, their families, and neighbours. In Britain, public funds to support medical research have also been rationalized, leaving both the caring and the research charities with a perceived threat to their independence of action, as they resist the task of simply picking up the bill for care or research which had been previously funded wholly or in large part by the state. At the very least, it has forced the medical philanthropies to redouble their efforts to publicize the importance of their activities to legislators and other public officials. Indeed, philanthropies have acquired a pressure-group function on behalf of their constituents, be they the research community, medical institutions, or the individuals suffering from a particular illness or disability. (➤ Ch. 50 Medical institutions and the state; Ch. 57 Health economics)

The voluntary sector is thus not likely to disappear from the medical scene. Nor was it ever meant to in countries with well-established voluntarist traditions. One of the chief architects of the British welfare state, William Beveridge (1879–1963), followed up his blueprint of post-war reconstruction (the Beveridge Report of 1942) with a monograph on *Voluntary Action* (1948). Existing charities and philanthropies have their own in-built institutional momentum, programmes, endowments, and employees with ambitions and careers at stake. They have shown themselves to be flexible in adapting appeals and agendas to changed circumstances. Tuberculosis charities branched out into other lung diseases as tuberculosis began to recede from Western society;[5] polio philanthropies moved into birth defects and other crippling diseases of childhood as immunization programmes made polio a rare disease (building on the success of the polio vaccines as a reason to redouble generosity). AIDS and other new health problems have spawned their own voluntaristic associations to provide care and support when public facilities have proved inadequate. Indeed, the proliferation of self-help groups, and voluntary AIDS charities such as the Lighthouse Trust in Britain has been a remarkable feature of the epidemic. (➤ Ch. 26 Sexually transmitted diseases) As the population structure of Western societies has shifted, conditions such as Alzheimer's Syndrome have become more prevalent. This disease has acquired philanthropic visibility, especially as scientists claim to be close to understanding its aetiology and therefore to be in a position to control it, retard its progress, or even prevent it. (➤ Ch. 46 Geriatrics) For the past century, 'cancer' has enjoyed a high philanthropic profile, aided by the widespread fear that its diagnosis provokes.[6] (➤ Ch. 25 Cancer) Multiple sclerosis and muscular dystrophy attack young adults and children and attract vigorous charitable giving; kidney diseases, mental disorder, and stroke do much less well.

The reasons for the relative appeal of the many collecting charities are complicated and historically contingent, although they are clearly connected to public fears and sympathies, the state of medical knowledge, and the effectiveness of the fund-raising exercises, among other factors. Tax laws in the United States have made charitable giving more directly attractive to the individual than those in Britain. Social ideologies of participation and self-reliance are probably important in explaining the greater continuing significance of voluntarism in English-speaking countries than in continental Europe.

Medical philanthropy has thus had a complex role in the support of both medical care and medical research, the former based on long-term traditions, the latter on more recent involvement. The remainder of this chapter will examine briefly each of these facets in turn.

PHILANTHROPY AND MEDICAL CARE

While most of the preceding section has been concerned with the financial side of philanthropy, the voluntarist tradition is also about donating time. Both within the hospital and outside of it, a good deal of unpaid activity has long been channelled into the medical enterprise. Despite the tangible careerist gains that consultant medical staff traditionally derived from their hospital appointments, these were in the voluntary sector, technically unpaid, and so encased in the trappings of philanthropy. Nursing functions were equally complex: nursing orders continued to operate in many places, and Florence Nightingale (1820–1910) provided a symbol for charitable activity during and after the Crimean War (1854–6). Almost £50,000 was collected in memory of her service, and although nothing to do with Nightingale was ever straightforward, the Nightingale Trust Fund provided the financial backing for the nursing school at St Thomas's Hospital.[7] Earlier, nursing charities had provided for the gratuitous services of nurses for the poor. (➤ Ch. 54 A general history of nursing: 1800–1900)

From about the mid-nineteenth century, 'lady visitors' became more active within the hospitals.[8] These volunteers would sit with patients, read to them, and sometimes follow up the hospital episode with a home visit. Lady almoners became common slightly later, an innovation encouraged by the Charity Organisation Society, itself a powerful force in British voluntarism from its foundation in 1869.[9] Almoners, sometimes paid and sometimes volunteers, assessed patients' home situations and 'worthiness' as recipients of charity, and often arranged after-care. Women were also in the vanguard of home visitation schemes. The 'Bible Women' of Mrs Ellen Ranyard (1810–75) sold Bibles and offered domestic and health advice in the worst British slums.[10] In Chicago, Hull House (1899) was founded after the visit by Jane Addams (1860–1935) to a similar housing settlement in London, Toynbee Hall (1884).[11] The Salvation Army, founded by William Booth (1829–1912) in 1878, recruited thousands of 'officers' and 'soliders' of both sexes to its ranks. Booth's troops soon learned that hungry souls were difficult to save and that food is often the best medicine. From the turn of the century, milk depots – some funded publicly, some from private donations – began to distribute milk to babies and advice on infant care to mothers. (➤ Ch. 45 Childhood)

These instances – the tip of a veritable iceberg – remind us that health and welfare are inseparable, and that religion underwrote a good deal of nineteenth-century charity. (➤ Ch. 61 Religion and medicine) Voluntarism provided a socially acceptable outlet for the energies of thousands of middle-class women, and through the tradition's relationship with nursing and what became known as social work, the beginnings of occupational niches for women. (➤ Ch. 38 Women and medicine) The voluntarist tradition also helped catalyse the more formal involvement of the state in welfare activity, partly by increasing public awareness of the enormity of social deprivation and need, and sometimes by turning voluntarists like Beatrice Webb (1858–1943) into socialists. Born into wealthy circumstances, Webb developed a social conscience and, as a young woman, threw herself into good works. However, she became disillusioned with the paternalism and condescension towards their charges exhibited by many of those associated with the Charity Organisation Society, and with her husband, Sydney Webb (1859–1947), argued that poverty was best attacked not through piecemeal charity, but by creating a new economic reality where citizens would have rights to health and welfare services, and workers the control over their own destinies.[12]

The twentieth-century state has not, contrary to Webb's hope, made charities redundant; indeed, their number has continued to increase steadily. In many instances, the voluntary sector has managed to work in partnership with public agencies, and the 'educational' functions of many large modern charities include explicit presure-group activity, to encourage increased public allocation of resources in some particular direction. At the same time, medical philanthropies have remained fiercely independent, conscious of their own importance and wary of the anonymous face of state bureaucracy. This is seen particularly strikingly in the ethos surrounding the voluntary hospitals, which, until at least the inter-war period, enjoyed a major proportion of charitable giving in the field of health.

In both Britain and the United States, voluntary hospitals provided the core of medical care for a significant portion of the non-pauper population. By the last third of the nineteenth century, however, voluntary hospitals were under increasing financial pressure, as the hospitals themselves became more complex, employed more kinds of paid staff, and were being run more and more along business lines. At the same time, they had been founded as charitable institutions, devoted to providing free care to the worthy poor who required it, and many who supported them were reluctant for the hospitals to become tainted with too commercial an image. Through fêtes, bazaars, soirées, sermons, and dinners, worthy citizens were encouraged to give. Much of the emphasis was on local pride, and support for the local hospital, but national associations were also important in co-ordinating fund-raising and raising the collective profile of the hospitals. In Britain, the Hospital Sunday Fund co-ordinated collections at churches; a Hospital Saturday Fund encouraged waged workers to give something from their wage packets (received on Saturday). In the United States, the American Hospital Association (founded in 1899) was concerned with the public image of the voluntary institutions. A National Hospital Day, first held in 1921 (on Florence Nightingale's birthday), became an annual event.[13]

Linking famous names to hospital charity was a commonplace: local business people and national industrial magnates, religious leaders, and literary figures, and, in Britain, royalty and the aristocracy. The King Edward Hospital Fund for London, established while Edward VII (1841–1910) was still Prince of Wales, was one of the most successful, capitalizing on royal appeal and the ability of well-placed philanthropists to persuade various members of the royal family to participate in fund-raising events, as well as giving liberally themselves. A key figure in the fund was Sir Henry Burdett (1847–1920), who devoted his life to the management, advertising, and financing of hospitals throughout the English-speaking world. For Burdett, the charitable nature of the voluntary hospitals placed them apart from (and above) those which were publicly funded, and he worked to ensure their independence from state control, as well as seeing that King's Fund monies went directly to the hospitals' services for patients, rather than an attached medical school or research activities.[14]

Nevertheless, the inter-war years were difficult for the voluntary hospitals, and they began to appear much less philanthropic in their structures and outlooks, through the growth of pay-beds, third-party insurance payments, and salaried professional administrators and staff. The American Hospital Association was content in the 1930s to encourage the injection of public money into the voluntary system, as long as independence was not compromised, and the Second World War hastened, but probably did not cause, the nationalization of the British voluntary hospitals, which were already in deep financial straits. During the past half-century, voluntary or community hospitals have continued to exist in the United States, attracting funds and voluntary service, although business methods are used to run them. A 1976 legal ruling in Michigan on hospital tort liability recognized this: 'the modern hospital, whether operated by a city, a church, or a group of private investors, is essentially a business'.[15] The growth of government-sponsored payment schemes – Medicare and Medicaid – has further eroded the extent to which hospitals rely on voluntary donations to support them.

Although hospital giving has declined in relative importance, a vast array of other medical and welfare charities have continued to thrive. The blind, deaf, limbless, and ruptured have had their benefactors; charities for working-class housing, soup-kitchens, and public baths have had health as much in view as morals and economic efficiency. In the twentieth century, however, specific diseases have provided the most concentrated focus for non-hospital medical philanthropy. Tuberculosis charities were begun in late nineteenth-century America, to provide assistance and facilities for consumptives. Local, state, and national associations were formed, and when in the early 1900s the American National Red Cross, which was already interested in tuberculosis, joined with the National Tuberculosis Association in the sale of Christmas seals, charitable giving for relief of the disease increased dramatically. The International Red Cross Society, founded in 1864, had initially been concerned with the aid of sick and wounded prisoners in wartime, but its brief gradually expanded to many aspects of health, as well as the more familiar role of providing emergency relief to citizens in times of disasters. The sale of Christmas seals actually originated in Denmark in 1904, but hospital charities had used similar gimmicks even earlier. (➤ Ch. 59 Internationalism in medicine and public health)

A good many of the collecting charities continue to be focused on a single disease, organ, or system, and although the support of research has often become a high priority, both education and direct assistance are still part of the appeal. Mutual aid and support groups are often national in their organization, though more local in their work, and offer meetings, literature, and more tangible benefits for both the afflicted individual and the associated carers, for conditions as diverse as cystic fibrosis and colostomies, mental disorders and drug dependence, obesity and anorexia.

If hospitals have many business characteristics, so, in a sense, do the larger collecting charities, which have big advertising budgets and staffing levels, are bound by complicated legal statutes, and often dispense charity merely by paying professional health workers to practise their skills. Since health provision is one of the leading industries throughout the developed world, it is perhaps inevitable that the supporting charities should also reflect the commercialism that governs much of the medical establishment.

PHILANTHROPY AND MEDICAL RESEARCH

Many of the medical philanthropies support research as well as care; indeed, it could be argued that the caring functions represent the continuation of long-established patterns, whereas philanthropy played a decisive role in the creation of academic medicine in English-speaking countries. In Germany, medical research enjoyed substantial public investment from the mid-nineteenth century, and though the system was much admired by many foreign students who studied in the German-speaking lands between about

1850 and the First World War, in neither Britain nor the United States was much state patronage of either laboratory or bedside research forthcoming until well into the twentieth century. Rather, research-orientated medical scientists turned to individual wealthy philanthropists for support to endow chairs, build laboratories, and provide fellowships. (➤ Ch. 11 Clinical research)

The universities were the primary beneficiaries of this 'endowment of science' movement. A number of the British provincial civic universities attracted money from local industrialists, and there were several privately endowed chairs in physiology and other basic sciences before the end of the nineteenth century.[16] The novelist George Eliot (Mary-Anne Evans (1819–80)) established a studentship in memory of her companion George Henry Lewes (1817–78); and a more extensive fellowship scheme was established by the South African mining magnate Sir Otto Beit (1865–1930), in memory of his brother Alfred Beit (1853–1906).[17] (➤ Ch. 7 The physiological tradition) Among American universities, Harvard was particularly successful in attracting research philanthropy, but nothing quite matched the endowment by Baltimore railroad magnate and philanthropist Johns Hopkins (1795–1873) of a whole university, opened in 1876 and dedicated to research and advanced teaching. A hospital and medical school were central to Hopkins's vision, and although the latter was not fully operational until the 1890s, it attracted not only high-calibre staff and students, but also additional funds from later philanthropists.

It is no accident that these are examples of substantial sums donated by well-disposed individuals. The philanthropic general public was traditionally more concerned with care than research, and it was not until Louis Pasteur (1822–95) captured the public's imagination that grass-roots giving began to be directed towards medical science. The Institut Pasteur, opened in 1888, was, in a sense, his memorial, and was built and endowed by private donations from people from all parts of the world. Other Pasteur institutes were also established in areas of French influence, often with a mixture of private and public money. The British attempt to found a comparable research institute, named first after Edward Jenner (1749–1823), and then after Joseph Lister (1827–1912), would have faltered but for the large gift of Edward Guinness, 1st Earl of Iveagh (1847–1927); even so, the word 'research' was carefully kept out of the institute's name (the Lister Institute of Preventive Medicine), to avoid a backlash from antivivisection groups.[18]

Late nineteenth-century laboratory successes, especially in bacteriology and immunology, brought research to the fore, and even in Britain, the Imperial Cancer Research Fund, established in 1902, was able to use the loaded word 'research' within a collecting context. (➤ Ch. 10 The immunological tradition) More specifically, members of the Rockefeller dynasty, particularly John D. Rockefeller (1839–1937) and his son, John D. II (1874–1960), began to devote a large portion of their surplus wealth to health-related issues. This wealth came through oil, and though he had some of the hallmarks of a typical 'robber baron' of rampant American capitalism, the elder Rockefeller, a devout Baptist, always had philanthropy high on his list of priorities.[19] In addition to a number of overtly religious projects, the University of Chicago was an early major benefactor; in fact, Rockefeller money helped to transform it from an insignificant Baptist institution into a major secular research-orientated university. By the late 1890s, one of his trusted advisers, Frederick T. Gates (1853–1929) (himself a Baptist minister) convinced Rockefeller that furthering medical knowledge and improving standards of medical care were ideal ways of using his vast fortune to promote the betterment of humankind. Despite the fact that Rockefeller's personal physician at the time was a homoeopath, he gave Gates a free hand.

An early tangible result was the Rockefeller Institute of Medical Research (1901) in New York City, with laboratories and an attached hospital for clinical research.[20] It quickly established itself as a major force in American academic medicine, both as a training-ground and as a site where newsworthy research was produced, such as a serum therapy for epidemic spinal meningitis developed by Simon Flexner (1863–1946), the Director of the institute's laboratories, and a yellow fever vaccine. Flexner and his mentor, William H. Welch (1850–1934), Professor of Pathology at Johns Hopkins, enjoyed the confidence of the Rockefellers and encouraged the expansion of Rockefeller largesse in the direction of medical research and disease prevention.

A notable example of the latter was the Rockefeller-funded campaign to eradicate hookworm from the American South. This 'disease of laziness' affected many poor black and white southerners; it produced chronic anaemia, tiredness, and lethargy. Essentially a disease of poverty, spread through inadequate disposal of faeces and walking barefoot over infested ground, it was both treatable and preventable. Wickliffe Rose (1862–1931) headed the Rockefeller Sanitary Commission, which was charged with the task of investigating the disease's prevalence, and educating the public about its dangers and the ways in which it could be treated and prevented. Rose and his corps of sanitary inspectors treated some 700,000 individuals, held more than 25,000 public meetings, and distributed more than 2 million pieces of educational literature between 1910 and 1915, when the campaign was ended and the Commission absorbed into Rockefeller's International Health Board (IHB).[21]

The IHB was itself a potent symbol of the fact that, by the First World War, the whole world was Rockefeller's oyster. It extended the hookworm campaign into tropical areas around the globe, built on the success of the American hookworm initiative by placing malaria and yellow fever control on its agenda, and channelled Rockefeller money into schools and institutes of public health and of tropical medicine in many countries, including Britain,

Czechoslovakia, Poland, Denmark, Bulgaria, Yugoslavia, Spain, Turkey, Japan, Greece, India, Brazil, and the Philippines. A fellowship programme was started to enable public-health workers in countries without facilities to study abroad.[22] (➤ Ch. 24 Tropical diseases; Ch. 51 Public health; Ch. 52 Epidemiology)

Rose and the growing army of personnel employed to oversee the spending of Rockefeller wealth and to implement policies soon discovered that grassroots campaigns in impoverished countries could be frustrating, and although the yellow fever and malaria initiatives were continued during the inter-war years, investment in education and research proved more manageable. Training doctors could have a knock-on effect, and there was Rockefeller investment as far apart as University College Hospital London and the Peking Medical College in China. The latter was something of an experiment in seeing how far the provision of native doctors trained in Western medicine could improve the health of a people and infiltrate their consciousness with 'scientific' notions of health and preventive medicine. (➤ Ch. 32 Chinese medicine) In between Europe and Asia, Rockefeller philanthropoids keep a watching brief on the American medical scene, encouraging the best medical schools with bequests. The task of differentiating the good from the indifferent and positively bad was made easier by Abraham Flexner (1866–1959) with his famous exposé of 1910 on the state of American medical schools. (➤ Ch. 48 Medical education)

This survey, and another that Flexner (who was Simon's brother) conducted a couple of years later on British and European medical schools, were funded by the Rockefeller's chief rival in scientific philanthropy, Andrew Carnegie (1835–1918), a Scottish-born emigrant to America, who made a vast fortune in steel. Carnegie devoted but a tiny fraction of his philanthropic activity to medicine, although the life sciences did well out of him. Education, libraries, and world peace were the main targets of his largesse.[23] Nevertheless, Flexner's surveys on medical education made it easier for Rockefeller agents to identify appropriate medical institutions to invest in, and Flexner himself sat on several Rockefeller committees. In North America, Harvard, Johns Hopkins, Yale, Michigan, McGill, Washington (in St Louis), Rochester, and Vanderbilt universities were among the leading beneficiaries; in addition, the Rockefeller ideals of scientific medicine were furthered at University College London, St Bartholomew's Hospital Medical School; Cambridge and Edinburgh; Paris and Copenhagen; Utrecht and Stockholm.[24] High on the list of those ideals was the 'full-time system', Flexner's vision of a cadre of academic clinicians who devoted their time wholly to research and teaching, without the distractions of private practice.

The worldwide impact of Rockefeller money on medical research and education in the inter-war period was substantial; and although there was continued support of the Rockefeller Institute (now Rockefeller University), after the Second World War, Rockefeller philanthropy began increasingly to be diverted to other causes, including over-population, education, ecology, and world food supply. During the war, the American government became more actively concerned with both scientific and medical research, and in the years after 1945, the Government laboratories in Bethesda, Maryland, expanded into the massive National Institutes of Health (NIH), and large amounts of public money were channelled into research programmes in the universities and medical schools.[25]

American foundations continue to be active in the support of academic medicine. Some of the largest include the Commonwealth Fund, created in 1918 by the Harkness family;[26] and several named after or by the major benefactors, the Alfred P. Sloan Foundation, the Robert Wood Johnson Foundation, and the Josiah Macy Jr Foundation. More recently, the eccentric and reclusive businessman and film producer Howard Hughes (1905–76) left his vast fortunes to medical research. In general, though, the American medical philanthropies devote less than one-quarter of their investment income to research, and their research allocations are dwarfed by those of NIH. Rather, they have been concerned with areas where public money is perceived to be inadequate: medical education for minority groups; the hospice movement; health-policy studies; and the training of physician assistants. (➤ Ch. 55 The emergence of para-medical professions)

In Britain, the combined budgets of the medical research charities are roughly equivalent to that of the publicly funded Medical Research Council (MRC), and medical research consequently is much more dependent on the foundations and collecting charities. In the first half of the century, several private benefactors helped develop medical science and clinical research. The Sir William Dunn Trustees established departments of biochemistry and pathology in Cambridge and Oxford, respectively; and the first Viscount Nuffield (1877–1963), the automobile manufacturer, made several substantial bequests to the medical school at Oxford.[27] The two largest cancer charities, the Imperial Cancer Research Fund (1902) and the Cancer Research Campaign (1923) became rich enough to acquire and operate their own research laboratories, although the bulk of medical-research support is channelled through universities and medical schools. This has been the general policy of what has become the largest medical charity in Britain, the Wellcome Trust, created in 1936 by Sir Henry Wellcome (1853–1936), a pharmaceutical manufacturer. Wellcome's will left his business (now rather confusingly called the Wellcome Foundation plc) to trustees, with the instruction that they were to devote the profits to the support of medical research and the history of medicine.[28] The Trustees have supported research across a broad front, including tropical medicine, infectious diseases, and the neurosciences, and the recent prosperity of the parent company, combined with a flotation of a portion of its shares, have resulted in a significant increase in the Trust's disposable income within the past decade.

The activities of the various medical research charities have, since 1972, been loosely co-ordinated by the Association of Medical Research Charities (AMRC). This organization represents the 'private' research sector in discussions with the publicly funded MRC, and attempts to ensure that research funds are rationally distributed. The most important criterion for membership in the AMRC is that applications for research funds are peer-reviewed before grants are awarded.

During the past century, medical research has acquired a powerful image in Western society, and the humanitarian dimensions of medical care have continued to exert a compelling draw on the general public. As the collecting charities have become bigger, individual giving has become more anonymous. Nevertheless, both the collecting charities and the endowed philanthropies are so entrenched in the modern medical enterprise that their future in voluntaristic societies is secure.

NOTES

1 *The Association of Medical Research Charities Handbook, 1991–1992*, London, AMRC, 1991.

2 J. R. Wilson, *Margin of Safety*, London, Collins, 1963; B. D. Karl and S. N. Katz, 'The American private philanthropic foundation and the public sphere, 1890–1930', *Minerva*, 1981, 19: 236–70.

3 F. K. Prochaska, *Philanthropy and the Hospitals of London: the King's Fund 1897–1990*, Oxford, Oxford University Press, 1992.

4 R. M. Titmuss, *The Gift Relationship: from Human Blood to Social Policy*, London, Allen & Unwin, 1970.

5 R. H. Shryock, *National Tuberculosis Association, 1904–1954: a Study of the Voluntary Health Movement in the United States*, New York, National Tuberculosis Association, 1957.

6 J. T. Patterson, *The Dread Disease: Cancer and Modern American Culture*, Cambridge, MA, Harvard University Press, 1987; J. Austoker, *A History of the Imperial Cancer Research Fund 1902–1986*, Oxford and New York, Oxford University Press, 1988.

7 Monica Baly, *Florence Nightingale and the Nursing Legacy*, London, Croom Helm, 1986.

8 Charles Rosenberg, *The Care of Strangers*, New York, Basic Books, 1987; Geoffrey Rivett, *The Development of the London Hospital System, 1823–1982*, London, King Edward's Hospital Fund for London, 1986.

9 C. L. Mowat, *The Charity Organisation Society, 1869–1913*, London, Methuen, 1961.

10 F. K. Prochaska, *Women and Philanthropy in Nineteenth-Century England*, Oxford, Clarendon Press, 1980.

11 Kathleen McCarthy, *Noblesse Oblige. Charity and Cultural Philanthropy in Chicago, 1844–1929*, Chicago, IL, and London, University of Chicago Press, 1982.

12 Beatrice Webb, *My Apprenticeship*, 2 vols, Harmondsworth, Penguin, 1938.

13 Rosemary Stevens, *In Sickness and in Wealth. American Hospitals in the Twentieth Century*, New York, Basic Books, 1989.

14 See Prochaska, op. cit. (n. 3); and Rivett, op. cit. (n. 8).

15 Stevens, op. cit. (n. 13), p. v.

16 Peter Alter, *The Reluctant Patron, Science and the State in Great Britain, 1850–1920*, Oxford, Berg, 1987.

17 E. M. Tansey, 'George Eliot's support for physiology: the George Henry Lewes Trust, 1879–1939', *Notes and Records of the Royal Society of London*, 1990, 44: 221–40.

18 Harriett Chick, Margaret Hume and Marjorie Macfarlane, *War on Disease: a History of the Lister Institute*, London, André Deutsch, 1971.

19 J. E. Harr and P. J. Johnson, *The Rockefeller Century*, New York, Charles Scribner's Sons, 1988.

20 George W. Corner, *A History of the Rockefeller Institute, 1901–1953*, New York, Rockefeller Institute Press, 1964.

21 John Ettling, *The Germ of Laziness: Rockefeller Philanthropy and Public Health in the New South*, Cambridge, MA, Harvard University Press, 1981.

22 Raymond B. Fosdick, *The Story of the Rockefeller Foundation*, London, Odhams Press, 1952.

23 Robert E. Kohler, *Partners in Science. Foundations and Natural Scientists, 1900–1945*, Chicago, IL, and London, University of Chicago Press, 1991.

24 Howard S. Berliner, *A System of Scientific Medicine. Philanthropic Foundations in the Flexner Era*, New York and London, Tavistock, 1985.

25 V. A. Harden, *Inventing the NIH: Federal Biomedical Research Policy, 1887–1937*, Baltimore, MD, Johns Hopkins University Press, 1986.

26 A. McGehee Harvey and Susan L. Abrams, '*For the Welfare of Mankind': the Commonwealth Fund and American Medicine*, Baltimore, MD, and London, Johns Hopkins University Press, 1986.

27 Ronald W. Clark, *A Biography of the Nuffield Foundation*, London, Longman, 1972.

28 A. R. Hall and B. A. Bembridge, *Physic and Philanthropy: a History of the Wellcome Trust, 1936–1986*, Cambridge, Cambridge University Press, 1986.

FURTHER READING

Abel-Smith, Brian, *The Hospitals, 1800–1948*, London, Heinemann, 1964.

Andrews, F. Emerson, *Philanthropic Foundations*, New York, Russell Sage Foundation, 1956.

Berliner, Howard S., *A System of Scientific Medicine. Philanthropic Foundations in the Flexner Era*, New York and London, Tavistock, 1985.

Brown, E. Richard, *Rockefeller Medicine Men: Medicine and Capitalism in America*, Berkeley, University of California Press, 1979.

Checkland, Olive, *Philanthropy in Victorian Scotland. Social Welfare and the Voluntary Principle*, Edinburgh, John Donald, 1980.

Curti, Merle, *American Philanthropy Abroad: a History*, New Brunswick, NJ, Rutgers University Press, 1963.

Gunn, Selskar M. and Platt, Philip S., *Voluntary Health Agencies: an Interpretive Study*, New York, Ronald Press, 1945.

Jonas, Gerald, *The Circuit Riders: Rockefeller Money and the Rise of Modern Science*, New York, Norton, 1989.

Low, Sampson, Jr, *The Charities of London*, London, Sampson Low, 1863.

Owen, David, *English Philanthropy, 1660–1960*, Cambridge, MA, Harvard University Press, 1960.

Prochaska, Frank, *The Voluntary Impulse: Philanthropy in Modern Britain*, London, Faber & Faber, 1988.

Shryock, Richard S., *National Tuberculosis Association 1904–1954. A Study in the Voluntary Health Movement in the United States*, New York, National Tuberculosis Association, 1957.

Weaver, Warren, *U.S. Philanthropic Foundations: their History, Structure, Management and Record*, New York, Harper & Row, 1964.

Whitaker, Ben, *The Foundations: an Anatomy of Philanthropic Foundations*, Harmondsworth, Penguin, 1979.

64

MEDICINE AND ARCHITECTURE

Christine Stevenson

Architecture impinges upon medicine in two ways, which correspond to the maintenance of health, and its restoration. A building should not impair the health of its occupants, as when, for example, prefabricated concrete components turn out to let in water on assembly. More broadly, architects are asked to suggest ways that people, including those with mental and physical handicaps, can live and work in reasonable physical and psychological health in the close proximity that we demand. They also design types of buildings, notably the hospital, involved with the care of the sick.

There are limits to what architecture can do, or undo. It is population density itself, and not the buildings that enable it, which admits the gravest threats to human health; it is the invisible administrative cordons that are flung up in the face of disease that make the stoutest barriers. Aspects of this subject are therefore developed in other chapters. (➤ Ch. 49 The hospital; Ch. 51 Public health; Ch. 27 Diseases of civilization)

Because architecture is the art or science of building, its products by definition should be healthy: dry, sound, easily cleaned, and so forth. The built environment moves in and out of the foreground of medical thinking, but an architect's invocation of medicine can never be assumed to evince any serious engagement with it, or, for that matter, to have any effect on what was built. For example, the *Ten Books on Architecture*, by Marcus Vitruvius Pollio (writing *c.*25 BC), begins with a chapter on the education of the architect. This should include the 'study of medicine on account of the questions of climates . . . , air, the healthiness and unhealthiness of sites, and the use of different waters. For without these considerations, the healthiness of a dwelling cannot be assured.'[1] But Vitruvius also advocated the study of many other subjects, among them music, astronomy, and law (drains feature in the treatise as a potential source of nasty legal, not hygienic, problems):

the architect was, simply, to be of useful culture. The environment's influence on human health was a truism by Vitruvius's day and scarcely required his emphasis, but this is the only complete architectural treatise to survive from antiquity, and many architectural students who never read the Hippocratic *Airs, Waters and Places* and *Epidemics*, still study Vitruvius. The significance of clean air and water and healthy sites to his professional descendants may be taken for granted, just as medical writers like Galen (AD 129–*c*.200/210) would advocate the construction of wide streets and well-ordered buildings. (➤ Ch. 15 Environment and miasmata)

A sick person is put in a room apart; and then, perhaps, in an entirely separate house; and finally in a building for the sick alone. This progression could be that of a declining elder today: it is also the history of hospitals. The overwhelming majority of sick people in history who have not been cared for in their own houses have been nursed in someone else's, perhaps the doctor's. As late as the first decade of the twentieth century, the Swedish-Americans of Kansas City, Missouri, in the absence of a 'good Swedish boarding house'[2] opened a hospital for those coming to town to see a doctor. Trinity Lutheran Hospital was one of hundreds of small, sectarian or ethnic hospitals opened in the United States: purpose-built examples did not look much different from the converted houses in which, historically, most hospitals have found their first quarters.

On the other hand, a hospital's function has never been confined to the care of the sick. They were, and are, collegiate and self-perpetuating institutions that in many ways bind their patrons and populations, both staff and patients, to one another and to the wider world, as Lindsay Granshaw's article in this encyclopedia explains. (➤ Ch. 49 The hospital) These social operations can affect a hospital's size and outward appearance much more dramatically than its medical functions do: an obvious example is the way they reinforced the impressions of munificence, stability, and legitimacy which a sponsoring authority – whether a sixth-century king of Persia, an eighteenth-century lord provost of Edinburgh, or a twentieth-century American university – was anxious to cultivate.

THE HISTORY OF HOSPITAL ARCHITECTURE

To care for the sick was one of the joyful obligations of Christian hospitality and the hospital, like other welfare establishments, first appeared as a building in fourth-century Byzantium. With monastic infirmaries, we find the first hospital type in the West: these were usually long, aisled halls with a chapel at one end (some ruins were, understandably, later mistaken for those of churches). The beds, at right angles to the walls in the aisles, were typically screened, at first with curtains and later with wooden partitions, in a process afterwards repeated at civil hospitals: such arrangements were more private, and warmer. At some, as by 1500 in the infirmary for choir monks at Fountains Abbey (North Yorkshire), masonry walls were built to form private rooms with fireplaces, a development that probably turned the hall itself into a mere corridor. A larger infirmary could acquire a minutorium, for the recuperation of monks who had been bled (*minuti*), an apothecary's office and store, and an isolation ward, among other additions of a less specifically medical kind.

Sick-rooms were also attached to churches associated with miraculous cures. (➤ Ch. 61 Religion and medicine) St Dymphna could heal mental disorders, perhaps because of her martyrdom by decapitation. By the late fifteenth century, afflicted pilgrims at the site of her cult in Gheel, Belgium, were accommodated in rooms (still existing, in restored form) abutting the church. One room had a view of the altar, a modest illustration of the axis on which hospitals would be aligned for centuries. Jeremy Bentham (1748–1832) substituted the sight of a preacher for that of the elevation of the Host in his *Panopticon* (1791),[3] and rationalists would supplant both with a house for a chief physician, administration block, or, in a monolithic hospital, an operating theatre (or even an operating theatre/chapel combined). However, the principle of centrality remained constant, even when literal sight-lines were no longer possible. Symmetry was facilitated by the human race's division into two sexes (not a factor in the planning of conventual infirmaries).

Pious individuals and such secular organizations as guilds also founded hospitals. The most splendid of the surviving French medieval hospitals is the Hôtel Dieu in Beaune, founded in 1443 by the Chancellor of Burgundy, Nicolas Rollin. To its 'Grand-Salle des Malades' were soon added two other ranges, all grouped around a courtyard in a cloister arrangement that would have a long history.

Hospitals abounded in medieval Europe: for the fourteenth century, an estimate of one for every 1,000 inhabitants in many towns is thought to be reasonable.[4] Most were tiny and undistinguished, but after churches, hospitals were the most prominent urban public buildings, sites for individual or corporate patronage that also provided sculptors and painters with important commissions. More painters' than architects' names are known for the earlier period, but there is no reason to doubt that the latter were employed at prestigious foundations.

Through the gradual addition of wards terminating in a common altar, Florence's S. Maria Nuova (founded 1286) had assumed a cross-shaped plan by 1500, a form that had become standard for Italian hospitals over the course of the century. Its origin is unclear, but it spread through increasingly formal systems of reportage. During the planning of the enormous Ospedale Maggiore, Milan (started 1456), for example, Duke Francesco Sforza

(1401–66) asked his ambassadors to obtain details of the staffing, financing, and layout of S. Maria Nuova, and S. Maria della Scala in Siena, also cruciform. By this date, clearly, hospital architecture had become an identifiable subject for investigation, although one inseparable from hospital organization.

The plan by Antonio Averlino Filarete (c.1400–69) for the Ospedale Maggiore took the form of two crosses, one for each sex, separated by a large rectangular court with a chapel in the centre. The hospital (now part of Milan University) was four centuries in construction, but it was illustrated, and its practical and hygienic needs carefully explained, in Filarete's *Treatise* (written 1460–5), which circulated widely in manuscript. The Ospedale Maggiore and Rome's Ospedale di S. Spirito (1474–82) were the most influential examples of the cruciform type, which spread to England (the Savoy Hospital, finished 1517); Spain, where it was taken to perfection at the Hospital de Santa Cruz, Toledo (1504–14), and the Hospital Real, Granada (1511–22), and its New World colonies; and, in the seventeenth century, France and Germany.

Famous, too, was the vastness of the square plain enclosed by the arcades of the Lazaretto (1488) near Milan, for cases of infectious diseases like plague; such hospitals were always outside the city. From hundreds of cells behind the arcades, patients could see into the open, octagonal chapel in the centre of the huge court. Not until the nineteenth century was the lazaretto discarded as a mechanism for controlling the spread of disease from port to port, and even the last examples, such as the complex at Marseilles (1821–8) by M.-R. Penchaud (1772–1833) had chapels with deep porches on which Mass was celebrated in the sight of all.

During the Renaissance, the idea of hospitals so good that 'none is sent to them against their will', that 'nobody would not chuse ... to go thither, than lie sick at home'[5] was, literally, Utopian. But even Sir Thomas More (1478–1536) envisaged hospitals outside the town walls. This had not been the rule, with the exception of those for plague and leprosy victims. Ordinary medieval hospitals do not seem to have had a particular physical let alone symbolic place, even among town-dwellers increasingly aware of contagion and other dangers that accompanied urban congregations. Many hospitals were built just within the town walls, outside the centre, not necessarily because they were considered offensive, although they had neighbours like butchers' shambles that were, but because land was cheaper and more readily available there. Other typical neighbours were religious foundations. The outskirts were also where the poor settled, and they were the users of hospitals.

In the fifteenth century, however, both architects and lay people began to conceive of cities whose 'ideal' quality derived as much from symbolic planning as attention to Hippocratic injunctions about airs and waters. The first was Leone Battista Alberti (1404–72) in his *De Re Aedificatoria* (1452, fully pub. 1485), which incidentally specified that hospitals for contagious diseases should be built not only outside the city, but away from the public highways. (This became a commonplace. There was no attempt to conceal the practical advantage of cheap land.) Filarete's treatise elaborated the ways in which particular buildings and institutions were to interact, both aesthetically and functionally, with others and with the town as a whole. Both men agreed that hospitals should be beautiful, as well as commodious and sound, but criticism of over-elaborate 'houses for the poor' could also be heard. Hospitals were singled out by non-architects like the Spaniard Juan Luis Vives (c.1493–1540), whose *De Subventione Pauperum* (1525) was typical for its insistence that the poor and sick should be collected in special institutions, not only to ensure their spiritual and corporeal well-being, but also to stop them begging at church porches and otherwise rendering the city disagreeable, and to reduce the risk of contagion. Such theorists not only credited the cruciform plan with hygienic advantages, including ventilation (for whose sake the chapel was sometimes moved from the crossing-point), they invested it with the powers of separating different classes of inmates and facilitating surveillance: in both ways could it rectify the contagious and disorderly promiscuity of urban existence. Later architects inherited long traditions of concern with ventilation, contagion, the proper appearance of hospitals, and their discipline's potency in the face of social ills.

England's hospital architecture, so long disadvantaged by comparison with that in Catholic countries, was improved by a series of buildings and rebuildings that began with the Bethlem (1674–6, demolished c.1816) of Robert Hooke (1635–1702) and went on to include the Royal Hospitals of Sir Christopher Wren (1632–1723) in London, that at Chelsea for soldiers (1682–9), and its naval counterpart at Greenwich (started 1696). The founders of the English military hospitals (among which can be included the Royal Hospital at Kilmainham, near Dublin, the greatest seventeenth-century building in Ireland, started 1680 to a design by William Robinson, *fl.* 1643–1712) were spurred on by the example of the great Hôtel des Invalides in Paris (founded 1670) for old or disabled veterans. Designed by Libéral Bruant (c.1635–97), its four-storey ranges enclose a number of rectangular courtyards.

That the health of civilians, as well as old and disabled soldiers and sailors, was a state responsibility became a truism on the European continent during the eighteenth century, but this understanding did not embrace any enthusiasm for hospitals; if anything, the reverse was the case. The medical objections to hospital, as opposed to domiciliary, care centred on the simple, physical fact of the building, the necessarily rigid and unnatural enclosure it formed. Only some kinds of illness could suitably be treated under these conditions; in general, hospitals were relatively inflexible environments that could not be adjusted to the requirements of a particular patient in the way that the principle of individual specificity, on which therapeutics was based until the mid-nineteenth century, demanded: this complaint goes back to at least Celsus (25 BC–AD 50). Nor was a crude ward-distribution by kinds of disease, a principle almost as old, universal by the eighteenth century. Medieval foundations, coping with crumbling fabrics and chronic cash shortages, could no longer manage it, and at newer, purpose-built institutions like the Edinburgh Royal Infirmary (founded 1729) fiscal convenience and economies of scale seem to have dictated ward arrangements at first. In the 1780s, however, small fever wards, which could be easily cleaned and ventilated, were set up at Edinburgh: ward organization by diagnosis had already been a major feature of the proposals for the new Hôtel Dieu in Paris by Jacques-Réné Tenon (1724–1816) and others. It would lessen the chances of cross-infection, and facilitate the study of a disease through the comparison of its course in different cases, an idea that particularly appealed to Parisian 'hospital' and asylum medicine after the turn of the century.

The hospital was also an artificial environment, with diseases, most notoriously typhus, the 'hospital' or 'jail' fever, peculiar to itself and other closed institutions. (➤ Ch. 19 Fevers) Sick people emanate poisons, concluded Sir John Pringle (1703–82), and in sufficient concentration the resulting tainted atmosphere, when inhaled, causes this fever. The prophylactic was ventilation, which in effect opens up the hospital enclosure. The concept, and fear, of 'hospital diseases' resulted in a strangely anthropomorphic vision of buildings with 'inbred disease',[6] and 'traumatic'[7] and chronic infections. It survived the advent of germ theory: erysipelas, pyaemia, septicaemia, and gangrene were, and were known to be, commoner on hospital wards than elsewhere until the twentieth century. (➤ Ch. 16 Contagion/germ theory/specificity) While miasmatism held sway, scientific opinion advocated the construction of small wards and small hospitals: not only did every patient increase the concentration of toxins, large spaces were too difficult to ventilate. (➤ Ch. 15 Environment and miasmata)

By the end of the century, the European continentals had to grant that England, scarcely in the vanguard of medical science, was, with Scotland, peerless when it came to institutional planning and administration. London's medieval hospitals got new homes, and the 'voluntary' hospital movement later stimulated many foundations that typically rented and converted a house and then, when funds permitted, acquired purpose-built quarters. In keeping with the prevailing architectural idiom, these were Palladian in style and, mostly on the outskirts of towns, they resembled unpretentious villas. Unlike real Palladian houses, however, their storeys were often of equal heights and identical plans. This activity was matched only in Paris, where philanthropists founded and endowed small hospitals after disastrous fires at the Hôtel Dieu, the last in 1772.

As far as Paris was concerned, it was the Royal Naval Hospitals at Haslar, near Portsmouth (opened 1761), and Stonehouse, near Plymouth (completed 1765), that were of paramount significance. Both were huge, accommodating 2,000 and 1,200 patients, respectively, but both were laid out around courtyards, and Stonehouse moreover in the isolated pavilions that had come to be seen as the ideal, 'self-ventilating' type. Haslar's first senior physician was James Lind (1716–94), certainly a stickler for fumigation and ventilation in his eighty-four wards, but it was Stonehouse, possibly designed under the influence of Pringle's writings, that aroused the particular admiration of Tenon when he visited England in 1787, for he saw it as the near-embodiment of what he had been advocating for years.

Continental Europe architects trained in academies. This system not only facilitated the importation of other disciplines – the physician-scientist Jean-Baptiste Le Roy (d. 1800) read papers about ventilation to the architectural students – it accustomed architects to the translation of written briefs, set for competitive examinations, into graphic designs. The Hôtel Dieu fire of 1772 began a sixteen-year discussion, at first about its rebuilding, and then about hospital architecture in general, which embraced the French academies of sciences and architecture, as well as the church. Soon after the fire, the government asked the Académie des Sciences for advice. Le Roy, together with the architect Charles-François Viel (1745–1819), worked out a plan featuring parallel, single-storey ward-pavilions whose roofs had ventilation ducts. By 1788, more than fifty plans had been presented, among them that of the surgeon Antoine Petit (1718–94) for a giant wheel with ward-spokes radiating from a domed, ventilating hub (1774). A similar plan of 1785, by the architects Claude-Philippe Coquéau (1755–94) and Bernard Poyet (1742–1824), was studied by the science academy at Louis XVI's order, which indicates the seriousness of the business, as well as the apparent discounting of architecture unexamined by science. Poyet went on to help Tenon with the definitive pavilion plan, published in Tenon's *Mémoires sur les hôpitaux de Paris* (1788), the most important book about hospital construction for a century, and the culmination of one of the major events of the Enlightenment.

Tenon was the first to describe ward-pavilion hospitals as 'machines for healing'.[8] He and his colleagues believed that one machine, in mass production, would suffice: 'the best plan is unique and it must be able to produce everywhere the same solutions in response to the same demands'.[9] What Bruno Fortier has called the *banalisation* of hospitals,[10] their reduction to the infinitely reproducible pavilion, was underway, but it was a slow start. Not until the construction by Martin Pierre Gauthier (1789–1855) of the 'model' Hôpital Lariboisière in Paris (1839–54) was the perfect exemplar available. It would be widely admired, not least in England.

Meanwhile, the architectural academy was setting medal-competition subjects like an 'island lazaretto' (1784), whose brief specified widely separated pavilions, and a 'hospital for 1,200 beds' (1787), along with the usual triumphal arches and bridges. This typological, normative way of thinking was reinforced by the aims and methods of the Conseil des Bâtiments Civils and its equivalents in other European countries. These bodies were formed to identify and promote national building styles whose rationality and flexibility would permit their application to prisons, markets, abattoirs, hospitals, asylums, and lazarettos, to name only the building types of significance to public health: new social orders were to find immediate architectural expression. In turn, with such bureaucracies behind it, architecture regained some autonomy. In 1842, for example, the Conseil, exasperated with shifting therapeutic desiderata, authorized Emile-Jacques Gilbert (1793–1874), architect to the rebuilding of Charenton (started 1838), to complete the asylum as J. E. D. Esquirol (1772–1840) had planned it. The new chief physician, who had held up construction for months in the hope of replacing private rooms with dormitories, could *not* change the specifications at that point. Changes cost money.

Anglo-American architects, most trained by apprenticeship and self-employed, could scarcely look to academies or ministries. For them – and, in practice, for any architect actually on site – hospitals presented local, technical problems, not questions with a universal solution to be discovered after debate at the highest levels. They could advise a committee how to start building with erratic funding, or how an existing structure could be adapted to meet such new demands as a fever epidemic, or expanded to generate more income: public baths and cells for lunatics (almost invariably fee-paying) were popular schemes. And, since the voluntary hospitals also embodied collective civic charity, they could grant them a dignified (though always economical) monumentality. As Charles Bulfinch (1763–1844), the Architect of the Massachusetts General Hospital (opened 1821) in Boston, wrote to its directors in 1817, a hospital building should be 'ornamental to the town, and gratifying to the sight and feelings of each one, who may reflect that he has assisted in [its] endowment'. He recommended stone, not brick: it was more expensive, but required less maintenance and its 'richness' 'will allow of a less decorated stile of ornament'.[11] Indeed, hospitals were not supposed to look *too* grand, and thus give rise to the suspicion that money was being wasted. This practical consideration was reinforced by age-old notions of 'decorum'. The simple modesty of hospitals' façades corresponded to their inhabitants' demeanour (in theory) and social status.

More tacit conclusions about the building type have proved surprisingly durable. Many hospitals were constructed piecemeal, as the money came in. Robert Adam (1728–92) was told in 1791 that his plan for the Glasgow Royal Infirmary 'should be such that a part of it may be conveniently executed, and the other part, gradually carried on as the Demand may require, till the whole plan be fully executed':[12] such instructions were very common. In 1982, the British Department of Health and Social Security published the identical principle as the 'nucleus concept': that of building a hospital in phases, beginning with a 300-bed core that could function autonomously.

The written record suggests that architects working at this local, vernacular level had more to say about hospital façades, budgets, and construction schedules than about their plans, but perhaps, *pace* the French academy of sciences, there was not much to be said. When the US Congress passed a law authorizing the construction of permanent naval hospitals in 1811, 'that able engineer, Mr. Latrobe'[13] was employed to design them. Benjamin Henry Latrobe (1764–1820) made no bones about his lack of medical knowledge in his subsequent report (1814), but his statement that he chose small wards from his 'own conviction that [they were] the best in a medical point of view'[14] suggests what was undoubtedly true: medical theory was not yet beyond the grasp of an able engineer.

Nor was the technology of healthy building particularly recondite: no gentleman then demurred at designing his own home – or hospital – should he have a mind to do so. An architectural competition for the Derbyshire Infirmary yielded a 'considerable number'[15] of plans, but none to the satisfaction of the committee, whose members designed it themselves, afterwards employing a drawing-master to make the working plans. In 1807, the building site caught the lively eye of William Strutt (1756–1830), an intimate of Erasmus Darwin (1731–1802), the Bentham brothers, and Robert Owen (1771–1858). Strutt had already equipped his own and friends' houses with various ingenious gadgets: his ventilation and heating system was used at Derby and the West Riding Pauper Lunatic Asylum (Wakefield, Yorkshire), among other institutions. For architects and medical and lay trustees, the new science of 'domestic economy', comprising systems of heating, ventilation, water supply, and sewage disposal, was the most interesting and useful part of hospital design. Clearly illustrated books had newly become available, and Bulfinch – himself a Harvard graduate, a gentleman-architect – coloured a diagram of flues and underlined passages about the systems at Wakefield in his copy of Sylvester's book about the Derby Infirmary.

The American hospital governors' genial sense of superiority over the crowded, disease-soaked Old World – they did not have to wrestle with ancient town and hospital fabrics – did not prevent them from assiduous note-taking in Europe. Dr George Parkman write to his fellow Massachusetts

General trustees from Italy in 1812, advising them that there were few useful models there, but he later presented them with a book about the asylum in Nottingham. Charitable institutions had long been on tourist itineraries, and after 1800 'travel guides' to hospitals and asylums began to proliferate for the use of, among others, medical students intending to take up institutional appointments.

The charitable hospital was a useful vehicle for social advancement: it was customary for architects (like doctors) to donate their designs and in this way rank among the gentlemen-governors. By 1800, a few British architects enjoyed reputations as specialist hospital designers (plans were free, but architects staying with a project could reasonably expect to take a fee, perhaps as a contractor). In 1791, the Glasgow Royal Infirmary's building committee reported that it had written to an architect 'whose plans of Infirmaries had been executed with such success in different parts of England',[16] asking for a plan. This also, of course, reassured its promoters that the infirmary would benefit from experience. More significantly, perhaps, in 1807 the Parliamentary Select Committee appointed to inquire into the 'state of criminal and pauper lunatics' called the architect John Nash (1752–1835), who claimed to have designed three asylums, among other expert witnesses.

The bulk of eighteenth- and early nineteenth-century medical texts have nothing to say about hospital construction. Nevertheless, medical reformers almost invariably began their critiques of *institutions* with catalogues of deficiencies in existing *buildings*. Typical is the following, Tenon on the Hôtel Dieu:

> We have seen rooms so narrow that the air stagnates and is not renewed and that light enters only feebly and charged with vapours. . . . We have seen a room for convalescents on the third floor which could be reached only via the smallpox ward.[17]

This negativism, this seeming preference for demolition over specific, constructive suggestion, was deliberate. As the physician John Aikin (1747–1822) wrote, 'It does not belong to my profession to lay down an architectural plan for one of these buildings. . . . But by pointing out what to avoid, we in effect give rules what to aim at'.[18] Tenon *did* lay down a plan, but he also claimed only the right to guide, not design. He wrote to George Dance the younger (1741–1825), the architect of Newgate Prison and the rebuilt St Luke's Hospital (1782–7, demolished c.1965):

> My aim in this work is not to set myself up as an architect, nor to talk of the building and decoration of these houses of charity. . . . I have merely to consider hospitals in relation to the patient . . . and, in the art of curing, to discover general principles which might be applied in the construction (*formation*) and layout (*distribution*) of buildings designed for their assistance.[19]

'Decoration' was always left to architects, but the line between 'principles' and 'building' can be attenuated to the point of invisibility. A century later, there would be real confusions, still evident in the secondary literature, about the authorship of hospital designs.

The well-travelled John Howard (*c*.1726–90) could identify exemplars of planning and organizations from Leeds to Venice, and he provided relatively specific recommendations for construction in his *Account of the Principal Lazarettos in Europe*.[20] Like Tenon and the other medical travellers, he was oblivious to the appearance of hospitals. They described, rather, the relative placements of rooms, and ventilation and laundry systems, and noted patient numbers and the relative outcomes of operations. The building was judged by quantifiable effects.

Criticism of architecture *per se* centred on the simple fact that architects were trained to use space as economically as possible. As Latrobe wrote, 'with the limited fund of the hospital therefore, the first consideration in forming the design was to cover as little ground as possible'.[21] But, of course, the doctors wanted more ground per patient, not less. Denis Diderot (1713–84) claimed in the *Encyclopédie* article on hospitals that their design was too important to be left to architects, but objections were half-hearted on the whole, with the important exception of those concerning lunatic asylums.

THE DESIGN OF LUNATIC ASYLUMS

Institutions for the mentally ill present a special case because psychiatry's very rise as a profession was indissoluble from general, lay acceptance of the idea that the asylum was the proper receptacle for the lunatic, that madness required this special architecture. This was the only medical speciality to mount a sustained campaign against architecture – the rival competence in the programme of constructing nurturing environments constructed by humans – and the first to regard the building as an active therapeutic device, and not just something to keep out the rain while the doctors got to work. The mad-doctors' written briefs were of a length and specificity then unprecedented in the history of architecture. (➤ Ch. 56 Psychiatry)

Around 1800, burgeoning psychiatric professionalism coincided with the pressing need to remove lunatics from prisons and workhouses, part of a greater movement to reform and refine the administration of social welfare all over Europe and the Americas; and a concomitant interest in the design of 'reformed' residential institutions, particularly prisons, with an eye to the careful separation of different categories of inmate.

Hospitals were not central to the professional lives of most medical practitioners, and they were certainly peripheral to the great Enlightenment project of keeping entire populations healthy and reproducing. Mad-doctors, however, all advocated the construction of new asylums, even while castigating those in existence. Theirs were the loudest medical voices criticizing architecture: the problem was not with the institution, but with the botch that architects had, supposedly, made of its buildings. The asylum's plan was 'not at all a trivial thing to be left up to the architects alone',[22] wrote Esquirol in 1818; the same year, the phrenologist J. G. Spurzheim (1776–1832) exploded that the architect, 'fond of his art', 'likes to display . . . fine columns' but is completely 'ignorant of the human mind in its state of health and disease'.[23]

Carefully designed, purpose-built asylums would render redundant manacles and other forms of physical coercion and restraint. Such an institution was the Glasgow Royal Asylum (opened 1814) of William Stark (1770–1813). However, Stark's highly scientific radiating plan, for which he provided an intelligent justification on the basis of the separation of patients according to sex, class, and clinical state,[24] was too inflexible to accommodate facilities that shortly after became defined as desirable, among them a chapel, a billiard-room, and workrooms.

Stark's plan permitted central surveillance, but it was not, strictly speaking, 'panoptical'. Bentham's institutional archetype was rarely applied to asylum design: doctors suspected that it was expensive to build, difficult to ventilate, and encouraged laziness among staff. The Panopticon was itself influenced by earlier prisons, however, and prisons and asylums sometimes steered dangerously convergent courses. This was pointed out by Samuel Tuke (1784–1857) in his book on pauper lunatic asylums which compared the Glasgow Asylum with the new Ipswich County Gaol. The difference was that, once incarcerated, a prisoner stayed put, whereas asylum inmates should be able to graduate from one division to another depending on their 'capacity for rational enjoyment',[25] that is, their behaviour. Tuke accepted the large, public, pauper lunatic asylum as a necessary evil – his *Practical Hints* were published in connection with the architectural competition for the Wakefield asylum – but his name is associated with the other asylum archetype, the Friends' Retreat in York (opened 1792).

By then, associationalist psychology had thoroughly permeated architectural and psychiatric theory alike. No one was immune to the 'character' of the environment, and given lunatics' propensities for drawing faulty conclusions on the basis of external stimuli, their surroundings had to be unambiguously soothing. In particular, as John Bevans, the Retreat's architect, wrote, 'if the outside appears heavy and prison-like it has a considerable effect upon the imagination'.[26] The Retreat's anodyne, domestic appearance was carefully worked out by Bevans and Samuel's grandfather, William Tuke (1732–1822). It was inseparable from the idea of psychological therapy conducted within the spacious, clean home for the morally regenerating, surrogate family.

Thanks to the effectiveness of Samuel's illustrated *Description*,[27] and the cohesive cosmopolitanism of the Society of Friends, no fewer than five asylums explicitly influenced by the form of the Retreat opened in the next three decades in the United States, for example, and Americans still assume that psychiatric hospitals are what the American architect Frank Gehry (b. 1929) has called 'sweetie-pie Georgian mansions in the trees'.[28]

Europe, however, has a different asylum mythology. In 1961, Enoch Powell, Britain's Minister of Health, signalled his government's belief that the therapeutic philosophy embodied by the great nineteenth-century asylums was dated and discredited, and in so doing, described them unforgettably.

> There they stand: isolated, majestic, imperious, brooded over by the gigantic water-tower and chimney combined, rising, unmistakable and daunting, out of the countryside; the asylums which our forefathers built with such immense solidity.[29]

Charenton, Colney Hatch: they are huge, isolated outside the cities they served; they dominate the landscape from their heights, and all because they were planned to be self-enclosed and self-sufficient worlds, whose limits would not, prison-like, readily be apparent to their inmates. No less than the Retreat and its thousand (mostly private) successors, the European public regional asylums share a domestic ethos, but it is that of the extended family, the village or estate.

'Conceive a spacious building resembling the palace of a peer, airy, and elevated, and elegant, surrounded by extensive and swelling grounds and gardens',[30] begins a famous passage by the psychiatrist W. A. F. Browne (1805–85): the sort of palace envisaged was Blenheim, not Buckingham, and it is only appropriate that asylum gardens like that at Schleswig, Germany (completed 1820) were described as in the 'English', or picturesque, style, and that among the most admired devices at Charenton were the *sauts-de-loup*, or ha-has. The estate, with its home farm and various offices and outbuildings, all presided over by the agents of a benign and far-seeing landowner, presented an inspirational model for asylum directors, who never shed the dream of leading self-sufficient rural colonies, placed great stress on the therapeutic potency of repetitive, outdoor work, and sought to impart the rural virtues of self-discipline and taciturnity to the inmates. Many European asylums were built in a farmhouse-Italianate style. This had been developed around 1800 in France, where architect-archaeologists identified it as the primitive classical vernacular. The style was not only appropriate – 'moral therapy' had a strong whiff of Stoicism about it – its simplicity, and the readiness with which its elements could be combined lent themselves to a building type that was supposed to be as attractive and informal as possible.

TOWN-PLANNING AND PUBLIC HEALTH

Identical principles governed the hygienic construction of hospitals and cities, but hospitals led the way. According to Lewis Mumford:

> Perhaps the greatest contribution made by the industrial town was the reaction it produced against its own greatest misdemeanours; and, to begin with, the art of sanitation or public hygiene. The original models for these evils were the pest-ridden prisons and hospitals of the eighteenth century: their improvement made them pilot plants, as it were, in the reform of the industrial town.[31]

For all the eighteenth-century hospital's faults, it was better than many people's homes, 'the closeness and unwholesomeness of which is too often one great cause of their sickness',[32] as the preamble to the subscription list of the Westminister (London) Public Infirmary (founded 1719) had it.

There are many anecdotes to suggest that eighteenth-century city-dwellers would go to some lengths to avoid having a hospital as a neighbour: in Copenhagen in the 1780s, residents of one fashionable area even offered to club together to buy a hospital another site – far away. This was, however, an institution for lunatics and venereal-disease sufferers: Frederiks Hospital (opened 1757, now the Museum of Decorative Art), with a more salubrious population, had been built as one of the focal points of that very quarter. The constructions of the Edinburgh and Glasgow Royal Infirmaries similarly signalled those cities' embarkations on systematic town-planning schemes. It is therefore dangerous to generalize about their status in the neo-classical city: not all were regarded, like Paris's Bicêtre, as a 'receptable for all the most monstrous and vile things to be found in society',[33] a quotation that Michel Foucault used in his famous discussion of the *grande peur*.

However, many decayed medieval foundations were regarded as horrific reminders of a Gothic past, prime targets for institutional and urban reforms that would rehouse and possibly remove them to the outskirts, along with other unpleasant and unwholesome relics like prisons, fish-markets, slaughter-houses, and tanneries. Similarly, the walls that still surrounded so many Old World cities were regarded as barriers to the free circulation of air; they had certainly begun to inhibit expansion. Many came down or were incorporated into park-and-promenade schemes. Along with the promotion of commerce, public health – including public safety – was the desideratum behind eighteenth-century urban 'improvements'.

Innumerable quarters were tidied up, and some 'new towns', outstandingly that in Edinburgh, were laid out on grid plans that opened the buildings to light and air. Town-planning theory, with its emphasis on clearing congestion, had not advanced much in 1,800 years: Vitruvius was regularly quoted, and not least his passage advocating the embellishment of urban walks ('walking in the open air is very healthy') with 'green things', which emit 'refined and rarefied air'[34] that clears the vision and disperses superfluous humours. A century and a half of speculative development in London culminated in an enormously influential English vision of town-planning as 'the art of linking a set of Elysian scenes'[35] like that presented by Nash's Regent's Park (1821–30). Architects and doctors increasingly invested such scenes with physiological as well as psychological potency. Camillo Sitte insisted on the hygienic function of the urban park, which he called a 'sanitary green'.[36] Doctors too, notably Benjamin Ward Richardson (1828–96), began to compose in the venerable utopian genre.[37]

But houses were not, at first, targeted as sites for rebuilding or refurbishment, except by pioneer planners of co-operative, integrated industrial communities like Robert Owen (New Lanark, Scotland, 1815) and Charles Fourier (1772–1837) in France. Later manufacturers sponsored the building of model towns, and philanthropic bodies like the Peabody Trust (1862) made huge sums available for model tenement housing for the respectable working classes, which in general became a subject of keen interest for people including Napoleon III and Prince Albert.

How had the problem of mass housing achieved such unprecedented prominence? The period 1800–50 saw huge relative increases in urban populations all over the Western world. Newly available statistical data on mortality and morbidity rates were correlated with subjective observations of quarters and even individual streets that were overcrowded, filthy, poorly serviced, and shoddily built: Edwin Chadwick (1800–90) in his *Inquiry into the Sanitary Condition of the Labouring Population*, for example, sought to show how local atmospheric miasmata that caused the so-called 'epidemic' diseases were generated by such conditions.[38] (➤ Ch. 52 Epidemiology)

This concept, and the appropriate response, is well illustrated by Mary Shelley (1797–1851) in her scientific romance *The Last Man*. The novel is set at the end of the twenty-first century, when plague spreads inexorably towards the Republic of England. It is an 'epidemic', not 'what is commonly called contagious, like the scarlet fever, or extinct small-pox'; as such,

> its chief force was derived from pernicious qualities in the air, and it would probably do little harm where this was naturally salubrious... cleanliness, habits of order, and the manner in which our cities were built, were all in our favour.[39]

The traditional architectural responses to 'contagious' diseases – around 1820, the threat of yellow fever, thought to be 'contagious' on an unprecedented level, stimulated the last great lazaretto-construction programme, in France – were joined by wider-ranging measures to combat the epidemics. Cholera arrived in England five years after Shelley's novel was published, and, as William Guy (1810–85) later wrote,

> When the cholera did us the favour to pay us a visit (I speak seriously, it was a favour), we made preparation for its reception. We cleansed out many an Augean stable, set the scavengers to work in right earnest, whitewashed sundry houses, and showed a wholesome respect for the threatened invader.[40]

Cholera is not propagated by filth as such, but by bacterially infected water. This and comparable demonstrations neither impeded the cleansing of cities, nor its beneficial effects: after all, poor housing can be implicated in many non-communicable disorders although many links remain surprisingly resistant to experimental (as opposed to experiential) demonstration. (➤ Ch. 53 History of personal hygiene)

THE PAVILION-PLAN HOSPITAL

The discrediting of miasmatism similarly had little immediate effect on its other great architectural manifestation, the pavilion-plan hospital. It looks like nothing else: with it, the building type finally abandoned its ecclesiastical, monastic, and domestic antecedents.

> The 'pavilion system', as conceived by its advocates, consisted preferably of single storey, or failing this, two-storey ward blocks, usually placed at right angles to a linking corridor which might either be straight or enclosing a large central square; the pavilions were widely separated, usually by lawns or gardens. In the wards, complete cross-ventilation was achieved by opposite rows of tall, narrow windows reaching from floor to ceiling. Natural ventilation, from doors, windows and fireplace was the rule.[41]

Effectively an invention of the circle debating the reconstruction of the Hôtel Dieu in the 1770s and 1780s, with encouragement from the examples of the British naval hospitals, the pavilion plan was reintroduced to Britain after widely-admired French examples, in particular the Lariboisière, had been constructed.

After 1850, hospital design became inseparable from the wider questions of hospital size, siting, and control; town-planning and sanitary reform; and, ultimately, from the future of empires, in the form of their armies. Lay people, architects, doctors, and nurses allied to promote a single plan type, and, in its wake, the idea that hospital architecture was necessarily the province of highly specialized expertise.

Richardson, for his *Hygeia*, 'proposed to abandon "the old idea of warehousing diseases on the largest possible scale", and advocated a small hospital for every 5,000 people'.[42] Henry C. Burdett (1847–1920) pointed to the maldistribution of hospitals in London in an 1881 lecture to the Social Science Association, which hints that patients might be better served by placing hospitals under a degree of central-government control. Burdett's books include *Hospitals and Asylums of the World*, and he founded two periodicals on the subject.[43] Always, he encouraged hospital boards to look further and further afield for advice. He asked for £250 to advise on plans submitted for Glasgow's Victoria Infirmary. The directors' confidence in their own judgement was not completely undermined, however: they found someone to do it for 100 guineas.

Specialist journals like Burdett's *The Hospital* joined an increasing number of architectural periodicals, among them *The Builder*, published by George Godwin (1813–88). It would be difficult to overestimate the influence of Godwin, who began investigating for himself the fetid courts and alleys of England in the 1850s, and whose journal addressed every conceivable conjunction of medicine and architecture. The same period saw the formation of such specialized practices as those of Casimir Tollet (1829–99) in France and Henry Saxon Snell (1830–1904) in England. New specialities create their own histories: both men wrote books that combined historical surveys with gazetteers, like Burdett's, of existing buildings; all to demonstrate that the pavilion plan was superior to other types.[44] Saxon Snell's *Hospital Construction and Management*,[45] co-authored by a physician, claimed to be the first textbook on the subject in English: Gill W. Wylie, MD, had made no such claim in his *Hospitals: their History, Organization, and Construction*.

Florence Nightingale (1820–1910) wrote, famously, in her *Notes on Hospitals* that 'the very first requirement of a hospital is that it should do the sick no harm':[47] she adhered firmly to a miasmatic theory of contagion that Vitruvius would have recognized, and advocated the pavilion plan that for a century had been thought to admit maximum air circulation between and inside hospital wards. In this she was strongly influenced and encouraged by Godwin and the surgeon John Roberton (1797–1876). Dozens of hospital-construction committees asked for her advice: when Dr Thomas Williams of the Swansea Infirmary wrote to her in 1864, she replied that 'A hospital is almost as difficult a place [*sic*] of construction as a watch and there is no building which requires more special knowledge'.[48] In an echo of Chadwick's earlier dismissal of civil engineers as incapable of grasping the principles of 'sanitationism', she wrote that she could not honestly recommend more than two or three architects in the land.

More and more doctors interested themselves in hospital design. The surgeon Charles Hawkins, not a fan of the pavilion type (he thought it too expensive), described his plan for Queen Charlotte's Hospital, London, which he had shown at an architectural exhibition the year before, in a 1862 letter to the *Lancet*. John Marshall (1818–91), also a surgeon, read a paper to the National Association for the Promotion of Social Science in 1878 that advocated the construction of circular wards, an idea regularly taken up for twenty years. Remarkably, given their status in most hospitals only a century earlier, some doctors became their own architects, or so one must describe John Shaw Billings (1838–1913) at Baltimore's Johns Hopkins Hospital (1876–89), a pavilion-type exemplary for its attention to the 'total isolation and segregation of patient-care spaces . . . design details which maximize sunlight and cleanliness . . . and the continuous introduction of "pure" air through extensive provision for natural and mechanical ventilation and heating'.[49] No medical (as opposed to architectural) historian attributes Johns Hopkins to the project architect John Niernsee (1831–85), but it must be conceded that the detail and execution of the buildings meets the highest standards of his profession.

Pavilion hospitals are expensive, in both land and construction costs. On confined sites, they were amenable only to the most destructive kind of enlargement, filling in the spaces between the wards: this was the fate of St Thomas's Hospital, London, designed by Henry Currey in 1867, with six three-storey pavilions linked by a 900-foot corridor-spine. As early as 1864, they were demonstrated to reduce 'hospitalism' no more than other types; and the aetiology on which they were predicated was soon superseded by the findings of bacteriology. But only in the twentieth century was the pavilion type superseded by the more compact and economical ward-tower, in a return to the monolithic hospital. Nightingale's recommendations for the minimum volumes and areas of space for each patient and bed, respectively, were actually increased in Britain until the late 1930s; and features like external stairwells, intended to facilitate the circulation of air, likewise survived long after miasmatism was discredited.

Various reasons for the resilience of the pavilion plan can be adduced. Architects doubtless liked its typological distinctiveness, as well as sheer size and expense; clients, on the other hand, knew that with it they could play safe and build in stages. The 'spine-and-pavilion' and related 'extended courtyard' plans, two of a dozen current general-hospital subtypes, are still valued for the ease with which they can be enlarged (on suburban sites), and planted areas integrated. And, of course, it makes no difference to a building whether it is mephitic or germ-laden air that causes nosocomial (hospital) infections.

THE MODERN HOSPITAL BUILDING

Infections are still a serious problem, 'prolong[ing] the stay of between 4 and 10 per cent of patients, in all the developed countries'.[50] Furthermore, it is still not known whether preventive measures should focus on air, or people and objects, as the carriers of germs, and, in the face of the experimental difficulties involved, adherents of one or the other hypothesis can be ruled by extra-scientific considerations. Architects might encourage a client to think about 'airborne' routes, because then they are in a position to help, by providing airtight doors separating areas of differential pressure, with the operating room (OR) having the highest (and thence down through prep-room, clean corridor, dressing-room, disrobing-room, and outside corridor), and, for the instruments, 'clean' and 'dirty' routes to and from the OR. Elaborate experimentation that began in the 1960s seems to show, however, that the careful maintenance of aseptic techniques (with, perhaps, ultra-clean air blown on the table during high-risk surgery) will do as much or more to reduce infection. The airborne route is not the busiest one, and the patient's own body is a particularly fertile source of bacteria. This conclusion, at first 'greeted with incredulity'[51] was vindicated after further investigation, but also after an oil crisis (in 1973) that led many authorities to look again at hospital-construction costs. However, mechanical pressurization is still highly desirable in critical-care wards and other areas where airborne infection remains a problem. Certain patients can now be accommodated in isolation rooms with reversible systems: 'normally the pressure variable between the isolation room and the corridor favors keeping the patient's germs in the room, but for HIV patients – or any immunosuppressed patient – the relationship must be reversed to protect the patient from [the germs] in the corridor.'[52]

In this way, germ theory has affected the siting and design of the OR, and in comparable ways, hospital laboratories. On the wards themselves, its most important expression was the sealed, mechanically ventilated glass iso-lation cubicle, which became common in European and American children's hospitals after 1900. However, disquiet with the cubicles, and in general with ward routines that discouraged the children's free mixing with one another and their visitors, was expressed as early as the 1920s.

Psychological medicine is not a new element in general-hospital design and it is obviously one of particular interest to architects. Bulfinch wrote in 1817 that private rooms, which were 'much more agreeable to the domestic habits of our people'[53] were, when possible, preferable to wards at the Massachusetts General. The Americans' continuing preference for private rooms over open wards is today often ascribed to the machinations of insurance companies: but hospitals, surrogate houses, must be expected to differ from culture to culture in their nursing (as opposed to clinical) zones.

In general, accommodation for teaching, medical services, and medical specialities now form the core of a hospital building, the so-called 'clinical' zone; the wards are grouped around it. The story of twentieth-century hospi-tal design is one of a losing battle against the construction costs incurred by the ever-expanding clinical and administrative zones. An index that has become increasingly important is the ratio resulting when the gross area of the hospital is divided by the number of beds: it is expressed as M^2 : bed. The nineteenth-century ratio was typically 20 : 1; after the Second World

War this had risen to 75–80 : 1 in some countries.[54] Ward towers represent an attempt to get around this problem: an early example is University College Hospital, London (compl. 1906), by Alfred Waterhouse (1830–1905), in which four-storey ward-blocks rise from a single-storey base: these pavilions are themselves cruciform, to take maximum advantage of a confined site.

Hospital design is now a speciality in which architectural students can receive formal training, in addition to the more traditional routes of working in a specialized office, or winning a competition – and then telephoning around for advice. Every year, a very large number of periodicals and books are published, and conferences held about the subject. Architects do not require medical knowledge any more than they ever did, but equally they still have to understand hospital procedures, and the amount of technical data to be mastered has seen a geometric progression in the last century. Some, like regulations governing hospital electrification and humidification, vary between countries: these complex matters are increasingly left to subcontractors. And some factors, like examination and therapy routines (how long will a patient have to wait?) are individual to the hospital. For this reason, as well as in a reaction to the discipline's extremely technical nature, many hospital architects see themselves as mediators between various user-groups. Good ones will not assume that the hospital chief necessarily knows what is best for all the medical personnel, let alone the kitchen- and cleaning-staff.

To some extent, hospitals have finally acquired architectural- (as opposed to medical-) theoretical glamour. Given their accelerated rate of functional development, it is now thought to be unreasonable to expect architects to tailor a building to fit; they can only plan to accommodate change. This logical extension of an old understanding, along with the related ideas of 'expendability' and a universally available pop-technological culture, appealed to theoretically inclined architects in the 1960s. While 'Plug-in City' (1964–6) of Peter Cook (b. 1936), for example, necessarily remained on paper, standarized and almost infinitely accommodating hospital-building envelopes were constructed for what are in fact called 'plug-in departments'.

We are now fastidious about expendability and pop-technological culture, and anyway cannot always afford new, state-of-the-art hospitals. Old fabrics can be renewed, provided that standards applying to new buildings are relaxed, and that the hospital's location is still useful: it is an attractive notion, but many renovation costs are hidden until work begins. There are tens of thousands of historic hospital buildings in the world, and very few can hope for renovation, conversion to new uses, or legislative protection.

ACKNOWLEDGEMENTS

I am extremely grateful to the friends who commented on drafts of this article, and above all to Dale R. Brown, Peter Pawlik, and Jeremy Taylor, who helped me with their great knowledge, as historians and practitioners, of architecture and hospital planning in particular.

NOTES

1 Vitruvius, *The Ten Books on Architecture*, trans. by Morris Hicky Morgan, Cambridge, MA, Harvard University Press, 1914; repr. New York, Dover, 1960, I: i: 10.

2 Joan E. Lynaugh, 'From respectable domesticity to medical efficiency: the changing Kansas City hospital, 1875–1920', in Diana Elizabeth Long and Janet Golden (eds), *The American General Hospital: Communities and Social Contexts*, Ithaca, NY, and London, Cornell University Press, 1989, pp. 21–39; see p. 27.

3 Jeremy Bentham, *Panopticon; or the Inspection House: Containing the Idea of a New Principle of Construction Applicable to . . . Penitentiary-Houses, Prisons . . . and Schools* [etc.], 3 vols, London, T. Payne, 1791.

4 John Henderson, 'The hospitals of late-medieval and Renaissance Florence: a preliminary survey', in Lindsay Granshaw and Roy Porter (eds), *The Hospital in History*, Wellcome Institute Series in the History of Medicine, London and New York, Routledge, 1989, pp. 63–92; see p. 67.

5 From Gilbert Burnet's translation of More's *Utopia* (1516), London, 1684, pp. 92–3. Quoted in Edward P. de G. Chaney, ' "Philanthropy in Italy": English observations on Italian hospitals, 1545–1789', in Thomas Riis (ed.), *Aspects of Poverty in Early Modern Europe*, Alphen aan den Rijn, Sijthoff, 1981, pp. 183–217; see p. 183.

6 John Aikin's phrase, quoted by Guenter Risse, *Hospital Life in Enlightenment Scotland: Care and Teaching at the Royal Infirmary of Edinburgh*, Cambridge, Cambridge University Press, 1986, p. 23.

7 From a report prepared in Swansea after an 1876 outbreak of erysipelas and other infections: T. G. Davies, *Deeds Not Words: a History of the Swansea General and Eye Hospital 1817–1948*, Cardiff, University of Wales Press, 1988, p. 80.

8 He used the phrase *machines à guérir* in a MS now in the Bibliothèque Nationale: Barry Bergdoll, 'The architecture of isolation: M.-R. Penchaud's quarantine hospital in the Mediterranean', *AA Files*, 1987, 14: 3–13; see p. 12 n.

9 From the *Third Report* of the commission for the new Hôtel Dieu project (1787): *La Meilleure disposition est unique et elle doit offrir partout les mêmes secours aux mêmes besoins.* Quoted by Bruno Fortier, 'Architecture de l'hôpital', in Michel Foucault *et al.*, *Les Machines à guérir: aux origines de l'hôpital moderne*, Paris, Institut de l'Environment, 1976, pp. 71–86, see p. 75 n.

10 Ibid., p. 71.

11 Leonard K. Eaton, 'Charles Bulfinch and the Massachusetts General Hospital', *Isis*, 1950, 41: 8–10, on pp. 10–11.

12 Glasgow Royal Infirmary Minute Books HB 14/1/1, p. 25, minutes of the meeting of 19 July 1791.

13 William P. C. Barton, *A Treatise Containing a Plan for the Internal Organization and Government of Marine Hospitals, in the United States*, Philadelphia, PA, [for the Author], 1814, p. 3.

14 'Mr Latrobe's Report on marine hospitals', in ibid., pp. 111–20; see p. 112.

15 Charles Sylvester, *The Philosophy of Domestic Economy, as Exemplified in the Mode of Warming, Ventilating, Washing... Adopted in the Derbyshire General Infirmary*, Nottingham, H. Barnett, 1819, pp. iii, vii, 1–2.

16 Op. cit. (n. 12). The architect was 'Mr Blackburn', identified in the near-contemporary index to the Minutes as William Blackburn, now remembered for his *prison* designs.

17 Quoted by Erwin H. Ackerknecht, *Medicine at the Paris Hospital, 1794–1840*, Baltimore, MD, Johns Hopkins University Press, 1967, p. 133.

18 John Aikin, *Thoughts on Hospitals*, London, Joseph Johnson, 1771, p. 20; quoted in Barbara Duncum, 'The development of hospital design and planning', in F. N. L. Poynter (ed.), *The Evolution of Hospitals in Britain*, London, Pitman Medical 1964, pp. 207–29; see p. 211.

19 Letter in the Bibliothèque Nationale, quoted by Pinon, *L'Hospice de Charenton: temple de la raison ou folie de l'archéologie/The Charenton Hospital: Temple of Reason or Archaeological Folly*, trans. by Murray Wylie, Archives de l'Institut Français d'Architecture, Brussels, Pierre Mardaga, 1989, p. 39 n.

20 John Howard, *Account of the Principal Lazarettos in Europe*, 1789; 2nd edn, 1791.

21 Latrobe, op. cit. (n. 14), p. 112.

22 Jean Etienne Dominique Esquirol, 'Des établissements des aliénés en France et des moyens d'améliorer le sort de ces infortunés' (1818), repr. in *Des Malades mentales considerées sous les rapports médical, hygiènique, et médico-légal*, 3 vols, Paris, J.-B. Baillière, 1838, Vol. II, pp. 399–431, p. 421.

23 J. G. Spurzheim, *Observations on the Deranged Manifestations of the Mind, or Insanity*, London, Baldwin, Craddock & Joy, 1817, pp. 214–15.

24 William Stark, *Remarks on the Construction of Public Hospitals for the Cure of Mental Derangement*, Edinburgh, 1807; 2nd edn, Glasgow, James Hedderwick, 1810.

25 *Practical Hints on the Construction and Economy of Pauper Lunatic Asylums*, York, William Alexander, 1815; see pp. 17–18, 23–4.

26 Samuel Tuke quoted by Anne Digby, 'Moral treatment at the Retreat, 1796–1846', in W. F. Bynum, Roy Porter and Michael Shepherd (eds), *The Anatomy of Madness: Essays in the History of Psychiatry*, Vol. II: *Institutions and Society*, London and New York, Tavistock, 1985, pp. 52–72; see p. 54.

27 *Description of the Retreat, an Institution near York for Insane Persons of the Society of Friends*, York, W. Alexander, 1813.

28 Mark Alden Branch, 'A "village" of hope', *Yale Alumni Magazine*, November 1989, pp. 30–34; see p. 32.

29 Enoch Powell to the National Association of Mental Health, 9 March 1961, quoted in Sandra Barwick, 'The hidden heritage', *Independent Magazine*, 29 October 1988, pp. 45–50; see p. 47.

30 Andrew Scull (ed.), [W. A. F. Browne, *What Asylums were, are, and ought to be*, 1837] *The Asylum as Utopia: W. A. F. Browne and the Mid-Nineteenth Century Consolidation of Psychiatry*, Tavistock Classics in the History of Psychiatry, London and New York, Tavistock/Routledge, 1991, p. 229.

31 Lewis Mumford, *The City in History: its Origins, its Transformations and its Prospects*, London, Penguin Books, 1966, p. 541; orig. pub. 1961.

32 Duncum, op. cit. (n. 18), p. 207.

33 Louis-Sébastien Mercier, *Tableau de Paris*, Amsterdam, 1783, Vol. VIII, p. 2; quoted in Michel Foucault, *Madness and Civilization: a History of Insanity in the Age of Reason*, trans. by Richard Howard, Social Science Paperback series, London, Tavistock, 1971, p. 203.

34 Vitruvius, op. cit. (n. 1), V: ix: 5.

35 Alistair Rowan, 'Neo-classical town planning', in Arts Council of Great Britain, *The Age of Neo-Classicism*, Catalogue of the 14th Exhibition of the Council of Europe, London, 1972, pp. 656–60; see p. 659.

36 Camillo Sitte, *Der Städtebau nach seinen Künstlerischen Grundsätzen*, 1889.

37 Benjamin Ward Richardson, *Hygeia, or the City of Health*, 1875.

38 Edwin Chadwick, *Inquiry into the Sanitary Condition of the Labouring Population*, 1842.

39 Mary Shelley, *The Last Man*, London, Hogarth Press, 1985, pp. 167, 178; orig. pub. 1826.

40 W. A. Guy, *Unhealthiness of Towns, its Causes and Remedies*, London, Charles Knight, 1845, p. 25; quoted by Gerry Kearns, 'Cholera, nuisances and environmental management in Islington, 1830–55', in W. F. Bynum and Roy Porter (eds), *Living and Dying in London, Medical History* (suppl. 11), London, Wellcome Institute for the History of Medicine, 1991, pp. 94–125; see p. 94.

41 Anthony King, 'Hospital planning: revised thoughts on the origin of the pavilion principle in England', *Medical History*, 1966, 10: 360–73; see p. 360.

42 Quoted by Mumford, op. cit. (n. 31), p. 544.

43 Henry C. Burdett, *Hospitals and Asylums of the World*, 1891–3.

44 Casimir Tollet, *De l'Assistance publique et des hôpitaux jusqu'au XIXᵉ siècle*, Paris, 1889; *Les Édifices hospitaliers depuis leur origine jusqu'à nos jours*, 2nd edn, Paris, 1892; *Les Hôpitaux modernes au 19ᵉ siècle: description des principaux hôpitaux français et étrangers les plus récemment édifiés*, Paris, 1894.

45 Frederic J. Mouat and H. Saxon Snell, *Hospital Construction and Management*, London, J. & A. Churchill, 1883.

46 Gill W. Wylie, *Hospitals: their History, Organization, and Construction*, New York, 1877.

47 Florence Nightingale, *Notes on Hospitals*, 3rd edn, London, Longman, Green, 1863, p. iii; orig. pub. 1859.

48 Davies, op. cit., (n. 7), pp. 63–4.

49 Dale R. Brown, 'Medico-architectural determinism in 19th century hospital designs', unpublished paper delivered at the AAHM annual conference, 1991.

50 W. Paul James and William Tatton-Brown, *Hospitals: Design and Development*, London: Architectural Press, 1986, p. 69.

51 Ibid., p. 71.

52 Personal communication from Dale R. Brown, 1991.

53 Eaton, op. cit. (n. 11), p. 10.

54 James and Tatton-Brown, op. cit. (n. 50), p. 5.

FURTHER READING

L'Architecture des hôpitaux. Monuments historiques, April-May 1981, vol. 114.

Bergdoll, Barry, 'The architecture of isolation: M.-R. Penchaud's quarantine hospital in the Mediterranean', *AA Files*, 1987, 14: 3–13.

Diez del Corral, Rosario and Checa, Fernando, 'Typologie hospitalière et bienfaisance dans l'Espagne de la Renaissance. Croix grecque, panthéon, chambre des merveilles', *Gazette des Beaux-Arts*, 1986, 107: 118–26.

Donnelly, Michael, 'Representations of the asylum', and 'The architecture of confinement' in Donnelly, *Managing the Mind: A Study of Medical Psychology in Early Nineteenth-Century Britain*, London and New York, Tavistock, 1983.

Duncum, Barbara, 'The development of hospital design and planning', in F. N. L. Poynter (ed.), *The Evolution of Hospitals in Britain*, London, Pitman Medical, 1964, pp. 207–29.

Eaton, Leonard K., *New England Hospitals, 1790–1833*, Ann Arbor, University of Michigan Press, 1957.

Forty, Adrian, 'The modern hospital in England and France: the social and medical uses of architecture', in Anthony D. King (ed.), *Buildings and Society: Essays on the Social Development of the Built Environment*, London, Routledge & Kegan Paul, 1980.

Foucault, Michel, *et al.*, *Les Machines à guérir: aux origins de l'hôpital moderne*, Paris, Institut de l'Environnement, 1976.

Garnot, Nicholas Sainte Faire and Martel, Pierre (eds), *L'Architecture hospitalière au XIXe siècle: l'exemple parisien*, Les Dossiers du Musée d'Orsay 27, Paris, Éditions de la Réunion des Musées Nationaux, 1988.

Henderson, John, 'The hospitals of late-medieval and Renaissance Florence: a preliminary survey', in Lindsay Granshaw and Roy Porter (eds), *The Hospital in History*, Wellcome Institute Series in the History of Medicine, London and New York, Routledge, 1989.

James, W. Paul and Tatton-Brown, William, *Hospitals: Design and Development*, London, Architectural Press, 1986.

Jetter, Dieter, *Geschichte des Hospitals*, 6 vols to date, Stuttgart, Franz Steiner, 1966–.

Markus, Thomas A., 'Introduction' and 'Buildings for the sad, the bad and the mad in urban Scotland, 1780–1830', in Markus (ed.), *Order in Space and Society: Architectural Form and its Context in the Scottish Enlightenment*, Edinburgh, Mainstream, 1983.

Murken, Axel Hinrich, *Vom Armenhospital zum Großklinikum: die Geschichte des Krankenhauses vom 18. Jahrhundert bis zur Gegenwart*, Cologne, DuMont, 1988.

Pevsner, Nikolaus, 'Hospitals', in Pevsner, *A History of Building Types*, London, Thames & Hudson, 1976.

Pinon, Pierre, *L'Hospice de Charenton: temple de la raison ou folie de l'archéologie/The Charenton Hospital: Temple of Reason or Archaeological Folly*, trans. by Murray Wylie, Archives d'Institut Français d'Architecture, Brussels, Pierre Mardaga, 1989.

Prior, Lindsay, 'The architecture of the hospital: a study of spatial organization and medical knowledge', *British Journal of Sociology*, 1988, 39: 86–113.

Scull, Andrew, 'A convenient place to get rid of inconvenient people: the Victorian lunatic asylum', in Anthony D. King (ed.), *Buildings and Society: Essays on the Social Development of the Built Environment*, London, Routledge & Kegan Paul, 1980.

Taylor, Jeremy, *Hospital and Asylum Architecture in England 1840–1914: Building for Health Care*, London, Mansell, 1991.

Thompson, John D. and Goldin, Grace, *The Hospital: A Social and Architectural History*, New Haven, CT, and London, Yale University Press, 1975.

Vidler, Anthony, 'Confinement and cure: reforming the hospital, 1770–1789' in Vidler, *The Writing of the Walls: Architectural Theory in the Late Enlightenment*, Princeton, NJ, Princeton Architectural Press, 1987.

65

MEDICINE AND LITERATURE

Michael Neve

Few areas of the history of medicine, and medicine's place in culture, are as obscure and as liable to misconceived forms of interpretation, as medicine and its relationship to literature. Leaving aside the enormous question of how medicine and literature relate to each other in non-Western contexts, the issue contains a great variety of simple, internal difficulties.

Is it a matter of how medicine, or doctors, or experiences of doctoring, or the experience of agony, come to be represented *within* literature? Does literature in that sense provide a higher discourse – a truer experience of life's trials – than medicine itself, by housing medicine and explicating it? Or should medical texts be discussed as literary texts, even if this was not part of their historical genesis? Is it time to think of the Hippocratic Corpus, or *De Motu Cordis*, by William Harvey (1578–1657), as literary works, even (and this is sometimes proposed) as fictions? And what about medicine and the drama: is it perhaps in drama that medicine receives its fullest representation, including its fullest critique? Or is that, in turn, simply a lesser part of a greater story, the story that spells out the case (and it is after all a very old case) for drama as a form of medicine? There are numerous difficulties, tracing the connections between two vast areas of human effort that may not be easily twinned. Indeed, the desire to twin them may be an ambition more attractive to medical practitioners than to writers and artists. The historian G. S. Rousseau places the difficulty of medicine's relationship to literature with skill:

> In our century nothing has influenced the physician's profile more profoundly than the loss of his or her identity as the last of the humanists. Until recently, physicians in Western European countries received broad, liberal educations, read languages and literatures, studied the arts, were good musicians and amateur painters; by virtue of their financial privilege and class prominence

they interacted with statesmen and high-ranking professionals, and continued in these activities throughout their careers. It was not uncommon, for Victorian and Edwardian doctors, for example, to write prolifically throughout their careers: medical memoirs and auto-biographies, biographies of other doctors, social analyses of their own times, imaginative literature of all types. In twentieth-century America, the pattern has changed; only the most imaginative physicians can hope for this artistic lifestyle as a consequence of the economic constraints and housekeeping demands placed upon the doctor in a world where servants have disappeared. Also, the diminution of 'humanist' content in the training of physicians has lent an impression – perhaps falsely so but nevertheless pervasively – that medics are technicians, anything but humanists. As a by-product, it has nurtured a myth (already old by the eighteenth-century Enlightenment) that medicine is predominantly a science rather than an art. Both notions require adjustment if physicians hope to return to their earlier enriched, and probably healthier, role.[1]

The usefulness of this quotation is to remind us that the idea of including medicine with literature as part of high culture is not an ancient idea, but a humanist one: a conjunction attempted not in the classical age, but in the Renaissance. Bearing in mind the need to see the Hippocratic ideal of doctor as a craftsperson, not philosopher or theorist, it would seem increasingly inappropriate to see ancient medical texts as *literary*, in the modern sense. Indeed, to re-describe them in that way, for historical reasons, might be to rob them of an independent, and utilitarian, medical purpose, in the attempt to subsume them under the category of 'literature'.

The problem with Rousseau's interpretation is that it underestimates the continuity of the medical literary enterprise. Not only are there considerable numbers of physician/literateurs in the twentieth century: there always have been, at least since the classical age, and the more useful approach (having agreed this) might be to study the subject matter of literature and medicine, and what it reveals, rather than assume an opposition between them, or as a series of sporadic relationships, fluctuating through historical time. To propose a continuity of practice since the Renaissance would not, of course, involve thinking of medical texts as literature.

Treating medical texts as literature, rather than treating literature as a source of insight that medicine only partially rivals, leads in turn to an underestimation of the variety of interests in Renaissance humanism. It is customary to draw attention to the sixteenth- and seventeenth-century work of Thomas Campion (1567–1620) and Sir Thomas Browne (1605–82) as humanist all-rounders and doctors, and as writers with clear medical literary interests. While certainly establishing the point that the gentleman-physician of the late Renaissance was the figure who initiated the literature of ornate, sometimes medical, meditation on life and death, it is still not clear how far medicine determined the discussion, as against biblical and classical influences. Medical remarks take their place inside a larger discussion, allowing one to think of authors like Browne as inhabiting a common culture of learning that does not give medicine a special place, over other forms of knowledge.

The point about the reflections of Browne and of Campion is that they followed on from a prehistory of literary representations of medicine, above all in Chaucer (c.1342–1400) and in Rabelais (c.1494–1553), a prehistory that was a rougher trade and which used a less élitist philosophy. Chaucer, especially in the prologue to the *Canterbury Tales* and in the 'Nun's Priest's Tale', established a satirical, sardonic view of doctors, who were seen as close to quackery and even closer to a love of money. The theme of the quack, the pretender, the beneficiary from the suffering of others, was to remain a powerful motif right up to the nineteenth century. The more socially realistic the writer's method, the more vituperative the satire, from Chaucer to the stage representations of Ben Jonson (1572/3–1637). Rabelais, a monk and doctor, turned the merely satirical, the merely representational, into something quite different. And, strictly speaking, inimitable. *Gargantua and Pantagruel* (published in full in 1564) lambasts the worlds of bookish learned scholars, and the humanists who sought to replace them. Of course, his sympathies were with the moderns (hence the censoring of parts of the work as heretical); what Rabelais did, however, was to make the text a feast in itself, packed with gigantic excretions and massive gorgings, a book that invites being put to use for the wiping of arses. *Gargantua and Pantagruel* burst out of the limitations of theological wisdom, as giants of medical scatology.

But Rabelais was unique. It is difficult to propose a post-Rabelaisian tradition, where medicine appears *as* literature, on the strength of Rabelais alone. In truth, the doctor, as a literary figure, is not at the centre of Renaissance cultural work, despite the satirical onslaughts of Rabelais and Jonson. (Indeed, Rabelais might be putting his very brief medical education to the task of asking his readers simply to live to the full, before dying.)

This relative marginality, both of the literary physician, and representatives of the medical world, is well illustrated in the works of Shakespeare (1564–1616) Doctors in Shakespeare are rare creatures, bringing acumen and assistance. In *King Lear* and *Macbeth*, the doctor makes his first appearance as a psychologist, an observer of the terrible action, who attempts to bring small doses of relief. In Shakespeare, there is only so much a doctor can do ('Therein the patient/must minister to himself'). When being made a figure of fun, taking Dr Caius in the *Merry Wives of Windsor* as an example, the humour turns, not on his quackery, but on his French accent and general nervousness.

For Shakespeare, the power of drama itself provides the medicine – the experience of madness, or betrayal, or love, or all these – and the doctor, almost like the playwright, observes the action. But again, it would be a reduction, a lowering of sights, to argue that Shakespeare's literature is a form of medicine. Shakespeare's drama might be, but that involves the getting up and going to the play, a quite different act to the act of reading. To collapse 'drama' into 'literature' may be legitimate, but involves a loss of distinction that (especially for Romantic critics of Shakespeare) depoliticizes his drama. And the central point remains: doctors are not the centre of attention in Shakespeare. Ophelia goes mad entirely alone. The apothecary, in *Romeo and Juliet*, is a desperate man and bringer of death. In *Timon of Athens*, in *Troilus and Cressida*, in *Julius Caesar*, bodies are fought over, become diseased, decay and die. There is no cure.

The classical doctor, as journeyman, or the satirical representation of pre-Renaissance doctors, as quacks, are figures at the periphery of any literary representation. It is, however, the Renaissance gentleman-physician who initiates a literary style and makes visible, for the first time perhaps, a self-consciously 'literary' prose that includes medical interests. But the crucial point (especially for Thomas Browne) was that those were also forms of private meditation, deliberately ornate and paradoxical. They do not offer social accounts of doctors and their practice, or offer medical accounts of the social sphere as part of literary genre. The extension of this medical interest into the social comes with the Enlightenment and with the growth of the medical profession itself. Originating within an élite, the literature that included accounts of medicine as a social practice became diffused within eighteenth-century commercial society. (➤ Ch. 47 History of the medical profession)

The eighteenth century in Europe, and the maturing of commercial civilization, brought with it the forms of culture where the place of doctors in society (and medical texts that begin to describe societies as bodies, with inhabitants of societies as products of environmental forces) could flourish. Above all in the novel – and in medical texts that satirized the effects of both society and society's doctors – a new conjunction of medicine and literature took place. The relative absence of doctors in the cultural productions of the Renaissance began to give way, first to the essays of such as Thomas Browne, and then to the full-blown rendering of doctors and medical prognostics on social ills, from Molière (1622–73) to Mandeville (1670–1733), from the late works of Shakespeare to Samuel Johnson (1709–84).

The otherwise nebulous subject of 'medicine and literature' came to be far more palpable in the Enlightenment, when literary persons engaged with doctors, and where doctors took up critiques of their age through expressly literary means and genres. The common run of humanist reflection, often tinged with a form of twilight Christianity, gave way to a series of separate spheres, a reflection in turn of the professionalization of writing, and an increased specialization in medicine itself. There can be little doubt that the invention of a novel-based 'literature', in the eighteenth century, began to marginalize the philosophically inclined physician and a literary humanist. And yet, far from being a division, a separation, that generated silence, this was also the age when literature and medicine started to take a concentrated interest in each other.

Most easily seen in the novel (including the career of the character Partridge in *Tom Jones*, by Henry Fielding (1707–54) *Tom Jones*), the new force of the medical/literary discussion is exemplified in the work of individual authors: Denis Diderot (1713–84) and, above all, the Englishman Samuel Johnson. Johnson did not merely provide the reading public with biographical accounts of doctors (mostly translations of Latin eulogies, like that for Hermann Boerhaave (1668–1738)), but he also engaged with medical theories of the eighteenth century and came to see doctors as heroic (and, sometimes, the opposite) and even worthy of rememberance in verse.[2] Above all, for Johnson, the good doctor was free of that most pervasive of human faults, vanity. Johnson's poem 'On the Death of Dr Robert Levet', written in 1783, a year before Johnson's own death, is worth quoting in full, remembering that Levet was not a grand medical figure, not part of the élite that had penned the humanist reflections of the pre-Enlightenment:

> Condemned to hope's delusive mine,
> As on we toil from day to day
> By sudden blasts, or slow decline,
> Our social comforts drop away.
>
> Well tried through many a varying year
> See Levet to the grave descend;
> Officious, innocent, sincere,
> Of ev'ry friendless name the friend.
>
> Yet still he fills affection's eye,
> Obscurely wise, and coarsely kind;
> Nor, lettered arrogance, deny
> Thy praise to merit unrefined.
>
> When fainting nature called for aid,
> And hov'ring death prepared the blow,
> His vig'rous remedy displayed
> The power of art without the show.
>
> In misery's darkest caverns known,
> His useful care was ever nigh,
> Where hopeless anguish poured his groan,
> And lonely want retired to die.

No summons mocked by chill delay,
No petty gain disdained by pride,
The modest wants of ev'ry day
The toil of ev'ry day supplied.

His virtues walked their narrow round,
Nor made a pause, nor left a void;
And sure th' Eternal Master found
The single talent well employed.

The busy day, the peaceful night,
Unfelt, uncounted, glided by:
His frame was firm, his powers were bright,
Though now his eightieth year was nigh.

Then with no throbbing fiery pain,
No cold gradations of decay,
Death broke at once the vital chain,
And freed his soul the nearest way.

Like Alexander Pope (1688–1744), who had spoken of 'This long disease, my life', Johnson reworks the relationship of medicine to literature by casting the writer as a patient, a patient furthermore both sceptical of medicine and yet profoundly aware of good social doctoring as an exercise of virtue. Unlike Diderot, Johnson places the religious guide, the priest, as higher than all others in vocational terms, but he still brought in to general English writing and linguistic usage a heightened sense of medical terms, their place in general culture, and the doctor's career as one open to understanding and admiration. And Johnson, and his contemporaries, had a market for their views because of the sheer volume of Enlightenment writing on medical topics: diet, climate, regimen, manners. The expansion of commercial publishing and commercial doctoring may have meant fewer doctors dominating the production of literary medicine. But these social forces permitted a great expansion of medical theories and hence medical lives appearing in literature itself.

Johnson and Mandeville provide the best examples, in England, of the cross-fertilization between medicine and literature, but also the use of medical ideas to explore moral and social issues. Mandeville, especially in his *Treatise of the Hypochondriack and Hysterick Passions* (1711), initiated a medical sociology that surfaced in his ironic and subtle *Fable of the Bees* (1714). Such works flourished in a common culture of medical debate, with the commercial power of the patient often equalling any cognitive advantage that accrued to the doctor. Above all, medicine and literature produced powerful versions of satire, when working together, as if satirical responses to material claims constituted the most intelligent way of displaying literature's relationship to medicine. Bringing in a character – the patient in agony – who had not been seen in the humanist literature, the medical literature of the Enlightenment raised entirely new questions of subject matter and genre. (➤ Ch. 67 Pain and suffering)

The doctor in the literature of Shakespeare, Jonson, and Sir Thomas Browne is a complex figure, most esteemed when most sceptical and most derided when most ambitious. The Enlightenment sees a different doctor – more socially beneficial, more attentive in the understanding of patients, more involved in what might be called honest commerce rather than learned obfuscation. There are few literary precedents for the richness of the medical world of Henry Fielding, or for the way in which Samuel Johnson opened out the lay perception of doctors and the patient's relationship with them. In a long poem such as 'The Dispensary' (1699), by Samuel Garth (1661–1719), various positions are set out with regard to commercial medicine and the possibility of a medicine for the poor. Garth's own view seems to be that apothecaries were (once again) displaying greed in order to prevent the founding of a dispensary for the poor; he also indicates a personal, highly deferential attitude towards the aristocracy. Whatever the politics of Garth's poem, it marks an Enlightenment, and English, poetical concern with the social history of medicine of a particularly rich kind. Garth's work sits well alongside the productions of Fielding, and of Tobias Smollett (1721–71), whose *The Adventures of Roderick Random* (1748) is a detailed story of the vagaries of life in the naval medical service. Likewise, in his *The Expedition of Humphry Clinker* (1771), Smollett created a hero, Matt Bramble, who corresponds with his adviser and friend, Dr Lewis. Like the more famous literary contradictions of Laurence Sterne (1713–68), Smollett had a considerable European reputation, based on the wealth of detail that he brought to the story of eighteenth-century medicine, its practitioners, its patients, and their strange threads of connection. As with Johnson, the most innovative of these was undoubtedly the strength of feeling attached to medical displays of greed and deception (an old story), now allied to the possibility of intense respect and even veneration. A deal had been struck, and the literature of the eighteenth century described it. (➤ Ch. 34 History of the doctor–patient relationship)

The appearance of Romantic writings, and the expounding of Romantic ideas of creativity and its relationship with illness, broke the Enlightenment connection. Many Romantic authors seemed to make pathology the only basis for literary insight, and at various stages denounced the culture of the Enlightenment for being too accessible, too conventional. Instead, the poets in particular journeyed elsewhere: Wordsworth (1770–1850) into brief flirtations with revolution; Coleridge (1772–1834) into drugs; William Blake (1757–1827) into an imagination deemed insane; Byron (1788–1824) and Shelley (1792–1822) into libertinism and political radicalism. But the striking thing about Romantic posturing is that despite the violence of feeling that much of it displayed, the place of medicine in literature was rarely discussed. The eighteenth-century conjunction of medicine and society, and the literature that it generated, began to disappear. Exceptions to this, most strikingly Mary Shelley (1797–1851) in her novel *Frankenstein* (1818) and P. B. Shelley's interest in vegetarianism, clearly displayed eighteenth-century preoccupations. The age of Keats (1795–1821) is an age when medicine and literature come apart, to stay that way in the work of the sons of doctors, such as Gustave Flaubert (1821–80).

Romantic genius departed for other worlds, and the eighteenth-century patient, like Johnson, became the nineteenth-century exile or invalid. The dialectic was lost, a fact that has made life difficult for historians of medicine and literature. For example, acres of print had been given over to the tracing of medical influences in the poetry of John Keats, who was a medical student at Guy's Hospital in the year 1815–16. The pay-off from this long search is almost nil. (A recent study of Keats and medicine by Hermione de Almeida, shows exactly how not to write history.) Indeed, it might be said that part of Keats's purpose (contra the eighteenth-century) would be to keep illness, including his own tuberculosis, hidden from the doctor's sight. Literature, in Romanticism, becomes an enemy to science and medicine, at least in their invasive forms, and this had important implications for the nineteenth century.

Historians of medicine agree that it is in the nineteenth century that modern medicine comes into a recognizable form. The proliferation of hospitals, of medical schools, of professional bodies representing the interests of doctors and the hierarchical organization of the medical profession itself, all were features of the nineteenth century. These developments were accompanied by the emergence of a medicine that might reasonably be called 'scientific': based in the clinic, or the laboratory, and initiating the long journey into the minutiae of pathology and the body's parts. Cells, tissues, brain sections, the bacillus, the virus, the spirochaete, the chromosome, the gene: all these were opened to what has been called the 'clinical gaze'. If the medicine of the Enlightenment can be characterized as like natural history, with the doctor looking at external signs, it can also be characterized as a time when these external signs were comprehensible to the patient. Eighteenth-century medicine set limits to its ambitions, and developed a language of description that was often esoteric, but by no means always. Within the disputed area of doctor/patient relations, medicine as it appeared in literature was recognizable in terms of a common language.

The medical language of the nineteenth century jettisoned this external and collectively comprehensible element, and headed into the dark cave of the previously unexplored internal body and its world. This journey into the interior, accompanied as it was by the professionalization of medicine itself, snapped the Enlightenment cord. Individual human beings were now objects of medical attention, not participants in their own struggles in life. What was happening to them was not always something they could understand. Indeed, in one sinister interpretation of nineteenth-century medicine, what was happening to them was not always something that they ought to understand. The trained doctor, and especially the trained new kid on the block, the psychiatrist, were now looking into a patient who had become part of the doctor's conversation, not a part of his or her own. In one sense, Romanticism's greatest fears about doctors, as expressed in the remarkable plays of the young German medical student Georg Büchner (1813–37), were coming true, or so many believed. Büchner, who died of typhoid at the age of 24, forecasts a world of dissection, of investigation, of opening up the innocent, not least in his fragment *Woyzeck*, written between 1835 and his death. The obscure relations of medicine to literature in the age of Romanticism began to be posthumously vindicated in the century that followed, as a response to the rise of clinical medicine and the medicalization of the human sciences, especially philosophy. It is of interest here that *Woyzeck* was not published until 1879.

The growth of medical specialisms in the nineteenth and twentieth centuries, not least in psychiatry, neurology, and psychology, had enormous implications for medicine and literature. Indeed, these two areas of human culture could be said to have been locked in combat, or estranged, or at least involved in a *folie à deux*, ever since. First of all, medical science began to turn its new gaze on human personality and human creativity, in order to understand and illuminate them. Literary creation might now be understood, especially if it could be construed as a product of disturbance and mental illness. Perhaps James Joyce (1882–1941) was suffering a form of schizophrenic illness when writing *Finnegan's Wake*? Perhaps (as has been suggested recently) the mature philosophy of Ludwig Wittgenstein (1889–1951) was, in fact, a form of nonsense, a form of 'schizophrenese'? Works of art could be classified, from now on, with some of them conducive to health, others not. With the medicalization of models of creativity, with brains replacing minds, the literary creator was now part of the population of the clinic. (➤ Ch. 43 Psychotherapy; Ch. 56 Psychiatry)

Thus, literature, at least in the work of some of its greatest practitioners, now had to create conditions whereby it might escape the clutches of clinical attention. If humanism had given way to Enlightenment conversation, which, in turn, had given way to Romantic mysticism, medical/literary relations in the nineteenth century entered a medicalized landscape where doctors figured large but not always in a good light. The doctors repaid the compliment by seeing many artists as insane, and the two cultures made famous by C. P. Snow (1905–80) were born. Even more importantly, many writers decided to accept the medical model – that the world was itself like some giant hospital, riddled with disease and contagion – but would then proceed to make their own literary diagnoses as to how that had come about. If there is a subject that can be called medicine *in* literature, and its twin, literature *in* medicine, then it is the product, not of the unique hilarities and grotesquerie of François Rabelais in the sixteenth century (where people still search for such a conjunction), but in the literature and medicine of bourgeois Europe. Rabelais, with his humanist satire, his carnival, his gaiety of mind, was a law unto himself. In the culture of modern Europe, everybody was involved: patients, doctors, writers, bystanders, artists, and (the point is essential) past figures like Rabelais, who could now be 'understood' as coprophiliacs, or lunatics, or thought-disordered. The disease of life was everywhere, as medicine, and literature, had to show.

Indeed, the modern academic study of the relationship of medicine to literature is itself the product of the growth of medicalization in the nineteenth century. What was once the satire of Jonathan Swift (1667–1745) could now be construed as the product of a diseased mind. What was once an attempt by Friedrich Hölderlin (1770–1843) to restore Hellas to German literature, in the 1790s, and even up to his death in 1843, could now be understood as the exhausted fantasies of an enfeebled madman. As has already been suggested, medicine had appeared within literature as a subject, before the Enlightenment and, more completely, during the Enlightenment. In the nineteenth century, medicine started to become a means of explaining literature, or, at the very least, of explaining why certain literary works took the form that they did.

This new relationship amounted to more than the increased appearance of doctors as characters, in the novel or in the drama. In *Middlemarch* (1871–2) by George Eliot (1819–80), or *Madame Bovary* by Gustave Flaubert (1857), remarkable accounts of provincial medical life were rendered. In *Dr Thorne* (1858) by Anthony Trollope (1815–82), a country doctor risks his reputation to protect his dead brother's illegitimate child, introducing her to wealth and society and steering her to a successful marriage. Subsequent examples are too numerous to mention. And, of course, Victorians and Edwardian physicians might try their hand at literary work (essays, fictions, biographies) in order to insert themselves into the growing story of the doctor's place in society. But of greater importance, for medicine and literature, was the growth of those theories that sought to explain works of art from a medical point of view. As discussed by Roy Porter in his essay in this encyclopedia, (➤ Ch. 27 Diseases of civilization) nineteenth-century degenerationist theory, especially in the writings of Henry Maudsley (1835–1918) and T. B. Hyslop (1864–1933) in England, and Cesare Lombroso (1836–1909) in Italy, began to describe literary productions as products of disease. The work of

Edgar Allan Poe (1809–49), or the art of the pre-Raphaelites, the Expressionists, and Symbolists, all received attention in this way.

Literature became an epiphenomenon, something that could best be understood by scientific medicine. Indeed, in the work of Emile Zola (1840–1902), the novelist aspired to the condition of the heroic physician, regarding the writings of life and character as events in nature to be examined scientifically, in imitation of medical methodology, in this case the physiologist Claude Bernard (1813–78) in his *Introduction à l'étude de la médecine expérimentale* of 1865. While it is true that Zola did not regard Bernard's text as literature in itself, he sought to re-establish literature as a form of medicine. Realism was impossible without this aspiration.

Of course, there was a reaction – a literary reaction – against this crucial development, and it is one that still determines the vexed question of how to write about medicine and literature. Literature, much of the great literature of the modern age, became the product of writers who made themselves ill, who cast themselves as degenerate, in order to keep the independence of literature alive. And they particularly did this – Anton Chekhov (1860–1904) is a great example – if they were doctors, and sick doctors especially. In so doing, these doctor/authors and those who imitated them could be said to have attempted to restore literature to its humanist ascendency over medicine, or any idea of medicine as literature. Such authors restored to the story of literature and doctors a humanist sense that the heroic alternative was in danger of forgetting something central to human experience: that there is, usually, nothing that doctors can do.

Heroic accounts of social doctoring (the *locus classicus* in English may well be *The Citadel* by A. J. Cronin (1896–1981), published in 1937), or innovative scientific doctoring, as in the immunological examples of Sinclair Lewis (1885–1951) in his novel *Arrowsmith* (1925), were widely read and admired. In both these books, the true heroes are not the ambitious and the famous, but the doctor who is socially responsible to the patients and wary of therapeutic ambitions that cannot be realized. But even more influential than Lewis or Cronin, in terms of modern literature, were authors who took the story of the medicalization of the nineteenth-century secular sciences even further, to restore a sense of medicine's fundamental vanity in the face of certain death. Whether or not these writers – Marcel Proust (1871–1922), Anton Chekhov, Louis-Ferdinand Destouches (known as Céline; 1894–1961) – restored literature to its independent status is open to discussion. What they did do was restore pessimism to its classical status, and contradict the heroic Whiggism of much nineteenth-century medical self-imagining.

Proust, the son of a society doctor, Adrien Proust (d. 1903) produced in his *À la recherche du temps perdu* (1913–27) an account of time past allied to a uniquely detailed study of social degeneration, partly based on sexual perversion. Proust himself, once his adored mother had died in 1905, left society, to return, asthmatic, to a bed in a room lined with cork to keep out the noise. Venturing out, occasionally, at night, or sometimes to the seaside, he wrote feverishly, racing against time. His achievement, which remains entirely astonishing, was not simply to complete his task: the idea that literature and medicine can be separately discussed in such a work becomes pointless. Pathology, time, social detail, the 'illness' that the author himself inhabited: these constitute the materials of Proust's achievement, as they do, in very similar ways, for the philosopher Friedrich Nietzsche (1844–1900), who relocates philosophy within the proposition that embracing illness, in modern culture, forms the beginning of new kinds of health.

Anton Chekhov, probably the greatest dramatist since Shakespeare, was a doctor as well as a playwright. Chekhov portrays many doctors in his stories and plays, but all of them inhabit the hilarity and despair that would have been recognizable to the classical authors, even perhaps to the authors of the Enlightenment. Usually drunk, and usually aware that something terrible has happened or is about to happen, they are in the full consciousness that might be characterized as medicine's truest state of mind: hopelessness. Even the rise of scientific medicine, and the therapeutic revolutions of the late nineteenth century, left plenty of room for such ancient thoughts, and Chekhov's doctors, as well as Chekhov himself, show this in memorable ways. And Chekhov even came close to resolving the difficult matter of literature and medicine with an aphorism that might well serve for the entire discussion: 'Literature is my mistress, medicine my wife'.

The intermingling of medicine and literature in the nineteenth and twentieth centuries, and the way that testified to the extent of professional medicine's enlargement, could be said to have reached a particular height (or depth) in the work of Céline. Having trained and practiced as a doctor, Louise-Ferdinand Destouches took up his *nom de plume*, and his pen, to produce a medical/literary attack on modern civilization of the utmost vehemence, written in remarkable and memorable French prose. Céline set the terms for his fiction explicitly within medicine, having produced a biography of Ignaz Semmelweis (1818–65), the Hungarian-born doctor who (for Céline) understood and conquered puerperal fever, becoming, through the washing of hands in a solution of chlorinated lime, a hero of antisepsis in the era before bacteriology. Céline took this example as a paradigm case, both of the putrid and inept character of much human activity and, because of Semmelweis's subsequent victimization and madness, the likely fate for any pioneer of maternal and social health. (➤ Ch. 44 Childbirth) In his works, such as *Voyage au bout de la nuit* (1932) and *Mort à credit* (1936), Céline attacked society as if it was a poisonous cadaver, with the novelist as mortician and surgeon. Politically, he became explicitly anti-Semitic and a collaborator with the Vichy government during the Second World War. His novels returned, not to the styptic, neo-stoic silence of Chekhov's doctors, but to Swiftean satire, now backed up by a form of biological grotesque. His last novel (*Nord*, 1960) sees the whole of Europe as a decayed and poisoned hospital.

All three of these authors, Proust, Chekhov, and Céline, returned the novel and the drama to its earlier authority by reworking both illness and the models of literary medicine to a pitch that placed them outside the prevailing mode of Whiggish optimism. In so doing, they not only contradicted the 'heroic' style of narrative and biography favoured by doctor-authors themselves, they also made a new kind of literature, by taking in the medicalization of the human sciences and then creating a literature that transcended it.

This achievement, on behalf of sickness and writing about sickness, placed doctors back in the narrative, no longer as conquerors, but as full of doubt as the pre-bourgeois tradition has always seen them. Indeed, the doctor who was without a pair of other eyes to for assistance – the eye of the artist perhaps, or the detective – was partially sighted. This is the brilliant insight in the fiction of the medically-trained Arthur Conan Doyle (1859–1930). Disillusioned with life in general practice, Doyle wrote himself into the canon of world literature by inventing a male doubles team, Holmes and Watson, where the doctor is essential because helpfully unintelligent. Watson's ability to state the obvious allows Holmes and his lonely razor-sharp mind the companionship it would otherwise never have had (except perhaps in cocaine, and the playing of a violin). As the cultural historian Carlo Ginzburg has suggested, the doctor has to become a detective in the *fin-de-siècle*, just as the newly conceived psychoanalyst must look for clues where others see only irrelevance. Conon Doyle's male pair complete the innovations in the literary medicine of the modern age, by bringing together the clumsily honest doctor and the deviant, eagle-eyed observer, into an unbeatable combination. Doyle's achievement was to base this on the admission that what the doctor saw was never enough, and that no successful solution was possible without the assistance of the very degeneracy that mainstream medicine and criminal science was seeking to marginalize, classify, and, probably eliminate.

The medico-literary writing of the period before the Second World War reflected in its turn the uncertainties of medical science and the powerful sense of the relatively small advance made in the elimination of major diseases. Whether in the difficult area of 'diseases of the nerves', or tuberculosis, or smallpox, the major advances of the late twentieth century were not yet in existence. With the arrival of high-technology medicine and the disappearance of some diseases (smallpox, but not cholera or tuberculosis) the medical fiction of the recent period has reflected on different issues to those of the preceding decades. Long-term illness, above all cancer, has replaced both the incidence and the literature of sudden death. (➤ Ch. 25 Cancer) Hostility to the medical profession, perhaps at its height in the 1906 stage play *The Doctor's Dilemma* by George Bernard Shaw (1856–1950), became somewhat muted, with the impressive results achieved by antibiotics and with less acclaim, by the public-health movement. (➤ Ch. 51 Public health) At the same time, as with Céline, the medical metaphor became employed on an increasingly wide scale in the attempt to describe social and political illness. *Cancer Ward* (1968), by Alexander Solzhenitsyn, was the most important of these, with an entire society conceived as a deathly bureaucracy, housing insidious illness. Equally powerful was *The Plague* (1948), by Albert Camus, where the plague is a vision of German military occupation as viewed by a heroic doctor.

As for the literary expression of medicine and society, the critique of the profession *per se* has moved away from the documentary account of daily practice (which increasingly seems like an Edwardian genre) towards science fiction and futuristic dystopias. Stories where modern doctors appear as everyday heroes have been relegated to the highly popular romantic fiction associated with Mills & Boon. Partly dictated by the experience of National Socialist medicine, the medicine of the future appears trapped inside the politics of biotechnology, genetic engineering, secret plans for eugenical domination by nation-states. It is as if there is almost no fiction of daily general practice, only the literature of sinister post-modernism, lording it over a disconsolate and impecunious public sphere. This is the powerful theme of the novel *Time's Arrow* (1991) by Martin Amis (b. 1949). The arrival of (a few) Nobel-winning doctors has not been accompanied by a literature of public health, expressed in fiction. For public health, the literature of the present is the literature of political and journalistic controversy. For the medicine of high-tech research, the appropriate mode seems to be science fiction.

Recent writing on medicine and literature all reflect the influence of the nineteenth-century writers, in that the way they incorporated medicine into literature set the terms for subsequent debate. The endless discussion of 'two cultures', in this case science and the humanities, in fact conceals a great deal of interpenetration and co-mingling. But the vital point, once the two-cultures issue is laid to rest as just another Tweedledum and Tweedledee show, is that doctors and authors now compete over who can *write* 'better'. Skilled practitioners of the medical biographer's art – William Ober, above all – need no defending. In more controversial examples, of which the work of Oliver Sacks (b. 1933) is the most famous, the inclusion of literature (and music) within accounts of medical recovery can seem less accomplished. Indeed for certain critics, the work of Sacks provides perhaps the one example where medical case histories really do take on the quality of fiction. And yet

Sacks has an entirely deserved reputation for bringing up to a wide readership the imaginative excitement required to make sense of some bizarre and puzzling neurological phenomena, on behalf of the patient. His continual attempt to give these a wider cultural significance shows how far medicine and literature have become caught up since the Enlightenment. However, many modern practitioners do not have the time, or the inclination, to make literary constructions out of individual cases: many of their cases are routine, unglamorous, and socially explicable in matter-of-fact terms. Once again, this shows how the relationship of medicine to literature is explicated by the working life of the doctor-author, the nature of his or her specialization, and the judgement the clinician makes about an appropriate language of description. For many medical practitioners, the avoidance of a literary style might be a vital aspect of giving a good case history. For others, this might indicate a lack of imagination. The autobiography of the American doctor-writer William Carlos Williams, written in 1951, is a lovely meditation on this dilemma.

Given this, the dialectic of medicine and literature and the problems that beset it as a subject are unlikely to disappear. It is also the case that the work of the great nineteenth- and twentieth-century authors who absorbed medicine completely into their imaginative writing set precedents unlikely to be equalled. They restored to the argument the fact of death, however modern the hospital, however high the technology. Becoming ill in the process, the finest proponents of literary medicine kept the (fictional) Hippocratic Oath, at the very time when medicine itself was most in the grip of a dream of endless progress.

NOTES

1   G. S. Rousseau, 'Literature and medicine: towards a simultaneity of theory and practice', *Literature and Medicine*, 1986, 5: 152–81.
2   See J. Wiltshire, *Samuel Johnson in the Medical World*, Cambridge, Cambridge University Press, 1991.

FURTHER READING

Almeida, H. de, *Romantic Medicine and John Keats*, Oxford, Oxford University Press, 1991.
Beer, G., *Darwin's Plots: Evolutionary Narratives in Darwin, George Eliot and Nineteenth-Century Fiction*, London, Routledge, 1983.
Collins, J., *The Doctor Looks at Literature*, New York, George H. Doran, 1923.
Cousins, Norman, *The Physicians in Literature*, Philadelphia, PA, W. B. Saunders, 1982.
Crook, Nora, *Shelley's Venomed Melody*, Cambridge, Cambridge University Press, 1986.

Dewhurst, K. and Reeves, N., *Friedrich Schiller: Medicine, Psychology and Literature*, Oxford, Sandford, 1978.

Edgar, Irving, *Shakespeare, Medicine and Psychiatry: an Historical Study in Criticism and Interpretation*, London, Vision, 1971.

Levine, G., *The Realistic Imagination: English Fiction from Frankenstein to Lady Chatterley*, Chicago, IL, Chicago University Press, 1981.

Leavy, Barbara Fass, *To Blight with Plague: Studies in a Literary Theme*, New York, New York University Press, 1992.

Ober, W. B., *Boswell's Clap and Other Essays*, Carbondale, Southern Illinois University Press, 1979.

Peschel, Enid Rhodes, *Medicine and Literature*, New York, N. Watson Academic Publications, 1980.

Rousseau, G. S., 'Literature and medicine: the state of the field', *Isis*, 1981, 72: 406–24.

——, *Tobias Smollett: Essays of Two Decades*, Edinburgh, T. & T. Clark, 1982.

Smithers, D. W., *This Idle Trade: on Doctors who were Writers*, Tunbridge Wells, Dragonfly, 1989.

Soupel, S. and Hambridge, R., *Literature and Science and Medicine*, Los Angeles, CA, Clark Memorial Library, 1982.

Banks, Joanne Trautmann (ed.), *Healing Arts in Dialogue: Medicine and Literature*, Carbondale, Southern Illinois University Press, 1981.

Banks, Joanne Trautmann and Pollard, Carol (eds) *Literature and Medicine: an Annotated Bibliography*, 2nd edn., Pittsburgh, PA, University of Pittsburgh Press, 1982.

——, *Literature and Medicine*, Vol. I: *1982, to the Present*, Baltimore, MD, Johns Hopkins University Press.

Weissman, G., *The Doctor with Two Heads and Other Essays*, New York, Knopf, 1990.

Wiltshire, J., *Samuel Johnson in the Medical World*, Cambridge, Cambridge University Press, 1991.

66

WAR AND MODERN MEDICINE

Roger Cooter

INTRODUCTION

Few subjects in the history of medicine have been so poorly served as the relations between medicine and war. Although the belief that wars have acted as perverse handmaidens to medical progress has been often subscribed to, the character of this perversity has never been systematically analysed. So too, the notion of wars as 'watersheds' in the development of medicine is everywhere encountered, but the precise nature of such moments of change has largely evaded description. Despite – in part, perhaps, because of – warehouses of published and unpublished diaries and reminiscences by 'doctors at war' and 'surgeons at arms', extensive archives of medicine in the armed forces, and voluminous official medical histories (for every major war since the Crimean), serious research in this field has scarcely begun.

In fact, it is hard to think of another general area of history where the scholarship is so disproportionate to the available resources. In 1972, F. N. L. Poynter (1908–79), in a valuable (but far from definitive) bibliographical survey of British military medicine, observed that this was 'a field of study which has long been awaiting development'.[1] Notwithstanding subsequent complaints about the subject's neglect, however, and a half-dozen or so additional bibliographies, the world still waits. In the meantime, we have had chronicles of the organization of medicine in the armed forces, medical histories and bibliographies of particular wars, biographies of outstanding individuals, and articles on the importance of war to virtually every branch of medicine, surgery, and public health. But few have attempted to understand military medicine in its broader social, economic, and political settings, or even in its full medical context. Except for some studies of shell-shock during the First World War, in which theoretical and practical developments in psychiatry and psychology are linked to fundamental changes in society, economy, and culture,[2] one searches almost in vain for sustained socio-historical analysis of the relations between medicine and war.[3]

That the subject occupies such a negligible place in the history of medicine is odd. For whether or not one views war as central to Western civilization over the past two centuries, the fact remains that in major military undertakings since the late eighteenth century, organized units of health professionals have played an increasingly conspicuous part. Yet it would be wrong to proffer historical amnesia in explanation of the silence of scholars. As everywhere in history, explanatory power is less to be had from pathological reductions than from attention to historical contingencies. Although the latter cannot be fully examined here, they suggest that the reason for the silence of historians lies mainly in the social, intellectual, and professional contexts in which the academic history of medicine has been written.

For the early holders of chairs in the history of medicine in the late nineteenth century (mostly in medical schools in Germany), it was neither professionally politic nor intellectually desirable to ponder on war. Schooled in philosophy and trained in medicine, these historians tended to focus on medicine's classical origins and to approach their subject within an established framework of the history of ideas. Intellectual legitimacy might thus be granted to a fledgling sub-discipline in a way that was scarcely possible through the study of something as sordid, seemingly unintellectual, and vulgarly causal as the relationship between war and medicine. It may also be that in a context in which medicine was becoming not only increasingly impersonal, scientific, and surgical, but also bureaucratized – if not militarized – the need was all the more strongly felt to portray the nobility and humanity of medicine's past, rather than to reveal any kind of dependence on organized acts of violence.

As taken up by Fielding Garrison (1870–1935) and others in the first decades of this century, the history of medicine was written primarily in terms of the lives of 'great men'. Within this genre it was not inappropriate to direct attention to such 'pioneers' of military and naval medicine and surgery as Ambroise Paré (1510–90), Sir John Pringle (1707–82), John Hunter (1728–93), Sir Gilbert Blane (1749–1834), Baron Dominique-Jean Larrey (1766–1842), and Nicolai Pirogoff (1810–81). But the gaze was not meant to suggest that war might be a significant force in the shaping of medicine. On the contrary: since most of these men also rose to the top of civilian medical and scientific élites, their exaltation merely reiterated a professionally reassuring faith in 'self-development', 'individualism', 'shrewdness', and 'genius'. It is true that during the First World War, Garrison was led to an appreciation of the effects of war on medicine while preparing the second edition of his *Introduction to the History of Medicine*. In 1922, from his office in the Surgeon-General's Library, he wrote a historical survey of military medicine in which he subscribed to the view that war was a 'biological phenomenon' that always has and always will be with us.[4] But this interest in war was fleeting; for the most part, Garrison remained wedded, as he confessed, to the intellectualist history of medicine of 'the great German masters'.[5]

For different reasons, the next generation of academic medical historians was equally unattracted to the subject of war. Far more interested in the 'socialization' of medicine, historians such as Richard Shryock (1893–1972), Erwin Ackerknecht (1906–88), and George Rosen (1910–77) sought to elaborate what Henry Sigerist (1891–1957) identified as the essentially social nature of medicine. For them, war was not necessarily to be seen as a pathological phenomenon outside of, or disruptive to, the normal functioning of the social body. (Sigerist alone seems to have held to the view of war as a 'social disease'.) Rather, by virtue of its episodic nature, war was regarded merely as among the least suitable historical means for illustrating the integral nature of medicine to politics, economy, and culture. Of the ten books and over two hundred articles written by Rosen, for example, not one was to feature war in its title; few even approached the subject. For these historians, the study of medicine in relation to the fundamental socio-economic forces of industrialization and urbanization was thought to be much better served through the history of public health and hygiene, a topic so relentlessly pursued by them that the 'social history of medicine' came to be identified with little else. Within this history, moreover, important links between civilian and military involvements tended to be ignored or glossed over. (➤ Ch. 70 Medical sociology)

The present generation of historians of medicine, while inheriting much of their predecessors' intellectual outlook and social orientation, has had an important additional reason to shy away from the subject of war: Vietnam. In a context in which rock artist Edwin Starr could popularize the refrain, 'War! What is the good of war? Absolutely nothing!', few young scholars were anxious to pursue a conceivable contradiction to the idea of war as destructive of civilization, even if they were ignorant of the theses of Arnold Toynbee and John Nef.[6] Unsurprisingly, those few who focused specifically on the historical relations between war and medicine did so in order to articulate a radically anti-militarist line. In 1978, an impressive article by Howard Levy looked at the contradictions inherent in a profession supposedly devoted to saving life, yet which acted in the service of organized slaughter. Levy was thus to make sense of the involvement of military medical practitioners in explicitly counter-intelligence operations in Korea and Vietnam.[7] A decade later, a group of German historians further explored some of the ethical tensions and historical dilemmas surrounding medicine and war.[8]

They claimed to be motivated not by the atrocities of German doctors during the Second World War (which other historians were beginning to explore in depth),[9] but rather, by the then medically chic anti-nuclear movement. Among their naïve conclusions was that real discussion of the relationship between medicine and war only began with the anti-nuclear movement.

But these preliminary reconnaissances into the uncharted social and cultural terrain of medicine and war were the exceptions. Most medical historians in the 1970s and 80s, if they noticed the subject of war at all, demonstrated few signs of interest (unlike growing numbers of social, economic, and cultural historians). While not unwilling to admit to wars as watersheds, and grant some causality to war with respect to the history of hospitals, specialization, demography, and social policy, they could not imagine war competing with, say, the social impact of major plagues and epidemics, alternative medicine, or the rituals and interventions surrounding sex, birth, madness, childhood, ageing, and death. Subjects like these initiated and encouraged what studies of medicine and war were presumed only to discourage or retard: the investigation of the subtle and complex expressions of medicine's social relations. Surely medicine in war, like war itself, was dominated by a kind of reductionist *realpolitik*: naked power relations and the overt manipulations of bodies. Little wonder that prominent sociologists and archaeologists of medical knowledge and power paid war no heed.

Importantly, too, this was no place for women. Almost by definition, war was 'boy's own' stuff – indeed old boys' stuff – clearly preoccupied with great men, great battles, and great technical achievements. Only recently have feminists begun to explore this masculine heartland to decipher its implications for gender relations. The result is some of the best social and cultural commentary on war and militarism to date.[10] But few of these insights have been carried over into the history of medicine, notwithstanding the Nightingale industry and various reflective accounts of women doctors and nurses in wars from the Crimean to Vietnam. Alone in terms of feminist history is Anne Summers's recent study of military nursing between 1854 and 1914.[11] Summers's book is also one of the few to link the history of war and militarization, not just to feminist issues, but to the social history of medicine in general. As such, we shall return to it later when addressing the historical problematic of war and medicine.

In what follows, then, the aim is primarily historiographical and interpretive. To attempt seriously to cover all the conceivable relations between war and medicine, war upon war, would be an impossible task in the space available. So too, would be any attempt to move across and between the temporal and spatial zones of military and naval engagements with a view to exploring medical continuities and discontinuities. Indeed, to do justice to merely one therapeutic facet of medicine or to one professional branch of it during a single war within a single national context would be a formidable undertaking.

This chapter therefore mainly confines itself to Anglo-American sources and, whilst drawing on evidence from the Napoleonic wars to the Second World War, concentrates on the period between the American Civil War of 1861–5 and the 'Great War' of 1914–18, when both medicine and warfare were revolutionized technologically. This was also the period when the organization of military medicine was significantly reformed, although this development was by no means peculiar to the second half of the nineteenth century. Since antiquity, armies had had medical services of one sort or another, though they appear to have gone into decline by the Middle Ages. In the eighteenth century, as armies and navies became larger and more professional (with soldiers and sailors becoming waged rather than reliant on booty), the value of organized medical services in the maintenance of discipline, morale, and fighting power became increasingly clear.[12] In the face of epidemics, in particular, sanitary measures came to seem a necessary part of military equipage. Efficiency and troop morale came to be seen as further obtainable through co-ordinated planning in the handling of the battle wounded. By the Battle of Fontenoy in 1745, the French – the pace-setters in military organization – were already operating a system with *ambulances* (as temporary hospitals were called) located close to the front lines. Larrey's famous 'flying ambulances' in the Napoleonic wars simply extended the mobility of this arrangement.

Hand-in-hand with these organizational developments went the emergence of career structures and professionalization in military medicine. Force was added to this process, in particular, through the introduction of medical examinations for military recruits, an event which itself reflects the movement to more professionalized and disciplined armies and navies. More-stringent requirements for the entry of doctors themselves into the armed forces came to be imposed towards the end of the eighteenth century. Concurrent was the granting of relative rank to medical officers, though the granting of command authority and disciplinary functions to doctors was to be contested in many countries throughout the nineteenth century.

Neither the organization of military medicine nor professionalization within it were continuous processes, however. The years of relative peace after the Napoleonic Wars led to cut-backs in military budgets and to the quiessence, if not demoralization, of military medical personnel. Moreover, the vicissitudes of this branch of both the military and the medical professions differed considerably between one country and the next. Only towards the end of the nineteenth century – in particular after the Franco-Prussian War of 1870–1 – did a degree of uniformity prevail in the military medical bureaucracies of the Western powers. Managerial expertise came to the fore, although, even then, the staffing and resources of military medicine continued to prove unequal to the actual demands of battle.

The major wars between 1800 and 1945 are listed in Table 1. This also provides estimates of the number of deaths from disease and from wounds, and indentifies some of the medical problems associated with particular campaigns. Although the ratio of deaths-from-wounds to deaths-from-diseases is more or less accurate, the absolute numbers cited provide, at best, only a rough guide to the burdens that faced the medical profession during wars. Some belligerent states (or branches of their armed forces) failed to keep any such statistics, while others partly made them up and/or abstracted them in such a way that comparisons are now difficult to make. Also arbitrary is the distinction between 'killed' and 'died of wounds', not to mention that between deaths from 'diseases' and deaths from 'wounds' given the reality of wound infection. Knowledge of the latter may partly account for the fact that by the First World War, the category 'sick and injured' was tending to replace 'wounded' and 'diseased'. The 'sick and injured', moreover, were often made well enough to re-enter battle and, hence, re-enter the statistics as 'wounded', 'injured', or 'killed'. Among British troops during the First World War, 82 per cent of the 'wounded' and 93 per cent of the 'sick and injured' were eventually returned to some form of duty. The least certain of all these figures, though, are those on the number of combatants. Even where absolute numbers exist for particular sides, these are seldom reliable. Often, they include reservists who may not have actually experienced battle. In wars of long duration, the numbers of combatants might include those who only served for brief periods, and others who, having served briefly, then signed up anew (as frequently occurred during the American Civil War).

It is not, however, around these particular wars and their specific medical problems that this chapter rotates. It centres, rather, on one of the abiding themes in the folklore of medical history: the notion of war as good for medicine. In what follows, an exploration is conducted into the validity of this claim, with samples brought forward of evidence both for and against it. I then turn to question the evaluative exercise itself as a basis for conceiving the relations between war and medicine. As social and historical reasons explain the past neglect of the subject by scholars, so new interest in the social relations of medicine, I shall suggest, should encourage the pursuit of the history of war and medicine as a means to the further illustration of those relations.

THE MEDICAL AUDIT OF WAR

Virtually everything that has been written on the subject of war and medicine stresses that the former, for all its horrors, has brought benefit to the latter.

Table *1* Major wars and medical problems 1793–1945

War	Date	Combatants (000s)	Killed	Wounded	Battle casualties (000s)		Ratio of (a) to (b)	Particular problems
					(a) Deaths from diseases	(b) Deaths from wounds		
French Revolutionary and Napoleonic (British army only)	1793–1815	198 (mean av.)	16	70	194.0	8.0	24:1	fevers, diarrhoea, typhus, dysentery
Peninsular War (British under Wellington)	1808–14	64 (mean av.)	7	32.0	30.0	4.0	7.5:1	typhus, yellow fever
Crimean (French, British, and Russian)	1854–6	730	34	–	130.0	26.0	5:1	cholera, typhus; scurvy among French troops
American Civil	1861–6	2–3,000	118	–	344.0	63.0	5:1	typhoid, malaria, typhus, dysentery, diarrhoea, measles, smallpox
Franco-Prussian (Prussians only)	1870–1	1,100	17	–	15.0	11.0	1.36:1	typhoid; smallpox epidemic severest among the French
Russo-Turkish (Russians only)	1877–8	100	30	–	81.0	5.0	16:1	typhus, typhoid
Spanish-American (USA only)	1898–1902	172	–	–	3.0	0.8	3.75:1	typhoid, yellow fever, malaria
South African (British only)	1899–1902	500	–	–	14.0	7.5	1.9:1	typhoid
Russo-Japanese (Japanese only)	1904–5	1,350	76	–	36.0	17.0	2:1	typhoid
		650 (av.)	43	153	13.0	8.0	1.6:1	enteric fever, smallpox, diphtheria, cholera

First World War (British and Dominion troops)	1914–18	11,096 (includes non-battle casualties)	418 (+ 362 missing)	2,004*	113.0	167.0	0.67:1	largest proportion of injuries were to legs, head, neck, trunk, arms; other major problems included shell-shock, tetanus, gas-gangrene, gas-asphyxia, trench-foot
First World War	1939–45	5,896 (armed, auxiliary, and civil)	357	369	3.0	87.0† (RN and RAF only)	0.09:1	burns to airmen; multiple injuries from civilian bombing; 40 per cent of all discharges from the Army were for mental disorders

* 8,040,188 'sick or injured'

† includes deaths from drowning, suffocation, etc.

Sources: Louis C. Duncan, 'The comparative mortality of disease and battle casualties in the historic wars of the world', *Journal of the Military Service Institution of the United States*, 1914, 54: 141–77; S. Dumas and K. O. Vedel-Petersen, *Losses of Life Caused by War*, ed. by Harald Westergaard, Oxford, Clarendon Press, 1923; T. J. Mitchell and G. M. Smith, *History of the Great War: Medical Services: Casualties and Medical Statistics*, London, HMSO, 1931; Friedrich Prinzing, *Epidemics resulting from Wars*, ed. by Harald Westergaard, Oxford, Clarendon Press, 1916; W. F. Mellor (ed.), *Medical History of the Second World War: Casualties and Medical Statistics*, London, 1972.

Indeed, long before Leon Trotsky (1879–1940) announced that 'war is the locomotive of history',[13] medicine was considered one of the few real beneficiaries of this engine of progress. For exactly how long this implicitly militarist and overtly positivist notion has been around is not clear, and latter-day attributions to Hippocrates (c.450–370 BC) of the statement that 'war is the only school for the surgeon'[14] should be treated with caution on a number of counts. But by the mid-nineteenth century at least, the idea of war as providing valuable opportunities for both individual and general medical advance was being sustained even in the face of military-medical calamity. A British surgeon in the Crimean War (1853–6), for instance, while confessing that 'this war has, unfortunately, added little to our medical knowledge', yet felt compelled to insist that

> every such war *must* furnish some surgical facts which are worthy of being chronicled, and *must* afford the surgeon some lessons which, without adding to this knowledge much that is absolutely new, are yet worthy of being remembered. A great war, in short, is a great epoch in the onward march of surgical science, when the slowly elaborated teachings of civil life are tested on a grand scale in the presence of representatives from every school.[15]

The two world wars did much to reinforce this 'progress through bloodshed' thesis. In particular, they gave substance to the view that, by stimulating medical research, wars lead to significant advances in health care (thus concealing awkward questions about the 'normal' allocation of medical resources). The First World War, besides introducing blood transfusions, hastening developments in reconstructive or plastic surgery, stimulating work in the design of artificial limbs, and also launching aviation medicine, promoted research into wound-shock, shell-shock, and gas-asphyxia, among much else. In Britain, the consolidation of the Medical Research Committee (late Council) itself was one of the outcomes of the First World War. But above all, this positivist argument was clinched by the apparent transformations of medicine during the Second World War as a result of the introduction and mass production of the 'miracle drug' penicillin. (➤ Ch. 39 Drug therapies) Thereafter, as modern biomedicine entered its golden age, it became 'commonplace . . . to speak of the stimulation of medical progress by the demands of modern warfare, the good that cometh out of evil'.[16]

Like most such statements, the few attempts to generalize on the impact of war on medicine have mostly been made by doctors themselves, largely in the wake of the two world wars. Typically, as in chapters on war in medically authored histories of surgery, such accounts celebrate 'progress', in terms of the great men and great technical achievements supposedly called forth by war.[17] Or, as in the essay on 'The medical balance sheet of war' by Zachary Cope (1881–1974), a surgeon to St Mary's Hospital, London, and one of the editors of the British official medical history of the Second World War, the criterion for assessment rests, retrospectively, on the 'advance' of medical science.[18] Unsurprisingly, Cope was to locate on the positive side of his balance sheet every war since the Franco-Prussian, when antiseptics were first used on a large scale (by the Germans, not the French). Cope was also able to slip in the Crimean War, not (as he might have) on the basis of the use of anaesthetics, but rather on that of the reforms in army hygiene and nursing popularity ascribed to Florence Nightingale (1820–1910). It is further characteristic of this genre that, as in Cope's article, little is made of the medical accomplishments among the losing sides in wars. While a close connection is implied between a nation's medical science and its military might, the need to investigate the actual politics of medicine in war is effaced.

The currency of the notion of war as good for medicine does not, however, derive solely from the comments of the medical profession. Professional historians, too, have endorsed the view – albeit, with varying degrees of qualification, and usually only in the course of seeking to explain socio-medical and professional developments, rather than glorifying medico-technical achievements. Allan Mitchell, for example, examining the relations between physicians and patients in late nineteenth-century France, has identi-fied the Franco-Prussian War as crucial in exposing the maldistribution of doctors and the inadequacies in therapeutic and educational facilities.[19] One of the solutions to these problems, the promotion of more-specialized methods of treatment, is among the specific boons of wartime highlighted in the Anglo-American studies of Rosemary Stevens.[20] Her insistence that medi-cal specialization thrived during the two world wars, with the army acting as a 'filtering system for quality', has been particularized in recent scholarly studies of cardiology, orthopaedics, psychiatry, and rehabilitation medicine.[21] These studies elucidate how at least three of the four requirements for speciality development postulated by George Rosen in his classic work on specialization were fulfilled during the world wars: large groups of patients, specialized facilities, and the financial resources to support specialization. Only Rosen's fourth postulate, a technological focus or technological inno-vation, has come to be seen as wanting. Conceptual and organizational factors now appear to count for more.

Nor is it only in relation to specialization and professionalization that historians have perceived war as beneficial to medicine. The medical provision for, and the health and nutrition of, civilian populations during wartime has also been brought within the audit. In one of the few monographs specifically to address the question of the effects of war on public health, J. M. Winter has argued on the basis of life-expectancy figures that the health of the poorest section of British society was much improved during the First World War.[22] In concluding that the so-called residuum of British society never had it so good, Winter's thesis stands alongside that of the social-policy analyst Richard Titmuss, who viewed both world wars as having a positive effect on health and welfare.[23] Superficially, at least, this argument is given considerable strength in British history by reference to the formation of the Ministry of Health immediately after the First World War, and the National Health Service immediately after the Second World War.

In general, the outlooks of Winter and Titmuss are also in harmony with the familiar story of how recruitment for the Boer War encouraged various programmes in maternal and child health and welfare, school medical services, health visitors, and so on in the 'quest for national efficiency'.[24] (➤ Ch. 45 Childhood) Arguments for these causes (as well as for the eugenics movement) were bolstered by the lurid light cast on 'the people's health' during the recruiting for the First World War. The medical inspection of the recruits for the Second World War, however, directed more attention to mental health (partly as a result of the 'medicalization of mind' stemming from the 1914–18 experience with shell-shock). In the USA, the rejection of hundreds of thousands of draftees for psychiatric reasons is said to have been a major impetus to mental-health policy and to the evolution of psychiatry during the postwar years.[25] (➤ Ch. 56 Psychiatry) In Britian during the Second World War, the case for the systematic reform of health services was strengthened not only by revelations of the physical and mental state of the military recruits, but also by the poor state of health of many of the schoolchildren evacuated from London. Once again, war was to bring to light inadequacies and inequalities in health care.[26] Both world wars also abetted campaigns and legislative enactments against the spread of venereal disease, and did more besides: while soldiers and sailors were encouraged to use condoms, the medical profession, in their treatment of venereal disease (during the First World War), were led for the first time to an appreciation of chemotherapy.[27] (➤ Ch. 26 Sexually transmitted diseases)

Few historians of medicine today would fully endorse the 1919 claim of the physician Sir Thomas Clifford Allbutt (1836–1925) that the First World War transformed medicine from 'an observational and empirical craft to a scientific calling'.[28] But several historians have provided evidence supporting the view that the 1914–18 experience hastened the movement of science and technology to the bedside. One means to this end was the wartime development of the pharmaceutical industry, which became more intent on scientific and medical research. The industry's manufacture and commercialization of new and pirated products (such as the antisyphilitic drug salvarsan) were greatly accelerated as a result of ruptures in international trade agreements and the medical demands of the war.[29] Another means for the scientization of medical practice (which again raises the question of the allocation of resources in peacetime) was the wartime exposure of doctors to new or unfamiliar medical technologies, such as X-ray equipment and laboratories for pathology and bateriology. (➤ Ch. 35 The science of diagnosis: diagnostic technology; Ch. 11 Clinical research) According to the historian of medical technology Stanley Reiser, the First World War

> contributed greatly to the physician's respect for diagnostic laboratories, and created more demand. By 1918, nearly three hundred laboratories were established to supply analyses to physicians in the American Expeditionary Forces. The war provided many doctors with their first experience in the regular use of the diagnostic laboratory. Upon returning to private practice [in the USA], they encouraged the establishment of commercial laboratories, which have thrived vigorously up to the present.[30]

No less new to the majority of the medical profession during the First World War was the application of some of the principles of modern management to medical practice. The use of the medical record card, for instance, emerged as a routine part of everyday practice. The manner in which medicine came to be organized during the First World War also strengthened new professional values, even if, after the war, there was a general turning away from over-managerialized medicine as a result of practitioners' fears for their autonomy. Key concepts such as teamwork, continuity, hierarchy, and regionalism, for example, became stock-in-trade in the post-war reform vocabulary of medical politicians and planners, and were incorporated into such post-war schemes as those for primary healthcare centres, fracture clinics, and accident hospitals.[31]

Historians have directed little attention to the legacy of the gargantuan efforts at medical administration in the wars involving mass armies of volunteers and conscripts. But these managerial features may have been among the most important for civilian medicine. One overlooked example is the rise of organized ambulance services in most major towns in the Western world in the wake of the American Civil and the Franco-Prussian wars. The Civil War witnessed the innovations of Surgeon-General Jonathan Letterman (1824–72) for the systematic rapid rescue of the wounded, while the Franco-Prussian War afforded the first opportunity for the testing of the Red Cross and its affiliate ambulance organizations. Although primitive civilian services had existed before then for the conveying of sick and infectious patients, no organized system was available for the victims of accidents. War experience thus provided a model; indeed, military personnel were involved in the establishment of these civilian services. In Britain, Surgeon-General Sir Thomas Longmore (1816–95), the author of the first book devoted exclusively to the organization of ambulance transport – *A Treatise on the Transport of Sick and Wounded Troops* (1869), which was markedly influenced by Letterman – had his work enthusiatically taken up by the founders of the voluntarist St

John Ambulance Association (established in 1877).[32] Longmore himself was involved in the latter organization (as were several other military medical officers), and one of its key figures, John Furley (1836–1919), was to help in bringing out the second edition of Longmore's book in 1893. Although not all civilian ambulance services organized at this time – voluntary or rate-supported – were quite so committed as the St John Association to a military hierarchy of 'corps', 'divisions', and 'brigades', all of them drew upon such conceptions and practice. Thus the expanding cities with their myriad sources of industrial, domestic, and street accidents were divided into 'battle zones', each networked to medical headquarters and/or the police via 'telephonic' lines of communication.[33] Increasingly, during the dawn of the 'age of the masses', the standardizations and routinizations deemed necessary for the efficient medical operation of the mass army, and the technologies of transportation and information communication that enabled it, were seen as appropriate to the efficient operation of civilian society.

It would be absurd, however, to suppose that war was all good for medicine and its civilian and professional organization, and it would be wrong to suggest that this view has been universally endorsed. Medical authors themselves have expressed degrees of doubt and dissent, even in relation to supposed medico-technical advances. The US Army sanitarian and historian John Shaw Billings (1838–1913), for one, thought that the experience that eighteenth-century surgeons gained from the battlefield 'contributed little to the advancement of surgery'.[34] Garrison reflected in 1929 that, in contrast to the remarkable administrative achievements of the First World War, 'the medical innovations and inventions ... seem clever, respectable, but not particularly brilliant'.[35] And in 1946, in the flush of media enthusiasm for 'the miracles of modern military medicine', the welfare columnist Albert Deutsch opined in an article in the first volume of Rosen's *Journal of the History of Medicine and Allied Sciences*:

> The melancholy truth seems to be that wars generally have contributed but little to the progress of medical science. War undoubtedly does spread skills in medical practice as a result of the opportunities it gives doctors for operating on men in masses. It produces more surgeons, and improves their skills by practice.... Yet, in spite of the ballyhoo, I fail to recall a single medical discovery of primary importance that has come out of this or any war.[36]

More recently, many particulars of the war-as-good-for-medicine thesis have been contested by scholars – though, again, mostly in the course of the discussion of other things. The view entertained by Titmuss, for example, that the Second World War was the crucible for enlightened social welfare in Britain, has unequivocally been laid to rest in two recent volumes.[37] As these make clear, the formation of the National Health Service and other aspects of the post-war welfare state in Britain owed far less to the war than to the social and political developments of the inter-war period. In many ways, this revision forces greater weight to be attached to the First World War. Yet, at the level of social policy at least, it is generally agreed that one of the consequences of that war throughout the Western world was the dampening of pre-war social-welfare movements. Progressivism in America is said to have 'cracked and begun to crumble' before the war had ended, while in Britain, the promised 'land fit for heroes' rapidly fell to the axe of post-war austerity.[38]

Other arguments concerning the medical benefits of wartime have also failed the test of close scrutiny. With regard to Jay Winter's thesis, it has been pointed out that medical services during the First World War could have had little impact on the health of the civilian population in Britain, since few doctors were left in civilian practice.[39] The high pre-war incidence of complications in pregnancy and childbirth (such as puerperal fever) continued largely unchanged during the war, and standards of hospital care for civilians are known to have seriously declined.[40] (➤ Ch. 44 Childbirth) Weak and vulnerable social groups, such as the elderly and the mentally and physically handicapped, lost ground in the reallocation of scarce resources. As F. B. Smith has shown, the First World ('Great') War was anything but 'great' for sufferers from tuberculosis, especially those in British mental institutions. Indeed, tuberculosis, argues Smith, was 'probably the largest single cause of civilian casualties in all the belligerent nations'. In Germany, 280,000 people died from the disease, or one for every ten military casualties; in Britain, the mortality from this cause among young women reverted to its 1890 rate.[41]

In other European countries, too, the nutritional and other effects of the 1914–18 war on civilian populations were far from benign. In Germany, gout is said to have disappeared, but the flip side was an eightfold increase in rickets, hunger oedema, and other problems. (➤ Ch. 22 Nutritional diseases) In Russia, it was recorded that obesity, alcoholism, gout, gastritis, appendicitis, biliary disorders, and constipation all but disappeared, but there was a marked increase in enteritis, peptic ulcers, pyorrhoea, and arteriosclerosis.[42] Better known are the consequences of the privations caused by the Second World War, some of which are still coming to light, as in the long-term follow-up study of the childbearing decendants of the women who were born during the famine in Holland in the winter of 1944–5.[43]

Far less is known about the direct and immediate effects on public health and civilian medical services during other wars in other societies. That the effects could have been beneficial is doubtful, if only because fighting forces have traditionally been major carriers of disease, spreading infection in their wake.[44] That health and health care were probably much worsened seems more likely. In 1876, it was noted of the Turco-Serbian war, that the misery and suffering imposed on the native population were out of all proportion to the extent of the war. In words that have since become only too familiar, the suffering among civilians was described as 'something perfectly frightful'.[45]

Civilian health during most modern wars has usually further been hindered simply by the priority given to military medicine. Along with supplies of drugs and equipment, voluntary efforts and subscriptions on behalf of the sick and indigent have typically been patriotically redirected to the needs of troops. As physically disabled adults discovered during and after the First World War, without a military uniform their begging-bowls went empty. State funding for medical projects other than those deemed essential to military effort have also tended to be cut back. Money for the health programmes initiated by the New Deal of F. D. Roosevelt (1882–1945), for instance, began to disappear with the outbreak of the Second World War, and many of the programmes were terminated.[46] During the Russian Revolution of 1917 and the ensuing civil war of 1918–21, medical research virtually ceased; not only did doctors and scientists suffer the food shortages and the devastations of infectious diseases, but such basic working materials as paper, ink, gas, and electricity were in short and uneven supply.[47]

The belief that wars have had an immediate beneficial effect on the health and welfare of civilian populations may not be widespread for good reason. But what about the belief that, ultimately, wartime advances in therapeutics are incorporated into peacetime medicine, and that the practice of civilian medicine is significantly changed as a result? Here, first of all, it is important to note (in agreement with Deutsch) that few innovations have actually been war-born. Even the study of shell-shock – perhaps the nearest example of a war-born development – fails to pass muster when one considers the growing medical literature from the 1860s on 'railway spine' and 'traumatic neurasthenia'.[48] For the most part, war has accelerated research into old medical problems of military importance, the bulk of which are highly specific to that context and of little value outside it. The treatment of gunshot and shrapnel wounds, gas-asphyxia, gas-gangrene, and trench-foot, for instance, are rarely called for in peacetime. Wartime research priorities with obvious civilian applications, such as the treatment of fractures, flat foot, and venereal disease, have normally reverted to low status in peacetime because they are not very remunerative in private medical practice. Thus while war has sometimes caused new light to be cast on hitherto neglected patient populations (for example, the physically disabled) and on neglected problems (for example, the treatment of fractures), sustaining that impetus post-war has often been another matter. Moreover, as will be elaborated later in reference to the organization of hospitals, the transference from military to civilian medical contexts is seldom straightforward or unmediated by prevailing socio-economic and ideological conditions.

Often, too, in relation to the treatment of acute injuries, wartime conditions have been so different as to render the experience virtually irrelevant to peacetime, and vice versa. The need for urgency in wound treatment and amputations, for instance – well appreciated since the Napoleonic wars, and a major impetus to the development of front-line dressing-stations – was less essential in the controlled and eventually aseptic hospital environment with its anaesthetized patients. (➤ Ch. 42 Surgery (modern)) As noted during the Franco-Prussian War, 'errors may be committed by being too exclusively guided by the experience gained in civil hospitals'.[49] For instance, neurologists during the First World War found that their rule of thumb in civilian practice for assessing the gravity of a head injury – loss of consciousness – was often misleading with regard to gunshot wounds of the head.[50]

Moreover, because each of the wars mentioned here was substantially different medically and militarily from its predecessor, and because civilian medicine changed rapidly in the intervals between, the lessons of one were often of little value to the next. The experience of previous wars, in fact, could seriously deceive. A well-known example is the discovery by surgeons at the beginning of the First World War that the confidence they gained in the Boer War of the power of antiseptics to disinfect wounds was misplaced. In the bacteria-infested battlefields of Europe and Mesopotamia, unlike the Transvaal, nearly all wounds resulting from explosions were septic, and conventional treatment methods were impotent to check the progress of infection. Since the Franco-Prussian War, when the amputation rate on the wounded was brought down from its usual 30–40 per cent to 16.7 per cent, the rate had continued to fall – to as little as 0.5 per cent among the Japanese during the war with Russia in 1905.[51] But during the First World War, the rate soared to as high as 80 per cent of cases, until new methods of wound treatment could be found.[52] Previous war experience rendered the whole issue of wound treatment problematic at the start of the First World War; since greater mortality among troops had always resulted from non-combat causes, it was with disease prevention that military medicine was preoccupied – the more so as the practice of amputation diminished with the rise of conservative surgery during the latter decades of the nineteenth century. Although the Franco-Prussian and Russo-Japanese wars (from the victors' sides) signalled the possibly greater medical importance in future wars of wound treatment, the turn-of-the-century wars in South Africa and Spanish America reinforced an abiding faith in, and focus on, the importance of disease prevention.

Different, it might be thought, was the fate of those areas of medicine that were extensively professionalized through war. Surely the gains made by certain specialisms during wartime could not be lost simply by war's end? Yet this is very much the story of some of the specialisms that were first put on the medical map during the First World War when traditional power relations were weakened or eroded. While neurosurgery, plastic surgery, physical medicine, and rehabilitation, for instance, had to wait until the Second World War to have anything like the same market, orthopaedics found its progress checked even before the war had ended. During the war, it became organized around the treatment of fractures, but in July 1918 a special committee of the Royal College of Surgeons viewed with 'mistrust and disapprobation the movement in progress to remove the treatment of conditions always properly regarded as the main portion of the general surgeon's work from his hands, and place it in those of "Orthopaedic specialists".'[53] As a result, the orthopaedic desire for post-war control of fractures in civilian hospitals was stymied. Other would-be specialists were equally frustrated when they endeavoured to carve a niche for themselves in post-war civilian practice. Not only was the market glutted by demobilized medical practitioners, but it was difficult to establish or re-establish the informal patient referral networks with general practitioners upon which private consultancy depended.

If the argument for war benefiting specialists is less than clear-cut, the case for it advantaging general practitioners is even worse. The latter, when conscripted, had far less reason than specialists to regard war as enhancing their professional interests. Especially in countries where military service was not compulsory, or where, as in Britain, the medical profession were exempt from military service, the enforced disciplines, routines, and red tape of medicine in the military were regarded with considerable disdain. During the Crimean War, the British tried to institute a civilian medical staff corps within the army to carry out elementary nursing, dispensing duties, and ambulance work, but the members' lack of discipline soon led to the corps' abandonment.[54] As rediscovered during the First World War, 'civilian medical practitioners [were] . . . not in the habit of taking orders', let alone of carrying out instructions without being furnished with a reason.[55] Whereas specialists might delight in the wartime potentials for expert knowledge, and relish their greater autonomy in military hospitals over civilian voluntary ones (where their activities were controlled by lay managers), general practitioners were compelled to be underlings within the military medical hierarchy. Aware also that the worth of medical procedures during war was assessed differently than in peacetime, civilian doctors of all types sometimes bore only grudgingly the deviations from their ethical codes. (➤ Ch. 37 History of medical ethics; Ch. 47 History of the medical profession)

Finally, while less well-off practitioners may have welcomed the security of military service, most resented the loss of their civilian income as much as they resented the loss of their autonomy. For many ordinary doctors, the consequences of experiencing salaried-servant status may have cemented a distaste for 'socialized medicine'. The protective league that German doctors formed in 1901 to resist state intervention in medicine was mirrored among practitioners in other Western countries, and personal experience of state medicine under the military could have done little to alter that point of view. (The German doctors' anti-statist journal, the *Artzliche Mitteilungen*, continued publication until 1928.) Although partly as a result of enforced co-operative military medical experience during the First World War, some group practices emerged in Britain and America, none was state-funded or controlled. In America, the majority of physicians in such groups were not generalists, but specialists who needed such co-operation for survival.[56] (➤ Ch. 50 Medical instititions and the state)

THE VIEW FROM THE TRENCHES

The medical 'goodness' of war appears still less so when the vantage-point becomes that of the ostensible objects of military medicine: the troops. To ask what medicine in war did for them brings to the forefront the paradox of medicine in war – the fact that its primary goal is not to preserve health for the sake of individuals, but for the sake of destroying the might of others. Since participation in such acts of violence is often not the preferred choice of conscripts – nor that even of volunteers, the longer a war continues – their interests and those of the medical profession in war are fundamentally opposed. From the reluctant combatant's point of view, the more efficacious the medicine of war, the worse it is as a tool of exploitation. For the war-weary soldier, as has been remarked of those in the First World War, a 'comfortable wound was a very desirable passport off the battlefield'.[57] Thus a medical service that could quickly restore a soldier or sailor to fighting fitness was not universally admired. From the combatant's perspective, war is not good for medicine so much as medicine is good for war.

Wars such as the American Civil and the First World War exposed large numbers of men to modern medicine and dentistry for the first time: one by one, recruits were stripped for examination, measured, weighed, tapped, and interrogated. Along with the soldiers and sailors whose lives and limbs were spared by the skills of military surgeons, such men may have returned home from war with higher demands for and expectations of orthodox medicine than when they left. If so, here was a further wartime gain to the medical profession. But equally noteworthy is the basis for the troops' distrust of the agents of the enforced medicalization of military life. Not least was the fear of being made the subject of a medical experiment, whether conducted systematically or *ad hoc*. Like slaves, prisoners, and orphans, soldiers and sailors were traditionally easy prey. As early as 1587, Barnaby Rich (*c*.1540–1617) in his *Pathway to Military Practice* had seen the need to advise surgeons to 'worke according to arte, not practisinge newe experiments upon a poore souldier'.[58] However, given the number of available bodies in the military and the authoritarian conditions, the temptations to experimentation were irresistible. Examples range from the trial of indiscriminate venesection during the Peninsular Wars, to the compulsory use of mepacrine for malaria during the Second World War. For Zachary Cope, two of the plus factors of medicine in modern war were, first, the fact that the discipline of the forces renders it 'more easy to test any method or drug on a sufficiently large scale to endure a definite result'; and second, '[that] it is possible to introduce compulsion and in this way confirm by large-scale experiment that which had been previously proved on a smaller scale'.[59] Such candour in itself reflects how professional values with regard to human experimentation were strengthened by the Second World War and its memory. Although the Nuremberg Code of 1947, drafted in revulsion at the 'madness' of Nazi doctors, gave formal recognition to the doctrine of 'informed consent' in medical experiments on human subjects, the doctrine was not readily embraced by the medical profession, while the Nuremberg Code itself tended to give legitimacy to further 'reasonable' experimentation on humans.[60]

Another reason for combatants to be on their guard against the medical profession was in connection with malingering and the self-infliction of wounds. Both practices, when undertaken to contrive honourable discharges from the armed services, were punishable at the highest levels of military authority. In Britain they were among the crimes referred to in the Mutiny Act (annually revised since 1689), punishable by courts martial. It was not, however, until the early nineteenth century, for interrelated economic and professional reasons, that the detection of malingering became a military priority. During the Napoleonic Wars, it became apparent that alarming numbers of soldiers and sailors were obtaining disability pensions; indeed, in the aftermath of those wars, to the horror of the treasury, it was claimed that there were nearly as many men on such pensions as there were *in* the armed forces.[61] Although in France during these years, certain doctors, and even some hospitals, could be found 'to conspire in frauds or help create the symptoms of serious illness',[62] little such evidence exists for Britain. Partly in response to the treasury's concerns, and partly from an interest in improving job prospects in an overcrowded profession, civilian practitioners in Britain staked claims to expertise in the detection of malingering. Ever after, suspected malingerers ('skulkers' in navy talk) had to pit their wits against medical officers intent on their unmasking.

Given these interests in the detection of malingering, it is not surprising that troops sometimes resorted to drastic measures to outsmart the doctors. Sir George James Guthrie (1785–1856), the British Deputy-Inspector of Military Hospitals during the Napoleonic Wars, recollected a case in which a soldier swallowed a cork full of pins to produce haemoptysis (bloodspitting). More often, according to Guthrie, British soldiers resorted to the use of corrosive sublimate in order to simulate ophthalmia. The sublimate was so strong that the leeches afterwards used were poisoned.[63] French conscripts in Napoleon's army were said to be particularly ingenious; among their deceits was the introduction into their noses of the testes of cocks and the kidneys of hares so as to simulate polyps. More common were simulated 'back cases', lameness, blindness, deafness, paralysis, epilepsy, madness, and spermatorrhoea, many of which were detectable by the time of the American Civil War through the calculated medical use of anaesthetics: placed only half 'under', the suspected malingerer would be subjected to a battery of physical and mental tests designed to confuse and outsmart. Among reports of malingering during the First World War were cases of subcutaneous injections of irritating substances so as to induce abscesses. By then, the use of anaesthetics on suspected malingerers had been superseded by the use of 'a very strong faradic current', the mere suggestion of the forcible application of which (on the victims of shell-shock, among others) was proudly declared by medical experts to be 'almost infallible'.[64]

The self-infliction of wounds was often nearly as common as malingering. During the Franco-Prussian War, the London surgeon and future president of the Royal College of Surgeons William MacCormac (1836–1901) was 'astonished at the number of [French] soldiers who had got the end of their forefinger shot off'.[65] Again, during the war between Turkey and Serbia in 1876, the same observer lost count of the number 'of persons who have maimed themselves in the hand to avoid fighting'.[66] Such cases rarely tested the acumen of army and naval surgeons in the way that malingerers could, nor does it appear that the handling of these cases seriously tested the loyalties or ethics of medical officers. The latter were often so keen to prove their professional worth in the eyes of military disciplinarians that they were more outspoken on 'cowardice' than regular army officers.[67] For similar reasons, some medical officers during the first half of the nineteenth century defended the disciplinary value of flogging a practice which it was the duty of medical officers to oversee in order to guard against the feigning of reactions worse than those intended.[68]

It was often specifically in relation to malingering and self-mutilation that fundamental changes in military medicine were debated. Just as Florence Nightingale's denial that malingering existed among British troops in the Crimea helped her to muster support for the soldier-'victims' of a medically 'reactionary' War Office,[69] so one of the main arguments against dismantling the regimental system of the British Army was that the regimental surgeons were uniquely placed to detect malingerers. Regimental surgeons 'were by no means possessed of high professional knowledge, much less of general scientific acquirements, or university education' according to Wellington's

Surgeon-General, Sir James McGrigor (1771–1858), but they possessed an intimate knowledge of the troops that rendered malingering difficult.[70] More-centralized systems of military medical organization with high-ranking medical administrators at a distance were regarded as ineffectual from this point of view. Thus when it became necessary to introduce such systems, as during the American Civil War, new methods for detecting malingerers had to be devised. Chief among the solutions was the special hospital staffed by medical experts, such as that for neurology established in Philadelphia in 1863 under Silas Weir Mitchell (1829–1914) and his colleagues. 'Shock' victims were supposedly intended for this hospital, but the majority of the patients were cases of suspected malingering.[71] The military encouragement to cardiology, psychology, ophthamalogy, and otorhinolaryngology during the First World War was similarly much indebted to this disciplinary need. Clearly, the worth of such specialisms *to the military* was as much for their detective as for their corrective functions. This is not to deny, however, that the primary allegiance of the majority of medical officers involved in these and other branches of medicine may have been to the men under their care; distinctions need to be drawn between doctors identifying with the military establishment, and those who may have been doctors first and officers second.

RETHINKING THE RELATIONSHIP

To draw attention to malingering or, for that matter, to any aspect of the military interest in the health and welfare of troops is to highlight certain simple truths about war and medicine which tend to be masked in medico-centric accounts. Most evident is that the area of medicine that gains most from war is the institution of military medicine itself (here, as elsewhere, using the work generically, to include the navy). To it, above all, does war preach valuable 'lessons'. For those with professional stakes in the expansion of military medicine, it scarcely matters that a particular campaign may have been disastrous, medically as well as militarily; the greater the medical shortcomings of any war, the greater its potentially educative value for future wars and hence for bolstering military medicine. The unhappy tales of woe in the Crimea, in Cuba (during the Spanish–American War of 1898), and in the Transvaal, like the ill-fated Walcheren expedition of 1809 (abandoned as a result of the annihilation of over half of the 39,000 troops by malaria, dysentery, typhoid, and typhus),[72] were in this sense 'great events', for they provided powerful rationales for the reform and strengthening of military medicine, though reform itself was often another matter.[73] (➤ Ch. 19 Fevers)

Another basic point brought out by attention to malingering is that military medicine, whether pursued in peace or in war, is both product and agent of its political and economic time. This too is self-evident once we recall that the purpose of maintaining healthy troops is to win wars, the object of most of which has been to capture and control valuable lands and trade routes and/or defend economic ideologies. Since the eighteenth century at least, war at sea has mostly been economic warfare, the success of which has clearly been perceived to depend on the prolonged good health of sailors. Military medicine is also subject to rigorous budget constraints, which are politically determined. (➤ Ch. 57 Health economics)

Although little research has been conducted into the instrumental role of political economy in military medicine, the signs of it are everywhere. The title alone of the famous work by the British Inspector-General of Hospitals, Robert Jackson (1750–1827), *A Systematic View of the Formation, Discipline and Economy of Armies* (1804), provides one such clue. Moreover, as can be gathered from the contents of this work, Jackson harboured no illusions about why it was necessary to try and prevent soldiers and sailors from acquiring such disabling conditions and diseases as scurvy, typhoid, and yellow fever. Like others with commissions in military and naval medicine before and after him – from James Lind (1716–94) to Walter Reed (1851–1902) – Jackson was well aware that the ultimate purpose of military hygiene was to enable imperialist expansion. It was explicitly for this reason that towards the end of the nineteenth century the colonial powers funded, via their military establishments, some of the first and foremost schools of tropical medicine and public health. (➤ Ch. 24 Tropical diseases; Ch. 58 Medicine and colonialism)

The actual practice of medicine and surgery in the armed forces also needs to be viewed in terms of immediate political and economic forces. For example, as Colin Jones has illustrated in his scholarly overview of French military medicine from the time of Richelieu to Napoleon, it was above all economic expediency that encouraged French military surgeons under Napoleon to undertake the amputation of wounded limbs where, in many cases, conservative surgery might have sufficed.[74] The long and expensive hospital convalescence required for the conservation of limbs was deemed militarily unnecessary in a mass army of expendable conscripts. (Such was the context in which Larrey performed the first successful amputations at the hip.) In the different context of the First World War, however, where the value of conserving forces in the face of the wholesale slaughter was soon apparent, medical directives were modified accordingly:

> The primary objects of army hospitals [ran a British army memorandum of 1917] are to get the disabled, physically and mentally, fit to fight again; or, if this is not possible within a reasonable time, to return him to civil life at his highest possible value in the labour market, so that he may cost the public purse the less. If this can be more rapidly and effectually obtained by a relatively high scale of equipment (*e.g.*, orthopaedic surgery), or a larger personnel (*e.g.*, the nursing service), it may be more economical to provide them.[75]

Like the supposedly purely 'medical' function of medicine in war, the purportedly 'humanitarian' function is also open to political, economic, and ideological decipherment. Indeed, the origins of the veritable emblem of humanity in warfare, the Red Cross, owe less than is commonly imagined to the heart-rending experience of the Swiss Jean Henri Dunant (1828–1910) as he observed the sufferings of the wounded at the battle of Solférino in 1859. More crucial to what was to be agreed in Geneva five years later (as the historian John Hutchinson has shown) was the fact that the conditions set forth mutually suited the political interests of the belligerent states involved.[76] The yet-to-be-written history of the Red Cross in each of its different national contexts further suggests the role of complex political negotiations between conflicting military, medical, and philanthropic interests. We need not discount humanitarian impulses, but as with the role of leadership and ability in medical 'advance', their expression needs to be understood *within* history, not above it. To Gustave Moynier, for instance, who headed the International Committee of the Red Cross in Geneva from 1863 until his death in 1910, the object of the Red Cross movement was to raise the moral standards of common people and enable Europe to fulfil its 'civilizing mission' in the world. It is precisely because 'humanitarian aid' has been held to be above ideology in general and the politics of war in particular that it has often well served political ends, the medical-aid detachments to the Spanish Civil War being an obvious case in point.[77] (➤ Ch. 59 Internationalism in medicine and public health)

More overtly political is the history of the provision of welfare services for invalided ex-servicemen. Until the Second World War, when different legitimations of welfare came into play, the primary motive of nation-states in providing such services was to monitor and control the demobilized so as to prevent political revolt. For such purpose, the Hôtel des Invalides was established by Louis XIV in 1670, and the Chelsea Royal Hospital by Charles II in 1682. The involvement of the medical profession in such concerns was by no means necessarily passive. On occasions they exploited the threat of revolutionary activity among the war-disabled in order to further their own professional ends. Thus orthopaedic lobbyists in Britain during and after World War I deployed the rhetoric of social upheaval to persuade the government to set up rehabilitation centres under their control. (➤ Ch. 55 The rise of para-medical professions) Such rhetoric carried force, for, unlike more-traditional war victims (widows and orphans), the embittered war-wounded were capable of political pressure and violence (as recent studies of French and German veterans of the First World War have shown).[78]

Nor was this the only way in which medical practitioners were involved in such politics. Since they were invested with the power to decide whether an injury was war-related, there was a high degree of complicity with the state in the granting or refusing of disability pensions. In this connection, as in the detection of malingering, the role of doctors in wartime was comparable to their peacetime role in worker's compensation cases (the civilian territory for medical elaborations of malingering). It is no coincidence that Sir John Collie (1861–1935), one of few British medico-legal experts on malingering before 1914, was appointed to run the pensions arrangements for shell-shocked cases of the First World. This was 'only natural', as an obituarist remarked,[79] though, in fact, it was in the military that disability-based pensions and exemptions were pioneered.[80] (➤ Ch. 69 Medicine and the law)

In short, the view that 'best practice' in military medicine and welfare has been unambiguously driven by 'humanitarian' impulses is no easier to maintain than the notion that the therapeutics elaborated during wartime have conformed simply to what was most 'scientific' at the time. Yet it would be wrong to assume that this 'best practice' was always or only reducible to instrumental political and economic imperatives. Not only must different social and ideological contexts be taken into account in comprehending the acceptance or rejection of particular practices in wartime, but so too must the power of entrenched ideas and vested interests within the medical profession. The importance of the latter can be illustrated in connection with the treatment of wounds during the First World War, in particular with regard to the British Army's adoption of the method of Alexis Carrel (1873–1944) in preference to that espoused by the eminent 'immunologist' Almroth Wright (1861–1947). Carrel's method consisted of the irrigation of a wound with a strong germicide solution, notably that devised by the research chemist Henry Drysdale Dakin (1880–1952).[81] Although the Carrel–Dakin system was successfully 'sold' to the Army on the basis of how quickly and cheaply it could restore a soldier to fighting fitness, the price wasn't everything. The success of the sale rested as much on the fact that the system's disinfective principle fitted well with the reigning neo-Listerian paradigm in medicine. Wright's 'hypertonic saline system' (the so-called salt-pack method), on the other hand, was premised on anti-heroic 'naturalistic' principles: by applying a 'salt pack' to a wound, the body would be stimulated to generate its own antibacterial agents.[82] (➤ Ch. 10 The immunological tradition) Although the relative economics of Wright's system are unclear, and it is known that some medical officers tried out both approaches, its challenge to Listerian premises was enough to rule it out of court, literally through the major polemical attack on it by the leading advocate of Listerianism, Sir W. Watson Cheyne (1852–1932), who was then President of the Royal College of Surgeons. Perhaps metaphorically, too, Wright's system was destined to be marginalized, for in a context not just of war but of a war on Germans, it was difficult to establish rapport with a therapeutic system that sought to restore natural harmonies and equilibria rather than conduct organized violence on 'germs'. (➤ Ch. 16 Contagion/germ theory/specificity)

THE CALL TO CONTEXTS

By this point the limitations (if not the facile ahistoricity) of the 'war-as-good-for-medicine' thesis should be clear. Whether as forwarded by medical authors, narrowly in terms of advances in techniques and research, or as endorsed in different ways by historians, the thesis will be seen as equivocal at best. Although some aspects of medical knowledge and practice have obviously been accelerated and expanded by war, or altered, elaborated, and transformed, others have remained unaffected, while still others have been temporarily interrupted, demoted in political importance, marginalized, or halted altogether. Generalization is thus impossible. Quite apart from whether the perspective is that of patients or professionals, or whether the reckoning is made in the short or the long term, the worth of war for any aspect of medicine must be seen to vary according to the type of the war as well as to its time, place, duration, and – not least – its political and economic outcome. In selected cases – perhaps for selected periods – it might be possible to claim that medicine reaps in peace what it sows in war; but equally, it might be argued that medicine only reaps in war what it sows in peace, or that wars are but testing-grounds. Of only one thing can we be certain: that as research on different wars comes to be undertaken, there will emerge as many pro and con assertions regarding their effects on the medical profession and on medicine and health as currently exist for the non-medical social and economic effects of war.

But by now it might also be apparent that a part of the problem in trying to determine the relations between medicine and war lies with the question of 'effects' itself. A priori, the search for effects abstracts both war and medicine from the societies, economies, and cultures in which they are set, and assumes that the relationship between them is one of mechanical causal interaction. War is perceived as a force *sui generis*, and medicine merely as a recipient, passive or otherwise.

Now while it is true, if not a truism, that the conditions of war are in some respects peculiar, and may occasion responses in medicine different from those in peacetime, it would be ludicrous to suppose that war is wholly an extraneous phenomenon that merely periodically 'interrupts' the 'orderly progress' of society. To assume that medicine in war can be treated as if it were outside of society, or merely reactive to war, is not only to deny that war is part of a social process, but also to overlook that medicine itself is constitutive of the society and economy in which it is practised. Whatever else war and medicine may be, neither is autonomous.

It follows that the interactions of war and medicine will vary according to the practical and ideological nature of the medicine and the society at the time war occurs. To some extent, it also follows that the effects of war on medicine must ultimately be elusive, for if war and medicine are themselves parts of wider social processes, the impact of war on any aspect of medicine or professionalization can never be precisely calculated. Charles Rosenberg illustrates this point well in his comments on hospital reform in relation to the American Civil War. During that war, the unprecedented provision and organization of hospitals was regarded as 'a triumph of scientific rationality', and it was around this triumph that a reformist consensus crystallized. What 'could be made to work effectively during the stress of war', it was argued, 'could certainly be made even more efficacious in peacetime.' But the war was not responsible for this reformist ideology (which Rosenberg traces back to the 1840s); nor did the war privilege it permanently. Much of the wartime reform enthusiasm evaporated as fast as the military administration itself. What the heightened political and economic circumstances of the war enabled was a realization of a vision of the possible in hospital reform. After the war this vision could only be sustained within the longer-standing reform tradition, and it was to be subjected to the vagaries of macro- and micro-political and economic debate. Thus Rosenberg's finding: that the effects of the Civil War on hospital reform were 'substantial but elusive'.[83]

Almost exactly the same can be said with regard to hospital reformism in Britain and America during and after the First World War. (➤ Ch. 49 The hospital) The wartime organization of hospitals epitomized the ideology that had been gathering economic force since at least the 1880s. But in the austere economic context of post-war Britain, the main result was simply 'exposure without adequate action';[84] the medico-political ideals of co-ordinated planning, standardization, and so on, while strengthened, had to wait until the emergency conditions of the Second World War before they were effectively implemented in civilian medicine. In America, some of the changes were sooner, but the same point holds: that the war itself (as Rosemary Stevens has observed in her study of hospitals), 'was only part of the broader socioeconomic environment of medicine'.[85]

An assessment of the effects on medicine of any particular war requires the socio-economic contextualization of the prevailing civilian and military medicine. For the century between the Crimean and the Second World War, however, there is additional reason why the relationship between war and medicine cannot be readily cast in narrowly causal terms. Quite simply, this is because the boundaries between peace and war are not easily drawn for this period, and the relations between civilian and military medicine are blurred. As Titmuss reflected, breaking down was the assumption basic to a division between peace and war, namely, 'that war is an abnormal situation,

[and] that peace is – or ought to be – the normal lot of mankind'.[86] Although Western society was by no means in a state of constant war, it was increasingly 'militarized': not only were war and the preparations for it coming to be regarded as normal and desirable social activities, and military values and attitudes carried into civilian spheres, but, more fundamentally, society and economics were coming to be disciplined in accordance with military conceptions of efficiency.[87] The process was, in fact, dialectical, for as the size and scale of industrial production, philanthropic enterprise, and social 'disorder' grew, and more-disciplined systems of 'scientific management' were introduced, the more did military management appear as a model of efficiency. At a cultural level, as the boy scouts and similar movements make clear, moral, mental, and physical efficiency or robustness (for nations and individuals alike) was to be generated through the inculcation of military manliness.[88]

Some of the implications for medicine of some of the aspects of this process have been explored by Anne Summers. Identifying a new attitude to war in the mid-Victorian period as one in which war was becoming the business of the whole of society, and linking this to a new kind of citizenship, Summers traces the reflection of that citizenry within the history of nursing up to the time of the First World War. (➤ Ch. 54 A general history of nursing: 1800–1900) (In the uniforms of nurses, aspects of that militarization are still to be witnessed.) But the full history of the militarization of medicine has yet to be told. Even for continental Europe, where military medicine has been more central than in Britain and America, the relations of military to civilian medicine remain largely unstudied.

Here, we can do little more than note some of the more visible signs and symbols of the process as manifested towards the end of the nineteenth century in the English-speaking world, where, precisely because of weaker military traditions, the process of militarization was more marked. Indeed, one such sign of the process was the medical observation and lament of this difference. In a well-publicized lecture of 1903, for instance, specifically on the relations between the military and civilian medical services in Britain, a London physician dwelt enviously on the fact that:

> On the continent there is not that distinction between the military and civilian branches of the profession which exists here. Practically every civilian medical man has once been in the army and would merely revert to his former position in the event of war, while in terms of peace both work side by side in the large state hospitals. In Russia a large part of the civilian practice is in the hands of the military medical officers and their military hospitals would appear to play almost the same role that our large voluntary hospitals do in this country.[89]

Alongside statements such as this can be set the increased voluntary participation of practitioners in wars and in the reserve forces for war; their campaigns for the reform of the status, pay, and conditions of service of doctors in the army and navy; the unprecedented outpouring of reminiscences by doctors who had served in military campaigns since Waterloo; the cultivation of the image of medicine on the battlefield as the noblest expression of the 'gospel of humanity'; and, not least, the rewriting of civilian medicine (surgery, in particular) which emphasized its debts to military medicine.

Scarcely separable from these developments was the professionalization and increasing 'civilianization' of military medicine itself. By 1900, there were some fifty specialist military medical journals internationally,[90] and military medical associations were well represented in the likes of the American Medical Association, the British Medical Association, and the international congresses of medicine and surgery. Reflecting and hastening these developments was the rise to prominence within the international medical establishment of postgraduate military medical academies, such as that established in Washington, DC, in 1893 and that removed from Netley to London in 1902. It was in these schools that many of the world's leading bacteriologists and (what we would now call) immunologists and parasitologists were based: men such as Edmund A. Parkes (1819–76), the 'founder' of the modern science of hygiene; George Miller Sternberg (1838–1915), the leading American bacteriologist who was the founder of the school in Washington; Almroth Wright, to whom I have already referred (see p. 1559); and, in tropical medicine, David Bruce (1855–1931) and William Leishman (1865–1926), to name but a few. (➤ Ch. 11 Clinical research; Ch. 8 The biochemical tradition; Ch. 53 History of personal hygiene)

In view of these signs of the militarization of medicine, and in light of the latter context for bacteriology in particular, it is hardly surprising that military metaphors should have come to dominate medicine as a whole. That, even yet, each of our 'illnesses' must be *fought* (usually with the help of magic *bullets*, which we sometimes receive in the form of *shots*); that we *battle* AIDS by seeking the means to restore *defence systems*, just as we wage *war* on heart disease, and continue to run *campaigns* for research funding to *fight* such a dreaded *enemy* as cancer (*invasive, colonizing, destructive*), is but small testimony to the profundity and reach of the process. 'Biomilitarism', as one discourse analyst has labelled it, is now *the* language of modern biomedicine.[91] Only one other metaphor is as pervasive – that of the messages and codes of information technology – and even that draws heavily upon and conflates with military imagery. Thus the very conception of our bodies and, by extension, the medical acts upon them, remain well within the militarized social relations of medicine that emerged during the formative period of the making of modern medicine.

Clearly, then, there is need to think anew the relations between medicine and war. No longer can we continue to see them in a world apart from the rest of the history of society, economy, culture, *and* medicine, as merely causally interactive, largely self-contained, and mutually beneficial. Rather, as war comes to be seen (at least for much of the period focused on here), not as epiphenomenal, but as an epitome or apotheosis of the wider socio-economically informed process of militarization, so medicine must come to be seen as constitutive of that process, or as part and parcel of it. Pursued in these contextual terms, the history of medicine and war might reveal more than we have yet dared to imagine about the construction of disease entities, the structuring of medical institutions, and the daily practice of medicine as we know it. The call for research can be heard loudly.

NOTES

1   F. N. Poynter, 'The evolution of military medicine', in Robin Higham (ed.), *A Guide to the Sources of British Military History* London, Routledge, 1972, p. 591.
2   See Martin Stone, 'Shellshock and the psychologists', in W. F. Bynum, Roy Porter, and M. Shepherd (eds), *The Anatomy of Madness*, London, Routledge, 1985, Vol. II, pp. 242–71; Ted Bogacz, 'War neurosis and cultural change in England, 1914–22: the work of the War Office committee of enquiry into "shell-shock"', *Journal of Contemporary History*, 1989, 24: 227–56; Harold Merskey, 'Shell-shock', in German E. Berrios and Hugh Freeman (eds), *150 Years of British Psychiatry, 1841–1991*, London, Gaskell, 1991, pp. 245–67.
3   Aside from Howard Levy, 'The military medicinemen', in John Ehrenreich (ed.), *The Cultural Crisis of Modern Medicine*, New York, Monthly Review Press, 1978, pp. 287–300, I know of only one such attempt: Milton Roemer, 'History of the effects of war on medicine', Annals of Medical History, 1942, 4: 189–98. I am grateful to Mick Worboys for drawing this article to my attention. I was unaware of it when I wrote 'Medicine and the goodness of war', *Canadian Bulletin of Medical History*, 1990, 7: 147–59; which makes some of the same basic points.
4   Fielding Garrison, *Notes on the History of Military Medicine*, Washington, DC, Association of Military Medicine, 1922, p. 2.
5   Fielding Garrison, *Introduction to the History of Medicine*, 4th edn., Philadelphia, W. B. Saunders, 1929, p. 11.
6   A. Toynbee, *War and Civilisation* (selected by A. V. Fowler from Toynbee's *A Study of History*), London, Royal Institute of International Affairs, 1950; J. Nef, *War and Human Progress: an Essay on the Rise of Industrial Civilization*, London, Routledge, 1950.
7   Levy, op. cit. (n. 3).
8   Johanna Bleker and Heinz-Peter Schmiedebach (eds), *Medizin und Krieg: vom Dilemma der Heilberufe 1865 bis zum 1985*, Frankfurt, Fischer Taschenbuch, 1987.
9   See Michael Kater, *Doctors under Hitler*, Chapel Hill, University of North Carolina Press, 1989; Robert N. Proctor, *Racial Hygiene: Medicine under the Nazis*, Cambridge, MA, Harvard University Press, 1988; and Paul Weindling, *Health,*

Race and German Politics between National Unification and Nazism, 1870–1945, Cambridge, Cambridge University Press, 1989.

10 See R. Roach Pierson, 'Beautiful soul or just warrior: gender and war', *Gender and History*, 1989, 1: 77–86; Jean Bethke Elshtain, *Women and War*, Brighton, Harvester, 1987; and Cynthia Enloe, 'Beyond Steve Canyon and Rambo: feminist histories of militarized masculinity', in John R. Gillis (ed.), *The Militarization of the Western World*, New Brunswick, NJ, Rutgers University Press, 1989, pp. 119–40.

11 Anne Summers, *Angels and Citizens: British Women as Military Nurses, 1854–1914*, London, Routledge & Kegan Paul, 1988.

12 See Colin Jones, 'The welfare of the French foot-soldier from Richelieu to Napoleon', in *The Charitable Imperative: Hospitals and Nursing in Ancien Regime and Revolutionary France*, London, Routledge, 1989, pp. 209–40, Peter Mathias, 'Swords and ploughshares: the armed forces, medicine and public health in the late eighteenth century', in J. M. Winter (ed.), *War and Economic Development*, Cambridge, Cambridge University Press, 1975, pp. 73–90; Christopher Lloyd and Jack Coulter, *Medicine and the Navy, 1200–1900*, Vol. III: *1714–1815*, Edinburgh and London, E. & S. Livingstone, 1961; Neil Cantlie, *A History of the Army Medical Department*, Edinburgh and London, Churchill Livingstone, 1974, Vol. I. For an overview of the organization of military medicine since antiquity, see Charles Lynch, Frank W. Weed and Loy McAfee (eds), *The Medical Department of the United States Army in the World War*, Vol. I: *The Surgeon-General's Office*, Washington, DC, GPO, 1923.

13 Quoted in Arthur Marwick, 'The impact of the First World War on British society', *Journal of Contemporary History*, 1968, 3: 51–63; see p. 52.

14 Quoted in C. G. West, 'A short history of the management of penetrating missile injuries of the head', *Surgical Neurology*, 1981, 16: 145–9.

15 George H. B. Macleod, *Notes on the Surgery of the War in the Crimea with Remarks on the Treatment of Gunshot Wounds*, London, John Churchill, 1858, p. vii; emphasis added.

16 Francis Watson, *Dawson of Penn*, London, Chatto & Windus, 1950, p. 130. See also John Langdon-Davies, 'The war and medical progress', in Lord Horder (ed.), *Health and Social Welfare, 1945–1946*, London and New York, Todd Publishing, 1947, pp. 38–42.

17 Frederick F. Cartwright, 'Wars and wounds'; *The Development of Modern Surgery*, London, A. Barker, 1967, ch. 6: Owen H. Wangensteen and Sarah D. Wangensteen, 'Surgery of war', in *The Rise of Surgery*, Folkestone, Kent, Dawson, 1978, ch. 24. Similarly, see R. Scot Skirving, 'On the interaction between the war, the profession of medicine and the practitioner', *Medical Journal of Australia*, 27 December 1919, 547–51; and Brian Douglas, 'Armageddon reviewed: effects of the military on civilian medicine', *Pharos*, 1975, 38: 150–8.

18 Zachary Cope, 'The medical balance sheet of war', in *Some Famous General Practitioners and Other Medical Historical Essays*, London, Pitman Medical, 1961, ch. 10.

19 Allan Mitchell, 'Physicians and patients'. *The Divided Path: the German Influence on Social REform in France after 1870*, Chapel Hill, University of North Carolina Press, 1991, ch. 6.

20 Rosemary Stevens, *American Medicine and the Public Interest*, New Haven, CT,

Yale University Press, 1971, p. 127 ff; Stevens, *Medical Practice in Modern England*, New Haven, CT, Yale University Press, 1966, ch. 3.

21 Joel Howell, ' "Soldier's Heart" the Definition of Heart Disease and Speciality Formation early Twentieth-Century Great Britain', *Medical History* (suppl. 5), 1986, pp. 34–52'; Roger Cooter, *Surgery and Society in Peace and War: Orthopaedics and the Organisation of Modern Medicine, 1880–1948*, London, Macmillan; Glen Gritzer and Arnold Arluke, *The Making of Rehabilitation: A Political Economy of Medical Specialization, 1890–1980*, Berkeley, University of California Press, 1985; Berrios and Freeman, op. cit. (n. 2); Terry Copp and Bill McAndrew, *Battle Exhaustion: Soldiers and Psychiatrists in the Canadian Army, 1939–45*, Montreal and Kingston, McGill-Queen's University Press, 1990.

22 J. M. Winter, *The Great War and the British People*, London, Macmillan, 1985.

23 Richard Titmuss, 'War and social policy', in *Essays in the Welfare State*, 2nd edn, London, Allan & Unwin, 1963, pp. 75–87.

24 Geoffrey R. Searle, *The Quest for National Efficiency: a Study in British Politics and Social Thought, 1899–1914*, Oxford, Blackwell, 1971; Deborah Dwork, *War is Good for Babies and Other Young Children: a History of the Infant and Child Welfare Movement in England, 1898–1918*, London, Tavistock, 1987; Roger Cooter (ed.), *In the Name of the Child: Health and Welfare, 1880–1940*, London, Routledge, 1992.

25 Gerald N. Grob, .'The lessons of war, 1941–45'.*From Asylum to Community: Mental Health Policy in Modern America*, Princeton, NJ, Princeton University Press, 1991, ch. 1

26 Richard Titmuss, *Problems of Social Policy*, in (*History of the Second World War, United Kingdom Civil Services*), London, HMSO, 1950.

27 Allan M. Brandt, *No Magic Bullet: a Social History of Venereal Disease in the United States since 1880*, 2nd edn, New York, Oxford University Press, 1987. See also Suzanne Buckley, 'The failure to resolve the problem of venereal disease among the troops in Britain during World War I', in Brian Bond and Ian Roy (eds), *War and Society: a Yearbook of Military History*, London, Croom Helm, 1977, Vol. II, pp. 65–85.

28 T. C. Allbutt, 'Medicine in the twentieth century [a BMA address of 1919]', in *Greek Medicine in Rome with Other Historical Essays*, London, Macmillan, 1921, 542.

29 Jonathan Liebenau, *Medical Science and Medical Industry, the Formation of the American Pharmaceutical Industry*, London, Macmillan, 1987, ch. 8; and Michael Robson, 'The British pharmaceutical industry and the First World War', in Liebenau (ed.), *The Challenge of New Technology: Innovation in British Business since 1850*, Aldershot, Gower, 1988, pp. 83–105.

30 Stanley Joel Reiser, *Medicine and the Reign of Technology*, Cambridge, Cambridge University Press, 1978, p. 143.

31 See Watson, op. cit. (n. 16), ch. 7, esp. p. 145 on the origins of the Dawson Plan. See also Daniel Fox, *Health Policies, Health Politics, the British and American Experience, 1911–1965*, Princeton, NJ, Princeton University Press, 1987; Charles Webster, 'Conflict and consensus: explaining the British health service', *Twentieth Century British History*, 1990, 1: 115–51; and Roger Cooter, 'The meaning of

fractures: orthopaedics and the reform of British hospitals in the inter-war period', *Medical History*, 1987, 31: 306–32.

32 Nigel Corbet-Fletcher, *The St. John Ambulance Association: its History and its Part in the Ambulance Movement*, London, St John Ambulance Association, 1930; J. Clifford, *For the Service of Mankind: Furley, Lechmere and Duncan, St John Ambulance Founders*, London, Hale, 1971; and John Furley, *In Peace and War: Autobiographical Sketches*, London, Smith, Elder, 1905.

33 See G. J. H. Evatt, *Ambulance Organisation, Equipment, and Transport*, London, William Clowes, 1884.

34 J. S. Billings, 'The history and literature of surgery', in F. S. Dennis, *System of Surgery*, New York, 1895, Vol. I, pp. 17–144.

35 Garrison, op. cit. (n. 5), p. 790.

36 Albert Deutsch, 'Some wartime influences on health and welfare institutions in the United States', *Journal of the History of Medicine and Allied Sciences*, 1946, 1: 318–29.

37 Harold Smith (ed.), *War and Social Change: British Society in the Second World War*, Manchester, Manchester University Press, 1986; Arthur Marwick (ed.), *Total War and Social Change*, London, Macmillan, 1988. See also Alan S. Milward, *The Economic Effects of the Two World Wars on Britain*, London, Macmillan, 1972, pp. 22–4, *passim*.

38 Allen F. Davis, 'Welfare, reform and World War I', *American Quarterly*, 1967, 19: 516–33; David French, *British Economic and Strategic Planning, 1905–15*, London, Allen & Unwin, 1982; and Paul B. Johnson, *A Land Fit for Heroes: the Planning of British Reconstruction, 1916–1919*, Chicago, IL, University of Chicago Press, 1968.

39 Linda Bryder, 'The First World War: healthy or hungry?', *History Workshop Journal*, 1987, 24: 141–55. However, purported improvements in health in the face of diminished medical personnel constitutes a part of the paradox that Winter (op. cit. (n. 22), p. 138) seeks to explain.

40 Brian Abel-Smith, *The Hospitals, 1800–1948*, London, Heinemann, 1964, chs 16 and 17; and Virginia Berridge, 'Health and medicine', in F. L. M. Thompson (ed.), *The Cambridge Social History of Britain 1750–1950*, Vol. III: *Social Agencies and Institutions*, Cambridge, Cambridge University Press, 1990, p. 222.

41 F. B. Smith, *The Retreat of Tuberculosis, 1850–1950*, London, Croom Helm, 1988, p. 222.

42 Cited in John D. C. Bennett, 'Medical advances consequent to the Great War, 1914–1918', *Journal of the Royal Society of Medicine*, 1990, 83: 738–42. See also Richard Wall and Jay Winter (eds), *The Upheaval of War: Family, Work and Welfare in Europe, 1914–1918*, Cambridge, Cambridge University Press, 1988; and L. Margaret Barnett, *British Food Policy during the First World War*, London and Boston, MA, Allen & Unwin, 1985.

43 See L. H. Lumey, 'Obstetric performance of women after *in utero* exposure to the Dutch famine', unpublished Ph.D. thesis, Columbia University, 1988: discussed in Irvine Loudon, 'On maternal and infant mortality 1900–1960', *Social History of Medicine*, 1991, 4: 29–73; see pp. 43–4.

44 Freidrich Prinzing, *Epidemics Resulting from Wars*, ed. by H. Westergaard, Oxford, Clarendon Press, 1916. See also William H. McNeill, *Plagues and People*, Har-

mondsworth, Penguin, 1979; and Alfred W. Crosby, *America's Forgotten Pandemic: the Influenza of 1918*, Cambridge and New York, Cambridge University Press, 1989.

45 William MacCormac, 'Ambulances of the Turkish and Serbian armies', *British Medical Journal*, 14 October 1876: 504.

46 John Duffy, *The Sanitarians: a History of American Public Health*, Urbana and Chicago, University of Illinois Press, 1990, p. 262.

47 W. Horsley Gantt, 'The medical profession, soviet science and soviet sanitation: part II', *British Medical Journal*, 5 February 1927: 235.

48 See Edwin Morris, *A Practical Treatize on Shock after Surgical Operations and Injuries, with Especial Reference to Shock Caused by Railway Accidents*, London, Robert Hardwicke, 1867; and Wolfgang Schivelbusch, 'The accident', in *The Railway Journey: the Industrialization of Time and Space in the 19th Century*, Leamington Spa, Berg, 1986, ch. 8.

49 William MacCormac, *Notes and Recollections of an Ambulance Surgeon, Being an Account of Work Done under the Red Cross during the Campaign of 1870*, London, J. & A. Churchill, 1871, p. viii.

50 'Discussion on gunshot wounds of the head', *British Medical Journal*, 20 November 1915: 747–9; and Percy Sargent, 'Some lessons of the war applied to spinal surgery', *Proceedings of the Royal Society of Medicine*, 1920, 13 (3): 17–27.

51 S. Dumas and K. O. Vedel-Petersen, *Losses of Life Caused by War*, ed. by Harald Westergaard, Oxford, Clarendon Press, 1923, pp. 94–5; Thomas Longmore, *Amputations: an Historical Sketch*, Glasgow, Bell & Bain, 1876; and MacCormac, op. cit. (n. 49), p. viii.

52 C. S. H. Frankau, 'Gunshot wounds of joints', in W. G. Macpherson (ed.), *History of the Great War Medical Services, Surgery of the War*, London, HMSO, 1922, Vol. II, pp. 297–325; and Fred M. Albee, *A Surgeon's Fight to Rebuild Men: an Autobiography*, London, R. Hals, 1950, p. 100.

53 Royal College of Surgeons, 'Committee for Temporary Purposes', 1907–22, Vol. VI, p. 313 (MS, Royal College of Surgeons).

54 John Sweetman, 'The Crimean War and the formation of the Medical Staff Corp', *Journal of the Society of Army History Research*, 1975, 53: 113–19; Charles Macalister, 'The history of ambulance in warfare', *Liverpool Medico-Chirurgical Journal*, 1915, 35: 79–94, see p. 93; and Alan Ramsay Skelley, *The Victorian Army at Home*, London, Croom Helm, 1977, p. 42.

55 James W. Barrett, *A Vision of the Possible: What the R.A.M.C. Might Become. An Account of Some of the Medical Work in Egypt; Together with a Constructive Criticism of the R.A.M.C.*, London, H. K. Lewis, 1919, p. 170.

56 George Rosen, *The Structure of American Medical Practice, 1875–1941*, ed. by Charles Rosenberg, Philadelphia, University of Pennsylvania Press, 1983, p. 53.

57 John Keegan, *The Face of Battle: a Study of Agincourt, Waterloo and the Somme*, 2nd edn, London, Barrie & Jenkins, 1988, p. 240 n.

58 C. H. Firth, *Cromwell's Army*, London, Methuen, 1902; quoted in 'The army surgeon in Cromwell's time', *Medical Record*, 6 September 1902: 379.

59 Cope, op. cit. (n. 18), p. 169.

60 See Deutsch, op. cit. (n. 36), p. 318; David Rothman, *Strangers at the Bedside: a History of How Law and Bioethics Transformed Medical Decision Making*, New York,

Basic Books, 1991, p. 61, *passim*; Carolyn Faulder, *Whose Body Is It?: the Troubling Issue of Informed Consent*, London, Virago, 1985.

61 Hector Gavin, *On the Feigned and Factitious Diseases of Soldiers and Seamen etc; On the Means Used to Simulate and Produce Them; and On the Best Modes of Discovering Imposters*, 2nd edn, London, Churchill, 1843, pp. 12–14.

62 Alan Forrest, *Conscripts and Deserters: The Army and French Society during the Revolution and Empire*, New York and Oxford, Oxford University Press, 1989, p. 139.

63 Cited in William M. Keen, S. Weir Mitchell and George R. Morehouse, 'On malingering, especially in regard to simulation of diseases of the nervous system', *American Journal of the Medical Sciences*, 1864, 48: 367–94; see p. 367. See also Forrest, op. cit. (n. 62), pp. 136–7.

64 Donald C. Norris, 'Malingering', in *British Encyclopaedia of Medical Practice*, London, Butterworth, 1938, Vol. VIII, pp. 354–67; see p. 365.

65 MacCormac, op. cit. (n. 49), pp. 10–11.

66 William MacCormac, 'Ambulance of the Turkish and Serbian armies', *British Medical Journal*, 14 October 1876: 505.

67 Anthony Babington, *For the Sake of Example: Capital Courts-Martial, 1914–1920*, London, Leo Cooper (in association with Secker & Warburg), 1983, pp. xii, 59, *et passim*.

68 Peter Burroughs, 'Crime and punishment in the British Army, 1815–1870', *English Historical Review*, 1985, 100: 545–71; see p. 561.

69 Cited in the section on malingering in Joseph Janvier Woodward, *Outlines of the Chief Camp Diseases of the United States Armies as Observed during the Present War: a Practical Contribution to Military Medicine*, Philadelphia, PA, J. B. Lippincott, 1863, p. 325.

70 James McGrigor, *The Autobiography and Services of Sir James McGrigor*, London, Longman, Green & Roberts, 1861, pp. 175–6, 43–4.

71 S. Weir Mitchell, George P. Morehouse and William W. Keen, *Gunshot Wounds and other Injuries of Nerves*, Philadelphia, PA, J. B. Lippincott, 1864, p. 3.

72 T. H. McGuffie, 'The Walcheren expedition and the Walcheren fever', *English Historical Review*, 1947, 62: 191–202; R. M. Feibel, 'What happened at Walcheren: the primary medical sources', *Bulletin of the History of Medicine*, 1968, 42: 62–77.

73 Kate Elizabeth Crowe, 'The Walcheren expedition and the new army medical board: a reconsideration', *English Historical Review*, 1973, 88: 770–85; and Sweetman, op. cit. (n. 54).

74 Jones, op. cit. (n. 12), pp. 230–3.

75 P. Mitchell, *Memoranda on Army General Hospital Administration*, London, Baillière, Tindall & Cox, 1917, p. 1.

76 John Hutchinson, 'Rethinking the origins of the Red Cross', *Bulletin of the History of Medicine*, 1989, 63: 557–78; see p. 559.

77 See Jim Fyrth, *The Signal was Spain: the Aid Spain Movement in Britain, 1936–39*, London, Lawrence & Wishart, 1986.

78 Antoine Prost, *Les Anciens combattants et la société française, 1914–1939*, Paris, Presses de la Foundation Nationale des Sciences Politiques, 1977, 3 vols; and

Robert Weldon Whalen, *Bitter Wounds: German Victims of the Great War, 1914–1939*, Ithaca, NY, Cornell University Press, 1984.

79 *British Medical Journal*, 13 April 1935: 807–8. Collie's *Malingering and Feigned Sickness*, was published in London by Edward Arnold, 1913. Collie also wrote the preface to André Léri, *Shell Shock, Commotional and Emotional Aspects*, London, University of London Press, 1919.

80 Deborah A. Stone, *The Disabled State*, London, Macmillan, 1984, pp. 5 ff.

81 Alexis Carrel and G. Dehelly, *The Treatment of Infected Wounds*, trans. by Herbert Child, introd. by Anthony A. Bowlby, London, Baillière, Tindall & Cox, 1917.

82 Almroth E. Wright, 'On the treatment of infected wounds by physiological methods', *Lancet*, 17 June 1916: 1203–7; Wright, 'The question as to how septic war wounds should be treated. (Being a reply to polemical criticism published by Sir W. Watson Cheyne in the *British Journal of Surgery*.)', *Lancet*, 16 September 1916: 503–13.

83 Charles Rosenberg, *The Care of Strangers: the Rise of America's Hospital System*, New York, Basic Books, 1987, pp. 98–9.

84 Johnson, op. cit. (n. 38), p. 224 n; and Abel-Smith, op. cit. (n. 40).

85 Rosemary Stevens, *In Sickness and in Wealth: American Hospitals in the Twentieth Century*, New York, Basic Books, 1989, p. 81.

86 Titmuss, op. cit. (n. 23), p. 77.

87 See Michael Mann, *States, War and Capitalism: Studies in Political Sociology*, Oxford, Blackwell, 1988, p. 124; Alfred Vagts, *A History of Militarism: Civilian and Military*, London, Hollis & Carter, 1959, p. 453; and Michael Geyer, 'Militarization of Europe, 1914–1945', in Gillis, op. cit. (n. 10), pp. 78–9.

88 See J. A. Mangan and James Walvin (eds), *Manliness and Morality: Middle-Class Masculinity in Britain and America, 1880–1940*, Manchester, Manchester University Press, 1991; and Michael Roper and John Tosh (eds), *Manful Assertions: Masculinities in Britain since 1800*, London, Routledge, 1991.

89 V. Warren Low, 'The relationship of the military medical service to the civil profession', *Lancet*, 10 October 1903: 997–1001, see p. 999; *British Medical Journal*, 3 October 1903: 793–6.

90 See 'Medicine (military, periodicals and transactions of societies and congresses)', *Index Catalogue of the Library of the Surgeon-General's Office*, 1905, (2nd series), Vol. X, pp. 524–5.

91 Scott L. Montgomery, 'Codes and combat in biomedical discourse', *Science as Culture*, 1991, 12: 341–90. See also Susan Sontag, *Illness as Metaphor and AIDS and its Metaphors*, Harmondsworth, Penguin, 1991, pp. 65–72, 177–80.

FURTHER READING

(1) OFFICIAL HISTORIES (CHRONOLOGICAL)

A Medical and Surgical History of the British Army Which Served in Turkey and the Crimea during the War Against Russia in the Years 1854–55–56, 2 vols, presented to both houses of Parliament, London, 1858.

Medical and Surgical History of the Rebellion, 6 vols, prepared under the direction of Surgeon-General Joseph K. Barnes, US Army, Washington, DC, 1870–88.

Suzuki, S., *The Surgical History of the Naval War between Japan and China during 1894–5*, trans. from the original Japanese report under the direction of Baron Y. Saneyoshi, Tokyo, 1900.

Great Britain, War Office, *The Russo-Japanese War: Medical and Sanitary Reports from Officers Attached to the Japanese and Russian Forces in the Field*, London, HMSO, 1908.

The Medical Department of the United States Army in the World War, 15 vols in 17, prepared and pub. under the direction of Major-General Merrite W. Ireland, Surgeon-General of the Army, Washington, DC, 1921–9.

Macpherson, W. G. (ed.), *History of the Great War Medical Services*, 12 vols, London, HMSO, 1923–31.

Macphail, A., *The Medical Services: Official History of the Canadian Forces in the Great War: 1914–1919*, Ottawa, Department of National Defence, 1925.

Strott, G. G., *The Medical Department of the United States Navy in World War I*, Washington, DC, 1947.

The History of the Medical Department of the United States Navy in World War II, 3 vols, prepared under the direction of the Surgeon-General of the Navy, Washington, DC, 1950–3.

MacNalty, Arthur S. (ed.), *History of the Second World War: United Kingdom Medical Services*, 21 vols, London, HMSO, 1952–72.

Feasby, W. R., *Official History of the Canadian Medical Services: 1939–45*, 2 vols, Ottawa, Edmond Cloutier, 1953, 1956.

Link, M. M. and Coleman, H. A., *Medical Support of the Army Air Force in World War II*, Washington, DC, Office of the Surgeon-General of the US Air Force, 1955.

(2) BIBLIOGRAPHIES AND REFERENCE WORKS

Beckerling, Joan Letitia, *The Medical History of the Anglo-Boer War: a Bibliography*, Cape Town, University of Cape Town School of Librarianship, 1967.

Blanco, Richard L., 'Bibliographic essay on British military medicine, 1750–1850', in *Wellington's Surgeon-General: Sir James McGrigor*, Durham, NC, Duke University Press, 1974, pp. 223–7.

Breeden, James O., 'Military and naval medicine', in Robin Higham (ed.), *A Guide to the Sources of United States Military History*, Hamden, CT, Archon Books, 1975, pp. 317–45.

Garrison, Fielding H., *Notes on the History of Military Medicine*, Washington, DC, Association of Military Medicine, 1922.

Hoff, E. C. and Fulton, J. F. (eds), *A Bibliography of Aviation Medicine*, New Haven, CT, Yale Medical Library, 1942.

Joy, Robert J. T., 'Armed forces in the USA: medical services', in J. Walton, P. B. Beeson and R. B. Scott (eds), *The Oxford Companion to Medicine*, Oxford, Oxford University Press, 1986, pp. 73–9.

Poynter, F. N. L., 'The evolution of military medicine', in Robin Higham (ed.), *A Guide to the Sources of British Military History*, London, Routledge, 1972, pp. 591–605.

Stott, Rosalie, 'Medicine in the services', in Gerald Jordan (ed.), *British Military*

History: a Supplement to Robin Higham's Guide to the Sources, New York and London, Garland, 1988, pp. 525–51.

US National Library of Medicine, *Military Medicine*, Washington, DC, GPO, 1955 (reprint of the military section of *Index Catalogue of the Library of the Surgeon-General's Office*, 4th series, Vol. XI).

(3) SELECTED SECONDARY SOURCES

Adams, G. W., *Doctors in Blue: the Medical History of the Union Army in the Civil War*, New York, Schuman, 1952.

Ahrenfeldt, R. H., *Psychiatry in the British Army in the Second World War*, London, Routledge & Kegan Paul, 1958.

Benison, S., Barger, A. C. and Wolfe, E. L., 'Walter B. Cannon and the mystery of shock: a study of Anglo-American co-operation in World War I', *Medical History*, 1991, 35: 217–49.

Benton, Edward H., 'British surgery in the South African War: the work of Major Frederick Porter', *Medical History*, 1977, 21: 275–90.

Cantlie, Neil, *A History of the Army Medical Department*, 2 vols, Edinburgh and London, Churchill Livingstone, 1974.

Cassedy, James H., 'Numbering the North's medical events: humanitarianism and science in Civil War statistics', *Bulletin of the History of Medicine*, 1992, 66: 210–33.

Cooter, Roger, 'Medicine and the goodness of war', *Canadian Bulletin of Medical History*, 1990, 7: 147–59.

——, *Surgery and Society in Peace and War: Orthopaedics and the Organization of Modern Medicine, 1880–1948*, London, Macmillan, 1993.

Cunningham, Horace H., *Doctors in Gray: the Confederate Medical Service*, Baton Rouge, Louisiana State University Press, 1958.

Gillett, Mary C., *The Army Medical Department, 1775–1818*, Washington, DC, Center of Military History, 1981.

——, *The Army Medical Department, 1818–1865*, Washington, DC, Center of Military History, 1987.

Howell, Joel, ' "Soldier's Heart": the redefinition of heart disease and speciality formation in early twentieth-century Great Britain', in W. F. Bynum, C. Lawrence and V. Nutton (eds), *The Emergence of Modern Cardiology, Medical History*, suppl. no. 5, 1985: 34–52.

Hyson, John M., *The US Military Academy Dental Service: a History, 1825–1920*, West Point, NY, US Military Academy, US Army, 1987.

Hutchinson, John, 'World War I and the control of public health', in *Politics and Public Health in Revolutionary Russia, 1890–1918*, Baltimore, MD, Johns Hopkins University Press, 1990.

Jones, Colin, 'The welfare of the French foot-soldier from Richelieu to Napoleon', in *The Charitable Imperative: Hospitals and Nursing in Ancien Régime and Revolutionary France*, London, Routledge, 1989, pp. 209–40.

Keeffer, Chester Scott, 'Penicillin: a wartime accomplishment', in E. C. Andrus (ed.), *Advances in Military Medicine made by American Investigators Working under the Sponsorship of the Committee on Medical Research*, Boston, MA, Little, Brown, Vol. II, 1948.

Keevil, John, Lloyd, Christopher and Coulter, Jack, *Medicine and the Navy, 1200–1900*, 4 vols, Edinburgh and London, E. & S. Livingstone, 1957–63.

Laffin, John, *Surgeons in the Field*, London, J. M. Dent, 1970.

Lankford, N. D., 'The Victorian medical profession and military practice: army doctors and national origins', *Bulletin of the History of Medicine*, 1980, 54: 511–28.

Levy, Howard, 'The military medicinemen', in John Ehrenreich (ed.), *The Cultural Crisis of Modern Medicine*, New York, Monthly Review Press, 1978, pp. 287–300.

Mathias, Peter, 'Swords and ploughshares: the armed forces, medicine and public health in the late eighteenth century', in J. M. Winter (ed.), *War and Economic Development*, Cambridge, Cambridge University Press, 1975, pp. 73–90.

Roemer, Milton I., 'History of the effects of war on medicine', *Annals of Medical History*, 1942, 4: 189–98.

Shepherd, John, *The Crimean Doctors: a History of the British Medical Services in the Crimean War*, 2 vols, Liverpool, Liverpool University Press, 1991.

Shryock, Richard H., 'A medical perspective on the Civil War', *American Quarterly*, 1962, 14: 161–73.

Skelley, Alan Ramsay, 'The health of the rank and file', in *The Victorian Army at Home*, London, Croom Helm, 1977.

Sturdy, Steven, 'From the trenches to the hospitals at home: physiologists, clinicians and oxygen therapy, 1914–1930', in J. V. Pickstone (ed.), *Medical Innovation in Historical Perspective*, London, Macmillan, 1992, pp. 104–23, 234–45.

Summers, Anne, *Angels and Citizens: British Women as Military Nurses, 1854–1914*, London, Routledge & Kegan Paul, 1988.

Titmuss, Richard, 'War and social policy', in *Essays on 'the Welfare State'*, 2nd edn, London, Allen & Unwin, 1963, pp. 75–87.

——, *Problems of Social Policy (History of the Second World War, United Kingdom Civil Services)*, ed. by W. K. Hancock, London, HMSO, 1950.

Vess, David M., *Medical Revolution in France, 1789–1796*, Gainesville, University Presses of Florida, 1975.

Winter, J. M., *The Great War and the British People*, London, Macmillan, 1985.

67

PAIN AND SUFFERING

Roy Porter

Pain is one of the more puzzling, and neglected, topics of the history of medicine; there is not even an index reference under 'Pain', let alone an article devoted to it, in Roderick McGrew's excellent *Encyclopaedia of Medical History*. It is, however, central to the healer's art. Without pain, people would not commonly think themselves ill, convince others of their being sick (expressing pain is our main way of authenticating illness), or, by consequence, consult the doctor. Pain constitutes the alarm signal that typically precipitates the clinical encounter; and, not least, through the placebo power of the bedside manner, pain management has been central to workaday medical practice, past and present.

Yet pain has been a poor relation in the intellectual priorities of medicine, never achieving the status enjoyed by death in physiology, pathology, and disease theories. Medical philosophies have often treated it as epiphenomenal, a problem best left to patients themselves, or to the comforting ministrations of nursing staff, while the consultant attends to life-threatening lesions. Half a century ago, John Alfred Ryle (1889–1950), a founder of social medicine, contended that one of the unfortunate effects of the extension of laboratory-based scientific medicine had been further to push pain, downgraded as a subjective response, to the margins of the doctor's field of vision. He deprecated this tendency, and called for the intensified scientific study of pain, for both clinical and humanitarian reasons. The last generation has, in fact, seen a reawakening of medical interest in the nature of pain and the centrality of pain control in relieving the sick, including the founding in 1973 of the International Association for the Study of Pain.

LANGUAGES OF PAIN

Pain poses problems to the historian. Encouraged by its implicitly materialist metaphysic, the diagnostic procedures of modern medicine proceed on the assumption that pain is a determinate clinical phenomenon that can be linked, in principle and, hopefully, in practice, to specific lesions or disorders. Thus well-mapped patterns of pains in the region of the shoulder and the upper left side of the body will be reliable indications of angina. Medicine distinguishes these from other feelings of discomfort whose source is non-specific (emotional or psychological), even if they may idiomatically be termed 'heartache' or 'heartbreak'. Medicine has thus typically sought to distinguish pain from other sensations it might denominate as 'suffering'. Pain is deemed the special province of medicine; distress or misery in the wider sense coming primarily under the care of priests, friends, counsellors, and psychotherapists.

Presuppositions of this kind, that there is an authentic difference between the clinical and the colloquial connotations of pain, between pain as a specific disease symptom and (non-specific, non-localizable) suffering, have been basic to our modern medical outlook. 'Real pain, especially severe pain', argued the distinguished American physician, Walter Alvarez (1884–1978), 'points to the presence of organic rather than functional disease. On the other hand, a burning, or a quivering, picking, pricking, pulling, pumping, crawling, boiling, gurgling, thumping, throbbing, gassy or itching sensation, or a constant ache, or soreness, strongly suggests a neurosis.' Yet such distinctions are inherently problematic, not to say question-begging. For pain is irreducibly subjective. Whatever it may signal, or be an expression of, pain is felt, is a sensation (or, better, an experience), and is thus in the mind or in the psyche.

This dubious tendency to differentiate 'physical' and 'mental' pain, of course, provides a passport to the realm of what have been called, for the last century, psychosomatic disorders, conditions in which the sick person may feel the pains associated with organic disease (and may as a consequence demand surgery, etc.) but where no physical lesions are medically apparent. In some cases (hysterical paralyses, for instance) it may be easy for medicine to identify a disorder as psychosomatic; in others (migraine, for example) the distinction may trickle through our fingers like sand. There remain various current conditions – such as chronic fatigue syndrome or myalgic encephalomyelitis (ME) – where medicine is divided as to how to pigeon-hole the pain.

To the medical historian, the problems of understanding pain in the past are yet more complex. For one thing, the historian must take into account alternative mind–body metaphysics that cut the disease cake differently from our organic/psychosomatic polarization. For another, there is something ineffable, beyond recall, about the pains patients suffered in the past. The early Victorian writer Harriet Martineau (1802–76) took to her bed for five years, complaining of unbearable abdominal agonies. Were her troubles organic or psychosomatic? Miss Martineau, her personal physicians, and the wider medical profession, debated the issue extensively in person and in print. The historian cannot tell; in the end, it may not matter.

Attempts to draw clear-cut distinctions between pain as a disease sign or symptom and pain as non-specific suffering might, in any case, be anachronistic if applied to the humoralist medical philosophies dominant from antiquity to the eighteenth century. (➤ Ch. 14 Humoralism) Such views saw maladies in a holistic manner, and tended to view 'physical' and 'spiritual' events as a continuum or as two sides of the same coin. Even after the demise of humoralism and with the rise of the pathology of M. F. X. Bichat (1771–1802), clinicians routinely found themselves encountering clusters of chronic pain which they were unable to match against specific lesions. Nineteenth-century physicians and surgeons, unwilling to regard such symptoms as (merely) psychosomatic or marks of the malingerer, developed the idea of the 'syndrome' and deployed intermediate explanatory categories such as neuralgia, spinal irritation, or functional disorder.

There is a further reason why the history of pain and suffering presents severe historical problems. Pain can be an evanescent and indirect phenomenon, difficult to measure, and hard to verbalize, at least with any precision. As has often been remarked, feeling ill tends to reduce even the most articulate to states of mute misery or speechlessness. Reflecting sympathetically upon the hypochondriac's plight, Thomas Beddoes (1760–1808), the prominent Bristol physician, remarked that 'the hypochondria sufferer always finds language fails him, when he gives vent to his complaints'.[1] Whatever his words, they inevitably sounded inadequate or anticlimatic: 'He tells you he has heart-burn, dreadful flatulence', and so forth, but these were distant approximations to his actual sensations. And so, 'after vain and unsatisfactory efforts, his conclusion generally is, "In short you see before you, the most miserable wretch upon the face of the earth".' Beddoes put his finger on the problem. Words were perhaps well designed to represent tangible objects in the natural, external world. By contrast:

> language has not yet been adjusted with any degree of exactness, to our inward feelings. Hence medical reports, where these feelings come in question, stand a double chance of inaccuracy. The invalid, with whom the representation must originate, may express himself ill [sic!]; and the physician may misconceive him if he takes him simply at his word, or by trying to help him out may substitute his own ideas. How little then can we depend upon generalization of such obscure data![2]

In the light of such reflections, it could be argued that the most intense anguish is unsayable, supported, perhaps, by a modification of Wittgenstein's maxim: 'whereon it is impossible to speak, silence is not just golden but mandatory'. Certain philosophers of pain have argued that physical wounds or emotional injuries may be so terrible that to translate them into words (though not necessarily into screams or gestures) may indecently traduce and trivialize them: we talk of 'unspeakable' cruelties. With Nazi extermination-camp tortures in mind, George Steiner has contended that abominations may be so excruciating (physiologically and psychologically) as to be beyond the healing power of words and the redemptive capacity of art.[3] And, in her *The Body in Pain*, an exhaustive discussion of the place of pain in theodicies and secular metaphysics, Elaine Scarry has noted that Evil has been characterized in Judaeo-Christianity as possessing a capacity not just to maim and mutilate but to *silence* its victims, as classically with the raped woman who cannot or will not tell of her ordeal, or, more broadly, with the 'unmentionability' of certain diseases (in our century, notably cancer).[4]

Certainly, many codes of conduct, notably Stoicism, prescribe dignified silence, somatized into the stiff upper lip, in the face of pain, as proof of the mastery of mind over matter, of nobility of soul, and of the consolations of philosophy. Stereotypically, in patriarchal value-systems, men are meant to bear pain – on the battlefield, for instance – without flinching or complaint, whereas women are expected to betray their weakness in screams and tears (though certain recent studies in experimental psychology suggest that men bear pain less well than women).

Despite these ambiguities, the history of pain is no silent saga of dumbness and evasion. If, for their part, medical theorists have, as Ryle alleged, been slow to train their sights on the subject, other disciplines have been primarily devoted to explicating its theory and practice, its avoidance or infliction: criminal codes, torturers' manuals, penological systems, religious exercises, and sadomasochistic pornography, especially the writings of the Marquis de Sade (1740–1814). A powerful meditative tradition humoured the pleasures of melancholy.

Nor have ordinary sufferers been silent about their experiences of 'living pain'. The letters and journals of sick people from earlier centuries offer appalling documentation of griefs and anguish, the human *via dolorosa* in this 'vale of tears'. Some sources seem to indicate that, in earlier centuries, the language of pain was more limited in inflection. The seventeenth-century Derbyshire diarist William Tildesley suffered chronically from what may have been arthritis. His responses are laconic in the extreme, but may be no less expressive for that. On successive days he entered into his journal: 'June 15, In great payne; June 16, In paines alover; June 17 In great payne'. We sympathize with his agonies, and with his difficulties in expressing them.

Other writers have taken pains to cultivate far richer vocabularies for communicating their woes – perhaps because, psychologically speaking, a pain expressed may be a pain diminished or defused. It helps, we say, to get if off your chest, a conviction central to the Freudian endeavour to treat neurotic disorders with the 'talking cure'. (➤ Ch. 43 Psychotherapy) According to Freud (1856–1939), psychic problems, displaced and shelved by somatization, might be resolved by verbalization. To judge from the eloquent testimony of his correspondence, Samual Taylor Coleridge (1772–1834) must surely be one of the most articulate sufferers of all time. Colderidge's case adds a further perspective to the above-quoted observations of Beddoes, his close friend and political sparring-partner. For Coleridge was widely believed to be a hypochondriac, heaping imaginary maladies upon himself as a palliative for psychological guilt, on the principle that one pain drives out another; though, on the analogue of 'the boy who cried wolf', this endeavour perhaps proved hopelessly counterproductive. Such examples reveal profound ambivalences in our culture regarding the expression of suffering. Pain is experienced directly only by the patient. Its expression, in words or gestures, seeks psychophysiological discharge, but also hopes to elicit sympathy; the person adopting the sick role expects some secondary gain. But the stereotype of the *malade imaginaire* prominent from the eighteenth century – the patient whose disorders were fired by a 'warm imagination' – suggests that such a performance risked backfiring amongst a public on its guard against those making a career of pain. Too fluent a talent for articulating agonies excited fears that they were mere rhetoric or histrionics; greater sympathy was often granted to those who suffered in silence. In our culture, it is permissible to have a 'complaint', but not to be a 'complainer'.

This was reinforced by the view of Victorian physicians, particularly specialists in psychological medicine, that it was dangerous to allow patients to depict their pains too graphically, lest this encourage morbid introspection. Faced with patients who dwelt on their 'complaints', physicians advocated diversionary activities: riding, sport, fresh air, massage, and the notorious 'rest cure' developed in the United States by George Beard (1839–83) and Silas Weir Mitchell (1829–1914). Sent to a nursing-home to recover from a 'nervous breakdown', Virginia Woolf (1882–1941) was thus denied pen and paper, books and visitors, in the naïve hope of taking her mind off her troubles.

Without our traditional dread of public emotion and fear of talking, there may be something Anglo-Saxon about these fears (in Mediterranean cultures, the sick are more voluble about voicing their pains, without the suspicion of this being counterproductive). Though the English language has no want of pain words, cultural bias has encouraged reference to pain typically being couched in the preferred idiom of understatement. The English may reputedly be doubled up with pain, and have one foot in the grave, but will respond to health inquiries with a reassuring 'a bit under the weather' or 'a little off-colour'. Pain is clearly an embarrassing intrusion, not easily managed.

THE PHYSIOLOGY OF PAIN

Pain looms large in medical knowledge and practice. As the archetypal presenting symptom, it is bound to be pivotal to the art of diagnosis. Yet pain is not necessarily central to disease theories or therapeutic priorities, for it is perfectly possible, on paper if not by the bedside, to stipulate a radical distinction between pain and disease. Thus aches, cramps, sorenesses, smarts, stings, and other distresses may be experienced without any necessary connection to disease in some strict sense that might be 'objectively' gauged by counts of pathogen presence, functional impairment, or palpable lesions. There is nothing self-contradictory about the idea of a painless disease, though most would think the notion of pain-free illness involves a linguistic solecism, for sickness is generally regarded as coterminous with the experience of something being 'wrong'. (Of course, some illnesses are far more painful than others, cancer of the pancreas being excruciating, leukaemia more debilitating.) (➤ Ch. 12 Concepts of health, illness, and disease)

Down the centuries, pain has been the principal precipitant of medical encounters. By contrast, some degree of functional impairment – encroaching deafness, failing sight, stiffness of the joints – has commonly been suffered without initiating medical engagement, so long as excruciating or anxiety-arousing pain is absent. And every culture, subculture, and individual has a distinctive pain threshold, beneath which, by predilection or pressure, it is customary to bear discomfort (so the saying goes, to 'grin and bear it'). But unexpected pain, strange pain, erratic pain, searing pain, or intense or protracted levels of discomfort are the typical triggers speeding people into primary care, both in the hope of mitigating the distress, and on the assumption that pain itself is symptomatic of some deeper malady.

Within the protocols of traditional medicine, the physician would seek to discover what was wrong by 'taking the history': that is, soliciting from the patient a full verbal account of the complaint. (➤ Ch. 34 History of the doctor--patient relationship) The patient would recite the pain's profile: its nature, location, onset, duration, intensity, periodicity, quality (gnawing, burning, drawing, shooting, vice-like), and so forth. Prior to the nineteenth-century introduction of stethoscopes and opthalmoscopes, medicine possessed little diagnostic technology useful for mapping pains on to specific subcutaneous locations. As diagnostic aids, clinicians used oblique techniques, such as pulse-taking and the assessment of eye- and skin-colour. It was not routine practice to conduct systematic hands-on physical examinations. In mid-

Victorian England, Peter Latham (1789–1875) could still insist, 'not only degrees of pain, but its existence, in any degree, must be taken upon the testimony of the patient'. According to Michel Foucault (1926–85), in the nineteenth century the traditional question, 'What is the matter?', was to give way to the modern, 'Tell me where it hurts', or, in other words, there was a shift from focusing upon symptoms to the rise of a medicine of signs. (➤ Ch. 35 The art of diagnosis: medicine and the five senses; Ch. 36 The science of diagnosis: diagnostic technology)

In short, within the holistic medical philosophies inherited from the Greeks, internal pain, though by no means slighted, was treated as indicative of general constitutional malaise, resulting from some systemic humoral imbalance. In many disorders, pain was believed to have no fixed abode: 'flying gout', for instance, would unpredictably migrate from limb to limb. Hence the prudent therapeutic indication was, by means of bloodletting or counter-irritants (blisters), to divert the pain-centre away from the trunk, and especially away from the vital organs, towards the extremities. (➤ Ch. 40 Physical methods)

Only with the development of specialities such as neurology, of diagnostic aids like the X-ray, and of exploratory operations, did it become easy to index pain more precisely to specific locations and pathological events (toxins, joint degeneration). A significant step was the identification by F. J. V. Broussais (1772–1838) of inflammation as the source of all disease. Likewise, only more recently have differential diagnosis methods been developed, capable of matching, by elimination, particular presentations of pain against distinct disorders. This is especially crucial in the case of referred pain, where the epicentre is, for neurological reasons, dislocated from the seat of the lesion: for example, shoulder discomfort may arise from a ruptured spleen. In short, only recently has the physiology of pain itself become well understood. (➤ Ch. 7 The physiological tradition; Ch. 9 The pathological tradition)

Certain conceptual underpinnings came with the rise of nervous anatomy in the Scientific Revolution, thanks to key figures like Thomas Willis (1621–75), Marcello Malpighi (1628–94), and Giovanni Borelli (1608–79). (➤ Ch. 5 The anatomical tradition) Albrecht von Haller (1708–77) clarified the functional distinction between muscles (endowed with irritability, the property of contracting under stimulus) and nerves (which alone possessed sensitivity, the power to communicate feeling). Robert Whytt (1714–66), William Cullen (1710–90) and other Edinburgh eminences, John Hunter (1728–93) in London, and the Montpellier 'vitalists', especially Théophile Bordeu (1722–76), further explored the relations of sensation to the nervous system. Early in the nineteenth century, François Magendie (1783–1855) in France and Charles Bell (1774–1842) in Britain established the sensory/motor division of the spinal roots as fundamental to nervous organization.

Anatomists, meanwhile, drew upon the theory of the 'reflex arc' articulated as part of the Cartesian theory of the body machine. René Descartes (1596–1650) cited the instinctive withdrawal of a foot from a flame, to exemplify the mechanical nature of the workings of the organism. Heat impacted upon the skin, causing signals to be sent to the brain like a tug on a bell-rope. Pain was the ringing of the bell, a signal to trigger self-preservative action.

This representation of pain-production as a beneficial reflex mechanism, an alarm system, proved suggestive to Enlightenment thinkers. It reinforced their celebration of the functional perfection of the living organism. It confirmed that human behaviour was not random and inexplicable, but the product of regular and predictable economies of 'motivation': that is, what moved people to action. By analogy with the mechanical reflex, utilitarians such as the law-reformer Jeremy Bentham (1748–1832) argued that humans inherently reacted to the positive stimulus of pleasure and the negative sanction of pain (which he dubbed 'the only evil'). A science of motives was therefore feasible, making use of a 'felicific calculus'; and it could be turned into an applied science through environmental management. Judicious distribution of pleasurable and painful sensory inputs in controlled milieux (prisons, schools, and workhouses) would condition subjects to behave in desired and calculable directions. The sensationalist psychophysiologies of Enlightenment thinkers such as Claude-Adrien Helvétius (1715–71) thereby paved the way for modern behaviourism, above all the projects of Ivan Pavlov (1849–1936) and B. F. Skinner (1904–90).

Consolidation of the sensory–motor model of nervous organization rendered it conceptually easy, if, under laboratory conditions, often vastly tricky, for nineteenth-century experimental physiologists further to explore the relations between sensation and movement in the limbs and the workings of the central nervous system. Perhaps under the stimulus of phrenology, understanding of the localization of functions in the brain was slowly improved. In exquisite vivisection experiments (sometimes upon themselves), involving severing nerve fibres or the ablation of brain tissues, a succession of investigators, notably Pierre Flourens (1794–1867) (who was antipathetic to the idea of localization), Marshall Hall (1790–1857), Johannes Müller (1801–58), Claude Bernard (1813–78), David Ferrier (1843–1928), and, slightly later, Charles Sherrington (1857–1952) and Henry Head (1861–1940), laid bare the intricacy of the central nervous system's mechanisms for controlling sensation and activity. By the early twentieth century, the alterations in sensation and motion which, it had long been known, could be effected by severing spinal nerve roots, could be produced by ablations in the brain. Such discoveries suggested resolutions of many of the problems traditionally posed by pain.

The differential sensitivity to pain of various bodily parts had long puzzled observers: why were finger-tips or lips so much more responsive than the skin on the back? why was pain not felt immediately in diseased internal organs like the liver? Neurology demonstrated that these were functions of the differential distribution of nerve-endings. But pain itself seemed to possess a labile quality that did not easily square with the automatic responses implied by the simple reflex model. It was well known that bodily surfaces could become supersensitive to pain (hyperaesthesic: as in tickling), or unresponsive to it. A standard test for a demoniac in the witch-trials of the late Middle Ages and early modern period was insensitivity to pain, examined by applying a candle or sticking pins in the suspect. Nineteenth-century neurophysiology showed that such bizarre occurrences were authentic: not, of course, as the Devil's doings, but explicable in terms of abnormalities of brain functioning. The great neuro-anatomist Jean-Martin Charcot (1825–93), who concentrated in his later years on documenting the physiological inflexions of hysteria, experimented widely on the peculiar reactions of hysterics to pain stimuli, using hypnosis to induce anaesthesias and hyperaesthesias. Other investigators explored the phenomenon of the 'phantom organ' – 'pain' in an amputated limb – and, conversely, loss of sensation in a physiologically whole part: occurrences recently explored in Oliver Sacks's autobiographical *A Leg to Stand On* (1984). (➤ Ch. 21 Mental diseases)

Such advances in the understanding of protective mechanisms in their turn created fresh problems, physiological, psychological, and philosophical. If pain was one inflexion of the reflex response (so asked Enlightenment materialists such as La Mettrie (1709–51) and their nineteenth-century successors), could it, in any strict sense, be said to be the *cause* of activity? Or was it only its accompaniment, a noise in the machine? Pain, it could be argued, was not the motivation for withdrawing one's foot from the fire, but the psychological adjunct to the physical reflex of stimulus and response. Feeling and action were not linked as cause and effect but were *parallel* responses, the one, psychological; the other, physiological. Such arguments could be mobilized to suggest that man was nothing but a machine, and consciousness, the privileged Cartesian *cogito*, just a by-product and a bystander.

The claims that humans are wholly material beings, that mind is a function of brain, and that pain is a function of specific brain fibres, are naturally pregnant with consequences for medicine. Such views imply in practice that the key to pain lies in investigation of the biochemical and physiological activities of the brain. Thus, in a modern research tradition arising out of the investigations by Henry Dale (1875–1968) into the brain-modifying properties of substances such as ergot, the role of chemical neurotransmitters in pain inhibition has been demonstrated. To counter painful stimuli, endorphins (a form of neuropeptides) are spontaneously released to override the normal protective mechanisms of pain, for instance at times of great excitement or danger (thus explaining why soldiers often do not notice appalling wounds in the heat of battle). Such discoveries are, in turn, suggestive for the molecular modelling of drugs (for example, antihistamines). (➤ Ch. 8 The biochemical tradition; Ch. 11 Clinical research)

At a far cruder level, a school of psychosurgery prominent in the 1940s argued that the mental tortures suffered by psychiatric patients were produced by brain disturbance and might be treated by direct assault upon the frontal lobes. Lobotomies and leucotomies were designed to remove offending matter believed to be responsible for excess tension. Discovery that such intervention produced no specific cure, only a general loss of sensation (the 'zombie effect') led to the abandonment of such procedures. Far more sensitive brain operations nowadays are being developed as promising ways of dealing with otherwise-untreatable pain. (➤ Ch. 42 Surgery (modern))

By no means all schools of healing, however, have embraced biochemical and physiological theories of pain. By some, pain has continued to be viewed as positive proof of the primacy of the psychological (or even the spiritual) over the organic. The last century has seen energetic research into pain-inducing or -inhibiting conditions (hypnosis, trance, hysteria, voodoo, brain-washing), which champions of parapsychology claim defy explanation by reductionist physiology. And modern psycho-dynamics has touted its own solutions to such mysteries. Freud, who was confident he could distinguish physical from mental pain from the descriptive language used by patients, explained both 'hysterical' anaesthetizations and paralyses on the one hand, and, on the other, painful but diseaseless symptoms, like persistent coughs or discharges, as somatic conversions, consequent upon repression of primary psychological disturbance (for example, Oedipal trauma in infancy). The wisdom of the unconscious, or psyche, displaces unresolved emotional conflict or insupportable anguish (psycho-dynamic theorists allege), by translating them into more manageable, organic modes. Georg Groddeck (1866–1934) took the extreme position that all physical pain was, in reality, psychological, to be interpreted as a form of non-verbal language: thus neck pain implied a 'pain in the neck', alias nuisance. Similarly, Thomas Szasz has suggested that pain should be construed primarily psycho-sociologically, as a mode of communication well adapted to attracting attention in a highly medicalized society.[5]

Opponents counter that such 'psychological' explanations for pain are trivializing and false. Trivial, because pain is subjective – felt experience – by definition; false, in that the authentic neurophysiological basis of pain is being clarified by brain research. With neurological advance, the sufferings of many of Freud's hysterical patients could now be confidently diagnosed as stemming from an organic pathology.

The enduring value of 'psychological' theories, however, is that they draw us out to the wider contexts of philosophy, emotion, language, and personal significance, which give meaning to the study of pain. The mind–body interplay in pain generation continues to puzzle and provoke: there is still debate, for example, as to the varying role of different nerves in pain communication. Two hundred years ago, reflecting upon the sovereignty of the biological, the pioneer demographer, Thomas Malthus (1766–1834), remarked that intense concentration – such as that demanded by writing – could obliterate the pangs of toothache for a while, but not for good. Modern observations of the effects of shell-shock or hallucinatory drugs have confirmed the truth of this insight, but have not yet finally explained it.

CULTURES OF PAIN

It is axiomatic within medicine that pain is useful. Physicians and philosophers long ago concluded that if, in some carelessly designed Utopia, assault and battery, dog-bites and frost-bite, toxins and infections provoked no pain, survival would be jeopardized. Within the evolutionary biophilosophies developed in the generations after Darwin (1809–82) and Pasteur (1822–95), pain became viewed as a patho-physiologically normal and 'healthy' response to disease dangers, though the tendency for pain to be inordinately prolonged or agonizing poses problems for Darwinian adaptive-mechanism theories: is it not disproportionate to its functions?

Yet if, to the physician, pain is protective, it is also, to the common person, an evil, fearful and sinister. Faced with this double vision, philosophers have felt obliged to confront the problem of pain. A key aim of Epicurus (341–270 BC), for example, was to advocate a 'damage limitation' mode of living, designed to minimize self-inflicted exposure to pain: a simple life, minimizing expectations and ambitions, would offer fewest hostages to fortune. Contrary to the popular stereotype of the sybaritic Epicurean, the good life lay not in the pursuit of hedonism, but in the avoidance of heartache. The Stoicism of Marcus Aurelius (AD 121–180) and others similarly taught followers to rise above passions, appetites, and senses, which would only turn to pain.

The evil of pain may be construed as positive, or as a negative state of deprivation (for example, hunger pangs). Dualistic religious philosophies like Gnosticism and Manicheism have tended to interpret pain as the work of the Devil or some evil principle, exploiting the corruptions of the flesh. Platonists, by contrast, have been inclined to interpret pain as privation. As is evident from the Bible and the great Christian epics of Dante (1265–1321) and Milton (1608–74), Christians developed subtle arguments for justifying the painful ways of God to man. 'Pain is not in its nature an evil in the proper sense' argued William Gladstone (1809–98), 'nor is it invariably attended with evil as a consequence.'[6]

Orthodox Christian theology asserted that pain was not an integral design feature of Creation. It had entered the world through Original Sin at the expulsion from Paradise, when God laid His curse upon man, that he would henceforth be condemned to labour by the sweat of his brow; upon woman, that she would bring forth in pain; and upon humankind in general that disease and death would stalk the world. Thus pain is the divine penalty for disobedience, and a constant reminder of the turpitude of fallen man (an idea reinforced by etymology, 'pain' being derived from *poena*, Latin for 'punishment'). (➤ Ch. 61 Religion and medicine)

Down the centuries, preachers further asserted that God visited pain upon the sinful *en masse* in the form of plagues. Individuals were devoutly to bear affliction as a divinely ordained cross, in the assurance that it was integral to a providential plan of tribulation and purification. As Job's trials showed, the proper response to divinely inflicted adversity was to be long-suffering: to be a martyr to disease was no less glorious than to be a martyr to the infidel. Especially for Catholics, expiatory mortification of the flesh, with goads and hair-shirts, or by fasting, struck a blow for holiness, quelling carnal urges, and emancipating the spirit.

Yet caution was always urged upon the faithful, lest they fetishized pain, making a proud cult out of *homo dolorosus*. For charity also required the relief of pain. After all, Luke had been a physician, Christ had performed healing miracles, and, finally, what was promised in Heaven was not more agony, but bliss. Hence Christian apologists developed nuanced positions regarding medicine and its potential for pain conquest. Suffering was to be embraced as a gift of Providence, as a blessing indeed. Yet it was also to be alleviated by medical aid and charitable offices. These ambiguities, inlaid deep within Christian attitudes towards ill health, find echo in the casuistry of the churches' teachings towards war (just wars are holy; but the Christian should also turn the other cheek); towards the brute creation (all creatures great and small are God's, yet only humans have immortal souls, hence it is legitimate to inflict a degree of suffering upon animals to meet higher, human needs); and towards heretics (apostates may justly be tortured and executed, for truth's sake and the greater glory of God).

From medieval times, clergy embraced robust attitudes towards physical pain: sinful people were bound to be punished, temporally and eternally, by the God of wrath. With the coming of the Age of Reason, theologians constrained to propose more refined theodicies. Pain, many suggested, should be understood as but a 'partial evil' subserving (as Alexander Pope (1688–1744) phrased it) a 'universal good'. According to the evergreen *Natural Theology* (1802) of Archdeacon William Paley, 1743–1805), pain was a 'lesser evil', functional as a caution against a 'greater'. Today's twinge in the toes is a providential stop-sign, directing us to reduce alcohol consumption lest tomorrow we get gout.

More imaginative apologists speculated that God might have brought disease and deformity into the world out of sheer creative superfecundity. The existence of the blind and deaf, freaks and cripples, averred Soame Jenyns (1704–87), perhaps enriched Creation through enhancing the dazzling heterogeneity of types; or, at least, it served to fill every step on the Chain of Being. All that could exist, must necessarily exist: plenitude was aesthetically pleasing to the Supreme Being. Samuel Johnson (1709–84) treated Jenyns's wretched piece of special pleading for pain – the Devil's argument in disguise – with the contempt it deserved. Such apologetics, Johnson insisted, were tantamount to suggesting that the Almighty took sadistic 'delight in the operations of an asthma, as a human philosopher in the effects of the air pump'. They would chuckle 'at the vicissitudes of an ague'; and would find it 'good sport . . . to see a man tumble with an epilepsy, and revive and tumble again, and all this he knows not why'. The magnificent sting in the tail is, of course, Johnson's insinuation that Jenyns was vindicating divine justice by proving that God was no more callous in visiting humans with pain, than were men in their own cruelties to animals. Johnson insisted, however, that good could come out of pain: 'The mind is seldom quickened to very vigorous operations but by pain, or the dread of pain'.[7]

Enlightenment sensibilities rejected Christianity's apparent acquiescence in the inevitability of pain, and modern secular outlooks have given high priority to its minimization. If medievals thought of sickness and poverty as divinely ordained, modern governments feel obliged to seek their eradication. Traditional Christians craved the good death; moderns seek the prolongation of pain-free life.

In the nineteenth century, the ubiquity of pain became a prime argument of atheists. Faced with the suffering involved in the struggle for survival, Charles Darwin and other sensitive souls could no longer accept that the wise person automatically looked, as Pope had recommended, 'from Nature up to Nature's God'. Christian evolutionists had their riposte: God had programmed the sanction of suffering into the evolutionary economy so that the weak would be weeded out, and none but progressive specimens survive and thrive. For Darwin, the tenets of faith were no less painful than those of Nature. He could not stomach the 'cruel' Christian doctrine that unbelievers would be condemned to eternal hellfire. His Unitarian acquaintance, Harriet Martineau, was equally dismissive of the moral acceptability of Christian teachings on pain. Pieties about the beauties of suffering, she argued in her *Life in the Sick-Room: Essays by an Invalid* (1854) glamourized morbid self-pity and sapped the will to be well.[8]

In the secularizing shift from the theocentric to the homocentric universe, Enlightenment *philosophes* made the minimization of pain and suffering the keynote of their philosophy, notably, of course, utilitarians with their felicific calculus. The great cat-lover, Jeremy Bentham, for instance, urged an end to wanton cruelty towards animals, not on religious grounds, nor out of any precocious appreciation of animals' rights, but because animals were equally capable of suffering as humans. Advocates of the decriminalization of suicide argued that self-destruction was a legitimate escape from unnecessary and hopeless suffering. The modern case for voluntary euthanasia has proceeded along the same lines. (➤ Ch. 37 History of medical ethics)

In such developments, the medical profession was caught on the horns of a dilemma. Many doctors, like the Quakers John Coakley Lettsom (1744–1815) and Thomas Hodgkin (1796–1866), were distinguished humanitarian campaigners against judicial torture, duelling, militarism, the slave trade, imperialism, and other cruel abuses. On the other hand, medical progress seemed to hinge upon the tradition of experimental physiology discussed on p. 1582, and Victorian experimentalists became increasingly harassed by antivivisectionist campaigners for their alleged indifference to the pain they inflicted upon dumb animals, charges still levied by animal-rights activists, particularly when experimentation is conducted for lucrative but trivial purposes like cosmetic-testing. British experimenters tended to respond with a 'greater good' defence, claiming that they were careful to minimize pain by anaesthetizing animals wherever possible, and painlessly destroying them later. By contrast, certain nineteenth-century continental European physiologists appeared to uphold the Cartesian 'automaton' position on brute sensibilities, and flaunt a lofty indifference in the name of science. Since 1876, British legislation has codified procedures for pain control in vivisection experiments. (➤ Ch. 69 Medicine and the law)

PAIN AND PROGRESS

Has pain changed over time? There is agreement – witness 'Malthus's toothache' – that circumstances dramatically affect our experience of its intensity. Medical anthropologists and sociologists have demonstrated that different societies respond dissimilarly to 'painful' sensations. Thus some 'psychologize' more than others, while others 'somatize'. What an affluent New Yorker might take to a psychiatrist may be presented by a Mexican to his physician as an acute gastric upset or by a Chinese as chronic fatigue. Some cultures encourage florid rituals of wailing; as with screaming in labour, these may be effective coping strategies. Physical changes are experienced more or less painfully, according to wider contexts of meaning. In the West, according to medical anthropologists, women commonly experience symptoms of the menopause as painful, because it is a watershed, signalling status-deterioration. In other cultures, menopausal escape from fertility may presage social upgrading (an end to polluting menstruation, elevation to the standing of elder), and is therefore not attended by distressing symptoms. (➤ Ch. 29 Non-Western concepts of disease; Ch. 60 Medicine and anthropology)

It has often been asserted that the progress of civilization has been attended by increased sensitivity to pain: 'the savage does not feel pain as we do', judged Silas Weir Mitchell. (➤ Ch. 27 Diseases of civilization) This alleged phenomenon might be read positively, as witnessed by growing antipathy to wanton brutality and the mounting of campaigns against judicial torture, unnatural punishments, and cruel sports. Or it might be thought of negatively: a sapping of hardihood, a deplorable enfeebling of moral fibre and the capacity to endure. The eminent Victorian jurist James Fitzjames Stephen (1829–94) bemoaned such softening: 'that anybody should be in pain and not be immediately relieved – that sharp pain should ever be inflicted upon any one . . . shocks and scandalizes people in these days'.[9]

There are many imponderables. Is, for instance, the founding of Amnesty International testimony to the enhanced moral conscience of the twentieth century, or to the fact that torture is currently being employed by more regimes than ever before? Does the use of epidurals in labour mark the end, not before time, of a certain punitive streak amongst gynaecologists, or show that Western women have ceased to be prepared to experience their natural functions? (➤ Ch. 44 Childbirth)

In any case, direct evidence is utterly inconclusive. Attempts to calibrate degrees of fortitude shown by the sick down the ages against some scientific scale of suffering present insurmountable methodological and measuring problems. What is clear is that the human organism has plastic powers of adjustment to meet the challenges demanded of it. Historians are impressed by the habitual bravery of seventeenth- and eighteenth-century forebears when faced with unanaesthetized amputations, or the prospects of grisly death. But the fortitude seen in a modern field-hospital can match it. If less courage is generally shown today by civilian patients, it is probably because less is expected or demanded.

There have been some shifts, however, in the stance of the medical profession towards pain relief. Sedatives and narcotics had long been used to quell pain – mandragora and henbane (hyosciamine) in antiquity, and subsequently alcohol – but painkillers were not central to the *materia medica* of the classical or Renaissance physician. That situation was to change, and analgesics became more important in prescribing practice. This has partly been due to growing access to effectual drugs and materio-technical progress. From the seventeenth century, opium was easily available, the one truly effective sedative in the traditional pharmacopoeia. The emergent pharmaceutical industry of the nineteenth century developed major synthetic compounds: morphine (1806), codeine (1836), and, in 1892, acetylsalicylic acid – the humble aspirin. (➤ Ch. 39 Drug therapies)

But attitudes have collaterally changed as well. Though bedside practice may have been different, there is little sign that the Renaissance physician conceived of pain control as his prime vocation. Growing customer assertiveness probably changed that, as did competition from quacks, whose patter promised gentle, painless remedies. The art of pain management grew in esteem. From the eighteenth century, physicians began to calm the pangs of the dying with generous doses of laudanum and paregoric (opium in liquid form). And the nineteenth century saw the anaesthetics revolution. The idea, or its uptake, came tardily and slowly. To us, it is remarkable that, as late as the 1790s, Thomas Beddoes and Humphry Davy (1778–1829) could carry out detailed self-experimentation with nitrous oxide (laughing-gas) as a putative remedy for respiratory disorders, without seriously attempting to capitalize upon its remarkable anaesthetic properties. But by the 1840s, the gas was being used to aid dental extractions, and chloroform and ether were becoming employed in childbirth and internal surgical operations; the term 'anaesthesia' was itself coined by Oliver Wendell Holmes (1809–94) in the 1840s. Queen Victoria (1819–1901) had her son, Prince Leopold, delivered under chloroform in 1853, and distinguished practitioners such as James Simpson (1811–70) and John Snow (1813–58) gave the practice their blessing. The hypodermic syringe, invented in the same year, allowed the injection of narcotics.

Hypnosis has enjoyed an occasional vogue, as has acupuncture in more recent times (it has been shown to have a physiological effect, stimulating endorphin release). Cocaine came into use in the 1880s, popularized by Freud, amongst others; the safer novocaine was introduced for dentistry in 1905. From 1950, psychotropic drugs have transformed psychotherapeutics.

Initially, there were pockets of resistance, on moral and therapeutic grounds, from the medical old-guard, but patients voted with their feet. Childbirth by 'twilight sleep' became popular early in the twentieth century. Modern feminism has questioned the trend, reminding women of the undesirability of resigning control of their bodies. In fact, most practitioners were quickly converted to the benefits of anaesthetics. Calmer and more tractable patients let surgeons probe deeper, and take their time at the operating table. In the first half of the eighteenth century, William Cheselden (1688–1752) won renown for his skills as a lithotomist, because he could remove a bladderstone in two minutes, thereby minimizing excruciating pain. By high-Victorian times, operations under anaesthesia might take half an hour or more.

Critics of high-tech modern medicine such as Ivan Illich (b. 1926) have deplored this retreat from the head-on confrontation with pain. Such refusal to face reality, they allege, undermines self-management and personal control. He or she who cannot face pain will not be able to face death. Yet, as is amply shown by the liberal policy with morphine dosages followed in British hospices, the signs are that effective pain control can materially enhance the quality of life in the terminally sick. Successful pain management may be one of the more tangible and widespread, if less glamorous, triumphs of modern medicine.

NOTES

1 Quoted in Edward Shorter, *From Paralysis to Fatigue, A History of Psychosomatic Illness in the Modern Era*, New York, Free Press, 1992, p. 290.
2 T. Beddoes, *Hygeia*, 3 vols, Bristol, Phillips 1802–3, Vol. II, essay viii, p. 78. The following quotations from Beddoes come from the same place.
3 George Steiner, *Language and Silence*, New York, Atheneum, 1967; London, Atheneum, 1970.
4 Elaine Scarry, *The Body in Pain*, Oxford, Oxford University Press, 1985.
5 Thomas Szasz, *Pain and Pleasure. A Study of Bodily Feelings*, London, Tavistock, 1957.
6 Quoted in Martin Wiener, *Reconstructing the Criminal. Culture, Law and Policy in England, 1830–1914*, Cambridge, Cambridge University Press, 1991, p. 111.
7 Mona Wilson (ed.), *Johnson. Prose and Poetry*, London, Rupert Hart Davis, 1968, p. 365.
8 Harriet Martineau, *Life in the Sick Room: Essays by an Invalid*, 2nd edn, London, Moxon, 1854.
9 Quoted in Wiener, op cit. (n. 6), p. 178.

FURTHER READING

Bakan, C., *Disease, Pain and Sacrifice: Towards a Psychology of Suffering*, Chicago, IL, and Boston, MA, Beacon Publications, 1971.
De Moulin, D., 'A historical-phenomenological study of bodily pain in Western medicine', *Bulletin of the History of Medicine*, 1974, 48: 540–70.
Hodgkiss, A. D., 'Chronic pain in nineteenth-century British medical writings', *History of Psychiatry*, 1991, 2: 27–40.
Keele, K., *Anatomies of Pain*, Oxford, Blackwell Scientific Publications, 1957.
Kleinman, A., *Social Origins of Distress and Disease: Depression, Neurasthenia, and Pain in Modern China*, New Haven, CT, Yale University Press, 1986.
Lewis, C. S., *The Problem of Pain*, London, Centenary Press, 1940.
Morris, David B., *The Culture of Pain*, Berkeley, University of California Press, 1991.
Pernick, Martin S., *A Calculus of Suffering. Pain, Professionalism and Suffering in Nineteenth Century America*, New York, Columbia University Press, 1985.
Scarry, Elaine, *The Body in Pain*, Oxford, Oxford University Press, 1985.
Shorter, Edward, *From Paralysis to Fatigue. A History of Psychosomatic Illness in the Modern Era*, New York, Free Press, 1992.

Starobinski, J., 'A short history of bodily sensation', *Psychological Medicine*, 1990, 20: 23–33.

Steiner, George, *Language and Silence*, New York, Atheneum, 1967; London, Atheneum, 1970.

Szasz, T., *Pain and Pleasure. A Study of Bodily Feelings*, London, Tavistock, 1957.

Taylor, F. Kräupl, *The Concepts of Illness, Disease and Morbus*, Cambridge, Cambridge University Press, 1979.

Wall, Patrick D. and Melzack, Ronald, *The Challenge of Pain*, New York, Basic Books, 1983.

Wear, Andrew, 'Historical and cultural aspects of pain', *Bulletin of the Society for the Social History of Medicine*, 1985, 36: 7–21.

68

MEDICAL TECHNOLOGIES: SOCIAL CONTEXTS AND CONSEQUENCES

Harry M. Marks

'Disease', quipped a now infamous medical historian, 'does not exist. What does exist is not disease but practices.'[1] It is more difficult to deny the material reality of technology. Machines shine, watch silently ('monitor'), feed the body, and cleanse the blood. They measure what the body is doing, what it has done and, most mysteriously, peer inside what was once hidden: the heart, the womb, the brain.

The most direct route to the history of medical technology lies through the objects themselves: their appearances, design, and capacities. We have such histories for the longer-lived, more-common technologies – the microscope, the stethoscope, the X-ray machine – as well as for those of interest to particular parties – the cardiologist's electrocardiograph (ECG) or the assorted tools of the anaesthesiologist.[2] (➤ Ch. 36 The science of diagnosis: diagnostic technology)

Histories of devices and techniques provide essential information to the historian writing about the uses, meaning, or the social contexts and consequences of medical technology. One cannot meaningfully write about the slow development of blood transfusion without knowing that transfusions in the early twentieth century required a skilled surgeon to anastomose the donor's and recipient's blood vessels. Innovations in the cannulae used in 'direct' transfusions lowered the required level of surgical skill, but only the acceptance of stored blood made the surgeon's aid dispensable.[3] (➤ Ch. 42 Surgery (modern)) Similarly, so long as the string galvanometer of W. Einthoven (1860–1927) weighed 600 pounds and took five people to operate, electrocardiography was unlikely to find a place in routine hospital practice, much less in the physician's office.[4] Developments in medical science were no less dependent on technology. The images produced by the achromatic compound microscope of J. J. Lister (1786–1869), if not responsible for the efflorescence of the cell theory in the 1840s and 1850s, at least deserve credit for resolving doubt about the shape and structure of blood cells.[5] (➤ Ch. 6 The microscopical tradition)

A few historians have begun to explore the social implications of these technical histories: what skills and resources were needed to operate new equipment, how were new images or information interpreted, and how was access to new technologies regulated by cost, custom, convenience, or professional control? For the most part, the information needed to analyse how technologies were used, distributed, and controlled remains buried in the technical literature whose authors have at best limited interest in such questions.[6]

Writing on medical technologies remains dominated by the themes of the medical sociologist and policy analyst: technological innovation and diffusion, technology and the organization of medical work, the costs and social regulation of new technologies and the 'industrial-medical complex'.[7] Rather than report directly on this social-science literature, this chapter will explore several themes inspired by it:

1 the life histories of medical technologies;
2 technologies and medical work;
3 images and experiences of medical technologies; and
4 the social management of medical technologies.

The chapter will emphasize the recent (post–1850) history of medical machines, not because medicine prior to 1850 lacked devices, but because historians have written even less about the social place of medical machines in that era than in the one that followed it.

LIFE HISTORIES OF MEDICAL TECHNOLOGIES

Writing about medical technologies would be easier if we had a few life histories to analyse and compare. Most medical technologies began clinical life as research tools. Even the now commonplace thermometer began as a research instrument, used by C. A. Wunderlich (1815–77) to study the body's response to disease in the hopes of deriving a science of 'thermonomy'.[8] John Shaw Billings (1838–1913) found his thermometer of little use at Civil War bedsides.[9] By the 1880s, every physician was advised to carry one, not only to 'assist' in diagnosis but to 'aid . . . in curing people by heightening their confidence in you'.[10] The calorimeter, developed to study related metabolic processes in health and disease, remained principally a research tool.[11] Yet no one comparing Wunderlich's charts of temperature in typhoid patients with the later charts by W. Coleman and E. F. DuBois (1882–1959) of their basal metabolic rate would have easily predicted the thermometer's social success.[12]

Robert Frank, Joel Howell, and Ellen Koch have each argued that successful diagnostic technologies must provide clinically useful, *intelligible* information. The ECG, Frank argues, succeeded because it provided *less* information about heart function than other instruments, whose results were correspondingly more difficult to interpret clinically. Koch observes that physicians favoured ultrasound devices that produced X-ray-like images over instruments operating on different principles, whose unfamiliar images were difficult for physicians to comprehend, much less interpret.[13]

Clinical utility is as much a product of historical events as an inherent property of a technology. O. H. Robertson (1886–1966) operated a clinically successful blood-banking system used by American and British forces during the First World War. His accomplishment was praised by the British and then forgotten. Blood-banking was reinvented in the 1930s by a Soviet physician and a physician from Chicago.[14] According to Frank, clinical utility is (in part) socially produced. The ECG's value could only be established by advocates like Sir Thomas Lewis (1881–1945), who had the requisite enthusiasm for the product, sufficient patients on whom to assess and demonstrate the instrument's worth, and the opportunity to 'train their fellow clinicians in a new way of thinking and looking'.[15] Yet less successful innovations also had their champions: the calorimeter of F. G. Benedict (1870–1957) and Du Bois, the ballistocardiogram of Isaac Starr (1895–1989), and the gastric freezing device of Owen Wangensteen (1898–1981).[16] Technological success is multiply determined.

The life history of X-rays – arguably the most successful medical technology of the early twentieth century – illustrates how many elements enter into success. Widely reported by the German physicist Wilhelm Roentgen (1845–1923) in January 1896, the mysterious rays which could 'see through' solid objects were immediately promoted as popular entertainment, a technological marvel, and an icon of modern science.[17] Public lectures vied with scientific meetings in advertising the new technology to physicists, physicians, and the public. X-ray photographs of the human hand were among the more-dramatic demonstrations of the new device.[18] Curious physicians found the publicized demonstrations relatively easy to emulate. The basic elements of the device – a coil, a mercury interrupter, batteries, and a vacuum tube – were available in most physics laboratories:

> a local doctor or surgeon with a suitable case, usually a needle lodged in the patient's finger or foot, would seek the help of a science professor in the local college ... and together they would produce a radiograph.[19]

Commercial production of X-ray coils and tubes, begun in the year following Roentgen's discovery, made the devices even more widely available.[20]

Within a few months of Roentgen's announcement, enthusiasts in Britain, France, and the United States emerged to exploit the device's medical potential.[21] Philanthropists around the world, compelled by the widespread publicity, provided funds to install X-ray equipment in hospitals.[22] (➤ Ch. 63 Medical philanthropy after 1850) In Paris, the municipal government collaborated with the local trade unions to establish a series of autonomous radiological clinics, against the wishes of physician-radiologists.[23]

Medical, engineering, and commercial interests fuelled rapid technical progress, making the machines easier to use and broadening the range of clinical applications.[24] Yet the routine clinical use of X-rays lagged well behind the innovations reported in the medical and scientific press.[25] Radiographers were quick to demonstrate the instrument's capacity to visualize the soft tissues of the chest, the abdomen, and the uterus. In practice, the early devices appear to have been used principally to aid surgeons in locating and extracting foreign objects, or in treating various skin conditions.[26] Technical problems proved easier to transcend than medical conservatism. US army physicians, defending the adequacy of conventional physical diagnosis, rejected the routine use of chest X-rays to screen military recruits for tuberculosis in the First World War.[27] (➤ Ch. 35 The art of diagnosis: medicine and the five senses)

Although army doctors discouraged certain uses of X-rays, the First World War undeniably furthered medical radiology. X-ray screening for tuberculosis was rejected, but X-rays were widely used in diagnosing pneumonia and pleurisy as well as for surgical cases.[28] More than half the soldiers admitted to US army hospitals received diagnostic X-rays.[29] More important, the war stimulated the British and American X-ray industry, and encouraged the development of professional radiology. (➤ Ch. 66 War and modern medicine) In civilian practice, it had been common for surgeons and physicians to interpret their own X-rays. The military took its advice from radiologists, who set up schools to train medical specialists in roentgenological diagnosis. Physicians returned from the war more familiar with the clinical use of X-rays, and the services of radiologists in interpreting them.[30]

Few medical technologies had as auspicious a beginning as Roentgen's rays. The images of the body they produced fascinated the scientific and lay public from the outset. Radiological pioneers capitalized on the public's interest, while enlisting the aid of physicists and engineers in improving the technology. The accident of war stimulated further technical developments, while familiarizing more physicians with the uses of X-rays. Some of this success can be credited to the technology itself: the X-rays' utility, unlike that of the ECG or the ophthalmoscope, extended beyond that of a single organ and its diseases. Other factors were more circumstantial: in the United States, wartime experiences with X-rays were reinforced by the demands of the American College of Surgeons that accredited hospitals possess both X-ray equipment and the services of a professional radiologist.[31]

Historical narratives about medical technologies presume an account not just of what happened, but why it happened. Until we have more studies of technological successes and failures, we shall be handicapped in judging the truth of the histories being written.

TECHNOLOGY AND MEDICAL WORK

Some technologies are closely associated with specific medical specialities: X-rays and radiology, the laryngoscope and laryngology, anaesthesia equipment and anaesthesiology. The paradigm case is ophthalmology, as described by George Rosen. One of the first medical specialities, ophthalmology started when H. von Helmholtz (1821–94) developed an instrument – the ophthalmoscope – which could visualize the ocular fundus and direct attention to diseases of the eye.[32] As Rosen noted, ophthalmology's development in the United States depended on far more than an instrument: a prior conceptual orientation toward organ-based disease; a large, poor immigrant population with much eye disease; a geographically concentrated pool of practitioners; and ready access to European research and equipment.[33] Even so, few medical specialities fit the model so neatly. Organ-based specialities (for example, cardiology, gastroenterology) or those centred on specific clinical populations (for example, paediatrics, geriatrics) outnumber those rooted in mastery of a particular technology.

The specialist's sphere of activity, even when centred around technology, remained subject to revision. Rosen's laryngologists, who began by removing foreign bodies from the windpipe, soon extended their reach to the bronchi and the stomach. Thoracic surgeons, who initially sought the laryngologists' aid, were training their own residents in endoscopic technique by the 1930s. Gastroenterologists, in developing endoscopy, followed a similar path to technological autonomy.[34] Incursions on the laryngologists' field were based on more than claims to mere technical competence. Surgeons argued that their greater knowledge of chest disease better equipped them to interpret the information provided.[35]

Claims to know patients and diseases, not machines, generally underwrite physicians' rule over technologies. (➤ Ch. 34 History of the doctor–patient relationship) The early radiologists won out over competition from independent photographers and physicists, just as chemistry laboratories under the supervision of clinical pathologists came to dominate commercial laboratories run by chemists. (➤ Ch. 11 Clinical research) In both cases, physicians offered an interpretation of the *medical* significance of their products that non-medical competitors could not provide. As the sociologist Andrew Abbott has eloquently argued, professions gain control over markets by developing and pursuing such knowledge claims. Physicians' assertions of clinical competence are but a subset of professionals' assertions of cognitive expertise.[36] Technical competence *per se* plays a minor role in establishing medical jurisdiction over a technology. The radiological technician may master the operation of new CT scanning equipment far more quickly than the radiologist. It remains the radiologist who dictates the terms of the technician's work and defines the meaning of its products.[37]

Medical jurisdiction over the work of non-medical technical personnel is an established pattern in contemporary medical life. In the United States, there are currently more than six health-care professionals for every physician.[38] The division of labour in medicine is based on an old principle, with the same justification as elsewhere in society – economies of scale. The use of assistants, Wunderlich argued, permits the physician to determine:

> the temperature of every patient in a ward containing 20 beds . . . in less than an hour and much of this time can also be usefully employed in simultaneously making other observations.[39]

For Wunderlich, such delegation posed no threat, so long as the physician retained control over interpretation of the results.[40]

As many historians have shown, gender orders the medical division of labour. The physician's hands – anaesthetists, radiographers/radiological technicians, laboratory technicians – are predominantly female. Moreover, even in these highly technical occupations, they do the conventional women's work: explaining, comforting, touching. Yet the gendered organization of medical work precedes, casually and historically, particular technologies and the occupations associated with them.[41] Thus, as Davis suggests, the preference in the United States for (women) nurses to administer anaesthesia was largely determined by (male) surgeons who did not wish to share authority in the operating theatre with other doctors.[42] (➤ Ch. 38 Women and medicine)

Technological advances can destabilize an existing division of labour. Social scientists emphasize the ways in which new equipment challenges traditional professional roles.[43] Any change in a workplace may disrupt existing routines and roles. Whether those disruptions produce permanent realignments in the division of medical labour is less clear.[44] The packaging of drugs in pre-measured ampoules transformed intravenous (IV) drug administration from a 'minor surgical procedure' to a routine practised in any physician's office. Yet the effects on sales of IV drugs were probably greater than the marginal changes in physicians' activities and income.[45]

Some technical innovations do produce dramatic social effects. In the early

1900s, blood transfusions were an experimental procedure mastered only by an Alexis Carrel (1873–1944) or a George Crile (1864–1943) – a highly skilled surgeon able to sew the donor's vessel to the recipient's. Newly designed cannulae introduced in the following decade made the surgical hook-ups much easier (and less interesting) to perform; each city soon developed one or two specialists in the procedure, who were called as the occasion demanded. The adoption of blood-banking in the late 1930s – made possible by the use of anticoagulants – put an end to the emerging surgical speciality of 'transfusionists' needed to perform direct transfusions.[46] The expansion of clinical laboratory testing following the Second World War caused a substantial shift in the activities and self-image of clinical pathologists.[47] The introduction of tanked oxygen, on the other hand, apparently had little immediate effect. Nurses incorporated the administration of oxygen into their routine; it was decades before the ancillary profession of respiratory therapist was established.[48]

The effects of technical change on medical work depend in part on whose work is affected. As X-ray machines became easier to operate in the years after the First World War, medical radiologists faced increasing competition both from non-medical radiographers and other physicians who chose to interpret their own X-rays. Radiologists obtained the support of organized medicine in their efforts to regulate the work of non-medical radiographers. They were less successful in keeping other physicians from purchasing and interpreting their own X-rays.[49] The literature on technological change clearly instructs us that innovation presents repeated opportunities for changing the organization and content of medical work. It is less clear how, when, or why some possibilities become reality and others do not. (➤ Ch. 47 History of the medical profession; Ch. 55 The emergence of para-medical professions)

IMAGES AND EXPERIENCES

Contemporary writings on medical technology portray an ambiguous situation: technology empowers; technology oppresses. The dominant image represents the physician as a sorcerer's apprentice who has unleashed powers beyond his control. Nowadays, technology is said to 'reign' in the kingdom of medicine, subordinating even the physician to a 'technological imperative' that dictates the acquisition and use of ever more machines.[50] Other, more heroic, images of the physician, armed with technology, conquering disease, seem partially eclipsed.[51] At first glance, the picture of medical technologies run amok seems a response to recent developments: the life-extending powers of organ transplants and artificial respiration, the brave new world of prenatal diagnosis, or the simple ubiquity of machines in modern medicine. Yet behind the fear of thoughtless, imperious machines lies an older fear of unthinking physicians:

> For unless men keep ahead of their instrumental aids, these, to coin a word, will merely dementalise them, and but measurably lift the mass without in proportion advantaging the masters of our art.[52]

For technology's medical critics, whether writing in this century or the last, the danger lies mainly in the thoughtless use of machines by other physicians. Only the thinking physician, whose intellect rules the machine, is safe from being ruled by it. What appears initially as a critique of technology turns out, on further examination, to be a criticism of medicine's social order.[53]

The historical and sociological literature on medical technologies derives largely from the reporting of physicians. The patient's voice is muted in medical testimony; the patient's experience hard to locate in the medical record. It is easier to find out what was done than what was thought or felt.[54] The problem is compounded for technology. Patients are concerned about discomfort, pain and fear, recovery and dying, time and money. They do not generally focus on the machines that may cause discomfort, enable their recovery, or bankrupt their families.[55] (➤ Ch. 67 Pain and suffering)

Those patients undergoing long-term renal dialysis, however, are intimately acquainted with a medical technology. Individuals whose kidneys no longer function effectively require the aid of a machine to remove substances normally excreted in the urine.[56] In haemodialysis, patients must be connected several times a week to a machine which processes (dialyses) the blood, removing toxic waste substances and returning cleansed blood to the body. The machine connection is made through a surgically implanted shunt beneath the skin, establishing permanent links to the artery from which blood is drawn and the vein through which it is returned. Dialysis alters blood volume and the concentration of electrolytes and other regulatory chemicals. Patients routinely experience discomfort or headaches (from pressure and volume changes); nausea, fatigue, or muscular cramps (from chemical changes); or a sense of renewal and relief as the toxins are removed. Potentially life-threatening machine failures and user errors, while less common, are familiar experiences.[57]

For many patients, dialysis begins as an alien and unnerving experience: 'I expected the needles, I did not expect blood going through the pipes.'[58] Over time, patients become familiar with the procedure and its effects, but a sense of dependence on the machine remains:

> Always at the back of your mind there is the thought that you are really living on borrowed time. . . . You appreciate that while you got this [machine], something you weren't originally meant to have, by medical or modern science you got [it], then make the most of it.[59]

Unlike most other machine-dependent patients, individuals on dialysis are ambulatory as well as sentient, able to perceive, learn, and act on their knowledge.[60] Minor changes in routine or equipment problems instruct dialysis patients about *their* body's response to *their* machine. Yet physicians and nurses characteristically dismiss this knowledge, discounting patients' diagnoses of difficulties with supplies and equipment. Individuals who dialyse themselves at home are freer to manage iatrogenic problems without interference, while centre or hospital dialysis patients find their complaints are treated as evidence that *they* are the problem.[61]

Historians have adopted the term 'medicalization' to describe the expansion of physicians' activities and medical world views to new spheres of social life. The shift from home to hospital care, particularly in the case of childbirth, gave new influence to physicians' words and deeds.[62] (➤ Ch. 44 Childbirth) Medical technologies are similarly affected by the setting where they are used and the language used to communicate about them.

SETTINGS

The neo-natal intensive care unit (NICU) and amniocentesis stand as symbols of the new, high-technology medicine that has reshaped experiences of pregnancy and childbirth. In the NICU, physicians' values and judgements dominate, to the point of determining how and when parents can share in decision-making.[63] The genetic counsellors who explain the results of amniocentesis to pregnant women are no less imbued with medical values,[64] but so long as the women's decisions about what to do are made outside the clinic, medical advisers cannot decide for them.

LANGUAGE

Differences between the two settings are complemented by differences in the ruling language. The language of the NICU, a highly condensed shorthand used to communicate information and render decisions, excludes even the most technically competent parents from participation.[65] In genetic counselling, by contrast, conventional lay language retains some of its power. The counsellor's 'negative finding' (no abnormalities noted) becomes the woman's 'positive' finding: 'good news'. None the less, the dichotomous medical language (negative/positive, normal/abnormal) eliminates a broad range of concerns from parental consideration.[66]

Feminist scholars make the strongest case for considering technology as an independent force reshaping our experience, images, language, and concepts. Barbara Katz Rothman argues that the technology of prenatal amniocentesis has engendered a 'tentative pregnancy', in which women remain 'unsure whether they are "mothers" or "carriers of a defective fetus" '.[67] Those women notified of an abnormality face the choice of aborting or continuing to term, a choice given new meaning by the ultrasound image of the foetus as a separate entity. Without the technologies of ultrasound and amniocentesis, neither the uncertainty nor the dilemma would exist. Even women who escape this dilemma may find that the prenatal test redefines foetal viability and foetal age, both formerly anchored in bodily experiences. For advocates of prenatal screening, the technology solves a pre-existing problem – birth defects – thereby giving women an opportunity to avoid suffering and burdens. For Rothman, the technology imposes more than it empowers, fashioning new conflicts and burdens from circumstances it has produced.[68]

Rothman's exemplary analysis, based on detailed interviewing of pregnant women and their counsellors, does not readily capture events, images, and influences outside their experience. As Petchesky argues, the meaning of foetal images is multiply determined: by photographic and advertising traditions, by political struggles over abortion, as well as by the experiences of individual women.[69] And, as with other obstetrical technologies, women of different classes and circumstances may experience the technology of ultrasound differently.[70]

Historians have not probed deeply into how national, regional, ethnic, racial, and class differences affect the distribution of medical technology.[71] The concluding section, on the social management of medical technology, explores the causes and consequences of such variation in the contemporary world.

SOCIAL MANAGEMENT OF MEDICAL TECHNOLOGY

It is a truism of social investigation that economic status, standard of living, nutrition, health, and life expectancy will vary according to where one lives, one's occupation, race, gender, religion, and nationality.[72] Not surprisingly, the provision and use of medical technology also varies by country, region, race, gender, and socio-economic status. (➤ Ch. 70 Medical sociology)

Males over the age of 64 are three times more likely to receive dialysis if they live in the (former) Federal Republic of Germany (FRG) than in the United Kingdom (UK). Transplant rates in the UK, on the other hand, are double those in the FRG. Within the UK, individuals living in the Merseyside, East Anglia or north-east Thames regions are from 2.5 to 3 times more likely to receive dialysis than those living in Yorkshire or the west Midlands.[73]

African-Americans are half as likely as whites to receive coronary artery bypass surgery, even among patients hospitalized for coronary heart disease. Hospitalized women in Massachusetts and Maryland similarly receive less surgery than men for diagnosed heart disease.[74] Managers, professionals, and white-collar workers in Lyons are more likely to use radiologists and other specialists than blue-collar workers. French women from the professional and managerial classes or those with a university education are more likely to undergo ultrasound in pregnancy than others.[75]

Economics alone explains some of these differences. (➤ Ch. 57 Health economics) Western European countries are better provided with new technologies than countries in eastern Europe or Asia.[76] The United States exceeds other countries in the supply and use of most high-technology procedures and equipment. It has nearly eight times as many magnetic resonance imaging (MRI) and radiation therapy units per capita as Canada, and three times as many open heart surgery units. Twice as many coronary artery bypass operations (per capita) are performed in the United States as in most European countries, and there are twice the number of patients (per capita) on dialysis than elsewhere.[77]

Differences in medical culture play a role in distributing technology. Physicians from the United States have a much lower threshold than British physicians for recommending surgery for patients with coronary artery disease. Infants in Brazil and Puerto Rico are delivered by Caesarean section at rates well above even those of the United States. Danish, Swedish, German, and Dutch physicians apparently prefer vacuum-assisted deliveries, while the French and British do not.[78] The medical-care system also reproduces existing social inequalities. Use of medical technology may be governed by where one works or lives.[79] In some cases, concern for the economic health of domestic industries can override more-parochial medical demands to import new technologies.[80] (➤ Ch. 4 Medical care)

Few of these contemporary differences have been adequately investigated from a socio-historical perspective. Why should patients living in Alabama, Mississippi, Kentucky, and Tennessee receive two-thirds more open-heart surgery than individuals living in the wealthier, medically intensive, New England states? Do regional differences in the use of obstetrical technologies endure over time?[81] Because virtually all such studies are technology- or disease-specific, we know little about whether social and regional disparities in the supply of medical technologies are systematic or reflect local peculiarities of speciality training and supply. Inadequate data reinforce historians' reluctance to examine the contribution of medical care to social inequalities in health.[82] The most consistent finding is paradoxical: since the 1910s, middle- or upper-income women around the world have been at higher risk of more medical intervention during childbirth.[83]

Since the 1960s, most industrialized countries have spent an increasing proportion of national income on health care; the public share of health-care expenditure has also increased. It is widely believed that medical technologies have *something* to do with cost increases, despite both conceptual and practical difficulties in measuring their role.[84] Such developments have fuelled the long-standing conviction of academics, bureaucrats, and social reformers that medical technology, like other social goods, should be distributed by rational criteria.[85]

Agreement to distribute medical technology rationally does not produce consensus as to what constitutes a 'rational criterion'. Physicians emphasize clinical performance: does the technology improve biological function or survival, or, in the case of diagnostic technologies, does it provide useful information about function? Planners take an engineering approach: given a certain level of clinical performance, how many units are needed to serve a population of specific size and composition? Economists ask whether the monies spent would have a more productive use if invested elsewhere. (➤ Ch. 50 Medical institutions and the state)

Such characterizations are obviously ideal types. From the 1920s through to the 1960s, academic physicians, government officials, and social reformers in the USA and UK combined an engineering and clinical model, while economic evaluations have been increasingly influential since 1970. Normative economics now provides the *lingua franca* for an international community of academic physicians, social scientists, and planners.[86] Successful translation of technology assessments into practice is another matter.

Government restrictions on the production and use of medical technologies are weak in most countries, by comparison with policies regulating therapeutic drugs.[87] Even in Great Britain, with a centralized national health-care system, formal technology assessments are generally advisory rather than binding. Countries with more decentralized financing or delivering systems (for example, Canada, United States, France) offer fewer opportunities to control the supply and distribution of medical technologies.[88] Scrutiny varies with a particular technology's symbolic importance, its political vulnerability, and the policies of the responsible agencies.[89] The results do not reflect anyone's idea of 'rational allocation'.

Formal technology assessments delineate the limits of clinical knowledge and judgement, but information does not govern clinical practice.[90] Money and politics, by determining what is feasible, determine how and on whom technologies are used. British physicians have, in effect, rationed dialysis use by age, offering a clinical rationale for their reluctance to place patients aged over 65 on the procedure.[91] Heart patients in the Netherlands, cardiac surgeons in the United States, and radiologists in Britain have evaded official restrictions through politics and publicity. In the United States, families denied insurance authorization for organ transplants use network television to raise funds and locate organs.[92]

Medical care has always been rationed by social and economic criteria.

The novelty of the present situation lies in efforts to override conventional medical judgements about the value of new procedures and the selection of appropriate beneficiaries. Community groups in Oregon have recently debated which services should be offered by the state's Medicaid programme. AIDS activists in the United States have successfully challenged the procedures by which the Food and Drug Administration assesses new therapies. Such initiatives affect only small segments of medical-care recipients.[93] The vast majority of decisions to use medical technologies are still made at the bedside, by physicians using conventional medical (and social) criteria.[94] Yet as governmental involvement with medical-care policy intensifies, political opportunities to reassess clinical judgements broaden and increase.[95] Some commentators view the current ferment around medical technologies as a product of the technologies themselves, and their awesome capacities. I have argued here that the ferment is no less a product of our social and political arrangements for deciding about when, how, and for what reasons we will use our machines.

ACKNOWLEDGEMENTS

The author would like to thank Susan Bell, Peter Buck, Joel Howell, Stuart Leslie, Rosemary Stevens, and John Harley Warner for helpful information and advice, and JoAnne Brown for criticism and instruction beyond the call of friendship.

NOTES

1 François Delaporte, *Disease and Civilization. The Cholera in Paris, 1832*, Cambridge, MA, MIT Press, 1986, p. 6.
2 See Further Reading.
3 Bertram M. Bernheim, *Adventure in Blood Transfusion*, New York, Smith & Durrell, 1942, pp. 23–33, 119–121, 130–2; Louis K. Diamond, 'A history of blood transfusion', in Maxwell Wintrobe, *Blood, Pure and Eloquent. A Story of Discovery, of People, and of Ideas*, New York, McGraw Hill, 1980, pp. 674–8.
4 George E. Burch and Nicholas P. DePasquale, *A History of Electrocardiography*, San Francisco, Norman, 1990, pp. 30–5, 112–16. Weight and bulk aside, it was generally believed that the ECG equipment needed to be installed in a room with a reinforced concrete floor to reduce vibrations. Telegraph or telephone was used to transmit the impulses to the instrument, sometimes installed over a mile away. See M. J. G. Cattermole and A. F. Wolfe, *Horace Darwin's Shop. A History of the Cambridge Scientific Instrument Company*, Bristol, Adam Hilger, 1987, pp. 230–1. On the early development of the portable electrocardiogram, see Burch and Pasquale, *A History of Electrocardiography*, pp. 43–6.
5 R. H. Nuttall, 'The achromatic microscope in the history of nineteenth-century science', *Philosophical Journal*, 1974, 11: 71–9; Brian Bracegirdle, 'J. J. Lister and the establishment of histology', *Medical History*, 1977, 21: 187–91; Thomas

Hodgkin and J. Lister, 'Notice of some microscopic observations of the blood and animal tissues', *Philosophical Magazine*, 1827 (NS), 2: 130–8.

6 For examples of the new historiography, see the works by Audrey Davis, Joel Howell, Robert Frank, Edward Yoxon, and Ellen Breckenridge Koch, cited in Further Reading.

7 For recent reviews of these literatures, see Susan E. Bell, 'Technology in medicine: development, diffusion and health policy', in Howard E. Freeman and Sol Levine (eds), *Handbook of Medical Sociology*, 4th edn, Englewood Cliffs, NJ, Prentice-Hall, 1989, pp. 185–204; Julius A. Roth and Sheryl Burt Ruzek (eds), *The Adoption and Social Consequences of Medical Technologies. Research in the Sociology of Health Care*, Greenwich, JAI Press, 1986 Vol. IV; W. Richard Scott, 'Innovation in medical care organizations: a synthetic review', *Medical Care Review*, 1990, 47: 165–92; Institute of Medicine, Committee for Evaluating Medical Technologies in Clinical Use, *Assessing Medical Technologies*, Washington, DC, National Academy Press, 1985.

8 C. A. Wunderlich, *On the Temperature in Diseases: a Manual of Medical Thermometry*, London, New Sydenham Society, 1871, pp. 51–2. On the development and promotion of the thermometer in medicine, see Stanley Joel Reiser, *Medicine and the Reign of Technology*, New York, Cambridge University Press, 1978, pp. 110–21; Daniel M. Musher, Edward A. Dominguez and Ariel Bar-Sela, 'Edouard Seguin and the social power of thermometry', *New England Journal of Medicine*, 1987, 316: 115–17; Dominguez, Bar-Sela and Musher, 'Adoption of thermometry into clinical practice in the United States', *Reviews of Infectious Diseases*, 1987, 9: 1193–1201.

9 John Shaw Billings, 'Medical reminiscences of the Civil War', *Transactions of the College of Physicians of Philadelphia*, 1905, 27: 116.

10 D. W. Cathell, *The Physician Himself and What He Should Add to His Scientific Requirements*, reprinted New York, Arno Press, 1972, p. 18; orig. pub. 1882. Dominguez, Bar-Sela, and Musher, op. cit. (n. 8), p. 1199, report that charting of vital signs, including temperature was 'routine' by the early 1870s at the New England Hospital for Women and Children and the Massachusetts General Hospital.

11 Frederic L. Holmes, 'The intake-output method of quantification in physiology', *Historical Studies in the Physical and Biological Sciences*, 1987, 17: 235–70; William S. McCann, *Calorimetry in Medicine*, Baltimore, MD, Williams & Wilkins, 1924. According to McCann, calorimetry's clinical value was in regulating thyroxine dosage for those with hypothyroidism, and had also been used by Joslin and Benedict to establish the dietetic requirements of newly diagnosed diabetics; see pp. 52–5.

12 For criticisms of early temperature charts, see Reiser, op. cit. (n. 8), pp. 119–20.

13 Robert G. Frank Jr, 'The telltale heart: physiological instruments, graphic methods, and clinical hopes, 1854–1914', in William Coleman and Frederic L. Holmes (eds), *The Investigative Enterprise. Experimental Physiology in Nineteenth Century Medicine*, Berkeley, University of California Press, 1988, pp. 222–5; Joel D. Howell, 'The Rise and Fall of the Ballistocardiogram', unpublished MS, 1985; Ellen Breckenridge Koch, 'Process of innovation in medical technology:

American research on ultrasound, 1947 to 1962', unpublished Ph.D. thesis, University of Pennsylvania, 1990, pp. 133–6.

14 Geoffrey Keynes, *Blood Transfusion*, London, Oxford Medical Publications, 1922, p. 17; S. L. Wain, 'The controversy over unmodified versus citrated blood transfusion in the early 20th century', *Transfusion*, 1984, 24: 404–7. Robertson reportedly advised Bernard Fantus in setting up the blood bank at Cook County Hospital in Chicago. See J. Garrott Allen, 'O. H. Robertson – an inquiring mind: from blood bank to cutthroat trout', *Pharos*, 1985, 24: 25–7. Similarly, the 1952 polio epidemic in Copenhagen, which stimulated European efforts to develop mechanical ventilators, had little impact in the United States. See 'Historical background to automatic ventilation', in William Mushin, L. Rendell-Baker, Peter W. Thompson and W. W. Mapleson, *Automatic Ventilation of the Lungs*, Oxford, Blackwell Scientific Publications, 1980, pp. 206–11.

15 Frank, op. cit. (n. 13), pp. 274–5.

16 On the ballistocardiogram, see Howell, op. cit. (n. 13); on gastric freezing, see Harvey V. Fineberg, 'Gastric freezing – a study of diffusion of a medical innovation', in Committee on Technology and Health Care, Institute of Medicine, *Medical Technology and the Health Care System. A Study of the Diffusion of Equipment Embodied Technology*, Washington, DC, National Academy of Sciences, 1979, pp. 173–200.

17 On popularization of Roentgen's discovery for Britain, see E. H. Burrows, *Pioneers and Early Years. A History of British Radiology*, London, Colophon, 1986, pp. 15–17. For the United States, see Nancy Knight, ' "The new light": X-rays and medical futurism', in Joseph J. Corn (ed.), *Imagining Tomorrow. History, Technology and the American Future*, Cambridge, MA, MIT Press, 1986, pp. 10–34. For Canada, see J. T. H. Connor, 'The adoption and effects of X-rays in Ontario', *Ontario History*, 1987, 79: 92–107.

18 Pierre Pizon, *La Radiologie en France, 1896–1904*, Paris, L'Expansion Scientifique Française, 1970, pp. 13–14; Ruth and Edward Brecher, *The Rays. A History of Radiology in the United States and Canada*, Baltimore, MD, Williams & Wilkins, 1969, p. 13.

19 Burrows, op. cit. (n. 17), p. 20. A similar pattern of collaboration between physicians and physicists was reported in the United States: see Lynne Allan Leopold, *Radiology at the University of Pennsylvania 1890–1975*, Philadelphia, University of Pennsylvania Press, 1981, pp. 5–7; for Canada and the United States, see Brecher and Brecher, op. cit. (n. 18), pp. 59–60, 70–4. On construction of the devices, see Burrows, pp. 44–5.

20 On early instrument-makers see Burrows, op. cit. (n. 17), pp. 44–75; E. R. N. Grigg, *The Trail of the Invisible Light*, Springfield, IL, C. C Thomas, 1965, pp. 46–166.

21 For Britain, see Burrows, op. cit. (n. 17), pp. 79–94, 95–143. For France, see Pizon, op. cit. (n. 18), pp. 13–24, 44–56. For the United States, see Brecher and Brecher, op. cit. (n. 18), pp. 59–64, 70–80.

22 Burrows, op. cit. (n. 17), p. 76; Leopold, op. cit. (n. 19), p. 23; Rosemary Stevens, *In Sickness and in Wealth. American Hospitals in the Twentieth Century*, New York, Basic Books, 1989, p. 35.

23 Pizon, op. cit. (n. 18), p. 54. The Commonwealth of Pennsylvania supplemented

private funds to allow the University Hospital to purchase adequate equipment. Leopold, op. cit. (n. 19), p. 23.

24 On technical developments in France, see Pizon, op. cit. (n. 18), pp. 22, 28–34 (who is curiously silent on the commercial role). For developments in Britain and the US, see Burrows, op. cit. (n. 17), pp. 44–75; and on the US, see also Brecher and Brecher, op. cit. (n. 18), pp. 191–210.

25 Joel Howell, 'Early use of X-ray machines and electrocardiographs at the Pennsylvania Hospital', *Journal of the American Medical Association*, 1986, 255: 2320–2; Leopold, op. cit. (n. 19), p. 12; Burrows, op. cit. (n. 17), pp. 81, 86, 88; Frederick L. Hoffman, "The statistical experience data of the Johns Hopkins Hospital, Baltimore, MD, 1892–1911', *Johns Hopkins Hospital Reports*, 1916, 17: 344. Annual exams at these institutions were initially of the order of 100–400 per year, growing to 1,000 some time within the first decade of operation. Subsequent growth accelerated, with the number of exams growing by several thousand each year.

26 On early uses in clinical practice, see Burrows, op. cit. (n. 17), pp. 80, 88–90; Howell, op. cit. (n. 25), pp. 2320–1.

27 US Surgeon General's Office, *The Medical Department of the United States Army in the World War*. Vol. IX: *Communicable and Other Diseases*, Washington, DC, Government Printing Office, 1928, pp. 193–4. For the radiologists' view of the policy, see Ramsey Spillman, 'The value of radiography in detecting tuberculosis in recruits', *Journal of the American Medical Association*, 1940, 115: 1371–8. For earlier, less problematic military applications of the new technology, see Burrows, op. cit. (n. 17), pp. 194–217; *The Use of the Roentgen Ray by the Medical Department of the United States Army in the War with Spain*, Washington, DC, Government Printing Office, 1900.

28 On pneumonia, pleurisy, and empyema, see US Surgeon General's Office, op. cit. (n. 27), Vol. V: *Military Hospitals in the United States*, 1923, p. 255; Vol. IX: *Communicable and Other Diseases*, 1928, pp. 152–4; for surgery, see Vol. XI (Part 2): *Surgery*, 1924, pp. 206–7.

29 Ibid., Vol. I: *The Surgeon General's Office*, 1923, p. 471.

30 On growth of the British industry, see W. G. MacPherson, *History of the Great War Based on Official Documents. Medical Services. General History*. Vol. I: Medical Services in the United Kingdom, London, HMSO, 1921, p. 170. War contracts secured General Electric's place in producing X-ray equipment, and established the Coolidge tube developed there as the US standard. See George Wise, *Willis Whitney, General Electric and the Origins of US Industrial Research*, New York, Columbia University Press, 1985, pp. 176–9. The war also stimulated use of X-ray film over the harder-to-process and -handle glass plates. See Howell, op. cit. (n. 25), p. 2321.

On the role of radiologists in the First World War training and service, see US Surgeon General's Office, op. cit. (n. 27), Vol. I: *The Surgeon General's Office*, 1923, pp. 465–9; Vol. XI (Part 2): *Surgery*, 1924, pp. 206–7; MacPherson, op. cit. (n. 30), pp. 170–1.

31 Use of the bacteriological laboratory was promoted during the war with mixed success. Post-war growth in the number of US hospital laboratories, abetted by the American College of Surgeons, exceeded that of radiology departments. US

Surgeon's General's Office, op. cit., (n. 27), Vol. I: *The Surgeon General's Office*, 1923, pp. 291–6; Vol. IX: *Communicable and Other Diseases*, pp. 290–95; Vol. II: *Administration of the American Expeditionary Forces*, 1927, pp. 139–40, 197. On the ACS' role, see Stevens, op. cit. (n. 22), pp. 77–8.

In contrast to X-rays and clinical laboratories, the wartime promotion of nitrous oxide and oxygen anaesthesia, as administered by nurse anaesthetists, encountered continued resistance after the war. See W. D. A. Smith, 'A history of nitrous oxide and oxygen anaesthesia. Part XII: developments in America and nitrous oxide anaesthesia between world wars', *British Journal of Anaesthesia*, 1972, 44: 215–21; Virginia S. Thatcher, *History of Anaesthesia with Emphasis on the Nurse Specialist*, New York, Garland, 1984, pp. 96–103, 122–4.

32 H. Helmholtz, *The Description of an Ophthalmoscope*, Chicago, IL, Cleveland, 1916; orig. pub. 1851; George Rosen, *The Specialization of Medicine with Particular Reference to Ophthalmology*, New York, Froben Press, 1944.

33 Ibid., pp. 22–3, 30–7.

34 Rosen, op. cit. (n. 32), pp. 25–7; on gastroenterology and endoscopy, see Audrey B. Davis, 'Rudolf Schindler's role in the development of endoscopy', *Bulletin of the History of Medicine*, 1972, 46: 150–70; Joseph B. Kirsner, *The Development of American Gastroenterology*, New York, Raven Press, 1990, pp. 275–85. For a more technologically determinist account, see Martin A. Strosberg, 'Technological innovation, specialization, and speciality societies: the case of endoscopy', *Bulletin of the New York Academy of Medicine*, 1979, 55: 498–509.

35 Lyman H. Richards, 'Endoscopy at the crossroads', *Annals of Otology, Rhinology and Laryngology*, 1941, 51: 791–803.

36 Andrew Abbott, *The System of the Professions. An Essay on the Division of Expert Labor*, Chicago, IL, University of Chicago Press, 1988. On radiology, see Burrows, op. cit. (n. 17), pp. 18, 175–6, 178–85, 189–90; Gerald V. Larkin, *Occupational Monopoly and Modern Medicine*, London, Tavistock, 1983, pp. 61–91; Pizon, op. cit. (n. 18), pp. 52–5. According to Burrows, surgeons and other clinicians were far less willing to accept the medically trained radiologist's claim as an interpreter of X-ray images. Burrows, op. cit. (n. 17), p. 179.

On clinical laboratories and technicians in the US see William D. White, *Public Health and Private Gain. The Economics of Licensing Clinical Laboratory Personnel*, Chicago, IL, Maaroufa Press, 1979; for Britain, see Larkin, op. cit. (n. 36) p. 70.

37 Stephen R. Barley, 'Technology as an occasion for structuring: evidence from observations of CT scanners and the social order of radiology departments', *Administrative Science Quarterly*, 1986, 31: 78–108; Barley, 'The social construction of a machine: ritual, superstition, magical thinking and other pragmatic responses to running a CT scanner', in Margaret Lock and David Gordon (eds), *Biomedicine Examined*, Boston, MA, Kluwer Academic, 1988, pp. 497–539.

38 US Bureau of Labor Statistics, *Employment and Earnings*, 1991, 38: 185–9.

39 Wunderlich, op. cit. (n. 8), p. 78.

40 Wunderlich, op. cit. (n. 8), p. 75. Edouard Seguin, by contrast, advocated the democratization of thermometry so that more patients would recognize when they needed to consult a physician. See the essays by Musher *et al.*, op. cit. (n. 8).

41 Susan Reverby, 'Health: women's work', in David Kotelchuck, *Prognosis Negative. Crisis in the Health Care System*, New York, Vintage Books, 1976, pp. 170–83; Reverby, *Ordered to Care. The Dilemma of American Nursing, 1850–1945*, Cambridge, Cambridge University Press, 1987.
    See also Cynthia Cockburn, *Machinery of Dominance. Women, Men and Technical Know-how*, Boston, MA, Northeastern University Press, 1988, pp. 112–41, for an excellent discussion of the complexities of gendering and occupation. On emotional and communicative work in radiography, see ibid., pp. 122–3; Jeanne Guillemin and Lynda Lytle Holstrom, *Mixed Blessings: Intensive Care for Newborns*, New York, Oxford University Press, 1986, p. 174, for the interpretive work of nurses in the neonatal intensive care unit. The phrase, 'physician's hand', comes from Barbara Melosh, *The Physician's Hand: Work Culture and Conflict in American Nursing*, Philadelphia, PA, Temple University Press, 1982.

42 Audrey B. Davis, 'Anesthetist and anesthesiologist: technology in the social context of a medical and nursing specialty', *Transactions and Studies of the College of Physicians of Philadelphia*, 1989 (series 5), 11: 132–3.

43 See, along with the essays by Barley op. cit. (n. 37), Barbara A. Koenig, 'The technological imperative in medical practice: social creation of a "routine" treatment', in Lock and Gordon, op. cit. (n. 37), pp. 465–96; Cockburn, op. cit. (n. 41), pp. 112–41; Anselm Strauss, Shiznko Fagerhaugh, Barbara Suczek and Carolyn Wiener, *Social Organization of Medical Work*, Chicago, IL, University of Chicago Press, 1985, p. 67; Michèle Fallous, 'La révolution échographique', *Sociologie du travail*, 1988, 30: 301–11.

44 See Cockburn's discussion of radiographers and CT scanning, op. cit. (n. 41). CT scanning offers radiographers substantially reduced roles in both patient interactions and managing the machine. Yet because radiographers rotate between CT scanning and conventional radiography, no substantive 'deskilling' of the occupation has occurred.

45 Carl Voegtlin, 'The limitations of intravenous medication', *Journal of the American Medical Association*, 1922, 79: 421; Walton Forest Dutton, *Intravenous Therapy. Its Application in the Modern Practice of Medicine*, 2nd edn, Philadelphia, PA, F. A. Davis, 1925, pp. 138–40.

46 Diamond, op. cit. (n. 3), pp. 674, 677; Ronald H. Girdwood, 'Fifty years of an organized blood transfusion service in Scotland', *Scottish Medical Journal*, 1990, 35: 24–8. On Carrel and Crile, see Richard E. Rosenfield, 'Early twentieth century origins in modern blood transfusion therapy', *Mount Sinai Journal of Medicine*, 1974, 41: 626–7. For the history of one leading 'transfusionist' who happily continued a career in blood-banking, see Bernheim, op. cit. (n. 3).

47 Rue Bucher, 'Pathology: a study of social movements within a profession', *Social Problems*, 1962, 10: 40–51; Bucher and Anselm Strauss, 'Professions in process', *American Journal of Sociology*, 1961, 66: 325–34.

48 There was considerable medical resistance to the use of therapeutic oxygen generally, and tanked oxygen in particular. See Steven Sturdy, 'From the trenches to the hospitals at home: physiologists, clinicians and oxygen therapy, 1914–1930', in John V. Pickstone (ed.), *Medical Innovations in Historical Perspective*, London, Macmillan, 1992; Lynn Wyner White, 'Adopting commercial oxygen for medical use', *Respiratory Therapy*, 1979, 9: 30–2. For nursing and oxygen administration,

see Amy Frances Brown, *Medical Nursing*, Philadelphia, PA, W. B. Saunders, 1945, pp. 84–7. On the development of respiratory therapy, see White, 'Education of oxygen-treatment personnel 1928–48', *Respiratory Therapy*, 1979, 9: 35, 38–9.

49 G. V. Larkin, 'Medical dominance and control: radiographers in the division of labour', *Sociological Review*, 1978 (NS), 26: 843–58. On the difficulties of controlling competition from non-radiologist physicians in the US, see Peter Buck and Barbara Rosenkrantz, 'Healthy, wealthy and wise', unpublished MS. Gastroenterologists were similarly unsuccessful in controlling which physicians could perform gastroscopies, once simpler, safer endoscopes became available. Davis, op. cit. (n. 34), pp. 169–70.

50 Reiser, op. cit. (n. 8); Stewart Wolf and Beatrice Bishop Berle, *The Technological Imperative in Medicine*, New York, Plenum Press, 1980.

51 For earlier imagery of physician-researchers, see Charles Rosenberg, 'Martin Arrowsmith: the scientist as hero', in Rosenberg, *No Other Gods. On Science and American Social Thought*, Baltimore, MD, Johns Hopkins Press, 1976, pp. 123–31; John Burnham, 'American medicine's golden age: what happened to it?', *Science*, 1982, 215: 1474–9; Renée C. Fox and Judith P. Swazey, *The Courage to Fail. A Social View of Organ Transplants and Dialysis*, 2nd edn, rev., Chicago, IL, University of Chicago Press, 1978.

52 S. Weir Mitchell, *The Early History of Instrumental Precision in Medicine*, New Haven, CT, Tuttle, Morehouse & Taylor, 1892, p. 9.

53 Both the technological optimist, S. Weir Mitchell, and the technological pessimist, S. J. Reiser (writing eighty years later), offer a similar analysis of the dangers technologies pose to medical judgement. See Mitchell, op. cit. (n. 52), pp. 8–9; and Reiser, op. cit. (n. 8), pp. 227–31. The ability to use new technologies judiciously and with discrimination was a hallmark of mid-nineteenth-century views of professionalism in the United States, a tradition continued to the present. See Martin S. Pernick, *A Calculus of Suffering: Pain, Professionalism and Suffering in Nineteenth-Century America*, New York, Columbia University Press, 1985; Harry M. Marks, 'Ideas as reforms: therapeutic experiments and medical practice, 1900–1980', unpublished Ph.D. thesis, Massachusetts Institute of Technology, 1987. The social and cultural context for this ideology has been elegantly analysed for the case of Britain by Christopher Lawrence, 'Incommunicable knowledge: science, technology and the clinical art in Britain 1850–1914', *Journal of Contemporary History*, 1985, 20: 502–20.

54 Roy Porter, 'The patient's view. Doing medical history from below', *Theory and Society*, 1985, 14: 175–8.

55 Ann Oakley, *The Captured Womb. A History of the Medical Care of Pregnant Women*, New York, Blackwell, 1984, p. 161; James D. Campbell and Anne R. Campbell, 'The social and economic costs of end-stage renal disease. A patient's perspective', *New England Journal of Medicine*, 1978, 299: 386–92; Jennifer Wilson-Barnett, 'A review of research into the experience of patients suffering from coronary thrombosis', *International Journal of Nursing Studies*, 1979, 16: 185–7; Jennifer Jones, B. Hoggart, Josephine Withey, Kim Donaghue, and B. W. Ellis, 'What the patients say: a study of reactions to an intensive care unit', *Intensive Care Medicine*, 1979, 5: 89–92; David S. Shovelton, 'Reflections on an intensive therapy unit', *British Medical Journal*, 1989, 1: 737–8. Some first-person reports

place greater emphasis on machines than others: see W. L. C. Chilver, 'On being a patient in an intensive therapy unit', *Nursing Mirror*, 6 April 1978, 146: 33–5.

56 Steven J. Peitzman, 'From dropsy to Bright's disease to end-stage renal disease', *Millbank Quarterly*, 1989 (suppl. 1), 67: 16–32; Richard A. Rettig (with Ellen Marks), *Implementing the End-Stage Renal Disease Program for Medicare*, Santa Monica, CA, Rand Corporation, 1980; William Drukker, 'Haemodialysis: a historical review', in John F. Maher (ed.), *Replacement of Renal Function by Dialysis. A Textbook of Dialysis*, 3rd edn, Dordecht, Kluwer Academic, 1989, pp. 20–86.

57 The description here follows Uta Gerhardt and Marianne Brieskorn-Zinke, 'The normalization of hemodialysis at home', in Roth and Ruzek, op. cit. (n. 7), pp. 275–9. See also Alonzo L. Plough, *Borrowed Time. Artificial Organs and the Politics of Extending Lives*, Philadelphia, PA, Temple University Press, 1986, pp. 52–70, 86–100. Continuous ambulatory peritoneal dialysis, in which dialysis occurs without mechanical assistance, through an indwelling shunt in the abdomen, while avoiding some of the problems of haemodialysis, introduces others. Charles M. Mion, 'Practical use of peritoneal dialysis', in Drukker, op. cit. (n. 56), pp. 537–89. Studies are not yet available to indicate whether the absence of a machine hook-up alters the experiences of these dialysis patients.

58 Gerhardt and Brieskorn-Zinke, op. cit. (n. 57), p. 284; Peitzman, op. cit. (n. 56), p. 29.

59 Gerhardt and Brieskorn-Zinke, op. cit. (n. 57), p. 300.

60 Poliomyelitis patients with acute and chronic respiratory dysfunction report many of the same experiences as chronic dialysis patients. Joseph M. Kaufert and David Locker, 'Rehabilitation ideology and respiratory support technology', *Social Science and Medicine*, 1990, 30: 867–77.

61 Plough, op. cit. (n. 57), pp. 57–62, 96–100.

62 Charles Rosenberg, 'The therapeutic revolution: medicine, meaning and social change in nineteenth-century America', in Morris J. Vogel and Rosenberg (eds), *The Therapeutic Revolution. Essays in the Social History of American Medicine*, Philadelphia, University of Pennsylvania Press, 1979, pp. 3–26; Judith Walzer Leavitt, *Brought to Bed. Child-Bearing in America, 1750–1950*, New York, Oxford University Press, 1986, esp. pp. 171–212; Jean-Pierre Goubert (ed.), 'La médicalisation de la société française, 1770–1830', *Historical Reflections/Réflexions historiques*, 1982, 9: 3–304. For evidence of successful resistance to medical intervention in a 'medicalized' institution, see Nancy Schrom Dye, 'Modern obstetrics and working-class women: the New York Midwifery Dispensary, 1890–1920', *Journal of Social History*, 1987, 20: 551, 555–7.

63 Guillemin and Holmstrom, op. cit. (n. 41), pp. 169–225; Barbara G. Sonowitz, 'Managing parents on neonatal intensive care units', *Social Problems*, 1984, 31: 390–402.

64 Barbara Katz Rothman, *The Tentative Pregnancy. Prenatal Diagnosis and the Future of Motherhood*, New York, Penguin Books, 1987, pp. 159–64.

65 Guillemin and Holmstrom, op. cit. (n. 41), pp. 188–91. Even parents who learned to access the unit computers for information on their infant's status were excluded once physician-to-physician (or nurse) communications began.

66 Rothman, op. cit. (n. 64), pp. 159–65.

67 Rothman, op. cit. (n. 64), p. 7.

68 Rothman, op. cit. (n. 64), esp. pp. 96–105.

69 Rosalind Pollack Petchesky, 'Foetal images: the power of visual culture in the politics of reproduction', in Michelle Stanworth (ed.), *Reproductive Technologies. Gender, Motherhood and Medicine*, Minneapolis, University of Minnesota Press, 1987, pp. 57–80. Plough's account of renal dialysis, op. cit. (n. 57), incorporates ethnography of individual experience and epidemiological study of group survival with political-economic analysis of the technology.

70 Petchesky, op. cit. (n. 69); H. Gardent, J. Goujard, M. Fardeau and M. Crost, 'Analyse économique de la diffusion d'une innovation médicale: l'exemple du diagnostic prenatal par amniocentèse précoce', *Revue d'epidémiologie et santé publique*, 1984, 32: 88–96. On other obstetrical technologies, see Jennifer Beinart, 'Obstetric analgesia and the control of childbirth in twentieth-century Britain', in Jo Garcia, Robert Fitzpatrick and Marcia Richards, *The Politics of Maternity Care*, Oxford, Clarendon Press, 1990, pp. 121–6; Leavitt, op. cit. (n. 62), pp. 64–86, 198–208; Leavitt, 'Birthing and anesthesia: the debate over twilight sleep', *Signs*, 1980, 6: 147–64; Jonathan Lomas and Murray Enkin, 'Variations in operative delivery rates', in Iain Chalmers, Murray Enkin and Marc J. N. C. Kerise (eds), *Effective Care in Pregnancy and Childbirth*, Oxford, Oxford University Press, 1989, p. 1190.

71 But see, in addition to the works cited in n. 70, Pernick, op. cit. (n. 53).

72 Robert Woods and John Woodward, *Urban Disease and Mortality in Nineteenth-Century England*, New York, St Martin's Press, 1984; Simon Szreter, 'The importance of social intervention in Britain's mortality decline *c.*1850–1914: a re-interpretation of the role of public health', *Social History of Medicine*, 1988, 1: 1–37; Richard J. Evans, *Death in Hamburg. Society and Politics in the Cholera Years 1830–1910*, London, Penguin Books, 1987; Hallie Kinter, 'Determinants of temporal and areal variation in infant mortality decline in Germany, 1871–1933', *Demography*, 1988, 25: 597–609; Dominique Tabutin, 'La surmortalité féminine en Europe avant 1940', *Population*, 1978, 33: 121–48; Kenneth Sokoloff, *The Heights of Americans in Three Centuries: Some Economic and Demographic Indications*, Working Paper no. 1384, New York, National Bureau of Economic Research, 1984; Reynolds Farley and Walter R. Allen, *The Color Line and the Quality of Life in America*, New York, Oxford University Press, 1989; Victor Fuchs, *Who Shall Live? Health, Economics and Social Choice*, New York, Basic Books, 1974; Frans W. A. van Poppel, 'Regional mortality differences in western Europe: a review of the situation in the seventies', *Social Science and Medicine*, 1981, 15D: 341–52.

73 Thomas Halper, *The Misfortunes of Others. End-stage Renal Disease in the United Kingdom*, Cambridge, Cambridge University Press, 1989, pp. 23, 15, 25; Arnold S. Relman and Drummond Rennie, 'Treatment of end-stage renal disease. Free but not equal', *New England Journal of Medicine*, 1980, 303: 996–8, provides similar data on US variations.

74 Mark B. Wenneker and Arnold M. Epstein, 'Racial inequalities in the use of procedures for patients with ischemic heart disease in Massachusetts', *Journal of the American Medical Association*, 1989, 261: 253–7; Edward L. Hannan, Harold Kilburn, Jr, Joseph F. O'Donnell, Gary Lukacik, and Eileen P. Shields, 'Inter-

racial access to selected cardiac procedures for patients hospitalized with coronary artery disease in New York State', *Medical Care*, 1991, 29: 430–41; Earl Ford, Richard Cooper, Angel Castaner, Brian Simmons and Maxine Mar, 'Coronary arteriography and coronary bypass surgery among whites and other racial groups relative to hospital-based incidence rates for coronary artery disease: findings from NHDS', *American Journal of Public Health*, 1989, 79: 437–40; John Z. Ayanian and Arnold M. Epstein, 'Differences in the use of procedures between women and men hospitalized for coronary heart disease', *New England Journal of Medicine*, 1991, 325: 221–5.

75 Renée Serange-Fonterme, 'Les disparités sociales de consommation médicale', *Social Science and Medicine*, 1985, 21: 105; A. S. Poisson-Salmon, G. Breart, F. Maillard and C. Rumeau-Rouquette, 'Distribution of ultrasound during pregnancy in France between 1976 and 1981', *International Journal of Epidemiology*, 1987, 16: 235–7; Bruno Hubert, Beatrice Blondel and Monique Kaminski, 'Contribution of specialists to antenatal care in France: impact on level of care during pregnancy and delivery', *Journal of Epidemiology and Community Health*, 1987, 41: 327; Gardent, Goujard, Fardeau and Crost, op. cit. (n. 70).

76 G. P. Hanson, J. Stjernsward, M. Nofal and F. Durosinimi-Etti, 'An overview of the situation in radiotherapy with emphasis on the developing countries', *International Journal of Radiology, Oncology, and Biophysics*, 1990, 19: 1257–60; P. Bol, H. C. Grobben and E. Borst-Eilers, 'Aantallen coronaire bypass-operaties in Nederland en andere westerse landen', *Nederlands Tijdschrift Geneeskunde*, 1989, 133: 1869; Betty Wolder Levin, 'International perspectives on treatment choice in neonatal intensive care units', *Social Science and Medicine*, 1990, 30: 902.

77 Dale A. Rublee, 'Medical technology in Canada, Germany, and the United States', *Health Affairs*, 1989, 9: 178–81; Bol, Grobben and Borst-Eilers, op. cit. (n. 76).

78 Robert H. Brook, R. E. Park, Constance M. Winslow, Jacquelin B. Kosecoff, Mark R. Chassin, and J. R. Hampton, 'Diagnosis and treatment of coronary disease: comparison of doctors' attitudes in the USA and the UK', *Lancet*, 1988, 1: 750–3; Francis C. Notzon, 'International differences in the use of obstetric interventions', *Journal of the American Medical Association*, 1990, 263: 3286–91; Per Bergsjo, Eberhard Schmidt and Detlev Pusch, 'Differences in the reported frequencies of some obstetrical interventions in Europe', in J. M. F. Phaff (ed.), *Perinatal Health Services in Europe*, London, Croom Helm, 1986, p. 83.

79 Joel Weissman and Arnold M. Epstein, 'Case mix and resource utilization by uninsured hospital patients in the Boston metropolitan area', *Journal of the American Medical Association*, 1989, 261: 3755; Gardent, Goujard, Fardeau and Crost, op. cit. (n. 70), pp. 92–3; Ann Cartwright and Robert Anderson, *General Practice Revisited. A Second Study of Doctors and their Patients*, London, Tavistock Publications, 1981, pp. 150–3.

80 The French government may have restrained purchases of whole-body CT scanners until French instruments were available. See F. Fagnani, J. P. Moatti and C. Weill, 'The diffusion and use of diagnostic imaging equipment in France. The limits of regulation', *International Journal of Technology Assessment in Health Care*, 1987, 3: 531–43. The influence of national industrial policy and health-

care policy has been best studied for the case of pharmaceuticals. See Gary Gereffi, *The Pharmaceutical Industry and Dependency in the Third World*, Princeton, NJ, Princeton University Press, 1983, esp. pp. 202–43.

81 Robert L. Kennedy, Margaret A. Kennedy, Robert L. Frye *et al.*, 'Cardiac catheterization and cardiac surgical facilities. Use, trends and future requirements', *New England Journal of Medicine*, 1982, 307: 986–93; C. Rumeau-Rouquette and J. Llado-Arkhipoff, 'Analyse régionale des enquêtes', in Rumeau-Rouquette, Christiane du Mazubrun and Yvon Rabarison (eds), *Naître en France. 10 ans d'evolution, 1972–1981*, Paris, Doin Éditeurs, 1984, pp. 184–5.

82 See C. H. Lee, 'Regional inequalities in infant mortality in Britain, 1861–1971: patterns and hypotheses', *Population Studies*, 1991, 45: 55–65. For an approach with contemporary data, see Johann P. Mackenbach, Karin Stronks and Anton E. Kunst, 'The contribution of medical care to inequalities in health: differences between socio-economic groups in decline of mortality from conditions amenable to medical intervention', *Social Science and Medicine*, 1989, 29: 369–76.

83 Irvine Loudon, 'Obstetric care, social class, and maternal mortality', *British Medical Journal*, 1986, 293: 606–8; Stevens, op. cit. (n. 22), pp. 173–4; Beinart, op. cit. (n. 70); Marsha Hurst and Pamela S. Summey, 'Childbirth and social class: the case of cesarean delivery', *Social Science and Medicine*, 1984, 18: 621–31; Fernando C. Barros, J. Patrick Vaughan and Cesar G. Victora, 'Why so many Caesarean sections? The need for a further policy change in Brazil', *Health Policy and Planning*, 1986, 1: 19–29; Jeffrey B. Gould, Becky Davy and Randall S. Stafford, 'Socioeconomic differences in rates of Cesarean section', *New England Journal of Medicine*, 1989, 321: 233–9.

84 'Health care expenditure and other data', *Health Care Financing Review*, 1989 (suppl.): 121–2; Jonathan Brown and Harry M. Marks. 'Buying the future: the relationship between the purchase of physical capital and total expenditure growth in US hospitals', in US Department of Health, Education and Welfare, *Health Capital Issues. Papers Presented at the Health Capital Conference*, Washington, DC, Government Printing Office, 1981, pp. 27–46; Martin Pfaff, 'Differences in health care spending across countries: statistical evidence', *Journal of Health Politics, Policy and Law*, 1990, 15: 9.

85 Daniel M. Fox, *Health Policies, Health Politics. The British and American Experience, 1911–1965*, Princeton, NJ, Princeton University Press, 1986; Marks, op. cit. (n. 53).

86 Fox, op. cit. (n. 85); Daniel M. Fox, 'Health policy and the politics of research in the United States', *Journal of Health Politics, Policy and Law*, 1990, 15: 481–99; Stevens, op. cit. (n. 22), pp. 98–104, 193–9, 219–21, 227–8; Malcolm Ashmore, Michael Mulkay and Trevor Pinch, *Health and Efficiency. A Sociology of Health Economics*, Milton Keynes, Open University Press, 1989. An intellectual and institutional history of these movements, national as well as international, is yet to be written.

87 H. David Banta and Kerry Britain Kemp (eds), *The Management of Health Care Technology in Nine Countries*, New York, Springer, 1982; Institute of Medicine, op. cit. (n. 7), pp. 228–43.

88 Barbara Stocking, 'The management of medical technology in the United Kingdom', in Banta and Kemp, op. cit. (n. 87), pp. 10–27; Stocking, 'Strategies

for technology assessment and implementation in some European countries', *International Journal of Technology Assessment in Health Care*, 1986, 2: 19–26; Susan Bartlett Foote, 'Assessing medical technology assessment: past, present and future', *Milbank Quarterly*, 1987, 65: 59–80; Adam L. Linton and C. David Naylor, 'Organized medicine and the assessment of technology. Lessons from Ontario', *New England Journal of Medicine*, 1990, 323: 1463–7; Caroline Weill, Francis Fagnani and Christian LeFaure, 'The assessment of medical technology. The case of France', *International Journal of Technology Assessment in Health Care*, 1989, 5: 144–50; Pierre Durieux, Catherine Viens-Bitker, Dominique Jolly and Claudine Blum-Boisgard, 'Examples of the influence of evaluation on health policy', *Health Policy*, 1988, 9: 325–30. Even in Sweden, technology acquisition is decentralized and centralized technology assessment largely consultative. Christopher Ham, 'Governing the health sector: power and policy making in the English and Swedish health services', *Milbank Quarterly*, 1988, 66: 389–414. For a somewhat conflicting, but earlier, view of Sweden, see Erik H. L. Gaensler, Egon Jonsson and Duncan vB. Neuhauser, 'Controlling medical technology in Sweden', in Banta and Kemp, op. cit. (n. 87), pp. 167–92.

89   Barton J. Bernstein, 'The artificial heart program', *Center Magazine*, 1981, 22–41; Arthur L. Caplan, 'The artificial heart', *Hastings Center Report*, 1982, 12: 22–4; Michael J. Strauss, 'The political history of the artificial heart', *New England Journal of Medicine*, 1984, 310: 332–6; Richard A. Rettig, 'The politics of organ transplantation: a parable of our time', *Journal of Health Politics, Policy and Law*, 1989, 14: 191–227; Durieux, Viens-Bitker, Jolly and Blum-Boisgard, op. cit. (n. 88); Institute of Medicine, op. cit. (n. 7), pp. 53–69, 211–27; James P. Kahan, C. R. Neu, Glenn T. Hammons, and Bruce J. Hillman, *The Decision to Initiate Clinical Trials of Current Medical Practices*, Santa Monica, CA, Rand Corporation, 1985.

90   Linton and Naylor, op. cit. (n. 88); Jonathan Lomas, 'Words without action? The production, dissemination, and impact of consensus recommendations', *Annual Review of Public Health*, 1991, 12: 41–65; Marks, op. cit. (n. 53); Institute of Medicine, op. cit. (n. 7), pp. 176–210.

91   Halper, op. cit. (n. 73), pp. 120–40; Henry J. Aaron and William B. Schwartz, *The Painful Prescription. Rationing Hospital Care*, Washington, DC, Brookings Institution, 1984.

92   According to Stocking, the majority of body CT scanners in Great Britain before 1978 were purchased with private funds. See Stocking, op. cit. (n. 88), p. 20. On radiologists lobbying in Britain, see Ham, op. cit. (n. 88), p. 400. On the Dutch campaign for more heart-surgery facilities, see L. M. J. Groot, 'Medical technology in the health care system of the Netherlands', in Banta and Kemp, op. cit. (n. 87), pp. 150–66. For defiance of US Food and Drug Administration regulations governing medical devices, see Caplan, op. cit. (n. 89). On organ transplants, see Rettig, op. cit. (n. 89).

93   For recent overviews of developments in Oregon, see Charles J. Dougherty, 'Setting health care priorities. Oregon's next steps', *Hastings Center Report*, 1991, 21: 1–10; David C. Hadorn, 'The Oregon priority-setting exercise: quality of life and public policy', *Hastings Center Report*, 1991, 21: 11–16; David M. Eddy, 'What's going on in Oregon', *Journal of the American Medical Association*, 1991,

266: 417–20. On AIDS treatments and the FDA, see Harold Edgar and David J. Rothman, 'New rules for new drugs: the challenge of AIDS to the regulatory process', *Milbank Quarterly*, 1990, 68 (suppl. 1): 111–142. In neither case has the process ensured the full participation of those most affected.

94 It has been repeatedly shown that medical decisions do not reflect the decisions patients would make for themselves. See Barbara J. McNeil, R. Weichselbaum and S. G. Pauker, 'Fallacy of the five-year survival rate in lung cancer', *New England Journal of Medicine*, 1978, 299: 1397–1401; McNeil, Weichselbaum and Pauker, 'Speech and survival: tradeoffs between quantity and quality of life in laryngeal cancer', *New England Journal of Medicine*, 1981, 305: 982–87.

95 On the shaping of politics by medical policies, see Lawrence D. Brown, *New Policies, New Politics: Government's Response to Government's Growth*, Washington, DC, Brookings Institution, 1983.

FURTHER READING

For a general introduction to the specialized literature on the history of medical technology, see:

Davis, Audrey B., *Medicine and its Technology: an Introduction to the History of Medical Instrumentation*, Westport, CT, Greenwood Press, 1981.

'Medical technology', in Trevor I. Williams (ed.), *A History of Technology*, Oxford, Clarendon Press, 1978, Vol. VII, pp. 1316–62.

For works on specific technologies, see the following:

MICROSCOPES

Bracegirdle, Brian, *A History of Microtechnique*, Ithaca, NY, Cornell University Press, 1978.

Bradbury, S., *The Evolution of the Microscope*, Oxford, Pergamon Press, 1967.

Munro, Rachael M., *Towards a Social History of Microscopy in Victorian England*, Kensington, New South Wales, 1981.

Turner, Gerard L'E., *Essays on the History of the Microscope*, Oxford, Senecio, 1980.

STETHOSCOPES

Bishop, P. J., 'Evolution of the stethoscope', *Journal of the Royal Society of Medicine*, 1980, 73: 448–56.

Huard, Pierre, 'Evolution du stethoscope', in *Comptes Rendus. 106ᵉ Congrès Nationale des Sociétés Savantes*, Paris, Bibliothèque Nationale, 1982, fasc. 4, pp. 91–104.

ELECTROCARDIOGRAM

Burch, George E. and DePasquale, Nicholas P., *A History of Electrocardiography*, San Francisco, CA, Norman, 1990.

X-RAYS AND RADIOLOGY

Brecher, Ruth and Brecher, Edward, *The Rays. A History of Radiology in the United States and Canada*, Baltimore, MD, Williams & Wilkins, 1969.

Burrows, E. H., *Pioneers and Early Years. A History of British Radiology*, London, Colophon, 1986.

Glasser, Otto, 'The technical development of radiology', *American Journal of Roentgenology, Radium Therapy and Nuclear Medicine*, 1965, 36: 229–57.

Grigg, E. R. N., *The Trail of the Invisible Light*, Springfield, IL, Thomas, 1965.

ANAESTHESIA AND ARTIFICIAL RESPIRATION

'Historical background to automatic ventilation', in William Mushin *et al.*, *Automatic Ventilation of the Lungs*, Oxford, Blackwell Scientific, 1980, pp. 184–247.

Smith, W. D. A., *Under the Influence. A History of Nitrous Oxide and Oxygen Anaesthesia*, London, Macmillan, 1982.

Sykes, W. Stanley, *Essays on the First Hundred Years of Anaesthesia*, 3 vols, London, Churchill Livingstone, 1982.

Thatcher, Virginia S., *History of Anaesthesia, with Emphasis on the Nurse Specialist*, New York, Garland, 1984.

Thomas, K. Bryn, *The Development of Anaesthetic Apparatus*, Oxford, Blackwell Scientific, 1985.

Audrey Davis has pioneered in the new social history of medical technology:

Davis, Audrey B., 'Life insurance and the physical examination: a chapter in the rise of American medical technology', *Bulletin of the History of Medicine*, 1981, 55: 392–406.

——, 'Anesthetist and anesthesiologist: technology in the social context of a medical and nursing specialty', *Transactions and Studies of the College of Physicians of Philadelphia*, 1989 (series 5), 11: 123–34.

——, 'Rudolf Schindler's role in the development of endoscopy', *Bulletin of the History of Medicine*, 1972, 46: 150–70.

In addition to Davis's work, see the following examples of the new historiography:

Frank, Robert G. Jr, 'The telltale heart: physiological instruments, graphic methods, and clinical hopes, 1854–1914', in William Coleman and Frederic L. Holmes (eds), *The Investigative Enterprise. Experimental Physiology in Nineteenth-Century Medicine*, Berkeley, University of California Press, 1988, pp. 211–90.

Howell, Joel D., 'Machines and medicine: technology transforms the American hospital', in Diana Elizabeth Long and Janet Golden (eds), *The American General Hospital. Communities and Social Contexts*, Ithaca, NY, Cornell University Press, 1989, pp. 109–34.

——, 'Cardiac physiology and clinical medicine? Two case studies', in Gerald L. Geison (ed.), *Physiology in the America Context, 1850–1940*, Bethesda, MD, American Physiological Society, 1987, pp. 179–92.

Koch, Ellen Breckenridge, 'Process of innovation in medical technology: American research on ultrasound, 1947 to 1963', unpublished Ph.D. thesis, University of Pennsylvania, 1990.

Yoxen, Edward, 'Seeing with sound: a study of the development of medical images', in Wiebe E. Bijker, Thomas P. Hughes and Trevor J. Pinch (eds), *The Social Construction of Technological Systems. New Directions in the Sociology and History of Technology*, Cambridge, MA, MIT Press, 1987.

Much innovative work on medical technology has come from women's history. See, in particular:

Leavitt, Judith Walzer, *Brought to Bed. Child-bearing in America, 1750–1950*, New York, Oxford University Press, 1986.

Morantz, Regina Markell and Zshoche, Sue, 'Professionalism, feminism and gender roles: a comparative study of nineteenth century therapeutics', *Journal of American History*, 1980, 67: 568–88.

Oakley, Ann, *The Captured Womb. A History of the Medical Care of Pregnant Women*, New York, Basil Blackwell, 1984.

Ratcliffe, Kathryn Strother, *Healing Technology: Feminist Perspectives*, Ann Arbor, University of Michigan Press, 1989.

Stanworth, Michelle (ed.), *Reproductive Technologies. Gender, Motherhood and Medicine*, Minneapolis, University of Minnesota Press, 1987.

69

MEDICINE AND THE LAW

Catherine Crawford

Relations between medicine and the law are a persistent theme in Western culture. The urge to compare them, for example, seems endemic. In medieval Europe, the relative merits of the two secular learned professions were a popular topic of disputation. Scholars argued about which had the nobler aims, greater certitude, closer connections with the Divine, and more capacity to increase morality and happiness. In later centuries, comparisons focused on the types of reasoning each required, on differences in social status, and on the law's greater success in excluding outsiders from practice. More recently, medicine and law have vied for authority over aspects of insanity, death, and ethics. And in what might be considered a modern version of the medieval debate, scholars now compare the *power* of law and medicine in society. In Foucault's influential analysis, 'juridical power' (that of a sovereign) has, during the past few centuries, been overtaken in significance by 'bio-power' (the power of the norm), a process that has tended to enhance the power and importance of medicine. This development is plainly seen, for example, in the histories of suicide and homosexuality, where acts once considered merely illegal came to be seen as pathological.[1]

Law and medicine have interacted over the centuries in three main ways. First, medicine has assisted law for legal purposes, notably the detection of crime and the adjudication of disputes. Second, law has regulated medicine by imposing rules on healers. This category – medical law – includes licensing, malpractice, professional privileges and obligations, and the ethical standards in medicine that are backed by legal sanctions. Finally, law has supported medical aims through health legislation: laws enforcing practices of preventive medicine and sanitation, governmental provision and supervision of medical services, and regulation of the salubriousness of food and drink, medicines, and the environment.

The second and third kinds of relations between medicine and the law are discussed in other essays in this volume. (➤ Ch. 47 The history of the medical profession; Ch. 51 Public health; Ch. 37 The history of medical ethics; Ch. 61 Religion and medicine; Ch. 4 Medical care; Ch. 5 The anatomical tradition; Ch. 50 Medical institutions and the state) This chapter focuses mainly on the first type of medico-legal relations – that concerning the administration of justice.

Terminology in this area is varied. Early modern European usages included the Latin-derived 'forensic medicine' (*medicina forensis*, medicine of the forum) and 'medical jurisprudence'. Both came to be used interchangeably in Britain and America, along with the less common terms 'political', 'state', and 'juridical' medicine, often to cover the entire range of medico-legal relations. German coinages included 'medical police' (eighteenth century, see Ch. 51) and 'courtroom medicine' (*Gerichtsmedizin*, nineteenth century). The expression preferred in France from the eighteenth century, *médecine légale*, gradually gained wide currency, and in the 1960s the German and British medico-legal societies both recommended general adoption of that term (*Rechtsmedizin*, legal medicine). Although there is still some disagreement about the connotations of various terms, it is now usual to reserve 'forensic medicine' for medicine relating to law courts and regulatory bodies, and to use 'legal medicine' for the more comprehensive notion.[2]

In broadest terms, the history of forensic medicine is a story of medicalization – an expansion of medical authority into new social territory. The field's evolution has therefore reflected changing interests and approaches within medicine. The history and politics of the medical professions have also played an important part. Finally, because law is almost always the dominant party in law–medicine interactions, the role of medical expertise has varied greatly according to the needs and methods of different legal systems and governments. This essay considers the two major legal traditions of the West – Continental (Roman-canon law) and Anglo-American (common law) – but also touches on Talmudic law and makes comparative reference to China.

ANCIENT LEGAL MEDICINE

The earliest relations between law and medicine were essentially regulatory. References to medicine in ancient legal sources specify fees for various medical services and prescribe penalties for bad practice. The code of Hammurabi (Babylonian, *c.*1750 BC) applied the principles of compensation and retribution in kind: if a slave died while under medical treatment, the practitioner had to provide a replacement, whereas if the deceased were not a slave, the doctor was to lose a hand. In ancient Egypt, a healer who lost a (free) patient could be punished by death if he had deviated from the methods of treatment laid down in the sacred book of Hermes. It is not known whether medical assessors were involved in adjudicating such cases or whether these penalties were actually applied.[3]

In classical Athens, doctors provided expert opinion in trial proceedings, although such evidence was not required by law. Greek law was basically private in nature, and it was victims or their families who investigated and prosecuted crimes – even homicide – by bringing lawsuits. There is clear evidence that such litigants summoned medical men to testify in cases of injury or death, and that their testimony was given special credence. Doctors also attested to illness when, for example, a citizen sought to be excused from the duties of an elected office on grounds of ill health.[4]

Roman Egypt's expanding bureaucracy included officials who investigated cases of injury and violent death and submitted written reports on the facts and their causes. Administrative papyri dating from the first to the fourth centuries AD show that these officials often consulted medical men. There is little evidence of medico-legal practice elsewhere in the Roman Empire, but judicial use of the expertise of midwives was specified in late-Roman codifications. The code of Theodosius (438 AD) decreed that pregnant women could not be executed and that the fact of pregnancy should be established by midwives. The *Digest* compiled under Justinian (533 AD) indicated that when there was a dispute between a recently divorced couple over whether or not the woman was pregnant with the man's heir, she was to be inspected for pregnancy by three midwives.[5]

Several European law codes of the fifth to tenth centuries contained detailed provisions for *wergeld* – financial compensation for wounds according to their severity – and some implied the use of experts to classify injuries for this purpose. The laws of the Salian Franks, for example, required that wounds be assessed by 'men of proven skill'.[6] But it was among the Jews that legal medicine flourished most in pre-modern times. Jewish law affects nearly every aspect of life, and since Talmudic times medicine has been an important source of exemptions to its dictates. Medical or health considerations could justify suspending or modifying the observance of laws regarding the Sabbath, festivals, fasts, prayer, mourning, diet, circumcision, and numerous hygienic practices. (➤ Ch. 53 History of personal hygiene) The Talmud itself (compiled during the third to sixth centuries AD) relates several cases in which religious, civil, or criminal judgments were based on medical assessment; subsequent commentaries and rabbinical *responsa* gave much attention to the problems of what was called the 'doctor's trustworthiness' in matters affecting religious decisions. The prohibition against healing on the Sabbath, for example, could be ignored in cases of danger, and medical judgement as to what qualified as dangerous could be unreservedly followed. It was forbidden to wear amulets or to utter incantations, but both were permitted if they were medically indicated and their efficacy had been thoroughly proven. But,

above all, it was the complex laws of ritual uncleanness – especially menstrual
– that produced debate about the authority of doctors' opinions in ancient
and medieval Judaism. The Talmud contains a case in which rabbis were
asked whether two women with strange vaginal discharges were ritually
impure; the rabbis consulted doctors on whether the substances were conge-
aled blood, and the medical conclusion (apparently based on a solubility test)
was followed.[7]

MEDICINE AND PUBLIC ORDER IN MEDIEVAL AND EARLY MODERN TOWNS

The growth of towns in medieval Europe was accompanied by an increase
in both the regulation of medicine and the policing of crime; these two
activities became linked in official systems of wound registration by doctors,
which enhanced the ability of municipal governments to control violence.
The idea was to suppress private vengeance and to facilitate redress through
the law instead. In Venice, for example, a law of 1281 required medical
practitioners to report to the police all cases of wounds that appeared to have
been caused by violence; an account of the wound and a detailed prognosis
had to be submitted immediately if the injury was serious, and within two
days if not.[8] By means of this collaboration between medical men and the
law, acts of violence could be consistently brought to light and assailants
could be detained (thus preventing acts of revenge), wounds could be officially
recorded before death (thus preventing fraudulent additions to them after
death), and dying victims could be interviewed, all of which helped to make
any subsequent legal proceedings better informed and more just. The official
scrutiny of all injuries at an early stage by medical men also helped with one
of the commonest problems in early forensic medicine, that of deciding
whether someone wounded in a brawl or duel had died of his wounds or
from some other cause. Laws along these lines were enacted and enforced
in many European cities from the thirteenth century onwards. (Medico-legal
specialists in France today are still obliged to make detailed legal reports on
wounds treated in hospitals, as a matter of routine.)

European wound legislation often required attackers to maintain the victim
and pay for medical care until the cure was complete, an arrangement
conforming to the decree in Exodus that if a man inflicts an injury on his
neighbour, 'he shall cause him to be thoroughly healed' (often, from an early
date, rendered as 'he shall pay the doctor'). Municipal statutes in Bologna
dating from the thirteenth century empowered the city treasurer to confiscate
a convict's goods to pay for the medical assessment and treatment of the
victim's wounds by two doctors. Medieval Swedish laws required assailants

to provide their victims with a choice among three experienced surgeons; Irish law specified provision of 'food and leech'.[9]

These laws requiring routine medical inspection of the living wounded overlapped with the concerns and regulations of the medical communities themselves. Surgeons' guilds in medieval and early modern Europe typically required practitioners to report serious cases to guild officials without delay; this enabled the senior surgeons of the town to oversee treatment, thereby protecting the public against failures by inexperienced and incompetent practitioners, while providing worthy ones with some protection against malpractice actions.[10]

Midwives, too, performed policing functions in early modern Europe. Local regulations in German, French, and Scottish communities required them to report illegitimate births (to prevent abandonment) and to press unmarried women in the throes of childbirth for the names of the fathers (to secure financial support for the children); in seventeenth-century Nuremburg, midwives had to report miscarriages as well.[11] The oaths sworn by English midwives seeking a bishop's licence likewise included promises to extract the truth about paternity and to refuse requests for secret births.

Surgeons also examined corpses, both for secular authorities and for the Church, from an early date. Canon law decretals compiled in 1209 contain examples, such as a case where Innocent III (pope, 1198–1216) had to decide whether a blow given by a bishop in a fracas at Mass could have caused an eventual death (because if so, canon law did not permit the bishop to continue performing holy offices). The Pope had the body appraised by two surgeons and a physician, and ordered that the medical statement be publicly proclaimed.[12] Some towns had laws obliging magistrates to commission medical inspections of the body in all cases of alleged homicide; a statute of this kind was enacted in Freiburg between 1407 and 1411.[13] The code of criminal procedure promulgated for the Holy Roman Empire by Charles V (r. 1519–56) in 1532 specified that judges had to consult surgeons in all cases of suspected homicide, and midwives in suspected infanticides. This code, known as the Carolina, is considered as a landmark in the history of forensic medicine. It was imposed over a large part of continental Europe, and was widely imitated, as in the edict issued by Francis I (r. 1515–47) at Valence in 1536, which made examinations by medical experts mandatory in all cases of suspected homicide throughout France. However, the Carolina and the edict of Valence merely made obligatory and comprehensive what had been practised at least occasionally for centuries.

The actual dissection of bodies for legal purposes was practised in Bologna by the end of the thirteenth century. These forensic proceedings were probably the earliest human dissections since ancient Alexandria. It therefore seems likely that the renaissance of human anatomy in Bologna and other early university towns was stimulated by demand from the law. If so, it provides a striking illustration of how law and legal needs can provoke and shape, as well as merely make use of, the growth of medical knowledge.

MEDICO–LEGAL KNOWLEDGE

A brief survey of the early literature on legal medicine will give an idea of the range of medical questions that could arise in courts of law. The French royal surgeon Ambroise Paré (1510–90) published a short treatise for surgeons, *Traité des rapports* (1575), which explained how to report on the lethality of wounds, the signs of virginity in women, and the indications of death by lightning, smothering, drowning, apoplexy, poison, and infanticide; it also discussed the age limits to conception and explained how to differentiate between wounds given to a body when dead and alive. Assessing virginity was important because non-consummation of marriage was the most straightforward of the very few grounds for divorce under ecclesiastical law.

Whereas Paré was a surgeon who wrote his treatise in the vernacular, most early texts on forensic medicine were written in Latin by physicians or jurists. Giovanni Battista Codronchi (1547–1628) produced a comparable book for physicians, *Methodus testificandi*,[14] which added malingering and male impotence to Paré's topics. A guide for jurists on medico-legal matters was published in 1578 at Venice by Giovanni Filippo Ingrassia (1510–80), a Sicilian physician who taught at the University of Palermo; it included discussions of judicial torture and mutilation, deformity, frigidity, multiple birth, and the duration of pregnancy. *De Relationibus medicorum*, by another Sicilian physician and professor, Fortunato Fedele (1550–1630), was published in Palermo in 1602; it discussed public hygiene as well as the needs of the courts, as did *Medicus politicus* by the physician Roderigo da Castro (1541–1627).[15] (Forensic medicine remained linked with public health until the late nineteenth century.) Paulo Zacchia (1584–1659), principal physician to Innocent X (Pope, 1644–55) and medical adviser to the highest court of canon law, produced a massive compilation of sources and expert opinions on medical problems arising in secular and church courts: *Quaestiones medico-legales* appeared in seven volumes between 1621 and 1635.[16]

Texts on legal medicine continued to proliferate in continental Europe during the seventeenth and eighteenth centuries, especially in the German lands. A prominent theme in this literature is human reproduction, which is hardly surprising given the importance of inheritance in secular law, and given the fact that while it is women who bear children, property and privilege passed down the male line. Unfaithful wives could disrupt orderly inheritance by producing false heirs. Moreover, a childless woman whose husband died often stood to see his fortune go directly to collateral heirs unless she were pregnant by him, a situation that created an incentive for her to arrange a pregnancy after his death, without delay. Legal presumptions about the maximum possible duration of human gestation had been laid down in ancient times: the Roman Twelve Tables (449 BC) decreed that in cases of disputed paternity, the longest period of pregnancy that could be allowed was ten months, as did the Napoleonic Code in the nineteenth century. But there were many instances in medieval and early modern times in which longer periods, up to fourteen months, were accepted by the courts, often on a combination of evidence about the woman's virtuous character and medical testimony about the presence of special circumstances tending to prolong gestation. Paternity disputes remained intractable from a medico-legal point of view until the discovery of blood groups in 1900 made it possible to *disprove* consanguinity in many cases. Positive proof of paternity only became possible in the late 1980s with the development of genetic fingerprinting – a landmark in the history of relations between the sexes.

A problem that occupied an increasingly important place in early modern works on legal medicine was that of ascertaining whether a dead infant had been murdered, had died accidentally, or been born dead. A French edict of 1556 and an English statute of 1624 both enacted the presumption that an unmarried mother who concealed her pregnancy and labour was guilty of a capital crime in the event of the infant's death, unless there was evidence that the infant was stillborn. Similar legislation was imposed in other parts of Europe. These fierce laws reversed the usual legal presumption of innocence and consequently directed attention to the problem of what could constitute evidence of stillbirth. Signs of prematurity became important. Towards the end of the seventeenth century, a number of medical men on the European continent devised a mechanical test of live birth: following a physiological principle mentioned by Galen (AD 129–*c*.200/210), the dead infant's lungs were removed and placed in water. Floating was thought to indicate that the child had lived and breathed, inflating its lungs; sinking, that it had been born dead. The lung test was oddly reminiscent of the divinatory ordeal by water, in which an accused person who floated was guilty, whereas an innocent person would sink. This legal test was widely practised in Europe until the church abolished it in 1215, and it persisted thereafter in the practice of 'swimming' supposed witches. But the lung test also had a simple physiological rationale, and it became common in the eighteenth century for surgeons in Europe and America to perform it in cases of suspected infanticide.

Growing humanitarian sentiment in the eighteenth century was accompanied by public dissatisfaction with the harshness of the infanticide laws, which doubtless stimulated medical men to question the validity of the lung test. Concern for the plight of poor, unwed mothers is evident in the influential essay of 1783 by William Hunter (1718–83), 'On the uncertainty of the signs of murder in the case of bastard children', which argued that courts should *not* rely on medical evidence of live birth. Other medical men sought ways of making the lung test more reliable, and several refinements to it – involving precise measurements, weight ratios, and supplementary tests of the stomach and intestines – were developed in the late eighteenth and nineteenth centuries.[17]

LAW AND THE STATUS OF THE MEDICAL EXPERT

Hardly anything was written on legal medicine in England until two hundred years after the first wave of continental Europe publications. It was not uncommon for midwives, surgeons, and physicians to provide expert testimony in early modern English courts, and England did not lack learned medical culture, but writings on medico-legal subjects were rare in the Anglo-American world until the late eighteenth century. The main reason for this striking time-lag was the profound difference between the English and continental legal systems, which had begun to diverge in the thirteenth century. Whereas continental courts forged a learned legal system based on Roman law and canon law, England developed the existing common law and enlarged the traditional use of juries. Roman-canon law gave an important role to medical experts and tended to foster medico-legal science, whereas the common law privileged the opinions of lay people and was less hospitable to medical expertise.

There were no juries in the Roman-canon system: all cases were investigated and decided in inquisitorial fashion by professional judges. The power this gave to individual judges was offset by a complex law of proof designed to exclude subjective judgement as completely as possible from the process of adjudication. Judges had to fulfil minutely prescribed conditions deemed to provide a complete, rational proof before they could pronounce anyone guilty of a capital crime. The essential first step was to prove that a crime had been committed. In the case of homicide, a judge had to view the victim's body and establish by his own, legally privileged perception that a person had died by violence; this determination was considered too important to be established by witnesses, even medical ones. This meant that when a surgeon examined a corpse, he had to be given judge-like status beforehand for his observations to have legal significance; it was not legally possible for him to 'prove' part of the *corpus delicti* (the facts which constitute an offence) in the role of witness. Medical practitioners who assisted at continental Europe trials were therefore officials of the court, and as such, received fees. Their reports, too, had official status, for they were an essential part of the trial dossier. The formalized system of proof, with its demand for maximum certainty and minimum judicial discretion, meant that where medical assessment was potentially useful, it tended to be made mandatory.

Roman-canon legal procedure was built upon the principle of deference to expertise. All decisions of fact were made by professional jurists, whose reasoning was governed by comprehensive rules of inference which were spelled out in scholarly texts on legal proof. Medical facts were no exception, and because they, too, were meant to be decided on the basis of textual authority, there was a juristic demand in Roman-canon law systems for texts on *medico*-legal proof: that is, for texts on forensic medicine.

Other features of continental Europe legal procedure encouraged medico-legal science more directly. In France, for example, judicial decisions of both fact and law were routinely reviewed by superior judges, and difficult judgments were passed up through the hierarchy for consideration by higher courts; as part of this process of review, problematic *medico-legal* decisions could likewise be passed on to experts of higher standing. Some continental Europe systems provided for medico-legal difficulties to be sent directly to the highest medical authorities. The Carolina, following Italian practice, stated that whenever judges were in doubt, they were to get help from the nearest university. From the mid-sixteenth century, therefore, German courts sent formally-recorded trial proceedings to university law faculties, and, for a fee, the academics returned them with written opinions. It also became common practice from this time, on the basis of the same statute, for the courts to refer medical questions to university medical faculties, which issued collective judgments that were considered more or less binding. In German lands, difficult medico-legal problems were thus resolved by panels of professors at leading centres of medical teaching and research.

All this contrasted sharply with practice in early modern England, where decisions of fact were made by lay juries under a comparatively free system of proof. Medical investigation was nowhere obligatory, though it could be arranged by the coroner (the local official responsible for investigating sudden or suspicious deaths), by the parties, or by the magistrate conducting pre-trial proceedings (if any of these chose). But neither medical experts nor their findings had official status in English common law. Medical practitioners contributed to inquests and trials in the role of witness, and testified on much the same footing as other witnesses, frequently without payment and often *sub poena*. Their evidence was given orally and, like other testimony, it had only as much authority as the jury of lay people was willing to give it in each instance. Although questions of law were governed by precedent and resolved by judges, questions of fact – which included most medico-legal questions – were not. Any judgment that contained a determination of fact had to be given to a jury, which deliberated in private and did not ordinarily give reasons for its verdict. As legal rules of evidence gradually developed, judges could control what jurors heard, but not the way jurors *weighed* what they heard. There was no way that a learned doctrine of proof could be applied to factual decision-making in these circumstances, and consequently there was no demand for texts on proof, either legal or medico-legal. The unanimous opinion of twelve men under oath was supposed to provide an acceptable level of certainty.

The contrasting implications for expertise of the Roman-canon goal of rational certainty and the common-law standard of lay consensus are illustrated by their respective methods of discovering whether female felons who 'pleaded the belly' in stay of execution were truly pregnant. In continental Europe and Scottish trials, the decisions were made by midwives, who acted as court officials. In Anglo-American courts, however, until well into the nineteenth century, a special jury consisting of twelve local married women – the 'jury of matrons' – was sent to inspect such prisoners and to return a verdict.[18]

Because common-law trials were adversarial and there was no limit to the number of medical witnesses who could testify, contradictory medical evidence was not uncommon in Anglo-American courts. As well as being opposed by other doctors from the neighbourhood, a medical witness might encounter hostile cross-examination, and his status as a witness, whose role was essentially to respond to questions, put him and his profession at a disadvantage when they were challenged by a skilled lawyer on the latter's home ground. The result was that medical men in common-law countries tended to view medical witnessing as an unpleasant and unremunerative obligation, a circumstance that discouraged them from developing an interest in medico-legal work.

Scotland's legal procedure had features in common with both systems, and its inquisitorial style was more encouraging to specialization in forensic medicine than was Anglo-American procedure. The Scottish procurator fiscal was a trained lawyer responsible for both investigating and prosecuting crimes; he was thus more like a continental Europe judge than an English magistrate, judge, or coroner.[19] A Scottish medical professor interested in forensic medicine (such as Robert Christison, 1797–1881) could more easily become involved in medico-legal cases on a privileged and regular basis through collaboration with the procurator fiscal, than could a comparable aspirant in England (such as John Gordon Smith, 1792–1833), where responsibility for criminal investigations and prosecutions was much more decentralized.

The argument that medico-legal science was fostered by more rationalistic, expertise-based legal systems is supported by the Chinese case. China, a more thoroughly bureaucratic society than anything known in medieval Europe, produced in 1247 the first systematic treatise on forensic medicine, the *Hsi yuan chi lu* (the washing away of unjust imputations, or wrongs).[20] Written by the judge Sung Tzhu (1181–1249), it was part of a long-standing tradition of legal guides and medico-legal case-books for judges, which were created for the same reason as the Roman-canon legal literature in Europe: the need to regulate judicial decision-making closely in a juryless system run by a pyramid of officials.

The earliest evidence of medico-legal investigation in China, in the third century BC, comes from the state of Chhin, which had adopted the doctrines of the Legalist school of philosophy. The Legalists thought that the law should be written down in detail, leaving nothing to individual interpretation, and they placed great emphasis on quantification and on objective methods of adjudication. These features – common to Chinese Legalism and Roman-canon law – encouraged the appearance and growth of forensic medicine.[21]

The *Hsi yuan chi lu* contained detailed medico-legal doctrine, explaining, for example, how to differentiate among accidental, suicidal, and homicidal drowning and the disposal of an already-dead body in water. It also described medico-legal tests, such as the use of red light to reveal injuries. As early as the ninth century, corpses were examined in sunlight under red silk umbrellas because the red light made internal contusions appear on the surface of the body; it also made visible, on washed bones, a difference between damage that had been inflicted before and after death.[22] It was not until the nineteenth century that Chinese forensic medicine fell behind that of the West. (➤ Ch. 32 Chinese medicine)

After 1800, doctors in Britain and America became more interested in legal medicine. This was partly because developments within medicine were directing their attention independently to subjects that happened to be relevant to medico-legal work – to dissection, pathological anatomy, physiology, and analytical chemistry, and generally to methods of making medicine more objective and certain. (➤ Ch. 7 The physiological tradition; Ch. 9 The pathological tradition; Ch. 8 The biochemical tradition) Another factor was the contemporary drive to reform the medical profession and improve its reputation; forensic medicine had significance in this context because, unlike most medical practice, it was performed publicly, under challenging adversarial conditions. The regular profession was preoccupied in this period with suppressing quackery and incompetence, and was continually campaigning for legislation that would give it a legal monopoly on healing; the fact that doctors were seeking new levels of government protection was doubtless another factor in their frequent emphasis on what the medical profession, through the practice of forensic medicine, could do and was already doing for the state. Reform-minded editors of medical journals, such as Andrew Duncan (1773–1832) and Thomas Wakley (1795–1862), actively promoted the field, with some success. In 1831, the Society of Apothecaries required applicants for its licence to attend a course of lectures on the subject. Forensic medicine was made a compulsory part of medical education at Edinburgh University in 1833 and of all Scottish medical degrees in 1837, while in England, the Medical Witnesses Acts (1836 and 1837) established statutory fees for medical men who gave expert testimony at inquests or criminal trials.[23]

PSYCHIATRY AND THE LAW

Psychiatry has been a contentious area of medico-legal relations for most of the past two hundred years. (➤ Ch. 56 Psychiatry) The nineteenth century saw vigorous conflict in most Western jurisdictions between the medical and legal professions over the question of criminal responsibility. And although in recent decades the insanity defence has tended to become overshadowed by the civil liberties of mental patients as the most visible and controversial area of interaction between psychiatry and law, it remains a potentially explosive issue which, as in the 'Yorkshire Ripper' trial, periodically threatens to disrupt the social-administrative and political consensus that normally governs the treatment and disposal of mentally abnormal offenders.

The idea that the insane should not be punished for criminal acts is a venerable one, appearing in *Laws* by Plato (*c*.428–347 BC), the Babylonian Talmud, many early European codes and the early common law. In England, from the time of Hadfield's trial (1800) (see p. 1631) it became the practice for criminal trial juries to find special verdicts of 'not guilty by reason of insanity'. Sometimes there was legal discussion about how to define the boundary between criminality and insanity, but before the nineteenth century, the question was not treated as a particularly medical one. To be acquitted as irresponsible, an offender had to be totally mad, and the evidence and judgement of medical men on this point differed little from that of lay people. After 1750, however, the insanity defence became more common and, especially after about 1830, more likely to involve medical testimony. It was around this time that medical practitioners were acquiring a special interest in insanity, and becoming more confident of their ability to detect a 'partial' insanity, often imperceptible to lay people, which could entail inability to control criminal impulses.

After the controversial acquittal of Daniel McNaghten in 1843, the English Law Lords drew up a set of guidelines at the request of Parliament which formed the legal basis for assessing criminal insanity and responsibility for more than a century. Known as the 'McNaghten Rules', they specified that the criminal's mental state had to have been such that he or she either did not know what they were doing or did not know that it was wrong. This legal formula denied psychological medicine's claim that there were disorders of emotion and volition that could exist without any disorder of the understanding. (➤ Ch. 21 Mental diseases) However, lawyers, judges, and many lay people saw in the medical notion of partial insanity a determinism tending to undermine the assumption of free will on which the criminal law was based, and they considered it essential that the common-sense notion of individual responsibility for one's actions be preserved. Debates over trials involving the insanity defence thus expressed a basic conflict between legal and medico-psychological ways of thinking about human nature and conduct.[24]

Whereas Anglo-American law presented juries with a fairly clear-cut choice between responsibility and madness, continental Europe and Scottish legal systems provided for intermediate verdicts, which allowed *degrees* of responsibility to be recognized. Medical assessments of varying mental states could therefore be incorporated comparatively smoothly, despite the introduction of juries in many traditionally Roman-canon jurisdictions during the nineteenth century. The non-adversarial position of the experts consulted also helped to lessen medico-legal conflict. Even under these more inquisitorial conditions, however, murder trials involving the question of mental disorder created medico-legal controversy and sensation.

Special administrative frameworks for dealing with criminal lunatics were established in many countries during the nineteenth century. In England, after the uproar surrounding the acquittal in 1800 of James Hadfield, who had shot at King George III, the Criminal Lunatics Act (1801) was swiftly passed, empowering justices to detain indefinitely offenders acquitted on the grounds of insanity. Initially, these criminal lunatics were supposed to be kept at Bethlem, where Parliament funded space for them; eventually, a special asylum was opened at Broadmoor in 1863. The legislation of 1801 also provided for the detention of deranged persons who were thought *likely* to commit criminal acts, but it made no mention of consulting medical opinion.

During the nineteenth century, medical men in Western countries acquired some authority in the various procedures whereby the mentally disordered were incarcerated in public and private institutions. In France, civil legislation of 1838 made medical certification a necessary condition for asylum committal, while nevertheless vesting decisive authority in the hands of central government officials, magistrates, and the police. In England, the powers of the Metropolitan Commissioners in Lunacy to supervise the insane and to inspect asylums were extended to cover the whole country in 1845. The Commissioners included both doctors and lawyers, but the commitment framework remained essentially a legal one.

By the late nineteenth century, the idea of involving scientific experts in social policy generally and in the state's response to crime in particular had acquired considerable political influence in Europe and America. During the first two-thirds of the twentieth century, psychiatric expertise became an increasingly important part of social administration, and legislation on mental disorder came to reflect medical priorities. An example is the sex offenders legislation enacted in most American states during the 1930s and 1940s, which allowed – and, in some cases, still allows – the indefinite confinement and compulsory treatment of prisoners who had committed sexual offences that were either violent or involved minors. These statutes were based on contemporary confidence in the ability of psychiatrists and psychologists to identify distinct sexual psychopathology and to predict precisely who would behave in a sexually dangerous manner. This confidence now appears to have been misplaced. Recent research in Canada and the United States indicates that the majority of sex offenders are polydeviant, and that the legal concept of sexual dangerousness has no clinical validity.[25]

In 1922, legislation on infanticide was enacted in England which reduced that offence from murder to manslaughter when the 'balance' of the woman's mind had been 'disturbed' by giving birth; the Infanticide Act (1938) added lactation as a mitigating cause of mental disturbance for up to twelve months after the birth.[26] The Homicide Act (1957) introduced the plea of diminished responsibility in England, with the result that if a jury were convinced that an abnormality of mind had affected responsibility even to a small degree, any charge of murder would be reduced to manslaughter, allowing the judge almost complete discretion in sentencing. The plea of diminished responsibility created a middle ground between legal and psychiatric approaches to criminal responsibility, and effectively superseded the medically naïve McNaghten Rules: in order to make a psychiatric defence, it was no longer necessary to argue that a defendant was insane. The defence of 'insanity' has consequently rarely been used in England since 1957, and mentally disordered offenders have produced much less medico-legal argument than formerly. This has made the forensic psychiatrist in Britain less of a court-room protagonist and more of a clinician and administrator. However, in places where diminished responsibility has not been introduced, such as Canada and some parts of the United States, insanity remains an important psychiatric defence option, and a modified version of the McNaghten Rules is still applied; the issue therefore continues to generate complex medico-legal debate both in and out of the courtroom.[27]

In both Europe and America, however, the criminal justice side of forensic psychiatry has become less dominant in the twentieth century because other areas of legal-psychiatric practice have multiplied, including medical and life insurance, compensation for injury, psychiatric support for victims of violence and, above all, the rights and liberties of mental patients. This last area has grown dramatically since the publication in 1963 of Thomas Szasz's *Law, Liberty and Psychiatry: an Inquiry into the Social Uses of Mental Health Practices.*[28]

Szasz rejected the 'medical model' of mental illness, and argued that 'mental illness' was merely an ideological construct serving the interests of psychiatric imperialism and social control. Anti-psychiatry sentiment was fuelled also by influential sociological critiques of 'total institutions' and by the intense publicity given to the role of psychiatry in the repression of dissent in the Soviet Union. Recent legislation such as the Californian Lanterman–Petris–Short Act (1972) and the British Mental Health Act (1983) has greatly enhanced legal and institutional safeguards for patients' rights. Whereas in the nineteenth century, alienists represented a force for clemency against the terrible power of the death penalty, in the late twentieth century, contact between psychiatry and the law is exemplified more by use of the law to protect citizens against the power of psychiatry.

The patients' rights movement is not limited, however, to civil-libertarian matters such as improper confinement and the right to refuse treatment. In recent years, the use of compulsory commitment powers has declined, partly because of an increasing political preference for non-institutional, community-based psychiatric treatment. One result of the decarceration process has been a growth of concern among mental health workers and activists with the rights of the mentally disordered outside institutions to receive care and treatment, and this area of law is now growing rapidly.[29]

THE POLITICS OF EXPERTISE

During the nineteenth century, medicine came to play an increasingly important role in social administration, and medical expertise in general became the subject of recurrent political controversy. In England and Wales, the Births and Deaths Registration Act (1837) required the registration of all deaths; with the introduction soon after of medical certification of cause of death, and its gradual extension during the next fifty years to cover nearly all deaths, medical men were for the first time called upon by the community to play the key role in distinguishing 'natural' from 'unnatural' deaths. During the same period, national lunacy and public-health legislation conferred sweeping legal powers of entry, inspection, compulsory medical examination, treatment, commitment, and sequestration upon doctors acting in a variety of official capacities, which proved deeply offensive to civil libertarians, religious dissenters, feminists, and advocates of *laissez-faire*. Especially strong hostility was aroused in the community at large by the Vaccination Acts (1840 to 1871), which ordered universal vaccination, and the Contagious Diseases Acts (1864, 1866), which authorized the compulsory medical examination and treatment of women suspected of prostitution. (➤ Ch. 26 Sexually transmitted diseases)

In the courts, medical evidence was called upon with increasing frequency in a wide range of civil and criminal proceedings during the nineteenth century, and it became a persistent source of conflict both within the medical profession and between the medical and legal professions. Moreover, it posed problems of credibility for the medical profession, especially in the adversarial common-law jurisdictions of England and the United States. In civil cases, where large sums of money were often at stake, medical witnesses contradicted each other so frequently that their impartiality – upon which the claim to scientific objectivity depended – was widely called into question. Both doctors and lawyers expressed concern that expert witnessing was becoming an unscrupulous trade and bringing the profession into disrepute. Efforts to develop more reliable, authoritative expertise and more harmonious relations between the two professions led to the formation of co-operative organizations such as the medico-legal societies of New York (1867), Paris (1868), Massachusetts (1877), London (1900–1), and Berlin (1904), as well as innumerable round-table discussions and attempts to establish joint consultations, for example in pre-trial briefings.

The tensions and conflicts surrounding the expansion of medico-legal expertise were especially acute in the case of the Anglo-American coronership. During much of the nineteenth and early twentieth centuries, there was almost continual agitation in England and the United States for reform or, in some cases, abolition of the coronership. Although the power and importance of this medieval institution had declined considerably by the nineteenth century, coroners were still responsible for the investigation of sudden and suspicious deaths. Coroners, who were elected for life in England, did not have to have any medical or legal training (though in nineteenth-century England the majority were lawyers) and they did not have to consult medical experts. The fact that lay people and lawyers had almost complete authority to define the aims, scope, and methods of coroner's inquests was much complained of by medical men. Professional and public dissatisfaction led to various attempts at reform, but changes were relatively modest and slow. The 1860 Coroners' Act enlarged the scope of the inquest and freed the coroner from dependence on local magistrates. Further legislation in 1887 made the English coronership a salaried government post no longer filled by election. But the coroner still decided how 'medical' an inquest would be, and not until 1926 were coroners required to have either legal or medical qualifications. Even today, the controversy over the respective merits of a medical or legal coronership is by no means dead, while in recent years, the apparent secrecy and arbitrariness of some coroners' proceedings have once again occasioned public dissatisfaction with the English medico-legal investigative system.[30]

In the United States, the office was a highly political appointment, and as state, county and city governments changed, coroners came and went, so that

American coroners were less likely to have even the benefit of much experience. In 1877, the Massachusetts coronership was replaced by the office of Medical Examiner, but medical authority was still severely limited by the fact that the examiner could not perform an autopsy without permission from the District Attorney. New York introduced a medical-examiner system in 1918 that gave the incumbent more autonomy, but by the mid-1930s only a handful of cities and states had abolished the coronership. Medico-legal reformers claimed that lay coroners tended to select their physician-assistants according to social and political criteria rather than any relevant expertise, but even medical coroners and examiners were not exempt from charges of political bias and corruption.[31]

The continental Europe organization of legal medicine, the envy of many Anglo-American medico-legists since the early nineteenth century, was still the ideal for many of them in the 1930s and 1940s. By then, most European countries had one (or more) medico-legal institute where all aspects of legal medicine were practised, from forensic pathology and psychiatry to ballistics and serology, under a director who usually held a university chair in legal medicine. These scientifically unrelated subjects had been brought together because of their common usefulness to the law; it was a unity created entirely by legal needs. Part of the appeal of the institute-model for Anglo-American medical jurists lay in its provision for research, teaching, career structure, and a secure institutional base for their interdisciplinary speciality, which, with a few exceptions, had failed to find a secure niche in either the medical or legal faculties of British and American universities.

However, efforts to establish similar institutions in Britain and America during the inter-war years met with little success. By that time, the idea of an all-embracing, centralized medico-legal institute was making less sense scientifically because intense specialization had occurred in the relevant disciplines. Moreover, with the rapid growth in the early twentieth century of forensic sciences which often had little connection with medicine – such as forensic ballistics, psychology, fingerprint identification, and biochemical analysis – and the expansion of clinical forensic medicine (in criminal as well as civil matters), 'legal medicine' was becoming a more professionally, as well as scientifically, heterogeneous field. In England, separate forensic-science laboratories under the Home Office were created during the 1930s; by that time, hospital psychiatrists and prison medical officers were usually considered the best experts on forensic psychiatry, and general-hospital pathologists were becoming the obvious consultants on forensic pathology, while police surgeons were increasingly seen as having an important role to play in clinical medico-legal detection. The comprehensive institutes, which had developed in continental Europe in the nineteenth century and which reflected that period's vision of the all-round medico-legal expert, seemed much less appropriate in the mid-twentieth century because expertise had become more specialized and medico-legal practice more diversified and dispersed.

The two models also clearly embodied differing historical legacies. European medico-legal institutes reflect the more centralized and bureaucratic organization of continental Europe states, as well as the emphasis of Roman-canon law on expertise and impartial authority. On the other hand, the eclectic, sometimes less efficient investigative systems that have evolved in the Anglo-American world exemplify traditional common-law values of adversarial confrontation, 'free' (or partisan) selection of witnesses, and a democratic, decentralized pragmatism. Commentators in both medico-legal cultures have freely acknowledged and often wished to emulate the more advantageous features of the other.

Dissatisfaction has nevertheless been stronger in Anglo-American jurisdictions, where the difficulties that juries and adversarial procedure pose for expert testimony are a perennial topic of discussion. The arguments and the range of proposed solutions have not changed since the nineteenth century, but innovations are being tried. In 1975, United States federal legislation authorized judges to appoint court experts in non-criminal trials. However, this experiment has been pronounced a failure because so far judges have proved unwilling to exercise this power.[32] A step in another direction was taken in 1983, when Congress amended Federal Rule of Evidence 704 to restrict the admissibility of testimony by mental-health experts because of the frequency of 'competing expert witnesses testifying to directly contradictory conclusions' about a person's sanity. The sponsors of the amendment doubted jurors' ability to resolve such disagreements. Ongoing research is attempting to evaluate the competence of jurors to deal with expertise, and the effects of the adversary system on the quality of expert evidence and final decisions.[33]

Although medical expertise is now deeply entrenched in modern law and government, and the law–medicine clashes of the nineteenth century have given way to subtler negotiations and greater mutual respect, the contemporary medico-legal scene is still chronically subject to disputes about the value, authority, and even integrity of all kinds of expert testimony. Courtroom disputes between medical witnesses, and professional rivalries between different sorts of medical and scientific experts, have continued to undermine the positivist vision of science as a guarantor of justice. In Britain especially, medico-legal and, more recently, forensic-scientific evidence has been a focus of growing public disenchantment with criminal justice administration generally. At the same time, medico-legal expertise is clearly implicated in a general crisis currently affecting nearly all forms of expertise in advanced Western polities.[34]

In the late twentieth century, the areas of law–medicine interaction that attract most attention are medical law and bioethics. During the past two or three decades, doctor–patient relationships have undergone an unprecedented amount of legal scrutiny in litigation over matters such as medical negligence, informed consent, and access to resources within health-care delivery systems. (➤ Ch. 34 History of the doctor–patient relationship) At the same time, the 'cutting edges' of medical science have given rise to pressing legal questions of profound importance about abortion, surrogacy, *in vitro* fertilization, wrongful conception, wrongful life, organ transplantation, research on human subjects, euthanasia, doctor-assisted suicide, and the definition of death. In all these areas case law and legislation have burgeoned, and medical law has become a thriving field of academic study. (➤ Ch. 11 Clinical research; Ch. 42 Surgery (modern); Ch. 46 Geriatrics)

ACKNOWLEDGEMENTS

I am grateful to Michael Clark for generous assistance in preparing this essay, and to Vivian Nutton, Margaret Pelling, and Roger Smith for helpful comments on the text.

NOTES

1   Michel Foucault, *Discipline and Punish*, London, Allen Lane, 1977; Foucault, *The History of Sexuality*, Vol. I: *An Introduction*, New York, Random House, 1978; François Ewald, 'Norms, discipline, and the law', *Representations*, 1990, 30: 138–61. For the medicalization of the crime of suicide, see this volume, Ch. 61: 'Religion and medicine', p. 1449.

2   William J. Curran, 'The confusion of titles in the medicolegal field: an historical analysis and a proposal for reform', *Medicine, Science and the Law*, 1975, 15: 270–5.

3   Darrel W. Amundsen, 'The liability of the physician in Roman law', in H. Karplus (ed.), *International Symposium on Society, Medicine and Law, Jerusalem, March 1972*, Amsterdam, London and New York, Elsevier, 1973, pp. 17–31; see p. 17.

4   Darrel W. Amundsen and Gary B. Ferngren, 'The physician as expert witness in Athenian law', *Bulletin of the History of Medicine*, 1977, 51: 202–13.

5   Darrel W. Amundsen and Gary B. Ferngren, 'The forensic role of physicians in Ptolemaic and Roman Egypt', *Bulletin of the History of Medicine*, 1978, 52: 336–53; Jaroslav Nemec, *Highlights in Medicolegal Relations*, rev. and enl. edn, Bethesda, MD, US Department of Health, Education, and Welfare, 1976; Amundsen and Ferngren, 'The forensic role of physicians in Roman law', *Bulletin of the History of Medicine*, 1979, 53: 39–56; p. 47.

6   Robert P. Brittain, 'Origins of legal medicine: Leges Barbarorum', *Medico-legal Journal*, 1966, 34: 21–3.

7   Immanuel Jakobovits, *Jewish Medical Ethics: a Comparative and Historical Study of*

the Jewish Religious Attitude to Medicine and its Practice, New York, Bloch, 1959, 1975, pp. 232–7, *passim*; Julius Preuss, *Biblical and Talmudic Medicine*, trans. and ed. by Fred Rosner, New York, Sanhedrin Press, 1978.

8 Guido Ruggiero, 'The cooperation of physicians and the state in the control of violence in Renaissance Venice', *Journal of the History of Medicine*, 1978, 33: 156–66.

9 Alessandro Simili, 'The beginnings of forensic medicine in Bologna', in Karplus, op. cit. (n. 3), pp. 91–100, see p. 92; Nemec, op. cit. (n. 5), p. 20; John Cule, 'The court mediciner and medicine in the laws of Wales', in Chester R. Burns (ed.), *Legacies in Law and Medicine*, New York, Science History, 1977, pp. 26–51, see p. 53 n.

10 Madeleine Cosman, 'Medieval medical malpractice: the dicta and the dockets', in S. Jarcho (ed.), *Essays on the History of Medicine Selected from the Bulletin of the New York Academy of Medicine*, 1976, New York, Science History, pp. 71–96.

11 Merry Wiesner, 'Early modern midwifery: a case study', in Barbara A. Hanawalt (ed.), *Women and Work in Preindustrial Europe*, Bloomington, Indiana University Press, 1986, pp. 94–113; see p. 99.

12 Ynez Violé O'Neill, 'Innocent III and the evolution of anatomy', *Medical History*, 1976, 20: 429–33; see pp. 430–1.

13 Peter Volk and Hans Jurgen Warlo, 'The role of medical experts in court proceedings in the medieval town', in Karplus, op. cit. (n. 3), pp. 101–16; see p. 104.

14 Giovanni Battista Codronchi, *Methodus testificandi*, Frankfurt, 1597.

15 Fortunato Fedele, *De Relationibus medicorum*, Palermo, 1602; Roderigo da Castro, *Medicus politicus*, Hamburg, 1614.

16 Paulo Zacchia, *Quaestiones medico-legales*, 7 vols, 1621–35.

17 Robert P. Brittain, 'The hydrostatic and similar tests of live birth: a historical review', *Medico-Legal Journal*, 1963, 31: 189–94; Mark Jackson, 'New-born child murder: a study of suspicion, evidence, and proof in eighteenth-century England', unpublished Ph.D. thesis, University of Leeds, 1992.

18 James C. Oldham, 'On pleading the belly: a history of the jury of matrons', *Criminal Justice History*, 1985, 6: 1–64.

19 M. Anne Crowther and Brenda White, *On Soul and Conscience: the Medical Expert and Crime. 150 Years of Forensic Medicine in Glasgow*, Aberdeen, Aberdeen University Press, 1988, p. 12.

20 Sung Tzhu, *Hsi yuan Chi lu*, 1247.

21 Lu Gwei-Djen and Joseph Needham, 'A history of forensic medicine in China', *Medical History*, 1988, 32: 357–400; see pp. 368–9.

22 Ibid., pp. 378–9; see p. 379 n.

23 Catherine Crawford, 'A scientific profession: forensic medicine and professional reform in British periodicals of the early nineteenth century', in Roger French and Andrew Wear (eds), *British Medicine in an Age of Reform*, London and New York, Routledge, 1991, pp. 203–30.

24 Roger Smith, *Trial by Medicine: Insanity and Responsibility in Victorian Trials*, Edinburgh, Edinburgh University Press, 1981.

25 A. M. McFarthing, 'A survey of the social, legal, historical and "psycho-babble"

factors leading to sex offenders legislation in the areas of British common law heritage', *Medicine and Law*, 1990, 9: 1278–95.

26 Katherine O'Donovan, 'The medicalisation of infanticide', *Criminal Law Review*, 1984: 259–64.

27 Christopher M. Green and Laurence J. Naismith, 'A comparative perspective on forensic psychiatry in Canada and England', *Medicine, Science and the Law*, 1988, 28: 329–35.

28 Thomas Szasz, *Law, Liberty and Psychiatry: an Inquiry into the Social Uses of Mental Health Practices*, 1963.

29 Clive Unsworth, *The Politics of Mental Health Legislation*, Oxford, Clarendon Press, 1983.

30 Tony Ward, 'Coroners, police and deaths in custody in England: a historical perspective', in *The State of Information in 1984*, Working Papers in European Criminology, no. 6, European Group for the Study of Deviance and Social Control, 1984, pp. 186–215.

31 Julie Johnson, 'Speaking for the dead: Forensic scientists and American justice in the twentieth century', unpublished Ph.D. thesis, University of Pennsylvania, 1992.

32 Edward J. Imwinkelreid, 'The court appointment of expert witnesses in the United States: a failed experiment', *Medicine and Law*, 1989, 8: 601–9.

33 Ibid. pp. 604, 606 n.

34 Roger Smith and Brian Wynne (eds), *Expert Evidence: Interpreting Science in the Law*, London and New York, Routledge, 1989; David Nelken, 'The truth about law's truth', Faculty of Laws, University College London, Working Papers, no. 7 [n.d., *c*.1990].

FURTHER READING

Ackerknecht, E. H., 'Early history of legal medicine', *Ciba Symposia*, 1950–1, 11: 1288–1304, 1313–16. (Also in Chester R. Burns (ed.), *Legacies in Law and Medicine*, New York, Science History, 1977, pp. 247–69.)

Brookes, Barbara, *Abortion in England, 1900–1967*, London, Routledge, 1988.

Cawthorn, Elisabeth, 'Thomas Wakley and the medical coronership – occupational death and the judicial process', *Medical History*, 1983, 30: 191–202.

Clark, Michael and Crawford, Catherine (eds), *Legal Medicine in History*, Cambridge, Cambridge University Press, 1993.

Crawford, Catherine, 'The emergence of English forensic medicine: medical evidence in common law courts, 1730–1830', unpublished D.Phil. thesis, University of Oxford, 1987.

De Ville, Kenneth Allen, *Medical Malpractice in Nineteenth-Century America: Origins and Legacy*, New York and London, New York University Press, 1990.

Faden, Ruth R., Beauchamp, Tom L. and King, Nancy M. P., *A History and Theory of Informed Consent*, New York and Oxford, Oxford University Press, 1986.

Fischer-Homberger, Esther, *Medizin vor Gericht: Gerichtsmedizin von der Renaissance bis zur Aufklärung*, Berne, Huber, 1983. This is the most detailed study of continental Europe legal medicine between 1500 and 1800; it also provides a valuable account of the period before 1500.

Forbes, Thomas R., *Surgeons at the Bailey: English Forensic Medicine to 1878*, New Haven, CT, Yale University Press, 1985.

Harris, Ruth, *Murders and Madness: Medicine, Law and Society in the Fin de Siècle*, Oxford, Clarendon Press, 1990.

Havard, J. D. J., *The Detection of Secret Homicide: a Study of the Medico-Legal System of Investigation of Sudden and Unexplained Deaths*, London, Macmillan, 1960.

Keown, John, *Abortion, Doctors and the Law: Some Aspects of the Legal Regulation of Abortion in England from 1803 to 1982*, Cambridge, Cambridge University Press, 1988.

Macdonald, Michael and Murphy, Terence R., *Sleepless Souls: Suicide in Early Modern England*, Oxford and New York, Oxford University Press, 1990.

Moore, Michael S., *Law and Psychiatry: Re-thinking the Relationship*, Cambridge, Cambridge University Press, 1984.

Smith, Roger, 'The law and insanity in Great Britain, with comments on continental Europe', in F. Koenraadt (ed.), *Ziek of schuldig? Twee eeuwen forensische psychiatrie en psychologie*, Utrecht, Willem Pompe Instituut, 1991, pp. 247–81.

Walker, Nigel, *Crime and Insanity in England*, Vol. I: *The Historical Perspective*; Vol. II: *New Solutions and New Problems*, Edinburgh, Edinburgh University Press, 1968 and 1973, respectively.

70

MEDICAL SOCIOLOGY

David Armstrong

Medical sociology, as its name implies, is concerned with the relationship between medicine and society. The discipline itself is relatively young, but needless to say, the relationship between medicine and the social domain is much older, and indeed has been the subject of many historical studies, especially those falling within the area of social history. Yet while the latter is clearly a sub-discipline of history, medical sociology comes from a different root and approaches its problems with different theoretical and methodological concerns.

EARLY MEDICAL SOCIOLOGY

It is possible to trace a prehistory of medical sociology in the great nineteenth-century investigations of the health and welfare of the population, yet the subject itself would identify its roots as being located not in this effervescence of public health but in the twentieth-century development of the discipline of sociology. Of course, the founders of sociology are usually sought in that self-conscious period of the nineteenth century when the progress and development of societies became a topic of interest – figures such as Montesquieu, Comte, and Marx (1818–83) are often identified as the pioneers – but sociology proper did not really emerge until the early years of the twentieth century, when Emile Durkheim (1858–1917) in France was appointed to the first chair in the subject. Unlike Karl Marx, that other founder of sociology, Durkheim's concern with the social was not simply one facet of a more overarching economic and political analysis. For Durkheim, society was an object *sui generis* which merited its own approaches and methods. Indeed, Durkheim was concerned to distinguish the nascent sociology from its more boisterous sibling, psychology, by claiming that psychological phenomena ultimately had a social origin. Equally, Durkheim was intent on establishing the scientific credentials of this new subject by arguing that social 'facts' were susceptible to investigation through scientific method.

Durkheim was the author of several seminal books that firmly established the discipline of sociology and provided a variety of lines of enquiry which have persisted until the present day. His first book, *The Divison of Labour in Society*,[1] offered a theory of social change. He argued that pre-industrial society was characterized by a low division of labour in which individual identity was subsumed to that of the group. With the development of cities, the growth of population, and a concurrent increase in 'moral density', the division of labour expanded such that individual occupations were becoming increasingly specialized (particularly from the time of the Industrial Revolution). The effect of this was to create a society based on separateness rather than similarity: this meant that individual identity – and indeed the very word individualism – could emerge as an object of analysis. (➤ Ch. 27 Diseases of civilization)

The two stages in the evolution of social order, from 'mechanical solidarity' based on similarity to 'organic solidarity' based on differences, were poles of a continuum along which, according to Durkheim, societies were still travelling. This meant that while the pre-industrial form of social solidarity had for the most part disappeared, the new order based on individual interdependence was still unfolding. Indeed, in the second edition of the book, Durkheim commended the role of professions as bulwarks against the fragmentary forces at work in modern society.

Durkheim followed his first book with a treatise on scientific method entitled *The Rules of Sociological Method*,[2] which attempted to establish the research credentials of the new discipline. His third book, which has been of particular interest to medical sociologists, was an application of his theory of society and methodology to the problem of suicide.[3] This study can be claimed as the first major work in medical sociology.

In outline, following from his theoretical work on the division of labour, Durkheim proposed different types of suicide that depended on the degree of integration of the individual in the society: thus, at one extreme, altruistic suicide occurred when life was taken for the benefit of others, and at the other, egoistic suicide occurred when death was welcomed for more selfish reasons. Durkheim reasoned that the rate and type of suicide in any society would reflect on its degree of social integration. The latter might be estimated by looking at familial ties, type of religion, state of war, and so on. Examining contemporary suicide statistics in tables of three variables, Durkheim developed a primitive form of multivariate analysis to show that suicide rates did vary in different European societies according to his theory, and that the rate was indeed lower amongst 'integrated' groups such as the married, Catholics, and populations during wartime.

Suicide remains an important book. It has informed much subsequent work in sociology, epidemiology, and psychiatry, and its main findings have been confirmed in more recent studies. Its significance for sociology, however, lay beyond its status as a piece of shrewd epidemiological deduction. The book showed convincingly that social factors could be conceptualized, measured, and used, to interpret real-world events. In particular, the apparently very personal activity of committing suicide was shown to be socially patterned, indicating the powerful influence of wider social forces often outside the direct awareness of the individual.

POST-WAR BEGINNINGS OF THE DISCIPLINE

Despite the promise of Durkheim's seminal work at the beginning of the century, sociology made slow progress during the first half of the twentieth century. Surveys were sporadically carried out into various social problems and Mass Observation (in which a panel of 'ordinary people' kept detailed diaries) marked the beginning of an interest in the everyday activities of the average citizen. But social research only began to come into its own during the Second World War, when various surveys were used as government tools to monitor the effect of war on the population. For example, in Britain, the War-time Social Survey asked people about their experiences of illness; and in the United States, the classic study of the American soldier showed the way in which social phenomena could be carefully measured and analysed.[4] On the strength of these experiences, sociology seemed to offer expertise in measuring the characteristics of people that governments, and increasingly medicine, became keen to extend once the war was over. (➤ Ch. 66 War and modern medicine)

One of the earliest post-war problems to require a social science input was the failure of many people to avail themselves of population immunization programmes. For example, the Sabin and later the Salk vaccines provided an effective and safe technique for guarding against poliomyelitis, yet many parents did not respond to the invitation to bring their children for this simple procedure. An earlier age might have explained this in terms of fecklessness or ignorance, but the preventive medicine of the 1950s turned to psycho-social explanations. The major theory to emerge from this work was the Health Belief Model which, with various revisions, is still called upon to explain health-related behaviour.[5] Essentially, the Health Belief Model claimed that various measurable facets of individuals, such as their concern, motivation, and previous experiences, could be used to explain and predict their behaviour with regard to preventing ill health.

The Health Belief Model was primarily a psychological model of human behaviour and related mainly to preventive activities, but evidence began to accumulate of a parallel problem that sociologists rapidly made their own. To be sure, many people failed to use available preventive services, but of far greater consequence – and apparently even more inexplicable – many patients, when ill, chose not to seek medical attention.[6] A core assumption of medicine, indeed the basis of the 'medical model', was that when patients experienced the symptoms of illness, they would present these to the doctor, whereupon the doctor would look for the corroborative clinical signs to make an accurate diagnosis: but if patients failed to present their symptoms, even those that signified serious pathology, then physicians could not even begin their task. The search for the reasons why patients chose not to take their symptoms to the doctor ushered in a major body of investigations around this problem of 'illness behaviour', as Mechanic called it.[7] And in the following decade, during the 1960s, when it was discovered that patients also took many apparently trivial and inconsequential symptoms for medical advice, the field extended itself to the whole question of why patients did or did not choose to go to the doctor. (➤ Ch. 34 History of the doctor–patient relationship)

The chief method used for these investigations was the survey. Used intermittently during the nineteenth and early twentieth centuries, new refinements such as sampling techniques and their associated statistics made the survey a powerful tool: and who better to use it than the student of social life, the sociologist? Thus, the early history of medical sociology in the post-war years can be located around a new socio-medical instrument, which could explore not the individual body of the sick person, but the several bodies, some ill, some well, contained in the community.

The new medical sociology had the necessary tools to tackle an important problem; in addition, almost by default, it acquired some accompanying conceptual baggage. Post-war general sociology was dominated by a theoretical model called structural-functionalism (heavily influenced by Talcott Parsons (1902–79)), which emphasized consensus and order in social affairs. Later, this perspective was to be undermined by a more critical sociology, which questioned the existence and maintenance of social order, and stressed the importance of conflict in social activities. However, the first medical sociologists inevitably looked to structural-functionalism for a conceptual underpinning of their work.

In 1951, Parsons had published a collection of essays on 'the social system' which described how various components of society functioned as a part of the whole.[8] One of the essays advanced the idea of role reciprocity between doctor and patient: doctor–patient interaction was another of the many mechanisms through which social order and stability was maintained.

The specific social status given the patient in the interaction with the doctor was the 'sick role'. Parsons described two benefits and two obligations of those with sickness in modern society: they gained from being temporarily excused their normal social roles and from not being held responsible for their illness; and they were expected to want to get well and to comply with the appropriate medical authorities. Later critics of Parsons – and there were many – rejected this narrow formulation of the sick role. Its assumptions of consensus and harmony have become less popular as an explanatory framework in sociology theory; equally, it would seem that the sick role as described by Parsons ignores the plight of many patients with chronic illnesses who are unable to benefit from or fulfil one or more of its characteristics.

Nevertheless, for all its faults, the sick role still forms one of the conceptual building-blocks of medical sociology: it is attacked and criticized, but still cited. The historical significance of Parsons's concept was that it recast the doctor–patient relationship from a therapeutic encounter to an engagement of wider 'social control' mechanisms. The term, social control, has various usages in sociology – and perhaps a pejorative image outside – but for Parsons it was simply the glue that held society together. Illness was a deviant status and without appropriate control mechanisms over patient behaviour and motivation there was a potential risk to social stability. The interaction between doctor and patient was therefore part of the mechanism through which order was restored by giving the patient a specific set of expectations and actions that prevented disharmony. The doctor–patient relationship was essentially a social encounter, one event in a million similar events, which had social effects. Medicine, which for so long had stressed doctor–patient interaction as a therapeutic relationship, could now be challenged: unknown to the participant players, both were significant actors on a wider social stage.

The idea of the patient as a social actor corresponded well with the empirical problem of patients' behaviour which had been discovered in the early medico-social surveys. The notion of the sick role gave a conceptual basis for thinking about the apparent vagaries of patients' response to symptoms and medical intervention. The other themes in Parsons's original essay, namely the doctor's responsibilities in the medical encounter, were less well quoted, though they too represented a novel theoretical line of enquiry which was further developed in ensuing decades in terms of the role of the medical profession in society. (➤ Ch. 47 History of the medical profession)

Following the Parsonian model, the medical profession, like other professions, was construed as an essential component of harmonious social functioning. Echoing Carr-Saunders and Wilson's 1933 classic inter-war treatise on the medical profession,[9] social theorists saw the profession and its work as a form of ideal social organization. Here were a group of people drawn together by a commitment to the welfare of the public and sharing a common expertise: these two characteristics, namely a service ideal and an esoteric knowledge base, were the basis of any profession in society.[10] Questions then arose about exactly which occupational groups could be defined as professions and, for those aspiring to professional status, the steps that might be taken to achieve it.[11] But it was medicine that remained the archetypal profession against which all other claims had to be compared during the 1950s, and indeed for most of the 1960s.

By the end of the 1950s, the outline of the new discipline of medical sociology could be more clearly discerned. There was a 'problem' in the form of patient behaviour; there was a methodology – mainly survey techniques – which could usefully be used to investigate this problem; there were the beginnings of a theoretical base, particularly involving the sick role and the professions, which could be culled from more general sociological writings; and there were sociologists who were willing to begin to specialize in the social problems of medicine. These were necessary conditions for the emergence of the new discipline, or at least of another sub-speciality of general sociology: but the added ingredient which was to propel medical sociology to becoming the largest and most independent child of its parent discipline was medical patronage.

Organized health care has grown in size and extent throughout the twentieth century, but never as rapidly as during the latter decades. For many Western countries, upwards of 10 per cent of gross national product underpins medical care in all its forms. This has meant that medical sociology has emerged and grown during a period of remarkable expansion in medicine, with the result that it has benefited to a degree unmatched by any other branch of sociology. On its own, it is unlikely that the sociological insights of Parsons on the field of medicine would have had any more impact than his views on other institutions in society, and medicine would have remained simply another part of society that general sociologists occasionally explored. However, medicine recruited sociologists using the power and largesse that it enjoyed in increasing amounts after the Second World War. These sociologists came to see themselves as medical sociologists. Yet this patronage also had its costs, and a constant feature of the new discipline was the tension between the critical intellectual parentage of sociology and the more utilitarian resources and purposes of medicine.

The tension between these different loyalties of medical sociology has mostly manifested itself in the desire to develop and extend a conceptual and theoretical basis for the subject on the one hand, and the need to carry out those empirical studies on the 'real world', which might have more pragmatic implications. Already, at the beginning of the discipline, this tension was clear. Writing in 1957, Strauss made what has now become a classic observation: there was both a sociology *in* medicine and a sociology *of* medicine.[12] The sociology of medicine was a developing discipline based on that initial insight of Parsons, and building on the rediscovered classic work of Durkheim. As such, it treated medicine as simply another social institution through which society could be better studied. Sociology in medicine, on the other hand, was part and parcel of the medical enterprise. Certainly, it seemed much more oriented towards the patient's perspective than traditional medical practice, but it was still essentially concerned with the improvement of health services and the further amelioration of illness and disease.

This close relationship between medicine and medical sociology has continually proved rewarding and difficult. One gain for sociology has been the alliance with many critical or disaffected members of the medical community who have made significant contributions to a literature that medical sociologists are often inclined to call their own. And of course, medical sociologists have often felt privileged to be in a position to contribute directly or indirectly to patient welfare. But at times, this tutelage has proved too much for a self-professed critical discipline. How to study the golden goose in a critical way without jeopardizing the golden egg has offered the essential tension in which medical sociology has developed over the last few decades.

QUALITATIVE METHODS

Sociology and social anthropology have had a long and close relationship. In major theorists such as Durkheim and his nephew Marcel Mauss (1872–1950), they have shared a common heritage; and sociology has been particularly willing to borrow methodological techniques and conceptual frameworks from its sister discipline. While sociology started with a claim to skills in survey techniques, social anthropology professed the benefits of more-informal methods of data-gathering. Structured questionnaires were of little value in those pre-industrial societies so commonly studied by social anthropologists. In part, this was because of problems of translation and literacy, but also because the very posing of a specific question made assumptions about the respondent's world-view. Thus a question on the prevalence of headaches is meaningless if the culture does not construe head pains in this way. Anthropologists therefore developed more naturalistic, inductive methods to study alien cultures. Such methods started not with a question or hypothesis, but with a problem: the purpose of the investigation was then to gather fairly unstructured data by observation or interview, and from these 'induce' a hypothesis or statement about how things were. (➤ Ch. 60 Medicine and anthropology)

By the 1960s, it became apparent that many facets of Western culture were also alien and needed open-ended exploration using the anthropologist's ethnographic approach. Perhaps the two earliest classics in medical sociology to use this new approach were the studies of stigma and asylums carried out by Erving Goffman (1922–82).[13]

Goffman was unconcerned with the overall structures of society which had so preoccupied Parsons, nor did he turn to a questionnaire to elicit the world of the asylum inmate or of the stigmatized; after all, how could such a questionnaire be constructed without first knowing what these worlds contained? Instead, drawing upon a different theoretical tradition called symbolic interactionism,[14] Goffman focused on the everyday interactions between individuals, or social actors as they are called in this literature: the method he used was an ethnographic one, pioneered in non-industrial societies and tested during the inter-war years in some seminal work in Chicago on how people functioned 'on the street'.

Goffman obtained access to a long-stay mental hospital and simply observed. What he saw were various rituals and processes through which people were managed on a day-to-day basis. He recognized that individual identity was not compromised through some abstract structures of a distant society, but through the everyday interactions between different people and the meaning they gave their respective performances. This found an ideal illustration in the notion of stigma, which Goffman described as the discrepancy between real and virtual identities as people with their visible scars were processed remorselessly by others into having new self-perceptions. (➤ Ch. 56 Psychiatry)

Goffman's studies resonated with a recognition by sociologists that deviant behaviour existed not in the act, but in the eye of the beholder. There were no absolute 'abnormal' thoughts or deeds; rather, it was the labels that society gave to certain phenomena which determined their status.[15] Deviance was therefore established simply by the process of attaching a label to a behaviour: and clearly such labels were culturally relative in that they might vary from society to society and over time. Moreover, as Goffman's studies indicated, the labelling of certain behaviour or states as deviant could produce a 'secondary deviance' whereby the person's behaviour was changed to conform with the label.

The view that deviance in a society was a product of labelling, whether primary through the ascription of a label, or secondary through changes in behaviour, formed one of the cornerstones of the 1960s 'anti-psychiatry' movement. Many of its members were at least on the margins of medical sociology and deployed the theoretical arguments about the effects of labelling to good effect. At their most extreme, these suggested that all behaviour was inherently normal: it was psychiatrists, with their assumptions about what was socially acceptable – together with their institutionalized power-base – who produced mental illness by labelling people as either healthy or ill.[16] Several celebrated studies followed which pointed to both the apparent arbitrariness of psychiatric diagnosis and the debilitating effect of being given such a diagnosis, even provisionally.[17]

The lasting influence of the labelling perspective on mental illness, however, lay in the notion of secondary deviance, that people labelled as mentally ill gradually became ill or had their problems exacerbated by psychiatric treatment. Nowhere was this more apparent than in the large long-stay psychiatric hospitals which had survived almost intact from the nineteenth century. This is where reformers identified the damage done by incarceration and pressed for an open-door policy with more community care.[18]

The conceptual framework of labelling can claim at least some of the credit for this major shift in social and health policy. In addition, labelling has proved important in the field of disability, enabling the psycho-social problems experienced by the mentally and physically impaired – mainly brought about through the reactions of others – to be better understood and identified.[19] Indeed, the World Health Organization was sufficiently convinced of the importance of this perspective to introduce a now well accepted classification of impairment, disability, and handicap: impairment was the patient's biological deficit; disability was the degree to which function was affected; and handicap the extent of social problems, mostly brought about through labelling or the fear of labelling.[20]

If an outline of medical sociology was visible by the end of the 1950s, then its form was much more in evidence during the 1960s. This coming age of medical sociology was marked by the appearance of a specialized journal in 1960, the *Journal of Health and Human Behaviour*, its links with sociology being more confidently stated with its later retitling as the *Journal of Health and Social Behaviour*. In 1967, it was joined by *Social Science and Medicine*, which tried much more self-consciously to bridge the gap between medicine and its attendant socially oriented sciences.

CONFLICT PERSPECTIVES

In common with other areas of social life in the 1960s, the theme of conflict looms large in the theoretical development of medical sociology. The structural-functionalism of Talcott Parsons went into rapid decline and was replaced by 'conflict' theories (many strongly influenced by Marxism, in its varied forms) both within general and medical sociology. The new conflict perspective was increasingly critical of both the social and economic power of the medical profession, which seemed only to serve its own self-interest, and in turn to help perpetuate the remarkable inequalities in health status that successive surveys had identified.

From the Parsonian perspective, the medical profession had been seen as an important mechanism in the maintenance of social stability. Society had doctors because society needed doctors. The alternative thesis, that doctors existed because they had successfully wielded power in the market-place to seize a virtual monopoly of control over health-care provision, was an innovative thesis which began to gain ground.[21] This enabled the profession's past 'altruistic' acts, particularly those around licensing and registration, to be seen as less intended to 'protect the public' and more to squeeze out competition.

Perhaps the most significant break with the old sociology of the profession – which was said to have simply accepted the profession's own definition of itself – was the publication of Freidson's *Profession of Medicine* in 1970,[22] which suggested the medical profession's status was a product of political action in the widest sense. This thesis ushered in a series of new studies that 'exposed' the self-seeking aggrandizement of the profession – and at the same time caused many medical practitioners to regret employing and promoting these 'doctor bashers'!

Sociologists wishing to join this new wave of critical studies of the medical profession were attracted to historical sources for their research. The backdrop of most of these studies was the realization that the medical profession had managed to pull off an amazing feat: by the mid-twentieth century, it was extremely powerful but, unlike other commanding institutions of organized labour, the population had been persuaded that the medical profession's power was in the public interest. The roots of this achievement clearly went back to the nineteenth century, so that sociologists turned to historiographical sources, many of them secondary, to support their explanations of how medicine had succeeded. Most of these analyses focused on the marketplace. Medicine had succeeded in cornering the market for health care and it had demonstrated skilful 'occupational closure' through which new recruits to become health-care practitioners did so under the auspices of the profession, and alternatively qualified healers were driven out of business. But there were also a series of studies that examined less the political/economic ascendancy of medicine and more its cognitive triumph.

Again, in the Anglo-Saxon world at least, it was Freidson's *Profession of Medicine*, subtitled *A Study of the Sociology of Applied Knowledge*, that initially opened up a more cognitive approach to the study of medicine. Freidson tried to show that what medicine had achieved was the legitimate right to define who was ill and who was not, what was biologically abnormal and what was normal. He also claimed that 'illness may or may not have a foundation in biological reality, but it always has a foundation in social reality'. Of course, this claim had resonances in Parsons's twenty-year-old notion of the sick role – certainly all illness has a social dimension. The strong implication that it was possible for illness to exist only in social reality, without any biological correlates, was also unexceptional in view of the rhetoric of the 1960s anti-psychiatry movement: that was precisely their claim, that psychiatrists had used social judgements and not biological ones to identify/label mental illness.[23]

But there was also another more radical implication in Freidson's statement, namely that perhaps the biological reality of illness was actually irrelevant and that it was possible to perceive illness as wholly a social construct. Such an argument appears counter-intuitive: illnesses, especially those that result in death, must be fundamentally biological in nature because individuals are fundamentally complex biological machines. On the other hand, perhaps the very claim of the fundamental nature of the physical and biological realms, particularly in its relation to human identity, is part of the problem that needs to be explained. This potentially radical widening of the possibilities for critically evaluating medicine developed more fully during the following decade, but the ground was further prepared by two sociological studies that encompassed two hundred years of medical history.

In 1972, Johnson published a short monograph entitled *Professions and Power*,[24] in which he described three historical phases of professional organization: namely patronage, collegiate, and mediated. The basis for this division was his quasi-Marxist analysis of the relationship between professions as producers (of a service) and their clients as consumers. In any transaction between producers and consumers there is always an irreducible element of uncertainty, or indeterminacy, as he called it, which both sides struggle to control. In the eighteenth century, this indeterminacy in the medical consultation was largely controlled by patients because they tended to hold higher social and economic positions: thus the medical profession was organized under a system of patronage. During the nineteenth century, the medical profession seized control of the indeterminacy contained in medical knowledge as their work shifted to the new hospitals and their clients were drawn increasingly from lower social and economic strata. (➤ Ch. 49 The hospital) This enabled medicine to organize itself along self-governing collegiate lines. During the twentieth century, governments and other third parties (particularly insurance companies) have become more and more involved with the funding of health care; these agencies have thus begun to claim the right to control the indeterminacy factor by monitoring and influencing what doctors actually do in clinical situations. This represents the third phase of professional organization, namely third-party mediation. According to a recent study by Starr (see Further Reading) of the medical profession in the United States over the last two hundred years, this process may have almost reached the point where medicine has lost its former pre-eminence as an autonomous self-governing body able to define the nature of illness and what should be done about it. (➤ Ch. 50 Medical institutions and the state; Ch. 57 Health economics)

For Johnson, the key to professional organization was control over knowledge. Four years later, his colleague, Jewson, extended this analysis by examining the form of the knowledge itself under these different regimes of professional organization.[25] First, under patronage, or Bedside Medicine, as Jewson referred to it, the patient controlled the relationship such that medical practice was primarily based on the patient's view as expressed through symptoms. It was therefore the client's view of the world based on detailed recounting and classification of symptoms that was embodied in late eighteenth-century medical knowledge. (➤ Ch. 35 The art of diagnosis: medicine and the five senses)

With the advent of a collegiate system of professional control, a regime of Hospital Medicine came to dominate. Patients' views as expressed through symptoms were then subordinated to the doctor's perspective on illness, which was informed by pathology. A specific pathological lesion hidden within the body became the locus of illness, not the capricious movement of obscure symptoms. This meant that the patient had to defer to the doctor's knowledge of the true nature of illness, which occurred beyond immediate lay perception. Thus the relative relationship of activity and passivity between doctor and patient produced a system of medical knowledge, namely pathological medicine – with its concomitant clinical examinations and post-mortems – which, in its turn, reproduced the particular form of the doctor–patient relationship characterized by a subservient patient. This process was further extended in the late nineteenth and early twentieth centuries, according to Jewson, by the increasing reliance on Laboratory Medicine, in which the 'sick-man' became even further divorced from the immediate reality of his illness. (➤ Ch. 9 The pathological tradition)

Jewson's account of the shifts in medical knowledge described an increasing alienation of patients from their own illnesses through the imposition of the medical intermediary. His work thus belongs to that humanist (and at times, Marxist) trend in medical sociology which has seen itself struggling for patients' rights in the face of medical domination. This influence can also be seen in the discovery, or rediscovery, of major inequalities in health status.

Of course, looking to the past, it had long been apparent that poor people had worse health. Indeed, McKeown's seminal argument, summarized in his *The Role of Medicine*,[26] has pointed to the irrelevance of medicine and formal health care for most improvements in the health of the population, particularly the increase in life-expectancy since the mid-nineteenth century, and the major significance of nutrition, sanitation, and good housing, which were all intimately related to standard of living. (➤ Ch. 51 Public health) With the coming of the welfare state in many European countries, and general improvements in conditions of life, it had been anticipated that health inequalities based on deprivation would gradually disappear. Indeed, for a brief period in the 1960s, the notion of 'diseases of affluence' gained some ground. But using the results of surveys conducted by epidemiologists, government departments, and sociologists, it seemed clear that despite all the improvements in the standard of living during the twentieth century, the relative health statuses of different classes of the population either had been maintained or had even widened.[27] (➤ Ch. 71 Demography and medicine)

This phenomenon fitted the Marxist framework well. In the classic conflict between capital and labour, the latter was gradually immiserated: this damage to their material resources, in turn, had its effect on their health. The rise of the welfare state and general improvements in standard of living meant that progressive impoverishment was not the destiny of Western working classes, but nevertheless the data on health inequalities showed that for all this apparent improvement in their circumstances, the working class seemed to suffer much greater mortality and morbidity than their fellow citizens.[28] In part, this indictment was aimed at the class structure of modern societies, but in part it was also aimed at the providers of health care – from governments to medical practitioners – with their biases that consciously or unconsciously militated against working-class groups.[29] (➤ Ch. 72 Medicine, mortality, and morbidity)

Sociologists thus became concerned, as had epidemiologists before them, with measuring the health of the population so that the differences in health status of different groups – social classes, women, ethnic minorities, etc. – could be properly established. At first, it simply involved a close reading and secondary analysis of existing mortality data; but later, it moved into an examination of the features of the social and economic status of classes, women, and ethnic groups which might explain the apparent mortality differentials. There was some debate about the relative importance of these different factors, in particular whether health was damaged by material deprivation such as poor diet, inadequate housing, and paucity of resources in general, or by cultural factors such as the choices made by different groups of how to spend their income or in their attitudes to health and illness prevention. Both were no doubt important, and probably interrelated, but it was material factors that sociologists seemed to view as the most significant.

If material conditions did indeed relate closely to ill health, this would require additional resources to rectify. However, this proposition was advanced at precisely the same point at which the funding of health care was proving an almost bottomless pit. This led to a variety of alternative responses. In part, it was a question of becoming more effective and efficient with existing health-care resources, including the development of specific rationing mechanisms.[30] On the other hand, the need for additional resources could be challenged in terms of their consistent failure to solve the problems to which they were addressed. In a celebrated attack on the resources devoted to health care, Ivan Illich pointedly asked to what extent the seemingly never-ending health problems of the populations are a consequence of the provision of health care.[31] For Illich – and many critics of the New Right – it was the generous provision of health-care services (and indeed any welfare programme) that undermined the ability of individuals to cope with illnesses in the way that they were believed to have done in the past. Health services were not therapeutic, but iatrogenic. In consequence, people became increasingly dependent on the health system to sustain them through all life's minor as well as major tribulations. This perspective added an alternative voice to the usual chorus about the health-damaging effects of resource shortages: was pouring more resources into health care and offering a widening range of services always of value to patients? Certainly, the assumption of many doctors that more means better was not necessarily supported by the available evidence.

The argument that medicine might harm also resonated with further developments in relating the notion of 'social control', as laid out in Parsons's model of the doctor–patient relationship, more specifically to modern medicine. Far from control being exercised for patient welfare and wider social well-being, medicine seemed to be extending its interest and involvement into the minutiae of social life: not only were considerable medical resources available for the ill, but even the healthy were being persuaded that they were still 'at risk' and could usefully follow medical advice. The net effect was the increasing 'medicalization' of everyday life.[32] Medicine was seen to be replacing the role of the church and the law in policing the boundary between normal and abnormal. At its mildest, 'experts' took responsibility away from people, thereby rendering them more docile; at its most extreme, people were being controlled and manipulated by a subtle and potentially dangerous force.

SOCIAL FACTORS

The problem with mortality figures – and also with the rather limited morbidity data available – was that they were inherently crude and 'medicocentric' in their focus. Patients, as had long been recognized, saw the world differently and often seemed to have different views of health. Sociologists therefore began to look to alternative measures of health status which could encapsulate the patient's perspective. Some of the conceptual ground had been prepared by the recognition that impairment had a functional and social consequence that constituted an important part of the illness for the patient (see p. 1649);[33] but in addition, sociologists, often in collaboration with epidemiologists, began to develop 'subjective' health measures which would enable the patient's perspective to be incorporated into an understanding of the health of the population.[34]

The recognition that illness had an important social dimension that could be measured went hand-in-hand with a recognition that 'social factors' were important aetiological agents. The health inequalities of different social groups had alerted sociologists to the importance of 'group membership' for certain illnesses. In part, this could be explained in terms of the material resources available to group members or the culture of the group, but this failed to explain the often considerable variation in health status within the group itself. In a sense, social classes, genders, and ethnic minorities were too crude to tease out the social factors that produced illness in an individual.

Again working closely with social epidemiologists, medical sociologists began to explore the relationship between social factors and illness.[35] Some of this research was directed at uncovering the links between various facets of life-style and their health correlates,[36] particularly as this integrated with the needs of the growing health promotion and illness strategies of the 1970s and 1980s. Other research emphasized the importance of life events and social support. Psychologists had already reported on the effects of stress on health but, despite the initial promise, stress was proving remarkably difficult to define consistently across many studies. Life events, however, provided a more clearly defined personal 'insult' which could be studied. Observations of bereavement reactions had shown the powerful immediate effects of a negative life event, and work was pursued to explore the role of life events in psychiatric illness,[37] particularly depression, and in organic illness.[38]

One of the factors that seemed to ameliorate the effect of an unpleasant life event was a close social network. This finding was entirely congruent with Durkheim's early work on suicide, where again the risk seemed to be closely related to the social isolation of the individual. Thus there were firm grounds for believing that good social support might prevent illness, or at least reduce its impact.[39] Early survey work was promising, but as with stress research, definitions became a problem: what exactly was meant by social support? At first, it was measured by numbers of daily contacts with others, but this failed to take into account the quality of those contacts. But then, what was quality? If it was to be defined according to patient criteria – and that seemed sensible as it was the patient who was affected – then it was the person's perception of these relationships that was important. This led to the realization that it might not be the actual social-support network that was important, but the person's perception or belief that he or she had such a network. This would certainly help explain some of the observed differences in health status between those who described themselves as religious against those who did not, even allowing for different behaviours and contacts.[40]

Research into the role of different social factors in the aetiology of illness continues; it is complex both in research design and in the definition and measurement of these various rather nebulous social phenomena. But what this research has shown is the potential degree to which human illness can yield to explanation in psychological and social terms. That branch of sociology *in* medicine, which seemed to have succumbed to the pre-eminence of medicine, now seems to be beginning to take a leading role in directing medicine into new areas of research.

COGNITIONS

In the closing two decades of the twentieth century, health care has moved increasingly towards more social concerns – not least because of a crisis of funding in Western health-care systems and a rising consumerism. This has meant that many areas of medicine have developed a more social perspective, and the line that separates sociology in medicine and areas such as social epidemiology, social psychiatry, and primary health care has become increasingly blurred. This has meant that further opportunities have arisen for the development and extension of sociological methods into medicine itself, and for the recruitment of more sociologists. Sociology, from being the dangerous subject of the 1960s, is more frequently seen as a normal component of the range of skills and perspectives employed in medical research.

Yet perhaps in retrospect the area which will be seen to have been the most innovative during the 1980s and 1990s is the use of qualitative methods to explore cognitive issues. Studies during the 1970s of 'everyday life' were extended in the 1980s into a critical analytic tool. This perspective has been applied increasingly to medical environments and interactions to uncover the complex social processes going on. Perhaps many of the papers published in *Sociology of Health and Illness*, first published in 1979, best reflect this position.

These techniques have also been used to explore patients' experience of health and illness. Indeed, the problems of living with and experiencing illness have become important facets of the growth of research in medical sociology in recent years. It is no longer sufficient to study the social factors causing or surrounding diseases such as diabetes, epilepsy, or multiple sclerosis without exploring the actual experience of these illnesses by patients.[41]

This concern wtih patients' cognitions has also given the problem of illness behaviour a new lease of life. Anthropologists had observed that patients in pre-industrial societies had elaborate explanations, quite unrelated to the ideas of Western medicine, for why they became ill and what was the most appropriate treatment. Extension of this work to Western societies produced the realization that here too people used and depended on often sophisticated explanatory models for their illnesses, which were often at variance with 'offical' accounts.[42] For example, biomedicine explains an upper respiratory tract infection in terms of a virus, whereas most lay people seem to have ideas about draughts, wet hair, cold feet, etc., together with appropriate 'folk' remedies.[43] It thus became possible to begin to explain the 50 per cent of patients who fail to comply with medical instructions in terms of a failure of the doctor to identify the real underlying problem. Thus sociologists could advise doctors that part of the consultation should be spent eliciting and dealing with the patient's 'lay theories', as this cognitive need was an important dimension of many encounters.[44] (➤ Ch. 2 What is specific to Western medicine?; Ch. 29 Non-Western concepts of disease)

While sociologists expressed greater interest in patients' cognitions, there was a parallel move to examine medical cognitions critically. Medical knowledge had long seemed inviolable to sociological investigation: after all, it was highly technical and came under the trusteeship of 'science' as a form of 'privileged' knowledge. However, the exclusivity and epistemological superiority of scientific knowledge was itself under siege from the sociology of science, and the way was soon open for sociologists to invade the citadel of medicine.

There is a long and continuing debate within sociology about the exact role of knowledge in social processes. Mainly informed by a Durkheimian perspective, knowledge has been seen as a reflection of social forms. However, there have been repeated attempts to identify a body of knowledge which would somehow transcend the society from which it emerged: for example, the Marxist claim was always that workers had access to a more fundamental truth through their class position. Following the decline in religious belief in Western societies, it was scientific knowledge that managed to gain widespread social recognition of its privileged position. (➤ Ch. 61 Religion and medicine) Certainly, social factors might play a part in determining the time and circumstances of the discovery of new scientific facts, but the veracity of those facts was of a different order to the bias and values inherent in social knowledge. But the view that society could only influence the timing and appearance of scientific facts was challenged by the publication of Kuhn's *The Structure of Scientific Revolutions* in 1962.[45] Since then, the sociology of science has increasingly examined and challenged the claims of privilege that science has traditionally made.

This perspective has been applied to medical knowledge to argue that all medical categories, particularly diseases, are ultimately social 'constructions'. Diseases, being pathological processes, represent abnormal functioning, but abnormality cannot be identified in nature other than by using social criteria. Thus, all diseases somehow represent and reflect the various social patterns of their origin.

Jewson's argument (see p. 1652) that the extant form of medical cognition reproduced the social relations of production of that knowledge is an example of work in this vein, as is Foucault's *Birth of the Clinic*, first published in 1963 (but long in translation and even longer in recognition), as well as his later work.[46] Foucault's notions of power and surveillance have since been employed to explore the emergence of the current dominant biomedical model, which basically reduces illness to an intracorporeal biological lesion. The mechanisms of power, which are said to have pervaded Western society since the end of the eighteenth century, are used as a method of explaining the emergence of various facets of modern medical practice, particularly the hospital, post-mortem, and clinical examination. These techniques were used in the nineteenth century to 'discover' the human body. Parallel processes of exploring patient's talk have characterized much of twentieth-century medical development with a concomitant 'discovery' of the human mind and social relations.[47]

MEDICAL SOCIOLOGY AND THE HISTORY OF MEDICINE

The relationship of medical sociology to medical history might be described as that of a 'cognate discipline'. Its closest connection is with the social history of medicine, with which it shares the task of explaining various medical phenomena, often with seemingly similar methodological tools. Even so, there are significant differences between the two sub-disciplines.

Medical sociologists have tended to examine medical practice in the latter half of the twentieth century, although their interest has on occasion extended to the earlier parts of the century (when modern medicine and its associated health care apparently began its current phase of development), which has been more the preserve of the social historian. A very few medical sociologists have really invaded the historian's territory by going back as far as the late eighteenth and early nineteenth centuries to explore the origins of the current biomedical model.

Historians have applied traditional bibliographic methods to understanding the textured nature of medical events over the last two centuries, whereas sociologists have approached them in a more eclectic way. Medical sociologists first made their mark with quantitative studies, but more recently have emphasized the importance of qualitative approaches. These latter seem more in accord with many historical methods, which examine the empirical world and induce a more general statement or theory about what was happening. Indeed, the open-ended collection of speech 'data' might be carried out by sociologists or oral historians, and their analyses show similar logical patterns – though perhaps the sociologist's is more formalized.

However, sociologists have not extended this open-ended more qualitative method to historical material: when they have investigated historiographic data, it has been in a much more deductive manner, starting from some over-arching theoretical position. On these occasions, sociologists have opened up the texts knowing what they were looking for, whether it was evidence of class struggle, or occupational closure, or surveillance mechanisms. Some historians might make a similar explicit claim to a theoretical deductive schema, but many, like most ethnographers in sociology, would argue the virtues of theory emerging from the data rather than data being selected to fit the theory. Nevertheless, all research starts from some assumptions and arguably an atheoretical position may well harbour a closet Whig. The strength of medical sociology, it can be argued, is that these theoretical and methodological debates are part of the explicit agenda as different ways are explored to bring medicine more closely into focus. (➤ Ch. 4 Medical care)

NOTES

1　Emile Durkheim, *The Division of Labour in Society*, New York, Macmillan, 1933.
2　Emile Durkheim, *The Rules of Sociological Method*, Chicago, IL, Chicago University Press, 1938.
3　Emile Durkheim, *Suicide: a Study in Sociology*, London, Routledge & Kegan Paul, 1952.
4　K. Box and G. Thomas, 'The war-time social survey', *Journal of the Royal Statistical Society*, 1944, 107: 151; Paul Lazarsfeld, 'Expository review of "The American Soldier" ', *Public Opinion Quarterly*, 1949, 3: 337–404.
5　I. M. Rosenstock, 'Why people use health services', *Milbank Memorial Fund Quarterly*, 1965, 44: 95.
6　E. Koos, *The Health of Regionsville: What the People Felt and Did About It*, New York, Columbia University Press, 1954.
7　David Mechanic and E. H. Volkart, 'Illness behaviour and medical diagnosis', *Journal of Health and Human Behaviour*, 1960, 1: 86–94; Mechanic, 'The concept of illness behaviour', *Journal of Chronic Diseases*, 1962, 15: 189–94; I. K. Zola, 'Pathways to the doctor: from person to patient', *Social Science and Medicine*, 1973, 7: 677–89.
8　Talcott Parsons, *The Social System*, New York, Free Press, 1951.
9　A. M. Carr-Saunders and P. A. Wilson, *The Professions*, Oxford, Oxford University Press, 1933.
10　W. J. Goode, 'Encroachment, charlatanism and the emerging profession: psychiatry, sociology and medicine', *American Sociological Review*, 1960, 25: 902–14.
11　H. Wilensky, 'The professionalisation of everyone', *American Journal of Sociology*, 1964, 70: 137–58.
12　Robert Strauss, 'The nature and status of medical sociology', *American Sociological Review*, 1957, 22: 200–4.
13　Erving Goffman, *Asylums: Essays on the Social Situation of Mental Patients and Other Inmates*, London, Penguin, 1961; Goffman, *Stigma: Notes on the Management of Spoiled Identity*, London, Penguin, 1963.
14　A. M. Rose (ed.), *Human Behaviour and Social Processes: an Interactionist Approach*, London, Routledge & Kegan Paul, 1962.
15　E. Lemert, *Human Deviance, Social Problems and Social Control*, Hemel Hempstead, Prentice Hall, 1967; Howard S. Becker, *Outsiders: Studies in the*

Sociology of Deviance, London, Free Press, 1963; E. Schur, *Labelling Deviant Behaviour*, London, Harper & Row, 1971.

16 Thomas S. Szasz, *The Myth of Mental Illness*, St Albans, Paladin, 1962; David Ingleby (ed.), *Critical Psychiatry: the Politics of Mental Health*, London, Penguin, 1981.

17 D. Rosenhan *et al.*, 'On being sane in insane places', *Science*, 1973, 179: 250–8.

18 K. Jones and A. J. Fowles, *Ideas on Institutions: Analysing the Literature on Long-Term Care and Custody*, London, Routledge & Kegan Paul, 1984; though Scull argues the economic reasons for closing the mental hospitals: Andrew T. Scull, *Decarceration*, Englewood Cliffs, NJ, Prentice Hall, 1977.

19 R. A. Scott, *The Making of Blind Men*, London, Russell Sage, 1969; P. C. Higgins, *Outsiders in a Hearing World: a Sociology of Deafness*, London, Sage, 1980.

20 P. Wood, *Classification of Impairments and Handicap*, Geneva, World Health Organization, 1975; WHO, *International Classification of Impairments, Disabilities and Handicaps*, Geneva, WHO, 1980.

21 J. L. Berlant, *Profession and Monopoly: a Study of Medicine in the United States and Great Britain*, Berkeley, University of California Press, 1975; N. Parry and J. Parry, *The Rise of the Medical Profession*, London, Croom Helm, 1976.

22 Eliot Freidson, *Profession of Medicine: a Study of the Sociology of Applied Knowledge*, New York, Dodd Mead, 1970.

23 Peter Sedgewick, 'Mental illness *is* illness', *Salmagundi*, 1973, 20: 196–224.

24 T. J. Johnson, *Professions and Power*, London, Macmillan, 1972.

25 N. K. Jewson, 'Disappearance of the sick-man from medical cosmologies, 1770–1870', *Sociology*, 1976, 10: 225–44.

26 T. McKeown, *The Role of Medicine*, Oxford, Blackwell, 1979.

27 A. B. Hollingshead and F. C. Redlich, *Social Class and Mental Illness: a Community Study*, New York, John Wiley, 1958; P. Townsend and N. Davidson, *The Black Report*, London, Penguin, 1982.

28 L. Doyal, *The Political Economy of Health*, London, Pluto Press, 1979.

29 V. Navarro, *Medicine under Capitalism*, New York, Prodist, 1976; H. Waitzkin, 'Medicine, superstructure and micropolitics', *Social Science and Medicine*, 1979, 13: 601–9.

30 H. J. Aaron and W. B. Schwartz, *The Painful Prescription: Rationing Hospital Care*, Washington, DC, Brookings Institution, 1984.

31 Ivan Illich, *Medical Nemesis*, London, Caldar Boyars, 1974; Illich, *Limits to Medicine*, London, Caldar Boyars, 1978.

32 I. K. Zola, 'Medicine as an institution of social control', *Sociological Review*, 1972, 20: 487–504.

33 S. Katz *et al.*, 'The Index of ADL: a standardized measure of biological and psychosocial function', *Journal of the American Medical Association*, 1963, 185: 914–19.

34 S. Hunt *et al.*, *Measuring Health Status*, London, Croom Helm, 1986; I. McDowell and C. Newell, *Measuring Health Status: a Guide to Rating Scales and Questionnaires*, Oxford, Oxford University Press, 1987; J. G. Hollandsworth, 'Evaluating the impact of medical treatment on the quality of life: a 5-year update', *Social Science and Medicine*, 1988, 26: 425–34.

35 J. Cassel, 'The contribution of social environment to host resistance', *American Journal of Epidemiology*, 1976, 90: 171–200.

36 Mildred Blaxter, *Health and Lifestyles*, London, Routledge, 1990.

37 George W. Brown and T. Harris, *Social Origins of Depression: a Study of Psychiatric Disorder in Women*, London, Tavistock, 1978; B. S. Dohrenwend and B. P. Dorenwend (eds), *Stressful Life Events and their Context*, New York, Prodist, 1981.

38 Francis Creed, 'Life events and physical illness: a review', *Journal of Psychosomatic Research*, 1985, 29: 113–24.

39 L. F. Berkman and S. L. Syme, 'Social networks, host resistance, and mortality: a nine year follow-up study of Alameda County residents', *American Journal of Epidemiology*, 1979, 109: 186–204; S. A. Henderson, 'A development in social psychiatry: the systematic study of social bonds', *Journal of Nervous and Mental Diseases*, 1980, 168: 63–9.

40 F. V. Kasl and A. N. Ostfield, 'Psychosocial predictors of mortality among the elderly poor: the role of religion, well-being and social contact', *American Journal of Epidemiology*, 1984, 119: 410–23.

41 Mildred Blaxter, *The Meaning of Disability*, London, Heinemann, 1976; R. Fitzpatrick *et al.*, *The Experience of Illness*, London, Tavistock, 1984; G. Scambler and A. Hopkins, 'Being epileptic: coming to terms with stigma', *Sociology of Health and Illness*, 1986, 8: 26–43; R. Anderson and M. Bury (eds), *Living with Chronic Illness*, Boston, MA, Unwin Hyman, 1988.

42 A. Kleinman *et al.*, 'Culture, illness and cure', *Annals of Internal Medicine*, 1978, 88: 251–9; D. Blumhagen, 'Hypertension: a folk illness with a medical name', *Culture, Medicine and Psychiatry*, 1980, 4: 197–227.

43 Cecil Helman, ' "Feed a cold starve a fever" – folk models of infection in an English suburban community and their relation to medical treatment,' *Culture, Medicine and Psychiatry*, 1978, 2: 107–37.

44 David Tuckett *et al.*, *Meetings Between Experts: an Approach to Sharing Ideas in Medical Consultations*, London, Tavistock, 1985.

45 T. S. Kuhn, *The Structure of Scientific Revolutions*, Chicago, IL, Chicago University Press, 1962.

46 Michel Foucault, *The Birth of the Clinic: an Archaeology of Medical Perception*, London, Tavistock, 1963; Foucault, *Discipline and Punish: the Birth of the Prison*, Harmondsworth, Penguin, 1977.

47 David Armstrong, *Political Anatomy of the Body: Medical Knowledge in Britain in the Twentieth Century*, Cambridge, Cambridge University Press, 1983; Armstrong, 'The patient's view', *Social Science and Medicine*, 1984, 18: 737–44.

FURTHER READING

Armstrong, David, *Political Anatomy of the Body: Medical Knowledge in Britain in the Twentieth Century*, Cambridge, Cambridge University Press, 1983.

Arney, William R. and Bergen, Bernard J., *Medicine and the Management of Living: Taming the Last Great Beast*, Chicago, IL, Chicago University Press, 1982.

Atkinson, Paul, *The Clinical Experience: the Construction and Reconstruction of Medical Reality*, Farnborough, Gower, 1981.

Brown, George W. and Harris, T., *Social Origins of Depression: a Study of Psychiatric Disorder in Women*, London, Tavistock, 1978.

Fitzpatrick, R. *et al.*, *The Experience of Illness*, London, Tavistock, 1984.

Foucault, Michel, *The Birth of the Clinic: an Archaeology of Medical Perception*, London, Tavistock, 1963.

Freidson, Eliot, *Profession of Medicine: a Study of the Sociology of Applied Knowledge*, New York, Dodd Mead, 1970.

Goffman, Erving, *Asylums: Essays on the Social Situation of Mental Patients and Other Inmates*, London, Penguin, 1961.

Jewson, N. K., 'Disappearance of the sick-man from medical cosmologies, 1770–1870', *Sociology*, 1976, 10: 225–44.

Kleinman, Arthur, *Patients and Healers in the Context of Culture*, Berkeley, University of California Press, 1980.

McKeown, T., *The Role of Medicine*, Oxford, Blackwell, 1979.

Morgan, M., Calnan, M. and Manning, N., *Sociological Approaches to Health and Medicine*, London, Croom Helm, 1985.

Starr, Paul, *The Social Transformation of American Medicine*, New York, Basic Books, 1982.

71

DEMOGRAPHY AND MEDICINE

Richard M. Smith

INTRODUCTION

The mid-1950s constitute a phase in which a flow of publications witnessed both the emergence of a new historical sub-discipline within demography and a highly specific interpretation by a distinguished professor of social medicine of the causes of the great rise of population that began in the eighteenth century. Developments originating in that decade were to ensure that, thereafter, historical demography and medical history, or more precisely the social history of medicine, were to become fully intertwined, with very considerable mutual benefits.

In 1955, Thomas McKeown and R. G. Brown published a highly influential article denying or minimizing the medical contribution to the mortality declines which they regarded as largely responsible for population growth in eighteenth-century England.[1] The following year, there was published in France a technical research manual by M. Fleury and L. Henry, which laid out a method of deriving meaningful measures of demographic processes from ancient and often incomplete parish registers.[2] This small volume set in train a revolution both in methods adopted by, and findings accruing to, those researchers who were increasingly to be recognized as historical demographers. This chapter will review the context within which these two 'landmarks' occurred and how the subsequent development of historical demography has contributed to an understanding of the modern rise of population and, in particular, to the role played by falling mortality. (➤ Ch. 72 Medicine, mortality, and morbidity)

In the period following the Second World War, demography had grown significantly as a discipline and had done so in a climate of rising concern for understanding the reasons underlying rapid population growth in the less developed regions of the world. Such an interest was also indirectly stimulating the research of economic historians, who were seeking to improve their understanding of the demographic conditions against or within which industrialization had developed in the European past. The conditions applying in England were obviously the focus of their attention, given that country's primacy in experiencing so-called agricultural and industrial revolutions and associated increases in productivity. All participants in this debate assessed their evidence against the intellectual background of the global process of secular change known as the 'Demographic Transition'. This theory is generally considered to have been most comprehensively formulated in 1944 by F. W. Notestein, then Director of the Princeton Office of Population Research, at an international conference concerning world food supplies. It proposed that noteworthy population growth occurred during industrialization because fertility remained uncontrolled and high, whilst mortality declined on account of improved food supplies and personal living standards created by the 'industrial revolution', which subsumed other improvements in transport, agricultural output, public health and medical practice. Notestein supposed that 'the whole process of modernisation in Europe and overseas brought rising levels of living, new controls over disease and reduced mortality . . . mean while fertility was much less responsive to the process of modernisation.'[3] In Notestein's formulation, fertility's fall would be lagged behind that of mortality because of the deeply embedded behavioural patterns that buttressed high fertility to compensate for the heavy mortality that was assumed to afflict pre-modern societies. Eventually, however, the cumulative effects of industrialization and of all its social correlates undermined the norms of behaviour that served to sustain high fertility. When viewed within terms of this model, the 'modern rise of population' is an integral part of the Demographic Transition and falls within its second phase: the phase of declining mortality, but intransigently high fertility. Demographic Transition Theory is a classic evolutionary model of the kind that became so common in the natural and social sciences from the late nineteenth century. It is premissed upon a dogmatic notion of irreversible sequential change. As a demographic model, it was formulated within the classical theory of the determinants of population dynamics, which are conventionally associated with T. R. Malthus (1766–1834) and his intellectual peers. The theory in its initial construction treats both fertility and mortality as endogenously determined by the underlying economy and society and particularly sensitive to the quantity and price of food. Malthus's demographic theory, at least in its earliest versions, identified strongly with the 'positive check', which assumes a positive relationship between food-price changes and mortality. However, in later versions of his famous essay, Malthus came to emphasize the way in which the positive check might be superseded by a 'preventive check' if the incidence and age of marriage were sensitive to changes in the level of economic well-being.[4] It is apparent that these classical assumptions underpinning Malthus's approach to the determinants of mortality are readily detectable in the inter-war writings of such scholars as Talbot Griffith, Margaret Buer, A. M. Carr-Saunders, and Dorothy George, who all explained England's eighteenth-century mortality decline in terms of a range of prior social and economic changes, including the growth of medical knowledge and practice, improvements in social administration and public health, increased food production, and decreased consumption of alcohol.[5] It is noteworthy that these scholars in their approaches to the determinants of mortality change employed multi-factorial explanations.

Thomas McKeown, who undoubtedly should be regarded as an exponent of the classical position in the post-war period, continued to emphasize a particular variant of the positive check in his interpretation of the determinants of mortality and the primacy of mortality over fertility changes in driving the demographic motor of the eighteenth century. His ideas were developed in a number of individually and jointly authored essays, which were brought together in 1976 in his *The Modern Rise of Population*.[6] His argument depended very heavily on the returns of deaths classified by age and certified by cause that were available as a result of the implementation of a system of civil registration in England and Wales from July 1837. By disaggregating these data, he attempted to show that reductions in causes of death associated with airborne micro-organisms (especially tuberculosis) had contributed most to mortality decline from 1848 to 1971, followed, some considerable way behind, by causes associated with water- and food-borne organisms. Through a resort to argument by exclusion, McKeown built up his powerful thesis. He claimed that medical advances could not have been responsible for the decline of mortality since, apart from smallpox and diphtheria, most other diseases, which had by far the largest impact on the rise in life expectancy, were declining long before effective chemotherapy or other techniques of care were available to combat them. He applied much the same argument to the role played by sanitary and public-health measures which he saw as available only from the very late nineteenth century, although mortality decline long pre-dated their presence. (➤ Ch. 51 Public health) Furthermore, improvements in life expectancy that flowed from a decline in the incidence of causes linked with water- and food-borne micro-organisms were responsible for a small proportion of the mortality fall. Since he had shown that airborne micro-organisms accounted for the bulk of mortality decline in the nineteenth and twentieth centuries, McKeown felt confident that there was little place for processes that depended upon the spontaneous decline of pathogenic virulence or upon the reduced exposure to infection. As a consequence, resistance to infectious disease must have increased through an improvement of nutrition. His devastating critique of the case for eighteenth-century medical improvement may subsequently have caused some of his readers to lose sight of the fact that many of McKeown's predecessors, who were the subject of his attack, had also suggested a role for dietary improvements and greater predictability of the food supply in the mortality fall.[7]

It has recently been suggested that McKeown was really arguing not about the past, but about the present, since it could be contended that no one had ever claimed that medical treatment made a substantial impact on the European mortality decline.[8] In fact, it is possible to detect in his writings a tendency over time to depress the role he had been initially willing to allocate to medicine. In 1965, he was moved to identify at least three phases through which purposeful human intervention grew in significance in the determination of mortality: 'We conclude that the advance in health since the eighteenth century has been due to a rising standard of living from about 1770; sanitary measures, from 1870 and therapy during the twentieth century.'[9] In his celebrated Rock Carling monograph, *The Role of Medicine*, there was barely a place for medical therapy, for in the historic past he perceived in order of importance the determinants of health to be 'nutritional, environmental and behavioural'.[10] Indeed, he went so far as to claim that it had not proved necessary to understand the mechanisms of disease to control them, only to comprehend their origins and risk factors. Whether it is correct to perceive this position as a manifestation of McKeown's evident emphasis on the caring function of medicine as a counterweight to the hegemony of postwar medicine's perceived role as a 'curing' activity based upon high-tech, highly specialized hospital-based services is difficult to prove. It is, however, clear that his later writing on this topic came to be associated with a rather narrow standard-of-living determinism, indeed nutritional determinism.

McKeown's approach also became characterized by overt hostility towards many of the developments that were occurring and serving to create a self-conscious community of historical demographers. He was, of course, aware of the high hopes that demographers and economic historians were placing on parish registers in their investigations, but regarded them as unreliable sources for which too many allowances for under-registration and variability of recording of burials and baptisms from place to place had to be made. Such volatility in their data, he believed, made it impossible to infer national patterns from parish register-based case studies. McKeown remained instead committed to a method that assessed the reasons for mortality decline in the eighteenth century by extrapolating backwards in time from data revealed in the published reports of the Registrar General after 1837. For he wrote, 'if in the light of knowledge of the diseases that declined after 1838 it is concluded that specific measures of preventing or treating disease in the individual made no significant contribution to the reduction of the death rate by the nineteenth century, it seems reasonable to conclude that such measures are very unlikely to have been effective a hundred years earlier.'[11] Such a view of the eighteenth century was developed without specific reference either to demographic or nutritional evidence. This method led him inexorably to advocate the mortality declines of the eighteenth and nineteenth centuries as part of a unitary process – a secular trend that, once initiated, stretched over the following two centuries.

THE INSTABILITY OF MORTALITY

McKeown's calculated disregard of parish register based demographic research is perhaps surprising since, in the period prior to 1965 or 1970 when he was formulating his views about the primacy of nutrition, there had developed in France a school of historians who through their use of data on grain prices and death counts in parish registers had interpreted high mortality in the short run to be a direct product of high prices associated with harvest failure. In fact, by the early 1960s, the writings of French historians such as Jean Meuvret and Pierre Goubert on the *crise de subsistance* had achieved the status of classics.[12] Theirs was a mode of analysis for which Goubert's famous remark relating to the secular variations in mortality in the region of Beauvais in the late seventeenth and early eighteenth centuries stands as a leit motiv: 'The price of wheat almost always constitutes a true demographic barometer. The range and frequency of the fluctuations in grain prices control the size and frequency of the population crises. And these play a large part in determining population movements and even its size.'[13] The decline in the frequency of such crises could then be easily incorporated into demographic transition theory. Indeed, it was not difficult for the work of such economic-demographic historians to be subsumed within the argument of leading demographers, for instance Kingsley Davis who, in his survey of the Indian subcontinent in the first half of the twentieth century, believed he had found a characteristic pre-transitional population growth pattern in which the modest advances accumulated in 'normal' years only to be eliminated by recurrent crises that were principally related to subsistence.[14]

It is perhaps no coincidence that McKeown's first major essay on the modern rise of population coincided with the completion in 1955 of Karl Helleiner's magisterial conspectus of European population trends from the fourteenth to the eighteenth century, in which he had concluded that the eighteenth century saw a lessening of the frequency of mortality crises and a damping-down of the instabilities that had characterized earlier centuries.[15] However, Helleiner was not of the opinion that this instability was predominantly based upon variability in the adequacy of the food base, but emphasized variation in the intensity of epidemic disease that was autonomous of economy and society. Helleiner thought that it was of very great significance that genuine population growth finally became apparent in the wake of the disappearance of bubonic plague, the incidence of which could not be systematically correlated with subsistence short-falls. McKeown was sharply critical of such an approach, and clearly had Helleiner in mind when he wrote about those who were prepared 'even to attribute the remarkable growth of population before registration to the behaviour of a single disease'.[16] (➤ Ch. 52 Epidemiology)

THE TECHNICAL REVOLUTION IN HISTORICAL DEMOGRAPHY

While McKeown's position regarding the modern growth of population, in particular his denial of any significant medical contribution, was widely diffused, especially to an audience of medical historians, practitioners of social medicine, and epidemiologists, the parish registers came to be used by historical demographers in ways that were completely novel when contrasted with the earlier approaches to those sources which, with considerable justification, McKeown had regarded so suspiciously. The innovations were primarily directed towards solving a severe technical problem: the need to assemble information relating to both the number of vital events occurring in a population (for example, deaths among males aged five to nine) and the numbers within that age range 'at risk' to experience that event (that is, the actual number of males of that age in the population). After 1837 in England and Wales, the availability of periodic censuses and a system of civil registration of age-defined vital events enables the essential demographic 'stocks and flows' to be analysed.

Louis Henry, to his great credit, devised a technique that quickly came to be known in the English-speaking world as 'family reconstitution'; it depends on establishing links between events occurring to the same individual or to members of the same family. A burial register, for instance, that recorded the death of Thomas Swain is unlikely to lend itself to this technique, but one that records the burial of Thomas son of William Swain on a specified date is. When 'individuals' are distinguished from 'names', the life histories of families are drawn together from the time at which a marriage was initiated through to the deaths or marriages of the family members, and by drawing upon information contained in the life histories of other related families, the dates of baptism of the parents can be established and the later life histories of their children traced. A complete life history of any single family is not always (and in the English parish registers, rarely) possible because of the results of local migration. This tendency to construct a large number of incomplete life histories is not the problem it might at first sight appear, since Henry developed systematic rules to define when persons were in observation. 'Presence in observation' is defined in family reconstitution in differing ways according to the statistic sought and the information available. For instance, the date of passage out of observation of all the children to a marriage for the purpose of studying their mortality experience is the date of death of the first parent to die or, if that date cannot be established with reasonable certainty, the date of baptism of the youngest of the children in the family. To use a burial date as the delimiter of the period of observation when studying mortality would be to invite overweighting the final result with data drawn from families that experienced many child deaths. Henry formulated rules that are generally believed to have minimized the introduction of major distortions into the demographic rates thereby created. Henry's techniques were first applied to the registers of the Normandy parish of Crulai, and was soon thereafter 'anglicized' so as to take account of the distinctive characteristics of English registers by E. A. Wrigley, who applied the technique to the registers of the east Devon parish of Colyton.[17] These two communities – Crulai and Colyton – so Le Roy Ladurie suggests, have come to assume as distinctive a place in the minds of French and English demographic historians as do Rocroi and Waterloo, respectively, for the politico-military historians of these two countries.[18]

Of course, family reconstitution demands high-quality parochial registration, and only a minority of registers in fact reach the precise standards required for that technique to be applied. Even if the information is accurate and sufficiently complete, geographical mobility of the local population can limit findings to what is known as the 'reconstitutable minority'. For instance, in results reported in thirteen English parish reconstitutions completed before 1983, between 1600 and 1799 about 90 per cent of the legitimate live births could be used for the calculation of infant mortality, but only 16 per cent of the married women yielded births that could be employed to establish their age-specific fertility rates.[19] To date, several hundred reconstitutions have been undertaken from the parish registers of European countries. The largest number, and perhaps the most carefully undertaken, derive from France and England where there has been a very strict adherence to Henry's rules. Swedish research makes use of a remarkable system of annual (or periodic) listings of inhabitants, records of individual migrations, and literary skills that have been superimposed on to the parish registers in the husförhörslängder, which began in the late seventeenth century but were eventually organized from 1740 by the state.[20] Important German studies have taken advantage of the evidence in the Ortssipenbücher or genealogies, which are ready-made reconstitutions assembled by the parochial clergy for the Nazi government in Germany in the 1930s with the aim of establishing the racial purity of individuals.[21]

Significant applications of this technique to parish registers in southern Europe (Italy, Spain, and Portugal) are only just beginning, although important studies of registers were completed in the 1970s for communities in Hungary and Poland.[22] In general, the registers of eastern and southern Europe have been less effectively exploited and there is some reason to suppose that their quality may be lower when assessed against the demands made by this technique, particular before the late eighteenth century. Within western Europe, some unfortunate lacunae exist, particularly in countries with disparate religious allegiances; in Holland, a few Reform Church registers exist before the mid-seventeenth century, but Catholic registers rarely begin before 1700, and before the nineteenth century difficulties arise as a consequence of the lower-class practice of not using family names. In Scotland, while registers began to be kept in the 1550s, survival rates are low and the quality of record-keeping was poor. Irish registers survive in very small numbers and, while there are approximately 100 Catholic registers surviving from the eighteenth century, most state names only at baptism and marriage, precluding effective study of mortality.

Religious divisions or fragmentation also reduced the accuracy of registration in England after 1700. For instance, it has been estimated that about 9 per cent of all children in the 1780s and about 16 per cent in the 1820s came to be baptized by Nonconformist ministers; for burials, the short falls are about 5 per cent and 14 per cent, respectively.[23] None the less, Nonconformist groups have sometimes left records that reveal them to have kept exceedingly good registration systems which have been exploited by historical demographers. Baptismal practices in England were far from constant through time; in the sixteenth century, it was customary for baptisms to take place on or within a few days of birth, but by the 1790s, a gap of one month on average had arisen.[24] In that quite extensive interval, many infants died unbaptized, which means that the burial of unbaptized children often went unrecorded, making burial registration defective.

A technique known as biometric analysis of infant mortality, which exploits formal mathematical properties exhibited by deaths over the first year of life, can be applied to such deficient data to estimate the short-fall.[25] For England and Wales between 1750 and 1800, burials were at least 5 per cent deficient in number, and in the early nineteenth century this 'leakage' was even larger. Loss of vital events in the rapidly growing urban, industrial centres after 1750 were also considerable. In fact, the completeness of parochial registration declines so much that less than 75 per cent of all births and deaths were recorded by the Anglican clergy in the early nineteenth century. In France, the trend in the quality of recording tends to assume a completely opposite direction, with registers, especially those recording burials, being significantly incomplete until the late eighteenth century. In the English case it is, of course, noteworthy that corrections of registrational shortcomings are clearly necessary and especially at the point around which the debate over what McKeown regarded as the origins of the modern rise of population is most focused.

Family reconstitution is a technique that places heavy demands on the sources; it is time-consuming to perform and does not expose all aspects of the demographic behaviour of the majority of the population to view. It also tends to generate for individual communities, because of sample size requirements, demographic statistics covering blocks of times or cohorts that are rarely less than twenty-five years and frequently fifty years in duration. Consequently, finely tuned analysis of change through time is hard to achieve. It therefore generally provides the best coverage when the parish is large in area and rural, and where migration is modest; it is least successful in small urban parishes where population turnover is likely to be high, although it has in a few instances been successfully employed on certain urban communities in Europe (for example, Rouen and Geneva).[26] A limited or specially adapted form of reconstitution has usefully exploited registers for parishes in London and York, where the demographic findings are primarily confined to infant and child mortality and birth intervals of married women.[27] Estimations of adult mortality, marriage age, and age-specific marital fertility that enable distinctions to be drawn between migrants into towns and urban natives have not proven possible and confound any satisfactory attempt to measure what has come to be known as the 'urban grave-yard effect'.[28]

Notwithstanding certain of its limitations, family reconstitution has yielded many important findings, some of which I shall discuss, but it has not proven possible to use it to assess certain key issues relating to national population trends, and in the English case, to provide a satisfactory answer to the long-standing conundrum of whether the eighteenth-century rise of population owed more to movements in mortality or to fertility. Historians and demographers have long attempted to attack this problem by resorting to various forms of 'aggregative analysis' of parish registers. The technique in its essentials is straightforward, and involves using high-quality registers with reasonably continuous recording to establish annual and monthly series of counts of baptisms, burials, and marriages. The resulting series, particularly the differences between baptisms and burials, provide crude indicators concerning long-run population growth. From such counts it has proved possible to derive rough indices of natural increase and short-term variability of mortality and fertility through time. Large-scale aggregative data sets have been assembled for France and England; in France, a representative sample of 413 parishes has been analysed for the relatively brief period from 1740 to 1829. For England, the Cambridge Group for the History of Population and Social Structure established a set of 404 high-quality Anglican registers from the nearly 10,000 English parishes to reconstruct national demographic trends from 1541 (close to the point of the beginning of ecclesiastical registration) to the beginnings of civil registration in 1837.[29]

Work undertaken on the Cambridge 'sample' has proved to be of conceptual and methodological significance, since it has provided the raw material for the second major technical innovation in post-war historical demography. The raw data, much of which was collected by local volunteers, was subjected to quite intensive evaluation, and it received a variety of sytematically implemented corrections to remedy shortcomings caused by under-registration and biases in the sample. With these data, Wrigley, Schofield and Oeppen created a procedure termed 'back projection', which is a development that emerges from 'inverse projection', initially invented by R. D. Lee.[30] The principle of both back and inverse projection is that one begins with a known census population from which births and deaths in the previous years are subtracted and added respectively, enabling one to derive a population for that year. Such a procedure could be pursued to the beginning of an annual series of births and deaths, although it would be making the unrealistic assumption that there was no net migration. The Cambridge Group's 'back projection' takes migration into account. It begins with a census of proven accuracy and known age structure in 1871. If the English population had been closed over the period of 330 years leading up to 1871, and if the mortality of each birth cohort over this period was known, then successive inflation of survivors of a cohort at any census by an estimate of mortality over the cohort's life course should recreate the original birth cohort. If the estimated size of the birth cohort by this process is actually smaller than the observed births, deaths must have taken place outside the 'system' under observation. In fact, these missing deaths would relate to persons whose deaths occurred outside England and constitute a measure of net migration. These migrants are allocated to each time period by using a fixed-age schedule of migration, which assumes that the greatest propensity to migrate was between ages 20 and 35.

Inverse projection yields estimates of population size at five-year intervals. It is also possible to proceed to estimate age structures and to relate the estimated number of deaths, births, and marriages to these population totals to produce birth, marriage, and death rates. Since the publication of the results from the first application of this technique in 1981, it has been the subject of much interest and some critical comment. But it has received much general approval and the consensus is that the technique produces results that are reasonably robust.[31] However, it must be stressed that the method proceeds by making assumptions, some of which are open to dispute. In their pioneering application of this technique to evidence assembled from series of English vital events from 1541 to 1871, Wrigley and Schofield recognize this and have always regarded their findings as 'estimates' and not 'facts'. In all that follows in this present discussion, this fundamental point should be borne in mind.

Most observers would accept that in employing this technique on parish register based data for the period prior to establishment of a system of civil registration, demographic historians have revolutionized our understanding of the proximate causes of demographic growth in the eighteenth century. What is more, the increasingly sophisticated use of formal demographic tools on the data sets from other European countries for the period after $c.1750$ has significantly changed the terms of the debate to which McKeown first contributed in 1955.

LONG-TERM TRENDS IN MORTALITY: RESULTS FROM PARISH REGISTER STUDIES

The English demographic data set is the longest uninterrupted series to which both the techniques of family reconstitution and aggregative analysis via back projection have been applied. In that McKeown's thesis about the modern rise of population was developed largely, if not exclusively, with reference to England, I shall consider the consequences for his position of the findings from these relatively new but increasingly 'standard' techniques. Life expectancy at birth (e_0 – the average number of years a new-born baby may have been expected to live) certainly rose from a low point in the quinquennium centring on 1731 of 27.9 years to more than 40.2 years in that centring on 1836, the quinquennium within which civil registration was introduced. However, the gain implied by a stark comparison of these two points in time is somewhat illusory in so far as the value attaching to 1731 reflects the extremely severe mortality afflicting England in the late 1720s, when e_0 was only slightly above that for the quinquennium centring on 1561 of 27.8 and reflecting the terribly difficult years in the late 1550s which produced the very lowest value for the whole 330-year series. An e_0 of 36 or 37 would be more typical of the early eighteenth century and, when compared with values of $c.40$ years for the 1820s and 1830s, suggests that the mortality improvements, while by no means insignificant, were not of particularly great magnitude.

However, fertility was considerably more dynamic than mortality over the same period. The Gross Reproduction Rate (GRR, the average number of daughters that would be born to a woman during her lifetime if she passed through the childbearing ages experiencing the average age-specific fertility pattern) rose from 2.3 in the quinquennium centred on 1701 and, by that centred on 1816, had reached 3.06 with the bulk of the growth occurring after 1751. In the 1820s, the intrinsic rate of national growth in England had reached the heady heights of 1.5 per cent per annum. It is now clear that changes in fertility played a far greater role than changes in mortality in generating demographic growth on this scale, in the seventy to eighty years after 1750.[32] These findings could be amplified by use of evidence relating to female marriage age calculated from family reconstitutions, which, when set alongside estimates of proportions never marrying and illegitimacy (derived from an alternative aggregative series), suggest that almost three-quarters of the growth was the result of the rapid rise in fertility.[33]

While the role played by the fertility rise in the account of English population history produced by 'back projection' and strongly endorsed by family reconstitution provides vindication of the views of such scholars as Habbakuk, Krause, and Ohlin, and runs counter to those of McKeown and pre-war scholars such as Buer and Griffith (as well as the distinguished post-war analysts Helleiner, Glass, Chambers, and Flinn), it remains clear that there had been an amelioration of mortality for which explanations have to be provided.[34] Helleiner, Flinn, and Chambers had placed considerable emphasis on what they believed were significant reductions in the volatility of annual death rates, although they had come to feel that this stabilization of mortality could not be exclusively, or indeed primarily, caused by improvements in the adequacy of the food supply. Part of the reason for their scepticism derived from the fact that so many years of high mortality showed no association with years in which food prices were inflated and in which there were documented harvest failures. The English data derived from the 404-parish sample reveal a diminution in short-run variability in mortality from the seventeenth century. The mean deviation of the series of annual crude death rates declined, falling from 17.7 per cent in the quarter-century 1550–74 to reach 8.3 per cent in 1700–24. The fall through time was by no means smoothly distributed, and quarterly deviations from 1720–49 rose to 12.3 per cent before the preceding decline was resumed through the remainder of the eighteenth century. Brief crises also declined in England. In fourteen separate months between 1750 and 1799, mortality moved more than 25 per cent above a 25-year moving-average trend. In the next half century, it did so on just four occasions. Figures of steady decline should be compared with the fact that between 1650 and 1699 there were 55 separate months when a national monthly crisis can be detected.[35]

While fluctuations in annual mortality rates appear to have diminished elsewhere, they did not experience such a striking stabilization as was achieved in England. For instance, in France from 1800–49, the peak deaths for the half-century still averaged 13 per cent above the decadal medians, compared with a value of 7 per cent in England.[36] In all four of the Scandinavian countries, as well as Iceland, that were in possession of annual death rates in the early nineteenth century, volatility was even greater than in France.[37]

It is therefore necessary not to exaggerate the extent to which crisis mortality had disappeared, and of greater significance, perhaps, is the apparent absence of a spatially synchronized, pan-European 'stabilization' of mortality. Less is known of southern Europe, where there are currently no 'national' mortality series from *c.*1750–1850. There is, none the less, convincing evidence that in some Mediterranean societies, crisis mortality continued to be important well into the nineteenth century. For instance, the parish registers of central and southern Spain show these areas to have been struck by exceptionally severe epidemics between 1800 and 1804, which were worse than any crisis period since the late sixteenth century.[38]

While the patterns derived from the analysis of short-run instability in the death rate reveal certain consistencies, do they suggest any tendency towards there having been a sensitivity on the part of the death rate to short-run variations in the size of the harvest and the price of food? Investigation of systematic relationships between annual fluctuations in food prices and mortality rates has in the last two decades become a highly sophisticated econometric procedure. R. D. Lee has been an especially influential pioneer in the application of distributed lag models to this area of investigation, and in the 1980s many others followed in his footsteps by applying the technique to price and death series for various countries and regions in eighteenth- and nineteenth-century Europe. The technique facilitates calculation not only of the magnitude of the association between prices and deaths in the year in which the fluctuation occurred, but also in the four subsequent years, so that lagged relationships can be considered. Lee's work on English data from 1548 to 1834 has identified a systematic relationship between fluctuations in wheat prices and mortality, but it was noteworthy for being weak. In fact, only 16 per cent of the short-run variation in mortality was associated with price changes, and the bulk of this responsiveness was detectable in a relatively small number of years with extreme upward price fluctuations such as 1596/7, 1597/8, and 1545/6 (in order of severity).[39]

There was a decline in responsiveness of mortality after 1750, leading Walter and Schofield recently to state that 'although the connection between food price fluctuations and mortality was always weak, it was not until the mid-eighteenth century that it was entirely broken'.[40] What is notable is the existence of so many years when prices rose dramatically and mortality either remained impassively unresponsive or indeed fell. It is remarkable that in England in the 1690s, when food prices were exceedingly high in a run of very wet summers, there was no mortality rise. Indeed, while real wages in 1697/8 and 1698/9 were 22 and 21 per cent, respectively, below a 25-year moving average, the death rate in both years was marginally below, rather than above, average. The whole of north-west Europe was affected by the high food prices in the 1690s, but unlike England, this area did suffer significant accompanying rises in death rates.[41] Indeed, it would seem that for the period from 1677 to 1734, when comparisons can be made with England, 46 per cent of French deaths over age 5 were associated with grain-price movements. Only 24 per cent of non-infant deaths for the period 1675–1755 were associated with grain-price changes in England. Furthermore, in the year of the actual price shock, mortality was 30 per cent greater in France, compared with 11 per cent in England.[42] It is generally agreed that these lower elasticities of deaths in England prior to 1750 are to be explained by a better-balanced and perhaps more substantial diet, and a greater choice of substitutes for wheat, as well as a more responsive system of poor relief resting on the foundations of a fundamentally more productive agricultural system.[43] While the reasons for the contrasts between England and France may well be true, it should be noted that in all the European nations and regions for which distributed lag analysis has been undertaken (England, France, Italy, and Sweden), the late eighteenth century reveals a declining responsiveness of annual mortality rates to food-price changes. Furthermore, and perhaps more important, all time series reveal periods bearing relationships contrary to that expected; this has suggested to many the overriding importance of autonomous epidemic cycles that operated independently of food supplies.

While rather weak in appearance, the wider European tendency for mortality to stabilize over time, and for its short-term responsiveness to price rises to abate, might lead a committed disciple of McKeown to conclude that there is little in this evidence to suggest any feature that is fundamentally at odds with a nutrition-related theory of mortality decline. But what of the medium- to long-term relationship expressed not in terms of annual crude death rates, but in terms of life expectancy at birth and living standards? To date, the joint efforts of demographic and economic historians have not generated large bodies of data with which to test this relationship. Wrigley and Schofield's work based upon the English 404 parish sample has yielded striking findings when quinquennial values of e_0 are plotted alongside an 11-year moving average of real wages derived from the Phelps-Brown and Hopkins index. The surprise is that the two series suggest that they may well have been connected by an inverse relationship: life expectancy rose in the sixteenth century until the first quarter of the seventeenth, when real wages plummeted; the subsequent decline in life expectancy, which reached low points in the 1680s and 1720s, coincided with steadily rising real wages, while the substantial improvements in life expectancy after 1750 occurred against a background of falling real wages. If real wages are tied to trends in nutritional level, in particular for wage-earners whose share of the population increased over time, these data would appear to deny a direct link with mortality.[44] Massimo Livi-Bacci, in an important overview of these matters, while regretting the absence of comparable data sets extending over such a long period, is prepared to assert that, in general, periods of high mortality, such as the century after the Black Death and the seventeenth century, were phases of both high purchasing power for wage-earners and presumably of greater food availability per head. He therefore feels very confident in concluding that great epidemic cycles were largely independent of the state of nutrition of populations.[45] (➤ Ch. 22 Nutritional diseases)

ASSESSING MORTALITY'S AUTONOMY

Arguments of this kind have certainly proved attractive to those who wish to give serious consideration to accounts that starkly portray mortality as exogenously determined. Patrick Galloway, in particular, has made extensive use of distributed lag models over a large number of data series in which deaths can be related to temperature and rainfall recordings. He has forcefully suggested that periods of global warming (for example, 1670–1800) and cooling (for example, 1590–1670) are associated respectively with population growth and stagnation or actual decline.[46] However, while pre-industrial societies were undoubtedly vulnerable to climatic variation, the effect may have been more readily observable in the short term rather than the long term. For instance, the seasonality patterns of deaths in parish and civil registers bear witness to these influences, and in the temperate latitudes of the Northern hemisphere a late winter/early spring mortality peak is usually clearly apparent. Not surprisingly, this pattern reflects the fact that deaths from airborne infections reached a high point in late winter, while the peak season for intestinal infections was the late summer. We know too, that extremes of temperature had adverse consequences for mortality, although extremely hot summers seem to have been more devastating in their effect than the severe cold of the winter months. Age groups, of course, responded differently to these seasonal extremes. Overall death rates in England between 1664 and 1834 rose in the months of coldest temperatures with only limited lagged effects extending to subsequent months. This contrasts with deaths in especially hot summers, which also increased but did so in a much more protracted fashion over the month or two following the period of highest temperatures. It is thought that severe winter weather, which exacerbated mortality deriving from pneumonia, bronchitis, influenza, and other respiratory diseases, was especially serious in its impact on the elderly, who died very rapidly once they had contracted these infections. In contrast, hot summers killed infants and young children through digestive-tract diseases, which were debilitating and considerably longer in exacting their toll.[47] (➤ Ch. 18 The ecology of disease) These climatic effects were mediated through a wide range of other factors that could be either additive or multiplicative in their impact. Detailed research employing family reconstitution has detected such effects, which could exacerbate or dampen the risks of death. For instance, the impact of climate on infant mortality levels has been noted, but it has also proved necessary to control for the influence of such intervening variables as the length of the period of maternal breast-feeding, the season of birth and hence likely season of weaning, and the seasonal patterns of women's work. (➤ Ch. 45 Childhood) Recent work on the parish registers of the south-eastern counties of England has shown how height above sea level, especially in areas where malaria was endemic, could have striking effects on infant mortality rates.[48] In the warmer regions of southern Europe, such as Tuscany or Castile, where topographical change could be very great over relatively short distances, there were concomitant shifts in infant and child mortality rates that reveal the influence of seasonal extremes of temperature and the vulnerability of those born at high altitude in winter, or those who were weaned in the summer months at low altitudes.[49]

REINSTATING MORTALITY WITHIN SOCIETY AND ECONOMY

In reflecting on the impact of disease cycles and climate on mortality levels in the past, our attention has already been drawn to the work of those historians who regard mortality as in a very real sense autonomously or exogenously determined. This, for instance, is the premiss in certain highly regarded accounts of European demographic history which are ill-disposed to endogenous explanations of demographic change in which fertility is thought to display a highly elastic responsiveness to changes in the standard of living. Such a position is readily detectable in the attempts of R. D. Lee to specify the systemic qualities of European pre-industrial demographic regimes. Indeed, in a series of essays he has developed an interpretation of the demographic history of England from the fourteenth to the early nineteenth centuries, which presents it as fundamentally the acting-out of exogenous changes in mortality (the independent variable), which in turn determined changes in fertility, population size, and living standards.[50] Such a view is in part predetermined by a certain kind of econometric preference, as well as an overdependence upon the blunt weapon of the real wage as a convenient but not altogether realistic or satisfactory measure of social and economic well-being. It is now clear that arguments of this kind are provoking an increasingly vociferous counter-response from those who are suspicious of histories of mortality change that leave no place in the causal accounting for human agency. Such critics are not concerned to promote a return to a crude form of nutritional determinism, nor to allocate a heroic role for medical science as a catalyst for demographic change, but prefer to consider mortality shifts as deeply embedded in social structures or systems that cannot be represented by complex statistical manipulations of a few econometrically convenient variables. One distinguishable feature of this work is its attempt to move beyond an interpretation of mortality determinants that depends fundamentally upon the level of the real wage as the principal causal agent. Instead, particular attention is paid to the influences of society's spatial arrangements and their consequences for levels of exposure and resistance to infection through an evaluation of the impact of such parameters as regional ecological variability, population density, long-range human-migration flows, and patterns of short-distance human geographical mobility.

In recent years, examples of work couched in these terms have become readily available. Careful demographic research on the geographical incidence of plague, and in particular, the micro-geography of its occurrence within towns, streets, and households, has enabled historians such as Paul Slack to argue convincingly that quarantine controls in England and elsewhere in Europe deserve a prime place in any account of why plague was eventually eradicated as a major killer from the late seventeenth century.[51]

Work on metropolitan areas is increasingly revealing a disinclination to treat them in 'naturalistic' terms, which focus exclusively on their physical environment, the problem of their water supply and sewage disposal. For such an approach tends to over-emphasize the place of water- and food-borne gastric diseases in the metropolitan mortality regime. Through his use of the London Bills of Mortality and the detailed reconstitution of the registers of London Quakers, John Landers has radically changed our knowledge of London's demographic character in the late seventeenth and eighteenth centuries. He shows, contrary to the prevailing assumption, that mortality in London worsened dramatically after 1660, indeed after bubonic plague ceased to be a cause of death. The weekly Bills of Mortality enable Landers to track marked shifts in the seasonality of death. In particular, the decades around 1700 witnessed a substantial reduction in the relative numbers of summer burials and a corresponding increase in the numbers of those dying in the cold-weather months. Part of the change may have been correlated with a significant decline in mortality from an old established gastroenteretic condition ('griping of the guts'), but another contribution seems to be a growth in the significance of typhus and the bronchitis/influenza/pneumonia group of causes, which seems surprising given the high living standard and low prices of the time. However, while in general the pattern of London's mortality suggests it to have had a relationship with real wages that was as uncertain as that in the country at large, two diseases, smallpox and 'fevers,' displayed a strong positive statistical association with food prices. Such a relationship between smallpox and prices at first glance appears to be confusing, because it is widely believed that resistance to it was unaffected by nutrition. Migration behaviour provides a highly plausible explanation for the link. Smallpox was endemic and most likely universal as a childhood infection in eighteenth-century London, but Landers's reconstitution of the Quaker registers reveals that a quarter to a third of all smallpox casualties were aged 15 to 30, and almost all of these had recently migrated to London. It seems that conditions of stress associated with high prices led to enhanced movement to London of persons having no previous exposure to smallpox and hence no immunity. Similarly the waves of migrants and demobilized soldiers in an era of intensive large-scale military activity overseas created severe pressure on London's housing stock, which expanded inadequately with respect to demand over a good deal of the early and mid-eighteenth century. In fact, it is known that London's population increased throughout this period, but the physical expansion of the built-up area came to a halt. It is highly suggestive that the most marked manifestation of the 'autumn mortality peak' was to be found in the northern and western suburbs, where the sharpest decline in the quality of the housing stock occurred. Landers's work on London's epidemiological history in the century after plague's departure, based largely on various forms of aggregative analysis of the Bills of Mortality and reconstitution of Quaker registers, shows in striking fashion how mortality changes owed much to that city's place in the national and international migration system and to the economic forces that restricted the growth of the construction industry and the housing stock. In no sense would an account of London's mortality pattern after the Restoration be adequately captured by a simple-minded account of metropolitan unhealthiness with little room left for human agency.[52] (➤ Ch. 27 Diseases of civilization; Ch. 19 Fevers)

In his emphasis on concepts such as exposure, resistance to exposure, and boundedness, Landers has taken the analysis of mortality a considerable distance from McKeown's distinctive version of the 'positive check'. None the less, some other recent work that is based on changes in human height must be given very careful consideration, and obliges students of mortality change to look carefully at potentially strong links with living standards. Unlike much work using the blunt instruments of prices and wages, at first glance height data appear to be a rewarding indicator to employ in this quest, since they do seem to be a good predictor of nutritional status during childhood. Floud and Fogel are struck by the coincidence between improvements in child mortality after 1860 in Britain and the way that they match the evidence on heights, which began to rise with the birth cohorts of the 1860s. Taken together with the correlations established between height and subsequent mortality, the late nineteenth-century evidence appears to provide a compelling case for these researchers, who see the post-1860 mortality decline as linked to improved nutritional status.[53] However, it seems that this area of research has turned out to be a methodological and conceptual minefield. Care is definitely needed to distinguish between nutrition (food intake) and nutritional status (which also reflects the disease environment and is consequently susceptible to determination by public-health measures). For it is now firmly established that while low body weight increases a child's susceptibility to diarrhoea, extended bouts of diarrhoea tend to stunt growth and diminish the capacity to resist infection.[54] Consequently, a daunting task faces the researcher who wishes to distinguish between nutritional and public-health factors as determinants of life expectancy. As Schofield and Reher sensitively comment, in this area 'the gap between McKeown and his opponents may be more apparent than real'.[55]

This gap, however, may well be larger when the demographic evidence for periods prior to the 1830s is assessed. It is apparent from the English mortality series relating to expectation of life at birth and derived from back projection that mortality improved over the late eighteenth century. But what access to a series of this length also reveals, and of fundamental significance, is the deterioration in life expectancy that extended over most of the seventeenth and into the early eighteenth centuries. This deterioration of what is sometimes termed 'background' mortality, notwithstanding the increasing stability of annual and monthly death rates over the same period, has cast considerable doubt on the assumption so prominent in the thinking of the 1950s and 1960s, that a reduction in the volatility of a death-rate series automatically implied a rising life expectancy. Of equal significance is the finding that the improvement in life expectancy after 1750 and up to 1831 was equivalent to the net decline in life expectancy that had taken place over the preceding century and a half, so that the e_0 of the England of Victoria (r. 1837–1901) was at a level similar to that of Elizabeth (r. 1558–1603). We are obliged to ask whether the gain in mortality in the century from the early 1700s was truly secular. If it was not, at least in the English case, it is necessary to doubt whether the fall in mortality from the early eighteenth into the present century can be accurately treated as a unitary process in the fashion adopted by McKeown. In fact, Schofield has gone so far as to state that 'the improvement in mortality in the period 1750–1815 scarcely seems to be an integral part of the decisive and massive fall in the level of mortality that has occurred throughout Europe within the last hundred years'.[56] A similar recovery by 1800 to mortality levels last occurring in the late sixteenth century appears to characterize the only other truly lengthy data set available, which relates to Geneva.[57]

It is unfortunate that we lack other studies yielding measures of life expectancy that extend over both the seventeenth and eighteenth centuries. Evidence from family reconstitutions for individual parishes enables us to understand the structure of mortality changes revealed in their somewhat coarse form via back projection. They indicate that deterioration in life expectancy in England over the course of the seventeenth century was largely the product of rising infant and child mortality. Young children aged 1–4 suffered a rather greater and earlier rise in their mortality through the period from 1550 to 1740, with the sharpest deterioration in their life chances occurring before 1650. Their life chances improved significantly over the last half of the eighteenth century. Infant mortality rose less markedly through the seventeenth century, but then increased sharply in the late seventeenth and early eighteenth centuries, before falling quite markedly after 1740. Of particular interest is the finding that these trends, although not perfectly synchronized, are also detectable among the infants and young children of the English peerage. In this social echelon, the growth in infant mortality reached its peak in the quarter-century 1650–74, before falling back somewhat to experience an especially sharp decline after 1750. The similarity of these two trajectories, and the very notable fall in infant mortality among all social layers after 1750, suggests that a nutrition-based explanation of the trend is unlikely to prove acceptable.[58]

Reconstitution studies in England have revealed particularly high contributions of neonatal or endogenous infant mortality (days 0–28) to the overall rate in the first year of life. Prior to the mid-eighteenth century, the neonatal share is generally in excess of half of the total infant rate. However, in an amalgamated sample of communities, neonatal rates had fallen by almost 50 per cent from rates of approximately 100 per 1,000 to approximately 50 per 1,000 and, had not non-neonatal mortality risen somewhat, the net improvement over the late eighteenth century would have been even greater. The fall in neonatal mortality in the eighteenth century shadows a noteworthy decline in maternal mortality over the same period, from approximately 15 per 1,000 birth events in 1650–59 to 5.5 per 1,000 in 1800–49. In fact, the decline in maternal mortality was more marked than that of neonatal mortality, but there are grounds for supposing that we may be observing in both these developments the effects of changes in obstetrical practices and the management of the newborn.[59] These developments relating to mothers and their very young offspring reveal changes that may be said to run counter to one key strand in the McKeown thesis. (➤ Ch. 44 Childbirth)

The extent to which changes of age-specific mortality adopted similar trajectories in other European countries prior to and after the middle of the eighteenth century is at present largely a matter of speculation. In the period after 1750, when national demographic data of high quality become available in the Scandanavian countries (Sweden, Finland, Denmark) and for France (based on a sample of 413 communities), it is apparent that in all cases over the century prior to 1850, reductions in infant and probably child mortality were an important, indeed the dominant, component in national mortality declines, although they are far from perfectly synchronized. In all cases, the infant and child mortality rates started from levels in the mid-eighteenth century that were significantly higher than those to be found in England at the same date. By 1850, England was not particularly favoured by comparison with many of its northern and north-west European neighbours, although in the intervening period, massive urbanization and growing population densities served to elevate non-neonatal infant mortality rates. It is difficult to know whether analogous decreases in infant and child mortality occurred in other parts of Europe, such as Germany, Italy, and Spain, where information is still fragmentary although growing in quantity. Basing our judgement on the high overall mortality levels still prevalent in the middle of the nineteenth century (when expectation of life at birth was 30 or below), improvements over the previous century in these countries were likely to have been very modest.[60]

Work on parish registers generating results of the kind we have discussed immediately above is frustrating because of the limited information provided that bears directly upon causes of death. It is not until well into the nineteenth century that evidence on cause of death becomes readily available through systems of civil registration, although subject, of course, to the vagaries of unsystematic recording and variable diagnoses based on symptoms. In Sweden, however, a data set containing attributed causes of death is available, and one category that between 1750 and 1815 declined significantly is small-pox.[61] While such a trend is not necessarily generalizable to other parts of Europe, the fall in smallpox deaths and the improvements in child (not infant) mortality may well be connected. Such a connection McKeown acknowledged, although perhaps too grudgingly given his ignorance of the age-specific mortality changes occurring prior to 1837.

SPATIAL VARIATIONS IN MORTALITY AND THEIR SIGNIFICANCE

Another concern that demographers and population geographers increasingly show in their analyses is the growing recognition of wide regional differences in mortality at any given moment in time. Life expectancy, and especially infant and child survivorship, varied substantially within individual countries.[62] This was true of the seventeenth and eighteenth, as well as the nineteenth, centuries. Family reconstitution of English parish registers shows that infant mortality rates varied between the healthiest parish so far located, Hartland (north Devon), and the market town of Gainsborough (on the River Trent in Lincolnshire), by a factor of 2 to 3 throughout the seventeenth and eighteenth centuries. Such a difference between the two localities is still readily detectable when we compare the registration districts within which they are located immediately following the onset of civil registration in 1837.

Indeed, throughout the three-century period, life expectancy at birth in the north-Devon community rested close to 50 years, whereas that in Gainsborough was closer to 30, a difference that was hardly likely to be based on contrasting nutritional levels in the two populations.[63]

Contrasts of this kind are striking in England, particularly since it is supposed that breast-feeding patterns were remarkably invariant regionally and apparently relatively stable through time (if the changes in feeding practices that are so dramatically exhibited by higher social echelons and certain religious groups such as the Quakers are discounted). Family reconstitution has enabled historical demographers both to delve into the impact of breast-feeding on marital fertility and to observe its relationship with infant mortality. This is achieved by a means of detecting the extent of the period of post-partum non-susceptibility, which is considerably extended in the case of mothers who are breast-feeding. Two ways have been devised for estimating the duration of the period of non-susceptibility from reproductive histories of the kind generated by family reconstitution. One is to compare the interval between marriage and first birth and the following interval between first and second birth: the difference should reveal the extent to which the second birth interval is extended by non-susceptibility if breast-feeding is practised. Another way is to examine the relationship between length of birth intervals and the age of death of the child born at the beginning of the interval. Wilson's work on English family-reconstitution data shows that the non-susceptible period was 10–12 months from c.1550 to 1837, a duration that varied little from place to place and is compatible with breast-feeding that lasted well into the second year of the child's life.[64] Applications of these techniques to Belgian, French, German, and Swedish data reveal that there were very considerable regional differences in these countries in the length of the non-susceptible period. In non-breast-feeding areas such as Flanders and Bavaria, the non-susceptible period was as short as three or four months and mothers had very high fertility. Their offspring had very low survival prospects, since frequently infant-mortality rates were in the range of 350–400 per 1,000 – three times higher than many rural rates in England.[65]

To date, only a few demographic studies of infant mortality and breast-feeding have been able to set their findings alongside independent documentary evidence in which contemporaries make specific reference to actual practice. Work on Germany and Sweden in particular has, however, often succeeded in combining the two classes of evidence to great effect. Indeed, a particularly illuminating study of the northernmost Swedish parish of Nedertoneå has successfully shown the dramatic impact on infant mortality that followed from the attempts by state-trained midwives, newly arrived in the area, to convince mothers to breast-feed.[66] In this region, infant mortality had been over 400 per 1,000, because artificial feeding from birth was the practice. Of special interest in this study was the finding that in the initial stages of the change of practice, the lowest infant mortality was encountered among low-status, urban-domiciled families who quickly came into contact with the newly arrived, reforming midwives. The highest mortality continued to be encountered amongst the higher-status rural farmers, who held longest to the old ways. Such behavioural differences gave rise to patterns that ran counter to the orthodox view that high status and rural residence correlated strongly with low infant mortality. Notwithstanding the impressive findings that have flowed from the evidence suggesting a strong statistical association between breast-feeding and infant mortality, it is always necessary to control for other intervening variables which can serve to enhance or to depress the survivorship of the artificially fed infant. Historical demographers have not always been alert to these problems, and sometimes crudely reductionist accounts have been the results of attempts to explain spatial variability.[67]

CONCLUSION

In his consideration of mortality changes after c.1840, McKeown took little note of spatial variations. This must constitute a noteworthy blind spot in his analysis, for a very substantial part of the late nineteenth-century mortality decline was connected to the way in which the mortality gradient between urban and rural places was narrowed. The rapid and highly concentrated form of urbanization that came to characterize nineteenth-century Britain most likely had implications for the mortality consequences flowing from public-health measures, since it meant that once these reforms relating to sanitation, water supplies, and effective sewage removal had been efficiently organized and implemented, their ameliorative effects could be rapidly registered. Recent demographic studies of mortality change in the late nineteenth and early twentieth centuries have also given greater weight to the age-specific character of these shifts. Attention has been focused upon the persistently high rate of infant mortality until the turn of the century. In the late nineteenth century, 15–20 per cent of deaths in Britain occurred to those under the age of one year, with about 25 per cent contributed by those under 5 years. Continuous decline in infant mortality is not detectable until after the very late 1890s or 1900. Variations between urban and rural places in this period reflected the same ratios as had healthy and unhealthy places in the sixteenth and seventeenth centuries.[68] There were, of course, noteworthy differences in mortality by social class. Individuals such as Sir George Newman (1870–1948) and Sir Arthur Newsholme (1857–1943) were aware of the factors creating these rates, particularly the sanitary environment and its connection with epidemic diarrhoea, which was a major infant killer.[69] Recently, demographers have identified that in the 1890s, although non-diarrhoeal infant mortality was falling, mortality associated with diarrhoea rose through a sequence of unusually hot summers.[70] Further sanitary improvements and greater awareness of germ-free infant feeding do seem to have played major roles in driving down diarrhoeal infant mortality after 1900. It is noteworthy that the neonatal rate, which had fallen so sharply prior to 1830, had remained intransigent through the 1890s to the 1910s (at approximately 40–50 per 1,000), notwithstanding the considerable efforts to advance obstetric care and midwifery, *pace* McKeown.[71]

Recent emphasis has been given, as is now the case in the Third World, to the advantages that accrued both to mothers and their infants as controls on marital fertility served to reduce the size of completed families and widen the intervals between successive births.[72] The argument is that these changes, which were in train after 1870, enabled mothers to provide better care for fewer children. However, a detailed analysis of these links must await what may be another revolution in historical demography: the application of nominative linkage techniques to the civil registers, which, for statutory reasons, remain inaccessible to researchers in England and Wales. Until such research becomes possible, many of the arguments set out above remain plausible but unproven.

The discussion in this chapter reveals how demographic input into research on the history of mortality decline has widened our awareness of the array of factors, which may be important in isolation or amplified in conjunction with others, and which may have been not simultaneous, but sequential in their effect. It also emphasizes the advantages to be gained by looking at demographic data on a regional and local level, and above all, over a wide sweep of time. For generalizing from one country or projecting back through time from the better-known or more fully documented period to the less well known and data-deficient phase, which was the hallmark of McKeown's approach, now seems to have left his arguments severely exposed.[73] (➤ Ch. 70 Medical sociology)

NOTES

1 Thomas McKeown and R. G. Brown, 'Medical evidence related to English population changes in the eighteenth century', *Population Studies*, 1955, 9: 119–41.

2 Michel Fleury and Louis Henry, *Manuel de dépouillement et d'exploitation de l'état civil ancien*, Paris, Institut National d'Études Démographiques, 1956.

3 F. W. Notestein, 'Population – the long view', in T. W. Schultz (ed.), *Food for the World*, Chicago, IL, University of Chicago Press, 1945 pp. 36–57, see p. 39.

4 E. A. Wrigley, 'Elegance and experience: Malthus at the bar of history', in D. Coleman and R. S. Schofield (eds), *The State of Population Theory*, Oxford, Basil Blackwell, 1986, pp. 46–64.

5   G. T. Griffith, *Population Problems in the Ages of Malthus*, Cambridge, Cambridge University Press, 1926; M. C. Buer, *Health, Wealth and Population in the Early Days of the Industrial Revolution*, London, Routledge, 1926; A. M. Carr-Saunders, *The Population Problem*, Oxford, Oxford University Press, 1922; D. George, 'Some causes of the increase of population in the eighteenth century as illustrated by London', *Economic Journal*, 1922, 32: 325–52.

6   Thomas McKeown, *The Modern Rise of Population*, London, Edward Arnold, 1976.

7   See n. 5.

8   S. J. Kunitz, 'Explanations and ideologies of mortality patterns', *Population and Development Review*, 1987, 13: 379–408; and Kunitz, 'The personal physician and the decline of mortality', in Roger Schofield, David Reher and Alain Bideau (eds), *The Decline of Mortality in Europe*, Oxford, Oxford University Press, 1991, pp. 248–62.

9   Thomas McKeown, *Medicine in Modern Society*, London, Allen & Unwin, 1965.

10 Thomas McKeown, *The Role of Medicine: Dream, Mirage or Nemesis?*, London, Nuffield Hospitals Trust, 1976.

11 Thomas McKeown, 'Medical issues in historical demography', in Edwin Clarke (ed.), *Modern Methods in the History of Medicine*, London, Athlone Press, 1971, p. 60.

12 J. Meuvret, 'Les crises de subsistence et la démographie de la France d'ancien régime', *Population*, 1946, 1: 643–50; P. Goubert, *Beauvais et le Beauvaisis de 1600 à 1730*, 2 vols, Paris, S.E.V.P.E.N., 1960.

13 Goubert, op. cit. (n. 12), Vol. I, pp. 75–6.

14 K. Davis, *The Population of India and Pakistan*, Princeton, NJ, Princeton University Press, 1950.

15 K. F. Helleiner, 'The population of Europe from the Black Death to the eve of the vital revolution', in E. E. Rich and C. H. Wilson (eds), *Cambridge Economic History of Europe*, Cambridge, Cambridge University Press, 1967, Vol. IV, ch. 1. The essay was actually completed in 1955.

16 McKeown, op. cit. (n. 11), p. 70.

17 E. Gautier and L. Henry, *La Population de Crulai, paroisse Normande*, Paris, I.N.E.D., 1958; E. A. Wrigley (ed.), *An Introduction to English Historical Demography*, London, Weidenfeld & Nicolson, 1966; Wrigley, 'Family limitation in pre-industrial England', *Economic History Review*, 1966 (2nd series), 19: 82–109; Wrigley, 'Mortality in pre-industrial England: the example of Colyton, Devon, over three centuries', *Daedalus*, 1968, 97: 546–80.

18 E. Le Roy Ladurie, 'From Waterloo to Colyton', in *The Territory of the Historian*, Brighton, Harvester, 1979, pp. 223–34; first pub. in *Times Literary Supplement*, 1966.

19 E. A. Wrigley and R. S. Schofield, 'English population history from family reconstitution: summary results 1600–1799', *Population Studies*, 1983, 37: 159.

20 A.-S. Kälvemark, 'The country that kept track of its population: methodological aspects of Swedish population records,' in J. Sundin and E. Söderland (eds), *Times, Space and Man: Essays on Microdemography*, Stockholm, Almqvist & Wiksell, 1979, pp. 221–38.

21 J. E. Knodel, *Demographic Behaviour in the Past: Study of Fourteen German Village*

Populations in the Eighteenth and Nineteenth Centuries, Cambridge, Cambridge University Press, 1988.

22 R. Andorka, 'La prévention des naissances en Hongrie dans la région "Orman-sag" depuis la fin du XVIII siècle', *Population*, 1971, 26: 63–78.

23 E. A. Wrigley and R. S. Schofield, *The Population History of England: a Reconstruction*, London, Edward Arnold, 1981, ch. 5.

24 B. M. Berry and R. S. Schofield, 'Age at baptism in pre-industrial England', *Population Studies*, 1971, 25: 453–63.

25 E. A. Wrigley, 'Births and baptisms: the use of Anglican baptism registers as a source of information about the numbers of births in England before the beginning of civil registration', *Population Studies*, 1977, 31: 282–312.

26 Jean-Pierre Bardet, *Rouen aux 17e et 18e siècles: les mutations d'un espace social*, Paris, S.E.D.E.S., 1983; Alfred Perrenoud, *La Population de Genève du seizième au début du dix-neuvième siècle, étude démographique: structures et mouvements*, Geneva, Société d'Histoire et d'Archéologie de Genève, 1979.

27 R. P. Finlay, *Population and Metropolis: the Demography of London 1580–1650*, Cambridge, Cambridge University Press, 1981; C. Galley, 'Growth, stagnation and crisis: the demography of York 1561–1700', unpublished Ph.D. thesis, University of Sheffield, 1991.

28 A. M. van der Woude, 'Population developments in the northern Netherlands (1500–1800) and the validity of the "urban graveyard" effect', *Annales de démographie*, 1982, 55–75; A. Sharlin, 'Natural decrease in early modern cities: a reconsideration', *Past and Present*, 1981: 92, 175–80.

29 Dupâquier, *Histoire de la population française*, Vol. II: *De la Renaissance à 1789*, Paris, Presses Universitaires, 1989; E. A. Wrigley and R. S. Schofield, *The Population History of England 1541–1871: a Reconstruction*, London, Edward Arnold, 1981.

30 Wrigley and Schofield, op. cit. (n. 29), App. 15; R. D. Lee, 'Estimating series of vital rates and age structures from baptisms and burials: a new technique, with applications to pre-industrial England', *Population Studies*, 1974, 28: 495–512.

31 L. A. Clarkson, 'History will never be the same again', *Times Higher Education Supplement*, 5 February 1982, 483, p. 13; L. Henry and D. Blanchet, 'La population de l'Angleterre de 1541 à 1871', *Population*, 1983, 38: 781–826; R. D. Lee, 'Inverse projection and back projection: a critical appraisal and comparative results for England, 1539 to 1871', *Population Studies*, 1985, 39: 233–48.

32 Wrigley and Schofield, op. cit. (n. 29), ch. 7.

33 Wrigley and Schofield, op. cit. (n. 29), 240–4.

34 H. J. Habbakuk, *Population Growth and Economic Development since 1570*, Leicester, Leicester University Press, 1971; P. G. Ohlin, 'The positive and the preventive check: a study of the rate of growth of pre-industrial populations', unpublished Ph.D., thesis, Harvard University, 1955; J. D. Chambers, *Population, Economy and Society in Pre-industrial England*, Oxford, Oxford University Press, 1972; M. W. Flinn, *The European Demographic System 1500–1800*, Brighton, Harvester, 1981; D. V. Glass, 'Introduction', in Glass and D. E. C. Eversley (eds), *Population in History: Essays in Historical Demography*, London, Edward Arnold, 1965, pp. 1–22.

35 Wrigley and Schofield, op. cit. (n. 29), p. 317.

36 Alfred Perrenoud, 'The mortality decline in a long-term perspective', in T. Bengtsson, G. Fridlizius and R. Ohlsson (eds), *Pre-industrial Population Change*, Stockholm, Almqvist & Wiksell, 1984, pp. 41–69.

37 Ibid.

38 Vicente Pérez Moreda, *Las Crisis de Mortalidad en la España Interior: Siglos XVI-XIX*, Madrid, Siglo XXI de Espana Editores, 1980.

39 R. D. Lee, 'Short term variations in vital rates, prices and weather', in Wrigley and Schofield, op. cit., (n. 23), pp. 371–84, 392–401.

40 J. Walter and R. Schofield, 'Famine, disease and crisis mortality in early modern society', in Walter and Schofield (eds), *Famine, Disease and Social Order in Early Modern Society*, Cambridge, Cambridge University Press, 1989, p. 41.

41 M. W. Flinn *et al.*, *Scottish Population History from the Seventeenth Century to the 1930s*, Cambridge, Cambridge University Press, 1977; D. R. Weir, 'Markets and mortality in France 1600–1789', in Walter and Schofield, op. cit. (n. 40); and R. B. Outhwaite, *Dearth, Public Policy and Social Disturbance, 1550–1800*, Basingstoke, Macmillan, 1991.

42 P. R. Galloway, 'Basic patterns in annual variations in fertility, nuptiality, mortality and prices in pre-industrial Europe', *Population Studies*, 1988, 42: app., table 1, column headed 'R-sq'.

43 Walter and Schofield, op. cit. (n. 40).

44 R. S. Schofield, 'The impact of scarcity and plenty on population change in England', in R. I. Rotberg and T. K. Rabb (eds), *Hunger and History: the Impact of Changing Food Production and Consumption Patterns on Society*, Cambridge, Cambridge University Press, 1983, pp. 67–94.

45 M. Livi-Bacci, *Population and Nutrition: an Essay on European Demographic History*, Cambridge, Cambridge University Press, 1991. This was originally published in Italian as *Popolazione e Alimentazione: Saggio sulla storia demographia Europea*, Bologna, Società editrice il Mulino, 1987.

46 P. R. Galloway, 'Long-term fluctutions in climate and population in the pre-industrial era', *Population and Development Review*, 1986, 12: 1–24.

47 Wrigley and Schofield, op. cit. (n. 23), pp. 384–92; R. S. Schofield and E. A. Wrigley, 'Infant and child mortality in England in the later Tudor and early Stuart period', in C. Webster (ed.), *Health, Medicine and Mortality in the Sixteenth Century*, Cambridge, Cambridge University Press, 1979, pp. 61–95; L. Bradley, 'An enquiry into seasonality in baptisms, marriage and burials', Part III: 'Burial seasonality', *Local Population Studies*, 1971, 6: 5–31.

48 M. Dobson, ' "Marsh fever" – the geography of malaria in England', *Journal of Historial Geography*, 1980, 6: 357–90.

49 M. Breschi and M. Livi-Bacci, 'Saison et climat comme contraintes de la survie des enfants: l'expérience italienne au XIXème siècle', *Population*, 1986, 41: 9–36; D. S. Reher, *Familia, Polacion y Sociedad en la Provincia de Cuenca 1700–1900*, Madrid, Centro de Investigaciones Sociologicas Editorial Siglo XXI, 1988.

50 R. D. Lee, 'Population homeostasis and English demographic history', in R. I. Rotberg and T. K. Rabb (eds), *Population and Economy: Population and History from the Traditional to the Modern World*, Cambridge, Cambridge University Press, 1986, pp. 75–100; and Lee, 'Population dynamics of human and other animals', *Demography*, 1987, 24: 443–65.

51 P. Slack, *The Impact of Plague in Tudor and Stuart England*, London, Routledge & Kegan Paul, 1985.

52 J. M. Landers, 'Mortality and metropolis: the case of London 1675–1825', *Population Studies*, 1987, 41; and Landers, *Birth and Death in the Metropolis: Studies in the Demographic History of London, 1670–1830*, Cambridge, Cambridge University Press, 1992.

53 Robert Fogel, 'Second thoughts on the European escape from hunger: famines, price elasticities, entitlements, chronic malnutrition and mortality rates', National Bureau of Economic Research, Working Paper Series on Historical Factors in London Run Growth, 1989; R. C. Floud, K. W. Wachter and A. S. Gregory, *Height, Health and History: Nutritional Status in Britain 1750–1980*, Cambridge, Cambridge University Press, 1990.

54 P. G. Lunn, 'Nurtrition, immunity and infection', in Schofield, Reher and Bideau, op. cit. (n. 8), pp. 131–45.

55 R. Schofield and D. Reher, 'The decline of mortality in Europe', in Schofield, Reher and Bideau, op. cit. (n. 8), p. 11.

56 R. Schofield, 'Population growth in the century after 1750; the role of the mortality decline', in Bengtsson, Fridlizius and Ohlson, op. cit. (n. 36), p. 35.

57 Perrenoud, op. cit. (n. 36).

58 T.H. Hollingsworth, 'Mortality in the British peerage since 1600', *Population*, 1977, special number: 327. The speeding-up of infant mortality decline after 1750 may well have been aided by a resort to breast-feeding and the abandonment of wet-nursing by aristocratic mothers, although simultaneous improvements in child mortality from a date prior to the change of feeding habits implies that other influences were also at work. See V. A. Fildes, *Breasts, Bottles and Babies: a History of Infant Feeding*, Edinburgh, Edinburgh University Press, 1986, pp. 79–97.

59 Data presented by E. A. Wrigley at a meeting of the British Society for Population Studies on *'The Population History of England* – Ten Years On', held at the London School of Hygiene and Tropical Medicine, 20 June 1991; R. Schofield, 'Did the mothers really die? Three centuries of maternal mortality in "The World we have lost"', in L. Bonfield, R. M. Smith and K. Wrightson (eds), *The World We Have Gained: Histories of Population and Social Structure*, Oxford, Basil Blackwell, 1986, pp. 231–60.

60 Schofield and Reher, op. cit. (n. 55), p. 4.

61 G. Fridlizius, 'The mortality decline in the first phase of the demographic transition: Swedish experiences', in Bengtsson, Fridlizius and Ohlsson, op. cit. (n. 36), pp. 71–114. The impact of vaccination has sometimes been overplayed, and it has been argued, based on the English 'chronology', that the rise prior to 1700, especially in child mortality, was a consequence of the enhanced international movements of peoples in the sixteenth and seventeenth centuries, which increased the killing power, particularly of airborne infections, by allowing them to attack populations without, or with only limited, prior exposure. Progressively with the development of adverse ratios of susceptibles to non-susceptibles and genetic mutations, populations are thought to have acquired greater resistance, which would be displayed by falls in the mortality of those above the age of weaning. See W. H. McNeill, *Plagues and Peoples*, Oxford, Basil Blackwell, 1977;

and R. Schofield, review of McKeown's *Modern Rise of Population*, in *Population Studies*, 1977, 31: 179–81. Others doubt these arguments on the grounds that there was insufficient scope for genetic adaptation within the posited time scale. See R. Leowontin, *The Genetic Basis of Evolutionary Change*, New York, Columbia University Press, 1974.

62 O. Turpeinen, 'Infectious diseases and regional differences in Finnish death rates 1749–73', *Population Studies*, 1978, 32: 523–34; R. I. Woods and P. R. A. Hinde, 'Mortality in Victorian England: models and patterns', *Journal of Interdisciplinary History*, 1987, 18: 27–54.

63 Wrigley and Schofield, op. cit. (n. 19), pp. 175–83.

64 C. Wilson, 'The proximate determinants of marital fertility in England 1600–1799', in Bonfield, Smith and Wrightson, op. cit. (n. 59), pp. 203–30.

65 J. Knodel and E. Van de Walle, 'Breast feeding, fertility and infant mortality: an analysis of some early German data', *Population Studies*, 1967, 21: 109–31.

66 A. Brandstrom and J. Sundin, 'Infant mortality in a changing society: spatial variations in child care in Sweden 1820–94', in R. M. Smith (ed.), *Regional and Spatial Demographic Patterns in the Past*, Oxford, Basil Blackwell, 1992.

67 R. Lesthaeghe, 'The breast-feeding hypothesis and regional differentials in infant and child mortality in Belgium and the Netherlands during the nineteenth century', in Smith, op. cit. (n. 66).

68 R. I. Woods, P. A. Watterson and J. H. Woodward, 'The cause of rapid infant mortality decline in England and Wales 1861–1921. Parts I and II', *Population Studies*, 1988, 42: 343–66; and 1989, 43: 113–32.

69 George Newman, *Infant Mortality: a Social Problem*, London, Methuen, 1906; Arthur Newsholme, *The Elements of Vital Statistics*, London, Swan Sonnenschein, 1889.

70 Woods, Watterson and Woodward, op. cit. (n. 68).

71 I. Loudon, 'Deaths in childbed from the eighteenth century to 1935', *Medical History*, 1986, 30: 1–41; and Loudon, 'On maternal and infant mortality 1900–60', *Social History of Medicine*, 1991, 4: 29–74.

72 J. Hobcraft, J. W. McDonald and S. Rutstein, 'Child spacing effects on infant and early child mortality', *Population Index*, 1983, 49: 585–618; Alberto Palloni and Marta Tienda, 'The effects of breastfeeding and the pace of childbearing on mortality at early ages', *Demography*, 1986, 23.

73 A striking consideration of the very different patterns of demographic change exhibited by England, France, and Sweden between 1750 and 1850 is offered by Wrigley and Schofield, op. cit. (n. 23), pp. 245–8. Rising fertility in England, and rising mortality in Sweden were the leading proximate causes of population growth, but in France, fertility and mortality fell together to contain growth to modest rates. Obviously, other 'experiences' are being documented as historical demography advances as a sub-discipline.

FURTHER READING

Anderson, M., *Population Change in North-Western Europe 1750–1850*, Basingstoke, Macmillan, 1988.

Dupâquier, J., *Histoire de la population française*, Vol. II: *De la Renaissance à 1789*, Paris, Presses Universitaires, 1989.

Landers, J. M., *Birth and Death in the Metropolis: Studies in the Demographic History of London 1670–1830*, Cambridge, Cambridge University Press, 1993.

Livi-Bacci, M., *Population and Nutrition: an Essay on European Demographic History*, Cambridge, Cambridge University Press, 1991.

McKeown, Thomas, *The Modern Rise of Population* London, Edward Arnold, 1976.

——, *The Role of Medicine: Dream, Mirage, or Nemesis?*', London, Nuffield Hospitals Trust, 1976; Oxford, Basil Blackwell, 1978.

Rotberg R. I. and Rabb T. K. (eds), *Hunger and History: the Impact of Changing Food Production and Consumption Patterns on Society*, Cambridge, Cambridge Univeristy Press, 1983.

Schofield, Roger, Reher, David and Bideau, Alain, (eds), *The Decline of Mortality in Europe*, Oxford, Oxford University Press, 1991.

Slack, Paul, *The Impact of Plague in Tudor and Stuart England*, London, Routledge & Kegan Paul, 1985.

Smith R. M. (ed.), *Regional and Spatial Demographic Patterns in the Past*, Oxford, Basil Blackwell, 1992.

Szreter, S. R., 'The importance of social intervention in Britain's mortality decline *c.*1850–1914: a reinterpretation of the role of public health', *Social History of Medicine*, 1988, 1: 1–38.

Walter, John and Schofield, Roger (eds), *Famine, Disease and Social Order in Early Modern Society*, Cambridge, Cambridge University Press, 1989.

Woods, R. I., Watterson, P. A. and Woodward, J. H., 'The cause of rapid infant mortality decline in England and Wales 1861–1921. Parts I and II', *Population Studies*, 1988, 42: 343–66; and 1989, 43: 113–32.

Wrigley, E. A. (ed.), *An Introduction to English Historical Demography*, London, Weidenfeld & Nicolson, 1966.

Wrigley, E. A. and Schofield R. S., *The Population History of England 1541–1871: a Reconstruction*, London, Edward Arnold, 1981; Cambridge, Cambridge University Press, 1989 (first paperback edn with new introd.).

72

MEDICINE, MORTALITY, AND MORBIDITY

Stephen J. Kunitz

INTRODUCTION

My job in this final chapter, according to the editors' instructions, is to 'dissect the differences to the grand sweep of history which medicine has made'. The enormity, not to say presumption, of the task is diminished only slightly by limiting the discussion to mortality and physical morbidity. I shall leave aside considerations of psychiatric conditions, the Samaritan function that healers perform in every society of which I am aware, and the socially integrative role of healing that has been widely described. I shall also ignore definitional problems such as the differences between sickness and illness, and between sin and disease. I shall consider only the impact that individual healers caring for individual patients may have had that can be measured at the population level; and that which public functionaries concerned with the health of a population have had, also measured at the population level. Thus, if health-care technology is effective, but so limited in its accessibility or application as to have no discernible population-wide impact, I will not consider it, no matter how important it is in legitimating the role of science or the occupational status of practitioners. And if the drainage of a marsh was done to reduce exposure to the mosquito vectors of malaria, I will consider that a public-health measure. If, however, the drainage was carried out to increase the amount of arable land and malaria control was an unintended by-product, I will not consider that a public-health intervention.

My task includes the consideration of medicine's impact upon morbidity as well as mortality. Measurement of each is not without problems. In respect of mortality, for instance, something as taken-for-granted as age at death is not easily obtained from archaeological material or from contemporary non-literate peoples. Often, cause of death as well as of morbidity is not a straightforward determination cither. And the assessment of morbidity is by no means simple, as countless surveys of contemporary populations suggest. Whether one is sick or not is a far more subjective judgement than whether or not one is dead, although those of us who have faced large lecture halls may sometimes be uncertain of the vital status of our audiences – as no doubt they often are of us. The usual assumption is that as mortality rises or falls, so does morbidity. That is to say, case-fatality rates are constant. In respect of the major infectious diseases in the pre-antibiotic era, this was probably true. Since antibiotics have been widely available, that is no longer a valid assumption. And in respect of the non-infectious diseases, it may or may not be true, depending upon the disease and the period under consideration.

I shall proceed by first outlining the generally agreed-upon sequence through which human diseases have evolved. Then I shall consider at which places in the sequence personal- and public-health interventions seem to have had an impact upon mortality and morbidity at the population level. Finally, I shall deal briefly with fertility control as a special case of the impact of medicine.

THE EVOLUTION AND SPREAD OF INFECTIOUS DISEASES

It is generally agreed that infectious diseases have evolved in parallel with the transformation of human social organization and ecological adaptation from small hunting-foraging bands to sedentary agricultural societies of increasing size, to industrial societies. (➤ Ch. 18 The ecology of disease) The causes of death and disease that seem to have afflicted our earliest human ancestors were zoonoses, of which they were accidental hosts, or chronic infestations and infections that evolved along with them from our non-human primate ancestors.[1] Violence, both accidental and purposeful, accounted for many deaths and much disability. Judging by the evidence from the skeletal remains of early hunter-foragers, as well as from the investigations of contempory peoples, life expectancy at birth has been estimated to have been at least 20 and more commonly 25 to 30 years.[2]

The reasons for the shift from hunting-foraging in small bands to more sedentary agriculture have been a matter of much debate, but need not detain us here. For my purposes, it is the fact of the emergence of agriculture that is important, for it is associated with urbanization, crowding, and the unsanitary conditions these suggest, as well as with the evolution of density-dependent diseases specifically adapted to human populations. These are diseases such as smallpox, measles, and polio which, if the human host survives, cause life-long immunity and thus require populations of substantial size (perhaps

500,000 to a million) to become endemic. In smaller populations, the virus dies out and thus causes an epidemic outbreak when it is reintroduced after a cohort of new susceptibles has emerged. (➤ Ch. 27 Diseases of civilization; Ch. 52 Epidemiology)

The horrific epidemics caused by these diseases were one of the consequences of the emergence of large populations in the Old World. In the New World, in contrast, these same diseases did not evolve, perhaps because of the absence of domesticated animals from which they originally spread as zoonoses.[3] Whatever the reason, the impact on New World populations of these diseases when they were introduced by Europeans was catastrophic, though the magnitude of the population collapse is still a matter of debate. (➤ Ch. 58 Medicine and colonialism)

Despite the absence of density-dependent diseases in the New World, pre-industrial urban populations in the Old World and pre-Columbian urban populations in the New World had equally low life expectancy at birth, usually to the late teens or early twenties. Less densely settled and rural agricultural populations tended to have somewhat higher life expectancies.[4] That the pre-Columbian urban population of Teotihuacan had life expectancy as low as that of pre-industrial European cities and ancient Rome suggests that Old World epidemic diseases were not necessary to cause high mortality, and that endemic enteric and respiratory diseases were as lethal then as they continue to be in many less-developed countries at present.

The fact that life expectancy among hunter-foragers tended to be slightly higher than that of pre-industrial and pre-Columbian urban populations suggests that the rise of sophisticated civilizations was not accompanied in their early phases by improvements in health. Despite the existence of sewerage systems and aqueducts in Teotihuacan, Rome, and elsewhere, and despite the production in both the Old World and the New of increasingly sophisticated medical knowledge, the health of the populations as measured by survival did not improve. By these criteria, the passage of human societies from hunting-foraging to the high civilizations of antiquity was not accompanied by effectively applied medical knowledge. Indeed, even up to the early modern period, life expectancy at birth was not dramatically improved. In England in the seventeenth century, life expectancy at birth fluctuated between 28 and 40.[5] (➤ Ch. 71 Demography and medicine)

It was in the seventeenth and eighteenth centuries that life expectancy began to diverge dramatically among societies, increasing in some and remaining constant or decreasing in others, and it is from this time that the question of medicine's contribution becomes more compelling. To deal with this complexity, I have adopted a widely used classification to describe the impact of medicine on the trajectory of life expectancy in the so-called First, Second, Third, and Fourth Worlds.

THE EPIDEMIOLOGICAL TRANSFORMATION
OF THE FIRST WORLD

By First World, I mean western Europe, its overseas extensions in North America and Oceania, and Japan. This is a very heterogeneous collection. To simplify, I shall select examples rather than attempt to be comprehensive. I start with England, for more has been written about English population history, disease patterns, and medicine than about any other country of which I am aware.

I said on p. 1695 that life expectancy in England fluctuated widely right through the seventeenth century and clearly resulted from epidemics and pandemics that swept through the countryside at frequent intervals and super-imposed peaks of mortality on a high plateau of deaths from endemic diseases. This pattern changed during the eighteenth century, when the fluctuations dampened. By the second half of that century, an increase in life expectancy is discernible, which continued right through the nineteenth century. By the 1850s, the downward deflections in life expectancy had all but vanished. The explanation of the recession, first of epidemics and then of endemic diseases, and of the increase in life expectancy have been the subject of what has been called the standard-of-living debate. This has to do with whether the Industrial Revolution led to immiserization of the population or resulted in improvements in living conditions that were translated into gains in health and life expectancy. Those who argue that immiserization increased tend to explain increasing life expectancy by saying that public health had an important effect in counteracting deleterious consequences of the deterioration of living conditions.[6] Those who believe living conditions improved minimize the contribution of medical interventions.[7] (➤ Ch. 51 Public health)

I have argued elsewhere that it is important to distinguish between the recession of epidemics in the eighteenth century and of endemic diseases in the nineteenth.[8] To the degree that the spread of plague was controlled by the Habsburg *cordon sanitaire* along their border with the Ottoman Empire in the early eighteenth century, and that military medicine resulted in less spread of disease (especially typhus) from armies to civilian populations, it can be said that public health contributed importantly to the reduction of epidemics.[9] There is more debate about the impact of smallpox vaccination beginning in the early nineteenth century, but the weight of evidence now suggests that it did serve to make epidemics less severe and less frequent.[10] These three epidemic diseases (plague, typhus, and smallpox) are not made substantially more lethal if the victim is undernourished. Thus the standard of living, at least as measured by wages, is not likely to be the most powerful explanation of their recession. (➤ Ch. 19 Fevers)

On the other hand, endemic diseases such as tuberculosis and the diarrhoeas of infancy and childhood do seem to be made more severe by undernutrition (and conversely, diarrhoea makes malnutrition worse by damaging the absorptive capacity of the gut). Thus the recession of these diseases, in some instances, may be related to improvements in wages and increased purchasing power. It is quite clear, as McKeown has shown,[11] that there was little that personal physicians could do in the nineteenth century that was reflected in improved survival from the endemic diseases measured at the population level. (➤ Ch. 22 Nutritional diseases; Ch. 45 Childhood)

It is unfortunate that most of the debate has centred on England. The picture changes if we shift our focus to Japan and Germany, in both of which the standard of living as measured by per capita income remained lower than in England throughout the nineteenth century, and in which life expectancy improved dramatically.[12] Unquestionably, this was the result of public-health measures that were more readily organized in these two authoritarian societies than was possible in England. At the turn of the twentieth century, for instance, per capita income in Japan was about 12 per cent that of England and Wales, whereas life expectancy at birth was 43 and 45 years, respectively.[13]

Thus, in respect of the decline of infectious diseases in the First World up to the early twentieth century, it seems reasonable to say that care provided by personal physicians had virtually no impact, and that public health had an impact that was nowhere insignificant, but whose significance varied widely depending upon the political culture and economy of particular societies. As a perhaps excessively broad generalization, I would speculate that in societies such as England and its overseas extensions, which are characterized by a belief in individualism and, particularly during the nineteenth century, by a belief in the political philosophy of *laissez-faire*, a rising standard of living may well have been one of the important roads to lower mortality. In societies whose political culture is more authoritarian, bureaucratically organized public-health activities may have been the way reductions in endemic diseases were achieved. There was more than one route to the same end-point.

By the first decades of the twentieth century, mortality from endemic infectious diseases had receded in virtually all First World countries, and non-infectious causes of death and disability were becoming relatively, and in some instances absolutely, more significant. None the less, the development and diffusion of antibiotics in the 1930s and 1940s had a measurable and profound impact upon both mortality and morbidity, as did the development of immunizations for diphtheria, pertussis, and tetanus, and later polio and measles. (➤ Ch. 39 Drug therapies; Ch. 10 The immunological tradition) In the United States, there was an acceleration in the rate of decline of the age-adjusted death rate beginning in the 1930s,[14] and during the post-war years the spectrum of non-fatal diseases seen by physicians in office practice changed markcdly. For paediatricians, for example, this meant spending relatively more time dealing with the 'new morbidities', such as developmental, behavioural, and psycho-social problems, and relatively less caring for children acutely ill with severe infectious diseases.[15]

While there is little doubt that immunizations and antibiotics have had a profound impact upon the incidence and prevalence of infectious diseases in First-World populations, it is less clear what the impact of medicine has been on the non-infectious diseases. Moreover, since the past forty years is but a brief moment in the grand sweep of history with which I am concerned, a detailed consideration of this topic would be out of place. None the less, it is worth pointing out that a number of attempts have been made in several countries to compare the decline in deaths from causes thought to be amenable to medical interventions with those thought not to be amenable to interventions.[16] In virtually every instance, the rate of death from amenable causes, most of which were non-infectious, declined more rapidly than the rate from the non-amenable causes. The surprising increase in life expectancy among people in their eighties may be a reflection of our increasing ability to prevent death from a number of non-infectious diseases. (➤ Ch. 46 Geriatrics) The question of whether morbidity has increased or diminished as a result is one to which I shall return below (see pp. 1704–5).

THE RECESSION OF EPIDEMICS IN THE SECOND WORLD

I have argued thus far that, depending upon a nation's political culture, public-health measures have been of varying significance in reducing deaths from epidemic and endemic infectious diseases. In politically authoritarian societies, I have speculated, this has tended to be particularly true. In the Second World – that is, in the former Soviet Union and other eastern European and Balkan nations – it has also been the case. The USSR is surely the best example.

There is little doubt that mortality was declining, at least in European Russia, in the second half of the nineteenth century. From 1860 to 1910, the crude death rate fluctuated between 30 and 40 per 1,000, dropping to 29 around 1910. Life expectancy at birth in 1896–7 was 32.[17] It is futile to ask what would have happened to living conditions and life expectancy if the First World War, the Russian Revolution, and the civil war had not occurred. What did happen was social turmoil and political upheaval resulting in several years of famine, widespread epidemics, and loss of life on a scale beyond anything that had occurred since the Mongol invasions of the thirteenth century.

Considering the magnitude of the epidemic and political problems confronted,[18] the effectiveness of the response was truly impressive. Enthusiastic supporters of the Revolution, as well as less enamoured sceptics, were agreed on the basic facts.[19] Epidemics of typhus, relapsing fever, and smallpox were controlled; epidemics of plague (enzootic in various parts of Russia) were prevented; and endemic diseases such a trachoma, tuberculosis, typhoid, dysentery, malaria, and the venereal diseases were all dramatically reduced during the 1920s and 1930s. Accurate mortality and life-expectancy data are not available from the inter-war years. Life expectancy at birth in 1926–7 in the European part of Russia was estimated by Lorimer to have been 43 or 44 years (45–6 for females, 41–2 for males). In 1938–40, figures for all of the USSR are estimated to have been 480 for both sexes, 46.7 for males, and 50.2 for females. More recent estimates are of 37.5 years in 1927, 41.4 in 1938, and an astonishingly low 11.6 during the famine year of 1933. Crude death rates are estimated to have been about 23 per 1,000 in 1926–7 in the European part of the Soviet Union, and 20.7 for all of Russia in 1938–40.[20] Considering the turmoil and upheaval of those years, improvement in life expectancy and diminution in crude death rate from the pre-war years represents a significant accomplishment, for which public health is largely responsible.

But if the inter-war years exemplify what medicine is capable of accomplishing even under the most difficult conditions, the post-war years exemplify the limits of medicine when the prevailing diseases are non-infectious and the health-care system is starved of support. For example, according to Evgeni Chazov, Minister of Health of the USSR, the Russian health system's share of the national budget declined from 6.6 per cent in 1960 to 4.6 per cent in 1985. 'The increase in appropriations in absolute terms barely covered the expenditures resulting from population growth.'[21] The infrastructure of the system had been allowed to deteriorate or had not been modernized; training and incentives for health-care workers were inadequate; and diagnostic and therapeutic equipment, as well as pharmaceuticals, were not readily available.

The Russian population suffered mightily during the Second World War, and there is some evidence that people who survived have been at increased risk of death subsequently.[22] None the less, the failure of life expectancy to improve substantially over the past twenty years also reflects a failure of the Russian government and health-care system to significantly reduce alcohol and tobacco consumption; to effectively treat hypertension and thus prevent its sequelae; to alter dietary patterns in ways that might help prevent ischaemic heart disease; to control environmental pollution; and to deal adequately with the problem of infant mortality in the 1970s.[23] The evidence suggests that other eastern European countries have experienced something similar.[24]

The Second World thus exemplifies the enormous power that medicine has been able to exercise even under horrific conditions when the prevailing diseases are amenable to medical measures and the political and social context make action possible. It also exemplifies the limits of medicine when non-infectious conditions dominate the epidemiological regime and when prevention and cure require interventions that the society and/or its leaders are unable or unwilling to support.

MORTALITY IN THE THIRD WORLD: O DEBT, WHERE IS THY STING?

The same issues that I have discussed already arise when considering the Third World: the question of the efficacy of public and personal medicine in different political and epidemiological regimes, and the relative importance for improving health of socio-economic forces on the one hand, and technical interventions on the other. The Third World is enormously diverse, however, making generalizations difficult, though not impossible.

One of the observations that has been made repeatedly is that per capita income is positively correlated with life expectancy: the richer the population, the longer-lived it is. Clearly, rising income is associated with improving health. Since income and life expectancy have in general risen in Third-World countries in this century, disentangling the effect of medicine is particularly difficult, since more money buys not only more medical services but better housing, schooling, and food.

One ingenious and largely successful attempt to disentangle the effects of income and medicine has been provided by Samuel Preston,[25] who plotted life expectancies of a large number of national populations against per capita income in constant dollars at several periods in this century. There was, of course, an obvious association between income and life expectancy. More interesting, however, was the changing relationship. Holding income constant, life expectancy was higher in the more recent than in the more distant past. That is to say, a population with an income of $50 per capita in 1960 had higher life expectancy at birth than a population with an income of $50 per capita (in constant dollars) in 1900. Preston inferred that aid in the form of public-health technologies accounted for most of the change.

This is a plausible argument, but is of the same sort as the one McKeown attributed to Sherlock Holmes: 'When we have eliminated the impossible, whatever remains, however improbable, must be the truth.'[26] To be truly convincing, one would like to see as well a positive demonstration of the causal importance of any particular set of variables. There is some evidence of this sort. It has been widely observed that the very rapid falls in mortality rates which occurred after the Second World War had begun to slow in the 1970s.[27] This was not the result of an asymptotic effect in which life expectancy had risen so high that further increases had become very difficult to make. It seemed, instead, to be associated with economic stagnation and high levels of debt to international lending institutions.[28] In contrast, concessionary loans, which tend to be made for health and welfare projects, were positively related to rates of improvement of life expectancy.

Because these analyses are at the aggregate level and the details of the projects being supported are not known, one cannot assert too strenuously that an effect of international aid on the effectiveness of medicine has been demonstrated. On the other hand, case studies do indicate that primary health care has had a demonstrable impact on mortality in several settings in poor populations, thus increasing the plausibility of the causal relationship between concessionary loans and improved life expectancy.[29]

Yet another way to attempt to sort out the contributions to declining mortality of economic development on one hand and medicine on the other is by an analysis of deviant cases; that is, of countries that have both low income and high life expectancy, and those that have high income and low life expectancy. John Caldwell has done this, and examined especially closely Sri Lanka, Kerala State (in India), and Costa Rica, three relatively poor states whose populations have surprisingly high life expectancies. He concluded that:

> Unusually low mortality will be achieved if the following conditions hold: (1) sufficient female autonomy; (2) considerable inputs into *both* health services and education, both essentially of the modern or Western model, and with female schooling levels equaling or being close to male levels; (3) health services accessible to all no matter how remote, poor, or socially inferior to those providing them; (4) ensuring that the health services work efficiently, usually because of popular pressure (and, in addition, disciplining rural health workers by having a physician in charge); (5) providing either a nutritional floor or distributing food in some kind of egalitarian fashion; (6) achieving universal immunization; and (7) concentrating on the period before and after birth, usually by providing antenatal and postnatal health services and having deliveries performed by persons fully trained for this purpose, and by health visitors calling on households so frequently that they not only provide advice and services but also play a decisionmaking role in treatment (with decisions about infant treatment and survival after birth being, because of the institutionalized setting, almost completely out of parental hands).[30]

The results of these various studies all point in directions similar to those observed in previous sections: that medical interventions have made a contribution to improved life expectancy, which not infrequently has been independent of economic development; and that the socio-cultural and political context within which medicine operates is a major determinant of how effective it can be.

THE FOURTH WORLD

Fourth World is a term first coined in the early 1970s to describe indigenous, non-European peoples who have been displaced from their native lands by Europeans. In this broad sense, it is almost indistinguishable from much of the Third World. I use it here in a much more restricted sense to apply to those peoples who have been not simply colonized, but overwhelmed demographically by Europeans. Thus, I do not include black South Africans, for example, but I do include North American Indians, New Zealand Maori, and Australian Aborigines.

Life expectancy in the 1980s of these four groups of native peoples differed substantially: Australian Aborigines, 57.8; Canadian Indians, 68.4; New Zealand Maori, 66.5; and American Indians, 71.1.[31] Most striking is the low life expectancy of Aborigines; almost as striking is the relatively high life expectancy of American Indians. As in my previous examples, so here too I shall emphasize that medicine's benefits are only potential; that they are made actual by the context within which medicine both public and personal operates.

Turning first to the very low life expectancy of Aborigines, it is significant that they alone among these four indigenous peoples do not have treaties with the colonists. The result has been that until constitutional changes were made in the late 1960s, Aboriginal affairs were entirely under the control of state governments rather than the Australian Commonwealth government. State governments are much less likely than central governments to support the claims of indigenous peoples for land and services, as the experience of both American and Canadian Indians as well as the Aborigines indicates. State governments are much more directly in conflict with indigenous peoples over land rights and economic-development policy than are central governments. They view native claims as a threat to the tax-base of the state, as well as to the profits of corporations and private individuals, and are certainly disinclined to provide them with services.

Without treaties, indigenous peoples have little legal claim on the central government, however compelling their moral claims may be. This is not to say that treaties assure access to land and services; they simply increase the chances that claims will be recognized as legitimate by the central government with which the treaty was made. The reason central governments are more likely to be supportive of native rights than state governments is that they are in less direct conflict with natives over land rights and more likely to be influenced by reform-minded urban constituencies which are especially remote from battles over the use of natural resources. For the same reason, central governments have been more willing to provide services for native peoples as well. Historically, then, Aborigines have been especially deprived because the absence of treaties has brought them under the control of unsympathetic state governments rather than under the control of a somewhat less unsympathetic Commonwealth government. As a result, they have been deprived of both land and services until very recently.

There are, however, distinctions to be made among those nations that have signed treaties with indigenous peoples. Two are especially significant. First, both New Zealand and Canada have public provision of health care: New Zealand has a form of national health service; Canada has national health insurance. The United States has neither. Why, then, is life expectancy better for American Indians than it is for Maori and Canadian Indians? The paradox is more apparent than real. The very fact of universal entitlement has made both Canada and New Zealand less willing to provide special services to their indigenous peoples.[32] The United States, on the other hand, has provided health care to Indians on treaty reservations through the Indian Health Service precisely because there is no universal entitlement. This is a unique programme, whose sole obligation is the provision of personal and public preventive and curative services to a specially designated population.

The second distinction pertains to Canada and the United States. Indian administration involves both land and people. The latter has been emphasized less in Canada than in the United States, because in the latter the urban reform movement of the nineteenth century had a profound impact upon Indian policy. In Canada, where the equivalent movement was much weaker because cities were smaller, there was no comparable influence on Indian policy.[33] The result was virtually to ignore health and education services to Canadian Indians, a policy that was reinforced when universal entitlement to care was established and mistaken for universal access.

Like the examples in the previous section, these are at the aggregate level. It is thus worth pointing out that in the case of Indians, there is also evidence that particular programmes have had an impact on mortality. Most striking was the decline in tuberculosis deaths, as well as in the proportion of children with positive tuberculin skin-tests, after the initiation of tuberculosis control programmes in the 1950s. The dramatic decline in infant mortality to rates lower than the national average despite continuing widespread poverty and unemployment is another striking achievement. On the other hand, success has been virtually nil in preventing a substantial increase in the prevalence of non-insulin-dependent diabetes.[34]

Once again then, we see that medicine has been capable of having a profound impact upon mortality from infectious diseases, but that this does not occur in a vacuum. The context is crucial to success or failure.

MORBIDITY

The recession of infectious diseases which has benefited primarily women, infants, and children, has been accompanied by the emergence of chronic degenerative diseases, which has affected primarily the elderly. This transformation in disease regimes, what has been called the epidemiological transition,[35] has raised the insistent question of whether the prevalence of morbidity in the population has actually increased. The question has been asked even more insistently since it has been observed that in developed nations, life expectancy of people in their eighties has been increasing at an unexpectedly rapid rate.[36] Are people surviving now who in an earlier time would have died at younger ages and earlier in the course of their diseases? Are the survivors for the most part chronically ill and absorbing valuable resources that might better be turned to other purposes? (➤ Ch. 57 Health economics) And what role has medicine played in these developments?

Taking the last question first, it is clear that medicine has had a major impact on the recession of infectious diseases, through both prevention and treatment. The impact on the prolongation of life from the treatment of non-infectious, chronic, degenerative diseases is less clear. I am not referring here either to prevention of disease entirely or to definitive cure, neither of which has happened to a significant degree, but of amelioration and/or the postponement of death. There is no doubt that this has happened – most dramatically, of course, in our increased ability to maintain people in persistent vegetative states on life-support systems, and to transplant organs – but how much this has added to the prevalence of disability in any particular population is difficult to determine. (➤ Ch. 68 Medical technologies: social contexts and consequences; Ch. 42 Surgery (modern))

The issue regarding survival of people with chronic disabilities is twofold. First, as more people survive into old age, the age structure of the entire population changes.[37] With an increasing proportion of elderly people in the population, the total amount of chronic disease in the population is bound to increase, since chronic disability increases as a function of age. Second, however, is the question of whether the prevalence of disability is increasing more rapidly than the proportion of elderly people in the population. That is to say, is the age-specific rate of disability increasing over time? Are people in their eighties now less healthy than people of the same age-group were twenty years ago?

There are some optimists who believe that, through observing sensible preventive measures, it has already proved possible to compress morbidity more and more into the very last months of life.[38] There are pessimists who argue that medicine has simply delayed death, but has not prevented and cannot cure chronic diseases.[39] Hence, extension of life has been accompanied by a disproportionate increase in the prevalence of age-specific disability rates. Others believe that either genetic endowment,[40] the accumulation of physical insults throughout life,[41] or pre-natal environment plays a major role in the development of some or all chronic diseases.[42] These are susceptible in varying degrees to medical interventions and changes in personal behaviour, and their relative significance is as yet unknown.

Analyses of health-survey data from the United States and elsewhere have led several observers to conclude that extreme forms of disability are not increasing at a disproportionate rate as life expectancy has increased at older ages. For example, Crimmins, Saito and Ingegneri considered two measures of disability that have been used in the National Health Interview Survey in the United States: chronic activity-limiting conditions and bed disability. They concluded that:

> neither ... should be regarded as inherently more valid; the two definitions give us different information. Together they allow us to conclude that increases in life expectancy between 1970 and 1980 have been largely concentrated in years with a chronic disabling illness. However, while the number of years with a disabling illness has increased, the expected years spent outside an institution with disability so severe that one is confined to bed increased only slightly. In spite of the increases in long-term chronic disability, these findings allow us to discount the notion that advances in medical science are simply enabling us to spend increasing proportions of our lives as bed-ridden dependents.[43]

Thus, while medicine has undoubtedly contributed to some extent to the extension of life expectancy at older ages in developing nations, and while life extension has been accompanied by increases in the prevalence of chronic, activity-limiting conditions, it has not been accompanied by a significant increase in the proportion of moribund, bedridden elderly people in the population. It is also undoubtedly true, however, that the increasing prevalence of people with chronic, activity-limiting conditions does pose new responsibilities and burdens for individuals, families, and entire societies.[44]

FERTILITY

I have said that the epidemiological transition has particularly benefited women, infants, and young children. For women, the impact has been largely by making pregnancy, labour, and delivery safer. Broadly speaking, safety has been increased in two ways. First, the availability of antibiotics and blood-replacement therapy has significantly reduced maternal mortality rates, from 235–799 per 100,000 births in 1920 to less than 20 in the late 1980s.[45] Second, the availability of increasingly safe and effective methods of contraception has allowed for both increased intervals between births and for a decrease in the total number of births a woman has. Both have profound consequences for the health of women and their children, as well as for population structure more generally.

Perhaps most fundamental has been the change in age structure of populations with low birth rates. A decline in infant and child mortality is equivalent to an increase in birth rates. The consequence for population structure is a broad-based pyramid with a high proportion of young people. As fertility rates decline, however, the effect of declining infant and child mortality is more than counterbalanced, and ultimately the shape of the broad-based pyramid changes to become more columnar.[46] In such a population there is a high proportion of elderly people and a decreasing proportion of young people. The issues raised by this phenomenon are familiar: the potential bankruptcy of pension funds as money is drawn out by retirees more rapidly than it is replaced by young workers; the drain on health-insurance funds to care for an older and perhaps disproportionately sicker population; lack of employment opportunities for the young because jobs continue to be held by elderly incumbents; and so on.

A second change in population structure has to do with the better survival chances of women than men. Reductions in maternal mortality and birth rates do not account fully for this phenomenon, but they contribute substantially. (➤ Ch. 44 Childbirth) The result of these differences in survival have been that in developed societies, women outnumber men at all ages in adulthood. In old age, the difference is particularly noteworthy. Davies has written that, 'Old age in industrialized countries, is typically associated with widowhood, one-person families, reduced income and greater risk of poverty and institutionalization. As Paillat said, "In Europe, the population pyramid is being replaced by a column – like Nelson's column but with an elderly woman at the top of it!" '[47]

The degree to which the autonomy of women is being fostered by this numerical imbalance can only be guessed at. Clearly, however, increased availability of the means of controlling fertility and changes in the sex ratio of developed populations are working profound changes in domestic relationships, occupational structures, and in ideas of sexuality.

In the Third World, too, the availability of contraceptive technology has been viewed as a way to prevent overpopulation, ecological degradation, and increasing impoverishment. In the First and Second Worlds, it has often been argued, economic development and cultural change prepared women and men to use increasingly effective means of contraception as they became available. In poor countries, the attempt – successful in some places – has been to encourage limitation of fertility in order to make economic development possible. Thus in a vast and populous country like China, enforcement of the norm of one child per family, and the technological means to achieve it, may alter the society within only a few generations. As in the case of the means of death control, the context determines to a very large degree how effective 'medicine' can be, but there is no doubt that under certain circumstances medicine, in the form of fertility control, can have – and has had – profound consequences in First, Second, Third, and Fourth World populations.

CONCLUSIONS

I have said that medicine, both personal and public, has had a major impact upon the sweep of human history, but only in the past three or four centuries. In respect of the reduction of mortality and expansion of life expectancy, the effect has been through the control first of pandemics and epidemics, and then of endemic infectious diseases. The impact, if any, on chronic degenerative diseases has been much harder to measure, both because we know so relatively little about their aetiology and because their significance as a force to be reckoned with in human populations is so relatively new.

In addition to its impact upon mortality, medicine has had a profound impact upon fertility, permitting a significant reduction in birth rates at the same time as it has contributed substantially to an increase in child survival. The consequences have been momentous.

The age and sex structures of developed and developing societies have changed or are changing dramatically; and the extension of life has increased the prevalence of chronic disabilities in the populations of developed countries. The consequences of increased survival of children who would have died in past times is still a matter of speculation, but the notion of 'frailty' has been invoked to explain some of the increased prevalence of disabilities that some observers think has been shown.

Even more speculative are the consequences for social organization and sense of community which may be associated with the increasing certainty of full life-spans for most people in the First World. Arthur Imhof has written:

> My theory – derived from observations of traditional European societies – is that the uncertainty of life at the time of the old mortality pattern *forced* our ancestors to develop strategies in which more durable values, such as the enduring prestige of a prosperous farm, were placed at the center of one's thoughts and actions instead of an individual EGO. Only after the change from the old to the new mortality pattern with its far more certain, more reliable, and longer life span resulting in a quasi-guaranteed duration of any single EGO, could the traditional non-egocentered world be, and in fact rather quickly was, abandoned and replaced by an EGO-centered one, as has been so predominant in the Western World for several years now.[48]

I have been at pains to point out that medicine as an isolated activity has not caused all these conditions. The context within which medicine operates determines its effectiveness or ineffectiveness. This is true whether one is considering the most intimate domestic arrangements, such as the ability of a mother to influence the expenditure of resources for medical care, or the ability of governments to spend money on health services rather than armaments. If medicine as an activity has 'caused' the changes I have described, it has been as a necessary rather than sufficient cause. That is to say, the changes would not have occurred without the technology of public and personal health services, but the mere fact that such technologies are available is not sufficient. The socio-political and cultural context is crucial, both in allowing medicine to develop institutionally and in permitting its successful transplantation to settings in which it has not emerged spontaneously.

NOTES

1 A. Cockburn, *The Evolution and Eradication of Infectious Diseases*, Baltimore, MD, Johns Hopkins Press, 1963; W. H. McNeill, *Plagues and Peoples*, New York, Penguin, 1976.

2 M. N. Cohen, *Health and the Rise of Civilization*, New Haven, Yale University Press, 1989, pp. 100–2.

3 McNeill, op. cit. (n. 1).

4 R. Storey, 'An estimate of mortality in a pre-Columbian urban population', *American Anthropologist*, 1985, 87: 519–35. M. D. Grmek, *Diseases in the Ancient Greek World*, Baltimore, MD, Johns Hopkins University Press, 1989, pp. 101–5.

5 E. A. Wrigley and R. S. Schofield, *The Population History of England 1541–1871: a Reconstruction*, London, Edward Arnold, 1981, p. 230.

6 S. Szreter, 'The importance of social intervention in Britain's mortality decline 1850–1914; a re-interpretation of the role of public health', *Social History of Medicine*, 1988, 1: 1–37.

7 T. McKeown, *The Modern Rise of Population*, New York, Academic Press, 1976; McKeown, *The Role of Medicine*, London, Nuffield Provincial Hospitals Trust, 1976.

8 S. J. Kunitz, 'Speculations on the European mortality decline', *Economic History Review*, 1983, 36: 349–64; Kunitz, 'Making a long story short: a note on men's height and mortality in England from the first through the nineteenth centuries', *Medical History*, 1987, 31: 269–80.

9 M. Flinn, *The European Demographic System 1500–1820*, Brighton, Harvester Press, 1981.

10 A. J. Mercer, 'Smallpox and epidemiological-demographic change in Europe: the role of vaccination', *Population Studies*, 1985, 39: 287–307; J. H. Mielke, L. B. Jorde, P. G. Trapp, D. L. Anderton, K. Pitkanen and A. W. Eriksson, 'Historical epidemiology of smallpox in Aland, Finland: 1751–1890', *Demography*, 1984, 21: 271–95; Pitkanen, Mielke, and Jorde, 'Smallpox and its eradication in Finland: implications for disease control', *Population Studies*, 1989, 43: 95–111.

11 McKeown, op. cit. (n. 7).

12   S. B. Hanley, 'Urban sanitation in preindustrial Japan', *Journal of Interdisciplinary History*, 1987, 18: 1–26; S. R. Johansson and C. Mosk, 'Exposure, resistance and life expectancy: disease and death during the economic development of Japan, 1900–1960', *Population Studies*, 1987, 41: 207–35; Mosk and Johansson, 'Income and mortality: evidence from modern Japan', *Population and Development Review*, 1986, 12: 415–40.

13   Johansson and Mosk, op. cit. (n. 12), p. 217.

14   W. McDermott, 'The absence of indicators of the influence of its physicians on a society's health', *American Journal of Medicine*, 1981, 70: 833–43; McDermott, 'Social ramifications of control of microbial disease', *Johns Hopkins Medical Journal*, 1982, 151: 302–12.

15   S. J. Kunitz, 'The historical roots and ideological functions of disease concepts in three primary care specialities', *Bulletin of the History of Medicine*, 1983, 57: 412–32.

16   D. D. Rutstein, W. Berenberg, T. C. Chalmers, C. G. Child, A. P. Fishman and E. B. Perrin, 'Measuring the quality of medical care; a clinical method', *New England Journal of Medicine*, 1976, 294: 582–8; J. R. H. Charlton and R. Velez, 'Some international comparisons of mortality amenable to medical intervention', *British Medical Journal*, 1986, 292: 295–301; J. P. Mackenbach, 'Mortality and medical care', unpublished Ph.D. thesis, Erasmus University, Rotterdam, 1988; K. Poikolainen and J. Eskola, 'The effect of health services on mortality: decline in death rates from amenable and non-amenable causes in Finland, 1969–1981', *Lancet*, 1986, 1: 199–202.

17   B. A. Anderson, *Internal Migration during Modernization in Late Nineteenth-Century Russia*, Princeton, NJ, Princeton University Press, 1980, p. 38; G. Hyde, *The Societ Health Service: a Historical and Comparative Study*, London, Lawrence & Wishart, 1974, p. 242.

18   S. G. Solomon and J. F. Hutchinson, *Health and Society in Revolutionary Russia*, Bloomington, Indiana University Press, 1990.

19   Among the former was H. Sigerist, *Socialized Medicine in the Soviet Union*, New York, W. W. Norton, 1937, pp. 208–37. Among the latter was F. Lorimer, *The Population of the Soviet Union: History and Prospects*, Geneva, League of Nations, 1946, pp. 120–5.

20   Ibid., p. 125; E. Andreev, L. Darsky and T. Kharjkova, 'Reconstruction of the 1933 famine in the USSR shows that life expectancy dropped to 11.6 years', *Population Network Newsletter, Popnet*, 1991, 19 (spring). International Institute for Applied Systems Analysis, Laxenburg, Austria. Also reported in *Population and Societies*, January 1991, 253, Institut National d'Études Demographiques, Paris.

21   E. Chazov, 'The people's health is society's wealth', report of the USSR Minister of Health at the All-Union Congress of Physicians, 17 October 1988, Moscow, Novosti Press Agency, 1989, p. 5.

22   R. H. Dinkel, 'The seeming paradox of increasing mortality in a highly industrialized nation: the example of the Soviet Union', *Population Studies*, 1985, 39: 87–97.

23   C. Davis and M. Feshbach, *Rising Infant Mortality in the USSR in the 1970s*, series P–95, no. 74, Washington, DC, Bureau of the Census, US Department of Commerce, 1980; J. Dutton Jr, 'Changes in Soviet mortality patterns, 1959–77', *Population and Development Review*, 1979, 5: 267–91; E. Jones and F. W. Grupp,

'Infant mortality trends in the Soviet Union', *Population and Development Review*, 1983, 9: 213–46; Z. A. Medvedev, 'Negative trends in life expectancy in the USSR, 1964–1983', *Gerontologist*, 1985, 25: 201–8; B. A. Anderson and B. D. Silver, 'Sex differentials in mortality in the Soviet Union: regional differences in length of working life in comparative perspective', *Population Studies*, 1986, 40: 191–214; R. Cooper and A. Schatzkin, 'Recent trends in coronary risk factors in the USSR', *American Journal of Public Health*, 1982, 72: 431–40; Cooper and Schatzkin, 'The pattern of mass disease in the USSR: a product of socialist or capitalist development?', *International Journal of Health Services*, 1982, 12: 459–80; Cooper, 'Rising death rates in the Soviet Union: the impact of coronary heart disease', *New England Journal of Medicine*, 1981, 304: 1259–65; Cooper, 'Smoking in the Soviet Union', *British Medical Journal*, 1982, 285: 549–51.

24　P. A. Compton, 'Rising mortality in Hungary', *Population Studies*, 1985, 39: 71–86; P. Jozan, 'Some features of mortality in Hungary in the postwar period; the third stage of the epidemiologic transition', in M. Kokeny (ed.), *Promoting Health in Hungary*, Budapest, Central Statistical Office, 1987; D. P. Forster and Jozan, 'Health in Eastern Europe', *Lancet*, 1990, 335: 458–60.

25　S. Preston, *Mortality Patterns in National Populations*, New York, Academic Press, 1976.

26　McKeown, op. cit. (n. 7), p. 129.

27　D. Gwatkin, 'Indications of change in developing country mortality trends: the end of an era?', *Population and Development Review*, 1980, 6: 615–44.

28　R. Sell and S. J. Kunitz, 'The debt crisis and the end of an era in mortality decline', *Studies in Comparative International Development*, 1986–7, 21: 3–30.

29　D. Gwatkin, J. R. Wilcox and J. D. Wray, *Can Health and Nutrition Intervention Make a Difference?* Washington, DC, Overseas Development Council, 1980.

30　J. C. Caldwell, 'Routes to low mortality in poor countries', *Population and Development Review*, 1986, 12: 171–220, see p. 208.

31　Indian Health Service, *Trends in Indian Health*, Division of Program Statistics, Office of Planning, Evaluation and Legislation, Public Health Service, Department of Health and Human Services, Rockville, MD, 1989; Ministry of National Health and Welfare, *Health Indicators Derived from Vital Statistics for Status Indian and Canadian Populations, 1978–1986*, Ottawa, September 1988; E. W. Pomare and G. M. deBoer, *Hauora, Maori Standards of Health: a Study of the Years 1970–84*, special report series 78, Wellington, Department of Health, 1988; N. Thomson, 'Inequalities in aboriginal health', unpublished MPH thesis, University of Sydney, 1989.

32　The same is true in Australia, which also has national health insurance, further adding to the difficulties of providing special services to Aborigines.

33　J. Guillemin, 'The politics of national integration: a comparison of United States and Canadian Indian administrations', *Social Problems*, 1978, 25: 319–32.

34　S. J. Kunitz, *Disease Change and the Role of Medicine: the Navajo Experience*, Berkeley, University of California Press, 1983.

35　A. Omran, 'The epidemiologic transition': a theory of the epidemiology of population change', *Milbank Quarterly*, 1971, 49: 509–38.

36　S. J. Olshansky and A. B. Ault, 'The fourth state of the epidemiologic transition: the age of delayed degenerative diseases', *Milbank Quarterly*, 1986, 64: 355–91.

37   This is also a function of declining fertility, as discussed on p. 1696.

38   J. F. Fries, 'Aging, natural death, and the compresion of morbidity', *New England Journal of Medicine*, 1980, 303: 130–5; Fries and L. M. Crapo, *Vitality and Aging*, San Francisco, W. H. Freeman, 1981.

39   E. M. Gruenberg, 'The failure of success', *Milbank Quarterly*, 1977, 55: 3–24.

40   P. R. J. Burch, *The Biology of Cancer: a New Approach*, Baltimore, MD, University Park Press, 1976.

41   J. C. Riley, *Sickness, Recovery and Death*, Iowa City, University of Iowa Press, 1989.

42   D. J. P. Barker, C. Osmond, P. D. Winter, B. Margetts and S. J. Simmonds, 'Weight in infancy and deaths from ischaemic heart disease', *Lancet*, 9 September 1989, 577–80; Barker and C. Osmond, 'Inequalities in health in Britain: specific explanations in three Lancashire towns', *British Medical Journal*, 1987, 294: 749–52; Barker and Osmond, 'Infant mortality, childhood nutrition, and ischaemic heart disease in England and Wales', *Lancet*, 10 May 1986: 1077–81.

43   E. M. Crimmins, Y. Saito and D. Ingegneri, 'Changes in life expectancy and disability-free life expectancy in the United States', *Population and Development Review*, 1989, 15: 235–67, see p. 255. See also K. G. Manton, 'Changing concepts of morbidity and mortality in the elderly population', *Milbank Memorial Fund Quarterly/Health and Society*, 1982, 60: 183–244.

44   D. Callahan, *Setting Limits: Medical Goals in an Aging Society*, New York, Simon & Schuster, 1987; Callahan, *What Kind of Life? The Limits of Medical Progress*, New York, Simon & Schuster, 1990; M. Gilford, (ed.), *The Aging Population in the Twenty-First Century: Statistics for Health Policy*, Washington, DC, National Academy Press, 1988.

45   I. Loudon, 'Maternal mortality: 1880–1950. Some regional and international comparisons', *Social History of Medicine*, 1988, 1: 183–228.

46   A. J. Coale, 'The effects of changes in mortality and fertility on age composition', *Milbank Memorial Fund Quarterly*, 1956, 34: 79–114.

47   A. M. Davies, 'Epidemiology and the challenge of ageing', *International Journal of Epidemiology*, 1985, 14: 9–19.

48   A. E. Imhof, 'Planning full-size life careers: consequences of the increase in the length and certainty of our life spans over the last three hundred years', *Ethnologia Europea*, 1987, 17: 5–23, see p. 16 (italics in original).

FURTHER READING

Caldwell, J. C., 'Routes to low mortality in poor countries', *Population and Development Review*, 1986, 12: 171.

Cohen, M. N., *Health and the Rise of Civilization*, New Haven, CT, Yale University Press, 1989.

Flinn, M., *The European Demographic System 1500–1820*, Brighton, Harvester Press, 1981.

McKeown, T., *The Modern Rise of Population*, New York, Academic Press, 1976.

McNeill, W. H., *Plagues and Peoples*, Harmondsworth, Penguin Books, 1976.

Omran, A. R. 'The epidemiological transition', *Milbank Memorial Fund Quarterly*, 1971, 49: 509–38.

INDEX

Major references are printed in bold type.

Abbe, Ernst, development of microscope
    106, 112
Abbott, Andrew 1365, 1597
Abbott, Carlisle general practitioner
    1377–8
abdomen
    in medieval human dissection 82
    surgery 964, 981, 993–4, 998, 1001,
        1005, **1008–10**, 1008–10, 1010,
        1191
Abel, John 929
    isolation of adrenaline 487, 927
Abel-Smith, B. 1313
Aberdeen
    Royal Infirmary 99–100
    University, sale of medical degrees 99
Abernethy, John 981
aborigines, Australian **1702–3**
Aborigines Protection Society 1438–9
abortion 505, 853, 854, 855, 878, 1429,
    1461, 1601, 1637
    septic 1059, 1061, 1067
abscess 966
Academia Naturae Curiosorum,
    Ephemerides 977
Académie des Sciences, Paris 298, 1501,
    1503
Académie Royale de Chirurgie, Paris 973
    Mémoires 977
Académie Royale de Médecine, Paris
    620, 1239, 1336
accessory food factors 466
    see also vitamins

acclimatization *see* colonialism; ecology of
    disease; tropical diseases
accoucheurs *see* men-midwives
acetylcholine 144, 494, 929, 931
acetylsalicylic acid 1589
Achard, Charles, on 'diabetes of bearded
    women' 507
Achenwall, Gottfried, social statistics
    1235
Ackerknecht, Erwin H. 37, 348, 414,
    416, 444, 1186, 1538
Acland, Sir Henry Wentworth 111
acquired immune deficiency syndrome
    see AIDS
acromegaly 500
Acts of Parliament (UK)
    Aliens Act (1905) 594
    Anatomy Act (1832) **99–100**, 172, 981
    Apothecaries' Act (1815) 1053, 1134,
        1188
    Births and Deaths Registration Act
        (1837) 1633
    Cancer Act (1939) 550, 1380
    Contagious Diseases Acts (1864, 1866,
        1869) **568–9**, 903, 1138, 1248,
        1258, 1633
    Coroners' Act (1860) 1619, 1634
    Criminal Lunatics Act (1801) 1631
    Cruelty to Animals Act (1870) 131,
        134
    Education Act (1870) 1080
    Education (Provision of Meals) Act
        (1906) 1081, 1082

Homicide Act (1957) 1632
Infanticide Act (1938) 1632
Interments Act (1852) 1244
Local Government Acts (1858, 1872)
    1247, 1248
Lunatics Act (1845) 1361
Medical Act (1858) 898, 1053, **1134–5**
Medical Act Amendment Act (1886)
    1053, 1135
Medical Witnesses Acts (1836, 1837)
    1630
Mental Health Act (1983) 1633
Midwives Acts (1902, 1936) 1063,
    1067, 1324
Mutiny Act (1689 etc.) 1544
National Health Service Act (1946)
    224, 1257, 1384
National Health Service Act (1990)
    1385, 1387
Nuisances Removal and Diseases
    Prevention Acts (1848, 1855–63)
    1244, 1247
Opticians' Act (1958) 1343
Plague Act (1604) 1233
Poor Law Amendment Act (1834)
    1193, 1212, 1242, 1245, 1247,
    1309, 1317, 1323, 1375, 1376
Professions Supplementary to
    Medicine Act (1960) 1344, 1345
Public Health Acts (1848, 1858, 1875)
    1244, 1245, **1246–9**, 1375
Registration Act (1836) 1240
Russell Gurney Enabling Act (1876)
    898–9
Sanitary Act (1866) **1247–8**
Sewage Utilization Act (1867) 1247
Vaccination Acts (1840–71) 1248,
    1633
Venereal Diseases Act (1916) 573
Water Act (1852) 1245
Acts of US Congress
    Chamberlain-Kahn Act (1918) 570
    Hill-Burton Act (1946) 1383
    Insurance Act (1936) 1340
    National Cancer Act (1971) 538, 540,
        551
    National Disease Control Act (1938)
        574
    Pure Food and Drug Act (1906) 1140
    Sheppard-Towner Act (1921) 1086
acupuncture 17, 728, 729, 731, 733, 742,
    744, 748, 749, 1589

Adam, Robert, architect of Glasgow
    Royal Infirmary 1502
Adams, Duncan, study of thyrotoxic
    patients 499
Addam, Jane, founder of Hull House
    (Chicago) 1484
addiction, psychotherapy 1043–4
Addison, Thomas, Addison's disease
    485, 487, 491, 494, 496, 508, 927–8
adenomas 500, 501, 504, 509
adenosine tri-phosphate (ATP) 145, 165
Adler, Alfred 1038–9
    Neurotic Constitution 1038
    *Study of Organ Inferiority and its
        Psychical Compensation* 1038
adrenal cortex **506–9**
    Conn's syndrome 509
    cortisone therapy **508–9**
    Cushing's disease **507–8**
    hormone excess syndromes **506–7**
    surgery 1000
adrenal glands 485, 492, **494–6**, 927–8
    cancer 507
adrenal hyperplasia 506, 507, 508
adrenal medulla 509
adrenalectomy 506, 507–8, 1000, 1007,
    1014
adrenaline 146, 487, 490, 491, 494, 502,
    509, 927, 928, 931
Adrian, Edgar Douglas, 1st baron
    Adrian, physiology of nervous system
    137, 142–3
Aesculapius (Graeco-Roman healing
    god), cult of 52–3, 54
Africa *see* colonialism; ecology of disease;
    tropical diseases
ageing *see* geriatrics
agglutinins 196
agricultural societies 360–1, 756, 1694–5
    diseases 585–5
    health care 48, 635, **637–40**
agriculture
    19th-century 1664
    colonial 1418–19
ague 320, 321, 341, 343, 395, 917
Ahrun of Alexandria, *Pandects* 689
AIDS 202, 309, 354, 375–6, **575–80**,
    598, 1225, 1257, 1258, 1280, 1429,
    1563, 1604
    charities 1483
    diagnosis 576–8
    therapy 579

Aikin, John 1504
air-pump 304
air-ventriculography 1017
al Ḥārith ibn Kalada 681, 688
Al-Anon 1044
al-Bukhārī 707
al-Jāhiz 684, 688
al-Jurjānī 702
al-Kutubī, *Things of which Physicians dare not be Ignorant* 706
al-Majūsī *see* Haly Abbas
al-Ma'mun, caliph of Baghdad 692, 693, 694–5
al-Mas'udī 694
al-Matawakkil, caliph of Baghdad 695, 697, 699
al-Nābigha al-Dhubyāanī 681
al-Razi *see* Rhazes
al-Suyūtī 706
al-Ṭabari, *Paradise of Wisdom* 699
al-Zahrāwī 704, 714
Albee, F.H., motor bone-saw 1012
Albert, Prince-Consort 1509
Alberti, Leone Battista, *De Re Aedificatoria* **1499**
Albertini, Ippolito Francesco
  clinical records **32**
  use of palpation 812
Albigensians 1451
albinism 413, 426
Albright, Fuller, hyperparathyropidism 504
Albucasis 701
  De Chirurgia 965–6
Albury, William Randall xi, **249–80**
alchemy 58, 155, 338, 769–70, 893, 916, 1094, 1160
Alcoholics Anonymous 1043
alcoholism 417, 420, 476, 619, 622
Alderotti, Taddeo, Bologna medical professor 1121
Aldersgate Dispensary 1188
aldosterone 492, 508
aldosteronism (Conn's syndrome) 509
Alexander, Franz Matthias
  mind-body relationship 1042
  specificity theory of psychosomatic medicine **452–4**
Alexander III, the Great, king of Macedon 942
Alexander of Tralles 55, 682, 687

Alexandria 53, 687, 855, 942, 967, 1119, 1154, 1422, 1427, 1623
alexines 162, 163
Algeria, French rule 1394–5, 1397, 1398
Alibert, J.L. 350
alkaloids 919, 920, 921, 923, 924, 931
alkaptonuria 166, 425
Allbutt, Sir (Thomas) Clifford 218, 221, 1546
allergies 195–6, 415, 509, 597
Allgemeine Zeitschrift für Psychiatrie 1362
Alma Ata, International Conference on Primary Health Care 1429, **1431–2**
Almeida, Hermione de 1527
almoners, hospital 1341, 1484
alternative medicine 598, 795
  see also non-Western theories; unorthodox medical theories
Alvarez, Walter, on pain 1575
Alzheimer, Alois, Alzheimer's disease 375, 597, 1103, 1109, 1111, 1483
ambulance services, in wartime 1547
ambulatory surgery 1005, 1006
amenorrhoea 488, 500, 507
American Anthropological Association 1440
  Society for Medical Anthropology 1446
American Anthropologist 1440
American Cancer Research Society 548
American Cancer Society 539, 550, 1480
American College of Surgeons 1338, 1595–6
American Ethnological Society 1440
American Folk-Lore Society 1440
American Gastroenterological Association 210
American Heart Association 210, 1480
American Hospital Association 1341, 1486
  Patient's Bill of Rights **875–6**
American Institute of Homeopathy 611
American Journal of Physiology 132
American Medical Association 180, 555, 615, 616, 625, 874, 1137, 1142, 1337, 1378, 1382, 1563
  Council on Medical Education 1168, 1172, 1339, 1341
  ethics code (1847) 865, **868–9**, 872
American Neurological Association 1365
American Occupational and Physical Therapy Association 1331, 1339

American Optometric Association 1337
American Orthopaedic Association 1012
American Osteopathic Association 625
American Physiological Society 132, 134,
    135
    Handbook of Physiology 134
American Psychiatric Association 450,
    1367
American Psychoanalytic Association
    1367
American Psychosomatic Society 453
American Revolution (1775–83) 171,
    894, 1357
American School of Osteopathy 623
American Society of Biological
    Chemistry 155
American Society of Clinical
    Investigation 213
American Society of Clinical Pathologists
    1338
American Society for the Control of
    Cancer 549, 550
American Society for Experimental
    Pharmacology and Therapeutics
    929–30
American Society of Medical
    Technologists 1341
American Society of Radiologic
    Technologists 1331
American Surgical Association 995
*American Yearbook of Anaesthesia and
    Analgesia* 1001
Americas *see* colonialism; ecology of
    disease
amino acids 431, 432
Amis, Martin, *Time's Arrow* 1533
Ammon, Otto 428
Amnesty International 1588
amniocentesis **1600–1**
amoebiasis 360, 512, 532
amputation 60, 679, 963, 964, 967,
    970–1, 977, 978, 993, 1006, 1012,
    1123, **1550**, 1557, 1582, 1588
    effect of antisepsis 988
    first under anaesthesia 986
Amsterdam 97
    barber-surgeons' guild 1128
    register of lithotomies 977
    tropical hygiene institute 520
amulets 59
amyl nitrite 923
anaemia

malarial 385
nutritional 479–80
pernicious 209, 214, 480, 931
anaesthesia 32, 66, 112, 234, 261–2, 877,
    981, **984–6**, 992, 998, **1001–2**, 1015,
    1018, 1191, 1545, 1551, 1555, 1589,
    1592, 1596
    acupuncture 742, 748
    in animal experiments 136
    in childbirth 986, 1064, 1065, 1589
    endotracheal intubation 1001, 1019
    epidural 1588
    in intensive care 1005
    intratracheal insufflation 987
    intravenous/intramuscular 1001
    local 924, 931, 986–3
    lumbar 1014
    patients' fear 996
anaesthetics 920, 922, 924, 931
    *see also under names of anaesthetic
        substances*
analgesia 924, 986, 1064, 1588
anaphylaxis 195, 202
Anastasius of Balad 689
Anastasius of Sinai 690
anatomia sensata (Massa) 86
anatomia sensibilis (Berengario) 86
anatomy 5, 50, **81–101**, 81, 826–7, 1580
    19th-century **99–100**
    academic 82, 83–4, 85–6, 89, 93, 94,
        95
    ancient Greek **391–2**
    as basis of rationality in medicine **82–6**,
        89, 93–5
    comparative 255, 975, 1436, 1437,
        1438
    early modern reform **86–90**
    in Enlightenment **93–6**
    in Galen's work 86–7
    historiography **94–5**
    in Middle Ages **81–4**
    non-Western concepts 652–4
    in Renaissance 83, **84–6**, 296, **1123–4**,
        1160, 1623–4
    surgical 92, 96–7, 967, 971
    Vesalian 58, **86–8**, 971, 1160
    see also dissection
anatomy, morbid *see* morbid anatomy
anatomy, pathological *see* pathological
    anatomy
anatomy schools, private 95, **99–100**,
    103, 973

ancestral displeasure, as cause of disease 735, 743

Anderson, Elizabeth Garrett
  founds London School of Medicine for Women 900
  Paris medical doctorate (1870) 898

Anderson, Sir Edmund 1459

Andral, Gabriel, revives humoralism 282

Andrews' Liver Salts 1304

androgens 491, 492, 505, 506, 507

androsterone 146, 505

angina pectoris 205, 451, 923

angiography, cerebral 1017

angiotensin 492

aniline dyes, as microscopical staining agents 114

Animal Chemistry Club **156–7**

animal experimentation *see* vivisection

animal heat 121, 156, 157, 159

animal magnetism/electricity 125, 129, 447, 620, **1030–1**

animal models, in nutrition research 456, **474–81**

animals
  cancers 545, 546
  domestication, and spread of human infections 360, 361, 368, 373, 375, 377, 636, 1695
  humane treatment 1295, 1587
  rights 879–80, 1587
  surgery 128

animism 96, 443
  in Arabic-Islamic medicine 679–80, 683
  Stahl's 124

ankylostomiasis 1401

Anna O. (Bertha Pappenhheim) 448, 1034

Annales médico-psychologiques 1360

Annales School of historians 27

Annals of Medicine and Surgery 157

Annals of Surgery 995

Annual Reviews of Physiology 132

antelope, role in trypanosomiasis 358

anthrax 113, 193, 198, 328, 329, 1268, 1272, 1274

Anthropological Society of London 1443

anthropology, medical 9, 15–16, 22, 28, 36, 49, 564, **634–60**, 962, 1037, 1064, 1069–70, 1301–2, 1394, 1397, **1436–48**
  19th-century **1436–40**

early 20th-century **1440–3**
  indigenous health care **1407–10**
  late 20th-century **1443–5**
  see also folk medicine

anthropology, social 1647, 1656

anti-psychiatry movement **1366–8**, 1632–3, 1650–1

anti-slavery movement 897, 898, 1436, 1438

anti-vitalism, in Western tradition 21

anti-vivisectionists 903, 936, 1488, 1587

antibiotics 67, 199, 205, 235, 625, 877, **933–4**, 1002, 1006, 1019, 1107, 1280, 1305, 1694, 1697–8, 1705
  resistance of microbes 377, 933–4
  in venereal disease 574

antibodies 193, 1023
  natural 194–5
  reactions to antigens 196
  role in inflammation 110

anticoagulants 1004, 1005, 1021, 1598

anticontagionism 322–3, 517, 519

antigens 192, 196, 198

antihistamines 137, 195–6, 505, 1583

Antinomians 1451

Antiochus of Ascalon, astrologer 287–8

antiscorbutic factor 475–6

antisepsis 66, 208, 262, 328, 877, 932, **988–91**, 996, 999, 1191, 1545
  in childbirth 1057, 1058, 1059, 1060, 1061

antiseptics 1551

antitoxins 162, 194–5, 208, 924, 925, 930, 936, 1074, 1082, 1213, 1278
  immunity **196–7**

Antonio de la Ascension, description of scurvy 467

anxiety 595, 1040, 1441

aorta, stenosis 1020

apes
  anatomy 81, 86–7
  role in human evolution 357

apothecaries 60, 97, 98, 783, 784, 868, 891, 918, 1120, 1122, 1125, 1126, 1128, 1207, 1208, 1332, 1347, 1374, 1472

appendicitis 187, 994, 996, 1002, 1005–6, 1009, 1013

Appleby, Andrew 35

Appollonia, St 1456

apprenticeship 1151, 1159, 1162, 1163, 1164, 1216, 1347

in early civilizations 50
medieval medical pracitioners 1122
surgeons 57, 969, 973, 1158–9
see also guilds
Aquinas, St Thomas 1455
aquired immune defficiency syndrome *see*
AIDS
Arab-Islamic medicine 6, 16, 121, 155,
205, 315, 364, 393–4, **676–727**, 805,
853, 915, **945–7**, 1155, 1408, 1454–5
early Islamic medical discussions
682–6
formal medical tradition **686–707**
hospitals 55, 696, 699–70, **715–17**,
1182, 1469
influence on India 769, 771–2
medicine in society **708–17**
surgery 704, 714, **965–8**
traditional substrate **678–82**
Arabic language 771
early medical texts 55, 83, 85, 296
Hippocratic and Galenic texts 182,
281, 282, 288–9
translation movement 281, 676–7,
691–7, 698, **702–3**, 946–7, 965,
1121, 1156, 1455
Arawaks, Caribbean, European disease
epidemics 369
Arbuthnot, John, *Essay concerning the
Effects of Air on Human Bodies* 305
Arceo, Francisco 970
archaeology 634, 730, 756–7
Archagathus, bloodletting regime 943
architecture, medicine and 8, **1495–519**
hospital architecture **1495–519**
modern buildings **1512–14**
pavilion system 990, 995, 1191,
1476, 1501, **1510–12**
lunatic-asylum design **1505–7**
town-planning **1508–10**
*Archiv für die gesamte Physiologie der
Menschen und der Tiere* 132
Archiv für die Physiologie 132
Archiv für klinische Chirurgie 995
Archivo di Ortopedia 1011–12
Aretaeus of Cappodocia 440
describes ascites and tympanites 805
describes diabetes 487
Aristotelianism 1455
Aristotle 84, 313, 389, 391, 414, 689,
695, 706, 805, 1154, 1155
on castration 485

categories 82
classification principles 344
concept of soul 95, **250–1**
embryology 391
logical writings **249–50**, 253, 255
natural philosophy 87, 88, 91, 120,
121, 155, 1121, 1157
Problems 287
virtue ethic **855–6**
Armstrong, David xi–xii, **1641–62**
Armstrong, George, paediatrician 1188
Army and Navy Medical Boards 99
Arnim, Bettina von 896
Arnold, David xii, 517, **1393–416**
(ed.), *Imperial Medicine and Indigenous
Societies* 38
Arnold, Thomas, nosology 349
Arnold of Villanova, *De Conservanda
Inventute et Retardanda Senectute* 1290
Arnott, Neil, sanitary reformer 1242
Arnozan, Xavier 488
Arrhenius, Svante August 163, 196
arsenicals *see* Salvarsan
art
of diagnosis 5, 6, 784, **801–23**
medicine as **3–11**, 64
arteriosclerosis 1098, 1103
arthritis 368, 789, 840, 1013, 1111
rheumatoid 368, 497, 508
Arthus, Maurice, local anaphylaxis 195
Artzliche Mitteilungen 1553
Ascaris see roundworm
Ascheim
pregnancy test 146, 496
Selmar, on gonadotrophins 147
Aschoff, Ludwig, cellular pathology 187,
188
ascites 805, 810
Asclepius 687, 858, 951, 1120, 1471
Aselli, Gaspari 90–1
discovery of lymphatic system 541
asepsis 66, 67, 328, **987–92**, 995, 996,
998, **999**, 1013, 1074, 1191–3, 1303,
1551
in childbirth 1057, 1058, 1061
Ashley, Lord *see* Cooper, A.A.
Asia *see* Chinese medicine; colonialism;
Indian medicine; non-Western
medicine
asphyxia 261
aspirin 924, 1589
Association for the Advancement of

Radiology and Physiotherapy (UK) 1338–9
Association of American Medical Colleges 1169
Association of American Physicians 209–10, 213, 214, 215
Association Française pour l'Étude du Cancer 548
Association Générale des Médecins de France 1137
Association of Medical Research Charities (UK) 1480, 1492
Association of Medical Technologists (US) 1336
Association of Occupational Therapists (US) 1336
Association of Physicians of Great Britain and Ireland 215–16
Association for the Study of Internal Secretions 497
Assyria 585
Astbury, W. 164
asthma 195–6, 412, 414, 451, 509, 610, 621, 929
astrology 33, 57, 59, 85, 287, 338, 769, 770–1, 803, 893, 948, 1461
asylums 442, 1030, 1184, 1211, 1350, 1453, 1475, 1648
    lunatic 1357–65, 1505–7, 1631
Atebrin 932
atheists 1586
Athens 363, 391
    (classical) legal system 1621
    plague (4th cent. BC) 586
athletes, regimen in classical Greece 52, 956
Athlone, Earl of, Committee on Postgraduate Medical Education 218
Atkins, H.J.B., breast cancer therapy trial 1007
Atkinson, Edward, on schistosomiasis vector 530
Atkinson Morley Hospital 843
atomism 313, 319, 320
ATP see adenosine tri-phosphate
Atropa belladonna (deadly nightshade) 917, 920
atropine 921, 923, 929, 931
Auchincloss, Hugh sr. 790
Auenbrugger, Leopold, thoracic percussion 787, 814–15, 819, 828

Auer, John, intratrachael insufflation 987, 1001
Augustinian brothers 55–6
Aurelianus, Caelius 440, 1120
Aurelius, Marcus 1584
auscultation 64, 178–9, 348, 787, 794, 805, 811–13, 816, 829, 830, 834, 842, 877, 1187
    see also stethoscope
Australia
    aborigines 1702–3
    colonization 372, 1394, 1397
    yellow fever 33
Australophines 357
'auto-pharmacology' (Dale) 145
autoimmune diseases 499, 500, 503, 575–80
autopsies see dissection, human
Avenzoar 966
Avery, Oswald Theodore, DNA as carrier of genetic information 212, 1279
Avicenna 29, 288, 676, 700–1, 703, 710, 711, 717, 915, 946, 967
    Canon 55, 81, 700, 701, 702, 704, 705, 771, 965, 1121, 1157
    on mental diseases 440, 447
Avignon, Black Death (1348) 1473
Axelrod, J. 137
Ayurvedic medicine see Indian medicine
Azande, Evans-Pritchard's studies 647, 1442–3
Aztecs 368, 369, 370, 1403
    use of drugs 1408–1

Babbitt, Edwin Dwight, spinal manipulation 621
Babington, William 156
Baby M, lawsuit (1988) 879
Babylon 586, 963, 1620, 1630
    healing rituals 50
Bachstrom, Friedrich, observation of scurvy 469
Bacon, Francis
    1st baron Verulam 91, 315
    experimental method 122, 343, 346
    History of Life and Death 1097
    on political economy 1234
Bacon, Roger, De Conservatione Juventutis 1094–5, 1290
bacteriology 104, 162, 183, 184, 187, 192–4, 202, 208, 257–8, 325, 329–30,

349, 352, 473, 597, 793, 924-2,
931-5, **987-92**, 1060-1, 1074-5,
1082, 1099, 1103, 1167, 1169, 1192,
1221, **1254-6**, 1265, 1273-5, 1278,
1283-6, 1302, 1399, 1418, 1419,
1488, 1563
  contributions of microscopy 102,
  112-15
  culture techniques **113-14**, 193
  immunity **198-9**
  tropical diseases 519-20, 523
  see also contagion
Baghdad 55, 205, 689, 693, 698, 700,
1155, 1156, 1182
  Bayt al-Ḥikma 693, 695, 697
Baglivi, Giorgio 343, 345
Bagnold, Enid Algerine (Lady Jones)
1312
Baikie, William, quinine prophylaxis
1405
Bailey, C.P., cardiac surgery 1020
Baillie, Matthew 99, 605
Baillou, Guillaume de, on cosmic
influences in epidemics 1265
Bailly, Jean Sylvan, astronomer 620,
1031
Baker, Robert xii, **852-87**
Baker, S. Josephine, child welfare
schemes 1077-8, 1083-5
Baker, William Morrant 133
Bakewell, Robert 423
Bakey, Michael E. de, bypass surgery
1021
balance
  health as 665, 666-7
  of humours see humoralism
  natural 70, 254, 738, 743, 940, 946
Balfour, Arthur James 420
Balint, Michael 791
ballistocardiogram 1594
balsam 1408
Baltimore, David, discovery of reverse
transcriptase 546
Baly, Monica 1314
  William 133
Balzac, Honoré de 1133
  Country Doctor 415
Bamberg surgery (MS) 966
Bancroft, Joseph, Filaria bancrofti 514
Bang, Oluf, on virus chicken leukaemia
544-5

Banting, Sir Frederick Grant, discovery
of insulin 137, 146, 166, 491, 928
Baptists, philanthropy 1488-9
Bárány, R. 137
Barbados, epidemic constitution 298
barber-surgeons 784, 891, 961, **968-72**,
973, 977, 981, 1122-3, **1125-8**, 1130,
1133, 1159, 1332, 1347
barbers 55, 57, 60, 968, 972, 1128
  see also United Company of Barbers
  and Surgeons
barbiturates 924
Barcroft, Sir Joseph, respiratory
physiology 140, 141
Bard, Samuel, medical ethics 865
Barker, Lewellys 211-12
Barnard, Christiaan, first heart transplant
1023
Barnes, Mary 1367
barometer 297, 304
Barrie, Sir James Matthew, Peter Pan
1073
Bartholin, Caspar 92-3
Bartholin, Thomas 92-3, 97
  Anatomia Renovata 95
Bartholomaeus Anglicus 440
bartonellosis (Carrion's disease) 367
Bary, Anton de 329
Basedow, Carl Adolph von, Basedow's
disease 486, 1010
Bastian, Henry Charlton 113
Bateson, William
  introduction of genetics 425-6
  Mendel's Principles of Heredity 426
baths/bathing see hydropathy
Battey, Robert 488
battle injuries see war; wounds
Bayer Co. 931, 932
Bayle, Antoine Laurent Jessé 177
Bayle, Gaspard Laurent 176
  chest examination technique 828
Bayliss, Sir William Maddock
  endocrine research **145-7**, 489
  isolation of secretin 166
  physiology of digestion 138
  Principles of General Physiology 133
Bazalgette, Sir Joseph William 1245
BCG vaccine (tuberculosis) 199, 202,
1429
Beach, Wooster
  American Practice of Medicine 613
  founder of eclecticism **613-14**, 626

Beale, Lionel 110
Beard, George Miller 1365
  on degenerationism 593
  'rest cure' 1578
Beatson, George, on advanced breast
  cancer 488, 506
Beauchamp, Thomas 875
Beaufort, Margaret, Countess of
  Richmond and Derby 890
Beaulieu, Jacques de, lateral cystotomy
  979
Beaumont, William, physiology of
  digestion 138, 209, 884
Béclard, Pierre Augustin 177
Beddoe, John, *Races of Britain* 1438
Beddoes, Thomas
  Hygëia 1303
  on hypochondria 1576, 1578
  nitrous oxide research 1589
  on tuberculosis 592
Beecher, Henry 225, 877
  on abuse of patients in experiments
    874, 876
  on medical ethics 226
  Physiology of Anaesthesia 1002
Beers, Clifford, Mental Hygiene
  Movement 1044
Beeson, Paul 4, 213–14, 220, 221
behaviour
  deviant 1648–9
  psychotic neurotic **439–45**
  see also neuroses
behaviourism 1581
Behring, toxin-antitoxin reaction 162,
  193
Behring, Emil von 197, 199, 203
  diphtheria and tetanus immunization
    197, 201, 789
  humoralist theory of immunity 194
  hypersensitivity 195
Beijerinck, M.J., on tobacco mosaic
  disease 199
Beit, Alfred 1488
Beit, Sir Otto, Beit Fellowships 1488
Beiträge zur klinischen Chirurgie 995
Békésy, G. von 137
Bell, John 981
Bell, Joseph 834
Bell, Sir Charles 621, 981
  Bridgewater Treatise on human hand
    1455
  neurophysiology 1580

Bellers, John, on health of towns 1235
Belleville Dispensary, Paris 1072
Benedetti, Alessandro 85
Benedict, Francis Gano, calorimeter
  1594
Benedict of Nursia, St 54
Benedict, Ruth, American anthropologist
  1441, 1442
Benedict, St 1450
Bengal Famine (1943) 465
Bennett, John Hughes 111
  description of leukaemia 351, 543–4
Benoiston de Châteauneuf, F.J.V. 1240
benoxaprofen 936
Bentham, Jeremy 1242, 1506, 1581,
  1587
  anatomy reform 100
  calculus of utility 862, 880
  Panopticon 1497
Benthamites 322
Bentinck, Lord William Cavendish,
  Indian education reforms (1835) 773,
  1174
Benzi, Ugo, *consilia* 947
benzoic acid 921
Berengario da Carpi, Jacopo 89
  anatomia sensibilis 86
  anatomical text **84–6**
Bérenger-Féraud, L., internal fixation of
  fractures 1012
Bergmann, Ernst von 991, 997, 1017
Bergmann, Max 154
Bergonie, J.A., radiotherapy 553
Bergström, S.K. 138
beriberi 164, 352, 353, 371, 373, **472–4**,
  475, **476–7**, 512, 1401
Berkowitz, Edward 1214
Berlin 99, 105, 207, 895, 897
  Institute for Infectious Diseases
    (Koch) 194, 520
  surgical clinic 981
  Virchow's institute 182
Bernadette of Lourdes, St 1456
Bernard, Claude 65, 130, 140, 185, 188,
  266, 919, 1138
  on human experimentation 871
  on internal secretions 485, **1102**
  *Introduction to the Study of Experimental
    Medicine* **128–9**, 185, 1530
  on life and death **258–9**, 261, 263, 264,
    269
  milieu intérieur 139, 488

physiological research **126–9**, 138, 1187, 1581
work on curare 351, 919
Bernard of Gordon 440
Berne, Eric, transactional analysis 1044
Berne University, women medical graduates 898, 899
Bernheim, Hippolyte 1034, 1036
  Hypnotism, Suggestion, Psychotherapy 1033
  Treatise on the Nature and Uses of Hypnosis 1032, 1036
Bernouilli, Daniel and Jean 1265
Bernstein, Julius, permeable membrane theory 148
Berson, Solomon, insulin radioimmunassay 493
Bert, Paul, respiratory physiology 140
Bertillon, A.L.J. 548
Berzelius, Jöns Jakob, biochemical research 157
Best, Charles Herbert
  discovery of insulin 146, 166, 491, 928
  purification of heparin 1005
Bethlem Royal Hospital 1184, 1355, 1499, 1631
Bethune, Norman, humanitarian surgeon in Spain and China 1420
Bevan, Aneurin 1196
Bevans, John, architect of York Retreat 1506
Beveridge, William
  Beveridge plan 1196
  Voluntary Action 1483
Bhāvamiśra 768
Bhela Samhitā 760
Bible 694, 1484, 1584–5
  on insanity 1460
  on leprosy/lepers **530–1**, 1232, 1263
  New Testament 691, 1480
  Old Testament 586, 690, 693–4, 879, 940, 1263, 1450, 1622
Bicêtre, Paris 870, 1099, 1360, 1508
Bichat, M.F.X. 127, 176, 177, 181, 918, 1576
  autopsies 255
  definition of 'life' 253
  General Anatomy 177
  Pathological Anatomy 177
  tissue theories **104**, 125, **348–9**, **541–2**, 975, 981, 1132
  Traité des Membranes 104, 177

Bidloo, Govert 92
Biedl, Artur 490
Bieling, Richard 203
Biggs, Hermann, diphtheria antitoxin programme (NY) 1082–3
Biggs, Thomas R. 211
bile, black and yellow *see* humoralism
Bilharz, Theodor Maximilian 529
bilharzia *see* schistosomiasis
Billings, John Shaw 1548, 1593
  plan for Johns Hopkins Hospital 1512
Billroth, Theodor 184, 552, 1014
  gastro-intestinal surgery 1008, 1191
  pathology of tumours 182
  surgical statistics 993, 1014
Bills of Mortality
  Chester 1268
  London 300, 587, 1234–5, 1265, **1268, 1679–80**
Bilsius (de Bils), Ludovicus 92
Binns, Joseph, surgical casebook 972
bioassay, hormone 496
Biochemical Journal 154
Biochemical Society 135, 154
Biochemische Zeitschrift 154
biochemistry 66, **153–68**, 207, 209, 217, 282, 445, 793–1, 1017
  19th-century **156–63**, 184–5
  20th-century **163–7**
  origins 153
  professionalization **153–4**
  proto-biochemistry **155–6**
  see also chemistry; clinical research; drug therapies; physiology
bioethics **870–81**, 1176, 1636–7
biological tests, for poisons 930
biomedicine, *see* Western medicine
biometrics 1275
biopsy 116, 187, 219, 496, 500, 997, 1005, 1016
biotechnology 494, 555
Bird, Golding 157
birth rate 1074–5, 1084, 1101
  see also demography
birth trauma, as cause of neurosis 1037–8
birth-attendants, *see* men-midwives; midwives
Bismarck, Otto von 1078, 1136, 1384
Black Death (1347–51) 296, 365–6, 586, 685, 708–9, 1122, 1232, 1264, 1451, 1458, 1473
Black, Joseph, pneumatic chemistry 305

Black, Sir James, discovery of beta-
blockers 138
blackwater fever 386
Blackwell, Elizabeth 1143
first woman doctor in USA 894, 897,
903
founds New York Infirmary for
Women and Children 900
Blackwell, Emily, pioneer physician 897
Blackwell, Henry 897
Blackwell, Samuel 897
bladder
cancer 556, 1016
catheterization 815, 963
bladder-stone 412, 952, 962, 1015, 1589
bladder-stone
diagnosis 815
empiric operators 997, 1015
surgery 55, 60
see also lithotomy
Blake, William 1460, 1526
Blalock, Alfred
artificial ductus arteriosus 1020
role of blood loss in shock 1000
Blane, Sir Gilbert 1537
Blasius, Jan 97
blastema see cell theory
Bleuler, Eugen, academic psychiatrist
1039, 1366
blistering 64, 1580
Blizard, William 981
blood
circulation 21, 139–40, 731, 737, 918,
949, 972, 1127
discovery 9, 59, 91, 122, 282
extracorporeal 1002, 1005, 1020
pulmonary 88, 89, 122, 705
coagulation 187, 1021
in humoralism 51, 155, 284, 285, 286
and transmission of AIDS 575–6, 577
blood groups 164, 427, 431, 432, 1000
blood pressure 123, 487, 492, 509, 927,
951, 1002
blood transfusion 122, 503, 509, 972,
1000, 1067, 1451, 1544, 1592, 1598,
1705
blood-banking 1594, 1598
blood vessels 122, 123
microscopic research 110
bloodletting 20, 59, 60, 64, 347–8,
391–3, 397, 400, 403, 479–80, 516,
552, 605, 607, 611, 614, 616, 628,

666, 786, 917, 939, **940–51**, 961,
964–1, 966, 979, 1100, 1123, 1141,
1285, 1404, 1554, 1580
in ancient Greece and Rome **940–51**
in Broussais' regime 260–1, 263, 350
in Chinese system 728, 731
Islamic theories **945–7**
Blue Cross System (US) 1373, 1382–3
Blumenbach, Johann, on vital properties
124
Boas, Franz, American anthropologist
1437, **1440–1**, 1442
Bodin, Jean 1205
body
in Chinese system 734–5
concept in Greek medicine 34–5,
51–4, 82, 88
fundamental faculties 82
holistic conception 665–6
as machine see mechanism
sickness and soul **1450–2**
vital forces 96
body systems **79–229**
body-snatchers 99–100, 172, 981
body/mind relationship see mind/body
Boehme, Jakob 1295
Boer Wars (1880–81; 1899–1902) 420,
1256, 1318, 1542, 1546, 1551
unfitness of recruits 1078, 1084, 1086
Boerhaave, Hermann 97, 252, 253, 256,
343, 981, 1129, 1162, 1524
Aphorisms 398
on cancer causation 541
diagnosis **810**, 815, 817
on fevers **397–9**
on functional body systems 123–4
mechanical theory **94–6**
on melancholy 441
Bogar, founder of Siddha medicine 769
Bohr, Christian, respiratory physiology
140–1
Boisseau, F.G. 177, 178
Boissier de Sauvages, F. see Sauvages
Bologna 812, 816, 968
forensic medicine 1622
medieval medical curriculum **1121–2**,
1156, 1157, 1158
origins of human dissection **81–6**
renaissance anatomy 84, 1623–4
surgery 966–7
Bombast von Hohenheim, Theophrastus
Phillippus Aureolus see Paracelsus

Bond, C.E. 221
bone-marrow, transplantation 1024
bone-setters 49, 55, 57, 59, 65, 622–3, 638, 955, 978, 997, 1122
bones
  anatomy, in Galen 86–7
  diseases 504, 966
  grafting 1012
  implantation 1022
  surgery 859, 994, 996, 1006
  tumours 181
  X-ray diagnosis of deformities 840
  see also orthopaedics
Bonet, Théophile, *Sepulchretum* 170
Bonney, Victor, obstetrician 1063, 1065
Bonnot de Condillac, Etienne, association theory 441
Boorde, Andrewe
  Breviary of Health 1289
  Compendyous Regyment or a Dyetary of Healthe 948
Boorse, Christopher 240
Booth, Sir Christopher xii **205–29**
Booth, William, founder of Salvation Army 1484
Bordet, Jules
  complement fixation test 196, 573
  on immune haemolysis 196
Bordeu, Théophile de 484, 1457, 1580
Borelli, Giovanni 94, 1580
  on heartbeat 96
Borgognoni, Hugo 967
Borgognoni, Teodorico 967
Borrel, Amédée, viral aetiology of cancer 544, 546
Bosanquet, Nick xii, **1373–90**
Bostock, Bridget, faith-healer 1456
Bostock, John *the younger* 157, 159
Boston
  Board of Health 1250–1
  Lying-in Hospital 1190
  nursing 1310
Boston Medical Police 865
botany 180, 181
  botanical gardens 772, 1160, 1162
  botanical practitioners 612, 613–14, 616, 626
  cell theory in plants 105, 106, 109
  inheritance studies 425, 426, 429
  photosynthesis 156, 163, 165
  plant physiology 120, 156, 161–2
  plant therapies *see* herbalism

Bottini, E., prostate surgery 1015
botulism 201
Bourgeois, Louise, French midwife 891, 892
Bourke, John G., *Scatalogic Rites of All Nations* 1302
Bouteiller, Marcelle 663
Boveri, Theodor 107
  somatic mutation theory 545
Bovet, Daniel 137
  antihistamines in asthma 195–6
  discovery of succinylcholine 1001
Bowditch, H.I., *The Young Stethoscopist* 833
Bowditch, Henry P., Harvard physiologist 208
Bower manuscript 770–1
Boyden, Stephen 34
Boyer, Alexis, surgeon at Paris Charité 980
Boyle, Robert 298, 956, 1162, 1463–4
  air experiments 304
  physiological work 122
Bracegirdle, Brian xii–xiii, **102–19**
brachydactyly 425, 426
Bradford Education Authority, child nutrition study 1081
Bragg, Sally xxvi
Brahms, Johannes 1009
Braid, James 1033
  on hypnotic state 447–8
  Neurorypnology, or the Rationale of Nervous Sleep 1032
brain 1139
  anatomy, Galenic *rete mirabile* 86
  biochemistry 166
  blood circulation 998
  catheterization 1018
  control of hypothalamic hormones 493
  cranio-cerebral topographies 1017
  death **271–2**, **877–8**, 1024
  degeneration 1363
  diagnosis of function 1003–4
  effect of syphilis 567
  fever 941
  localization 1032, 1581
  microscopic anatomy 112
  new diagnostic technologies 844
  in old age 1103
  pain mechanism 1581
  shock therapy 20
  surgery 1583

thought as function 1457
tumours 1017
see also mental diseases; nervous system
Brain, Peter 393
Brain, Walter Russell, 1st baron Brain 1342
Brande, William Thomas 156
Brandt, Allan M. *No Magic Bullet* 30
Brandt, Allan M. xiii, **562–84**
Bray, Francesca xiii, **728–54**
Brazil
  AIDS epidemic 376
  beriberi outbreaks 373
  homoeopathy 634
breast
  cancer 488, 497, 506, 537, 540, 543, 552–3, 558, 1000, 1007, 1014
  surgery 181, 993, 994, 996
  see also mastectomy
breast-feeding 498, 1075, 1077, 1079, 1678
  and decline in infant mortality **1684–5**
  and natural immunity 195, 1075
Brendel, W., shock-wave lithotrity 1016
Breslau University 186
Bretonneau, Pierre, on continued fever 401
Breuer, Josef 448–9
  respiratory physiology 142
  (with Freud) *Studies on Hysteria* 448, 1034
Bricker, E.M., bladder carcinoma surgery 1016
Bridget of Sweden, St, healing miracles 891
Brieger, Gert H. xiii, **24–44**
Brieux, Eugene, *Les Avaries* 571
Bright, Richard, Bright's disease 207, 351
Briquet, Pierre, *Traité clinique et thérapeutique de l'Hystérie* 447, 448
Brissot, Pierre, bloodletting 948–9
British Association for the Advancement of Science 134, 1439, 1440
British East India Company 1173
British Empire 1318, 1417
  abolition of slavery 1397, 1400
  Cancer Campaign 549, 551–2
  see also colonialism
British Heart Foundation 220, 1480, 1481
British Journal of Surgery 995

British Medical Association 134, 1108, 1137, 1248, 1341, 1344, 1377, 1380, 1403, 1563
Board of Registration for Medical Auxiliaries **1339–42**
  on therapeutic experimentation 874
British Medical Journal 216, 223, 1087, 1336–7, 1342, 1344, 1376–7
British Optical Association 1331, 1337
British Pharmacological Society 135
British Pharmacopoeia (1858) 773
British Psychoanalytical Society 1041
British Roentgen Society 553
British Society of Chiropodists 1331
British Society of Physiotherapists 1331
British Society of Radiographers 1331
Brittain, Vera Mary 1312
Broadmoor Hospital 1631
Brock, Sir Russell, valvulotomy 1020
Brock, William H. xiii **153–68**
Brodie, Sir Benjamin Collins *the elder* 156
Bromfield, William 98
Brompton Hospital 1019, 1189
bronchitis 388, 1679
Broussais, F.J.V. 182, 257, 619, 950, 1580
  Examen des Doctrines médicales et des Systèmes de Nosologie 350
  life theories 256, 257, 259
  medical philosophy **350–1**
  therapeutic regime 260–1, 263
Brown, Alexander Crum, chemical structure and drug action 921, 923
Brown Animal Sanatory Instutution 142
Brown, Antoinette 897
Brown, Horace Tabberer 161–2
Brown, John, Brunonianism 256, 257, 260, 282, **347–8**, 400, 605
Brown, John and Lesley 878–9
Brown, Langdon *see* Langdon-Brown
Brown, Louise Joy, 'test-tube baby' 878–9
Brown, M.S. 214
Brown, R.G. 1663
Brown, Theodore M. xiii, **438–62**
Brown-Séquard, Charles Edouard 485
  'rejuvenating' hormone therapy 146, 1102
Browne, W.A.F., psychiatrist 1507
Browne, Sir Thomas 1521–2, 1523, 1526

Religio Medici 1449
Brownlee, John, quantification of
  infectivity 1275
Bruant, Libéral, design for Hôtel des
  Invalides 1499
Bruce, Sir David 215, 514, 1563
brucellosis 358
brucine 919
Bruck, Carl, diagnosis of syphilis 573
Brücke, Ernst von 129
Brunner, Johann 488
Brunschwig, A., treatment of pelvic
  cancer 1014
Brunschwig, Hieronymus, *Buch der
  Wundartzney* 970
Brussels, School of Tropical Medicine
  520
bubble-oxygenator 1021
Buchan, William, *Domestic Medicine*
  1297–9
Buchheim, Rudolf, pharmacology
  professor at Dorpat 920
Buchheim, Rudolf chloral hydrate
  research 922
Buchner, Eduard
  discovery of alexines 162
  discovery of zymase 160, 162
Buchner, Georg, *Woyzeck* 1528
Buchner, Hans, bactericidal properties of
  body fluids 194–5
Buckle, H.T. 421, 427
Bucknill, John Charles, (with Tuke)
  Manual of Psychological Medicine 444
Bud, Robert 539
Budd, George, scurvy research 469–70
Budd, William
  on fevers **403–5**
  germ theory 325, 1272
Buddha 760
Buddhism
  Chinese 728–9, 745
  Indian 758–9
Budin, Pierre, infant welfare scheme
  1075, 1076, 1079
Buer, Margaret 1665
Buffon, Georges-Louis 344
  'balance of nature' concept 254, 256
  degenerationist theory 1440
Builder 1511
Bulfinch, Charles, architect of
  Massachusetts General Hospital
  1502, 1503, 1513

Bullein, William, *Government of Health*
  1290
*Bulletin de l'Association Français pour
  l'Étude du Cancer* 548
Bullock, William, on adrenal virilism
  506–7
Burdett, Sir Henry 1486, 1510
  hospital administration 1319–20, 1377
  Hospitals and Asylums of the World 1511
  The Hospital 1322, 1511
Burdon-Sanderson, Sir John Scott,
  physiological research 130, 133, 140
Burghölzi asylum 1366
burial, premature 253, 254, 261, 272
Burke, William 100
Burnet, Frank Macfarlane 195, 202
  immunological nature of organ
  rejection 1023
Burney, Frances, account of mastectomy
  558
burns, skin-graft treatment 1022
Burnstock, G., ATP as neurotransmitter
  145
Burroughs Wellcome & Co. 929, 930
Burton, Robert 1288
  Anatomy of Melancholy 440, 451, 1289,
  1460
Busch, Hans Walter Hugo 117
Butler, Benjamin 1251
Butler, Josephine Elizabeth 569, 894,
  902, 903, 908
Buxton, Thomas Fowell 1438
Bynum, William F. xi, **3–11**, **335–56**,
  809, 1269, **1480–94**
bypass surgery 1021
Byron, George Gordon, 6th baron 1526
Bywaters, E.G.L. 219
Byzantium 1155, 1182, 1496
  Empire 686, 688, 691, 694–5
  medical care 54–5, 83
  preservation of culture 85

Cabot, Richard 187–8
  on cross-disciplinary diagnosis
  management 845
caesarean section *see* childbirth
caffeine 919
Cagnati, Massilio, *De Sanitate Tuenda*
  1290
Cagniard-Latour (de la Tour), Charles,
  fermentation chemistry 160
Cairns, Sir Hugh 220

Cairo 529
  Geniza 714
Caius, John 1161
calcitonin 492, 500
calculi *see* bladder-stone; gallstones;
  kidney-stones
Calcutta Medical College 1174, 1403
Caldwell, John 1701
California, Lanterman-Petris-Short Act
  (1972) 1633
Calmette, L.C.A., BCG vaccine 199
calorimeter 1594
Calvinism 1451, 1458
Cambridge Group for the History of
  Population and Social Structure
  1671–2
*Cambridge History and Geography of
  Disease* 4, 29
Cambridge Scientific Instrument Co.
  131
Cambridge University 97, 99, 131, 161,
  162, 218, 220, 221, 890, 899, 1121,
  1125, 1161, 1190
  Balfour Chair of Genetics 420
  Dunn benefaction 1490
  Physiological Laboratory 130, 132, 142
  St John's College 1182
  Trinity College 130
cameralism 1237
Cameron, Ewen, advocacy of vitamin C
  556
Campbell, Alfred Walter, *Histological
  Studies on the Localisation of Cerebral
  Function* 112
Campbell, Dame Janet Mary, reports on
  maternal mortality 1061
Campion, Thomas 1521, 1522
Camus, Albert, *The Plague* 1533
Canada *see* colonialism
Canadian Medical Association 1137
Canano, G. Battista 92
cancer 8, 181, 182, 193, 197, 201, 214,
  292, 326, 375, 412, 414, 485, 495,
  537–61, 597, 610, 789, 994, 1016,
  1100, 1106, 1483, 1533
  20th-century research **543–7**
  carcinogens **556–8**, 597, 598
  congenital susceptibility 432, 434
  historiography **536–9**
  hospitals 537, 547–8, 555
  humoral theories **540–1**
  institutional visibility **547–52**

pathological anatomy **541–2**
public fears 537–8, 547, **558–9**
therapeutics **552–5**
  chemotherapy 554, 932, 1004, 1014,
    1022
  gene therapy 20, 506
  radiotherapy 523–4, **548–50**, 1004,
    1014, 1016, 1022
  tumour diagnosis *see* tumours
  *see also and under names of organs/
    systems*; surgery
Cancer Research Campaign 551, 1480,
  1490
Canetti, Elias 785
Canguilhem, Georges 240, 820
canine distemper 200, 361
cannibalism, as cause of kuru 214, 1444
Cannon, Walter Bradford 187–8, 243,
  452
  on adrenaline secretion 490
  on meiosis 107
  theory of homeostasis 128, 492
  Wisdom of the Body 139
  X-ray examination of gut 139
Cantor, David xiii–xiv, **537–61**
Capdevila, J.G., venous autografting
  1022
capillaries 110, 122
  17th-century descriptions 103
Caplan, Arthur L. xiv, **233–48**
Caraka Saṃhitā 759, **760–9**
carbolic acid 988, 991
carbon dioxide, as cooling agent in
  cryosectioning 116
carbon monoxide 351
carcinogens *see* cancer
carcinoma 504, 507, 543, 993, 997, 1008,
  1009, 1015
cardiology 20, 68, 209, 349, 1098, 1100,
  1556
  cardiac arrest 509
  cardiac arrhythmias 215
  cardiac catheterization 68, 214, 219,
    223, 1021
  modern technologies 20, 844
  pacemakers 1006, 1110
  surgery 140, 1004, **1020–1**
  transplantation 1024
  see also heart
cardiovascular physiology **139–40**
  see also blood circulation
carditis 819–20

care *see* medical care
Caribbean 370
  colonization 1397, 1404
  slave trade 369
  yellow fever epidemics 33
Carlsberg Brewery, Denmark 163
Carlson, A.J., physiology of digestion 138
Carlyle, Thomas 592, 618, 953
Carmichael, Ann 29, 36
carmine, as staining agent in microscopy
  108
Carnegie, Andrew, Carnegie Foundation
  1141, 1169, 1176, 1480, 1490
Carolina Code (1532) 1623, 1627
carotene, as precursor of vitamin A 165
Carpenter, Kenneth J., *History of Scurvy
  and Vitamin C* 30
Carpenter, Kenneth J. xiv **464–83**
Carpenter, M. 1325
Carpentier, Alain, cardiac surgery 1021
Carr-Saunders, A.M. 1645, 1665
Carrel, Alexis 1021, 1022, 1598
  Carrel-Dakin wound treatment 999,
    1559
  open-heart surgery 1020
  transplantation and suturing research
    201, 995
Carrion, Daniel 884
  Carrion's disease *see* bartonellosis
Carter, Angela, *Sadian Woman* 907
Cartesians *see* Descartes
Cartier, Jacques 1396
Casal, Gaspar 471
case histories 32–3, 187, 205, 315, 730,
  744, 784, 830, 831, 972, 977, 1045,
Caspersson, Torbjörn Oskar, electronic
  imagery 108
Casserius, Julius 92
Castelain, Jean Pierre 673
castration *see* gonadectomy
Castro, Roderigo da, *Medicus politicus*
  1624
CAT/CT *see* computerized axial
  tomography
cataract 729, 764, 964, 968, 977, 1101,
  1351
  pre-senile 425
cataract-couchers 55, 62
catecholamines 496, 509
Catell, H.W. 841
Catherine I, the Great, empress of Russia
  892

Catholic Hospitals Association (US/
  Canada) 873
Catholicism 588, 1463, 1464, 1585
  asceticism 1450
  charity 1469, **1473–7**
  confession 1029
  cult of saints 1456, 1497
  defence of Galenism 87, 88
  Eucharist 1450
  exorcism 1459
  healing miracles 1456–7
  hospitals 1453–4
  and medical ethics 875, 878–9
  and medical traditions 8, 87
  missions 1419
  opposition to consanguinity 423
  treatment of insane 1356
Cattani, Giuseppona, antitoxin research
  193–4
cattle plague 322, 1266–7, 1272
cauterization 965, 966, 970
Cavallo, Sandra 1185
Cavendish, Margaret, Duchess of
  Newcastle 893
Caventou, Joseph Bienaimé
  development of morphine 918–19
  isolation of alkaloids 919
Cawley, Thomas, on diabetes 488
Céline (pseud. of Louis-Ferdinand
  Destouches) 1530, **1531–2**, 1533
cell theory 65, **104–9**, 118, 148, 179–81,
  208, 258–9, 263, 326, 1187, 1593
  abnormal cytology 116, 182–3
  blastema concept 105, **180–1**, 542
  cell as unit of life 105, 112
  cytoplasm 109, 494
  and death 269–70
  of immunity 194
  membranes 148–9
  microscopic elucidation **104–9**
  mitochondria 109
  nucleus 166, 179, 194, 430
    division (mitosis) **106–7**
    structure 105, 106, 108
  pathology 109–10, 182–3, 186, 192,
    282, 327, 351–2, **542–4**, 1138
  protoplasm 106, 160–1, 194
  specificity 182
  and virology 202
  see also chromosomes; nucleic acids
Cellier, Elizabeth, English midwife 892

Celsus, Aulus Cornelius *De Medicina*
963–4
Celsus, Aulus Aurelius Cornelius 1500
kidney-stone operation 979
Central Midwives' Board 1324
Centralblatt für Chirurgie 995
cerebral angiography 214
Chaderton, Laurence 1458
Chadwick, Sir Edwin 322, 588, 864,
1212, 1214, 1240, **1244**, 1246, 1247,
1299, 1303, 1511
New Poor Law (1834) 1242, 1273
*Report on Sanitary Condition of the
Labouring Population* **1242–3**, 1509
Chagas, Carlos, Chagas' disease 367,
522, 528
Chain, Sir Ernst Boris 574
isolation of penicillin 933
Chalmers, Lionel, *Account of the Weather
and Diseases of South Carolina* 298
Chambaud, Ménuret de 252
Chamberlen family, obstetrical forceps
893, 1052
Chambers, J.D. 1674
Chambéry, Archbishop of, on
consanguinity 417
Chapin, Charles, US public health
reformer **1254–5**
Charcot, Jean Martin 417, 791
on hysteria 448, 1033, 1036, 1045,
1365, 1457, 1582
On Senile and Chronic Diseases 1100
Charenton, Paris 1502, 1507
Chargaff, Erwin 154
chemistry of nucleic acids 166
Charité, Berlin 1187
Charité, Paris 401, 447, 980, 1075, 1166
charity (before 1850) 531, 855, 1169,
1176, 1296, 1319, 1325, **1452–4**,
1469–79
16th–17th centuries **1473–5**
18th–19th centuries 61–2, **1476–8**
in China 729, 745
hospitals 1053, 1056, 1061–2, **1181–6**
Middle Ages **715–16**, **1470–1**
role of women 890–1
Charity Commission (UK) 1317, 1481
Charity Organisation Society (UK) 1317,
1484, 1485
charlatans *see* empirics
Charles the Bold, duke of Burgundy 970
Charles I, king of Spain 369

Charles II, king of England 1265, 1301,
1558
Charles V, Holy Roman emperor,
Carolina Code 1623
Charles XIII, king of Sweden 956
Charnley, John, low-friction arthroplasty
1013
Chastenet, Jacques de, marquis de
Puységur, animal magnetism 1030
Chaucer, Geoffrey, *Canterbury Tales* 1522
Chauliac, Guy de 967–4, 1122
Chirurgia Magna 968
Chavunduka, Gordon, *Traditional Healers
and the Shona Patient* 1443
Chazov, Evgeni 1699
Chekhov, Anton 1530, 1531, 1532
Uncle Vanya 1137
chemical theories *see* Paracelsus
chemistry 59, 916, 919
applied to medicine **921–4**
and cancer aetiology 545
colloidal state **160–1**
dissolution of calculi 1017
pathological **184–5**
physiological 58–9, 123, 130, **140–1**
endocrine system **145–7**, 496
neurotransmission **141–5**
pneumatic 304–5, 324, 325
synthetic 475, 476, 494, 497, 501, 505,
508, 922, 927
see also biochemistry; iatrochemistry
chemists and druggists 60
chemotherapy 67, 197, 262, 538, 554,
924–6, **931–3**, 936, 1004, 1014, 1019,
1022, 1546, 1665
see also drug therapies
Chervin, Nicholas, anticontagionism 323
Cheselden, William 97
lateral cystotomy 979
lithotomy 1589
Chest, Heart and Stroke Association
1480
Cheyne, George
English Malady 591
Essay of Health and Long Life 1295–6
on nervous disorders 589, 590
Cheyne, Sir W. Watson, Listerian
surgeon 1559
Chicago
Institute of Psychoanalysis 452
University 213
chickenpox 362, 375

Child Health Organization 1085
childbirth 6, 807, 893, **1050–71**, 1549,
  1588, 1623
  18th-century maternal care **1051–3**
  19th-century maternal care **1053–7**
  20th-century 796–7, **1061–6**, 1602
  abnormal 1050, 1051, 1052, 1440
  anaesthesia 986, 1064–5, 1589
  caesarean section 679, 980, 1013,
    1064, 1475, 1602
  in China 731, 742
  control of haemorrhage 931, 1061,
    1067
  in Koran 683
  lying-in hospitals 1051–2, 1055–8,
    1061–2, 1065, 1185, 1190
  in primitive societies 48, 49, 50
  as ritualized social event 59, 1050
  role of medical practitioners 1050–2,
    1053–7, 1060, 1063–4, 1066–8
  ultrasound diagnosis 844, **1600–1**,
    1602
  see also midwives; mortality (maternal
    and perinatal); puerperal fever
childhood 365, 369, 372, 373, 738, 864,
  1072–91, 1697–8
  comprehensive welfare systems
    1084–6, 1546
  development of paediatrics 1073–4
  French initiatives 1072, **1074–6**,
    1078–9, 1080
  infant welfare in UK **1078–80**, 1485
  infant welfare in USA **1076–8**
  paediatric hospitals 1073, **1188**, 1190
  psychoanalysis 1038, 1041–2, 1042,
    1045, 1105
  schools health movement **1080–4**,
    1087, 1546
Children's Bureau (US) 1062
Children's Hospital of Philadelphia 1073
chimney-sweeps, and scrotal cancer 556
China 1425, 1426, 1620
  ancient 362
  bubonic plague 364, 365
  Christian missions 1419–20
  population control 1706
Chinese language 728, 748–9
Chinese Medical Commission 746–7
Chinese Medical Missionary Association
  746–7
Chinese medicine 4, 6, 16, 17, 20, 50–1,
  604, **728–54**, 767, 915, 929, 1429

diagnosis **739–40**
forensic medicine **1628–9**
gi 21, 731, **735–40**, 741, 742
health and disorder **738–9**
influence on West 729, 734, **745–9**
macrocosm and microcosm **734–7**
medical corpus **730–4**
physiology 731, 736, **737–8**
san jiao system 732, 739
six warps theory 732, 739
social relations of healing **743–4**
therapy **740–3**
wu xing (Five Phases) theory 17, 732,
  733, 734, 736, 737
yin/yang theory 17, 732, 733, 734, 736,
  737, 739, 740
see also acupuncture
Chinese texts
  A-B Canon 734
  Bencao Gangmu 732
  Canon of Problems 731–2
  Canon of the Pulse 734
  Divine Husbandman's Materia Medica
    731, 732
  Inner Canon 731, 732, 734, 739
  Treatise on Cold Damage Disorders 731,
    732, 739
  Yellow Emperor's Inner Canon of
    Medicine 728
Chipault, Antoine, neurosurgery 1017
chiropody 1217, 1239, 1331, 1340, 1341,
  1345
chiropractic 65, 604, 620, **624–6**, 955,
  1217, 1330, 1339
Chirurgische Bibliothek 977
Chittenden, Russell H. 154, 208
chloral hydrate 922
chloroform 920, 922, 986, 1589
chlorosis 479, 592
cholecalciferol (vitamin D3) 492
cholecystectomy 1005
cholecystitis 994
cholecystography 1009
cholera 30, 37, 114, 142, 192, 193, 196,
  198, 322, 325, 326, 327, 349, 353,
  374, 377, 512, 517, 520, 588, 924,
  1192, 1262, 1264, 1269, 1272–3,
  1298, 1399, 1401, 1421, 1424, 1451,
  1509–10
  epidemics (1832, 1848–49) 611, 613,
    1241–2, 1252–3
cholesterol 950

Christian, Henry Asbury, on conversion hysteria 449
Christian Science 621, 1462
Christian Union, London 1439
Christianity 288, 683, 685–7, 956, 969, 1264, **1449–68**
absorption of Hippocratic Oath 855
Arabic translations of texts **691–3**, 709
attitude to human dissection 81
baptism 951
and bloodletting 945
charity 54–6, 901–2, 1153, 1155–6, 1181–5, 1184, 1317, 1319, **1452–6**, **1469–79**, 1496
controversies on evolution 1436–7
healing doctrine 1407, 1464
healing miracles 54, 55, 891, 955, 1029, 1452, 1497
on hygiene 1292–3
ideas of life-span 1093, 1095, 1290
influence on medical care 54, 57, 1122, 1125
internal disputes 689–90
and medical institutions **1452–6**
salvation of soul 54, 57, 252, 263–4, 651, 1450–2, 1456
sin and suffering 234, 318, 589, 1252–3, 1296, 1357, 1449, 1451, 1458, 1464, **1584–6**
on witchcraft/possession **1458–9**, 1464
see also Bible; missionaries; religion
Christie Hospital, Manchester 547
Christina, queen of Sweden 892
Christison, Robert 1628
investigation of *Physostigma venenosum* 921
Christ's Hospital 1184
chromic acid, as hardening agent in microscopy 108
chromosomes 107, 432
abnormal 429–30, 433, 506
and cancer aetiology 545
sex 107, 430–1
chronic fatigue syndrome see myalgic encephalomyelitis
Chubin, D.E. 538, 539, 540
Church, O.M. 1325
Church Missionary Service 1419
chyle 91, 393
Ciba Foundation 1480
Cicero, *De Senectute* 1092

cinchona 341, 343, 374–5, 397, 398, 400, 605–6, 917, 920, 1408
Cipolla, Carlo 29, 1458
Civiale, J., lithotrity 1015
Civil Rights Movement 1175
Civil War
American (1861–65) 213, 611, 621, 897, **1251**, 1318, 1376, 1540, 1541, 1547, 1553, 1555, 1556, 1561, 1593
American (1861–66) 1542
English (1642–51) 1126, 1461
Russian (1918–21) 1550, 1698
Spanish (1936–39) 1000, 1420, 1558
Civilian Sanitary Commission (US) 1251
civilization
discontents **594–6**
diseases of 6, 311, 359, 361, 362–3, 368, 373, 375, 400–1, **585–99**, 640–1, 1694–5
facts of epidemiology **585–8**
as ideology **589–94**
modern problems **596–9**
see also public health
Cixous, Helene, feminist psychoanalyst 1044
Clapham sect 1437, 1438
Clark, Alfred Joseph, on drug action/receptors 930
Clark, Alonzo 180
Clark, Sir James 1243
Claude, A. 138
cleanliness see hygiene, personal
Clement VI, pope 1473
Clement XI, pope 1267
Clements, Forrest E. 642
Cleveland, Grover 559
Cleveland Clinic, Ohio 1021
climate see colonialism; meteorology; tropical diseases
Cline, Henry 981
clinical endocrinology **497–509**
clinical medicine 60, 63–4, 153, 181, 184, 186, 187, 353–4
see also hospitals
clinical records see case histories
clinical research 6, 7, 8, **205–29**, **543–7**
19th-century **207–9**, **1215–16**
20th-century **210–27**
early history **205–7**
ethical considerations **225–7**
role of philanthropy **1487–92**
in UK **215–25**

in USA 209–15
Clinical Science 222
clinical trials 193, 934, 1197, 1223, 1269, 1277
    doubly-blinded 794
    randomized 223, 1007
Clinique infantile 1072
Clot, A.B., anticontagionism 323
clothing, hygienic 1289
Clowes, William, on syphilis 970
club-foot *see* tenotomy
Cnidos 53, 90, 1154, 1156
cobalamin 480
cobalt, in cancer therapy 554
Cobb, Stanley 452
cocaine 923, 924, 931, 986, 1014, 1589
codeine 921, 1589
codes/codification *see* ethics
Codronchi, Giovanni Battista, *Methodus testificandi* 1624
Coffey, R.C., bladder carcinoma surgery 1016
Coffin, Albert Isaiah, Coffinism 1462
Cogan, Thomas, *Haven of Health* 1290
Cohen, Henry 336
Cohn, Ferdinand 329
Cohnheim, Julius Friedrich 185, 186
    on inflammation 183–4
    on pus formation 110
cold, common 383, 388
Cold War 1224
Cole, Rufus I 211, 212
Cole, Warren Henry, cholecystography 1009
Coleman, William 1594
    Yellow Fever in the North 33
Coleridge, Samuel Taylor 1526, 1578
Collège de France, Paris 128, 185, 1102
College of Speech Therapists (UK) 1344
Collegium Internationale Chirurgiae Digestivae 1009
Collie, Sir John, on malingering 1559
Collip, James, research on insulin 491
colloidal state chemistry 160–1
Colney Hatch asylum 1507
Cologne, barber-surgeons' records 972
Colombo, Realdo 89
    on pulmonary circulation 88
    on 'venous artery' 90
colonialism, medicine and 8, 37, 38, 302–4, 322–3, 634, 772, 1269, 1302, 1393–416, 1436, 1438, 1454, 1557
    acclimatization 1291
    disease control programmes 512, 515, 522, 525–8, 530, 1398–9, 1405
    epidemics and public health 1398–9, 1401–3
    health care for natives 1398, 1400–1, 1402, 1404, 1405–6, 1417–19
    impact of endemic diseases on colonizers 366, 370–1, 374, 513, 515–18, 521, 1396–7, 1418
    impact of European diseases on natives 366–71, 372, 377,515, 517–18, 522–3, 1695
    medical workers and colonial expansion 1395–8
    missions/philanthropy 1417–20
    Western/indigenous medicine relationships 1406–10
    see also slave trade; tropical diseases
colonic irrigation 620
Columbia (NY)
    College of Physicians and Surgeons 790
    Presbyterian Medical Center 452, 865
    University 430
Columbus, Christopher 471, 563
Colyton (E. Devon), demographic study 1669
coma, irreversible 875, 877
Commission for the Study of Ethical Problems in Medicine (US) 876
Committee for Freedom of Choice in Cancer Therapy 555
Commonwealth Fund (US) 1480, 1490
Community Chest (US) 1480
community medicine 70, 1600
    care of the elderly 1109
Company of Spectacle-Makers, London 1331–2
Company of Surgeons (1745–1800) 98, 1063, 1126
comparative anatomy *see* anatomy
complement fixation text 196
computer
    data processing 845–7
    use in imaging technologies 844–5
computerized axial tomography (CAT) 207, 235, 749, 794, 843–4, 1003, 1018, 1597
Comte, Auguste 256, 351, 1641
concepts of health
    contemporary society 233–6

disease as abnormality 243–4
illness and disease 7, 233–48
normativism v. non-normativism
    246–7
proponents of normativism 244–6
relationship between the concepts
    238–43
scope of medicine 236–8
in Western tradition 18–20, 234–5
see also ideas of life and death
Condorcet, M.J.A.N. de Caritat, marquis
de 1457
on prolongation of life 1099
Confucianism 728, 743, 744, 745
Conn, Jerome, Conn's syndrome 509
Conolly, John, moral therapy at Hanwell
asylum 1361
Conrad, Joseph 416
Conrad, Lawrence I. xiv, 676–727, 1182
Constantine I, the Great, Roman
emperor 1452
Constantinople 686, 687, 766, 1155–6,
1421–2
Pantokrator Hospital 1181–5
Plague of Justinian (AD 542) 364
Constantinus Africanus 440
constitutional and hereditary disorders 8,
116, 164, 192, 312, 412–37, 444, 592,
1255–6, 1363
consanguinity 423–5
constitution concept 413–16
degeneration concept 416–18, 592–5
heredity concept 418–19
impact of Mendelism 425–7
impact of molecular genetics 430–3
methodology and tuberculosis debate
427–30
nature-nurture controversy 421–3
perfectibility and hereditarianism
419–21
consumerism 1296, 1656
consumption see tuberculosis, pulmonary
contagion 113, 159, 296, 338, 400, 403,
685, 1060, 1264–7, 1267, 1271, 1274,
1298, 1420–1, 1498, 1499, 1509
contagion/germ theory/specificity
309–34
concept of specificity 315–16
concepts of contagion 311–15
contagion theories 316–30
17th–18th centuries 320–1
19th century 321–30

classical period 316–18
Middle Ages 318
Renaissance 318–19
definition 310
contagionism 33, 37, 588, 979
contagious diseases, see under names of
diseases
contraception 166, 497, 574, 1110,
1429–30, 1461, 1686, 1705–7
oral 505–6
controversies
anatomical 86–8, 93
cellular vs. humoral theory of immunity
194, 196
nature-nurture 421–3
in psychosomatic medicine 452–3
Cook, Harold J. xiv, 939–60
Cook, James, Pacific voyages 372
Cook, Peter, architect 1514
Cooper, Anthony Ashley, 7th earl of
Shaftesbury 1243, 1244, 1361
Cooper, J., pulmonary transplantation
1024
Cooper, Sir Astley Paston 157, 980
Cooter, Roger xiv, 1536–73
Cope, Sir (Vincent) Zachary 1544–5,
1554
Enquiry into Medical Auxiliaries
(1949) 1341–2
Copernicus, Nicolaus 319
Coptic language 686
Coquéau, Claude-Philippe, French
architect 1501
Corey, Robert Brainard 164
Cori, C.F. 137, 165
Cori, G.T. 137
Cormack, A.M., first CAT scanning
machine 843
Cornaro, Luigi, Trattato de la Vita Sobria
1095, 1292
cornea, transplantation 1024
Cornelis ab Hogelande 91
Cornell Medical Center 452
coronary arteriography 1021
coronary artery disease 789, 1602
coronary revascularization 1021
coronership 1634–5
Correns, Carl 425
Cortes, Hernan do 1396
Cortez, Hernan 369
corticosteroids 498, 508

corticotrophin 491, 492, 495, 501, 507, 508
cortin 491, 508
cortisol 491, 492, 503, 507, 508
cortisone 491–2, 501, 506, 507, **508–9**, 1000, 1023
Corvisart des Marest, J.N., baron 176, 178, 828
  Diseases and Lesions of the Heart and Great Vessels 827
  on heart disease 260, 349, 350
  pathogenic effects of natural imbalance 256–7
Cos 53, 90, 286, 1154, 1156
  see also Hippocrates
cosmology 283, 1160
cottage hospitals 1194
Council for International Organizations of the Medical Sciences (CIOMS) 1431
Council of Trent (1545–63) 1474–5
Councilman, William 188
Counter-Reformation 902, 1453, 1474–5, 1476
Cournand, André Frédéric, cardiac catheterization 137, 214
Cowasgee, patient in first Hindu-method rhinoplasty operation 765
cowpox 162, 320, 361, 1279
Cox, Alfred, BMA secretary 1377–8
Cox, Harald, typhus research 200
Cranach the Elder, *Fountain of Juventa* 1094
cranium, in medieval human dissection 82
Crawfoord, C., resection of stenosis of the aorta 1020
Crawford, Albert, isolation of adrenaline 487
Crawford, Catherine xiv–xv, **1619–40**
Creighton, Charles 29
cretinism 415, 417, 480, 481, 485, 494, 495, 498, 1010
Crichton, Alexander, *Inquiry into the Nature and Origin of Mental Derangement* 442
Crick, Sir Francis, structure of DNA 108, 166, 431, 492
Crile, George Washington 997–8, 1598
  muscle relaxation technique 1001
  physiological surgery 998
  role of blood loss in shock 1000

Crimean War (1854–56) 569, 1318, 1484, 1536, 1539, 1542, 1544, 1545, 1552, 1555, 1556, 1561
criminology *see* law and medicine
Crimmins, E.M. 1705
Cronin, A.J., *The Citadel* 1530
Crook Report on Opticians (UK; 1952) 1342
Crosby, Alfred 369
  Ecological Imperialism 34
  The Columbian Exchange 34
crowd diseases *see* diseases of civilization; epidemiology; public health
Crulai (Normandy), demographic study 1669
Crusades 56, 1156
Cruso, Thomas 765
Cuba, yellow fever 200, 526, 1253, 1274
Cullen, William 820, 1165, 1580
  diagnosis 807–8
  fever theories **399–400**
  First Lines of the Practice of Physic 346, 348, 808
  health as equilibrium 282
  on insanity 441–2, 447
  Materia Medica 605
  on nervous diseases 347
  nosology 300, 320–1, **346–7**, 447, 808
Culpeper, Nicholas, *Herbal* 1097
culture, medicine and 27, **1393–416**
Culver, Charles 245
cupping 917, 966
curare 128, 351, 919, 921, 925, 929, 930, 1001
Currey, Henry, architect to St Thomas's Hospital 1512
Currie, James, cold-water bath treatment 406
Curtin, Philip 1299, 1404
  Death by Migration 38
Curtis, Alva, leader of physio-medicalism 613
Curzon, Lord George Nathaniel, viceroy of India 1406
Cushing, Harvey William 220, 1014, 1382
  Cushing's disease and syndrome 501, **507–8**
  neurosurgery **1017**
  on pituitary tumours 500
Cushny, Arthur Robertson, geometrical properties of drug receptors 930

Cuvier, Georges 1438
  on life/death relationship **255–6**, 259
cyclosporine 1023
cyclotron 554
cystic fibrosis 432
cystoscope 1015
cysts, ovarian 993
cytology *see* cell theory
cytosurgery 115

Dakin, Henry Drysdale, Carrel-Dakin
  wound treatment 999, 1559
Dale, Sir Henry Hallett, physiology of
  nervous system 137, 144, 145, 929,
  1582
Dale, William 427
Dam, H. 137
Damerow, H.P.A., German psychiatrist
  1362
Dance, George *the younger*, architect of
  Newgate Prison 1504
Dandy, W. 1014
  pneumoencephalography 1017
Danielli, J., permeable membrane theory
  148
Danis, R., on fracture healing 1013
Dante Alighieri 1584
Daremberg, Charles Victor 24
Dareste, Camille 422
Darlington, Cyril Dean 313
Darwin, Charles Robert 412, 594, 953,
  1440
  animal/vegetable protoplasm 161
  evolutionary theory 268, 1437, 1439,
    1441, 1584, 1586
  on inbreeding 423–4
  Origin of Species 105
  view of death 259
Darwin, Erasmus 586, 809, 820, 1457,
  1503
Darwin, George, statistical research on
  consanguinity 424
Darwin, Leonard, eugenist 594
Darwinism 153, 194, 235, 242, 316, 328
Dastre, Albert, on natural death 264,
  269, 270, 271
Daughters of Charity, nursing order
  1475, 1477–8
Davaine, Casimir Joseph, on anthrax 113,
  1274
Davies, A.M. 1706
Davies, C. 1310, 1321

Davies, Emily 898
Davis, Andrew Jackson, spiritualist 621
Davis, Audrey B. 1597
Davis, Joseph Barnard, anthropologist
  1438
Davis, Kingsley 1667
Davson, H., permeable membrane theory
  148
Davy, Sir Humphry 156
  nitrous oxide experiments 1589
Davy, John 156
Dawson, Bertrand Edward, Viscount
  Dawson of Penn 218, 1195, 1382
Day, George, *Treatise of Diseases of
  Advanced Life* 1102
Dazille, Jean, *Observations générales sur les
  Maladies des Climats chauds* 303
DDT 197, 377, 407, 525–6
de Bils, L. *see* Bilsius
deaf-mutism 424–5
death 20–1, 1589
  apparent 261
  causes 81, **1693–4**
  clinical signs 252, 253, 257–8, 261,
    271–2
  definition 650–1, 877, 1024
  ideas of life and 7, **249–80**
  in non-Western theories 650–1
  sudden/suspicious 1619, 1634
  see also demography; mortality
Declaration of Helsinki (1964) 226
Declaration of Independence (US; 1776)
  868, 1237, 1357
deficiency diseases **464–83**
  see also under names of diseases
definitions
  contagion/infection/miasma 305–6,
    309, 314
  death 650–1, 877, 1024
  folk medicine 661
  health/disease concepts 236, 239,
    240–7
  'illness' in non-Western theories
    648–9
  irreversible coma 877
  life/death **249–72**
  medical care 45, 46
  medical education 1151
  nature (in biomedicine) 18
  para-medical **1329–30**
  pathology 169
  physiology 120

state/medical institutions **1205-7**
Defoe, Daniel 1267
degeneration 415-16, 420, 423, 433,
572, 1255, 1437, 1440, 1529, 1530-1
concept **416-18**, **593-6**
national 1074-5, 1078
psychiatric theories 1363
degenerative diseases 1219, 1444,
1704-5
Delaporte, François 30
DeLee, Joseph Bolivar, 'prophylactic
forceps operation' 1065
dementia
paralytica 215
praecox 1365-6
pre-senile 1103
senile 1102, 1108-9, 1111
demography and medicine 3, 6, 31-2,
35-6, 69-70, 300, 352, 1219, 1221,
1231, **1234-5**, 1238-40, 1315-16,
1320, 1422, **1663-93**
family reconstitution **1668-73**
instability of mortality **1667-8**
long-term mortality trends **1673-7**
mortality within society/economy
1678-3
spatial variations in mortality **1683-5**
see also colonialism; ecology;
epidemiology; mortality
dengue 512
Denis, Jean-Baptiste, blood transfusion
972
Denman, Thomas, midwifery treatise
1052
Denoon, Donald 531, 1404
dentistry 986, 1085, 1330, 1340, 1347,
1422, 1553, 1589
professionalization 1334, 1337
deoxycorticosterone 491, 508
deoxyribonucleic acid (DNA) 212,
431-2, 433, 492, 546
as carrier of genetic information 1279
double helix structure 108, 147, 166
recombinant 494, 555
Department of Health and Social
Security (UK) 1503
depression 21, 591, 595, 597, 1111, 1655
see also manic-depression
Depression (economic; 1931) 1382
Derbyshire Infirmary 1503
Desault, Pierre Joseph 176
introduction of bedside teaching 976

Descartes, René 91
Cartesianism 59, 1457, 1582, 1587
De Homine 124
Discourse on Method 1097
dualism 95, 443, 738
mechanistic philosophy 124, 1462,
1581
Destouches, Louis-Ferdinand see Céline
Deutsch, Albert 1548, 1558
Deutsch (Detre), Ladislas 194
Deutsch, Felix 452
Deutsche Gesellschaft für
Rassenhygiene 421
Deutsche Zeitschrift für Chirurgie 995
diabetes 1703
insipidus 488, 500, 501
mellitus 128, 146, 451, **487-8**, 496-7,
502-3, 597, 928, 1005, 1103, 1111,
1221
diagnosis 60, 66, 196, 336-7, 405, 496,
509, 573, 999, 1003, 1017
in Chinese medicine 731, 732, **739-40**
in geriatrics 1102, 1106, 1108
history-taking 784, 789, **792-5**, 801,
806, 808, 829, 842, 1165, 1579
in Indian medicine 768, 769
inspection of excreta 765, 768, 769,
784, 804-5, 806, 819
in medieval Islam 714
in non-Western theories 654-5
observation 784, 786, 806-8, 812, 817,
819, 829
patients' role 18, 63, 64, 66, 784,
789-90, **791-5**
physical examination 64, 178-9, 784,
787-9, 794, **808-13**, 828-5, 842,
1579
diagnosis, art of 5, 6, 784, **801-23**
18th century **806-18**
19th century 66, **818-20**
early history 46, 60, **802-5**
Middle Ages and Renaissance **805-6**
Diagnosis Related Groups (DRGs) 1198,
1387
diagnosis, science of 7, 127, 140, 207,
787-9, 794, **826-51**, 1165, 1546-7
anatomical thinking **826-7**
image **839-45**, 997, 1346
number/graph **833-9**
printout **845-7**
sound **828-33**, 1594, **1601**, 1602

Diagnostic and Statistical Manual of the American Psychiatric Association 1029
diagnostic techniques, *see under names of instruments and techniques*
diagnostic technologies **826–51**, 1005–6, 1010, 1015–12, 1018, 1021, 1143
see also under names of procedures/ technologies
dialysis *see* kidneys
diarrhoea 345, 396, 637, 760
  epidemic 1075, 1079, 1083
  infantile (summer) 1278, 1429, 1667, 1681, **1685–6**, 1696–7
  tropical 522, 531
diazepam 1001
Dick, George and Gladys Rowena (née Henry), scarlet fever antitoxin 197
Dickens, Charles 592, 1310
  Nicholas Nickleby 1072
Diderot, Denis 1476, 1524, 1525
  Encyclopédie 1128, 1350–1, 1505
  Rêve d'Alembert 1457
Dieffenbach, Johann Friedrich 981
  inverted suture technique 992
  tenotomy 993
diet 939, **940–51**, 1288, 1294
  in ancient Greece and Rome **940–5**, 1232, 1235, 1285–6
  in diabetes 502–3
  in early Chinese medicine 731
  Hindu 762–3
  Islamic theories **945–7**
  in old age 1096, 1097, 1102, 1104
  in pernicious anaemia 214, 931
  unorthodox regimes **618–20**, 622
  see also nutrition; regimen
dieticians 1345
Dietrich, Justina, Prussian midwife 892
digestion 156, 157, 612
  and nutrition 157, 159, 163
  physiology 125, 136, 137, 138
digestive system *see* gastro-intestinal system
digitalis 789, 917–18, 920, 930, 1101, 1102
Dionis, Pierre 972, 977
Dioscorides 682, 699, 703, 707, 1120
diphtheria 142, 193, 194, 196–7, 208, 321, 362, 363, 589, 597, 789, 924, 1082–3, 1138, 1254–5, 1278, 1429, 1665, 1697
disability 237, 238, 1226, 1549, 1550

age-specific 1704–5
disease
  biological basis 30
  Chinese theories **738–9**
  concepts 6–7, 18–20, **233–48**
  ecology of 6, **357–81**
  historiography **29–32**
  influence of environment **292–308**
  localization theory 176, 971, 987, 997, 1032, 1165, 1283, 1351
  see also nosology; pathology
diseases *see* civilization; endocrine; mental; nutritional; sexually transmitted; tropical
diseases, *see also under names of diseases*
dislocations 963, 964, 966, 971, 977, 1012
dispensaries 32, 61, 1188, 1189, 1477
  colonial (mobile) 1402, 1407
Dispensatorium Pharmacopoearum (Lyons, 1546) 916
Disraeli, Benjamin 1243
dissection, animal 81, **86–7**, 88, 391, 712, 1121
  see also vivisection
dissection, human 57, 58, 99, 176, 296, 1157, 1164, 1165
  in 18th century 62, 63, 97
  for cause of death 81, 170, 820, 826, 828, 830, 831–2, 967, 1098, 1100, 1122, **1623–4**
  Christian/Muslim attitude 712, 1456
  decline of 92
  in hospitals **171–6**, 188, 1187
  for localizing disease 170, 975–6
  origins **81–4**
  preservation techniques 92
  in private schools 97–8
  public 85–6, 89
  Renaissance **84–8**
  supply of cadavers 90, 99–100, 172–3, 981, 1161, 1187, 1478
  Vesalian **86–8**, 1160
Dissenters 1451
Dittel, J. von 1015
divination 49, 50, 55, 638, 735, 744, 770
DNA *see* deoxyribonucleic acid
Dock, George 186
  critique of X-ray diagnosis 842
doctor-patient relationship 4, 6, 67, 84, 225, 238, 353, **783–800**, **1644–5**, 1652

in ancient societies 47
at deathbed 263
in China **742–4**
confidentiality 1224
evidence in medical records 32
impersonality in high-tech milieu 68,
 70, 793–4
legal aspects 1636–7
in medieval Arab-Islam 714
modern period **787–92**, 1220
patient alienation 794–5
patient power 796–7, 1131, 1132
patient-as-person 791–2, 793–4, 794
physician dissatisfaction 795–6
post-modern period **792–7**
social conventions **815–18**, 828, 832
traditional period **783–7**
in Western tradition 18–20
see also diagnosis; ethics; psychiatry;
 psychotherapy
Dodds, Sir (Edward) Charles, production
 of stilboestrol 146–7, 505
Dogmatists 1120
Doisy, Edward Adalbert, criteria for
 hormone identification 137, 146
Doll, Sir Richard, on smoking and lung
 cancer 224, 1278
Dols, Michael 37
Domagk, Gerhard, discovery of Prontosil
 932, 1066
domestic medicine see family medicine
domiciliary nursing **1324–5**
Donath, Julius, mechanism of haemolysis
 196
Donders, F.C., standards of visual acuity
 1332
Doniach, Deborah, on thyroiditis 495
Donné, Alfred 180
Donne, John 313
Donovan, Charles, on kala azar 514
dopamine 493
Doré, Gustave 592
Dorpat University, pharmacology chair
 919–20
Douglas, James 94
 diagnosis of hernia 815
Dowbiggin, Ian 417
Down, John L.H., Down's syndrome
 429–30, 433
Doyle, Sir Arthur Conan 416, 834, 1532
Draper, Mrs, midwife to Queen
 Charlotte 893

dreams 49, 445, 449, 1366
 Freud's work 1035
Dreyer, Georges 199
DRGs see Diagnosis Related Groups
dropsy 336, 688, 786, 808–9, 812,
 917–18
 epidemic 476–7
Drosophila 107, 430
drug receptors 930
drug therapies 4, 8, 66–7, 145, 311,
 702–3, 704, 714, **915–38**, 984, 1009,
 1109
 19th-century **918–26**
  applied chemistry **921–4**
  origins of pharmacology **918–21**
 20th-century **926–36**
  physiological agents as drugs **926–9**
  purity of drugs 934–6
  science of drugs **929–31**
 in antiquity 51, 55, 915
 Renaissance/Enlightenment **916–18**
 scientific basis for drug use **918–19**
 in surgery 1001–2, 1004
 unorthodox **604–16**
 see also and under names of diseases;
  chemotherapy
drug-addiction 239, 354, 376
 and spread of AIDS 577
druggists 1134
drugs 60, 155, 156, 789, 793, 924–5,
 1408
 adrenergic blockers 509
 anti-inflammatory 508, 625
 antibacterial 924–6
 biotransformation 922
 Chinese 729, 730, 731, 732, **741–2**,
  745, 748, 749
 Indian 757, 758, 760, 762, 768–9, 775
 international standardization 1428
 intravenous administration 1597
 mode of action 930
 psychotropic 445, 904, 905, 1044,
  1046, 1108, 1366–7, 1368, 1589
 side effects **934–5**
 specifics 60, 262, 341, 343
 synthetic 67, 923
 see also and under names of drugs and
  hormones; antibiotics
Dryander (Eichmann), Johannes 85
Du Bois, E.F. 1594
 calorimeter 1594

Du Bois Reymond, Emile, electrical nature of nervous impulse 125, 129
Du Laurens, André *see* Laurens
dualism *see* mind/body dualism
Dubé, Paul, *Médecin des Pauvres* 1296
Dubos, Jean and René, *The White Plague* 30
Dubos, René 473
Dubost, Charles, resection of aneurysm of aorta 1020
Duchenne muscular dystrophy 432
Duclaux, Emile 195
Duden, Barbara 32–3
Duffy, John 33
Dufour, Léon, baby welfare clinic 1078
Dujardin, Félix, protoplasmic theory 161
Dumas, Jean Baptiste André 159
Dunant, Jean Henri, founder of Red Cross 1422, 1558
Dunbar, Helen Flanders, *Emotions and Bodily Changes* 452–3
Duncan, Andrew jr. 1188, 1629
use of thoracic percussion 819–20
Duncan, William, Liverpool medical officer of health 1244
Dunhill, Thomas, thyroid surgery 499
Dunn, Sir William, Cambridge and Oxford benefactions 154, 221, 1490
Dupuytren, Guillaume 980, 981
Durand-Ferdel, C.L., *Traité des Maladies des Vieillards* 1100, 1102
Durkheim, Emile 1351, 1442, **1641–2**, 1647, 1655, 1657
Rules of Sociological Method 1642
Suicide **1642–3**
Dutch Medical Association 880
Duvé, C.R. de 138
dwarfism 501
Dwork, Deborah xv, **1072–91**
dyestuffs industry 923
Dymphna, St 1497
dysentery 364, 523, 530, 917, 1251, 1264, 1318
amoebic 360, 512, 532
dysmenorrhoea 1013

East India Company 772
Eberhard im Bart, duke of Württemburg 1289
Eberth, Carl Joseph, typhoid bacillus 405
Eccles, Sir John E., physiology of nervous system 137, 144

ECG *see* electrocardiograph
eclecticism 604, **613–14**, 615, 616, 627
ecology of disease 6, 34, **357–81**, 1232
15th-century exploration/colonization **366–9**
16th-century slave trade **369–71**
17th–18th centuries **371–3**
19th-century **374–5**
20th-century **375–7**
disease and human evolution **357–63**
Graeco-Roman period 363
Middle Ages **363–6**
see also environment and miasmata
economics 92–3
laissez-faire 322, 903, 1633, 1697
Third World debt 1700–1
economics, health 8, 27, 68–9, 70, 188–9, 224–5, 233, 236, 1144, **1176**, 1210–11, **1212–13**, 1220, 1222–3, 1226–8, 1433, 1482–3, 1656
cancer funding 550–1
finance
(1760–1860) **1374–5**
(1860–1914) **1375–8**
(1910–48) **1379–82**
(1910–65) US **1382–4**
(1945–79) UK/Europe **1384–5**
budgeting, and insurance **1373–90**
(post-1979) **1385–8**
geriatrics 1110, 1111
technologies 844, **1601–4**
see also hospitals, budgets
Eddy, Mary Baker
founder of Christian Science 621
Science and Health 1462
Edelstein, Ludwig 854, 855
Edinburgh 173
Dispensary 1188
Hospital for Women and Children 900
new town 1508
Royal Infirmary 32, 806, 807–8, 819, 1185, 1500, 1508
University 98, 99, 126, 130, 180, 346, 447, 468, 807, 861, 864, 898, 900, 921, 950, 976, 981, 1294, 1580, 1629–30
Cullen's teaching 124–5
histology courses 111
Edison, Thomas 553
education *see* medical education; surgeons; women
Edward VII, king of England 1486

Edwards, A.T., pulmonary resection
1019
Edwards, Robert, *in vitro* fertilization
878–9
EEG *see* electroencephalograph
Egaz Moniz, A.C. de
cerebral angiography 1017
leucotomy 1018
Egypt 691, 695
ancient 50–1, 360, 585, 756, 942, 963,
1437, 1620–1
cholera outbreak (1883) 114
Coptic language 686
Pan-Arab Quarantine Board of Health
37, 1233, 1421, 1427
schistosomiasis 529–30
Ehrlich, Paul 114, 195, 208, 930
'chemical bullets' 163, 262, 925–6
discovery of Salvarsan 572, 574, 789,
926
humoralist theory of immunity 194,
196
physiology of nervous system 137, 144,
925
Eichmann, Johannes *see* Dryander
Eijkman, Christiaan, beriberi research
473–4
Eijkman, E. 137
Einthoven, Willem
ECG 215
string-galvanometer 137, 140, 1592
elderly *see* geriatrics
Electra complex 1036
electricity 324
animal *see* animal magnetism
in nervous system 142–3, 148
electro-surgery 1017
electrocardiograph (ECG) 32, 140, 215,
222, 223, 837, 847–8, 1106, 1592,
1594–5
electroencephalograph (EEG) 847, 877,
1043
electron microscope *see* microscopy
elements (earth, air, fire, water), in
humoral theory 612
Eleonora, Duchess of Troppau 893
elephantiasis *see* filariasis
Eli Lilley Company 928
Elias, Norbert, *Civilizing Process* 1300
Eliot, George (pseud. of Mary Anne
Evans) 1488
Middlemarch 1529

Elizabeth, countess of Kent 893
Elizabeth of Hungary, St, curative
miracles 891
Elizabeth I, queen of England 892, 1474,
1681
Ellermann, Vilhelm, on virus chicken
leukaemia 544–5
Elliotson, John, scurvy research 469
Elliott, T.R. 224
Ellis, Sir Arthur 217
Ellison, Edwin, Zollinger-Ellison
syndrome 504–5 ,
Elmquist, Rune, construction of heart
pacemaker 1006
Elsberg, C., neurosurgeon 1018
Elyot, Sir Thomas, *Castel of Health* 1289
embolism 1005
embryology 180, 181, 542
in plants 106
emetics 786, 917, 918, 1100, 1285
emetine 918
Empedocles of Acragas 283, 284, 285
emphysema 1100, 1102
empiricism 1126, 1127, 1128
empirics 55, 57, 59, 62, 85, 555, 565,
666, 744, 763, 968, 971, 977, 979,
1014, 1122–3, 1130, 1136, 1141,
1152, 1154–5, 1207, 1209, 1294,
1351, 1374, 1589
empyemia 963, 1019
encephalitis 368
Encyclopédie 61, 252, 419, 1128, 1350,
1505
endocrine diseases/edocrinology, *see also*
names of diseases, organs and
hormones
endocrine diseases/endocrinology 8, 67,
185, **483–510**, 927, 997, 1000, 1003,
1004, 1106
clinical syndromes **498–508**
development **490–98**
drug treatment **496–7**, 499, 501, 1014
mechanisms **494–5**
origins **483–9**
status of clinical endocrinology **497–8**
surgery **1009–10**, 1010–11
endocrine system, physiology **145–9**, 185
Endocrinology 498
endorphins 748, 1582–3, 1589
endoscopy 1005, 1011, 1016, 1596
energy, law of conservation 129

Engel, George, biopsychosocial approach
to disease 454
'English Hippocrates' *see* Sydenham, T.
Enthoven, Alain 1387
environment 51–2, 311, 317, 321, 342,
416, 587–8, 597–8, 988–9, 1232,
1239–40, 1285, 1287, 1291
carcinogenic factors 557–8
in humoralism 289
and miasmata 292–308, 1263, 1298,
1302
air as cause of disease 304–6
in Hippocratic Corpus 293–4
medical meteorology 296–300
medical topography and geography
300–2
Middle Ages/Renaissance 296
New World 302–4
work, and health 1213–14, 1222
see also architecture; ecology of disease
enzymes 137, 160–5, 489
in cancer research 546
defects 495
specific enzyme theory 160
eosin 789
ephedrine 929
Epicurus/Epicureanism 313, 1584
epidemic constitution 297–8, 301, 312,
342, 397, 400, 402, 1263, 1265, 1421
Epidemiological Society 1262, 1273
epidemiology 8, 30–1, 36–7, 113, 223–4,
349, 362–3, 465, 638, 739, 1209–10,
1219, 1221, 1262–82, 1401–3,
1693–711
16th–18th centuries 1264–9
19th-century 1269–75
20th-century 1275–80
in antiquity 1263–4
historiography 33–4
influence of environment 292–308
Middle Ages 1264
statistical method 1262, 1265–6,
1269–73, 1275–7
see also contagion; ecology of disease;
internationalism; public health
epilepsy 31, 284, 285, 412, 414, 439,
446, 941, 942, 1422, 1459–60
epizootics 1266–7, 1272, 1273
Erasistratus 286, 392, 393
on regimen 942–3
Erdheim, Jacob, on multiple endocrine
disorders 495

ergot 920, 931, 1582
ergotism 363
ergotoxine 929
Erhard, Hans Werner, psychotherapy
1044
Erickson, Milton H., on hypnosis 1041
Erlanger, Joseph 137, 143
Erxleben-Leporin, Dorothea Christiane,
Prussian pioneer physician 895–7
erysipelas 321, 979, 1060, 1061
erythropoietin 503
eserine 921, 929, 931
Eskimos, antiscorbutic diet 464, 470, 475
Espine, Marc d' 353
Esquirol, J.E.D. 1502, 1506
moral therapy 1359
ether
as anaesthetic 922, 985–6, 1001
as cooling agent in cryosectioning 116
ether theory (physics) 93
Etheridge, Elizabeth, *The Butterfly Caste*
30, 31
ethics, medical 3, 8, 69, 225–7, 615,
743–4, 763, 852–87, 1121, 1455,
1619
20th-century 870–81, 1110, 1538
animal rights 879–80
bioethecal critique 875–6
brain death 877–8
consent/refusal of therapy 873–41
in vitro fertilization 878–9
medical technology 876–7
mercy-killing 880–1
Physician's Oath 872–3
transplantation 1023–4
ancient virtue ethics 856–9
codification, 19th-century 868–70
Gregory's contribution 861–3
Hippocratic *Oath* 52, 852–62
Middle Ages and Renaissance 83, 861
Percival's contribution 864–8
see also experimentation, human;
Nuremberg Code
ethno-psychiatry 671
ethnography *see* anthropology
Ethnological Society of London 1439
Ettling, John *The Germ of Laziness* 30, 31
eudiometer 305
eugenics 419–21, 594, 872, 1255–6,
1304, 1546
Eugenics Society 594

Euler, Ulf Svante von, on
  neurotransmitters 137, 492, 929
European Journal of Physiology 132
European revolutions (1848) 894, 897–8
Eurotransplant 1023
Eustachio, Bartolomew, criticizes
  Vesalius 87–8
euthanasia 857–9, 872, 880–1, 1587,
  1637
Evans, Sir Charles Arthur Lovatt (ed.),
  Principles of Human Physiology 133
Evans, Herbert 491
Evans, Richard, *Death in Hamburg* 30, 37
Evans, Warren Felt, 'mind cure' 621
Evans-Pritchard, Sir Edward E. 647
  *Witchcraft, Oracles and Magic among the
  Azards* 1442–3
evolution 241–2, 316, 328, **1436–8**,
  1439, 1585
  role of disease **357–63**
exercise, therapeutic 956, 1286, 1290
exorcism 50, 57, 59, 656, 735, 1459,
  1460
  in Christianity 55
experimental medicine *see* clinical
  research; physiology
experimental method **126–8**, 205–6,
  1163–7
  Bacon's 122, 343, 346
Experimental Physiology 132
experimentation, animal *see* vivisection
experimentation, human 138, 202–3,
  206, 1223, 1637
  informed consent **873–41**
  Nazi atrocities 202–3, 225, **871–2**,
    1087, 1232, 1538, 1554, 1577
  on war recruits 1553–4
exploration/colonization *see* colonialism
Expressionists 1530
eye 129, 137, 620
  microscopic anatomy 112
  in occultism 313
  see also ophthalmology
Eyler, John 33
Eyre, Edward John, governor of Jamaica
  1439
Eyseneck, Hans J. 1045

Faber, Knud 341
Fabricius ab Aquapendente,
  Hieronymus, anatomy **88–9**, 93, 980
Fagge, C. Hilton, typhoid research 405

Faith Assembly (Indiana), childbirth
  records **1069**
faith healing 769, 1029–30
Falconer, William, *Influence of the Passions
  on the Disorders of the Body* 451
Falloppio, Gabriele, criticizes Vesalius
  87–8
Falret, J.R., psychiatrist 444
family medicine 18–19, 21, 47, 48, 233,
  670–2, 795, 1130, 1452
  in 17th century 58–9
  in classical Greece and Rome 51–4
  impact of sexually transmitted diseases
    571–2
  in primitive societies 638
family planning *see* contraception
family reconstitution **1668–77**, 1677–8,
  1679–80, **1681–4**
family therapy 1043
famine 35, 465, 586, 1698
Farabee, William Curtis, inheritance
  studies 425, 426
Farley, J. 529, 530
Farmer, John Bretland 107
Faroe Islands, measles epidemic 1270–3
Farr, William 33, 34, 1273, 1274
  laws of epidemics **1271**
  social statistics 1057, **1240–1**, 1375
  statistical nosology 324–5, 352–3, 588
Fedele, Fortunato, *De Relationibus
  medicorum* 1624
Federal Drugs Agency 555–6, 874
Feldenkrais, Moshé, impact of body on
  psyche 1042
Feldman, William Hugh, use of
  streptomycin in tuberculosis 933
Félicie, Jacqueline, lay healer 1122
Felix, Arthur, Vi antigen 198
Félix, C.F., anal fistula operation 972–3
Fellowship of Surgeons 969
feminism *see* women's rights movement
fenestration 1011
Fenwick, Mrs *see* Manson, Ethel
Ferenczi, Sándor 1037, 1038, 1041
  on anxiety 1040
fermentation 153, 156, 159, 160, 162,
  165, 192, 258, 262, 314, 324, 325,
  327, 328, 353, 988
Fernel, Jean
  disease classification 340
  Medicina 170
  'physiologia' 120

Férran, Jaime 198
Ferrier, Sir David, neurophysiology 1581
fertility 501, **1705–7**
  see also demography
fertilization 107
  in vitro (IVF) **878–9**, 1637
fever
  continued 321, 322, 399, 400–4, 807,
    1266, 1273
  essential 349, 352, 354
  intermittent 321, 322, 341, 516, 605–6
  malignant 1298
  pestilential 1264–5
  relapsing 321, 404, 406
  spotted (petechial) 399, 402
fevers 46, 297, 320, 349, 364, **382–411**,
    586, 1269, 1679
  19th-century **400–6**
  Boerhaave and followers **397–9**
  classification 321, 337, 338, 340, 341,
    344–5
  Cullen's influence **399–400**
  in Galen **393–4**, 955
  in Hippocratic Corpus **382–91**
    malarial **384–7**
    seasonal influence 388–90
    treatment 390–1
  hospitals 1309, 1376, 1377
  humoral theory 286
  Sydenham's concepts **394–7**
  tropical 514, 515, 518
  typhus and typhoid **401–6**
  unorthodox theories 605–6, 612, 613
fibre, as primary body unit (Boerhaave)
    94
Ficino, Marsilio, *Liber de Vita* 1289
Fick, Adolf, cardiac output 140
Fielding, Henry 1526
  Tom Jones 1524
filariasis 364, 370, 512, 514, 519, 531
Finke, Leonhard Ludwig, medical
    geography 301–2
Finland, famine (1696) 586
Finsen, Nils 214
Fischer, Emil 162, 163
  nature of proteins 163–4
Fischer, Johann Bernard von, *De Senio*
    1098
Fisher, Irving, economist 1254, 1375–6,
    1385
Fisher, R.A., *Design of Experiments* 223
fistulas 60

anal 815, 972–3
ano-rectal 993
vesico-vaginal 1013
Fitz, R.M., appendicitis 1008
Flagg, P.J., *Art of Anaesthesia* 1002
flame photometer 148
Flaubert
  Gustave 1133, 1527
  Madame Bovary 1529
Fleck, Ludwik 203
Fleidner, Theodore 902
Fleming, Sir Alexander, discovery of
  penicillin 933
Flemming, C.F., German psychiatrist
    1362
Flemming, Walter, *Zellsubstanz, Kern und
  Zelltheilung* 107
Fletcher, Sir Walter Morley 221, 222
Fleury, M. 1663
Flexner, Abraham, medical education
  reform 186, 212, 217, 219, **1141–3**,
    1169, 1176, 1378, 1382, 1490
Flexner, Simon 212, 1279, 1490
  experimental epidemiology 1277
  serum therapy in spinal meningitis
    1489
Fliarete, Antonio Averlino, plan for
  Ospedale Maggiore (Milan) 1498,
    1499
Fliedner, Theodor, influence on
  Florence Nightingale 894
Flinn, M.W. 1674
Flint, Austin 209
  *Treatise on the Principles and Practice of
    Medicine* 445
Florence
  healing guild (1293) 1122, 1183, 1207
  medical college 1124
  public health 29, 1458
  Renaissance hospitals 1183–4, 1185
  S. Maria Nuova 1183–4, 1497
Florey, Howard Walter
  1st baron Florey 574
  isolation of penicillin 933
Floud, R.C. 1680
  et al., *Height, Health and History* 35
Flourens, Marie Jean Pierre
  chloroform experiments 922
  neurophysiology 1581
Floyer, Sir John, on cold-bathing 1294–5
Flügge, C., asepsis 991
Foerster, O., neurosurgeon 1018

foetus
  human status 879
  malformation 935
  monitoring 1069
  pre-natal diagnosis 1598, **1600–1**,
    1602
Fogel, Robert 1680
folacin 480
Foley, A. xxvi
folk medicine 6, 20, 47, 54, 55, 57, 59,
    70, 613, **661–75**, 1656–7
  18th-century decline 61, 62
  in ancient societies 48–50
  in Arab-Islam **679–86**, 687, 697
  in classical Greece and Rome 51–4
  in early China 730
  flexibility of traditional systems **667–9**
  holistic concepts and traditional
    therapies **665–7**
  therapies **670–1**
  see also anthropology
follicle-stimulating hormone 147, 491,
    501
Fontana, Felice, eudiometer 305
Fontenoy, Battle of (1745) 1540
food see diet; nutrition
Food and Drug Administration (US)
    1604
Foot, Jesse 975
foraminifera 161
forceps, obstetrical 62, 893, 1051, 1052,
    1064, 1065
Ford, John 529
Ford Foundation 1385
Foreest, Pieter van 341
forensic medicine see law and medicine;
    lawsuits
Forestier, J., cerebral radiology 1017
Forlanini, C., artificial pneumothorax
    1017
formaldehyde, as fixing agent in
    microscopy 108
Forms of medicine, in Western tradition
    15–16
Forssmann, Werner, cardiac
    catheterization 137, 884
Forster, Robert 27
Fortes, Meyer, social anthropologist
    1442, 1443
Fortier, Bruno 1501
Foster, Sir Michael 130, 139, 142, 154,
    1441

founder *Journal of Physiology* 132
  Text Book of Physiology 133
Fothergill, John Milner
  Diseases of Sedentary and Advanced Life
    1102–8
  meteorological records 298
Foucault, Michel 27–8, 173, 240, 348,
    876–7, 1258, 1368, 1508, 1580, 1619
  Birth of the Clinic 27, 1657–8
  Histoire de la Folie 27
Fountains Abbey, N.Yorks 1497
Fourcroy, Antoine François de, comte
    159
Fourier, Charles, French architect 1509
Fourier, J.B.J. see Villot and Fourier
Fournier Alfred, syphilologist 571
Fournier, Jean, on anthrax 1268, 1270
Fox, Daniel M. xv, **1204–30**
Fox, Sir Theodore (Fortescue) 1343–4
Fracastoro, Girolamo 29
  contagion theory 296, 310, 313, 319,
    326, **1264–5**, 1267
  *De Contagione et Contagionis Morbis et
    Curatione* 340
  on syphilis 564
fractures 966, 971, 994, 999, 1006, 1012,
    1101, 1547, 1550, 1552
  callus healing 1013
  compound 978, 988, 999
  early treatments 963, 992
  internal fixation 1012, 1013
  observation by SEM 118
  skull 964, 1017
  X-ray diagnosis 840
Francis I, king of France 1623
Franco, Pierre 971
Franco-Prussian War (1870–71) 420,
    920, 994, 1074–5, 1084, 1086, 1364,
    1540, 1542, 1545, 1547, 1551, 1555
Frank, Johann Peter 173–4, 254, 1209
  medical police **1236–7**
Frank, Robert 1594
Frankland, Sir Edward, metabolism
    research 264
Franklin, Benjamin 206, 620, 1031
  advocates fresh-air bathing 954–5
Franklin, Rosalind Elsie, structure of
    DNA 166
Fraser, Sir Francis 217, 218, 219, 220
Fraser, Henry, beriberi research 474
Fraser, Thomas, isolation of eserine 921,
    923, 930

Frazier, C., neurosurgeon 1018
Frederick the Great, king of Prussia 895
Frederick III, emperor of Germany,
    laryngeal carcinoma 997
Frederick III, Holy Roman emperor
    1122
Frederiks Hospital, Copenhagen 1508
Freiburg University 187, 188
Freidson, Eliot, *Profession of Medicine*
    1650–1
Freind, John 1266
French Anti-Cancer League 549
French, Lady Essex, founder of Massage
    Corps 1333
French Revolution (1789–99) 98, 171,
    176, 301, 591, 816, 894, 902, 975,
    1165, 1208, 1210, 1269, 1353, 1355,
    1477–8
    Committee on Mendicancy 1237
    Committee on Salubrity 1237
    effect on medical profession 63,
        1131–3, 1186
    French, Roger xv, **81–101**
Frerichs, Friedrich von 488
Freud, Anna
    child analysis 1038, 1041–2
    Ego and Mechanisms of Defence 1038
Freud, Sigmund 347, 417, 907, 1044,
    1045, 1046, 1441, 1461, 1583, 1589
    Civilization and its Discontents 595–6
    Essays on Theory of Sexuality 1036
    Interpretation of Dreams 1035, 1366
    Moses and Monotheism 1037
    'On Narcissism' 1042
    psychoanalysis 445, 448–9, **1033–9**,
        1366, 1578
    on sexuality **1034–40**
    Token and Taboo 1037
    (with Breuer) *Studies on Hysteria* 448,
        1034
Freudians/neo-Freudians 452, **1039–42**
Frey, Max von 211
Friedman, Milton, economist 1385
Friedmann, Friedrich, tuberculosis
    vaccine 199
Friedreich, Johannes, organicist
    psychiatrist 443
Friendly Societies (Great Britain) 31
Frölich, Theodor, infantile scurvy
    research 474–5
Fromm, Erich, neo-Freudian
    psychoanalyst 1040–1

Frosch, Paul 199
Frost, Hampton 1279
Frugard, Roger *see* Roger of Palermo
Fry, Elizabeth 894, 1311, 1314, 1319,
    1454, 1476
    founds Sisters' Institute of Nursing
        902
Fuller, E., prostate surgery 1015
fungi 325–6, 327
Funk, Casimir, 'vitamines' 165, 475
Furley, John 1548

Gaddum, Sir John Henry, biological
    assay 930
Gaffky, Georg 405
Gajdusek, Carlton, on kuru 214, 1444
Galen 7, 84, 90, 91, 94, 243, 414, 759,
    771, 855, 963, 1119, 1283, 1284,
    1292, 1496
    Anatomical Procedures 84
    anatomy 86–7, 121, 805
    Ars Medica 1287–8
    on cancer 540–1, 552
    concept of soul 251–2
    De Sanitate Tuenda **1286–7**, 1290
    De Sectis 82
    diagnosis **804–5**
    fever theories 337–8, **393–4**, 955
    humoral theory 282, **286–90**, 315, 319,
        1232
    influence on Arab-Islamic medicine
        682, 687–8, 691, 693, 696, 699,
        701, 703
    on medical education 83, **1154–7**
    on mental diseases 440, 447
    Methodus Medendi 964, 967
    On Different Kinds of Fever 337–8
    On Maintaining Health 1094
    On the Use of the Parts 84
    public dissections 83, 85–6, 89
    regimen and bloodletting **943–5**, 948
    'seeds of disease' 295, 1263
    Vesalius's criticisms **86–8**, 90
Galenic medicine/Galenism 5, 83,
    89–90, 155–6, 171, 316, 339–40, 603,
    676, 709, 729, 965, 967, 971, 1101,
    1123–4, 1126–7, 1156, 1160, 1162,
    1283, 1294, 1456, 1460–1
galenicals 970
Galileo Galilei 862
    first thermometer 834
Gallagher, Nancy 37

Galloway, Patrick 1677
gallstones 840, 1005, 1008, 1016
Galton, Sir Francis
  eugenist 420, 422, 594, 1255, 1275,
    1439
  Natural Inheritance 421
Galvani, Luigi, animal electricity
  research 125, 129
galvanometers 207
Gamarnikow, E. 1313
ganglioneuromas 509
gangrene 321, 963, 978, 979, 984, 1550
Gann 548
Garcia, Manual, invention of
  laryngoscope 1011
Garnier-Chabot, Jeanne, founder of
  Oeuvres du Calvaire 547
Garrison, Fielding Hudson 24, 1548
  Introduction to the History of Medicine
    1537-8
Garrison, William Lloyd 897
Garrod
  on alkaptonuria 425
  Inborn Errors of Metabolism 166-7, 215,
    433
  Sir Archibald Edward 217
Garth, Sir Samuel, 'The Dispensary'
  1526
gas-asphyxia 1544, 1550
gas-gangrene 1550
Gaskell, Walter Holbrook
  cardiovascular physiology 139
  neurophysiology 143-4
Gassendi, Pierre, mechanical philosophy
  1162
Gasser, J.S. 137, 143
gastrectomy 505, 552, 1002
gastric secretions, chemistry 125
gastrin 490, 493, 504
gastro-enteropancreatic tumours **504-5**
gastro-intestinal system **136-9**, 178
  cancer 537, 1008, 1009
  Galen's theories **943-4**
  hormones 493, 927
  Pavlov's research 136, 137, 138, 266-7
  Réaumur's work 125
  role of pancreatic juice 128
  surgery 992, 994, 996, 998, **1008-10**
  see also digestion
gastroenterology 1596
gastroenterostomy 1008
Gates, Frederick T. 212, 1489

Gaub, Jerome 96
  De Regimine Mentis 451
Gauss, Carl Friedrich
  Gaussian curve 350-1
  social statistics 1235
Gauthier, Martin Pierre, architect of
  Hôpital Lariboisière, Paris 1502
Gay Men's Health Crisis (NY) 579
Gehry, Frank 1507
Gelfand, Toby xv-xvi, **1119**
General Board of Health (UK) 1246
General Medical Council 1134-5, 1137,
  1168, 1217, 1337, 1339
General Nursing Council 1324
General Optical Council 1342
general practitioners 8, 98, 784, 1112,
  1134-6, 1142, 1171, 1188, 1196-7,
  1373, 1381, 1552
  establish cottage hospitals 1193-4
  as family doctors 1384, 1387
  origins 62
  role in childbirth 1054, 1063-4,
    1066-8
generation 88, 320
  see also spontaneous generation
genes 107, 429, **430-4**, 492
  abnormal 164, 166
  and cancer 546-7
  'mapping' 430-1, 432, 433
  therapy 20, 434, 554-5
genetic counselling 1600
genetic fingerprinting 1625
genetics *see* constitutional and hereditary
  disorders
Geneva 1558
  Conventions **1422-4**
Geneva Medical College (NY) 897, 898
Gengou, Octave, complement fixation
  test 196, 573
Gentile da Foligno 81
Geoffroy, Jean, '*Goutte de Lait de
  Belleville*' 1072
Geoffroy Saint-Hilaire, Etienne 1438
geography
  medical 29, 37, **300-2**, 353, 514-15,
    518, 1269
  see also colonialism; demography;
    environment
George, Dorothy 1665
George III, king of England 1352, 1631
George IV, king of England 893
George V, king of England 219

Gerhard, William Wood 179
  typhus/typhoid research 401–2
geriatrics 6, 8, 69, 187, 253–4, 270,
  1092–115, 1219, 1226, 1287, 1384,
  1549, **1704–6**
  18th-century **1098–9**
  19th-century **1099–103**
  20th-century **1103–12**
  early theories **1092–4**
  Middle Ages and Renaissance **1094–6**
  in primitive societies 359, 636, 638
  Scientific Revolution **1096–7**
germ theory 113–14, 162, 194–5, 234,
  262, 302, **309–34**, 337, 353, 374, 416,
  427, 518–20, 523, 531, 623–4, 789,
  1138, 1141, 1191, 1274, 1283, 1399,
  1451, 1513
  meiosis 107
  of wound infection **987–92**
German Roentgen Society 553
German Surgical Society 1007
Germanin 932
Gerrard of Cremona 394
Gersdorff, Hans von, *Felthuch der
  Wundartzney* 970
Gert, Bernard 245
Gertrude of Helfta, abbess 890
Gesner, Conrad 88
Gestalt therapy 1043, 1442
Gevitz, Norman xvi, **603–33**
Geyer-Kordesch, Johanna xvi, **888–914**
gi see Chinese medicine
giantism 500
Gibbon, J.H., extracorporeal circulation
  1021
Gibraltar, yellow fever epidemic (1828)
  33, 1274
Giessen University 896
Gilbert, Emile-Jacques, architect of the
  Charenton 1502
Gill, C.A. 394
Gilman, Sander L. xvi, **1029–49**
Ginsberg, Carlo 1532
Gisborne, Thomas 881
  *Enquiries into the Duties of Men in the
    Professions* 865–7, 870, 871
Gladstone, William Ewart 1584–5
Glasgow 988–9
  Royal Asylum 1506
  Royal Infirmary 202, 544, 1503, 1504,
    1508
  University 99, 900, 1108

Victoria Infirmary 1511
Glass, D.V. 1674
Glasse, Robert, research on kuru 1444
glaucoma 1011
Glenelg, Lord *see* Grant, Charles
Glenny, Alexander 197
Gley, Eugène, on parathyroids 486
globular theory of tissues 104
Glover, Mary 1459
glucagon 503
Gluck, Themistokles 1012
  bone implantation 1022
glyceryl trinitrate 923
glycosuria 502
Gnau, medical tradition 634
Gnosticism 155, 1451, 1584
god/gods 915
  in ancient Greece and Rome 52–3
  in early societies 50, 362
Godwin, George, *The Builder* 1511
Godwin, William 419
  on prolongation of life 1099
Goelicke, André 94
Goffman, Erving 1358, 1648
goitre **480–81**, 483, 485, 495, **498–90**,
  993, 994, 1017
  exophthalmic 486, 499
  surgery 1000, 1010
  toxic *see* hyperthyroidism
Goldberger, Joseph, pellagra research
  472, 477
Goldblatt, Harry 492
Goldstein, Jan xvi, 214, **1350–72**
Golgi, Camillo 137
  Golgi bodies 109
  on nerve structure 112
gonadectomy 146, 485, 488, 489, 505,
  506
gonadotrophins 147, 491, 496, 501
gonads 490, 491, 495, **505–6**
gonorrhoea 198, 523, 572, 1263
  specificity 567–8
Goode, J. and J.D. 673
Goodenough, Sir William Macnamara,
  Committee on Medical Education
  (1942–4) 218
Goodwyn, Edmund 253
Goodyear, James 33
Gordon, Alexander 1052
  on contagiousness of puerperal fever
  1060

Gorgas, William Cedric, mosquito
eradication campaign 406, 526, 1279
Gosāla, Makkhali 758
Goubert, Jean-Pierre 1302, 1667
gout 336, 342, 345, 412, 414, 415, 590,
610, 840, 921, 1103, 1234, 1549
'flying' 354
Graefe, Albrecht, ophthalmologist 1011
Graefe, Carl Ferdinand von 981
Graham, Evarts Ambrose
cholecystography 1009
pneumonectomy 1019
Graham, James, unorthodox therapist
1296
Graham, Sylvester, Grahamism 65, 619,
622, 626, 1462
Graham, Thomas, colloidal state
research 160–1
Graham, Thomas, unorthodox
hydropathist 955
gram stain technique 114
Granada, Hospital Real 1498
Grand Tour, medical students' 97, 130,
175
Granit, R. 137
Granshaw, Lindsay xvi, 1180–203, 1496
Grant, Charles, Baron Glenelg 1438
Grassi, G.B., discovers mosquito vector
of human malaria 514, 520
Gratarolo, G., treatise on health 1289
Gratian 969
Graunt, John 33
Natural and Political Observations 1265,
1268
social statistics 1209, 1234–5
Graves, Robert James, Graves's disease
486, 1010
Gray, A.L., radiotherapy in bladder
carcinoma 1016
Great Ormond Street Children's
Hospital 1073, 1189
Greatrakes, Valentine, 'the stroker'
955–6, 1456, 1463–4
Greatzius, on differential diagnosis
808–9, 812
Greek language 693, 694, 695, 696, 703,
1123
decline 686–7
Greek medicine (classical) 34–5, 51–4,
82, 84–8, 155, 192, 281–5, 292–3,
297, 300, 302, 304, 306, 313, 363,
366, 1119, 1154, 1181, 1291

cult of Aesculapius 52–3
diet/regimen 52, 940–5, 956
disease classification 169
importance of Hippocratic Oath 855–9
influence on Arab-Islamic system 682,
687, 698, 706
insanity 1459–61
regimen 51–2, 951–8, 954, 1284–7
surgery 963–4
see also Hippocrates; Hippocratic
Corpus/medicine; humoralism
Green, Joseph Reynolds 161
Greenfield, William Smith, on Hodgkin's
disease 486, 544
Greenwood
Major 34
science of medical statistics 1232,
1275–8, 1279
Greenwood, Major 1262
Gregory, Annabel 35
Gregory, James, input/output
measurements 806
Gregory, John
Lectures on the Duties and Qualifications
of a Physician 861, 865
medical ethics 861–3, 864, 865, 869,
871, 873, 876, 877
Gregory, William 159
Grew
Nehemiah, on Epsom salts 953
quantitative social analysis 1234
Grey, Charles, 2nd Earl Grey 335
Grey, Lady 335
Griesinger, Wilhelm 1032
Pathologie und Therapie der psychischen
Krankheiten 443–4, 1363–4
Griffith, Harold Randall, clinical use of
curare 1001
Griffith, Talbot 1665, 1674
Grijns, Gerrit, on beriberi 474
Griscom, John H., Sanitary Conditions of
the Labouring Population of New York
1252
Grmek, Mirko D., Disease in the Ancient
Greek World 34–5
Grocers' Company, apothecaries'
separation (1617) 1126
Groddeck
George 452
psychological explanation of pain 1583
Gross, R.E., ligature of patent ductus
arteriosus 1020

group therapy 1043–4
Grove, John, germ theorist 326–7
growth hormone 491, 492, 493, 494, 500, 501, 502
Gruber, Max von 405
 antigen/antibody reactions 196
Grünpeck, Joseph 563
Guérin, J.M.C.
 BCG vaccine 199
 social medicine 1245
Guildhall Conference on Feeding School Children (1905) 1081
guilds, healing 56, 1122, 1123, 1124, 1125, **1126–30**, 1132–3, 1153, 1156, 1158, 1163, 1164, 1207, 1208, 1217, 1221, 1331–2, 1350, 1472, 1623
 see also barber-surgeons
Guillemin, R. 138
Guinness, Edward, 1st earl of Iveagh 1488
Guinter, Joannes 84
Gujarat Ayurveda University 774
Gula (Babylonian healing goddess) 50
Gull, William, on cretinous state 485
Gully, James Manby, hydropathist at Malvern 618, 953
Gussow, G. 531
Gusthart, Hume's physician 809, 814
Guthrie, Sir George James, on malingering 1554–5
Guy, William Augustus, medical statistician 1273, 1509
Guybert, Philibert, Traicté de la Conservation de Santé 1296
Guyon, F. 1015
Guy's Hospital 98, 207, 894, 980, 1185, 1439, 1453, 1527
 histology courses 111
gymnastics, remedial 939, **955–7**, 1290, 1345
gynaecology 832, 998, **1013–14**, 1065
 Chinese theories 738

Habbakuk, H.K. 1674
Habsburg Empire 1236, 1237
Hackett, C.J. 368
Hadcock, R.N. 1184
Haddon, Alfred Cort, Torres Straits expedition 1441, 1442
Hadfield, James, criminal lunatic 1631
Haeckel, Ernst
 cell theory 161

'dysteleology' 268
haematology 479
haematoxylin 108, 789
haemodialysis see kidneys
haemoglobin 432
 in anaemias 479
 chemistry 166
haemoglobinuria 196
haemolysis 196, 386
haemophilia 412
haemorrhage 470, 971, 978, 979, 985, 994
 cerebral see stroke
 post-partum 931, 1061, 1067
haemorrhoids 284, 393, 679, 813, 963, 966, 993
haemostasis 509, 964, 965, 991, 998, 1010, 1018
Haffkine, Waldemar, cholera vaccines 198
Hahn, Johann Sigmund, On the Power and Effect of Cold Water 617
Hahnemann, Samuel
 Chronic Diseases 610
 founder of homoeopathy **604–12**, 613, 614, 623, 626
 Materia Medica Pura 607, 609
 Organon of Rational Medicine 607, **609–12**, 620
Haight, C., pneumonectomy 1019
Haldane, John Scott, respiratory physiology 140
Haldane, Richard Burdon, Viscount Haldane, Commission on University Education 215–16, 219
Hales, Stephen 1236
 blood circulation experiments 123
 pneumatic chemistry 305
Hall, G. Stanley, psychologist 1040
Hall, Marshall, neurophysiology 621, 1581
Halle
 epidemic constitution 298
 University 97, 895, 1455
Hallé, Jean Noel 1239
Haller, Albrecht von 94, 483, 975
 anatomia animata 95–6
 concepts of sensibility/irritability **124–5**, 128, 1580
 De Partibus Corporis Humani Sensibilibus et Irritabilibus 124
 on death 252, 253

Elementa Physiologiae 95
Primae Linae Physiologicae 124
Halley, Edmond, social statistics 1235, 1265
Halliburton, William Dobinson 133
Halsted, William S. 210, 998, 1191–2
cocaine research 1014
introduction of surgical gloves 991, 1014
radical mastectomy 552, 1014
Haly Abbas 289, 676, 701, 703, 704, 717
Complete Medical Art 700
Libri Pantechni 965
Hamburg
cholera epidemics (1830–1910) 30, 37
tropical medicine institute 520
Hamer, William Heaton, statistics of measles epidemics 1275
Hammersmith Hospital 553–3
Postgraduate Medical School 218–19, 220
Hammurabi, king of Babylon 963
legal code 1620
Hannaway, Caroline xvii, **292–308**
Hansen, G.H.A., identification of leprosy bacillus 514, 530–1
Hanwell County Asylum 1361
Harden, A. 165
Hardenberg, Karl August von, founds Bayreuth asylum 1361
Hardy, G.H., Hardy-Weinberg equilibrium law 427
Hardy, William Bate 109
Hare, William 100
Harington, Sir Charles Robert, thyroxine research 490, 927
Harington, Sir John 947
Harken, Dwight Emery, cardiac surgery 1020
Harriman, Mrs J. Borden, philanthropist 1077
Harris, Elisha 1251
Harris, F. Drew, St Helen's milk depot 1079
Harris, Geoffrey W., pituitary function research 147, 493
Harris, Vincent Dormer 133
Harris, Walter 949–50
Harrison, Lawrence Whitaker 573–4
Hartley, David, association theory 441
Hartline, H. 137
Hartwig, Gerald W. 37, 531

Hārūn al-Rashīd, caliph of Baghdad 692, 696, 716
Harvard Scientific Co. 131
Harvard University 131, 187, 188, 208, 213, 897, 899, 981, 1107, 1490
endowments 1488
Medical School 874
'A definition of irreversible coma' 877
tropical diseases chair 520
Harvey, Gideon, *Diseases of London* 587
Harvey, William 91, 95, 96, 123, 296, 319, 892, 1096, 1162
De Motu Cordis 122, 1123, 1520
discovery of blood circulation 9, 59, 88–9, 206, 282, 396, 949, 972
on generation 88
Hashimoto, Hakaru, description of struma lymphomatosa 500
Hassall, A.H., *Microscopical Anatomy of the Human Body* 111
Hata, Sahachiro, discovery of Salvarsan 926
Hatchett, Charles 156
Hawaii, effects of colonization 372
Hawkins, Charles, plan for Queen Charlotte's Hospital 1511
hay fever 195
Haycraft, J.B. 1304
Haygarth, John 1236
environmental survey 588
smallpox inoculation 1236
study of Chester Bills of Mortality 1268
Head, Sir Henry, neurophysiology 1581
health, illness and disease, concepts of 7, 18–20, **233–48**
Health Belief Model **1643–4**
health care *see* medical care
health economics *see* economics
Health of Munition Workers Committee (UK) 1276
Heart 222
heart 918
artificial 1023
cardiovascular physiology 89, 91, 122, **139–40**
disease 260, 375, 451, 481, 598, 789, 827, 829–30, 951
in Hippocratic medicine 251
injury 1019, 1020
in old age 1100, 1101, 1106

as seat of soul (Aristotle) 121
see also cardiology
heart-lung machine 1020
heartbeat 96, 215, 392, 398, 487
in diagnosis *see* pulse
Heberden, William *the elder*, description
of angina pectoris 205
Hédon, Edouard, endocrine research
488
Heidegger, Martin 1367
Heim-Voegtlin, Marie, Swiss pioneer
physician 901
Heinroth, J.C.A.
Lehrbuch der Störungen des Seelenlebens
1356–7
on mental diseases 443
Heister, Lorenz, *Chirurgie* 970
Helleiner, Karl **1667–8**, 1674
Hellenism 688
in Renaissance **84–6**, 87
Helmholtz, Hermann L.F. von 148
invention of ophthalmoscope 1011,
1166, 1167, 1332, 1596
law of conservation of energy 129, 207
helminthology 519, 520, 523, 529–30
Helmont, J.B. van 319, 949
on fermentation 258
iatrochemistry 156
theory of disease **339–40**, 341, 540–1
Helsinki, Declaration of *see* World
Medical Association
Helvétius, Claude-Adrien, psycho-
physiology 1581
hemlock 920
Hench, Philip Showalter, steroid
treatment 137, 214, 508
Henderson, John 1183
Henderson, Lawrence Joseph 67
Henke, Adolphe 785
Henle, Friedrich Gustav Jacob
Allgemeine Anatomie 111
cancer theory 542
on miasma and contagion 326, 1271
Henry, Louis, family reconstitution 1663,
1668
Henry IV, king of France 89
Henry VIII, king of England 423, 1125,
1473
heparin 1005, 1021
hepatitis 202–3, 364, 368
Heraclitus of Ephesus 283, 284

herbalism 17, 49, 55, 57, 156, **638–40**,
657, 916, 1140, 1151, 1462
heredity *see* constitutional and hereditary
disorders
Hering, K.E.R., respiratory physiology
142
Herman, Paul, *Museum Zeylanicum* 772
hermaphroditism 506
hernias 815, 962, 964, 971
empiric operators 55, 60, 62, 968, 977,
979, 1122, 1351
modern surgery 1005–6, 1009
strangulated 979
Herodicus 858–9
Herodotus 1154
Herophilus 90, 392
regimen/bloodletting 939, 942
herpes 1263
Herrgott, François-Joseph, maternal
welfare clinic 1075
Hertcloup, C.L.S., lithotrity 1015
Herter
Christian Archibald 212
founder *Journal of Biological Chemistry*
155
Hertwig, Wilhelm August Oscar 107
Hertz, Henriette 896
Hervey, John, Baron Hervey of Ickworth
1295
Hess, W. 137
Hessen, Boris 25
Heusch, Luc de 656
Heussmeyer, K. 1087
Hewson, William, microscopical
preparations 111
Heyer, Gustave, *Das körporisch-seelische
Zusammenwirken in den
Lebensvorgangen* 451
Heymans, C. 137
Higham, John 27
Hildegard von Bingen, abbess 890
Hill, Archibald Vivian 137
Hill, John, *The Construction of Timber* 103
Hill, Sir Austin Bradford 223–4, 934
occupational health 1277, 1279
on smoking and lung cancer 223–4,
1277
Hill, Sir Leonard Erskine 133, 1276
Hillary, William, epidemic constitution of
Barbados 298
Himsworth, Sir Harold 224
Hindu medicine *see* Indian medicine

Hinduism 16, 759, 762, 771, 803–4,
1174, 1291, 1408
Hinshaw, H.C., use of streptomycin in
tuberculosis 934
Hinton, J., mastoiditis operation 1011
hip-replacement 1005
Hippocatic Corpus, *Airs, Waters, Places*
284, **293–4**, 387, 414, 1232, 1233,
1499
Hippocrates 5, 6, 25, 36, 51–2, 82,
282–3, 286, 337, 363, 391, **393–5**,
616, 699, 759, 915, 941, 964, 966,
977, 1292, 1350, 1544
on ageing 1092–3
on cancer 540, 552
Hippocratic Corpus 29, 53, 152, 283–4,
296–7, 363, 413–14, 696, 819, 941,
1120, 1262
Affections 185, 284
Airs, Waters, Places 1496
Ancient Medicine 35, 284, 383, 941,
942, 1286
Aphorisms 336
De Capitis Vulneribus 963
De Ulceribus 963
Diseases 285, 287
on environment **293–5**
Epidemics 9, 296, 386–8, 391, 859–60,
876, 1263, 1496
fevers **382–91**
malarial 384–8
seasonal influences 388–90
treatment 390–1
Generation 285
Humours 284
mental diseases 285, 439, 440
Nature of Man 285, 286, 287, 295, 383,
389
Oath 52, 206, 697, 763, **852–6**, 861,
870, 873, 876, 1119, 1121, 1154,
1533
On Joints 856, 860
physiology 120, 121
Precepts 859, 876
Regimen in Acute Diseases 391, 941
Regimen in Health 284, 941, **1285–6**
Sacred Disease 284, 285, 439, 941, 942,
1120
The Art 859–60, 860, 878
The Heart 251
virtue ethic **859–61**, 862
Hippocratic medicine 52, 55, 58, 81, 83,

96, 225, 253, 287, 304, 316, 320,
336–8, 341, 349, 1132, 1156, 1266,
1283, 1459, 1521
diagnosis **802–4**, 805
diet/regimen **941–3**
see also humoralism
Hiroshima 557
Hirsch, August, *Handbuch der historisch-
geographischen Pathologie* 29, 302, 429,
480, 481
Hirschfelder, Arthur D. 211
hirsutism 507
His, Wilhelm, bundle of His 140
histamine test 509
histamines 145
role in inflammation 110
histochemistry 115
histocompatibility 431, 432
histology 109, 130, 179, 189
in diagnosis 181, 997
literature **110–12**
origin of term (Mayer) 104
see also tissues
historiography 36–8
anatomical 94–5
of cancer **537–40**
medical 9, **24–44**, **1537–8**
history-taking *see* diagnosis
Hitler, Adolf 595, 1087
HIV **575–80**, 1225, 1258, 1513
Hobbes, Thomas 856
Leviathan 862
Hodgkin, Sir Alan L., membrane
experiments 137, 148
Hodgkin, Thomas 1587
founds Aborigines Protection Society
1438–9
Hodgkin's disease 544, 554
microscopy 104, 179
Hoff, Jacobus Hendricus van't 163
Hoffman, Frederick 548
Hoffmann, Erich, identification of
Spirochaeta pallida 572–3
Hoffmann, Friedrich 94, 97, 282, 605,
808
cancer/inflammation theory 540
epidemic constitution of Halle 298
on mental diseases 446
Hofmann, Caspar 93
Hogben, Lancelot 1275
Holbach, Paul Heinrich Dietrich, baron
d' 1457

Holcombe, L., *Victorian Ladies at Work*
1312
Hölderlin, Johann Christian Friedrich
1529
holistic medicine 70, 203, 282, 290, 454,
665–7, 956–7, 1334, 1462, 1576,
1580
see also Chinese medicine; humoralism
Holmes, Oliver Wendell 594–5, 1589
criticism of unorthodox systems 610,
611
on puerperal fever 1060
Holmes-Sellors, Sir Thomas,
valvulotomy 1020
Holst, Axel, scurvy research 474–5
Holst, Valentin, on treating 'whole'
patient 791
Holy Roman Empire 890
code of criminal procedure 1623
Home, Sir Everard 156
homeostasis 282, 492
Cannon's theory 128
Homo erectus 357, 359
Homo sapiens 357
Homo sapiens sapiens 357–8
homoeopathy 65, 66, 281, 314, **604–13**,
620, 627, 634, 774, 936, 1139, 1141,
1143, 1213, 1398, 1462, 1489
docrine of the psora 611
infinitesimal dosage 606–7, 609–10
similia similibus principle 65, 606, 609,
611
homosexuality 237, 238, 239, 245, 354,
376, 1619
Hood, Wharton, on value of bone-setting
622–3
Hooke, Robert 118
design for Bethlem Royal Hospital
1499
first description of cells 103
Micrographia 102
physiological work 122
Hooker, Worthington 610
on doctor-patient relationship 790
Physician and Patient 615, 970
hookworm 30, 31, 358, 360, 364, 370,
523, 530
eradication programmes 1253, 1489
Hôpital des Enfants Malades, Paris 1073
Hôpital Lariboisière, Paris 1502, 1510
Hopkins, B.E. 197

Hopkins, Donald R., *Princes and Peasants*
30
Hopkins, Sir Frederick Gowland 164–5,
222, 225
anti-neuritic vitamins 137
biochemistry chair (Cambridge) 154
Hopkins, Johns 1488
see also Johns Hopkins University
Hoppe-Seyler, Ernest Felix Immanuel
153, 162
vital phenomena/putrefaction analogy
258
Horder, John 792
hormone receptor sites 147
hormone replacement therapy (HRT)
497, 505
hormones 92–7, 145–6, 163, 166, 185,
282, **483–510**, 1000
laboratory determination 1003
see also under names of hormones
sex 146–7, 166, 485–6, 488, 491,
496–7, 501, **505–6**, 905, 928, 1102
steroid 147, 166, 214, 491, 493, 494,
496, 498
synthetic 494, 497, 501, 505, 508, 927
therapeutic use **926–8**, 1004, 1016
Horney, Karen, neo-Freudian
psychoanalyst 1040
Horsley, Sir Victor 215
neurosurgery 1017
thyroidectomy 486
Horwitz, Abraham, director of Pan-
American Sanitary Bureau 1422
hospice movement 1465, 1590
Hospital 1511
Hospital Association 1323
hospital fever *see* typhus
Hospital Information Systems 847
Hospital Saturday Fund 1194, 1486
Hospital Sunday Fund 1486
hospitals 7, 19, 32, 38, 54–6, 348, 973–4,
1006, **1180–203**, 1561
18th-century 61–2, 98, **1185–9**
19th-century 63–4, 126, 975–6,
980–2, **1187–94**, 1195
20th-century 68, **1194–8**
ancient/medieval **1181–4**, **1452–4**,
1469–71
autopsies 100, **171–6**, 188, 1187
budgets 1180, 1194, 1215, 1226,
1373, 1376–7, 1382–3, 1384, 1387,
1486, 1513

Chinese 729, 745
clinical education 127, 1155–6,
    1160–70, 1182, 1188
colonial 1402–3, 1407
early modern 57–8, **1184–5**, 1473,
    1474
French post-Revolution *see* Paris
governance 1196–7, 1210–11,
    1214–15, 1223
high-tech 832, 1376–7, 1595, 1666
infections 994, 998, 1002, **1191–2**,
    1198, **1498–9**, **1510–14**
Islamic 55, 696, 699–700, **715–17**
special 537, 547–8, 555, 1051, 1055,
    1057–8, 1065, 1073, 1185, **1189**,
    1309, 1477
see also architecture; clinical research;
    nursing; voluntary hospitals
Hôtel des Invalides, Paris 1499, 1558
Hôtel-Dieu, Beaune 1497
Hôtel-Dieu, Paris 976, 980, 1156, 1187,
    1500, 1501, 1504, 1510
Hounsfield, Sir Godfrey (Newbold), first
    CAT scanning machine 843, 1003
housing charities 1486–7
Houssay, Bernardo, Houssay
    phenomenon 137, 502
Howard, George, 7th earl of Carlisle
    1243
Howard, John 1235
    *Account of the Principal Lazarettos in
    Europe* 1505
Howell, Joel 32, 1594
Howell, W.H., *Textbook of Physiology* 133
HRT *see* hormone replacement therapy
Hubbard, John Perry, ligature of patent
    ductus arteriosus 1020
Hubel, David, physiology of nervous
    system 138, 143
Hubert, St 1456
Hudson, E.H. 366, 368
Huebner, Robert, viral oncogene theory
    546–7
Hufeland, Christian Wilhelm, *Art of
    Prolonging Life* 1098
Hufnagel, C., heart-valve implantation
    1021
Huggins, Charles Brenton, on hormone-
    dependent tumours 214, 506, 1016
Hughes, Howard, medical research
    endowment 1490
Hugo, Victor, *Les Misérables* 1072

Hull House, Chicago 1484
human genome project 432, 433
human immunodeficiency virus *see* HIV
humanism 394, 1528–9
    medical 860, 863, 864, 866, 867,
        876–8, 880–1
    Renaissance 1160–4, 1290, 1521
    recovery of ancient texts **84–5**, 1160
Humboldt, Wilhelm von 207
Hume, David 322, 809, 814, 862, 864
humoralism 5–6, 51–2, 55, 64, 121, 155,
    171, 243, **281–91**, 293–4, 296–7, 304,
    317, 338, 341–2, 827, 917, 987, 1124,
    1187, 1576
    17th-century 59–60
    ageing process 1093, 1098, 1101
    Ayurvedic doctrine 759, 764, 771
    cancer theory **540–1**, 552
    in cellular pathology **181–2**
    disease as imbalance 155, 169–70,
        243, **281–4**, 336, 590, **940–4**, 946,
        964–5, 1283, 1285, 1580
    elements 612
    flexibility of system **287–90**
    in folk medicine 667, 669
    Galenic theory 282, **286–90**, 315, 319,
        393, 783, 787, 964–5
    Hippocratic theory **283–7**, 295, 337
        fevers **382–91**
    humours (blood, phlegm, yellow and
        black bile) 55, 116, 284, 285, 382,
        414
    in Islamic medicine 707
    Middle Ages/Renaissance 57–8, 282
    non-naturals 52, 55, 88, **288–9**, 293,
        312, 343, 451, 946–8, 1232,
        1287–8
    seasonal cycle of disease **284–6**, 290,
        293–4, 296, 382, 388–90
    Sydenham's adoption 396–7
    theories of immunity 194, 196
Ḥunayn ibn Isḥāq 394, 691, **693–7**, 699,
    710, 711, 712
    Isagoge 289
    Medical Questions and Answers 288–9,
        704
    Ten Treatises on the Eye 698, 702, 704
Hunt, James, founder of Anthropological
    Society of London 1439, 1443
Hunter, John 111, 175, 176, 181, 485,
    490, **974–5**, 981, 1128, 1537, 1580
    cancer/inflammation theory 177, 541

diagnosis of Hume's liver tumour 809, 814
on life principle 124
museum 103, 110, 174
on syphilis 567
Treatise on Blood, Inflammation and Gunshot Wounds 110, 177, 974
Hunter, John and William, private anatomy school 98, 99, 100, 103, 973
Hunter, William 92, 974
midwifery practice 903, 1052, 1128
'On the uncertainty of signs of murder in bastard children' 1626
hunter-gatherer societies 358–60, 368, 589, 1694, 1695
health care 48, 635–6
Huntington's chorea 432
Huss, Magnus, *Alcoholismus Chronicus* 417
Hutcheson, Francis 862
moral sense theory 868
Hutchinson, John 1558
Hutchinson, Sir Jonathan, on heredity 412, 414–15, 416, 419
Hutchison, Robert, on neuroblastomas 509
Huth, Alfred 424
Hutterites, childbirth records 1069
Huxham, John, medical meteorology 298, 398
Huxley
Sir Andrew F., membrane experiments 137, 148
Thomas Henry 1135, 1439
hydronephrosis 996
hydropathy 65, 604, **616–19**, 622, 626–7, 939, **951–2**, 1106, 1294
hydrothorax 808
hygiene 304
hospital 988, 990, 995
infant 1079, 1080
military and naval 60–1, 398–9, 517
social 571
see also civilization; public health; sanitation
hygiene, personal 6, 61, 369, 516, 563, 617, 988, 1232, 1237, **1283–308**, 1622
19th-20th centuries **1300–5**
classical period to 18th century **1284–300**
see also hydropathy

hypercalcaemia 504
hyperglycaemia 502
hyperinsulinism 497
hyperparathyroidism 496, 497, 504, 1000
hyperpituitarism 500
hyperplasia 495, 504
adrenal 506, 507, 508
hypersensitivity 195
hypertension 502, 504, 509, 597, 1106, 1110
hyperthyroidism 451, 486, 499, 501, 1010
hypnosis 447, 620, **1032**, 1041, 1045, 1582, 1589
hypochondria 447, 592, 1525, 1576, 1578
hypodermic syringe, invention of 1589
hypoglycaemia 504
hypogonadism 501, 505
hypophysectomy 491, 500, 506, 508, 1000, 1007
hypophysis 1017
hypopituitarism 495, 500, 501, 505
hypotension, artificial 1018
hypotensive drugs 931
hypothalamus 492, 493, 494, 495, 500, 1017
hypothermia, artificial 1002, 1018, 1020
hypothyroidism 487, **498–9**, 501, 1010
Hyslop, Theophilus Bulkeley 1529
hysterectomy 552, 1005, 1014
hysteria 338, 342, **445–50**, 452, 592, 595, 610, 792, 906, **1033–35**, 1036, 1045, 1139, 1365, 1441, 1457, 1459, 1525, 1582, 1583
heredity as a factor 417

iatrochemistry 155–6, 258, 441, 603, 949, 953, 1160, 1294
theory of tumour formation 540–1
iatromechanism 1126, 1160, 1162, 1294, 1461–5, 1580–1
see also mechanism
iatrophysical school 603
Ibn Abī Shayba 707
Ibn Abī Uṣaybi'a, *Pristine Sources of Information on the Classes of Physicians* 706
Ibn al-Bayṭār 703
Ibn al-Jazzār 705
Ibn al-Nafīs, commentary on Avicenna's *Canon* 705

Ibn al-Quff, *Pillar sustaining the Art of Surgery* 704
Ibn Bakhtīshū', founder of first Islamic hospital 710, 716
Ibn Buṭlān, *Proper Pursuit of Health* 704–5
Ibn Darayd 710
Ibn Ilyās, *Mansurian Anatomy* 702, 712
Ibn Jazla 705
Ibn Māsawayh 712
Ibn Qayyim al-Jawzīya 707, 717
Ibn Riḍwān 710
Ibn Sīnā *see* Avicenna
Ibn Sinān 712
Ibn Ṭufayl 709–10
Ichikawa, Koichi, cancer research 556
ideas of life and death 7, **249–80**, 328, 329
  as contraries **264–72**
  as correlatives **254–60**
  opposition of life and death **249–50**
  as possession and privation **250–4**
  therapeutics and correlative death **260–4**
illegitimacy 894, 1623, 1674
Illich, Ivan 598, 1465, 1589, 1653–4
  Limits to Medicine 598
  Medical Nemesis 1144
illness, concepts of 7, 18–20, **233–48**
Imhof, Arthur 34, 1707
Imhotep (Egyptian healing god) 50
immune deficiency diseases 202
  see also AIDS
immunity 358, 366, 368
  antibacterial **198–9**
  antitoxic **196–7**
  antiviral **199–201**
  natural 194–5, 361, 369, 1399, 1404
  of survivors 362, 363, 365, 370, 372, 657
  tumour 546
immunization 227, 924, 1082, 1234, 1255, 1268, 1697, 1698
  mass 1429
immuno-suppressive drugs 1023
immunology 162, 164, **192–204**, 316, 329, 996, 1488, 1563
  19th-century **192–4**
  20th-century **195–203**
  cellular vs. humoral theory 194, 196
  'immune system' concept 192
  and nutrition 35–6, 194–5

toxin-antitoxin reaction 193, 194, 196, 197
  and transplantation **201–2**, 1023
immunotherapy 20, 202, 554–5
Imperial British East Africa Co. 1417
Imperial Cancer Research Fund 220, 548, 549, 551–2, 1480, 1488, 1490
imperialism *see* colonialism
implants 1012
  heart valves 1021
Incas 368, 369, 370, 1403
incontinence 1111
Index Medicus 454
India
  ancient 360, 362
  British 1395, 1397, 1406–7, 1418, 1420
    public health 1398–9, 1402–3
    Royal Commission on Sanitary State of the Army 1401
  bubonic plague 364, 365
  endemic cholera 374
  sanitary reform 517, 518, 525
Indian Medical Service 1398, 1403, 1418
Indian medicine 6, 16, 17, 50–1, 362, 717, **756–79**, 1173, 1429
  astrological medicine **770–1**
  Ayurvedic medicine 17, 21, 604, 729, **759–69**, 770–1, 773–5, 1173, 1408–9
    basic tenets **761–3**
    change and continuity **767–9**
    inoculation **766–7**
    practice **763–4**
    source texts **760–1**
    surgery **764–6**
  contemporary picture **773–5**
  early heterodox ascetics **758–9**
  foreign influences **771–3**
    British **772–3**
    Islamic 771
    Portuguese/Dutch 772
  influence on China 729
  prehistory and the Indus Valley **756–7**
  Siddha medicine **769–70**
  Vedic texts **757–8**
  Yunani system 769, 771, 773, 1173, 1410
Indian Medicine Central Council Act (1970) 774
Indians
  North American **1702–3**

see also colonialism
Industrial Revolution 400, 974, 988, **999**, 1642, 1664, 1696
industrialization 126, **1315–19**, 1453, 1454
infanticide 855, 893, 894, 896, 1623, **1625–6**, 1632
 in primitive societies 359, 636, 638
Infantile Paralysis Foundation (US) 1481
infants 60–1, 568, 1005, 1600
 deficiency diseases 465, 470, **488–90**, 481
 morbidity 1075
 sexuality 449
 welfare **1072–80**
  in France **1072, 1074–6**
  in UK **1078–80**
  in USA **1076–8**
 see also breast-feeding; mortality
infections see contagion; environment and miasmata; hospitals; immunity
infectious diseases see and under names of diseases; epidemiology; public health
infertility 245
infirmaries 62, 890, 902, 1193, 1196, 1453, 1477, 1496
inflammation 110, 187, 194, 260, 320–1, 392, 400, 401, 619, 950, 974, 984, 985, 1580
 and cancer 540, 541, 542, 543
 Cohnheim's theory 183–4
influenza 201, 322, 361, 362, 363, 364, 375, 1264, 1401, 1677
 pandemic (1919) 1170, 1278, 1425
Ingenhousz, Jan
 eudiometer 305
 plant chemistry 156
Ingram, Vernon 432
Ingrassia, Giovanni Filippo, forensic medicine 1624
inheritance, medico-legal aspects 1624–5
 see also constitutional and hereditary disorders
Innocent III, pope 1623
Innocent X, pope 1624
inoculation see smallpox
insanity, legal aspects 1619, **1630–2**, 1636
 religious **1459–61**
 see also mental diseases; psychiatry
insecticides 197, 524, 525–6, 1428
insemination, artificial 879

Institute of Medical Laboratory Science (UK) 1336
'institutes' of medicine 94, 96, 120, 122, 171, 397
Institution of Civil Engineers 1245
instruments
 meteorological 297, 299, 303, 304, 305
 see also microscopy; surgical instruments
Institut de Médecine Coloniale, Paris 520
insulin 146, 214, **490–91**, 492, 493, 497, 502, 508, 928, 931, 1221
 synthesis 164, 494, 496, 503
insulinoma 504
insurance
 and cancer deaths 548–9
 health 66–9, 997, 1143, 1196–8, 1213, 1222–3, **1373–88**
 medical lawsuits 553
 social 1257, 1433
  German system 66–7, 1213, **1379–80**
intensive care 68, 847, **1005**, 1600
interferon 554–5
internal medicine 81, 82, 83, 93, 178, 793, 1130, 1158
 physicians' monopoly 83, 97–8
 surgeons' aspirations 97–8
International Association of Cancer Victims and Friends 555
International Association of Endocrine Surgeons 1009
International Association of Gerontology 1107
International Association for the Study of Pain 1574
International Business Machines (IBM) 1021
International Conference on Primary Health Care (Alma Ata) 1429, **1431–2**
International Congress of Human Genetics 434
International Congress of Hygiene and Demography 1082
International Congress of Medicine 266
International Congress of Physiological Societies 135
International Guiding Principles of Biomedical Research involving Animals (1985) 880

International Hahnemannian Association 612
International Hepatobiliary and Pancreatic Association 1009
International Pharmacological Congress 135
International Statistical Congress (1853) 353
International Union of Physiological Societies 135–6
internationalism 175, 178, 1002, 1009, 1174, 1256, **1417–35**, 1444–6
  Alma Ata Declaration **1431–2**
  general principles **1432–4**
  OIHP and League of Nations **1424–5**
  Red Cross and Geneva Conventions **1422–3**
  religions missions/philanthropy **1417–20**
  Sanitary Conferences **1420–2**, 1424, 1427
  versus nationalism 1211, 1218, 1232
  see also World Health Organization; World War II
intestinal lesions see Peyer's patches
intestines see gastro-intestinal system
iodine deficiency, in thyroid disease 179, 189, 481, 485, 490, 494, 498–9
iodine therapy, for goitre 498, 499
  pre-operative 1010
ions 148–9
ipecacuanha 917, 918, 920, 1408
Iran, bubonic plague 364
Iraq 364, 691, 695
Ireland, potato famine (1840s) 404, 465
iridectomy 1011
iridology 620, 795
iron, in anaemia 479–80
irreversible vegetative state (IVS) **875**, 877
irritability 1580
  Broussais' concept 260
  Haller's concept 124, 128
Isenflamm, Jacob 792
Ishaq ibn Imram 440
Isidore of Seville 1155
Islamic medicine see Arab-Islamic medicine
islets of Langerhans 487–8, 491, 493, 495, 502
Israel, J., stenosis of the ureters 1015
IVF see fertilization

IVS see irreversible vegetative state

Jaboulay, M., autonomic nervous system surgery 1018, 1022
Jackson, Elizabeth, accused of witchcraft 1459
Jackson, James Barnard Swett 180
Jackson, James jr. 401
Jackson, Robert, *Systematic View of the Formation, Discipline and Economy of Armies* 1557
Jacobi, Abraham, American paediatrician 898, 899
Jacobi, Maximilian, organicist psychiatrist 443
Jacobson, Edith, neo-Freudian psychoanalyst 1040
Jacyna, Stephen 544
jail fever see typhus
Jamaica, black farmers' revolt (1866) 1439
James, William, psychologist 1040
James II, king of England 892
Janov, Arthur, primal therapy 1044
Jansenists 1029–30
Janzen, John M. 656, 1445
Japan 365
  beriberi outbreaks 373, 472–3
  Great Smallpox Epidemic (735–37) 364
  influence of Chinese medicine 729
  kanpo system 745–6, 747
  night-blindness 488
  schistosomiasis 529–30
Jarcho, Saul 32
Jardin du Roi, Paris 1162
Jaspers, Karl, German psychiatrist 1364
Jaucourt, Chevalier de 252
jaundice 345, 386
Java, cinchona plantations 374
Jefferson, Thomas 9, 1237, 1250
Jehovah's Witnesses 1451
Jelliffe, Smith Ely 452, 1366
Jenner, Edward, cowpox vaccination 9, 162, 192, 206, 372, 606, 729, 745, 766, 1279, 1404, 1409, 1488
Jenner, Sir William, study of continued fever 402–3
Jenyns, Soame 1586
Jesuits 1454, 1475
Jesuit's Bark see cinchona
Jesup North Pacific Expedition 1440

Jesus Christ 955, 1156, 1461–2
  healing miracles 54, 1452, 1471, 1585
  as 'physician' 1029
  virgin birth 690
Jews/Judaism 54, 682–3, 709, 715, 1036,
  1181, 1450, 1458, 1471
  educational discrimination 901, 1142,
    1159, 1175
  legal system **1621–2**
  migration of scientists (1930s) 154,
    1001
  Nazi persecution 595, 1087
  ritual cleansing 951, 1622
  Talmud on bloodletting 945
Jewson, N.D. 814, 1651–2, 1657
Jex-Blake, Sophia Louisa 894, 899, 902
  Berne medical doctorate 898
  founds London School of Medicine
    for Women 900
Johannitius *see* Hunayn ibn Ishaq
Johannsen, Wilhelm, genetic studies 430
John of Alexandria, commentary on
  Galen's *De Sectis* 82
John of Arderne 1122
John, king of England 954
John, St 298
Johns Hopkins University 208, 210, 211,
  213, 927, 991, 995, 1141, 1169,
  1191–2, 1255, 1479, 1488, 1490
  medical school and hospital 210,
    215–16, 219, 568, 1014, 1141,
    1143, 1512
  School of Hygiene and Public Health
    524, 1278
Johnson, A.O., quack 555
Johnson, G. Enid, clinical use of curare
  1001
Johnson, James, *Influence of Tropical
  Climates on European Constitutions* 516,
  1291, 1397
Johnson, Lyndon B. 1198
Johnson, Richard 1301
Johnson, Robert Wood, Foundation 1490
Johnson, Samuel 1523, 1526, 1586
  Dictionary 412
  'On the Death of Dr Robert Levet'
    1524–5
Johnson, T.J., *Professions and Power* 1651
joints
  replacement 1012, 1013
  surgery 1006

Jones, Agnes, Nightingale-trained nurse
  1319
Jones, Colin xvii, 1187, 1453, **1470–3**,
  1557
Jones, Ernest, founder of British
  Psychoanalytical Society 1041
Jones, Henry Bence 157
Jones, Mary, nursing pioneer 1319
Jones, Sir William 772
Jones, William Henry Samuel 387
Jonson, Ben 1522, 1526
Jordanova, L.J. 1209
Jorden, Edward, *Suffocation of the Mother*
  1459
Joseph II, Holy Roman emperor 1477
Joubert, Laurent 662
Journal of Anatomy and Physiology 132
Journal of Applied Physiology 132
Journal of Biological Chemistry 155
Journal of Cancer Research 548
Journal of the Chemical Society 154
Journal of Clinical Endocrinology 498
Journal of Clinical Investigation 213, 214
Journal of General Physiology 132
Journal of Health and Human Behaviour
  1649
Journal of Health and Social Behaviour
  1649
*Journal of History of Medicine and Allied
  Sciences* 1548
Journal of Neurosurgery 1018
Journal of Physiology 132, 154
Journal of Psychosomatic Research 453
*Journal of Public Health and Sanitary
  Review* 1273
Journal of State Medicine 1079
Joyce, James, *Finnegan's Wake* 1528
Judaeo-Christianity 1450, 1451, 1471,
  1577
Judaism *see* Jews
Julius Hospital, Würzburg 786
Jundīshāpūr (S. Persia) 688, 709, 710,
  715
Jung, Carl Gustav 1044, 1438, 1461
  collective unconscious 1039
  'life force' 1038
Jurin, James, statistical study of smallpox
  1268
jurisprudence *see* law
Justinian I
  Byzantine emperor 686
  Digest 1621

Kahn, Reuben Laidlaw, flocculation text 196
Kaiserswerth school for nursing deaconesses 1193, 1454, 1476
Kakar, Sudhir 771
kala azar 512, 514
Kalahari bush people, disease levels 585
Kantian principles 65
Kaposi's sarcoma 575
Karrer, P., structure of vitamin A 165
Katz, Sir Bernard 137
Kay-Shuttleworth, James Phillip, sanitary reformer 1242, 1247
Keats, John 1527
Keefe, Frank 550
Kellogg, John Harvey 1304, 1463
Kendall, Edward Calvin 137, 214, 491
    isolation of thyroxine and cortisone 927, 1000
Kendrew, J.C. 166
Kennaway, E.L., polycyclic hydrocarbons as carcinogens 556
Kennedy, Ian M. 225, 876
Kent, A.F. Stanley, cardiovascular physiology 140
Kenya and Uganda 1417, 1419
Kern, Vincenz von 981
Kernberg, Otto, child psychologist 1042
Kerr, James, school doctor 1081
ketosis 502
Kew Gardens, Jodrell Laboratory 161, 162
Khālid ibn Yazīd 688–9
kidney-stones 840, 979, 1000
kidneys 1483
    artificial 1022
    Bright's disease 207, 351
    dialysis 503, 1022–3, 1110, 1386, 1599–600, 1602
    failure 502, 503, 504
    in old age 1102, 1103
    transplantation 1023, 1386
    tuberculosis 1015
    see also Addison's disease
Kieser, Dietrich George, treatment of insane 1031
King, Richard, founder of Ethnological Society of London 1439
King Edward's Hospital Fund for London 550, 1377, 1481, 1486
King and Queen's College of Physicians, Dublin 899

King's College, London 469, 1190
King's College Hospital 1190, 1319
king's evil see scrofula
Kiple, Kenneth F., (ed.) Cambridge History and Geography of Disease 4, 29
Kiple, Kenneth F. xvii, 357–81, 585
Kipling, Rudyard 1406
Kirkbride, Thomas, case records 33
Kirkes, William Stenhouse 133
Kirklin, John, extracorporeal circulation 1021
Kitasato
    Shibasaburo 193, 208
    toxin-antitoxin reaction 162
Kitson-Clark, George S.R. 1248
Klarman, H., economist 1385–6
Klein, Edward Emanuel 114
Klein, Melanie 1041
    on female psychology 1040
    Psychoanalysis of Children 1038, 1042
Kleinman, Arthur xvii, 15–23, 671, 744
Klinefelter, Harry Fitch, Klinefelter syndrome 430–1, 506
Kneipp, Sebastian, Bavarian hydropathist 619, 953
Knights of St John 55
Knobloch, Tobias 90
Knoll, Max, electron microscope 117
Knowles, D. 1184
Knox, Robert 100, 516
    Races of Man 1438
Koch, Ellen 1594
Koch, Robert 114, 194, 208, 1136, 1274, 1421
    on cholera 374
    germ theory 113, 352, 990, 1192, 1274
    humoralist theory of immunity 194
    postulates 193, 315, 326, 329
    tropical disease studies 519, 525, 528
    on tubercle bacillus 195, 199, 350, 427–8, 429, 789
Kocher, Theodor 991, 998, 1005, 1017, 1191
    Chirurgische Operationslehre 993
    introduces sterilizable sutures 992
    Kocher's clamp 991, 1010
    thyroid function research 995, 1010
    thyroid gland surgery 214, 485, 490, 494, 994, 997, 1010
Koettlitz, Reginald, scurvy 470
Köhler, August, ultraviolet microscopy 108

Kohut, Hans, child psychologist 1042
Kolesov, Vasilii, bypass surgery 1021
Kolff, Willem Johann, artificial kidney machine 1023
Kolle, Wilhelm, cholera vaccine 198
Kölliker, Rudolph Albert von 111
  Manual of Microscopic Anatomy 112
Koran 677, 682, 683, 684, 690, 692, 696, 699, 706
Korea 746
  influence of Chinese medicine 729
  women and medicine 744
Korean War (1950–53) 1538
Kraepelin, Emil 444
  study of pre-senile dementia 1103, 1365–6
Krafft, C. 1009
Krafft-Ebing, Richard von 444–5
  psychiatric theory of degeneration 1363
Krankenkassen 67
Krause, Fedor, neurosurgery 1017
Krause, P., barium diagnosis of alimentary tract 1009
Krebs, Ernest, laetrile cancer treatment 555
Krebs, Sir Hans 153, 154, 166
  Krebs Cycle 165
  respiratory physiology 137, 142
Kroeber, Alfred, American anthropologist 1442
Krogh, August, respiratory physiology 137, 141
Kruif, Paul de, *Microbe Hunters* 790
Kuhn, Franz, intratracheal insufflation 987, 1001
Kuhn, Richard, synthesis of vitamin A 165
Kuhn, Thomas S., *Structure of Scientific Revolutions* 25, 1657
Kühne, W. 154
Kuhnke, LaVerne 37
Kunitz, Stephen J. xvii, **1693–711**
Küntscher, G.B.G., intramedullary nails in fracture repair 1013
kuru 214, 1444
Küster, E. von, surgical treatment of hydronephrosis 996
Kuznets, Simon, economist 1385
kwashiorkor 371, 481
kymograph 129, 207

La Mettrie, Julien Offray de 1582
  L'Homme Machine 1457
laboratory assistants 1336, 1338, 1341
Lacan, Jacques, neo-Freudian psychoanalyst 1041, 1044
lactation *see* breast-feeding
lacteals 91, 93
Ladies' National Association against the Contagious Diseases Acts 569, 908
Ladies' National Association for the Diffusion of Sanitary Knowledge 902–3
Laënnec, R.T.H. 176, 177, 181, 182, 187, 787, 1187
  cancer nosology 542
  diagnosis of phthisis 350, 830–1
  stethoscope 206, **828–9**, 831–2, 1132
  Treatise on Mediate Auscultation **178–9**
laetrile (unorthodox cancer treatment) 555 6
Lagueste, Edouard, endocrine research 488
Laidlaw, Sir Patrick Playfair, distemper vaccine 200
Laing, Ronald David 1043
  anti-psychiatry movement 1367
laissez-faire
  in 18th-century Britain 61–2, 592, 1236, 1355
  in 18th-century France 1129, 1131
  in 19th-century economics 322, 903, 1633, 1697
Lake, John 298
Lamarckianism 419–20, 421, 433
Lambert, Sir John 1248
Lambotte, A., osteosynthesis 1012
Lancet 159, 1080, 1342, 1343, 1344–5
Lancisi, Giovanni, on cattle plague 1267
Landers, John, demographic study of London Quakers **1679–80**
Landsteiner, Karl, blood groups 164, 196, 1000
Landy, David 30
Lane, A., internal fixation of fractures 1012
Lane, William Arbuthnot, on autointoxication 1304
Lanfranc, *Chirurgia Magna* 967
Langdon-Brown, Sir Walter Langdon, endocrine research 491
Langenbeck, B.R.C. von, cleft palate operation 993

Langenbeck, C.J.M. 981
Langerhans, Paul, islets of Langerhans 487–8, 491
Langley, John Newport 132, 133
  physiology of digestion 138
  physiology of nervous system 143–4, 925
language, importance in medicine 27–8, 194
Laplace, Pierre-Simon de, marquis 159
  probability theory 1269
  social statistics 1235
Larkin, Gerald xvii–xviii, **1329–49**
Larrey, Dominique Jean 1537, 1540
  amputation technique 1557
  triage policy 870
laryngology 1596
laryngoscope 832, 1596
larynx
  cancer 994
  extirpation 997
  surgery 1008
lasers, in surgery 1004, 1021
Lasker, Albert Davis 550
Lasker, Mary, philanthropist (cancer charities) 550–1
Last, Murray xviii, **634–60**
Lateran Council (1215) 1452
Latham, Peter, on patient's role in diagnosis 1580
Latham, Robert Gordon
  Descriptive Ethnology 1438
  Natural History of the Varieties of Man 1438
Latin culture, Pliny's role 8, 69
Latin language 703, 785, 861, 966, 969, 1121, 1123, 1157
  anatomical terminology 85
  use in medical texts 57, 83, 87
Latrobe, Benjamin Henry 1503, 1505
laudanum 916, 917, 1589
Laurens, André du 89–90, 440
  criticizes Vesalius **87–8**
  Discourse of the Preservation of Sight . . . and of Old Age 1096
Lauth, Thomas 94
Laveran, C.L. Alphonse, identifies protozoan as malarial parasite 406, 514, 519
Lavoisier, Antoine Laurent 620, 918, 1031
  chemistry of oxygen 305

respiration research 156, 159
law and medicine 8, 69, 83, 100, 840, 930, 1126, 1197, 1209, 1219, **1619–40**
  in antiquity **1620–2**
  causes of death 81, 170, 967, 1122
  early modern period **1622–4**
  medico-legal knowledge **1624–6**
  in medieval Arab-Islam 714–15
  politics of expertise **1633–7**
  psychiatry **1630–3**
  status of medical experts **1626–30**
  see also ethics; lawsuits
Lawrence, D.H. 596
Lawrence, Ghislaine xviii, **961–83**
Lawrence, Susan C. xviii, **1151–79**
Lawrence, William 421
lawsuits
  against obstetricians 1068–9
  concealment of pregnancy 894
  conception/gestation/parturition 892–3
  hospital tort liability 1486
  illegal practice 555, 1126
  irreversible vegetative state 875
  malpractice 794, 1126, 1623
  mercy-killing 880–1
  New York optometrists 1247
  Rose v. College of Physicians 1126
  surrogate motherhood 879
  X-ray misuse 553
lay healers 233–4, 451, 662, 665–6, 670–3, 744, 902, 1130, 1133, 1136
  in ancient societies 48–9
  female see women
  medieval 55, 890–2
Laycock, Thomas 414
lazarettos 56–7, 318, 564, 890, 1183, 1232, 1233, 1453, 1471, 1472, 1498, 1509
Le Boë, Franciscus de (Sylvius)
  clinical medicine 1162
  iatrochemistry 156
Le Roy, Jean-Baptiste 1501
Le Roy Ladurie, E. 1669
Leade, Jane (née Ward), mystic 894
League of Nations 1423, **1424–5**, 1427
Leake, John, midwifery treatise 1052
Lebert, Hermann, cancer cell theory 181, 182
Leclerc, Daniel 94
Lee, R.D. 1672, 1675, 1678

Lee, Richard, American anthropologist 1445

Lee, Robert, accoucheur 1054

Leeuwenhoek, Antoni van 92, 94, 206–7, 208, 320
microscopy 102–3, 105

Legalist philosophers 1629

Lehmus, Emilie, founder Berlin polyclinic 900–1

Leiden University 94, 96–7, 123, 126, 397–8, 861, 864, 971, 1294
'proto-clinic' **1161–2**
rise of medical school 92–3

Leiper, Robert T., on schistosomiasis vector 514, 530

Leipzig University 85
physiological institute 1140

Leishman, Sir William Boog 514, 1563

leishmaniasis 358, 367, 512, 514, 531

Leith Hospital 900

Leitz, microscope-makers 115

Lemaire, François Jules, antiseptic properties of carbolic acid 988

Lempert, Julius, fenestration technique 1011

Leonardo da Vinci, on 'natural' death 1096

Leoniceno, Niccolò, criticizes Pliny's anatomy 87

Leopold, Prince 1589

Lepore, Michael 790

leprosaria *see* lazarettos

leprosy 318, 360, 364, 366, 412, 512, 514, **530–1**, 563, 564, 565, 680, 715, 1122, 1263, 1429, 1458, 1471, 1472

leptospirosis 198, 358

Leriche
autonomic nervous system surgery 1018
physiological surgery 998
R. 1012

lesions 346, **348–53**, 1187
intestinal *see* Peyer's patches

Letterman, Jonathan, on evacuation of battle casualties 1547

Lettsom
founds Aldersgate Dispensary 1188
John Coakley 1587

leucotomy 1018, 1583

leukaemias 351, 543–4, 546, 557, 558
childhood 554

Levan, Albert, chromosome research 430

Lever, John Charles Weaver, accoucheur 1054

Lever, William Hesketh, 1st viscount Leverhulme 1303

Leverhulme Trust 1480

Levet, Robert, Samuel Johnson's elegy **1524–5**

Levi-Montalcini, R. 138

Lévi-Strauss, Claude, French anthropologist 1440

Levy, Howard 1538

Lévy-Bruhl, Lucien, French anthropologist 1442

Lewes, George Henry 421, 1488

Lewin, Kurt, T-group therapy 1043

Lewis, G. 634

Lewis, Henry Sinclair 1530

Lewis, Milton 38

Lewis, Sir Thomas 158, 206
clinical research 220, 221, 222–3
ECG 215

Lexer, E., venous autografting 1022

Lichtenberg, A. von, first retrograde pyelogram 1015

Liddell, Howard S. 1045

Liébeault, Auguste Ambroise, *Concerning Sleep and Analogous States* 1032, 1033

Liebig, Justus von **157–60**, 923
Animal Chemistry 159, 160
chemical explanations of pathology/physiology 324–5, 327
Chemistry of Agriculture 159–60
fermentation/putrefaction theories 159, 160
on origins of death 258, 264
preparation of chloral hydrate 922

Liebreich, Oscar, work on chloral hydrate 922

Liehrsch, Bernhard 784

life and death, ideas of 7, 121, **160–1**, **249–80**

Lighthouse Trust 1483

Lilienfeld, Abraham 33

Lillehei, Clarence Walton, extracorporeal circulation 1021

Linacre, Thomas 1290

Lind, James 1501, 1557
Essay on Diseases incident to Europeans in Hot Climates 303, 516
naval hygiene campaign 1236
scurvy research 206, 468–9, 475
Treatise of the Scurvy 1397

Lindbergh, Charles, pump for
extracorporeal circulation 1020
Lindenbaum, Shirley, research on kuru
1444
Ling, Pehr Henrik, Swedish gymnastics
system 956
Linnaeus, Carolus
'balance of nature' concept 254, 256
botanical/zoological taxonomy 320,
344–5
Flora Zeylanica 772
Genera Morborum **344–5**
Systema Naturae 345
Linton, Ralph, American anthropologist
1442
Lionetti, R. 673
lipid metabolism 214
role of pancreatic juice 128
Lipmann, F.A. 137
Lipowski, Z.J., holistic theory of disease
454
Lister Institute 1276, 1488
Lister, Joseph, 1st baron Lister 104, 110,
113, 208, 262, 933, 1191, 1303, 1488,
1559
antisepsis 328, **988–91**
germ theory 325
Lister, Joseph Jackson, achromatic
compound microscope 208, 1593
aplanatic foci principle 104, 112
Lister, Thomas Henry 1240
Liston, Robert 980
first amputation using anaesthesia 986
literature
Arab-Islamic **691–7**, **701–8**
Chinese classical tradition **730–4**
health advice **1289–90**
medicine and 8–9, 416, 571, 907,
1520–35
medico-legal 1624–5
obstetrical 1052
physiological **132–4**
surgical 961, 966–8, 970–1, 974, 977,
980, 995, 1001–2
lithium 1044, 1367
lithotomy 963, 964, 971, 977, 979, 1123,
1589
lithotrity 1009, 1015, 1016
Little, Clarence C. 550
Little, E. Graham 216–17
Little Mothers' Leagues 1078, 1086
liver 91, 165, 175, 353, 393

biopsy 219
cancer 558
in carbohydrate catabolism 128
cirrhosis 597
glucose synthesis 485
in malaria 385–6
surgery 1023
transplantation 1023
Liverpool
local public health acts 1244, 1375
School of Tropical Medicine 520, 521,
528
University, biochemistry chair 154
Livi-Bacci, Massimo 1676–7
Livingstone, David 1396, 1419
Lloyd-George, David 1380
Loane, M., *Englishman's Castle* 1325
lobotomy 1583
Local Government Board (UK) 1248,
1249
localization of disease *see* disease
Lock Hospital 1185
Locke, John 868
association theory 441
Some Thoughts concerning Education
1295
theory of natural rights 856, 862
Loeb, Jacques 132
on natural death 269, 270
Loeb, Leo, principle of biological
individuality 201–2
Loeb, Robert Frederick 793
Loeffler, F.A.J. 193, 199
Loewenstein, E. 197
Loewi, Otto, physiology of nervous
system 137, 144, 929
Lohmann, Karl 165
Lolimbrāja, *Vaidyajīvana* 761
Lombroso, Cesare 594, 1529
atavism in criminals 429
London
Great Plague (1665–66) 297, 371, 397,
1126, 1233
medical profession **1125–7**
population 1238
private anatomy schools (18th century)
97–9, 100, 103, 973
Royal Commission on University
Education 216–17
University 216–17, 218–19, 469
see also University College London

London Bills of Mortality *see* Bills of Mortality
London Cancer Hospital *see* Royal Marsden Hospital
London County Council 218, 219
London Epidemiological Society 1243, 1262
London Fever Hospital 402, 403, 404
London Hospital 217, 221, 1185, 1276, 1314, 1322, 1324, 1453
London Missionary Society 1419
London Pharmacopoeia (1824) 784–5
London School of Hygiene and Tropical Medicine 223, 520, 521, 524, 1262, 1276, 1277, 1279
Longmore, Sir Thomas, *Treatise on the Transport of Sick and Wounded Troops* 1547–8
Longoburgo, Bruno 967, 968
Looss, Arthur, schistosomiasis research 529–30
Lorenz, Ottoker 428
Lorimer, F. 1699
Lösch, Friedrich, identification of *Entamoeba histolytica* 514
Loudon, Irvine S.L. xviii, **1050–71**
Louis, P.C.A. 1187, 1216
on contagious agents 1272
Recherches sur les Effets de la Saignée 950
statistical methods 207, 403, 918, 1166, 1240, **1269–71**, 1273
study of typhoid 401, 403, 405
Louis XIV
king of France 972, 1358, 1474, 1558
Louis XV, king of France 973, 1164
Louis XVI, king of France 1031
Louis-Philippe, king of France 1360
Louise de Marillac, St, founder of Daughters of Charity 1475
Loux, Françoise xix, **661–75**
Lovatt-Evans, Sir Charles 223
Lower, Richard
blood transfusions 972
physiological work 122
Lowie, Robert, American anthropologist 1442
Lu Xun, Chinese physician 747
Lubbock, Sir John 424, 1439–40
Lucas, Keith, nervous impulse 142, 193
Lucas, Prosper, *Traité philosophique et physiologique de l'Hérédité naturelle* 418–19

Luckes, Eva Charlotte, matron of London Hospital 1314, 1322, 1324
Lucretius 338
atomism 313, 317, 319
Ludwig, Carl, physiological research 126, **128–30**, 211
Luke, St 1451–3, 1585
Lumley, John, 1st baron Lumley, founder of Lumleian lectures 89
Lundy, John Silas, intravenous anaesthesia 1001
lungs
in anaesthesia 1001
blood circulation 88, 89, 122, 705
cancer 224, 537, 557, 1019, 1278, 1280
Morgagni's research 175
in old age 1102
role in infection 324
surgery 1002, **1018–20**
transplantation 1024
lupus 214
luteinizing hormone 491
Luther, Martin 607, 1124, 1473
Lutheran Church 1454
Lyautey, Hubert 1406
lying-in hospitals *see* childbirth
lymphatic system 541, 810
lymphocytes 201, 202, 576
lymphomas 542, 544, 546, 554, 993
Lyons, M.I. 527

McBurney, C. 1009
McCollom, Elmer Verner, vitamin A research 165, 478
MacCormack, Carol xix, **1436–48**
MacCormack, Sir William 1555
MacDonald, Michael, *Mystical Bedlam* 32–3
MacDowall, Robert John Stewart 133
McDowell, Ephraim, ovariotomy 981
MacEachern, M. *Hospital Organization and Management* 1383
Macewen, Sir William, neurosurgery 1017
McGann, S. 1314
McGee, L.C., bio-assay technique 146
McGrew, Roderick E., *Encyclopedia of Medical History* 4, 1574
McGrigor, Sir James 1556
Machiavelli, Nicolò 1205
Mackenzie, Sir James, polygraph 215

Mackenzie, Sir Morell, laryngologist 997
McKeown, Thomas 31–2, 36, 1305,
    1697, 1700
  demographic theory 1663, 1668, 1671,
    1673, 1674, 1676, 1680, 1681–3,
    1685, 1686
  Modern Rise of Population **1665–6**
  Role of Medicine **1652–3**, **1666–7**
McKinley, William, assassination 842
Maclachlan, Daniel, *Treatise of the Disease
    and Infirmities of Advanced Age* 1102
Maclean, Charles, anticontagionism 323
Maclean, Una 1443
Macleod, John James Rickard, insulin
    research 137, 491
MacLeod, Roy and Lewis, Milton,
    Disease, Medicine and Empire 38
McNeill, *Plagues and Peoples* 34
McNeill, William 37
Macy, Josiah jr., Foundation 1490
Madras Courier 767
Madsen, Thorvald, whooping-cough
    vaccine 198
Magendie, François 7, 127, 128, 621,
    919, 922, 1580
  physiology of nervous system 142
  study of poisons 918
Maggs, Christopher xix, **1309–28**
magic/supernatural 22, 49–50, 59, 591,
    643–6, 769, 770, 771, 802, 803, 915,
    970, 1406, 1408, 1442, 1457, 1464,
    1476
  in Arabic-Islamic medicine **679–85**,
    687
  in Chinese medicine 735, 743
  disease causation 296, 311, 312
  in Indian medicine 758
  see also folk medicine; non-Western
    concepts of disease
Magnan, Valentin, psychiatric theory of
    degeneration 1363
magnetic healing 604, 620–1, 622, 623,
    624, 628
magnetic resonance imaging (MRI) 207,
    794, 844, 877, 1602
Magnus, Albertus 1455
Mahādevadeva, Hindu physician 771
Mahler, Margaret, *On Human Symbiosis*
    1042
Mahoney, John F., penicillin treatment
    of syphilis 574
Maimonides, Moses 451, 711

Maitland, Charles, smallpox inoculation
    1236
malaria 162, 320, 324, 360, 363, 364,
    372, 374–5, 415, 472, 512, 513, 514,
    515, 516, 518, 523, **524–6**, 786, 789,
    917, 926, 1234, 1250, 1398, 1404,
    1405, 1429, 1444, 1489–90, 1554
  Anopheles transmission 215, 384, 386,
    406, 519–20
  benign tertian 386, 387, 394
  falciparum 360, 366, 370, 384–5, 386,
    387
  in Hippocratic Corpus **384–8**, 403,
    406
  malignant tertian *see* falciparum
  Plasmodium parasites 358, 925
  quartan 385, 395, 396, 397
  quotidian 385
  vivax 373
malingering **1554–6**, 1559, 1624
Mall, Franklin 210, 211
Malpighi, Marcello 94, 1580
Malthus, Thomas Robert 1584, 1587
  demographic theory 1235, **1664–7**
  Essay on the Principle of Population 1099
Manchester
  cholera outbreak (1849) 1272–3
  Royal Infirmary 864–5
  nurse training 1321
Mancuso, Thomas, nuclear radiation
    research 557
Mandeville, Bernard 1523
  Fable of the Bees 1525
  *Treatise of the Hypochondriack and
    Hysterick Passions* 1525
Mandl, Felix, parathyroid surgery 504
mandragora 920
mania 338, 439, 440
manic-depressive psychosis 1044, 1367
Manicheism 690, 691, 692, 693, 1451,
    1584
manipulative medicine **620–6**, 1332
Manson, Ethel (Mrs Fenwick)
  Nursing Record 1322
  nursing reform 1312, 1319–20
Manson, Sir Patrick 215, 514, 518,
    519–21, 1411
  Tropical Diseases 512
Mantoux, Charles 199
Maoris 1395, 1402, **1702–3**
marasmus 371, 465, 481
Marburg, human dissection in 85

Marcet, Alexander John Gaspard 157, 159
Marcuse, Herbert 1041
Mareschal, Georges 973
Marey, E.J.
  sphygmograph 837, 838–9, 845
  thermograph 838
Maria Theresa, empress of Austria 892, 1098, 1237
Marie, Pierre, on acromegaly 500
Marie Curie Cancer Relief Fund 550
Marine, David, iodine therapy of goitre 498
Marine Hospital Service (US) 1254
Mark, St 298
Marks, Harry M. xix, **1593–618**
Marsden, William, founder Royal Marsden Hospital 548
Marseilles, lazaretto 1498
Marscilles, plague 1233, 1234
Martin, Archer John Porter 165
Martin, Henry Newell 135, 208
  cardiovascular physiology 139
Martin, Sir James Ranald, British physician in India 1410
Martin, Lillien J., founder Old Age Counselling Centre 1105–6
Martineau, Harriet 903, 1576
  Life in the Sickroom 1465, 1586
Marx, Karl 1641
  Marxism 592, 594, 1649, 1652–3, 1657
Māsarjawayh of al-Baṣra 689
mass spectograph 1002
Massa, Niccolò 89
  anatomia sensata 86
Massachusetts, coronership **1634–5**
Massachusetts, Eye and Ear Infirmary 1190
Massachusetts, General Hospital 452, 845, 1019, 1502, 1503–4, 1513
massage 742, 744, 765, 1332, 1333
Mastalier (Mastalíř), Joseph Johan, Vienna paediatrician 1189
mastectomy 552, 558, 1002, 1014
mastoiditis 1011
masturbation 591
materia medica *see* drug therapies; drugs
materialism 443, 1032, 1463, 1582
  biomedical 21
maternal care *see* childbirth
maternal mortality *see* mortality

maternal welfare 60, 61, 1075, 1077, 1079, 1085, 1086, 1546
mathematics 207
  in mechanism 95–6
  see also statistics
Matrons' Association 1323
Matthew, St 54
Maudsley, Henry, founder Maudsley Hospital 594, 1364, 1529
Maulitz, Russell C. xix, **169–91**, 213–14, 539
Mauss, Marcel 1647
Mayas 368
Mayer, A.F.J.C., *Ueber Histologie* 104
Mayo, Charles 499
Mayo Clinic 491, 499, 504, 507–8, 556, 843–4, 927, 934, 1000, 1001, 1021
Mayo, William 504
Mayow, John, physiological work 122
ME *see* myalgic encephalomyelitis
Meakins, H.C. 218
measles 200, 359, 361, 362, 363, 364, 365, 369, 375, 405, 531, 698–9, 1264, 1271, 1275, 1429, 1694, 1697
measurement
  physiological 123
  see also pulse; temperature
mecanotherapy 956
Mecca 683, 769
Mechanic, David 1644
mechanism 59–60, 91, 126, 264, 1162
  Boerhaave's 94, 95–6
  Borelli's 94
  Descartes' 124, 1581
  in Enlightenment 93–5
  Newtonian 93, 94
  see also iatromechanism
Mechthild of Magdeburg, abbess 890
Medawar, Sir Peter Brian 192
  immunological nature of organ rejection 1023
  skin-grafting research 202
Medicaid 1198, 1387, 1486, 1604
medical anthropology *see* anthropology
medical auxiliaries *see* para-medical professions
medical care 6, **45–77**
  17th century **58–60**
  18th century **60–3**
  19th century **63–7**
  20th century **67–70**
  before 4000 BC **48–51**

classical Greece and Rome 51–4
healing framework 45–7
Middle Ages 54–7
Renaissance 57–8
role of philanthropy 1484–7
medical education 7, 19, 171, 816,
  1151–79
  16th-17th centuries 1159–63
  18th-century 32, 178, 828, 1163–6
  19th-century 1166–70, 1215–16
  20th-century 793, 1170–7, 1219,
    1223, 1276
  before 1500 1153–4
  clinical 1129, 1132–4, 1160–70, 1182,
    1188
  Flexner reforms 186, 212, 217, 219,
    1169, 1490
  in medieval Middle East 710–13
  in physiology 127–31
  in tropical medicine 520–22
  women's 890, 895–901
  see also anatomy; clinical research;
    dissection; medical profession;
    universities
medical ethics see ethics
medical historiography 9, 24–44
medical institutions and the state see state
medical laboratory technologists 1345,
  1346
medical literature see literature
medical officers of health 1244, 1248–1,
  1256, 1257
medical philanthropy see philanthropy
medical police 61, 588, 1136, 1209,
  1236–7, 1620
medical profession 4, 16, 20–2, 743–4,
  1119–50, 1645–6, 1649–51
  19th-century 99–100, 127, 177,
    1134–8, 1246–7
    Britain 1134–6
    international trends 1136–8
    20th-century US 1138–43
  early modern period 59, 60, 1124–5,
    1455
    in London 1125–7
    in Paris 1127–8
  Enlightenment 60–2, 171–2, 179,
    1128–31
  forensic medicine 1629–30, 1633–4
  impact of science 18, 1163–7
  incomes 1374, 1377–8, 1379, 1384,
    1385, 1552
  influence of French Revolution
    1131–3
  intraprofessional divisions 8, 21,
    814–17, 968–76, 1053, 1120,
    1122–3, 1128–4, 1158, 1335, 1598
  licensing/regulation 6–57, 99, 1120,
    1122–6, 1129, 1132–3, 1139–42,
    1168, 1207–8, 1210–12, 1217–18
  Middle Ages 56, 709–11, 713–16,
    1120–3, 1472–3
  origins 51–4, 1119–50
  Renaissance 1123–4
  and society 1649–50, 1651
  specialization 210, 1008–24, 1073–4,
    1107–8, 1110, 1139, 1163, 1171–3,
    1189, 1212, 1238, 1528, 1545,
    1551–2, 1580, 1596–7, 1635–6
  and the state 1196, 1207–24, 1257
  in USA 209–15, 1138–43
  see also doctor-patient relationship;
    ethics; para-medical professions;
    physicians; surgeons
medical records see case histories
Medical Research Committee (1913–20)
  220–1, 1276
Medical Research Council 220, 222,
  924, 1197, 1275, 1276, 1277, 1490,
  1492, 1544
  Clinical Research Board 224
  Clinical Research Centre (Northwick
    Park) 222
  epidemiological analysis of clinical
    problems 223–4
  medical uses of radium 549
  randomized clinical trials 223
  on therapeutic experimentation 874
Medical Research Fund 221
Medical Research Society 222
Medical Review of Reviews 1104
Medical Society of London 1188
medical sociology see medical care;
  sociology
medical specialization see specialization
medical technologies see technologies
Medicare 1198, 1383, 1387, 1486
medicine
  as art/science 3–11
  historiography 24–44
Mediterranean 366, 369
  bubonic plague 364, 365
  climate 388
  disease pool 363

early civilizations 53, 915
expansion of Islam 686
medieval trade in drugs 55
quarantine 1232, 1264
meiosis 107
melancholy 338, 388, 390, 413–14, 439,
440, 447
in humoralism 285
Mellanby, Sir Edward 217, 224
Mellerstadt 85
Melosh, B. 1310
Meltzer, Samuel James 213
intratrachael insufflation 987
membranes
pathology 177–8
physiology **148–9**
men-midwives 62, 893, 903, **1050–2**,
1126, 1128
Mendel, Gregor, on inheritance 107,
425–7, 428, 429, 430, 433, 434
Mengele, J. 1087
meningitis, cerebrospinal 198, 199, 201
Menninger, Karl A., Menninger
Foundation 1461
menopause 494, 505, 1101, 1106,
1587–8
menorrhagia 808
menstruation 284, 393, 479–80, 498,
618, 666, 1101, 1450
mental diseases 8, 38, 166, 338, **438–62**,
567, 786, 797, 955, 1108, 1111, 1133,
1139, 1483, 1497
emotional factors in somatic disease
450–5
functional neuroses **445–50**
Galen's view 287
psychotic and severely neurotic
behaviours **439–45**
sociogenic explanation 591–2
see also psychiatry; psychotherapy
Mental Hygiene Movement 1044
Menzies, Sir Frederick 219
mepacrine 1554
Merck Drug Company 923
Mercurialis, Hieronymus, De Arte
Gymnastica 1290
mercury 1102
as purgative 917
in treatment of syphilis 58, 565–6, 628,
916, 970
mercy-killing 880–1

Mering, Joseph von, diabetes research
488
Merrem, O.C.T., pylorectomy 1008
Merriman, Sam, accoucheur 1054
Mesmer, Franz Anton, mesmerism 447,
620, **1030–1**, 1032, 1036, 1042, 1462
Mesopotamia 360, 695, 756, 942
medical care 50, 51
surgery 963
metabolic rate 496, 499
hormonal influence 494
metabolism 163, 165–6, 264–5, 489, 490,
491, 492, 494
Bernard's research 128
inborn errors 495
lipid 214
measurement of 123
specific enzyme theory 160
theory of disease 1000, 1004, 1012
metastasis 1003, 1014, 1023
mechanism 542–3
Metchnikoff, Elie
cellular theory of immunity **194**, 196
life/death theories 268, 270
phagocytic action of white corpuscles
110
Prolongation of Life 1102
meteorology, medical 36, 293, **296–300**,
311, 312, 398, 415, 564, 587–8, 1239,
1263, 1288, **1677–8**
Methodism (philosophy) 317, 591, 1120
Methodism (Wesleyan) 621, 1294, 1460
methonium compounds 1001
Metropolitan Asylums Board 1376
Metropolitan Commissioners in Lunacy
1631
Metropolitan Health of Towns
Association 1243
Metropolitan Life Insurance Co. 549
Metzler, Samuel James, intratrachael
insufflation 1001
Meulenbeld, G.J. 768, 769
Meuvret, Jean 1667
Mexico 370, 467
Spanish conquest 1403, 1404
Meyer, Adolf, clinical psychiatrist 444
Meyerhof, Otto 153
carbohydrate metabolism 165
respiratory physiology 137, 142
Meynert, Theodor, brain pathology 444
miasmata 400, 427, 988, 1243, 1271,
1273, 1274

concept 159, 295, 310, 1509–10
theory of disease 113, **304–6**, 588,
  1399
see also environment
Michigan University 210, 213
microbiology 65, 183, 192, 262, 374,
  375, 377, 519, 789, 790, 924–2,
  934–5, 1008
see also germ theory; putrefaction
microscopy 8, 18, 65, 66, 92, **102–19**,
  123, 125, 130, 160, 161, 187, 206–8,
  309, 320, 326, 374, 542, 1008, 1141,
  1593
  19th-century **104–9**, 127, **179–83**
  20th-century **114–19**
  early history **102–4**
  electron microscope 102, 108, 109,
    115, **116–18**, 545
  importance to life sciences 102, 106,
    176–7, **179–83**
  light microscope 115, 116, 117,
    118–19
    aplanatic foci 104, 112
    fluorescence techniques **115–16**
    phase contrast 115
  literature 103, **110–12**
  observation of living material **115–16**,
    119
  specimen preparation 103, 106, 108,
    109, **114–18**
    cryosections 116
    fixing 108
    metallic impregnation 109, 112
    mounting 106
    sectioning 106, 109, 116, 117
    staining 106, 108–9, 114, 115, 789,
    925
  see also bacteriology; cell theory;
    morbid anatomy
microsurgery 1004, 1011, 1018
microtome 116, 117, 789
Middle East *see* Arabic-Islamic medicine
Middlesex Cancer Research
  Laboratories 548
Middlesex Hospital 547, 1185, 1453
  physiology course 133–4
Midelfort, Christian Frederick, family
  therapy 1043
midwives 59, 638, 742–3, 893, **1050–6**,
  1062–5, 1067, 1122, 1126, 1151,
  1429, 1621, 1684–5
  community 1380

lay 48, 49, 50, 55, 57
  'policing' function 1623, 1628
  professionalization **891–2**, 896, **903–4**,
    1320, 1322, 1325
  see also men-midwives
Midwives' Institute 1320, 1322
Miescher, Friedrich 166
Migraine Trust 1480, 1481
migration, role in disease spread 363–4
Mikulicz-Radecki, J. von 991, 997, 998,
  1191
  aseptic technique 991
  electric oesophagoscope 1008
Milan
  Lazaretto 1498
  Ospedale Maggiore **1497–8**
  quarantine system (14th-century) 1232
milieu intérieur concept (physiology) 128
military medicine and hygiene 173, 304,
  398–9, 517, 523–4, 529, 970, 978,
  1129, 1236, 1251, 1299, 1317–18,
  1398, 1753
  control of prostitution **568–71**
  see also war and modern medicine
milk depots 1072, **1076**, 1485
Millie, Shan xxvi
Milne-Edwards, Henri, globular theory
  of tissues 104
Milton, John 1584
mind *see* mental diseases; psychiatry;
  psychotherapy
mind/body dualism 59, 67, 70, 95, 418,
  443, 738, 1449, 1462, 1486
mind/body relationship 18, **450–5**, 591,
  1042, 1357, 1368, 1575, 1584
Ministry of Health (UK) 1276, 1379–80,
  1546
  reports on maternal mortality 1061–2,
    1062
Minkowski, Oskar, diabetes research 488
Minoan civilization 954
Minot, G.R. 214, 222
Mirsky, A. 164
Miskawayh 710
missionaries 917, 1173, 1419, 1454
  in China 730–1, 746–7
  in India 773
  medical services 1407, **1417–20**, 1475,
    1482
Mississippian peoples, pre-Columbian
  368
mistletoe 342

Mitchell, Allan 1545
Mitchell, Juliet, feminist psychoanalyst 1044
Mitchell, Silas Weir 791, 1556, 1588
  on degenerationism 593
  'rest cure' 1578
  treatment of neurasthenia 1365
mitochondria, and respiration 109
Mitscherlich, Eilhard, life/putrefaction theory 258
Mitscherlich-Nielsen, Margarete, feminist psychoanalyst 1044
Mitteilungen aus den Grenzgebieten der Medizin und Chirurgie 997
Miyairi, K., schistosomiasis research 530
M'Naghten, Daniel, M'Naghten Rules 1630, 1632
Modell, M. 792
Modena, epidemic constitution 298, 301
Mohr, Fritz, *Psychophysische Behandlungsmethoden* 451
Moivre, Abraham de, *Annuities upon Lives* 1265
molecular biology 153, 163–5, 166–7, 220, 221, 431, 492, 498, 546, 1583
molecular genetics **430–3**, 434, 494
Molière (pseud. of Jean Baptiste Poquelin) 917, 1127, 1523
monasteries 695, 729, 890, 965, 1120, 1153, 1450, 1454–5, 1471–2, 1477
  Buddhist 745, 758–9
  dissolution 1184, 1473
  infirmaries **54–6**, **1452–4**, 1496–7
  survival of ancient texts 965
Mondeville, Henri de 83, 967–8
Mondino de' Luzzi 85
  Anathomia 81, 967
  and origins of human dissection 81, 82
Moniz, Egaz 214
monkeypox 361
monotheism, *see under names of religions*
Monro, Alexander *primus* 98, 976
Monro, Thomas, physician to Bethlem 1355
Montagu, Lady Mary Wortley, smallpox inoculation 192, 320, 766, 1236, 1267
Montaigne, Michel de 952
Monte, Giambatista, clinical lectures at Padua 1161
Montesquieu, Charles de Secondat, baron 1641

Montpellier 53, 87, 90, 94, 96, 125, 966, 967, 968, 1096, 1121, 1127, 1580
  école de santé 178, 1131
  medieval medical curriculum 1157, 1159
Moore, Benjamin, founder *Biochemical Journal* 154
Moore, J.E. 107
Moore, Thomas 165
Moorfields (Royal Ophthalmic) Hospital 1189
moral therapy *see* psychiatry
morality and disease 589–90
  urban vices 588
  see also Christianity; sexually transmitted diseases
Moran, Lord *see* Wilson, C.M.
morbid anatomy **171–6**
  18th-century **172–6**
  microscopic elucidation **109–10**
  in Renaissance 58, 170
  see also dissection, human
morbidity 1509, 1654, **1693–711**
  19th-century 1316
  20th-century 69–70
  child 1076
  infant 1076, 1083, 1278
  influence of work environment 1210, **1213–14**, 1222
morbus Gallicus see syphilis
More, Sir Thomas 1498
Morel, Benedict Augustin 593
  Traité des Dégénérescences **416–18**, 1363, 1366
Moreno, Jacob Levy, group therapy 1043
Morgagni, G.B. 176, 181, 605
  clinical records 32
  De Sedibus et Causis Morborum **174–5**, 348, 811–12, 826, 975, 1098, 1165
  pathological anatomy 205
  physical examination **810–13**, **816–19**
Morgan, John 1128
  Morgagni's influence 175
Morgan, Thomas Hunt
  genetic studies 430
  work on *Drosophila* 107
Morganroth, Julius 196
Moritz, Karl Philip 1031
Mormons 1463
Moro, Ernst 199
Moro, Marie Rose 671

Morpeth, viscount *see* Howard, G., 7th
  earl of Carlisle
morphine 608, 921, 1064, 1589, 1590
morphology 123, 328
  Vesalian 88
  Virchow's 184
Morris, C., synthesis of vitamin A 165
Morse, Edward S., 'Latrines of the East'
  1302
Morse, Robert 875
mortality 69–70, 548–9, 1226, **1234–5**,
  1239, 1240, 1270–3, 1299, 1375,
  1399, 1509, 1654, **1693–711**
  child 1052, 1076, 1681–2, 1706
  First World **1696–8**
  Fourth World **1702–3**
  infant 1083, 1085, 1238, 1265, 1276,
    1278, 1323, 1677–8, **1682–6**, 1703,
    1706
  influence of work environment 1210,
    1213–14, 1222
  maternal 868, 892, 1011, 1013,
    1057–61, 1065–9, 1429, 1705–6
  perinatal 1058, 1061, 1062, 1068,
    1069, 1478, 1682
  Second World **1698–700**
  Third World **1700–1**
  see also demography; ecology of
    disease; epidemiology
Morton, W.T.G., first use of ether
  anaesthesia 986
Moscow Scientific Institute for
  Experimental Apparatus and
  Instruments 1004
mosquitoes 519
  eradication campaigns 200, 406–7,
    520, **524–7**, 1253, 1279, 1405,
    1420
  Stegomyia 406
  vector of malaria (*Anopheles*) 373, 384,
    386, 406, 514, 519–20, 1275
  vector of yellow fever (*Aedes aegyptae*)
    360, 370, 514, 526, 1274, 1279
Mosso, Angelo, respiratory physiology
  140
motherhood, surrogate 879
Motor Neuron Association 1480
Motulsky, A.G. 433
Moulin, Anne Marie 192, 194
Moulin, Daniel de 817
Mount Vernon Hospital, Hampstead 221
moxibustion 731, 741

Moynier, Gustave 1558
MRI *see* magnetic resonance imaging
Muḥammad 684, 685, 688
  'Medicine of the Prophet' 683, **706–7**,
    717
Muhammad Ali, Egyptian quarantine
  system 1233
Mulder, Gerrit Jan, definition of proteins
  163, 165
Müller, Anton, psychiatrist 786
Muller, Hermann Joseph, mutagenic
  properties of X-rays 545
Müller, Johannes 182, 1581
  cell theory 105, 106, 542
  Elements of Physiology 132–3
  histopathology 180–1, 182
  theory of specific nerve energies 129
Muller, Ludwig von 216
multiple sclerosis 598, 1483
Multiple Sclerosis Society 1480
Mumford, Lewis 1508
mumps 362, 364, 369
Murchison, Charles, fever theory 404,
  405
Murdock, G.P. 642
  Ethnographic Atlas 643–4
Murphy, James Bumgardner, role of
  lymphocytes 201
Murphy, John Benjamin 1009
  Murphy's button 992, 1009
Murphy, W.P. 214, 222
Murray, George Redmayne, thyroid
  research 215, 487
Murray, J., kidney transplantation 1023
Murray, Joseph Edward 214
Murray, M. John 390–1, 393
muscarine 920, 928
muscles 124, 128
  electrical theory of function 125, 129
  in Galen's demonstrations 83
  oxidation of carbohydrates 165
  relaxation in surgery 1001
  therapeutic exercise 956
muscular dystrophy 1483
museums
  Hunterian 103, 110, 174, 974
  microscopy collections 103, 110, 115
  pathological 174, 175
Muslims *see* Arab-Islamic medicine
Mussolini, Benito 1087
Mu'tazila 692–3, 695

myalgic encephalomyelitis (ME) 596,
598, 1575
myelography 1017
Myers, Charles Samuel, anthropologist
1441, 1442
myotonic dystrophy 432
myxoedema 485–6, 927, 997, 1010
transplantation treatment 487

Naegeli, C.W. 161
Nagasaki 557
Napier, Richard 440
case records 33
psychotherapy 1460
Napoleon I (Bonaparte) 176, 827, 870,
1099, 1135, 1208, 1270, 1555, 1557
Napoleon III 1509
Napoleonic Code 1625
Napoleonic Wars (1793–15) 1542
Napoleonic Wars (1800–15) 469, 1134,
1239, 1540, 1551, 1554–5
narcissism 1042
narcosis, surgical 1002
narcotics 1001, 1464, 1588, 1589
Nascher, Ignatz
geriatrician 1103–5
Geriatrics 1104
Longevity and Rejuvenescence 1103
The Aging Mind 1104
Nash, John, architect 1504, 1509
Nasse, Friedrich, organicist psychiatrist
443
Nathan, Tobie 671
National Association for the Promotion
of Social Science (UK) 1243, 1248
National Association for the Study and
Prevention of Tuberculosis (US) 210
National Asthma Campaign (UK) 1480
National Cancer Institute (US) 539, 551,
554
National Health Service (UK; 1948) 550,
1067–8, 1085, 1108, 1110, 1111,
1197, 1227, 1340, 1384–5, 1481,
1546, 1548
Family Doctor Charter (1965) 1384
Trusts (1990) 1387
see also Acts of Parliament (UK)
National Hospital for Nervous Diseases,
London 1189
National Institute for Medical Research
(UK) 929, 930

National Institutes of Health (US) 213,
874, 1176, 1223, 1254, 1490
National Insurance Scheme (UK; 1911)
1213, 1380
National Kidney Research Fund (UK)
1480
National Radium Trust and Commission
(UK) 549–50
National Tuberculosis Association (US)
1487
natural childbirth 1064–5
natural philosophy see philosophy
nature 88
balance see humoralism
biomedical definition 18
healing power 21, 57, 64, 66, 96, 253,
260, 403, 607–8, 1462
Protestant view of God's presence in
87, 88
nature-nurture controversy 421–3
naturopathy 66, 604, 616–20, 626, 774,
795
Naturphilosophie 126, 316, 605, 1356,
1363
Naunyn, B. von 997
naval medicine and hygiene 58, 97–8,
304, 398–9, 467–9, 970, 1236, 1254,
1397, 1501, 1510, 1557, 1753
Nazis
human experiments 202–3, 225–6,
871–2, 1087, 1232, 1538, 1554,
1577
persecution of scientists 929, 1038
racial hygiene policy 595–6, 1000,
1304, 1669–70
Neanderthal Man 357
Near East 59
early societies 50, 53, 360
see also Arabic-Islamic medicine
Nebuchadnezzar II 1460
Needham, Joseph 733
Nef, John 1538
Negroes 1439
constitution 413
medical education 897
Neher, E., patch-clamping of membranes
138, 149
Neisser, Albert L.S.
discovery of gonococcus 568
syphilis diagnostic test 196, 573
Nelson, Horatio, viscount 469
neolithic age, medical care 50

Neosalvarsan 573, 926
nephrectomy 503, 1015
nephrology 207
Nernst, Walther Hermann, electrolyte
    chemistry 148
nerve fibres 124, 128
    microscopic examination 108
nerves 111–12, 207
    in Galen's demonstrations 83
    sensory and motor properties 128
    structure 112
nervous disorders 346–7, 349, 589–91,
    595, 620, 1189
    Linnaeus's classification 345
    see also mental diseases
nervous system 125, 214, 346, 488, 489,
    490, 1033, 1139
    anatomy 1580–1
    autonomic 143–4, 492, 920, 1018
    degenerative disorders 597
    integrative functions and chemical
        mediation 141–5
    neuromuscular junction 129, 919
    neurons 142, 143, 144, 493
    in old age 1100, 1103, 1111
    physiology 141–5, 1579–84
    surgery 996, 1002, 1006, 1010,
        1017–18, 1552
    see also neurology; neurotransmission
Netherlands
    18th-century medical profession 817
    famine (1944–45) 1549
    influence on Indian medicine 772
    Public Health Committee 873
Nettleton, Thomas, statistical study of
    smallpox 1267–8
Neuberg, C., founder Biochemische
    Zeitschrift 154
Neuburger, Max 24
neuralgia 592, 1576
neurasthenia 592, 792, 1139, 1365
    traumatic 1550
neuroblastomas 509
neuroendocrine system 493–5
Neurological Society of London 425
neurology 1139, 1365, 1555, 1580, 1582
neurophysiology 1003
neuroses 347, 907, 1034–5, 1042, 1044,
    1046, 1441, 1578
    cultural context 1039
    experimental 1045
    functional 445–50

sexual origin 1036–9
neurosurgery see nervous system
neurosyphilis 1103
neurotransmission 137, 141–5, 492, 494,
    495, 928–9, 1582
Neve, Michael xx, 1520–35
New England Hospital for Women and
    Children 900
New England Journal of Medicine 429, 874
New Guinea see Papua New Guinea
New Hospital for Women (London) 900
New Orleans
    tropical medicine 520
    yellow fever outbreaks (1853, 1905)
        33, 1279
New Poor Law see Poor Law
New World 302–4, 471, 1498
    see also colonialism; ecology of disease
New York
    quarantine authority 1250
    sanitary reform 1252
New York American 1104
New York Association for Improving the
    Condition of the Poor 1077
New York Cancer Hospital 547, 558
New York City Health Department
    Child Hygiene Division 1077–8, 1083
    schools health programme 1082–3,
        1084
New York Herald Antitoxin Fund 1082–3
New York Hospital 1188
New York Hospital for Diseases of the
    Skin 1190
New York Infirmary for Women and
    Children 900
New York Medical School 1104–5
New Zealand
    colonization 372, 1395, 1397
    Maori affairs 1702–3
    public health 1402
Newgate Prison 1504
    gaol fever 1236
Newman, Charles E. 814
Newman, Sir George 1085, 1685
News in the Physiological Sciences 132
Newsholme, Sir Arthur 1685
Newton, Sir Isaac 343, 344, 1162
    mechanism 94, 1461
    Newtonianism 93, 95
    Optics 93
    Principia 25, 343
Newton, Thomas 855

Ngubani, Harriet, *Mind and Body in Zulu Medicine* 1443
niacin 477–8
Nicaragua 1420
Nicholls, Frank 98
Nicolle, Charles 200
Nicolson, Malcolm xx, **798–821**
nicotine 920, 923, 925
Niel, Marie Claude 673
Nierensee, John, American architect 1512
Nietzsche, Friedrich W. 592, 596, 1531
Nigeria, Sopona smallpox cult 1408
night-blindness 468, 478
    congenital 426
Nightingale, Florence 894, 906, 1484, 1486, 1539, 1545, 1555
    advocacy of pavilion system 995, 1191, 1511
    medical reform 901, 902, 903
    Notes on Hospitals 1511, 1512
    nursing reform 995–6, 1193, 1311, 1312, 1318, 1319, 1322, 1325, 1376, 1454, 1476
Nightingale Trust Fund 1484
Nijinski, Vaslav 1460
Nissen, R., pneumonectomy 1019
nitrous oxide 922
    as anaesthetic 261, 922, 986, 1589
Nitze, M. 1016
    invention of cystoscope 1015
Nixon, Richard 538, 551
NMRI *see* nuclear magnetic resonance imaging
Nobel Prize in Physiology or Medicine 136, 137–8, 214–15, 222, 490, 995, 997, 1001, 1016, 1018
Nolan, P. 1325
Nomarski, G.X. 115
non-naturals *see* humoralism
non-Western medicine 16–17, 20, 21
    concepts of disease 6, **634–60**
        analytical models **646–56**
        anatomy/physiology/pathology **652–4**
        defining illness **648–51**
        therapeutics **654–6**
        changing systems **656–8**
        evolutionary models **635–41**
        typologies of medical concepts **641–6**

    see also Arab-Islamic medicine; Chinese medicine; Indian medicine
nonconformists 894, 897, 898
    see also under names of sects
Noorden, Carl von 791
noradrenaline 144–5, 492, 494, 495, 509, 929
Nordau, Max 594
Normanby, marquis of 1243
Norton, J. Pease 1254
Norway, deaf-mutism 424–5
nosology 5, 169, 173, 174, 300, 303, 316, 320–1, 324, **335–56**, 447, 542, 567, 588, 784, 1187
    18th-century **343–8**
    19th-century **348–53**
    classical tradition **336–8**
    early modern ontological disease concepts **338–40**
    Sydenham's contributions **340–3**
    syndromes, clinical **353–4**
    see also fevers
Notestein, F.W. 1664
Nothnagel, Hermann 791
Novocain 924, 1589
nuclear magnetic resonance imaging (NMRI) 1003, 1010, 1018
nucleic acids 107, 108, 164, 166, 431, 546
    see also DNA; RNA
nucleus *see* cell theory
Nuffield Chair of Medicine (Oxford) 220
Nuffield Foundation 1480, 1481, 1490
Nuremberg Code (1948) 226, **871–2**, 873, 880, 1554
Nuremberg War Crimes Tribunal (1945–6) 226, 871
nursing 4, **901–9**, 1143, **1193**, **1309–28**, 1562, 1598
    before industrialization **1313–15**, **1453–4**
    industrial influence **1315–19**
    modern **1319–24**
    Nightingale reforms *see* Nightingale, F.
    psychiatric and domiciliary **1324–5**
    religious communities 1453–4, 1472, **1476–8**, 1484
    training/professionalization 894, **1309–11**, 1314, **1320–4**, 1334
Nursing Record 1322
Nussbaum, Johann von, abdominal surgery 1191

nutrition 67, 207
  chemistry of foodstuffs 157, 159, 163
  impact of crop introductions 370–1,
    373
  infant 1072, **1074–80**, 1484–6
  and mortality decline 35–6, **1665–8**,
    1675–7, 1679–81, **1684–5**, 1697
  schoolchildren **1080–2**, 1087
  of typhoid patients 405–6
  see also diet
nutritional diseases 5, 6, 163, 359, 361,
  463–82, 512, 586, 1549
  animal models and the vitamin concept
    474–81
  early ideas on diet and health 466
  famine 35, 465, 586, 1698
  see also under names of diseases
  specific deficiency diseases **466–74**
Nutton, Vivian xx, 29, **281–91**, 337, 1182
nyctalopia *see* night-blindness

Oath
  Hippocratic *see* Hippocratic Corpus
  Physician's (Geneva 1948) **872–3**
Ober, William 1533
Oberlin College, Ohio 897
observation *see* diagnosis
obstetrics *see* childbirth
occult, influence on contagion 319
occupational medicine 556, 558,
  1213–15, 1222, 1266, 1268, 1270,
  1276, 1277–0, 1297
occupational therapy 1333–4, 1336,
  1341, 1345
Odericus of Genoa, *De Regenda Consilium*
  1289
Oedipus complex 1035, 1036, 1583
oesophagus, cancer 1019
  resection 1008
oestradiol 146, 491, 505
oestrin 146
oestriol 146, 505
oestrogens 491, 492, 505, 506
  anti- 501
  synthetic 147, 505, 927
oestrone 146, 505
Oeuvre de la Maternité, Nancy 1075
Oeuvres du Calvaire 547
Office International d'Hygiène Publique
  (OIHP) 1424–5
Ohlin, P.G. 1674
Olby, Robert C. xx, **412–37**

Old Age Counselling Centre, San
  Francisco 1105
Oliver, George, endocrine research 146,
  487, 489, 491
Olmstead, Frederick Law 1251
onchocerciasis 370, 531, 1428
oncology *see* cancer; tumours
ontological theory of disease 315,
  336–42, 346, 350, 352
oophorectomy *see* ovariotomy
open-heart surgery **1020–17**, 1020
ophthalmia 568, 1555
ophthalmology 698, 702, 704, 986, 1004,
  1011, 1337, 1340, 1422, 1556, 1596
  hospitals 1189, 1190
ophthalmoscope 832, 837, 1011, 1166,
  1331, 1332, 1579, 1595, 1596
opium 606, 760, 761, 916, 917, 918, 920,
  1588
opticians 104, 1331, 1337, 1339, **1342–3**
optometry 1238, 1331, 1337, 1347
orchidectomy 488
Ord, William, on myxoedema 485
Orfila, Joseph, *Traité des Poisons* 919
organ transplantation *see* transplantation
organelles 118
Organization for Economic Co-operation
  and Development (OECD) 1374,
  1385, 1426
organotherapy 146, **486–7**, 489, 497
Oribasius 55, 965, 1155
Orta, Garcia d', *Coloquios dos Simples* 772
orthopaedics 1002, **1011–13**, 1189,
  1552, 1558
  surgery 1006
orthoptics 1345
Osborne, John, midwifery treatise 1052
Osiris 29
Osler, Sir William 405–6
  on Addison's disease 487
  at Johns Hopkins 209, 210, 211, 212,
    568
  at Oxford 215, 216, 218, 219, 220
  Principles and Practice of Medicine 449
osmic acid, as fixing agent in microscopy
  108
osmotic pressure 148
osteitis fibrosa cystica 503
osteomyelitis 994
osteopathy 65, 604, 620, **621–6**, 627,
  1140, 1217, 1330, 1339
osteoporosis 505, 1106

Ostwald, Friedrich Wilhelm 163
O'Sullivan, Cornelius, enzyme research
    161–2
otorhinolaryngology **1011**, 1556
otoscope 1011
Ottoman Empire 371–2, 1236, 1422,
    1696
ovarian ablation 506
ovaries 490, 491, 494
    hormones 146, 147, 491, 492, 505,
        506, 927
ovariotomy 488, 506, 981, 993–4, 1013
Overton, C.E., osmotic pressure studies
    148
Owen, Robert 1503, 1509
Oxford Companion to Medicine 4
Oxford University 97, 99, 122, 890, 899,
    1121, 1125, 1160, 1163, 1190
    clinical research 211, 215, 216
    Dunn benefaction 1490
    histology courses 111
    medical education 218, 219, 220
    Waynflete physiology chair 130, 142,
        206
oxygen, discovery 305
oxytocin 491, 493
Ozanam, Frédéric, founder Society of
    St-Vincent-de-Paul 1477

Pacini, Filippo, description of cholera
    vibrio 325, 1421
Padua 88, 971, 1158
    18th-century medical profession 816
    clinical teaching 1129, **1160**
    economic decline 92–3
    human dissection 85, 1157, 1160
    Morgagni's work 174–5, 205, 812,
        1165
    Renaissance 84, 1129
    statutes 85–6
    surgery 966–8
paediatrics **1073–4**, 1086–7, 1189, 1698
Pagel, Julius Leopold 24, 899
Pagel, Walter 339
Paget, Dame (Mary) Rosalind,
    professionalization of midwifery 1320
Paget, Sir James 133, 622
    on histology 111
    on hospital hygiene 988
pain and suffering 6, 20, 46, 234, 345,
    669, 861, **1574–91**
    in childbirth 1064, 1065

cultures **1584–7**
language **1575–9**
physiology **1579–84**
progress **1587–90**
psychological theories 1577, **1583–4**
surgical 984
in Western tradition 18–20, 21
see also anaesthesia
Painter, T.S., genetic studies 430
Palade, G. 138
palaeolithic age *see* Stone Age
palaeopathology 563, 564, 585
Paley, William, *Natural Theology* 1585–6
Palladius 687
Palmer, Daniel David, founder of
    chiropractic **624–6**
Palmer, Richard 1233, 1290
palpation 787, 794, 801, 802, 805,
    809–10, 811–12, 813, 814, 818
Pan-American Sanitary Bureau 1422,
    1424, 1427
Pan-Arab Quarantine Board of Health
    37, 1233, 1421, 1427
Panama Canal 406, 526, 1253, 1279
pancreas 489
    cancer 504–5, 1009
    hormones 146, 166, 214, 487–8, 491,
        501–3, 928
    physical examination 811
    physiology 138, **145–6**
    transplantation research 1022
    tumours 504–5
pancreatectomy 502
pancreatico-duodenectomy 1009
Pandolfi, Mariella 671
Pangaea 359, 367, 372
Panum, Peter Ludvig, study of measles
    epidemic 1270–1
paper chromatography 165
Pappenhheim, Bertha *see* Anna O.
Pappworth, Maurice Henry 226
    on abuse of patients in experiments
        874
Papua New Guinea 531
    kuru epidemic 214, 1444
para-amino-salicylic acid (PAS) 933–4
para-medical professions 1171, 1192,
    1329–49, 1597
    early history 8, **1336–7**
    inter-occupational relationships
        1336–45
    inter-war years **1338–40**

post-1945 **1340–8**
Paracelsians 60, 156, 1127
  drugs 93
  rejection of anatomy 94
Paracelsus 7, 58, 93, 155–6, 319,
  338–41, 541, 603, 916, 1124, 1162,
  1437
  religious philosophy 1461, 1462
  on surgery 970
paracetamol 924
paralysis 610, 919, 921, 1583
parasites 327, 352, 353, 357–8, 360, 371,
  480
  intestinal 368
  life-cycles 326
  malarial 384–6
    Plasmodium falciparum 384–5
    Plasmodium malariae 385
    Plasmodium vivax 384, 386
parasitic infections *see* tropical diseases
parasitology 1280, 1563
parathyroid glands 486, 490, 493, 495,
  503–4, 928
parathyroidectomy 504
Paré, Ambroise 58, 892, 980, 1537
  amputation technique 970–1, 978
  Traité des Rapports 1624
  wound treatment 970–1
Paris 84, 89, 126
  demographic study (1821) **1239–40**
  école de santé (19th-century) 1099–100,
    1131–2
  école de santé (19th-century) 178, 1101
  hospitals (post-Revolution) 173, 176,
    179, **1187**, 1190, 1283, 1352,
    1501–3
  medical profession (early modern)
    1127–8
  medical school (Middle Ages) 967,
    1121, 1123, 1157, 1159
  medical school (post-Revolution) 63,
    127, 173, 207, 255, 348, 787,
    816–17, 950, 967, 975–6, 981, 1162
  Museum of Natural History 255
  private anatomy schools 97, 98, 100
  Radium Institute 548
  women medical graduates 898, 899,
    1143, 1175
Paris Medical Gazette 1245
Park, Katharine 29
Park, Mungo 1396

Park, William Hallock, diphtheria
  antitoxin programme (NY) 1082–3
Parke, Davis & Co. 146
Parkes, Edmund A. 1410, 1563
Parkinson's disease 597
Parkinson's Disease Society 1480
Parkman, George, trustee of
  Massachusetts General Hospital 1503
Parr, Thomas 1096
Parran, Thomas jr., campaign against
  venereal disease 550, 574
Parry, Caleb Hillier, on exophthalmic
  goitre 486
Parsons, Talcott, medical sociologist
  1644–5, 1646, 1647, 1648, 1649,
  1650
particles, in natural philosophy 91–2, 93
PAS *see* para-amino-salicylic acid
Pasteur Institute, Paris 162, 192, 208,
  268, 519, 932, 1488
Pasteur, Louis 208, 933, 1060, 1192,
  1302, 1303, 1488
  on anthrax 1274
  cellular theory of immunity 194
  fermentation research 113, 160–2,
    192–3, 988
  on fowl pest 193
  on fungi 325
  germ theory 327, 352, 988, 1138, 1274
  on putrefaction 257–8, 328, 988, 1191
  on rabies 199, 328, 789, 790, 1218,
    1274
  on specificity 328–9
pasteurization 327
patch-clamping (membrane physiology)
  138, 149
pathological anatomy 184, 255, 256, 349,
  350, 789–90, 793, 984, 996, 998,
  1132, 1165, 1351
  19th-century **176–85**, 196–9
  of cancer 541–2
  importance of microscope **179–83**
Pathological and Bacteriological
  Laboratory Assistants' Association
  (UK) 1336
Pathological Society (UK) 1338
pathology
  18th-century **174–6**
  19th-century 126, **176–85**
  and hospital expansion 63–4
  microscope as authority **179–83**

pathological physiology and
  chemistry 123, **184–6**
  Virchow's role **181–4**
  20th-century **186–9**
  ancient and modern 169–70
  'general' **170–1**
  international medical tradition 175–6
  non-Western concepts **652–4**
  surgical **1005–6**
  see also clinical research; disease/
    diseases; morbid anatomy; morbidity
pathology xix, 6, 94, **169–91**
pathophysiology 186, 341, 342, 346, 783,
  787, 984, 999, 1000, 1019, 1584
patients 59, 60, 84, 998, 1654
  in clinical research 208–9
  difficult 786–7, **1643–5**, 1656–7
  fear of surgery 996
  female see women
  hospital 998, 1186, 1192–7
  importance in medical history 25–6
  legal rights **873–5**, 1633
  and new technologies 20, **1599–600**
  role in diagnosis 18, 63, 64, 66, 740,
    801, **813–15**, 819, 829–30,
    1579–80
  role in modern health care 70, 71
  in Western tradition 18–19
  see also doctor-patient relaionship;
    ethics; medical care
Paton, Sir William Drummond
  Macdonald, research on methonium
  compounds 1001
Patterson, J.T. 538, 539
Patterson, K. David 37, 531
Paul of Aegina 55, 440, 687
  Epitome 965
Paul, John R., A History of Poliomyelitis
  30
Paul, St 88, 288, 1465
Pauling, Linus Carl
  advocacy of vitamin C 166–7, 556
  chemistry of haemoglobins 166
  DNA 166
  protein chemistry 164
pavilion system see architecture
Pavlov, Ivan Petrovich 488, 1581
  on conditioned reflex 1045
  physiology of digestion **136–8**, 266–7,
    270–1
Payen, Antoine 160
Paynel, Thomas 1289

Payr, E. 998
Peabody Trust 1509
Pearse, Everson 493
Pearson, Karl, biometrics 1275
Pecquet, Jean 91
Peek, Sir Henry, philanthropist 1081
Peking Union Medical College 747,
  1174, 1419, 1490
pellagra 30, 31, 371, 373, **471–2**, 475,
  476, **477–8**
Peller, Sigismund 539
Pelletier, Pierre Joseph
  isolation of alkaloids 919
  study of poisons 918
Pelling, Margaret xx, 37, **309–34**
Peloponnesian War (431–404 BC) 363
Pemel, Robert, Help for the Poor 1296
Penchaud, M.-R., architect of Marseilles
  lazaretto 1498
penicillin 793, **933–5**, 936, 999, 1067,
  1107, 1170, 1198, 1544
  in syphilis therapy 573, 574, 581
Peninsular War (1808–14) 1542, 1554
Pennsylvania Hospital 1188
  treatment of maniacs 1357
Pennsylvania University 213, 400
Pentecostalists 1465
Pepper, William, on neuroblastomas 509
Pepys, Samuel 1301
perception, in Foucault's work 27
Percival, Thomas 852, 861, 869–70, 876
  codification of medical ethics **864–8**,
    871, 874
  Medical Ethics **865–8**, 873, 1455–6
  Medical Jurisprudence 865, 867
percussion 64, 178–9, 348, 787, 794,
  805, 810, 812, 816, 834, 842
  thoracic 814–15, 819–20, 828
Pereira, Jonathan, physician/chemist 920
perfectibility and hereditarianism 419–21
pericardectomy 1020
Perkin, Sir William H., synthetic
  dyestuffs industry 923
Perls, Frederick, Gestalt therapy 1043
Pernick, Martin 32, 33
Perry, William 1437, 1441
Pershing, John Joseph 1333
Persia 688, 699–701
Persian language 676, 677, 771
personal hygiene see hygiene
Persoz, Jean François 160
Peru 370

Spanish conquest 1403
Peruvian Bark *see* cinchona
PET *see* positron emission tomography
Petchesky, Rosalind Pollack 1601
Peter, St 288
Peterson, Eleanor 894
Petit, Antoine 1501
Petit, J.L. 974
  amputation technique 978
Petrarch 917
Petri, Julius Richard 114
Pettenkofer, Max von 1212
Petty, Sir William 33, 1209
  Political Anatomy of Ireland 1234
  quantitative social analysis 1234
Peyer, J.C., Peyer's patches (typhoid)
  401, 402, 405
Peyronie, François de la 973
Pfalz, Liselotte von der 950
Pfeiffer, Richard Friedrich Johannes 405
Pflüger, Eduard F.W.
  Archiv für die gesamte Physiologie der
    Menschen und der Tiere 132
  cell theory 161
pH scale 163
phaeochromocytomas 497, 509
phantom limb phenomenon 1582
pharmaceutical industry 145, 874, 923,
  1197, 1546, 1588–9
  British 929–30
  controversies on patents 146
  Indian 769
  US 925–6
pharmacology *see* drug therapies
pharmacopoeias 916
pharmacy 184, 891, 915, 966, 1053,
  1129, 1330, 1422
  emergent profession 918
phenacetin 924
phenol *see* carbolic acid
phenylketonuria 166
Philadelphia 401, 402
  smallpox epidemic (1871–72) 1376
philanthropy (after 1850) 8, 212–13,
  220–1, 523–4, 903, 1317–11, 1325,
  1480–94
  cancer funds 537–8, **547–8**, 551–2
  child welfare 1073, **1076–8**, 1080–1
  forms and functions **1480–4**
  internationalism **1417–20**
  and medical care **1484–7**
  and medical research **1487–92**

US sanitary reform 1252
philanthropy (before 1850) *see* charity
Philiscus 386, 389
Philistion of Locris 286
philosophy 1154–5
  ancient Greek 855, 856–9
  British empiricism 419, 1126
  Enlightenment 862, 1128–31, 1583,
    1586–7
  existentialism 1043
  Indian tradition 761–2
  medical
    Forms 15–16
    Foucault's influence 27–8
    fundamental faculties 82
    Western concepts 18–20
    see also mechanism; mind/body
      dualism; soul
  Methodism 317, 591, 1120
  moral 1437
  natural 87, 88, 91, 96, 313, 320,
    338–40, 341, 343, 1356
    Aristotelian 87–8, 91, 120–1, 155,
      1121, 1157
    as basis of theoretical medicine 90
    Chinese theories **734–7**
    Galenic 155, **943–5**
    Harvey's 88
    in Middle Ages 83, 84
    new theories **90–6**
    Newtonian 93, 95
    in Renaissance 87
  Sophism 52
phlebotomists 59, 60, 680–1, 1129
phlebotomy *see* bloodletting
phlegm *see* humoralism
phobias 1045
photography 843
photomicrography 118
photosynthesis *see* botany
phrenicotomy 1019
phrenitis 336, 342
phrenology 421, 442, 1032, 1457, 1506,
  1581
phthisis 350, 586, 830–1
physical examination *see* diagnosis
physical methods 6, 51–2, 58, 348, 917,
  939–60
  bloodletting and dietetics **940–51**
  rubbing, stroking and gymnastics
    955–3
  water-bathing *see* hydropathy

physicians 56, 57, 60, 62, 1120, 1207, 1208
  academic **82–6**, 89, **93–5**, 171–2, **1152–6**, 1455, 1472
  élite 783–6, 805, 814, 890–1, 947–8, 961, 969, 971, 1122, 1124–7, 1133, 1135–6, 1175, 1347
  and literature **1520–35**
  as scientists 789–92, 794, **1138–44**
  social status **785–7**, 1051, 1131
  in Western tradition 18–19, 21
  see also internal medicine; medical profession
Physick, Philip Syng 981
physics 93, 207, 919
  and bodily function 59
  quantification of air 304
  social **1238–41**
  see also technologies
physio-medicalism 613
physiognomy 287
physiological agents as drugs **926–9**
physiological chemistry *see* biochemistry
Physiological Reviews 132
Physiological Society 134, 135
physiological surgery **998–1001**
physiology 5, 94, **120–52**, 296, 827, 918
  19th-century **126–31**
    Britain in 1870s **130–1**
  20th-century **131–49**
  in ancient world 121, **391–2**, **941–5**
  in Chinese medicine 731, 736, **737–8**
  in Enlightenment **123–5**
  experimental tradition **126–8**, 1138
  non-Western concepts 652–4
  of pain **1579–84**
  professionalization **126–8**, **131–6**
  in Renaissance **122–3**, **1123–4**
  see also and under names of physiologists and body systems; clinical research; Nobel Prize
physiotherapy 1331, **1332–3**, 1336, 1338–9, 1345, 1422
Piccolomini, Archangelo, Catholic view of anatomy 88
Pick, Daniel 416, 420
Pietism 896
Pincus, Gregory, oral contraception 505
pineal gland, in Cartesianism 1457
Pinel, Philippe 786, 1187
  moral therapy 442–3, 870, **1352–7**, 1359

Nosographie Philosophique **348–9**
pathology 178
Traité médico-philosophique sur l'Aliénation mentale 349, 1352
Pinker, Robert 1195
pinta 367, 368, 563
pinworm 358, 360
Pirogov, Nikolai Ivanovich 1537
  Pirogov medical society 1137
Pirquet, Clemens, on allergy 195, 199
Pitcairne, Archibald 94
Pitt, R. Margaret, Vi antigen 198
pituitary cachexia (Simmonds' disease) 501
pituitary gland 145, 490, 491, 495, 497, **500–501**, 502–3
  ablation 1014
  in Cushing's disease 507
  hormones 147, 492, 493, 928
  tumours 494, 496, 500, 505
pituitary infarction (Sheehan's syndrome) 501
Pius XII, pope, on resuscitation (1958) 875
Pizarro, Gonzalo 369
placebo effect 18, 19, 20, 47
plague 30, 57, 296, 297, 318, 319, 322, 326, 340, 358, 363, 371, 377, 397, 512, 522, 531, 587, 690, 1268, 1276, 1291, 1301, 1399, 1401, 1402, 1421, 1424, 1498, 1696, 1699
  bubonic 36, 364, 365, 372, 396, 586, 686, 1209–10, 1232–5, 1264, 1458, 1668
  Near East pandemic (AD 541–749) 684
  Pasteurella pestis vaccine 198
  see also Black Death
plants *see* botany
Plasmaquin 932
plastic surgery 765, 993, 996, 1022, 1106, 1544, 1552
Plato 6, 706, 878, 1154
  Laws 1630
  Republic 856–8
  Timaeus 286, 287, 336
  virtue ethic 855, 856
Platonism 155, 1584
Platter, Felix 440
pleurisy 284, 336, 397, 941, 948–9
Pliny *the elder*, anatomy 87

Plummer, Henry, on hyperthyroidism 499
Plunkett, Miss, empiric cancer-curer 555
pneumococci 1279
pneumoencephalography 1017
pneumonectomy 1002, 1019
pneumonia 198, 212, 367, 388, 403, 523, 531, 941, 1100, 1107, 1677
Pneumocystis carinii 575, 576
pneumothorax, artificial 1017
podiatry *see* chiropody
Poe, Edgar Allan 1530
poisons 81, 314, 351, 758, 853, 854, 919
    biological tests 930
    in physiological experiments 918
    therapeutic use 262, 921
Poland, typhus epidemic (1919) 1424
Policard, A. 1012
police, medical *see* medical police
poliomyelitis 30, 368, 375, 545, 1429, 1481, 1694, 1697
    immunization 201, 1483, 1643
politics 323, **1693–711**
    and child welfare 1074–6, 1078, 1087
    and degenerationism 420
    and health 8, 33, 60–1, 63, 236–7, 372–3
    medical 1245–6, 1270
    see also public health; state
Politzer, A., otorhinolaryngologist 1011
Pollender, Franz Aloys Antoine, on anthrax 113
Pollich, Martin 85
Pollio, Marcus Vitruvius, *Ten Books on Architecture* **1495–6**
pollution 321, 328, 329, 597
    carcinogenic effects 558
Polybus 286, 389–90
polycystic kidney disease 432
polygraph 215
polyps, nasal 963
Pompeii 951, 980
poor
    domiciliary care **1325–6**
    impact of epidemics 399, 404
    living conditions and disease **318–22**, 586, 1078–9, 1212, 1236, 1238, 1241–2, 1298
    medical care 58, 61, 62, 866–7, 1184, 1193–4, 1198, **1210–12**, 1222, 1453, 1454
    self-help **1297–9**

and spread of AIDS 577
as subjects for dissection 100, 1187–8
see also architecture; charity; childhood; philanthropy
Poor Law (New System, 1834) 1193, 1212, 1242, 1245, 1247, 1309, 1317, 1323, 1375–6
Poor Law (Old System, 1601) 1474
Pope, Alexander 1525, 1585
Popjay, surgeon-apothecary 785
population *see* demography
Portal, Antoine 94
    palpation technique 809
Porter, Dorothy xx–xxi, 31, 588, **1231–61**
Porter, Roy xi, **3–11**, 26, 31, **585–600**, 809, 814, **1449–68**, 1529, **1574–91**
Portugal
    exploration/colonization 366, 371, 374, 1417, 1419
    influence on Indian medicine 772
    plague epidemics 371, 372
positron emission tomography (PET) 844, 1003
Post, John, *Food Shortage, Climatic Variability, and Epidemic Disease* 36
post-partum sepsis 793
Postgraduate Medical School *see* Hammersmith
Postma, Geertruide, mercy-killing 880
potassium, in membrane physiology 148, 149
potato, importation from New World 371, 373
Pott, Percivall 977
    on scrotal cancer 556
Powell, Enoch 1507
Power-Cobbe, Frances 902, 903
Poyet, Bernard, pavilion plan 1501
Poynter, F.N.L. 219, 1536
practolol 936
Praxagoras of Cos 392
pre-Raphaelites 1530
pregnancy 498, 1549, **1600–1**, 1602, 1705
    and AIDS 577, 580
    anaemia 480
    diagnosis 146, 496, 813
    legal aspects 894, 1621, **1623–5**, 1627
    prevention *see* contraception
    toxaemia 1061
prehistory
    Indus valley 756–7

surgery 962
premenstrual syndrome 245
Premuda, Loris 809
Prentice, Caroline xxvi
Prentice, Charles, optometrist 1337
Presbyterians 1451, 1461
Presocratic philosophers 283
pressure manometer 165
Preston, Samuel 1700
Price, Jonathan xxvi
Prichard, James Cowles 1439
    Analysis of Egyptian Mythology 1437
    concept of hereditary constitution
        413–14, 416
    racial studies 1437–8
    *Researches into the Physical History of
        Mankind* 1437
Priessnitz, Vincent, hydropathy 65,
    617–19, 626, 953
Priestley, James, radical adrenalectomy
    507–8
Priestley, Joseph
    plant chemistry 156
    pneumatic chemistry 305
priests
    at deathbed 263–4, 271, 1464
    forbidden to shed blood 969, 1158,
        1452, 1472
    role in medical care 49–50, 59, 234,
        638, 735, 744, 969, 1130, 1356,
        1452, 1475, 1476
primates
    role in AIDS spread 376
    role in human evolution 357
Princeton Office of Population Research
    1664
Pringle, Sir John 398, 809, 817, 1500,
    1501, 1537
    military hygiene campaign 1236
Pringle, Sir John 807
Prins, Gwyn 38
printing, invention, impact on education
    1159
prison reform 894, 903
private anatomy/medical schools 95,
    99–100, 103, 973, 1130
private hospitals 1194, 1195
procaine 1001
*Proceedings of the Association of American
    Physicians* 214
Procopius 364
progesterone 146, 491, 505, 506

prolactin 491, 493, 500
prolactinoma 501
prolongation of life **267–72**
Prontosil 793, 932, 1066
prostaglandins 494
prostate gland
    cancer 497, 506, 1000, 1016
    hypertrophy 488, 1015
prosthesis 978, 1024
    femoral 1013
    heart valves 1021
prostitution 894, 896, 908, 1399, 1633
    control **568–71**, 580, 1138
proteins 166
    decomposition 162
    nature of 163–4
Protestant/Catholic 'correspondencies'
    96–7
Protestantism 588, 894, 898, 902, 1044,
    1159, 1184, 1365, 1454, 1456, 1463,
    1473–6
    cleanliness ethic 990
    and medical traditions 87–8
    missions 1454
    view of health and moral character 234
    see also Reformation
Protozoa 115, 358, 514, 519, 520, 925–6,
    932
Proust, Adrien 1530
Proust, Marcel 1530, 1532
    Recherche du Temps perdu 1530–1
Prout, William
    founder *Annals of Medicine and Surgery*
        157
    physiological chemistry **157–9**, 163
Provincial Medical and Surgical
    Association 1137
Prudential Insurance Co. 548
Prussian Royal Academy of Sciences 889
psyche *see* psychotherapy
psychiatric social workers 1340
psychiatry 19, 21, 22, 38, 349, 417, 793,
    906, 1033, 1139, 1232, **1350–72**,
    1460–1, 1505, 1546, 1648–9, 1655
    19th-century **1363–6**
    20th-century **1366–8**
    and the law **1630–3**
    moral therapy 442, 870, 1031, 1350,
        1352–7, 1363
    nursing **1324–5**
    see also asylums; civilization; mental
        diseases; psychotherapy

psychoanalysis 445, **448–50**, 452,
  1033–9, 1366–7, 1442
psychology 1436, 1438, 1556, 1641–2,
  1644, 1655
  associationist 441–2, 1506
  and pain 1577, **1583–4**
psychopathologies 907, 1045, **1631–2**
psychopharmacology 445, 904, 905,
  1044, 1046, 1108, 1366–7, 1368,
  1589
psychoses 1046
  senile 1103
psychosomatic disorders 591, 596,
  905–6, 1575–6, 1583
psychosomatic medicine **450–5**
Psychosomatic Medicine 452–3
psychosurgery 214, 1018, 1583
psychotherapy 21, 451, 620, 792, 797,
  1029–49, 1105, 1578, 1589
  18th-century **1030–1**
  19th-century **1032–3**
  20th-century **1037–46**
  neo-Freudians **1039–42**
  in non-Western theories 640, 657
  see also psychoanalysis
ptomaines 162
puberty 498
public health 8, 22, 28, 31, 115, 163,
  708–9, 747, 902–3, 990, 1198, 1209,
  1231–61
Public Health 1249
public health
  19th-century 309, **321–3**, 327, 988,
    1238–56
    social physics **1238–41**
    UK reform **1241–9**, 1273
    US reform **1250–5**
  20th-century **1256–8**
  early history **1232**
  Enlightenment 60–1, **1234–8**
  environment **292–308**
  historiography **36–8**
  internationalism **1417–35**
  work environment **1213–14**, 1222
  see also architecture; childhood;
    civilization; hygiene; sanitation;
    sexually transmitted diseases
public health officers *see* medical police
puerperal fever 321, 328, 924, 987,
  1055–6, **1058–61**, 1191, 1549
  drug therapies 1066–7
Pullan, B. 1184

pulse 123, 605, 1232
  in Chinese medicine 21, 739–40
  in diagnosis 345, 346, 392, 398, 765,
    768–9, 784, **804–6**, 818
Punnett, R.C., 'Mendelism in relation to
  disease' 426–7
purgation 20, 289, 347, 397, 552, 607,
  611, 614, 786, 917, 920, 979, 1102,
  1141, 1404
Puritans 93, 1459
Purkinje, Johan Evangelista
  on animal tissues **105–6**
  'protoplasm' 106
Purves, Herbert, study of thyrotoxic
  patients 499
pus *see* suppuration
Putnam, Mary, first Paris female medical
  graduate 898
putrefaction 159, 160, 257–8, 262, 313,
  314, 321, 322, 324, 327, 328, 990
Puusepp, Lyudvig Martinovich,
  neurosurgery 1017
pyaemia 321
pyelography, intravenous 1015
Pylarini, Giacomo, smallpox inoculation
  1267
pylorectomy 1008
pyocyanase 933
pyrethrum 525

quacks *see* empirics
Quain, Jones, *Dictionary of Medicine* 352
Quakers 894, 900, 1031, 1188, 1235,
  1252, 1314, 1319, 1354, 1436, 1438,
  1454, 1461, 1507, 1587
  family reconstitution **1679–80**, 1684
quarantine 37, 318, 322–3, 372, 587,
  1122, 1210, 1232, 1242–3, 1251,
  1255, 1263, 1264, 1267, 1271, 1458,
  1696
  international co-operation **1421–3**,
    1433–4
  of prostitutes 570, 571
*Quarterly Journal of Experimental
  Physiology* 132
Quarterly Journal of Medicine 216
Queen Charlotte's Hospital 1511
Queen Margaret's College, Glasgow 900
Quekett, John Thomas 110
  Lectures on Histology 111
  *Practical Treatise on the Use of the
    Microscopy* 111

Quervain, F. de
  appendicitis study 1009
  breast cancer statistical study 1007,
    1014
  fracture treatment 999
Quesnay, François 1128, 1129, 1130
Quetelet, L.A.J.
  probability theory 1270, 1275
  social statistics 350–1, 422, 1235, 1238
Quimby, Phineas Parkhurst, magnetic
    healer 620–1, 1462
quinine 789, 917, 919, 923, 925, 926,
    1102, 1418
  prophylaxis 516, 518, 525, **1403–5**
Quinlan, Joseph 875
Quinlan, Karen, IVS lawsuit **875**, 878
Qur'ān see Koran
Qusṭā ibn Lūqā, Christian physician 698,
    705, 707

Rabelais, François 1529
  Gargantua and Pantagruel 1522
rabies 100, 142, 328, 669, 789, 790,
    1138, 1218, 1274, 1456
race **1436–48**
  concept 1441
  diversity 1440
  mono- versus polygenesis debate
    1437–9
  Prichard's studies 1437–8
racism 517, 531, 594–5, 1406–7, 1436,
    1669–70
  educational discrimination 901, 1142,
    1175
  racial hygiene 1304
Radcliffe-Brown, A.R.
  Natural Science of Society 1442
  study of Andaman Islanders 1442
Rademacher, Johann, on physicians'
    poverty 785–6
radiation, and cancer causation 557
radiography 501, 1331, 1338–9, 1341,
    1345, 1595, 1598
radioimmunoassay 214, 493, 496, 499,
    501
radioiodine, in thyroid therapy 496, 497,
    499
radioisotopes 165–6
  in metabolism research 492
  in physiological research 148
radiology 877, 999, 1333, 1336–7,
    1338–9, 1595, 1596–7, 1598

  cerebral 1017
  radiotherapy 496, 497, 500, 501, 506,
    550, 553–4, 996, 1602
    in cancer 548, 549–50, 553–4, 1004,
      1014, 1016, 1022
Rafinesque, Constantin 614
railway spine 354, 1550
Raleigh, Sir Walter 917
Ramalingaswami Report (1980) 774
Ramazzini, Bernardino
  on cattle plague **1266**
  Diseases of Workers 1266, 1268, 1297
  epidemic constitution of Modena 298,
    301
Ramon, Gaston Léon 197
  flocculation test 196
Ramon y Cajal, Santiago 112, 137
Ramon y Cajal, Santiago y Cajal, defines
  neuron 142
Ramsbotham, Francis, accoucheur 1054
Ranchin, François, *Opuscula Medica*
    1096–7
Rand Corporation 1386
Rank, Otto, *Incest Motif in Poetry and
    Legend* 1037
Ransford, Oliver 1405
Ranters 1451
Ranum, Orest 27
Ranvier, Louis Antoine
  Leçons sur l'Histologie du Système nerveux
    112
  Traité des Maladies des Vieillards 1100
Ranyard, Ellen, organizer of 'Bible
    Women' 1484
Rather, L.J. 539
rationality in medicine, anatomy as basis
    82–6, 89, **93–5**
Rau, Johannes, lateral cystotomy 979
Read, Grantley Dick, *Natural Childbirth*
    1065
Read, Richard, on melancholy 441
Reagan, Ronald 559
Réaumur, René, digestion experiments
    125
Recklinghausen, Friedrich von 183, 186
  description of osteitis fibrosa cystica
    504
rectum
  cancer 993, 1009
  surgery 1004
Red Crescent 1423

Red Cross **1422–4**, 1428, 1431, 1487, 1547, 1558
Redfield, Robert 634
Reed, Walter 1557
  vector and virus of yellow fever 406, 514, 526–7, 1279
Referee 1080
reflexology 620, 795
Reformation 318, 1159, 1184, 1185, 1453, 1456, 1463, 1473–4, 1476
Reformed Medical Society 613
Regan, Thomas 880
Regent's Park, London 1509
regimen 939, **940–5**
  in ancient Greece and Rome 1232, 1235
  in humoralism 55
  in old age 1094, 1095, 1097, 1098, 1104, 1293
  see also hygiene, personal
rehabilitation 1111, 1334, 1552
Reher, D. 1681
Rehn, Ludwig
  hyperthyroidism 486
  suturing of heart injury 1020
Reich, Wilhelm 596
  theory of mass neurosis 1042
Reichstein, Tadeus 137, 491
Reil, Johann Christian
  Archiv für die Physiologie 132
  moral therapy 1356–7
Reiser, Stanley Joel xxi, 809, **826–51**, 876, 1547
'rejuvenation' 146, **486–7**, 505, 927, 1102
relapsing fever 358, 522, 1699
religion and medicine 6, 16–18, 158, 234, 312, 339–40, 941, 951, **1449–68**
  alternatives **1461–3**
  body, sickness and soul **1450–2**
  Christianity and medical institutions **1452–6**
  conflict **1456–9**
  monotheism in Western tradition 16–18
  primitive societies 49–50, 52–3
  religious insanity **1459–61**
  secularization **1463–5**
  see also under names of religions/sects
Remak, Robert, cell theory 180
Rembrandt 1128
Remusat, Charles de 420

renal failure *see* kidneys
renin 492
replacement surgery 1004–5, 1006, 1012, 1016, 1021, 1023, 1110
  see also transplantation
resection 984, 993, 994, 1006, 1008, 1009, 1012, 1019
respiration 122
  mitochondria and 109
respiratory system 1678–9
  physiology **140–1**, 142
respiratory therapists 1598
'rest cure' 1578
resurrectionists *see* body-snatchers
resuscitation 253, 261, 271, 875, 877
retina 112
  in colour vision 129
retinoblastoma 432, 434
retinopathy 502
Rettig, R.A. 538, 540
Reverby, S. 1310
Reverdin, J.L. 1010
  skin-grafts 1022
Revue Antropologia Medica 673
Revue des Maladies Cancéreuses 548
Rhazes 7, 676, 695–6, **699–701**, 703, 706, 710, 711
  Liber Medicinalis ad Almansorem 965
  On Smallpox and Measles 205, **698–9**
Rheede, Heinrich von 772
rheumatic fever 917
rheumatism 187
rhinoplasty 765–6, 767
riboflavin 478
ribonucleic acid (RNA) 147, 546, 547, 576
Ricettaria Fiorentino (1497) 916
Rich, Barnaby, *Pathways to Military Practice* 1553
Richards, Dickenson Woodruff 137, 214
Richards, Evelleen 539–40
Richardson, Sir Benjamin Ward 1273
  Hygëia 1303, 1509, 1510
Richelieu, Armand, duc de 1557
Richer, P.M.L.P., on hysteria 1457
Richet, Charles, anaphylaxis concept 195
Richter, A.G. 977
rickets 412, 475, **478–9**, 586, 1012, 1549
rickettsiae 196, 200
Rickman, Mary, carditis patient 819–20
Ricord, Philippe, venereologist 567

Rieder, H., radio-opaque contrast media
diagnosis 1009
Riffel, Alexander 428
Riis, Jacob August 1073
Riley, James 31, 587, 1299
rinderpest 361
Ringer, Sidney, Ringer's solution 139
Riolan, Jean *the younger* 90
criticizes Vesalius 87–8
Rippere, Vicky 289
Risse, Guenter B. xxi, 32, **45–77**
Riverius, Lazarus 94
Rivers, W.H.R. **1441–2**, 1443
Instinct and the Unconscious 1441
Medicine, Magic and Religion 1441
RNA *see* ribonucleic acid
Roberton, John, advocacy of pavilion
system 1511
Roberts, Oral 1465
Robertson, Oswald Hope, blood-banking
pioneer 1594
Robinson, William, design for Royal
Hospital, Kilmainham 1499
Rocha-Lima, Henrique da, typhus causal
agent 200
Rockefeller Foundation 213, 221, 523–4,
529, 746, 1141, 1174, 1419–20,
1480–2, **1488–91**
hookworm eradication programme
1253, **1489–90**
Institute for Medical Research 210,
212–13, 217, 219, 221, 987, 1020,
1277–1, **1489**
International Health Division 1276,
1420
mosquito control projects 406–7, 525
support for biochemistry 154
Yellow Fever Commission 527
Rockefeller, John D. 212, 1169, 1176,
1488–9
Rockefeller, John D. (II) 1488–9
Rockefeller University 132, 1490–1
Roe, Daphne, *A Plague of Corn* 30
Roemer, Milton I. xxi, **1417–35**
Roentgen, Wilhelm Conrad, X-rays 207,
839–41, 1166, 1192, 1218, 1336,
1594–5
Roentgen Society (UK) 1336
Roentgen Society (US) 1336
Roger Frugard of Parma 968
Practica Chirurgiae 966
Roger II, Norman ruler of Sicily 1122

Rogers, Carl Ransom, encounter group
therapy 1043
Rogers, Lina, first US school nurse 1083
Rogers, Sir Leonard
Fevers in the Tropics 523
mass cholera vaccination 198
Roitt, Ivan, on thyroiditis 495
Rokitansky, Carl von 791
humoral theory 282
pathological theory **181–2**, 542
Roland of Parma 966
Roller, C.F.W., German psychiatrist
1362
Rollin, Nicholas, chancellor of Burgundy
1497
Roman Empire 366, 369, 686, 1119,
1155, 1284, 1621
baths 951–2, 954
diet/regimen **940–5**, 956
disintegration 54, 1471
epidemics 363, 586
humoralism as dominant medical
theory 281, 287
importance of Hippocratic Oath
855–6, 861
medical care **53–4**
valetudinaria 54, 1155, 1181
see also Galen
Roman-canon law **1626–7**, 1628, 1629,
1631, 1636
Romanticism 126, 180, 591, 605, 896,
956, 1031, 1033, 1356, 1362, 1363
literature **1526–18**
Rome
classical *see* Roman Empire
Ospedale de S. Spirito 1498
Römer, Paul, serum antitoxin estimation
195
Roosevelt, Franklin Delano 1481, 1550
Roosevelt, Theodore 1254, 1375
Rose, J. 1314
Rose, Wickliffe, head of Rockefeller
Sanitary Commission 1489–90
Rose, William, lawsuit (1704) 1126
Rosen, George 25, 26, 34, 1209, 1538,
1545, 1548, 1596
Rosen, Samuel, stapes mobilization
technique 1011
Rosenberg, Charles 1561
Cholera Years 30, 31, 37
Rosettie, Joseph 96
Ross, Sir Ronald 1411

Mosquito Brigades 524–5
mosquito transmission of malaria 215,
   406, 514, 519–20, 1405
   probability theory 1275
Ross, Walter 539, 540
Rost, F. *Die Pathophysiologie des Chirurgen*
   999
Rothman, Barbara Katz 1600–1
Rothman, David J. 1362
Rothstein, W.G. 628
roundworm 360
Rous, Peyton, on chicken sarcoma 545
Rousseau, G.S. **1520–2**
Rousseau, Jean-Jacques 173, 596, 856
   Emile 1354
   on 'noble savage' 589
Roussel, Théophile, pellagra research
   471
Roux, Pierre Paul Emile 520
   diphtheria antitoxin 1082
   immunological research 162, 193–4
Royal Anthropological Institute of Great
   Britain and Ireland 1439, 1442
Royal College of Midwives 1322
Royal College of Nursing 1324
Royal College of Obstetricians and
   Gynaecologists 1063
Royal College of Physicians of London
   (founded 1518) 97, 99, 468, 557, 784,
   786, 1053, 1063, **1125–7**, 1130, 1159,
   1196, 1207, 1342, 1461
   anatomy lectures 89
   dissections 92
   Harvey's anatomical demonstrations
      96
   monopoly of internal practice 93
   pharmacopoeia (1618) 916
Royal College of Surgeons of England
   (est. 1800) 111, 412, 1053, 1063,
   1126, 1134, 1168, 1552, 1555, 1559
   Hunterian Museum 103, 110, 170,
      975
   registration of élite dentists 1337
Royal Commission
   on Health of Towns (1843–5) 1243–4
   on Marriage Law (1848) 423
   on Sanitary Administration (1868)
      1248
   on the Sanitary State of the Indian
      Army (1859) 517
   on Venereal Disease (1913) 573
Royal Hospital, Kilmainham 1499

Royal Hospital for Diseases of the Chest
   1189
Royal Hospitals (Chelsea and
   Greenwich) 1499, 1558
Royal Marsden Hospital 547, 1189
Royal National Orthopaedic Hospital
   1189
Royal Naval Hospitals (Haslar and
   Stonehouse) 1501
Royal Sea Bathing Hospital, Margate
   1188
Royal Society of London (est. 1660) 96,
   142, 156, 222, 297–8, 917, 975, 1130,
   1234, 1236, 1265, 1267–8
   dissemination of Leeuwenhoek's work
      103
   Philosophical Transactions 132, 977
   Proceedings 132
Royal Society of Medicine 426
   'Stethoscope versus X-ray' (debate,
      1945) **842–3**
Royal Statistical Society 1243, 1273
Royal Victoria Hospital, Netley 1410
Rubner, Max, conservation of energy 265
Rufus of Ephesus 440, 695, 709
Rumsey, Henry 1246
Runciman, Jean V. xxvi
Rush, Benjamin 348, 442, 868, 1237
   Account of the Body and Mind in Old Age
      1098
   anticontagionism 323
   fever theory 400
   on history-taking 829
   medical ethics 865
   *Medical Inquiries upon the Diseases of the
      Mind* 1357
Ruska, Ernst, electron microscope 117
Russell, Lady 868
Russell, Lord 1246
Russia
   Revolution (1917) 1550, 1698–9
   typhus epidemic (1919) 1424
   see also Civil War
Russo-Japanese War (1904–5) 1542,
   1551
Russo-Turkish War (1877–78) 1542
Rutherford, John 817
   on patient observation 807
Ruysch, Frederick 94, 97
Ryle, John Alfred
   on pain 1574, 1577
   social medicine 596–6

Sabin, Albert Bruce, poliomyelitis
vaccine 1643
Sacher-Masoch, Leopold von 907
Sacks, Oliver **1533–4**
    A Leg to Stand On 1582
Sade, Donatien
    Justine 907
    marquis de 1577
Saʾid al-Andalusī 688
St Bartholomew's Hospital 215, 217,
    218, 219, 220, 221, 1184, 1490
St Cecilia Hospital, Leiden 398
St Côme, Paris 972–3, 1164
St George's Hospital 975, 1185, 1453
St John Ambulance Association 1547–8
St John's Hospital for Diseases of the
    Skin 1189
St Joseph's Hospice 550
St Luke's Hospital 550, 1504
St Mark's Hospital for Diseases of the
    Colon and Rectum 1189, 1190
St Martin, Alexis, Beaumont's
    experimental subject 138, 884
St Mary's Dispensary for Women 900
St Mary's Hospital 216, 1544
St Nazaire, yellow fever epidemic (1861)
    33, 1274
St Paul's Infirmary (NY) 1190
St Peter's Hospital 1189
St Rose Free House for Incurable
    Cancer (NY) 547
St Thomas's Hospital 221, 980–1, 1156,
    1184, 1189, 1195, 1512
    Nightingale Training School 1193,
        1376, 1484
    physiology department 141
St Vitus's dance 342
Sakmann, B., patch-clamping of
    membranes 138, 149
Śākyamuni, Gautama 758
Salas, Ismael, pellagra research 471
Salerno
    animal dissection 81
    Articella 1156
    medical school 82–3, **966–8**, **1120–2**,
        1156–7
    Regimen Sanitatis 946–7, 1094, **1288–9**
Sali, Pietro 1289
Saliceto, Gulielmus da (William of
    Salicet) 967
salicylates 917

Salk, Jonas Edward, polio vaccine 201,
    1643
Salkowski, Ernst, immunization with
    toxoid 197
salmonella infections 258, 360
Salpêtrière, Paris 1099–100, 1187, 1365
Salvarsan 262, 572, 574, 789, 926, 931,
    1546
Salvation Army 1484
Samuelsson, B. 138
san jiao system *see* Chinese medicine
Sanctorius *see* Santorio, S.
Sandström, Ovar, description of
    parathyroids 486
Sanger, Frederick, synthesis of insulin
    164, 492
Sänger, M., transverse uterotomy 1013
sanitation/sanitary reform 360, **372–4**,
    405–6, 1234, 1665
    18th-century 1237
    19th-century UK **1211–12**, 1226,
        1242–50, 1272–3, 1375
    19th-century US **1250–5**
    in colonies **1398–9**, 1404
    international conferences **1420–2**
    tropical 38, 516–17, **522–6**
    women's contributions **901–3**
    see also civilization; public health
Sanskrit 695, 703
    Ayurvedic literature **759–69**, 770
    Vedic texts 757–8
Santo, Mariano 971
    kidney-stone operation 979
Santorio, Santorio, measurement of
    human functions 123, 205–6
Sarapion *see* Serapion
sarcomas 543, 545
    Kaposi's 575
Sartre, Jean-Paul 1367
Sasanian Empire 686, 688, 710
Sauerbruch, Ernst Ferdinand
    artificial hand 999
    negative pressure chamber 1019
Saunders, Cicely, founder of St Joseph's
    Hospice 550
Saunders, John Cunningham, founder of
    Moorfields Hospital 1189
Sauvages, François Boissier de 96, 820
    nosology 300, 320, **345–6**
    Nouvelles Classes de Maladies 345–6
Savoy Hospital, London 1498
scabies 565

scanning electron microscope (SEM)
116, 117, 118
scarlet fever 197, 321, 403, 606, 1058,
1061
Scarry, Elaine, *Body in Pain* 1577
Schäfer, Edward *see* Sharpey-Schafer
Schally, A. 138
Schaudinn, Fritz, identification of
Spirochaeta pallida 572
Scherrenmuller, Bartholomäus, *Regimen*
1289
Schick, Bela, Schick test 195
Schiff, Moritz, thyroid experiments
485–6
Schiller, Friedrich 888
Schimmelbusch, Kurt, bactericidal effect
of steam 991
schistosomiasis 359, 360, 370, **512–14**,
522, **529–30**, 1428
schizophrenia 353, 595, 1018, 1366,
1367
Schlatter, Carl, total gastrectomy 552
Schleiden, Matthias Jakob, cell theory
105–6, 179, 180
Schmeiden, V., pericardectomy 1020
Schmiedeberg, Oswald, pharmacology
professor at Strasbourg **920–2**, 930
Schmiedt, E., shock-wave lithotrity 1016
Schnitzler, Arthur, *Liebelei* 907
Schoenheimer, Rudolf 154
radioactive isotopes 165–6
Schofield, R.S. 36, 1675, 1681
demographic study of English parish
registers **1672–3**, 1676
schools health movement **1080–4**, 1087,
1379, 1422, 1430, 1546
Schopenhauer, Arthur 596
Schultze, Max, on retina 112
Schwann, Theodor
blastema concept 181
cell theory **105–6**, 109, 111, 179–80,
542
fermentation chemistry 160
Mikroskopische Untersuchungen 105
Schwarz, Oswald, *Psychogenese und
Psychotherapie körperlicher Symptome*
451
Schweitzer, Albert 1419
science
of diagnosis **826–51**
medicine as **3–11**, **789–92**, **1138–44**
Scientific Revolution (16th-17th

centuries) 7, 155, 339, 806, 1096–7,
1160, 1162, 1580
Scientologists 1042
scintigraphy 1003
scopolamine 1064
Scott, Sir Henry Harold, *History of
Tropical Medicine* 37–8, 529
Scott, Robert Falcon (1902 expedition)
470
Scott, Sir Ronald Bodley 4
Scribonius Largus 855
scrofula 412, 587, 679, 955–6, 1464,
1476
scrotum, cancer 556
scurvy 5, 30, 164, 206, 352, 353, 412,
467–71, 475, 481, 587, 1251
infantile 470, 474–5
Seamen's Hospital Society 1272
seasons, cyclic effect on health 284–6,
290, 293–4, 296, 382, 388–90, 394–5,
397
Sebright, Sir John 423
secretin 166, 489, 490, 493
sedatives/narcotics 918–19, 920, 923,
1588
Sedgwick, Peter 240
Sedgwick, William, US public health
reformer 1254
Seguin, Edward, medical thermometry
837–9
Seimens, H.W. 422
self-experimentation 205, 214, 567,
605–6, 871, 884, 918–19, 921, 922,
986, 1102, 1589
self-help *see* family medicine; poor
Selmi, Francesco, research on ptomaines
162
Selye, Hans, on 'diseases of adaptation'
597
SEM *see* scanning electron microscope
Semmelweis, I.P., puerperal fever 328,
987–8, 990, **1059–60**, 1191
Semon, Felix, on thyroid degeneration
485, 486
Semple, David, anti-typhoid vaccine 198
Senebier, J., plant chemistry 156
Seneca, on assisted suicide 855
senile dementia *see* dementia
senility *see* geriatrics
Sennert, Daniel, on genesis of tumours
541

Senning, Ake, implantation of heart
  pacemaker 1006
sensibility 1580
  Haller's concept 124
Sequeira, James, on adrenal virilism
  506–6
sera 66, 194, 195, 197, 198
Serapion, St 855
Sergius of Resh-'Ayna 688
Sertürner, Friedrich, isolation of
  morphine 918–19
Seton, Elizabeth Bayley, founder Sisters
  of Charity 1478
Seven Years' War (1756–63) 398
Seventh Day Adventists 1463, 1464
Severinus, Marcus Aurelius, *De Recondita
  Abscessuum Natura* 971
sex
  abnormalities 506, 591, 595
  chromosomes 107
  determination 430
  and pituitary gland 147
  see also hormones
sexuality 1042
  childhood 1035, 1036
  Christian attitudes 1461
  female 907–8, 1035, 1036
  Freud's work 1034–5, 1036, 1038,
    1039, 1040
  infantile 449
  male 1035, 1036, 1040
  psychopathology **1631–2**
sexually transmitted diseases **561–83**
  impact on families 571–2
  public health approaches 573–4,
    575–9
    control of prostitution **568–71**
  as social stigma 564, 566, 579
  specificity of gonorrhoea and syphilis
    567–8
  treatments
    early **564–5**
    modern **572–5**
  see also AIDS; gonorrhoea; syphilis
Sforza, Francesco, duke of Milan 1497–8
Shakespeare, William 1526, 1531
  portrayal of doctors **1522–3**
  Tempest 421
shamanism 49–50, 638, 640, 728, 744,
  769, 771, 1440
Shannon, James 550
Shanti Project (San Francisco) 579

Sharp, Jane, English midwife 892
Sharpey, William 130
Sharpey-Schafer, Sir Edward Albert 130
  (ed.) *Textbook of Physiology* 133
  endocrine research 146, 487, 489, 491
  Essentials of Histology 133
Shastid, Thomas, Illinois frontier
  physician 786–7
Shattuck, Lemuel, US public health
  reformer 1212, 1252
Shaw, George Bernard 1137
  Doctor's Dilemma 162–3, 797, 1533
Sheehan, Harold, Sheehan's syndrome
  501
shell-shock 449, 1536–7, 1544, 1546,
  1550, 1555, 1559, 1584
Shelley, Mary
  Frankenstein 1527
  The Last Man **1242**, 1509
Shelley, Percy Bysshe 1527
Sherrington, Sir Charles Scott 133, 1581
  Mammalian Physiology 134, 142
  on neural degeneration 143
  physiology of nervous system 137,
    141–2
Shimkin, Michael 539, 540, 544
shock 998
  anaphylactic 145
  kidney damage 1023
  surgical 985, 998, **1000**
  traumatic 1033
  see also shell-shock
Short, Thomas
  medical statistics 1299
  meteorological records 298
  New Observations on the Bills of Mortality
    1268
Shorter, Edward xxi, **783–800**
Shrewsbury, J.F.D., *A History of Bubonic
  Plague in the British Isles* 30
Shryock, Richard Harrison 25, 26, 538,
  1538
Shumway, N., heart transplantation 1023
Sicard, J.A., cerebral radiology 1017
sick poor *see* poor, medical care
sickle-cell anaemia 164, 431, 432, 433
Siddha medicine **769–70**
Siebold, Adam Elias von, obstetrician
  786
Siebold, Charlotte and Regina von,
  doctorates in obstetrics 896
Siena, S. Maria della Scala 1498

Sigerist, Henry Ernest 25, 38, 538, 1222, 1538
  Landmarks in the History of Hygiene 25–6
signatures, doctrine of 338, 339, 667
signs, doctrine of 916
Siler, J.F., pellagra research 472
Silesia
  hydropathy 617–18, 953
  typhus epidemic 1245–6, 1270
silkworms, muscardine disease (Henle's research) 113
Simmonds, Morris, Simmonds' disease 501
Simon, G. von, first nephrectomy 1015
Simon, Sir John 1214, 1243, 1244, **1246–8**, 1258
  English Sanitary Institutions 1273
  Necessaries of Health (Blue Books) 1247
Simpson, Sir James Young
  chloroform anaesthesia 922
  first use in childbirth 986, 1589
Sims, George R. 1080
Sims, J. Marion
  on gynaecological examination 832
  vesico-vaginal fistula repair 1013
sin and suffering 735, 743
  see also Christianity
Sinān ibn Thābit ibn Qurra 710, 712–13
Singer, Charles Joseph 24
Singer, Peter 876, 880
Sipple, John, on multiple endocrine disorders 496
Siraisi, Nancy 29
Sisters of Charity, nursing order 1453–4, 1478
Sisters' Institute of Nursing 902
Sitte, Camillo, *Der Städtebau nach seinen künsterlischen Grundsätzen* 1509–10
Sivin, Nathan 734
six warps theory *see* Chinese medicine
skin
  diseases 1123, 1189, 1190
  infections 636, 1082, 1083
  structure 94
skin-grafting 201, 202, 765–6, 1012, 1022
Skinner, B. Frederick, behaviourist 572, 1045
Skoda, Joseph 791
skull
  fractures 964, 1017

  see also trephination
Slack, Paul 1289, 1679
  Impact of Plague in Tudor and Stuart England 30
slave trade 366, 372, 515, 1408, 1409–10, 1439
  abolition 1397, 1400
  role in spread of diseases **369–71**
Sleeman, Sir William Henry 773
sleeping sickness *see* trypanosomiasis
Sloan, Alfred P., Sloan Foundation 1481, 1490
Sloan Kettering Institute 551, 874
Sloane, Sir Hans 1236
Slyke, Donald D. Van 212
smallpox 30, 205, 214, 318, 320, 321, 324, 342, 359, 361–7, 369, 371–2, 375, 396, 399, 403, 405, 512, 517, 586, 868, 1209, 1234, 1262, 1264, 1269, 1376, 1399, 1401, 1665, **1679–80**, 1683, 1694, 1699
  eradication 1279, **1428–0**, 1430
  impact on indigenous populations 1403
  inoculation 192, 199, 320, 362, 746, **766–7**, 1236, **1267–8**, 1271, 1409, 1451
  Jenner's cowpox vaccine 9, 162, 192, 206, 372, 606, 729, 745, 766, 1279
  Rhazes' work 698–9
  vaccination 202, 320, 766–7, 924, 1136, 1271, 1273, 1404–5, 1409, 1451, 1696
Smellie, William, midwifery treatise 1052
smells
  as cause of disease 304–6, 309, 314, 404, 588, 1236, 1243, 1300
  see also miasmata
Smith, Adam 1130, 1135
  Wealth of Nations 1351
Smith, Edward 163
Smith, Edwin, papyrus 963
Smith, F.B. 1218, 1549
  People's Health 1312
Smith, Sir Grafton Elliot 1437, 1441
Smith, John Gordon 1628
Smith, Joseph, founder of Mormon Church 1463
Smith, Nathan, on typhoid in New England 403, 405
Smith, Richard M. xxi–xxii, **1663–93**
Smith, Sydney 335

Smith, Theobald, toxin-antitoxin
immunization 197
Smith, Thomas Southwood, sanitary
reformer 322, 1242, 1244
Smith, Virginia 1294
Smithy, Horace Gilbert, cardiac surgery
1020
Smollett, Tobias, *Humphry Clinker* and
Roderick Random 1526
Snell, Henry Saxon, *Hospital Construction
and Management* 1511
Snow, Charles Percy 1528
Snow, John 1589
on cholera 1272–3, 1375, 1421
germ theory 311–12, 325
social Darwinism 592, 594, 596, 1255,
1304, 1406
social medicine movement 596–7
social physics **1238–41**
Social Science Association 1510, 1511
Social Science and Medicine 1649
Socialist Medical Association 1278
Société d'Anthropologie 422
Société Ethnologique de Paris 1439
Société Internationale de Chirurgie 995,
1010
Société Internationale de Chirurgie
Orthopédique 1012
Société Royale de la Médecine 1130,
1299
meteorological/topographical surveys
299, 301
society, medicine in **1117–392**
Society of Apothecaries of London 898,
1053, 1134, 1168, 1629
Society of Chiropodists 1336
Society of Friends *see* Quakers
Society of General Physiologists 132
Society for the Improvement of Animal
Chemistry 156
Society for Investigating the Nature and
Cure of Cancer 547
Society of Medical Officers of Health
1249
Society of Neurological Surgeons
(Philadelphia) 1018
Society of Optometists (NY) 1331
Society of Radiographers (UK) 1339
Society for the Registration of Nurses
1320
Society of Trained Masseuses 1336
sociobiology 596

Sociology of Health and Illness 1656
sociology, medical 454, **1039–41**,
1641–62
19th-century **1641–3**
cognitions **1656–8**
conflict perspectives **1649–54**
early 20th-century **1643–7**
and medical history 26–8, 31–2,
1658–9
medical technologies, social contexts
1593–618
qualitative methods **1647–9**
see also concepts of health, illness, and
disease; medical care
Socrates 856
sodium, in membrane physiology 148,
149
sodium-potassium ATPase 149
Solzhenitsyn, Alexander, *Cancer Ward*
1533
Somanowitch, Rosalie, Berne medical
doctorate 898
somatostatin 493, 494
Sones, Frank Mason jr., coronary
arteriography 1021
sonography 1003
compound 1016
Sontag, Susan 539
Sophia Dorothea, queen of Frederick
William I 893
Sophists 52
Soranus of Ephesus, *Chronic Diseases* 440
Sorbonne, Paris 264, 1187
Soubirous, Bernadette *see* Bernadette of
Lourdes
soul 443
Aristotle's concept 95, 121, **250–1**
at death 263–4
in Buddhism 728–9
in Cartesianism 59, 95
Galen's concept 251
in Judaeo-Christianity 54, 57, 95–6,
252, 651, **1450–2**, 1450, 1585
as life force 21
in non-Western theories 645
in Stahl's animism 94, 124
sound, in diagnosis **828–33**
Sourdille, M.L.J., fenestration technique
1011
South Africa *see* Boer Wars
Souttar, H., commissurotomy for mitral
stenosis 1020

Spain
  colonization 366, 370, 374, 467, 471,
    1403, 1407, 1408, 1419
  plague epidemics 371
  see also Civil War
Spallanger, Henri, tuberculosis vaccine
  199
Spallanzani, Lazzaro, on digestion 125
Spanish American War (1898–1902)
  1542, 1551, 1556
spas 953, 1294, 1300
  Bath 952, 953
  Gräfenberg 617–18, 953
  Malvern 618, 953
specialization 1139, 1163, 1171–3,
  1350–1
  cancer 547–52
  geriatrics 1107–8, 1110
  legal medicine 1635–6
  nursing 1324–5
  paediatrics 1073–4, 1086–7, 1698
  psychiatry 1350–2, 1354, 1359, 1364,
    1367, 1460, 1505
  surgery 1008–24
  tropical medicine 520–22
specificity 309–34, 352
  of gonorrhoea and syphilis 567–8
  Koch's concept 193, 208, 329
spectacles 102, 1095, 1331, 1340
  see also opticians; optometry
speech therapy 1333, 1341, 1344
Spencer, F.C., bypass surgery 1021
Spencer, Herbert 1135
Sperry, R. 138
sphygmograph 837, 845
Spiegel, Adriaan van der 92
spinal irritation 1576
spinal manipulation see chiropractic;
  osteopathy
spinal meningitis 621
spine
  catheterization 1018
  tumours 1017
  X-ray examination 1017
spiritualism 621
spontaneous generation 104, 310, 313,
  325, 326, 328
Spurgeon, Charles Haddon 1465
Spurzheim, J.D., phrenologist 1505
Sri Lanka, Ayurvedic system 17
Stahl, Georg Ernst 252, 605, 893, 1455
  animist philosophy 94, 124

cancer/inflammation theory 541
  rejects iatrochemistry 156, 158–9
  vitalism 443
Stalin, Joseph 1106
Stannard, David 372
Stannius, F.W., cardiovascular
  physiology 140
Stanton, Ambrose Thomas, beriberi
  research 474
Stark, William, architect of Glasgow
  Royal Asylum 1506
Starling, Ernest Henry 216
  Elements of Human Physiology 133
  endocrine research 145–6, 147, 489,
    927
  isolation of secretin 166
  Law of the Heart 139
  physiology of digestion 138
Starr, Edwin, rock artist 1538
Starr, Isaac 1594
Starzl, T.E., liver transplantation 1023
state, health care schemes 66–7, 68–9,
  1099, 1213, 1257, 1379–80
state, and medical institutions 8, 1204–30
  16th-18th centuries 1207–10
  19th-century 1210–18
  20th-century 1218–28
  definitions 1205–7
  see also economics; hospitals; public
    health; war
statistics 64, 207, 243, 300, 323, 350–1,
  353, 403, 1195, 1422
  Billroth's surgical clinics 993
  in biological tests 930
  breast cancer 1007, 1014
  epidemiological 1262, 1265–6,
    1269–73, 1275–7, 1299, 1375
  Farr's statistical nosology 324, 588
  in heredity studies 422, 424, 427–8
  Louis' work 207, 403, 918, 950
  social 1234–5, 1238–41, 1644
  see also demography; mortality
stature, effect of nutrition 35, 361
Staudinger, H., protein chemistry 164
steam, sterilization 991
Steenbock, H. 165
Stein, H.F. Karl vom 1361
Steiner, George 1577
stenosis
  aortic 1020
  pulmonary 1020
Stephen, Sir James Fitzjames 1588

Stephens, James 1438
Steptoe, Patrick Christopher, *in vitro* fertilization 878–9
stereology 118
sterilization, compulsory 1256
Sternberg, George Miller 1563
Sterne, Laurence 1526
steroids *see* hormones
stethoscope 178–9, 206, 350, 815, 816, 826, 827, **828–9**, 831–2, 833, 837, 842–3, 877, 975, 1100, 1132, 1187, 1579, 1593
Stevens, Rosemary 1545, 1561
Stevenson, Christine xxii, **1495–519**
Stevenson, Lloyd 406
Stewart, Alice, on foetal abnormalities 557
Stewart, Dugald, moral philosophy 1437
stilboestrol (synthetic oestrogen) 147, 505, 927
Stiles, Charles Wardell 1253
Still, Andrew Taylor, founder of osteopathy **621–5**
stillbirth 81, 743, 1625
Stockholm, Central Institute of gymnastics 956
Stockman, Ralph 479
Stoicism 1577, 1584
Stone Age 49, 756
Stone, Lucy 897
Stone, Sarah, midwife 1051
Storch, Johannes, case records 33
Stowe, Harriet Beecher 897
Strasbourg University 186, 920, 970
école de santé 178, 1131
Straus, Nathan, infant welfare scheme 1076, 1077
Strauss, Paul 1076
Strauss, Robert 1646
streptococci 1060–1, 1066
streptomycin 199, 223, 933–4
stress 491, 1655
Stricker, Salomon, *Handbuch der Lehre* 112
Strickland, Stephen 538, 540
string-galvanometer 140, 1593
stroke 1098, 1100, 1104, 1106, 1111, 1483
dietary factors 481
stroking 939, **955–6**
Stromeyer, Georg Friedrich Ludwig 785
tenotomy 993

struma lymphomatosa 499–500
Strumpell, Adolf, on emotional factors in disease 450, 451
Strutt, William, inventor 1503
strychnine 918, 919, 921
Studer, K.E. 538, 539, 540
succinylcholine 1001
succussion 813
Sudhoff, Karl Friedrich Jakob 24
suffering *see* pain and suffering
suicide 591, 595, 854, 896, 1451, 1464, 1587, 1619, **1642–3**
Sullivan, Harry Stack, on anxiety 1040
sulphanilamide 924, 932, 934
sulphonamides 793, 999, 1002, 1066, 1067, 1107, 1280, 1305
Summers, Anne 1539, 1562
Sung Tzhu, *Hsi yuan chi lu* **1628–9**
supernatural *see* magic
suppuration 110, 181, 184, 326, 963, 967, 971, 1012
surgeon-apothecaries 784, 973–4, 1130, 1134
as general practitioners 62
Scottish 98
surgeons 1120, 1125, 1126, 1127–2, 1207, 1208, 1472, 1623
aspire to practise internal medicine 97, 970, 1130
dissections 84, 89, 971
education 57, 83, **99–100, 966–8**, 971–6, 980–1, 994, 1129, 1158–9
élite 961, 967–8, 972–3, 974, 980, 982, 1127–8, 1130, 1135, 1136, **1163–5**
relations with physicians 83, 89, 94, 814–15, 968
see also barber-surgeons; guilds
Surgeons' Company of London *see* Company of Surgeons
surgery (modern) 8, 20, 66, 112, 140, 188–9, 219, 500–501, 503–4, **984–1028**, 1191, 1195, 1221, 1551, 1602
(1846–1910) **985–98**
(1914–60) **998–1004**
physiology/pharmacology **998–1003**
heroic 993–4, 998, 1002–3, 1004, 1013–14, 1015, 1018, 1019
post-1960 **1003–24**
impact of technology 843–7, **1003–7**
specialization **1008–24**

see also anaesthesia; *and under names of surgeons and operations*; antisepsis; asepsis
surgery, professionalization 58, 988, **994–8**
surgery (traditional) 6, 8, 51, 57, 81, 172, 178, 854–6, **961–83**, 1190–1
  18th-century **972–80**
  ancient/classical **962–5**
  conservative 970, 977–8, 981
  early 19th century **980–2**
  early modern 60, **968–72**
  Indian 758, 762, **764–6**, 773
  literature 961, 966–8, 970–1, 974, 977, 980
  medicine/surgery relationship **968–76**
  medieval and Arabic 82, 704, 961, **965–8**
  see also anatomy; barber-surgeons
surgical instruments 60, 62, 701, 970, 979, **980**, 990, 1011
  Albucasis' 966
  Paré's 58
  sterilization 990, 991
Susloya, Nadezhda, first Zurich female medical graduate 898
Suśruta Saṃhitā 759, **760–69**, 773, 801, 803
Sutherland, E.W. 137
Sutherland, John, statistical study of Manchester cholera outbreak 1272–5
Sutler, Henry, disobedient patient 786–7
Sutton, Daniel and Robert, Suttonian inoculation system 1236
Sutton, Walter Stanborough, on nature of genes 107
sutures 963, 964, 978, 992, 995, 1004
  intestinal 992
  vascular 1021
Svendberg, T., ultracentrifuge 164
Swammerdam, Jan 97
swamp fevers 1267
Swansea
  Infirmary 1511
  yellow fever epidemic (1865) 33, 1274
sweating sickness, English 340, 586
Sweden 108
  demographic research 1669
  diagnostic technologies 1016
  forensic medicine 1622–13
  health reform (18th-century) 1237
  remedial gymnastics system 956, 1332

Swedenborg, Emanuel, Swedenborgianism 1462
Swieten, Gerhard L.B. van 807
  Boerhaave Aphorismes de Cognoscendis et Curandis Morbis 810
  Oratio de Senum Valetudine tuenda 1098
  physical examination **810–13**, 816–19
Swift, Jonathan 1529
swine influenza 369, 377
Switzerland
  Arbeitsgemeinschaft für Osteosynthesefragen 1013
  foundation of Red Cross 1422–3
  women's medical education 898, 899, 901
Sydenham, Thomas 7, 60, 93, 205, 296–7, 316, 324, 325, 1127, 1187
  on chlorosis 479
  epidemic constitution 297, 312, **1265–6**
  on fevers 320–1, **394–7**, 398, 1266
  Medical Observations 395
  on mental diseases 441, 446, 447, 590
  theory of disease **340–3**, 345
Sylvester, Charles 1503
Sylvius, criticizes Vesalius **87–8**
Sylvius, F. *see* Le Boë, F. de
Sylvius, Jacobus 84, 85, 87, 90
symbolism 445
  in primitive societies 1443–4
Symbolists 1530
Synge, Richard Laurence Millington 165
syphilis 30, 58, 197, 296, 318, 319, 340, 363, 368, 371, 377, 412, 416, **562–84**, 586, 587, 610, 768, 926, 970, 1263, 1546
  diagnostic test 196, 201, 573
  non-venereal 360, 367, 368, 563
  origins **562–5**
  prophylaxis 571
  specificity 567–8
  therapies 58, 262, **565–6**, 572–4, 581, 628, 789, 916, 926, 931, 970, 1546
  Wunderlich's temperature observations 835
Syriac language 685, 686, 688–9, 691, 693, 694, 695, 696, 703, 704
  Book of Medicine 682
Szasz, Thomas 240, 878, 1368, 1583
  Law, Liberty and Psychiatry 1632–3
Szent, Gÿrgyi, A. 137

tachycardia 605
Tacuinum Sanitatis **1288–9**, 1300
Taine, Hippolyte 416
Takaki, Kanehiro, beriberi observation 472–3
'talking cure' *see* psychotherapy
Talmud 945, 1450, 1620
  laws **1621–2**, 1630
Tamils, Siddha system 769–70
Tansey, E.M. (Tilli) xxii, **120–52**
Taussig, H., artificial ductus arteriosus 1020
Tavel, E., pressure steam sterilization 991
Tavernier, Jean Baptists, baron d'Aubonne 773
Taylor, Zachary 1252
technologies 8, 16, **18–21**, 32, 68, 188–9, 206–7, 235, 1197, 1226, 1376, 1546–7
  in childbirth **1068–9**, 1070
  diagnostic **826–51**, 1580
  ethical aspects **876–7**
  impact on surgery **1003–7**, 1016, 1017, 1023
  prolongation of life 272, 1110
  social contexts **1593–618**
  see also under names of instruments and procedures
telescope 122
TEM *see* transmission electron microscope
Temin, Howard, discovery of reverse transcriptase 546
Temkin, Owsei 348, 816, 817
  The Falling Sickness 31
temperance movement 619, 622, 903, 1288, **1292–4**, 1296
temperature measurement 123, 740, 806–7, **834–9**
  in typhoid **405–6**
  see also thermometer
Temple, Sir William 412
Tennyson, Alfred, 1st baron 618, 953
Tenon, Jacques-René 1504, 1505
  design for Hôtel-Dieu, Paris 1500, 1501
  Mémoires sur les Hôpitaux de Paris 1501
tenotomy 993, 1012
Terence Higgins Trust (London) 579
testicular hormones 146, 488, 491, 927, 1102
  testosterone 146, 491, 505

tetanus 193, 197–8, 303, 924, 979, 1429, 1697
Teutonic Knights 55
thalidamide 935
Thames, River, pollution 588, 1272, 1421
Thane, Pat xxii, **1092–115**
Theiler, Max, yellow fever vaccine 200
Theodosius, legal code 1621
Theophilus of Edessa 689
Theorell, A. 137
theories of life, health and disease **233–59**
therapeutics 20–1, 38, 58, 64, 347–8, 784
  19th-century 32, **789–92**
  20th-century **793–7**
  in ancient societies **46–7**
  Arab-Islamic 678–9, 706–7, 713, 714–15
  Chinese **740–3**
  in classical Greece 52, **390–1**
  and death **260–4**
  Indian 768, 769
  in non-Western theories **654–6**
  Paracelsian *see* Paracelsus
  patients' consent **873–4**
  in Renaissance 58, **916–18**
  see also drug therapies; physical methods; unorthodox medical theories
Theresa of Avila, St, healing miracles 891
thermograph 838
thermometer
  alcohol 398
  clinical 123, 350, 806, **834–9**, 1593
  meteorological 297, 299
Thewlis, Malford W., *Geriatrics* 1105
thiamin 476
Thiérry, François 471
Thiers, Abbé 662
Thiers, Joseph, on 'diabetes of bearded women' 507
Third World 37, 478, 480, 513, 526, 529, 589, 598, 1280
  Christianity 1464
  family medicine 70
  life expectancy and economics **1700–1**
  population growth 1573–4, 1686, 1706
  public health problems 28, 36
  spread of AIDS 577–8, 598
Thirty Years' War (1618–48) 93

Thom, Douglas A., behavioural therapy 1045
Thomas, E.D. 214
Thomas, Keith 1295
Thomas, William, *Longevity in Man* 1099
Thompson, Clara, Ferenczi's analysand 1040
Thompson, Sir Henry, on bladder tumours 1015
Thomson, John 177
Thomson, Samuel
    New Guide to Health 613
    Thomsonianism 65, 604, **612–13**, 626, 628, 1139–40, 1462
Thomson, Thomas 157
thorax 1189
    in medieval human dissection 82
    surgery 1002, **1018–21**
thorocoplasty 1017–18
Thrace 301
threadworm 358
thrombolytic drugs 1021
thrombosis 181, 1005
Thucydides 363
Thurnam, John, anthropologist 1438
thymus 111, 484
thyroid gland 480–81, **484–5**, 492, **498–90**, 927, 928, 995
    cancers 500, 557
    function and metabolic rate 494
    radioiodine investigation 492, 496
    surgery 214, 215, 485, 490, 986, 994, 996, 997, **1010**
    see also goitre
thyroidectomy 486, 494
thyroiditis 494, 500
thyrotrophin 491, 492, 498, 499, 500
thyroxine 489, 492, 498, 500, 502, 927, 1000
Tiburtius, Franziska
    founder Berlin polyclinic **900–1**
    Zurich medical doctorate 898
Tierney, R. 1318
Tiersch, C., skin-grafts 1022
Tildesley, William, diarist 1577
Timoni, Emmanuel, smallpox inoculation 1267
Tissot, Simon André 95
    Avis au Peuple sur la Santé 1297
    on nervous disorders 589, 590, 591
tissue culture 116, 430, 545, 1012
tissues **105–6**, 181, 348–9, 1187

Bichat's theories **104**, 125, **348–9**, **541–2**, 975, 981, 1132
    globular theory 104
    origin of cancers **542–4**
    pathology 99, 104, 109, **177–81**, 619
    see also histology
Titmuss, Richard 1546, 1548, 1561
Tizzoni, Guido 193–4
Tjio, Joe Hin, chromosome research 430
tobacco 1429–30
    carcinogenic effects of smoking 224, 557, 597, 598, 1278, 1280
    hazards of passive smoking 1258
    introduction into England 917
tobacco mosaic disease 199
Todaro, George, viral oncogene theory 546–7
Todd, Dr, microscopy collection 110
Toledo, Hospital de Santa Cruz 1498
Tollet, Casimir, French architect 1511
'Tom', experimental subject 138
Tomes, Nancy 32–3
tonsillectomy 963, 966, 1002
tooth-drawers 49, 55, 57, 666, 1122
Topley, W.W.C., experimental epidemiology 1277
topography, medical **300–2**
Topping, C.M., introduction of microtome 789
Torres Straits expedition 1441
Torti, Francesco, clinical records 32
Tours, Moreau de 594
towns
    medicine and public order **1622–4**
    planning **1508–101**
    see also civilization; public health
toxicology *see* poisons
toxin/antitoxin reaction 193–4, 196–7, 925
toxins, titration 196
Toynbee, Arnold 1538
Toynbee Hall, London 1484
tracheo-bronchial anastomosis 1019
tracheotomy 994
trance/possession 22, 49
transmission electron microscope (TEM) **116–18**
    preparation techniques 117
transplantation 487, 497, 503, 505, 984, 995, 1004, 1006, **1021–4**, 1451, 1464, 1603, 1637
    bone-marrow 214, 1024

cornea 1024
ethical issues **1023–4**
heart 1023
kidney 214, 1022, 1023
liver 1023
lungs 1019, 1024
organ donation 877
role of immune system **201–2**, **1023**
tissue 984, 1006, 1022
veins 1022
see also skin-grafting
Trapham, Thomas, *Discourse on the State of Health of the Island of Jamaica* 1396–7
Traube, Moritz, fermentation chemistry 160, 162
trauma 1547–8
in early societies 51
psychological effects 448
see also war
Travers, Benjamin, *Physiology of Inflammation and the Healing Process* 110
Tréfouël, Jacques, discovery of sulphanilamide 932
trench-foot 1550
Trendelenburg, Friedrich, endotrachael intubation 1001
trephination 60, 962, 963, 964, 977, 986–7
Treponema pallidum 573, 926
treponematoses 167–8, 358
see also pinta; syphilis; yaws
Trevan, John William, biological assay 930
tri-iodothyronine 927
Tribondeau, L., radiotherapy 553
triiodothyroxine 492
Trindlay, James 765
Trinity Lutheran Hospital, Kansas City 1496
Triolo, Victor 539
Troeltsch, A.T. von
invention of otoscope 1011
mastoiditis operation 1011
Tröhler, Ulrich xxii, **984–1028**
Trollope, Anthony 1310
Dr Thorne 1529
tropical diseases 4, 6, 36–8, 215, 303–4, 322, **512–36**, 1489–90
as medical speciality **520–22**
prevention and control **524–31**

see also and under names of diseases; colonialism; ecology of disease; fevers; internationalism
Trotsky, Leon 1544
Trotter, Thomas 589, 590
View of the Nervous Temperament 347
Trousseau, Armand, psychological factors in disease 451
Tryon, Thomas 1295, 1788
Trypaflavin 932
trypanosomiasis 358, 367, 512, 514, 522, **527–9**, 926, 931, 932
tryptophan 477
Tschermak, Erich 425
tsetse fly, role in trypanosomiasis 358, 528–9
tuberculin 199, 202, 427, 1275, 1278
tuberculosis 30, 114, 178, 193, 197, 201, 321, 326, 352, 353, 360, 363, 364, 366, 367, 373, 377, 393, 420, 485, 494, 523, 531, 548, 558, 586, 589, 592, 597, 636, 994, 996, 1006, 1100, 1102, 1262, 1273, 1379, 1428, 1527, 1696, 1703
and AIDS 576
antibiotic therapy 231, 933
bacillus 195, 199, 350, 427–8, 429, 789
bovine 585
charities 1483, 1487
heredity debate **427–30**
kidney 1015
mortality 1057, 1058, 1268, 1269, 1276–7, 1549, 1665
pulmonary 223, 350, 388, 399, 412, 414, 587, 832, 1018, 1043, 1595
vaccination 199, 202, 1429
Tuffier, W., dilatation of aortic stenosis 1020
Tuke, Daniel Hack, (with Bucknill) *Manual of Psychological Medicine* 444
Tuke, Samuel 1506
Description of the Retreat 1355, 1507
Tuke, William 1506
asylum reform 1031
moral therapy 1354, 1355
Tulane University, tropical medicine school 520
Tumouri 548
tumours 494, 495, 509, 815, 984, 985, 993
adreno-cortical 1000

bladder 1015
brain 1017
diagnosis 181, 187, **812–30**, 1018
gastro-enteropancreatic **504–5**
immunity 546
liver 807, 809, 1023
localization 1003
neck 986
pituitary 500–501, 505
skin 966, 993
spinal 1017
turalaemia 358
Turck, Leopold, *De la Vieillesse* 1101
Turco-Serbian War (1876) 1549–50, 1555
Turin, early modern hospitals 1185
Turkey
medical MS collections 703–4
origin of smallpox inoculation 766–7
Turkish language 676, 677
Turner, Henry, Turner syndrome 430–1, 506
Turner, Victor, symbolism among Ndembus of Zambia 1443–4
'twilight sleep' 1064, 1589
twins, in heredity studies 422–3, 428
Tylor, Edward 1440
tympanites 805, 808, 810
typhoid 196, 198, 321, 327, 349, 360, **401–6**, 589, 597, 786–7, 789, 924, 1238, 1251, 1262, 1272, 1318, 1593
typhus 30, 200, 202, 321, 322, 349, 363, 369, 371, 375, 377, 399, 400, **401–6**, 465, 587, 589, 789, 1170, 1236, 1238, 1245–6, 1262, 1270, 1277, 1424, 1500, 1679, 1696, 1699

Uckermann, Vilhelm, on deaf-mutism in Norway 424–5
Uganda, trypanosomiasis epidemic 528
Ugrāditya, *Kalyāṇakāraka* 764
ulcers 60
gastro-intestinal 451, 597, 1004–5, 1008, 1009
rectal 813
skin 1022
tropical 523
Ullmann, E., autotransplantation experiments 1022
Ullmann, Manfred 696
Ulster religious revival (1859) 1460
ultracentrifuge 164, 165

ultrasound 794, 1594, 1601, 1602
in diagnosis 844
Unani medical system 717, 769, 771, 773, 1173
unconscious 1034, 1035, 1039, 1045
collective 1039
see also psychoanalysis
Unger, E., transplantation research 1022
Unitarianism 1586
United Company of Barbers and Surgeons (1540–1745) **97–8**, 969–70, 973, 1126
United Nations **1425–6**, 1427, 1432
Educational, Scientific, and Cultural Organization (UNESCO) 1431
International Children's Emergency Fund (UNICEF) 1424, 1426, 1429, 1432
International Refugee Organization 1426
universities 57, 99, 966, **1163–70**, 1207, 1208
in 19th-century Germany 65, 207, 211, 216, 919–21
in early modern Italy **1124–59**
medieval 56, **82–4**, **1120–3**, 1129, **1152–8**, 1207, 1208, 1454–5
philanthropic endowments 154, 220–1, 1488, **1490–1**
Renaissance **84–6**, **1159–63**
women's admission **896–901**, 1175, 1455
see also and under names of universities; medical education
University College Hospital, London 221, 222, 223, 224, 980, 1514
University College London 130, 133, 216, 486, 487, 489, 490, 1190, 1437, 1441, 1490
unorthodox medical theories 6, 64–5, **603–33**, 1139–40, 1217, 1462
drugging systems **604–16**
manipulative medicine **620–6**
natural healing **616–20**
see also under names of theories/regimes
unorthodox medicine 124, 234, 615–16, 625–6
cancer treatments 555–7
syphilis cures 565
unorthodox practitioners *see* empirics
Unschuld, Paul U. 16, 731–2, 734
urbanization *see* civilization; public health

Ure, Alexander, benzoic acid treatment
  of gout 921
ureters
  catheterization 1015
  stenosis 1015
urogenital surgery 1002, 1004, 1006
urology 996, **1015–17**, 1189, 1351–2
uroscopy 765, 768, 769, 784, 805, 806,
  819
'Urwa ibn ai-Ward 681
US Atomic Energy Commission 557
US Centers for Disease Control 579
US Public Health Service 874
Ussing, H.H., permeable membrane
  theory 148–9
USSR, epidemics **1698–700**
uterus
  anatomy 1052
  cancer 1014
  see also hysterectomy
utilitarianism 322, 327, 1242, 1581, 1587

vaccination 162, 320, 329, 527, 1247,
  1375, 1489
  compulsory 1248, 1633
  see also and under names of diseases;
    immunity
vaccines 66, 193, 196, 198–9, 235, 546,
  924–5, 1221, 1223, **1274–8**, 1280,
  1428, 1489, 1643
  defective 202–3
vagotomy 1009
vagus nerve 928
  role in digestion 138
Vaillard, Louis 488
Valence, edict of (1536) 1623
valetudinaria 54, 1155, 1181
Valsalva, Antonio Maria, rectal
  examination 813
valvulotomy 1020
Vanderkemp, John, first medical
  missionary in Africa 1419
Vane, Sir John 138
van't Hoff, J.H. see Hoff
Variot, Gaston, infant clinic 1072, 1075,
  1077, 1078, 1079
Varnhagen, Rahel 896
Varro 317
  'seeds of disease' 295
vasopressin 404, 491, 492, 493, 501
Vaugn, Victor C., US public health
  reformer 1254

Veatch, Robert, bioethicist 852, 875, 881
Vedic texts, medicine in 757–8, 759
vegetarianism 65, 619, 940, 1294, 1295,
  1296, 1462, 1463, 1527
venereal diseases 318, 420, 587, 970,
  1123, 1138, 1185, 1399, 1508, 1546,
  1550
  van Swieten's description **810–11**
  see also sexually transmitted diseases
Venice
  forensic medicine 1622
  physicians/surgeons guild 1207
  quarantine system 1232, 1264
Verona University 966–7
Vesalius, Andreas 58, 174, 296, 319,
  1161
  Fabrica 85, 92, 971, 1123, 1160
  morphology 88
  refutes Galen's anatomy **86–8**, 90
Vesling, Johan 93
veterinary medicine 242–3, 1264, 1266,
  1272, 1422
  physiology 127
Vicq d'Azyr, Félix, statistical survey of
  France 1299
Victoria, queen of England 896, 1589,
  1681
Viel, Charles-François, French architect
  1501
Vienna 987, 1060
  Allgemeines Krankenhaus 1191
  children's hospital 1189
  clinical medicine 1140
  hospital reform 1477
  University 260, 814–15, 1033, 1042
Vietnam War 27, 551, 1529, 1538
Vigarello, George, Concepts of Cleanliness
  1300
Vigo, Giovanni da 970
Villermé, Louis René 1212, 1270
  social statistics **1238–40**
Villot, Frédéric and Fourier, J.B.J.,
  Recherches statistiques sur la Ville de
  Paris 1239
Vincent de Paul, St 1453, 1475
  Society of 1477
Vines, Sydney Howard 161
Vīrasiṃha, astrological physician 770
Virchow, R.L.K. 36, 111, 174, 187, 188,
  258, 264, 282, 351, 992, 997, 1136,
  1216

cellular continuity concept 110, 181, 542–3

cellular pathology 109, **182–4**, 186, 1138, 1187

Cellularpathologie 110, 208, **351–2**, 987

on leukaemia 351

'political medicine' 1245–6, 1249, 1270

on syphilis 567

Virchow's Archiv 543

virginity, medico-legal assessment 1624

virilism 506–7

adrenal 495

virology 202, 376–7

theories of cancer aetiology 544, 545–7

viruses 196, **199–201**, 314, 352, 358, 527, 1274, 1279, 1656

retroviruses 546, **576–580**, 1225

Visconti, Bernabò and Gian Galeazzo, quarantine system (14th-century Milan) 1232

vision, unorthodox strengthening 620

vital power (*qi*) *see* Chinese medicine

vital principle (Van Helmont) 339

vitalism 21, 96, 129, 156, 158–9, 326, 443, 975, 1101, 1580

vitamin concept, research on animal models **474–81**

vitamins 373, 930, 931, 950

A 165, 478, 950

B 480, 931, 950

C 30, 137, 166–7,464, 475–6, 482, 540, 950

D 479, 492, 504, 950, 1012

K 137

Vitruvius 1508

Vives, Jean Luis, *De Subventione Pauperum* 1499

vivisection 83, 107, 110, 122–3, 125, 127–9, 131, 134, 136, 138–9, 148–9, 185, 193, 201, 205, 266–7, 304, **485–8**, 491, 927, 928, 972

anaesthesia experiments 986

animal rights 879–80

behaviour experiments 1045

drug trials 918, 919, 922, 934–5

experimental epidemiology 1277

surgery 992, 1012, 1020, 1022, 1023

transplantation

in cancer studies 545

in endocrine research 497, 505

Voegtlin, Carl 211

Voelker, F., first retrograde cystogram 1015

Volhard, Franz, observation of patients 788

Volkmann, Richard von, abdominal sugery 1191

Volney, Constantine 1237–8

Volta, Alessandro, electrical theory of muscle function 124, 125

voltage clamp (membrane physiology) 149

Voltaire (pseud. of François-Marie Arouet) 1476

voluntarism **902–3**, 1311, 1319, 1454, 1476, **1484–7**, 1547–8, 1550

voluntary hospitals 173, 1055–6, 1129, 1193, 1195, 1196, 1197, 1309, 1323, 1374–5, 1377, **1382–4**, 1387, 1481, **1485–7**, 1500, 1502

Voronoff, Serg, on glandular grafts 1106

Vries, Hugo de 425

Wachter, Kenneth 35

Wagner-Jauregg, Julius, dementia paralytica therapy 215

Wakefield Asylum 1506

Wakley, Thomas 159, 1629

Waksman, Selman Abraham, discovery of streptomycin 933

Wald, G. 137

Wald, Lilian 1083

Waldeyer, Wilhelm, cancer theories 543

Waller, Augustus, electrocardiograph 140

Walter, J. and Schofield, R. (eds), *Famine, Disease and the Social Order* 36

Walter, John 1675

Walton, John *et al.* (eds), *Oxford Companion to Medicine* 4

Wangensteen, Owen, gastric freezing device 1594

war and medicine (pre-1800) 1540

18th-century 173

ancient Greece and Rome 51, 54

surgery 978

see also wounds

war and modern medicine 27, **1536–73**

contexts **1560–4**

malingering **1554–6**, 1559, 1624

medical audit **1541–53**

nursing 1317–18

re-thinking the relationship **1556–60**

shell-shock 449, 1536–7, 1544, 1546,
    1550, 1555, 1559, 1584
  treatment of troops **1553–6**
  unfitness of recruits 420, 549, 1085–6
  wound management 994, 1550–1,
    1559
  see also Red Cross
Warburg, Otto 153, 165
  carbohydrate metabolism 165
  respiratory physiology 137, 142
Warner, John Harley 32, 628
Warner, Margaret Humphreys 33
Warnock, Mary, Report on *in vitro*
  fertilization (1984) **878–9**
Warren, John Collins 981
  first use of ether anaesthesia 986
Warren, Marjorie, rehabilitation of
  geriatrics 1107
Warren, Mary Ann, feminist philosopher
  879
Wassermann, August von, Wassermann
  reaction 196, 203, 573
water cure *see* hydropathy
Waterhouse, Alfred, architect of
  University College Hospital 1514
Watson, F.S., perineal prostatectomy
  1015
Watson, James D., structure of DNA
  108, 166, 431, 492
Watson, John Broadus, phobia treatment
  1045
Wear, Andrew xxii, 26, **1283–308**
Weatherall, Miles xxii–xxiii, **915–38**
Weatherall, Sir David 220
Weaver, W. 154
Webb, Beatrice and Sidney 1222, 1485
Weber, Frederick Parkes 791
Weber, Max 20
Weber, Sir Hermann David 791
Webster, John 1461
Wedekind, Frank, *Lulu* 907
Weed, Lawrence L., computerization of
  clinical data 846
Weinberg, Wilhelm, Hardy-Weinberg
  equilibrium law 427, 428–9
Weindling, Paul xxiii, **192–204**, 420
Weismann, August
  on heredity 422, 428
  on life/death 268
Welbourn, Richard Burkewood xxiii,
  484–511
Welch, William H. 210–11, 1489

welfare *see* childhood; philanthropy
welfare state 1482–3, 1548
  see also National Health Service (UK);
    state
Wellcome, Sir Henry Solomon xxvi, 1490
Wellcome Foundation plc 1490
Wellcome Research Laboratories, Sudan
  520
Wellcome Trust 220, 1480, **1491–2**
Wellington, duke of 1555
Wells, H.G. 416
Wells, Horace, first use of nitrous oxide
  as dental anaesthetic 986
Wells, Sir Thomas Spencer
  clean surgical technique **987–8**, 990
  ovariotomy 994, 1013
wergeld 1621
Wermer, Paul, on multiple endocrine
  disorders 495
Wertheim, E., radical hysterectomy 552,
  1014
Wesley, John 1288, 1301
  performs exorcism 1460
  Primitive Physick 1294, **1296**, 1462
West Indies *see* colonialism; ecology of
  disease
West Riding Pauper Lunatic Asylum
  1503
Western medicine 7
  conflicts with indigenous systems 37,
    38
  humoralism as basis 281–2
  ideas of life and death **249–72**
  influence of Chinese system 729, 734,
    745–9
  origins in Greece 84–6
  specific attributes **15–23**
    concepts of disease/health 18–20,
      233–48
    emphasis on individual **21–2**
    Forms **15–16**
    heroic therapies **20–1**
    monotheism **16–18**
Western Reserve University, Ohio 897,
  898
Westminster
  Margaret Beaufort's hospital 890
  Public Infirmary 1508
  Sydenham's observation of fevers
    394–7, 399
Westminster Hospital 1185, 1453

Whipple, A.O., pancreatico-
duodenectomy 1009
Whipple, George 214
whipworm 360
white corpuscles 110
role in inflammation 183–4
White, Ellen, leader of Seventh Day
Adventists 1463
White, William, orchidectomy 488
White, William Alanson, psychoanalytic
treatment of schizophrenics 1367
Whitehead, A.N. 1442
WHO see World Health Organization
whooping-cough 198, 362, 1429
Whytt, Robert 96, 1580
on nervous diseases 447
Widal, Georges Fernand Isidor,
diagnostic test for typhoid 405
Wiesel, Torsten, physiology of nervous
system 138, 143
Wilberforce, William 618, 1437, 1438
Wilcox, W.F. 1265
Wilder, Russell, on pancreatic tumours
504
Wilkins, Maurice, structure of DNA 166
Wilkinson, Lise xxiii, **1262–82**
Wilks, Samuel, on Hodgkin's disease 544
William of Salicet see Saliceto
Williams, Cicely Delphine, identification
of kwashiorkor 481
Williams, J. Whitridge, on natural
childbirth 1065
Williams, Thomas 1511
Williams, William Carlos 1544
Willis, Francis, physician to George III
1352, 1353
Willis, Thomas 170, 1580
on mental diseases 441, 446, 447
willow bark (source of salicylates) 917
Wills, Lucy, on anaemia of pregnancy
480
Wilson, C. 1684
Wilson, Charles McMoran, 1st baron
Moran 1196
Wilson, Edmund Beecher, Wilson's
disease 432
Wilson, James, hydropathist at Malvern
953
Wilson, Leonard G. xxiii, **382–411**
Wilson, P.A. 1645
Wilson, William G., alcoholism therapy
1043

Winchester Infirmary 1185
Winckelmann-Kirch, Maria, astronomer
889
Wind, Paul de, Dutch physician/surgeon
817
Winnicott, Donald Woods, child
psychologist 1042, 1044
Winslow, C.-E.A. 1265
Winter, J.M. 1545–6, 1549
Winterbottom, Thomas, *Account of the
Native Africans of Sierra Leone* 1397
Winternitz, Milton, social medicine 596
Wintringham, Clifton, meteorological
records 298
Wiseman, Richard, *Several Chirurgical
Treatises* 972
witchcraft/possession 893, **1458–9**,
1582, 1625
Withering, William, *Account of the Foxglove*
917–18
Wittels, Franz, psychoanalyst 791
Wittgenstein, Ludwig 1528, 1577
Wittkower, Eric 453
Witts, L.J. 220
Wöhler, Friedrich 159, 160
Wolf, Alexander, group therapy 1043
Wolff, Harold 452
Wolff, Jacob 540
Wollaston, William Hyde 157
Wolsey, Thomas, cardinal 1125
women, longevity 1101
women and medicine 6, 28, 38, 744,
888–914
17th-18th centuries **892–4**
doctors **895–901**, 1142, 1152, 1175
domestic role 571, 889, 892, 896, 906
lay healers 48, 59, **890–2**, 902, 1122
Middle Ages to 17th century **890–2**
para-medical careers 618, 1087,
1332–3, 1336, 1597–8
as patients 790, 811, 812–13, 818,
828, 832–3
psychology 905–7, 1040
public health reform **901–3**
religious vocation 1453–4, **1476–8**,
1484
sexuality 1035, 1036
voluntarism 890–1, 894, 899, 902–3,
1484–7
see also childbirth; midwives; nursing;
prostitution
Women's Co-Operative Guild 1079

Women's Medical College of Pennsylvania 900
Women's Physical Therapy Association (US) 1336
women's rights movement 894, 896, 898, 908, 1044, 1175, 1589, 1600
  first convention (Seneca Falls, NY; 1848) 897
Woolf, Virginia 1578
Woolley, Ann, *Pharmacopolinum Muliebris Sextus* 893
woolsorters' disease 1268–9
Worboys, Michael xxiv, **512–36**
Wordsworth, William 1526
work environment, and health **1213–14**, 1222
workhouses 100, 1193, 1196, 1242, 1358, 1376, 1505
World Bank 1386
World Federation of Societies of Anaesthesiology 1002
World Health Organization (WHO) 481, 524, 1174, 1257, 1279, 1374, **1422–3**, 1425, **1427–31**, 1432, 1444, 1649
  AIDS programme 576, 579
  International Classification of Diseases 450
  malaria eradication programme 526
  Programme: Health for All 1386
  smallpox eradication 199
World Medical Association 1431
  Declaration of Helsinki (1964) 226, 874, 880
  Physician's Oath (1948) **872–3**
World War
  anxiety neuroses 1441
  casualties 1194–5, 1196, 1333, 1541
  control of sexually transmitted diseases **570–711**, 573
  influence on child welfare **1084–5**
  internationalism **1425–7**
  maternity services 1067
  medical advances 1170, 1544–5, 1556, 1595
  mental health of recruits 1546
  organization of medical services 1312, 1547
  para-medical professions 1333, **1340–1**
  surgery 984, 1000, 1001
  unfitness of recruits 420, 549, 1085–6
  US medical services 1382

war crimes **871–2**, 1087, 1538–9
wound treatment **999**
World War I 115, 132, 135, 142, 186, 197, 198, 200, 212, 221, 235, 262, 375, 523, 596, 1276, 1536, 1537, 1540, 1543, 1548–50, 1552–3, 1557–9, 1561
World War II 36, 67, 68, 115, 148, 149, 154, 200, 222, 235, 373, 377, 407, 449, 524, 527–8, 529, 933, 1107, 1232, 1491, 1532, 1540, 1543, 1548, 1550–2, 1561, 1699
worms *see* helminthology
wound-shock 1544
wounds 81, **999**, 1123
  debridement 994
  early treatments 51, 54, 961, 963, 964, 966, 967
  gunshot 58, 137, 1550, 1551
  infection 262, 933, **987–92**, 999
  open treatment 988
  primary healing 964
  second-intention healing 967
  self-inflicted 1554, 1555
  stapling 1004
  suturing *see* sutures
  war injuries 58, 970–1, 974, 978
  see also antisepsis; asepsis
Wren, Sir Christopher 297–8
  architect of Royal Hospitals (London) 1499
Wright, Sir Almroth Edward 1563
  prophylactic vaccination 196, 198
Wright, Samson, *Applied Physiology* 133–4
Wrigley, E.A., demographic study of English parish registers 1669, **1672–4**, 1676
wu xing (Five Phases) theory *see* Chinese medicine
Wujastyk, Dominik xxiv, **756–79**
Wunderlich, Carl A. 184, 350
  medical thermometry **405**, **834–9**, 1593, 1597
  On the Temperature in Diseases 834–9
  psychological factors in disease 451
Wundt, Wilhelm, associationist psychiatrist 1039, 1044, 1045
Würzburg
  Physico-Medical Society, *Proceedings* 840
  University 182

Wylie, Gill W., *Hospitals* 1511

X-rays 188, 1015, 1017, 1166, 1192,
    1218, 1336, 1339, 1346, 1376, 1547,
    1580, 1592, 1595, 1596, 1598
    in cancer therapy 548, 549, 550, 553,
        554, 996
    in diagnosis 139, 496, 550, **840-4**,
        992, 995, 997, 1002
    diffraction 164
    discovery 839-40, **1594-5**
    mutagenic properties 545
    in transplantation 1023
xerophthalmia 165

Yale University 208, 596, 1490
    Sheffield Scientific School 154
Yalow, Rosalind 214
Yamigiwa, Katsusaburo, cancer research
    556
Yarumchuck, William 539
yaws 303, 366, 367, 368, 512, 523, 531,
    563, 1401, 1428
Ye Tianshi, on heat-factor disorder 732
yellow fever 33, 200, 303, 322, 358, 360,
    370, 372, 374-5, 377, 406, 472, 512,
    515, 522, 524, **526-7**, 1209, 1250,
    1253, 1274, 1279, 1404, 1421, 1424,
    1489-90, 1509
    vaccine 527, 1489
Yersin, Alexandre
    diphtheria vaccine 193, 1082
    plague vaccine 198
yin/yang theory *see* Chinese medicine
York Retreat 1354, 1461, 1506, 1507
York University, economic survey
    (Quality Adjusted Life Year) 1386
Yorkshire Ripper 1630
Young, G.M. 1238
Young, H., prostate surgery 1015
Young, J.Z. 148
Young, W.J. 165
youth movements 1562
Yperman, Jan 967
Yule, Udny 426
Yūnanī medical system 1410
Yūnanī medical system *see* Unani

Zacchia, Paulo, *Quaestiones medico-legales*
    1624
Zakrzewska, Marie Elizabeth, pioneer
    physician 897, 900
Zande people (southern Sudan), illness
    theories 647
Zander, Jonas Gustaf Wilhelm,
    mecanotherapy 956
Zeiss, Heinrich 203
Zeitschrift für Krebsforschung 548
Zeitschrift für physiologischen Chemie 153
Zerbi, Gabriele
    anatomical text **85-6**
    on medical ethics 86
    on old age 1095
Zerbists 86
Zernike, Frits, phase contrast microscope
    115
Zhang Jieben, Chinese physician 736
Ziegler, Heinrich Ernst 428
Zimbabwe National Traditional Healers'
    Association 1443
Zinsser, Hans, *Rats, Lice and History* 30
Zoeller, Christian, tetanus immunization
    197
Zola, Emile 416, 1530
    L'Assommoir 1363
Zola, Irving 1445
Zollinger, Robert, Zollinger-Ellison
    syndrome 504-5
Zondek, Bernhard
    on gonadotrophins 147
    pregnancy test 146, 496
zoology
    inheritance studies 425, 426, 429
    taxonomy 255
Zoroastrianism 677
Zuckerman Report on Cancer Research
    (1972) 551
Zulus, concepts of illness 1443
Zurich
    surgical clinics 993
    University 898, 899, 900, 993
        women medical graduates 1143,
            1175
zymase 160, 162
zymosis 324, 325